W9-BLG-580

2019 Annual

ICD-10-PCS

The Educational Annotation of ICD-10-PCS

Procedure Index, Tables, and Appendices

CRAIG D. PUCKETT

Channel Publishing, Ltd.

Complete Official ICD-10-PCS Text, FY2019 Version
Effective October 1, 2018
as standardized by
U.S. DEPARTMENT OF HEALTH AND HUMAN SERVICES
CENTERS FOR MEDICARE AND MEDICAID SERVICES

ISBN: 978-1-946729-13-2

9 781946 729132

DISCLAIMER

Every effort has been made to ensure the accuracy and reliability of the information contained in this publication. However, complete accuracy cannot be guaranteed. The editor and publisher will not be held responsible or liable for any errors.

Corrections Identification and Reporting

In an effort to provide our customers with the best code books possible, Channel Publishing has added a "Channel Errata Page" for each of its ICD-10 code books on its web site: www.channelpublishing.com. These Channel Errata Pages will be updated whenever an error is identified. Check the appropriate web page periodically for any changes to your Channel Publishing ICD-10 code book.

In addition, if at any time you identify a potential error, please copy the page and fax/mail/e-mail it to: Channel Publishing, Ltd., Attn: ICD-10 Book Production Department, 4750 Longley Lane, Suite 209, Reno, NV 89502. FAX (775) 825-5633. E-mail: info@channelpublishing.com

ICD-10-PCS, FY2019 Version, Effective October 1, 2018

© 2018 CHANNEL PUBLISHING, LTD.

All rights reserved. This book is protected by copyright. No part of it, including but not limited to, the unique, distinctive graphic design and arrangement of the displayed information and other distinctive graphic elements that enhance the usefulness of this publication, may not be used, copied, imitated, replicated, or reproduced in any form or by any means, including photocopying, electronic, mechanical, recording, or utilized by any information storage and retrieval system without prior written permission from the copyright owner.

This edition contains the Complete, Official ICD-10-PCS Text, FY2019 Version as standardized by the U.S. Department of Health and Human Services, Centers for Medicare and Medicaid Services.

Published by CHANNEL PUBLISHING, Ltd., Reno, Nevada

Produced by Craig Puckett, Editor; Susan Dely, Assistant Editor;
Jo Ann Jones, RHIA, CCS, CPC-A, Editorial Assistant; Charisse Rose, Editorial Assistant;
Trey Puckett, Editorial Assistant

Printed in the United States of America

Additional sets may be ordered from Channel Publishing, Ltd., 4750 Longley Lane, Suite 209, Reno, Nevada 89502, 1-800-248-2882, www.channelpublishing.com

ISBN: 978-1-946729-13-2

Channel Publishing, Ltd.

Publishers of

"THE EDUCATIONAL ANNOTATION OF ICD-10-CM/PCS"

August 2018

Dear ICD-10 Colleague:

First, I would like to personally thank each and every Channel Publishing customer who has purchased and enjoyed our ICD-9-CM and ICD-10 coding products and services over these past 32 years.

Thank you for purchasing Channel Publishing's *2019 The Educational Annotation ICD-10-PCS* code book. I trust you will enjoy the new, innovative design, layout, and new, coder-helpful features that we have created for you. I would also like to thank everyone who shared their ICD-10 comments and suggestions over the years from our "Preparing for ICD-10" seminars eighteen years ago, to those of you who called or wrote in, and those who stopped by our booth at AHIMA. We listened and made note of those comments and suggestions to bring you what we believe is an excellent ICD-10-PCS code book, and at an incredibly low price.

In addition to this *2019 Educational Annotation of ICD-10-PCS* code book, I'd like to remind you about all our ICD-10 products and services. I strongly believe that the ICD-10 products and services we've developed will make this transition easier for you, both from a learning point of view and a budget point of view. Please visit our web site www.channelpublishing.com for details and sample content.

Once again, thank you for your purchase and I look forward to providing quality ICD-10 products and services to you in the years to come.

Sincerely,

Craig D. Puckett

Craig D. Puckett,
President, and Publisher

4750 Longley Lane, Suite 209 • Reno, NV 89502-5982 • (775) 825-0880 • Customer Service 1-800-248-2882 • FAX (775) 825-5633
WEB SITE: www.channelpublishing.com • E-MAIL: info@channelpublishing.com

You Asked for ...

AFFORDABLE ICD-10 CODE BOOKS

...we continue to deliver!!!

Hundreds of New Codes/Updates to ICD-10-CM & ICD-10-PCS

2019 ICD-10-CM

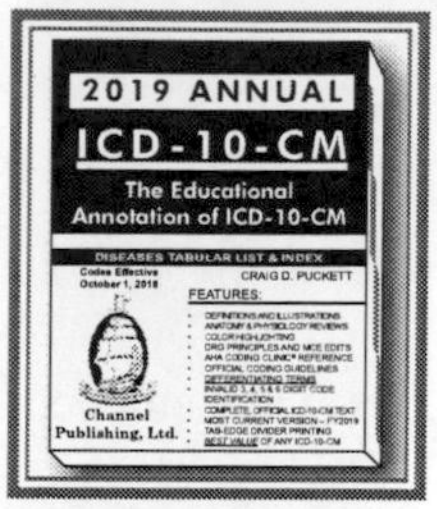

Low Price $79.95

2019 Annual Version
- Paperback bound
- Same content as SoftCover and Spiral

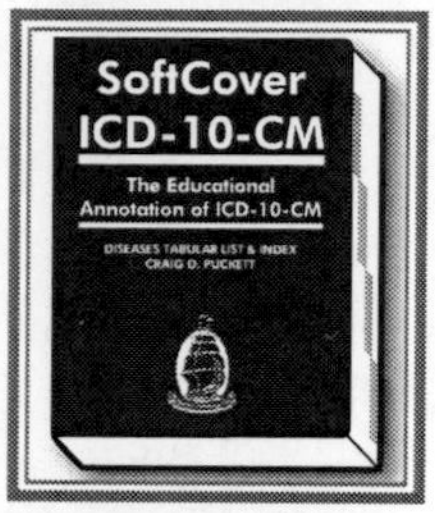

Low Price $89.95

Reusable Tab Set $17.95

2019 SoftCover Version
- Loose-leaf, updateable
- Same content as Annual and Spiral
- Optional tab-divider set

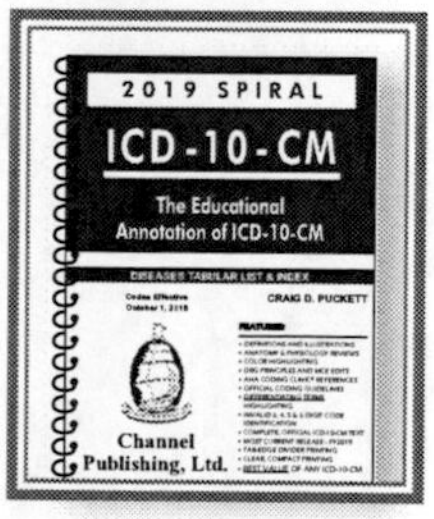

Low Price $84.95

with Tabs $99.95

2019 Spiral Version
- Spiral coil bound
- Same content as Annual and SoftCover
- Optional tab-divider set

ICD-10-CM ANNOTATED/ENHANCED FEATURES IN ALL THREE VERSIONS

- ✓ Color Highlighting of Text & Symbols
- ✓ Definitions
- ✓ Illustrations
- ✓ Anatomy Reviews
- ✓ Physiology Reviews
- ✓ DRG Principles
- ✓ Medicare Code Edits
- ✓ AHA Coding Clinic® Reference Notations
- ✓ Highlighted Term Differentiation
- ✓ Further use of Dashes (-)
- ✓ Further use of Placeholder "x"
- ✓ Excludes ❶ Graphic
- ✓ Excludes 1 and Excludes ❷ Key
- ✓ Highlighted 7th Digit Subclassifications
- ✓ Color Tab-Edge Printing
- ✓ 2019 Official Coding Guidelines
- ✓ Invalid Code Identification Symbols
- ✓ Complete, Official Text

Compare our Products/Features/Prices to others!!

See Web Site for Sample Pages

2019 ICD-10-PCS

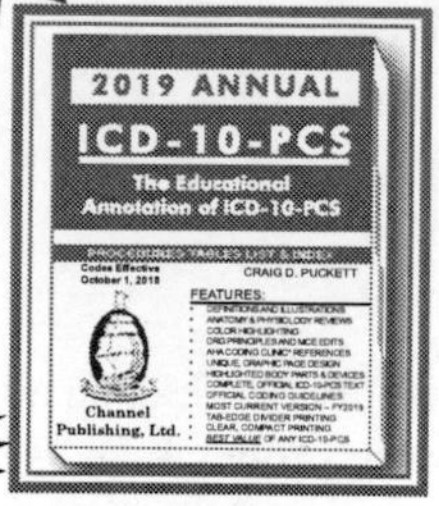

Low Price $69.95

2019 Annual Version
- Paperback bound
- Same content as SoftCover and Spiral

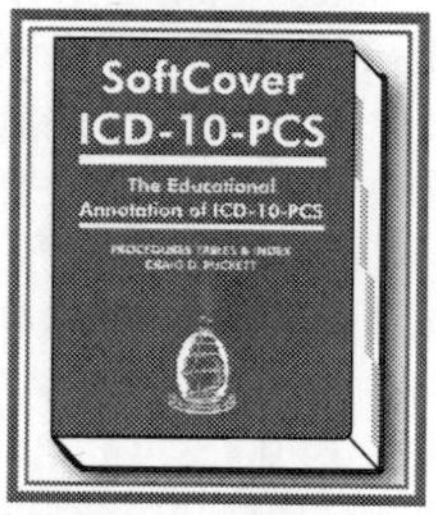

Low Price $79.95

Reusable Tab Set $17.95

2019 SoftCover Version
- Loose-leaf, updateable
- Same content as Annual and Spiral
- Optional tab-divider set

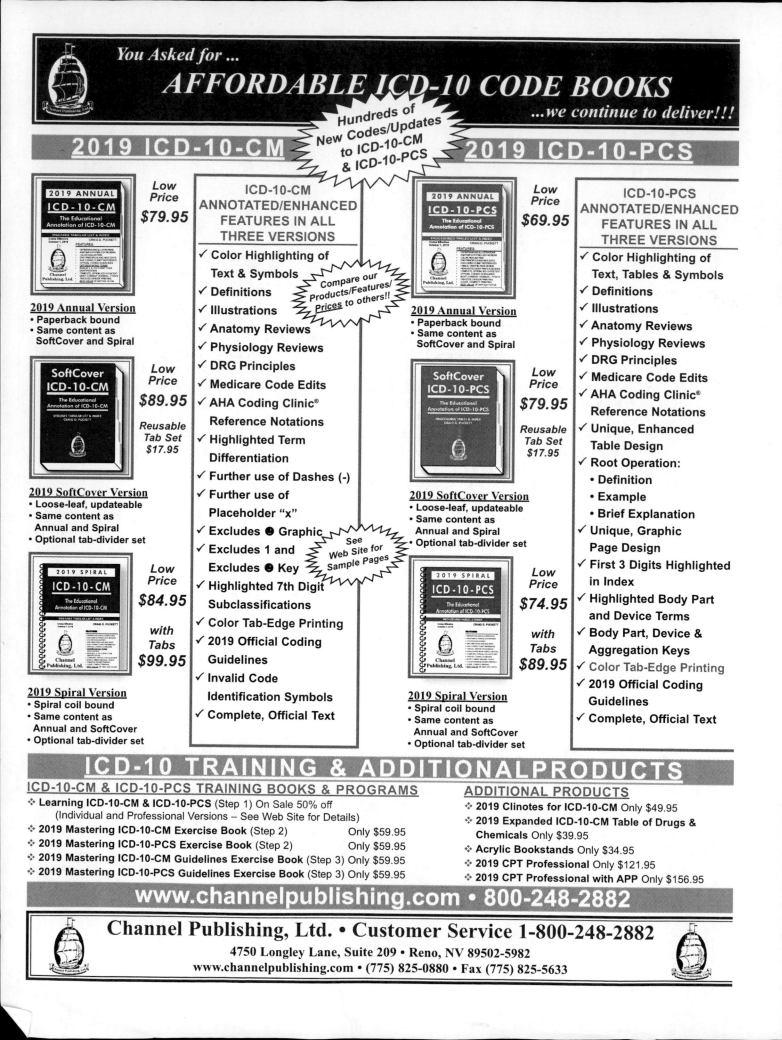

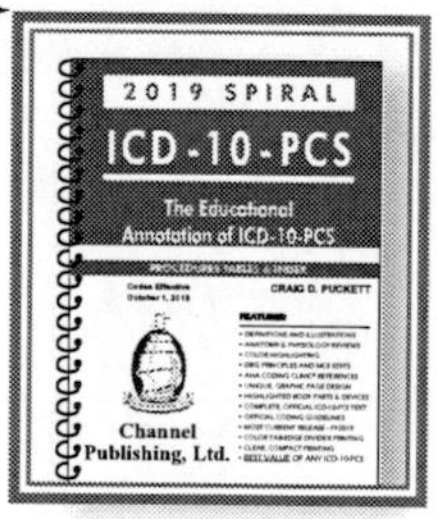

Low Price $74.95

with Tabs $89.95

2019 Spiral Version
- Spiral coil bound
- Same content as Annual and SoftCover
- Optional tab-divider set

ICD-10-PCS ANNOTATED/ENHANCED FEATURES IN ALL THREE VERSIONS

- ✓ Color Highlighting of Text, Tables & Symbols
- ✓ Definitions
- ✓ Illustrations
- ✓ Anatomy Reviews
- ✓ Physiology Reviews
- ✓ DRG Principles
- ✓ Medicare Code Edits
- ✓ AHA Coding Clinic® Reference Notations
- ✓ Unique, Enhanced Table Design
- ✓ Root Operation:
  - Definition
  - Example
  - Brief Explanation
- ✓ Unique, Graphic Page Design
- ✓ First 3 Digits Highlighted in Index
- ✓ Highlighted Body Part and Device Terms
- ✓ Body Part, Device & Aggregation Keys
- ✓ Color Tab-Edge Printing
- ✓ 2019 Official Coding Guidelines
- ✓ Complete, Official Text

ICD-10 TRAINING & ADDITIONALPRODUCTS

ICD-10-CM & ICD-10-PCS TRAINING BOOKS & PROGRAMS

- **Learning ICD-10-CM & ICD-10-PCS** (Step 1) On Sale 50% off (Individual and Professional Versions – See Web Site for Details)
- **2019 Mastering ICD-10-CM Exercise Book** (Step 2) Only $59.95
- **2019 Mastering ICD-10-PCS Exercise Book** (Step 2) Only $59.95
- **2019 Mastering ICD-10-CM Guidelines Exercise Book** (Step 3) Only $59.95
- **2019 Mastering ICD-10-PCS Guidelines Exercise Book** (Step 3) Only $59.95

ADDITIONAL PRODUCTS

- **2019 Clinotes for ICD-10-CM** Only $49.95
- **2019 Expanded ICD-10-CM Table of Drugs & Chemicals** Only $39.95
- **Acrylic Bookstands** Only $34.95
- **2019 CPT Professional** Only $121.95
- **2019 CPT Professional with APP** Only $156.95

www.channelpublishing.com • 800-248-2882

Channel Publishing, Ltd. • Customer Service 1-800-248-2882

4750 Longley Lane, Suite 209 • Reno, NV 89502-5982

www.channelpublishing.com • (775) 825-0880 • Fax (775) 825-5633

2018 ICD-10 FALL SALE ORDER FORM

Sale Prices Expire 12/31/18

1. CUSTOMER INFORMATION (Ship books to address below)

☐ Organization or ☐ Individual | ATTN: Name/Title/Dept. | Customer ID # | Order Date

Shipping Address (Street address required for FedEx delivery) | Telephone

City | State | Zip | E-Mail Address

2. ORDER INFORMATION

	PRODUCT — See Web Site for 2019 CODE BOOKS and Complete Product Descriptions	Quantity	Regular Price	Fall Sale Price	Total(s)
CODE BOOKS	**2019 ICD-10-CM, The Educational Annotation of ICD-10-CM**			Exp. 12/31/18	
	Annual Version ICD-10-CM (Paperback) (ISBN: 9781946729-**12-5**)		$79.95 ea.	—	
	Spiral Version ICD-10-CM (Spiral coil) (ISBN: 9781946729-**18-7**)		$84.95 ea.	—	
	Spiral Version ICD-10-CM with Tabs (Spiral coil) (ISBN: 9781946729-**19-4**)		$99.95 ea.	—	
	SoftCover Version ICD-10-CM (Vinyl cover, updateable) (ISBN: 9781946729-**14-9**)		$89.95 ea.	—	
	2019 Update ICD-10-CM (Full text replacement) (ISBN: 9781946729-**15-6**)		$63.95 ea.	—	
	Tab Set for ICD-10-CM (SoftCover only, reusable) (ITEM: TABCM)		$17.95 ea.	—	
	2019 ICD-10-PCS, The Educational Annotation of ICD-10-PCS				
	Annual Version ICD-10-PCS (Paperback) (ISBN: 9781946729-**13-2**)		$69.95 ea.	—	
	Spiral Version ICD-10-PCS (Spiral coil) (ISBN: 9781946729-**20-0**)		$74.95 ea.	—	
	Spiral Version ICD-10-PCS with Tabs (Spiral coil) (ISBN: 9781946729-**21-7**)		$89.95 ea.	—	
	SoftCover Version ICD-10-PCS (Vinyl cover, updateable) (ISBN: 9781946729-**16-3**)		$79.95 ea.	—	
	2019 Update ICD-10-PCS (Full text replacement) (ISBN: 9781946729-**17-0**)		$56.95 ea.	—	
	Tab Set for ICD-10-PCS (SoftCover only, reusable) (ITEM: TABPCS)		$17.95 ea.	—	
TRAINING	(Professional Version – Includes: PowerPoint Slides, Instructor's Manual, DVD set, Workbook & Code Book) (Individual Version – Includes: DVD set, Workbook & Code Book - CM-12 CEUs, PCS-20 CEUs)				
	Professional Version – Learning ICD-10-CM (Step 1) (ITEM: SBCM-P)		~~$599.95~~ ea.	$299.97 ea.	
	Additional Learning ICD-10-CM Workbook & Book Packages (ITEM: ACM19W)		$84.95 ea.	—	
	Professional Version – Learning ICD-10-PCS (Step 1) (ITEM: SBPCS-P)		~~$699.95~~ ea.	$349.97 ea.	
	Additional Learning ICD-10-PCS Workbook & Book Packages (ITEM: APC819W)		$74.95 ea.		
	Individual Version – Learning ICD-10-CM (Step 1) (12 CEUs) (ITEM: SBCM-I)		~~$299.95~~ ea.	$149.97 ea.	
	Individual Version – Learning ICD-10-PCS (Step 1) (20 CEUs) (ITEM: SBPCS-I)		~~$399.95~~ ea.	$199.97 ea.	
	2019 Mastering ICD-10-CM Exercise Book (Step 2) (ISBN: 9781946729-**24-8**)		$59.95 ea.	—	
	2019 Mastering ICD-10-PCS Exercise Book (Step 2) (ISBN: 9781946729-**25-5**)		$59.95 ea.	—	
	2019 Mastering ICD-10-CM Guidelines Ex Book (Step 3) (ISBN: 9781946729-**26-2**)		$59.95 ea.	—	
	2019 Mastering ICD-10-PCS Guidelines Ex Book (Step 3) (ISBN: 9781946729-**27-9**)		$59.95 ea.	—	
	The Last Word on ICD-10 (Step 4) (ISBN: 9781933053-**61-5**)		~~$69.95~~ ea.	$34.97 ea.	
OTHER	**2019 Clinotes for ICD-10-CM** (ISBN: 9781946729-**22-4**)		$49.95 ea.	—	
	2019 Expanded ICD-10-CM Table of Drugs & Chemicals (ISBN: 9781946729-**23-1**)		$39.95 ea.	—	
	Acrylic Bookstand ☐ **One-piece** (ITEM: BSOP) ☐ **Two-piece** (ITEM: BSTP)		$34.95 ea.	—	
	CPT® 2019 Professional Edition (ISBN: 978162202-**752-1**)		$121.95 ea.	—	
	CPT® 2019 Professional Edition and QuickRef app (ISBN: 978162202-**882-5**)		$156.95 ea.	—	

• OUTSIDE CONTINENTAL U.S.: Call for rates and shipping options. U.S. Dollars.
• EXPRESS SHIPPING: Call for delivery options and rates.

Fall Sale Prices Expire 12/31/18

Continental U.S. Shipping & Handling	
Less than $50	$7
$50-$99	$12
$100-$199	$19
$200-$299	$29
$300+	$39

Product Subtotal	
Shipping & Handling	
Nevada Res. Only Add Local Sales Tax	
Total Order Amount	

3. PAYMENT METHOD

☐ **Purchase Order (Attach copy)** ☐ **Check Enclosed**

☐ **Credit Card: MC, VISA, DISC, AMEX** (Charged date order received)

__ / __ Exp. Date | Sec. Code | Authorized Cardholder Signature

Billing Address (Street number or PO Box and Zip Code) ☐ Same as shipping

MAKE CHECKS PAYABLE AND MAIL TO:

Channel Publishing, Ltd.
4750 Longley Lane, Suite 209
Reno, NV 89502-5982
1-800-248-2882
(775) 825-0880
Fax (775) 825-5633
E-Mail: info@channelpublishing.com
Web Site: www.channelpublishing.com

Channel Publishing, Ltd.

THANK YOU FOR YOUR ORDER FS99088

TABLE OF CONTENTS

© 2018 Channel Publishing, Ltd.

INTRODUCTION TO ICD-10-PCS

THE INTERNATIONAL CLASSIFICATION OF DISEASES Tenth Revision Procedure Coding System (ICD-10-PCS) was created to accompany the World Health Organization's (WHO) ICD-10 diagnosis classification. The new procedure coding system was developed to replace ICD-9-CM procedure codes for reporting inpatient procedures.

Unlike the ICD-9-CM classification, ICD-10-PCS was designed to enable each code to have a standard structure and be very descriptive, and yet flexible enough to accommodate future needs.

This Introduction contains the following parts:

- What is ICD-10-PCS?
- ICD-10-PCS code structure
- ICD-10-PCS system organization
- ICD-10-PCS design
- ICD-10-PCS additional characteristics
- ICD-10-PCS applications

WHAT IS ICD-10-PCS?

ICD-10-PCS is a procedure coding system that will be used to collect data, determine payment, and support the electronic health record for all inpatient procedures performed in the United States.

History of ICD-10-PCS
The World Health Organization has maintained the International Classification of Diseases (ICD) for recording cause of death since 1893. It has updated the ICD periodically to reflect new discoveries in epidemiology and changes in medical understanding of disease.

The International Classification of Diseases Tenth Revision (ICD-10), published in 1992, is the latest revision of the ICD. The WHO authorized the National Center for Health Statistics (NCHS) to develop a clinical modification of ICD-10 for use in the United States. This version of ICD-10 is called ICD-10-CM. ICD-10-CM is intended to replace the previous U.S. clinical modification, ICD-9-CM, that has been in use since 1979. ICD-9-CM contains a procedure classification; ICD-10-CM does not.

The Centers for Medicare and Medicaid Services, the agency responsible for maintaining the inpatient procedure code set in the U.S., contracted with 3M Health Information Systems in 1993 to design and then develop a procedure classification system to replace Volume 3 of ICD-9-CM. ICD-10-PCS is the result. ICD-10-PCS was initially released in 1998. It has been updated annually since that time.

ICD-9-CM Volume 3 Compared with ICD-10-PCS
With ICD-10 implementation, the U.S. clinical modification of the ICD will not include a procedure classification based on the same principles of organization as the diagnosis classification. Instead, a separate procedure coding system has been developed to meet the rigorous and varied demands that are made of coded data in the healthcare industry. This represents a significant step toward building a health information infrastructure that functions optimally in the electronic age.

The following table highlights basic differences between ICD-9-CM Volume 3 and ICD-10-PCS.

ICD-9-CM Volume 3	ICD-10-PCS
Follows ICD structure (designed for diagnosis coding)	Designed/developed to meet healthcare needs for a procedure code system
Codes available as a fixed/finite set in list form	Codes constructed from flexible code components (values) using tables
Codes are numeric	Codes are alphanumeric
Codes are 3 through 4 digits long	All codes are seven characters long

ICD-10-PCS CODE STRUCTURE

Undergirding ICD-10-PCS is a logical, consistent structure that informs the system as a whole, down to the level of a single code. This means that the process of constructing codes in ICD-10-PCS is also logical and consistent: individual letters and numbers, called "values," are selected in sequence to occupy the seven spaces of the code, called "characters."

Characters
All codes in ICD-10-PCS are seven characters long. Each character in the seven-character code represents an aspect of the procedure, as shown in the following diagram of characters from the main section of ICD-10-PCS, called MEDICAL AND SURGICAL.

	Section	Body System	Root Operation	Body Part	Approach	Device	Qualifier
Characters of a PCS code	1	2	3	4	5	6	7

An ICD-10-PCS code is best understood as the result of a process rather than as an isolated, fixed quantity. The process consists of assigning values from among the valid choices for that part of the system, according to the rules governing the construction of codes.

Values
One of 34 possible values can be assigned to each character in a code: the numbers 0 through 9 and the alphabet (except I and O, because they are easily confused with the numbers 1 and 0). A finished code looks like the example below.

0 2 1 0 3 D 4

This code is derived by choosing a specific value for each of the seven characters. Based on details about the procedure performed, values for each character specifying the section, body system, root operation, body part, approach, device, and qualifier are assigned.

Because the definition of each character is a function of its physical position in the code, the same value placed in a different position in the code means something different. The value 0 in the first character means something different than 0 in the second character, or 0 in the third character, and so on.

Code Structure: Medical and Surgical Section
The following character explanations define each character using the code **0 L B 5 0 Z Z**, "Excision of right lower arm and wrist tendon, open approach" as an example. This example comes from the MEDICAL AND SURGICAL section of ICD-10-PCS.

Character 1: Section
The first character in the code determines the broad procedure category, or section, where the code is found. In this example, the section is MEDICAL AND SURGICAL.
0 is the value that represents MEDICAL AND SURGICAL in the 1ST character.

Character 2: Body System
The second character defines the body system—the general physiological system or anatomical region involved. Examples of body systems include LOWER ARTERIES, CENTRAL NERVOUS SYSTEM, and RESPIRATORY SYSTEM.
L is the value that represents the Body System, TENDONS in the 2ND character.

Character 3: Root Operation
The third character defines the root operation, or the objective of the procedure. Some examples of root operations are BYPASS, DRAINAGE, and REATTACHMENT. In the sample code below, the root operation is EXCISION.
B is the value that represents the Root Operation, EXCISION in the 3RD character.

© 2018 Channel Publishing, Ltd.

Character 4: Body Part
The fourth character defines the body part, or specific anatomical site where the procedure was performed. The body system (second character) provides only a general indication of the procedure site. The body part and body system values together provide a precise description of the procedure site.

Examples of body parts are KIDNEY, TONSILS, and THYMUS. When the second character is L, the value 5 when used in the fourth character of the code represents the right lower arm and wrist tendon.
5 is the value that represents the Body Part, LOWER ARM AND WRIST, RIGHT in the 4TH character.

Character 5: Approach
The fifth character defines the approach, or the technique used to reach the procedure site. Seven different approach values are used in the MEDICAL AND SURGICAL section to define the approach. Examples of approaches include OPEN and PERCUTANEOUS ENDOSCOPIC.
0 is the value that represents the the Approach, OPEN in the 5TH character.

Character 6: Device
Depending on the procedure performed, there may or may not be a device left in place at the end of the procedure. The sixth character defines the device. Device values fall into four basic categories:

- Grafts and Prostheses
- Implants
- Simple or Mechanical Appliances
- Electronic Appliances

In this example, there is no device used in the procedure. The value Z is used to represent NO DEVICE, as shown below.
Z is the value that represents the Device, NO DEVICE in the 6TH character.

Character 7: Qualifier
The seventh character defines a qualifier for the code. A qualifier specifies an additional attribute of the procedure, if applicable.

Examples of qualifiers include DIAGNOSTIC and STEREOTACTIC. Qualifier choices vary depending on the previous values selected. In this example, there is no specific qualifier applicable to this procedure.
Z is the value that represents the Qualifier, NO QUALIFIER in the 7TH character.

0 L B 5 0 Z Z is the complete specification of the above procedure: "Excision of right lower arm and wrist tendon, open approach."

ICD-10-PCS SYSTEM ORGANIZATION

The ICD-10-PCS system is organized in three parts: the Tables, the Index, and the Definitions.

Tables (see example below)
The Tables are organized in a series, beginning with section 0, MEDICAL AND SURGICAL, and body system 0, CENTRAL NERVOUS SYSTEM, and proceeding in numerical order. Sections 0 through 9 are followed by sections B through D and F through H and X. The same convention is followed within each table for the second through the seventh characters—numeric values in order first, followed by alphabetical values in order.

The following examples use the MEDICAL AND SURGICAL section to describe the organization and format of the ICD-10-PCS Tables.

The MEDICAL AND SURGICAL section (first character 0) is organized by its 31 body system values. Each body system subdivision in the MEDICAL AND SURGICAL section contains tables that list the valid root operations for that body system. These are the root operation tables that form the the system. These tables provide the valid choices of values available to construct a code.

The root operation tables consist of four columns and a varying number of rows, as in the following example of the root operation EXCISION, in the TENDONS body system.

The values for characters 1 through 3 are provided at the top of each table. Four columns contain the applicable values for characters 4 through 7, given the values in characters 1 through 3.

A table may be separated into rows to specify the valid choices of values in characters 4 through 7. A code built using values from more than one row of a table is not a valid code.

For the complete list of ICD-10-PCS Official Coding Guidelines, please refer to the Official Coding Guidelines following this Introduction.

See Tables above for Table explanation.

1ST - 0 Medical and Surgical (Section)
2ND - L Tendons (Body System)
3RD - B EXCISION (Root Operation)

EXCISION GROUP: Excision, Resection, Destruction, Extraction, (Detachment)
Root Operations that take out some or all of a body part.

EXCISION: Cutting out or off, without replacement, a portion of a body part.

Explanation: Qualifier "X Diagnostic" indicates excision procedures that are biopsies
Examples: Ganglionectomy tendon sheath wrist – CMS Ex: Liver biopsy

Body Part – 4TH			Approach – 5TH	Device – 6TH	Qualifier – 7TH
0 Head and Neck Tendon	8 Hand Tendon, Left	L Upper Leg Tendon, Right	0 Open	Z No device	X Diagnostic
1 Shoulder Tendon, Right	9 Trunk Tendon, Right	M Upper Leg Tendon, Left	3 Percutaneous		Z No qualifier
2 Shoulder Tendon, Left	B Trunk Tendon, Left	N Lower Leg Tendon, Right	4 Percutaneous endoscopic		
3 Upper Arm Tendon, Right	C Thorax Tendon, Right	P Lower Leg Tendon, Left			
4 Upper Arm Tendon, Left	D Thorax Tendon, Left	Q Knee Tendon, Right			
5 Lower Arm and Wrist Tendon, Right	F Abdomen Tendon, Right	R Knee Tendon, Left			
	G Abdomen Tendon, Left	S Ankle Tendon, Right			
6 Lower Arm and Wrist Tendon, Left	H Perineum Tendon	T Ankle Tendon, Left			
	J Hip Tendon, Right	V Foot Tendon, Right			
7 Hand Tendon, Right	K Hip Tendon, Left	W Foot Tendon, Left			

© 2018 Channel Publishing, Ltd.

Sections
ICD-10-PCS is composed of 17 sections, represented by the numbers 0 through 9 and the letters B through D, F through H, and X. The broad procedure categories contained in these sections range from surgical procedures to new technology.

The 17 sections are divided into three groups:
- Medical and Surgical Section
- Medical/Surgical Related Sections
- Ancillary Sections

Medical and Surgical Section
The first section, and the only section in the first group, MEDICAL AND SURGICAL, contains the great majority of procedures typically reported in an inpatient setting. As shown in the previous section discussing ICD-10-PCS code structure, all procedure codes in the MEDICAL AND SURGICAL section begin with the section value 0.

For a complete list of the Body Systems (Character 2) in the MEDICAL AND SURGICAL section, please see the Table of Contents located on page vi.

Medical/Surgical Related Sections
Sections 1 through 9 of ICD-10-PCS comprise the Medical and Surgical-related sections. These sections include obstetrical procedures, administration of substances, measurement and monitoring of body functions, and extracorporeal therapies, as listed below.

Section Value	Section Title
1	Obstetrics
2	Placement
3	Administration
4	Measurement and Monitoring
5	Extracorporeal Assistance and Performance
6	Extracorporeal Therapies
7	Osteopathic
8	Other Procedures
9	Chiropractic

In sections 1 and 2, all seven characters define the same aspects of the procedure as in the MEDICAL AND SURGICAL section.

Codes in sections 3 through 9 are structured for the most part like their counterparts in the MEDICAL AND SURGICAL section, with a few exceptions. For example, in sections 5 and 6, the fifth character is defined as duration instead of approach.

Additional differences include these uses of the sixth character:
- Section 3 defines the sixth character as substance.
- Sections 4 and 5 define the sixth character as function.
- Sections 7 through 9 define the sixth character as method.

Ancillary Sections
Sections B through D, F through H, and X comprise the ancillary sections of ICD-10-PCS. These seven sections include imaging procedures, nuclear medicine, and substance abuse treatment, as listed below:

Section Value	Section Title
B	Imaging
C	Nuclear Medicine
D	Radiation Therapy
F	Physical Rehabilitation and Diagnostic Audiology
G	Mental Health
H	Substance Abuse Treatment
X	New Technology

The definitions of some characters in the ancillary sections differs from that seen in previous sections. In the IMAGING section, the third character is defined as type, and the fifth and sixth characters define contrast and contrast/qualifier respectively.

Additional differences include:
- Section C defines the fifth character as radionuclide.
- Section D defines the fifth character as modality qualifier and the sixth character as isotope.
- Section F defines the fifth character as type qualifier and the sixth character as equipment.
- Sections G and H define the third character as a type qualifier.

Index
The ICD-10-PCS Index can be used to access the Tables. The Index mirrors the structure of the Tables, so it follows a consistent pattern of organization and use of hierarchies.

The Index is organized as an alphabetic lookup. Two types of main terms are listed in the Index:
- Based on the value of the third character (e.g., Root Operation, Root Type)
- Common procedure terms (e.g., Cholecystectomy)

Also included in the Index are the body parts identified in the Body Part Key and the devices identified in the Device Key.

Main Terms
For the MEDICAL AND SURGICAL and related sections, the root operation values are used as main terms in the Index. In other sections, the values representing the general type of procedure performed, such as nuclear medicine or imaging type, are listed as main terms.

For the MEDICAL AND SURGICAL and related sections, values such as EXCISION, BYPASS, and TRANSPLANTATION are included as main terms in the Index. The applicable body system entries are listed beneath the main term, and refer to a specific table. For the ancillary sections, values such as FLUOROSCOPY and POSITRON EMISSION TOMOGRAPHY are listed as main terms.

In the example below, the index entry "Bypass" refers to the MEDICAL AND SURGICAL section tables for all applicable body systems, including ANATOMICAL REGIONS and CENTRAL NERVOUS SYSTEM.

Bypass
Cavity, Cranial 0W110J-
Cerbral Ventricle 0016-

Common Procedure Terms
The second type of term listed in the Index uses procedure names, such as "appendectomy" or "fundoplication." These entries are listed as main terms, and refer to the possible valid Root Operations by using a "see" instruction, as shown in the following example.

Cholecystectomy
– *see* Excision, Gallbladder 0FB4-
– *see* Resection, Gallbladder 0FT4-

Definitions
The ICD-10-PCS Definitions contain the official definitions of ICD-10-PCS values in characters 3 through 7 of the seven-character code, and may also provide additional explanation or examples. The definitions are arranged in section order, and designate the section and the character within the section being defined.

The Medical and Surgical section body part value definitions refer from the body part value to corresponding anatomical terms. The Medical and Surgical section device definitions refer from the device value to corresponding device terms or manufacturer's names. The Substance value definitions in the Administration section refer from the substance value to a common substance name or manufacturer's substance name. These definitions are also sorted by common term and listed separately as the Body Part Key, Device Key, and Substance Key respectively.

The ICD-10-PCS Device Aggregation Table contains entries that correlate a specific ICD-10-PCS device value with a general device value to be used in tables containing only general device values.

© 2018 Channel Publishing, Ltd.

Tabular Order File

The ICD-10-PCS Order file contains a unique "order number" for each valid code or table "header," a flag distinguishing valid codes from headers, and both long and short descriptions combined in a single file.

The code descriptions are generated using rules that produce standardized, complete, and easy-to-read code descriptions.

ICD-10-PCS DESIGN

ICD-10-PCS is fundamentally different from ICD-9-CM in its structure, organization, and capabilities. It was designed and developed to adhere to recommendations made by the National Committee on Vital and Health Statistics (NCVHS). It also incorporates input from a wide range of organizations, individual physicians, healthcare professionals, and researchers.

Several structural attributes were recommended for a new procedure coding system. These attributes include:

- Multiaxial structure
- Completeness
- Expandability

Multiaxial structure

The key attribute that provides the framework for all other structural attributes is multiaxial code structure. Multiaxial code structure makes it possible for the ICD-10-PCS to be complete, expandable, and to provide a high degree of flexibility and functionality.

As mentioned earlier, ICD-10-PCS codes are composed of seven characters. Each character represents a category of information that can be specified about the procedure performed. A character defines both the category of information and its physical position in the code.

A character's position can be understood as a semi-independent axis of classification that allows different specific values to be inserted into that space, and whose physical position remains stable. Within a defined code range, a character retains the general meaning that it confers on any value in that position. For example, the fifth character retains the general meaning "approach" in sections 0 through 4 and 7 through 9 of the system. Any specific value in the fifth character will define a specific approach, such as OPEN.

Each group of values for a character contains all of the valid choices in relation to the other characters of the code, giving the system completeness. In the fifth character, for example, each significantly distinct approach is assigned its own approach value and all applicable approach values are included to represent the possible versions of a procedure.

Each group of values for a character can be added to as needed, giving the system expandability. If a significantly distinct approach is used to perform procedures, a new approach value can be added to the system.

Each group of values is confined to its own character, giving ICD-10-PCS a stable, predictable readability across a wide range of codes. In sections 0 through 4 and 7 through 9 of the system, for example, the fifth character always represents the approach.

ICD-10-PCS' multiaxial structure houses its capacity for completeness, expandability, and flexibility, giving it a high degree of functionality for multiple uses.

Completeness

Completeness is considered a key structural attribute for a new procedure coding system. The specific recommendation for completeness includes these characteristics:

- A unique code is available for each significantly different procedure.
- Each code retains its unique definition. Codes are not reused.

In Volume 3 of ICD-9-CM, procedures performed on many different body parts using different approaches or devices may be assigned to the same procedure code. In ICD-10-PCS, a unique code can be constructed for every significantly different procedure.

Within each section, a character defines a consistent component of a code, and contains all applicable values for that character. The values define individual expressions (open, percutaneous) of the character's general meaning (approach) that are then used to construct unique procedure codes.

Because all approaches by which a procedure is performed are assigned a separate approach value in the system, every procedure which uses a different approach will have its own unique code. This is true of the other characters as well. The same procedure performed on a different body part has its own unique code, the same procedure performed using a different device has its own unique code, and so on.

Because ICD-10-PCS codes are constructed of individual values rather than lists of fixed codes and text descriptions, the unique, stable definition of a code in the system is retained. New values may be added to the system to represent a specific new approach or device or qualifier, but whole codes by design cannot be given new meanings and reused.

Expandability

Expandability was also recommended as a key structural attribute. The specific recommendation for expandability includes these characteristics:

- Accommodate new procedures and technologies
- Add new codes without disrupting the existing structure

ICD-10-PCS is designed to be easily updated as new codes are required for new procedures and new techniques. Changes to ICD-10-PCS can all be made within the existing structure, because whole codes are not added. Instead, one of two possible changes is made to the system:

- A new value for a character is added as needed to the system
- An existing value for a character is added to a table(s) in the system

ICD-10-PCS update: PICVA

An example of how the updating of ICD-10-PCS works can be seen in the coronary artery bypass procedure called Percutaneous in-situ coronary venous arterialization (PICVA). This procedure is no more invasive than a percutaneous coronary angioplasty, but achieves the benefits of a bypass procedure by placing a specialized stent into the diseased coronary artery, through its wall into the adjacent coronary vein, and diverting blood flow through the stent into the artery past the blockage.

ICD-10-PCS was updated in 2004 to include an appropriate range of codes for the PICVA procedure (16 possible codes). This was accomplished simply by adding another row to the relevant table (as shown in the example below) containing two approach values for the non-invasive approach, two device values for the possible types of stent, and a single qualifier defining the coronary vein as the source of the new blood flow, as in the example below.

The values for characters 1 through 3 at the top of each table are:
0: MEDICAL AND SURGICAL (Section)
2: HEART AND GREAT VESSELS (Body system)
1: BYPASS: Altering the route of passage of the contents of a tubular body part

Body Part Character 4	Approach Character 5	Device Character 6	Qualifier Character 7
0 Coronary Artery, One Artery 1 Coronary Artery, Two Arteries 2 Coronary Artery, Three Arteries 3 Coronary Artery, Four or More Arteries	3 Percutaneous 4 Percutaneous Endoscopic	4 Drug-eluting Intraluminal Device D Intraluminal Device	D Coronary Vein

Structural integrity

As shown in the previous example, ICD-10-PCS can be easily expanded without disrupting the structure of the system.

In the PICVA example, one new value—the qualifier value Coronary Vein—was added to the system to effect this change. All other values in the new row are existing values used to create unique, new codes.

© 2018 Channel Publishing, Ltd.

This type of updating can be replicated anywhere in the system when a change is required. ICD-10-PCS allows unique new codes to be added to the system because values for the seven characters that make up a code can be combined as needed. The system can evolve as medical technology and clinical practice evolve, without disrupting the ICD-10-PCS structure.

ICD-10-PCS ADDITIONAL CHARACTERISTICS

ICD-10-PCS possesses several additional characteristics in response to government and industry recommendations. These characteristics are:

- Standardized terminology within the coding system
- Standardized level of specificity
- No diagnostic information
- No explicit "not otherwise specified" (NOS) code options
- Limited use of "not elsewhere classified" (NEC) code options

Standardized Terminology

Words commonly used in clinical vocabularies may have multiple meanings. This can cause confusion and result in inaccurate data. ICD-10-PCS is standardized and self-contained. Characters and values used in the system are defined in the system.

For example, the word "excision" is used to describe a wide variety of surgical procedures. In ICD-10-PCS, the word "excision" describes a single, precise surgical objective, defined as "Cutting out or off, without replacement, a portion of a body part."

No Eponyms or Common Procedure Names

The terminology used in ICD-10-PCS is standardized to provide precise and stable definitions of all procedures performed. This standardized terminology is used in all ICD-10-PCS code descriptions.

As a result, ICD-10-PCS code descriptions do not include eponyms or common procedure names. Two examples from ICD-9-CM are 22.61, "Excision of lesion of maxillary sinus with Caldwell-Luc approach," and 51.10, "Endoscopic retrograde cholangiopancreatography [ERCP]." In ICD-10-PCS, physicians' names are not included in a code description, nor are procedures identified by common terms or acronyms such as appendectomy or CABG. Instead, such procedures are coded to the root operation that accurately identifies the objective of the procedure.

The procedures described in the preceding paragraph by ICD-9-CM codes are coded in ICD-10-PCS according to the root operation that matches the objective of the procedure. Here the ICD-10-PCS equivalents would be EXCISION and INSPECTION respectively. By relying on the universal objectives defined in root operations rather than eponyms or specific procedure titles that change or become obsolete, ICD-10-PCS preserves the capacity to define past, present, and future procedures accurately using stable terminology in the form of characters and values.

No Combination Codes

With rare exceptions, ICD-10-PCS does not define multiple procedures with one code. This is to preserve standardized terminology and consistency across the system. Procedures that are typically performed together but are distinct procedures may be defined by a single "combination code" in ICD-9-CM. An example of a combination code in ICD-9-CM is 28.3, "Tonsillectomy with adenoidectomy."

A procedure that meets the reporting criteria for a separate procedure is coded separately in ICD-10-PCS. This allows the system to respond to changes in technology and medical practice with the maximum degree of stability and flexibility.

Standardized Level of Specificity

In ICD-9-CM, one code with its description and includes notes may encompass a vast number of procedure variations while another code defines a single specific procedure. ICD-10-PCS provides a standardized level of specificity for each code, so that each code represents a single procedure variation.

The ICD-9-CM code 39.31, "Suture of artery," does not specify the artery, whereas the code range 38.40 through 38.49, "Resection of artery with replacement," provides a fourth-digit subclassification for specifying the artery by anatomical region (thoracic, abdominal, etc.).

In ICD-10-PCS, the codes identifying all artery suture and artery replacement procedures possess the same degree of specificity. The ICD-9-CM examples above coded to their ICD-10-PCS equivalents would use the same artery body part values in all codes identifying the respective procedures.

In general, ICD-10-PCS code descriptions are much more specific than their ICD-9-CM counterparts, but sometimes an ICD-10-PCS code description is actually less specific. In most cases this is because the ICD-9-CM code contains diagnosis information. The standardized level of code specificity in ICD-10-PCS cannot always take account of these fluctuations in ICD-9-CM level of specificity. Instead, ICD-10-PCS provides a standardized level of specificity that can be predicted across the system.

Diagnosis Information Excluded

Another key feature of ICD-10-PCS is that information pertaining to a diagnosis is excluded from the code descriptions.

ICD-9-CM often contains information about the diagnosis in its procedure codes. Adding diagnosis information limits the flexibility and functionality of a procedure coding system. It has the effect of placing a code "off limits" because the diagnosis in the medical record does not match the diagnosis in the procedure code description. The code cannot be used even though the procedural part of the code description precisely matches the procedure performed.

Diagnosis information is not contained in any ICD-10-PCS code. The diagnosis codes, not the procedure codes, will specify the reason the procedure is performed.

NOS Code Options Restricted

ICD-9-CM often designates codes as "unspecified" or "not otherwise specified" codes. By contrast, the standardized level of specificity designed into ICD-10-PCS restricts the use of broadly applicable NOS or unspecified code options in the system. A minimal level of specificity is required to construct a valid code.

In ICD-10-PCS, each character defines information about the procedure and all seven characters must contain a specific value obtained from a single row of a table to build a valid code. Even values such as the sixth-character value Z, NO DEVICE and the seventh-character value Z, NO QUALIFIER, provide important information about the procedure performed.

Limited NEC Code Options

ICD-9-CM often designates codes as "not elsewhere classified" or "other specified" versions of a procedure throughout the code set. NEC options are also provided in ICD-10-PCS, but only for specific, limited use.

In the MEDICAL AND SURGICAL section, two significant "not elsewhere classified" options are the root operation value Q, REPAIR and the device value Y, OTHER DEVICE.

The root operation REPAIR is a true NEC value. It is used only when the procedure performed is not one of the other root operations in the MEDICAL AND SURGICAL section.

OTHER DEVICE, on the other hand, is intended to be used to temporarily define new devices that do not have a specific value assigned, until one can be added to the system. No categories of medical or surgical devices are permanently classified to OTHER DEVICE.

© 2018 Channel Publishing, Ltd.

ICD-10-PCS APPLICATIONS

ICD-10-PCS code structure results in qualities that optimize the performance of the system in electronic applications, and maximize the usefulness of the coded healthcare data. These qualities include:

- Optimal search capability
- Consistent character definitions
- Consistent values wherever possible
- Code readability

Some have argued that, in the world of the electronic health record, the classification system as we know it is outmoded, that classification doesn't matter because a computer is able to find a code with equal ease whether the code has been generated at random or is part of a classification scheme. While this may be true from an IT perspective, assignment of randomly generated code numbers makes it impossible to aggregate data according to related ranges of codes. This is a critical capability for providers, payers, and researchers to make meaningful use of the data.

Optimal Search Capability

ICD-10-PCS is designed for maximum versatility in the ability to aggregate coded data. Values belonging to the same character as defined in a section or sections can be easily compared, since they occupy the same position in a code. This provides a high degree of flexibility and functionality for data mining.

For example, the body part value 6, STOMACH, retains its meaning for all codes in the MEDICAL AND SURGICAL section that define procedures performed on the stomach. Because the body part value is dependent for its meaning on the body system in which it is found, the body system value D, GASTROINTESTINAL, must also be included in the search.

A person wishing to examine data regarding all medical and surgical procedures performed on the stomach could do so simply by searching the following code range: 0D*6***

Consistent Characters and Values

In the previous example, the value 6 means STOMACH only when the body system value is D, GASTROINTESTINAL. In many other cases, values retain their meaning across a much broader range of codes. This provides consistency and readability.

For example, the value 0 in the fifth character defines the approach OPEN and the value 3 in the fifth character defines the approach PERCUTANEOUS across sections 0 through 4 and 7 through 9, where applicable. As a result, all open and percutaneous procedures represented by codes in sections 0-4 and 7-9 can be compared based on a single character—approach—by conducting a query on the following code ranges:
[0 through 4,7 through 9]***0** vs. [0 through 4,7 through 9]***3**

Searches can be progressively refined by adding specific values. For example, one could search on a body system value or range of body system values, plus a body part value or range of body part values, plus a root operation value or range of root operation values.

To refine the search above, one could add the body system value for GASTROINTESTINAL and the body part value for STOMACH to limit the search to open vs. percutaneous procedures performed on the stomach: 0D*60** vs. 0D*63**

To refine the search even further and limit the comparison to open and percutaneous biopsies of the stomach, one could add the third-character value for the root operation EXCISION and the seventh-character qualifier DIAGNOSTIC, as follows: 0DB60*X vs. 0DB63*X

Stability of characters and values across vast ranges of codes provides the maximum degree of functionality and flexibility for the collection and analysis of data. The search capabilities demonstrated above function equally well for all uses of healthcare data: investigating quality of care, resource utilization, risk management, conducting research, determining reimbursement, and many others.

Because the character definition is consistent, and only the individual values assigned to that character differ as needed, meaningful comparisons of data over time can be conducted across a virtually infinite range of procedures.

Code readability

ICD-10-PCS resembles a language in the sense that it is made up of semi-independent values combined by following the rules of the system, much the way a sentence is formed by combining words and following the rules of grammar and syntax. As with words in their context, the meaning of any single value is a combination of its position in the code and any preceding values on which it may be dependent.

For example, in the MEDICAL AND SURGICAL section, a body part value is always dependent for its meaning on the body system in which it is found. It cannot stand alone as a letter or a number and be meaningful. A fourth-character value of 6 by itself can mean 31 different things, but a fourth-character value of 6 in the context of a second-character value of D means one thing only—STOMACH.

On the other hand, a root operation value is not dependent on any character but the section for its meaning, and identifies a single consistent objective wherever the third character is defined as root operation. For example, the third-character value T identifies the root operation RESECTION in both the MEDICAL AND SURGICAL and OBSTETRICS sections.

The approach value also identifies a single consistent approach wherever the fifth character is defined as approach. The fifth-character value 3 identifies the approach PERCUTANEOUS in the MEDICAL AND SURGICAL section, the OBSTETRICS section, the ADMINISTRATION section, and others.

The sixth-character device value or seventh-character qualifier value identifies the same device or qualifier in the context of the body system where it is found. Although there may be consistencies across body systems or within whole sections, this is not true in all cases.

Values in their designated context have a precise meaning, like words in a language. As seen in the code example which began this chapter, 0LB50ZZ represents the text description of the specific procedure "Excision of right lower arm and wrist tendon, open approach." Since ICD-10-PCS values in context have a single, precise meaning, a complete, valid code can be read and understood without its accompanying text description, much like one would read a sentence.

Please see the Appendices following the Ancillary Sections for further detailed information on ICD-10-PCS and its components.

© 2018 Channel Publishing, Ltd.

Channel Publishing's 2019 ICD-10-PCS Educational and Enhanced Features

Enhanced 2019 Features

Unique, Enhanced Table Design

The basic PCS tables have been significantly enhanced (graphic design) to help coders clearly and quickly identify the components of each PCS code table.

Inclusion of Example and Brief Explanation in PCS Table design

The addition of root operation examples and a brief explanation of the root operation (in addition to the root operation definition) helps coders understand each root operation without referring to a table in the appendices.

Unique, Graphic Page Design

The unique, graphic page design clearly identifies which PCS code tables are located on that page and helps coders stay focused on the particular root operation for that body system. In addition, code tables that are too extensive for one page have that continued information very clearly identified.

Highlighted First 3 Digits in Index

The first 3 digits of each code in the Alphabetic Index are in boldface type to help coders identify and search for the correct 3-digit PCS code table in the Tabular Table sections.

Highlighted Body Part & Device Terms

The body part and device terms in the index have blue screen bars placed over them to help coders more easily differentiate between standard index entries and the body part and device terms.

Body Part, Device & Device Aggregation Keys

The body part, device, and device aggregation keys (tables) are listed in separate appendices following the Tabular Table sections.

All 7 Characters Clearly Identified

All 7 characters of a PCS code are clearly identified in each PCS code table to help coders learn and properly select the appropriate character for each digit.

Tab-Edge Printing

Chapter-by-chapter, and section-by-section stair-stepped, tab-edge printing helps coders locate the correct section quickly.

Clear, Compact Typeface Printing

The use of a clear, compact typeface allows coders to clearly and easily locate and read all text in the Alphabetic Index and Tabular Tables.

Clear, Compact Guidewords at the Top of Each Page

The use of clear, compact guidewords allows coders to clearly and easily locate the correct page in the Alphabetic Index and Tabular Tables.

© 2018 Channel Publishing, Ltd.

Channel Publishing's 2019 ICD-10-PCS Educational and Enhanced Features

Educational Annotations

(Each Body System and Section)

Anatomy and Physiology Reviews
Anatomy and physiology reviews that help coders understand the anatomical structures and physiology of the various systems.

Illustrations
Anatomical illustrations with call outs of body parts.

Definitions
Medical definitions of common procedures written by a coder for coders.

AHA Coding Clinic® Reference Notations
Identifies AHA Coding Clinic® articles and Q&As (with descriptive title) that have relevant information for certain codes or code categories.

Body Part Key Listings
Identifies the Body Part Key listings specific for that body system or section.

Device Key Listings
Identifies the Device Key listings specific for that body system or section.

Device Aggregation Table Listings
Identifies the Device Aggregation Table listings specific for that body system or section.

Coding Guidelines
Lists the Official Coding Guidelines specific for that body system or section.

Tab-Edge Printing for Educational Annotations Pages
The Educational Annotations pages are identified by two digits in the screen bar: First digit – Section, Second digit – Body System.

Additional 2019 Features

Groups of Similar Root Operations
At the top of each table is a list of similar Root Operations that includes that table's Root Operation. The Root Operations in parentheses are Root Operations that are not included in that Body System.

Body System Specific Root Operation Examples
Each table identifies the CMS general Root Operation example and a Channel Publishing created Body System Specific example.

Medicare Code Editor Edits
Identifies codes that are edit-reviewed for age and sex-related discrepancies and coverage conditions.

Blue Color Highlighting of Graphic Design and Selected Text
Color highlighting of Index:
- Highlighted Body Part Key terms – Screened Blue
- Highlighted Device Key terms – Screened Blue
- Tab-Edge Printing – Blue

Color highlighting of Tables:
- Tables – Blue
- Root Operation Definitions – Blue
- Medicare Code Editor Edits – Blue
- Tab-Edge Printing – Blue

INTRODUCTION TO AHA CODING CLINIC® REFERENCE NOTATIONS

BACKGROUND

AHA Coding Clinic® is a registered trademark of the American Hospital Association. AHA Coding Clinic® Reference Notations is not a product of the American Hospital Association, and Channel Publishing, Ltd. is not affiliated with or endorsed by the American Hospital Association. The American Hospital coding website can be accessed at www.ahacentraloffice.org.

The AHA Coding Clinic® for ICD-10-CM/PCS is published quarterly by the American Hospital Association. The *Coding Clinic* is the official publication for *ICD-10-CM/PCS* coding guidelines and advice as designated by the four cooperating parties. The cooperating parties listed below have final approval of the coding advice provided in the *Coding Clinic*: American Hospital Association, American Health Information Management Association, Centers for Medicare and Medicaid Services, National Center for Health Statistics.

The *Coding Clinic* provides specific information and guidelines that are helpful for determining proper coding, and is used by CMS in reviewing claims. The goal of the *Coding Clinic* is to provide coding advice, official coding decisions, and news. It promotes accuracy and consistency in the use of ICD-10-CM/PCS. It offers coding guidelines and advice based on adherence to the statistical classification scheme of ICD-10-CM/PCS and the definitions specified in the Uniform Hospital Discharge Data Set (UHDDS).

INTRODUCTION

Channel Publishing has developed the AHA Coding Clinic® Reference Notations to help coders access the official coding advice found throughout all issues of the *Coding Clinic*. This information has been referenced in three ways: 1) at the Educational Annotations portion of each Body System/Section, 2) at the identified Coding Guideline, and 3) a categorical index of articles (see below) that are too broad in scope to be assigned to 1) or 2). Any comments regarding these reference notations should be directed to: *Coding Clinic* Reference Notations, c/o Channel Publishing, Ltd., 4750 Longley Lane, Suite 209, Reno, Nevada 89502.

GUIDANCE IN USE

Coders are encouraged to reference all relevant information contained in the *Coding Clinic* to promote the most accurate coding possible for their organization. It is important to understand the basic criteria for assigning the *Coding Clinic* Reference Notations. The basic criteria consists of: Assignment to codes with direct or indirect information concerning the proper use of each particular code, assignment to a code category when the information is relevant to all codes in that category, and assignment to codes where a coder might commonly attempt to use a code in error.

MISCELLANEOUS AHA CODING CLINIC® REFERENCE NOTATIONS INDEX

© 2018 Channel Publishing, Ltd.

MISCELLANEOUS AHA CODING CLINIC® REFERENCE NOTATIONS INDEX

© 2018 Channel Publishing, Ltd.

NOTES

© 2018 Channel Publishing, Ltd.

IMPORTANT NOTES REGARDING THESE PRINTED GUIDELINES

These guidelines are effective for the 2019 version (May 2018 posting) of ICD-10-PCS. A newer version may become available after this book has been printed. Coders should periodically check the Centers for Medicare and Medicaid Services (CMS) web site for the most current version. CMS Web Site: www.cms.gov

Some Body System specific Guidelines have been reprinted on the Educational Annotations pages for those Body Systems. However, they are not a substitute for using the entire set of Official Coding Guidelines.

Channel Publishing, Ltd.

2019 ICD-10-PCS Official Guidelines for Coding and Reporting

The Centers for Medicare and Medicaid Services (CMS) and the National Center for Health Statistics (NCHS), two departments within the U.S. Federal Government's Department of Health and Human Services (DHHS) provide the following guidelines for coding and reporting using the International Classification of Diseases, 10th Revision, Procedure Coding System (ICD-10-PCS). These guidelines should be used as a companion document to the official version of the ICD-10-PCS as published on the CMS website. The ICD-10-PCS is a procedure classification published by the United States for classifying procedures performed in hospital inpatient health care settings.

These guidelines have been approved by the four organizations that make up the Cooperating Parties for the ICD-10-PCS: the American Hospital Association (AHA), the American Health Information Management Association (AHIMA), CMS, and NCHS.

These guidelines are a set of rules that have been devel oped to accompany and complement the official conventions and instructions provided within the ICD-10-PCS itself. The instructions and conventions of the classification take precedence over guidelines. These guidelines are based on the coding and sequencing instructions in the Tables, Index and Definitions of ICD-10-PCS, but provide additional instruction. Adherence to these guidelines when assigning ICD-10-PCS procedure codes is required under the Health Insurance Portability and Accountability Act (HIPAA). The procedure codes have been adopted under HIPAA for hospital inpatient healthcare settings. A joint effort between the healthcare provider and the coder is essential to achieve complete and accurate documentation, code assignment, and reporting of diagnoses and procedures. These guidelines have been developed to assist both the healthcare provider and the coder in identifying those procedures that are to be reported. The importance of consistent, complete documentation in the medical record cannot be overemphasized. Without such documentation accurate coding cannot be achieved.

© 2018 Channel Publishing, Ltd.

Table of Contents

Conventions

A1

ICD-10-PCS codes are composed of seven characters. Each character is an axis of classification that specifies information about the procedure performed. Within a defined code range, a character specifies the same type of information in that axis of classification.

Example: The fifth axis of classification specifies the approach in sections 0 through 4 and 7 through 9 of the system.

A2

One of 34 possible values can be assigned to each axis of classification in the seven-character code: they are the numbers 0 through 9 and the alphabet (except I and O because they are easily confused with the numbers 1 and 0). The number of unique values used in an axis of classification differs as needed.

Example: Where the fifth axis of classification specifies the approach, seven different approach values are currently used to specify the approach.

A3

The valid values for an axis of classification can be added to as needed.

Example: If a significantly distinct type of device is used in a new procedure, a new device value can be added to the system.

A4

As with words in their context, the meaning of any single value is a combination of its axis of classification and any preceding values on which it may be dependent.

Example: The meaning of a body part value in the Medical and Surgical section is always dependent on the body system value. The body part value 0 in the Central Nervous body system specifies Brain and the body part value 0 in the Peripheral Nervous body system specifies Cervical Plexus.

A5

As the system is expanded to become increasingly detailed, over time more values will depend on preceding values for their meaning.

Example: In the Lower Joints body system, the device value 3 in the root operation Insertion specifies Infusion Device and the device value 3 in the root operation Replacement specifies Ceramic Synthetic Substitute.

A6

The purpose of the alphabetic index is to locate the appropriate table that contains all information necessary to construct a procedure code. The PCS Tables should always be consulted to find the most appropriate valid code.

A7

It is not required to consult the index first before proceeding to the tables to complete the code. A valid code may be chosen directly from the tables.

AHA Coding Clinic® Reference Notation(s) — Coding Guideline A7

Reconstruction, main index term .... AHA 14:2Q:p10

A8

All seven characters must be specified to be a valid code. If the documentation is incomplete for coding purposes, the physician should be queried for the necessary information.

A9

Within a PCS table, valid codes include all combinations of choices in characters 4 through 7 contained in the same row of the table. In the example below, 0JHT3VZ is a valid code, and 0JHW3VZ is *not* a valid code.

1ST- 0 Medical and Surgical 2ND- J Subcutaneous Tissue and Fascia 3RD- H INSERTION	EXAMPLE: Placement pacemaker generator INSERTION: Putting in a nonbiological appliance that monitors, assists, performs, or prevents a physiological function but does not physically take the place of a body part. EXPLANATION: None		
4TH Body Part	**5TH Approach**	**6TH Device**	**7TH Qualifier**
S Subcutaneous Tissue and Fascia, Head and Neck V Subcutaneous Tissue and Fascia, Upper Extremity **W Subcutaneous Tissue and Fascia, Lower Extremity**	0 Open 3 Percutaneous	1 Radioactive Element 3 Infusion Device	Z No Qualifier
T Subcutaneous Tissue and Fascia, Trunk	0 Open 3 Percutaneous	1 Radioactive Element 3 Infusion Device **V Infusion Pump**	Z No Qualifier

A10

"And," when used in a code description, means "and/or," except when used to describe a combination of multiple body parts for which separate values exist for each body part (e.g., Skin and Subcutaneous Tissue used as a qualifier, where there are separate body part values for "Skin" and "Subcutaneous Tissue").

Example: Lower Arm and Wrist Muscle means lower arm and/or wrist muscle.

A11

Many of the terms used to construct PCS codes are defined within the system. It is the coder's responsibility to determine what the documentation in the medical record equates to in the PCS definitions. The physician is not expected to use the terms used in PCS code descriptions, nor is the coder required to query the physician when the correlation between the documentation and the defined PCS terms is clear.

Example: When the physician documents "partial resection" the coder can independently correlate "partial resection" to the root operation Excision without querying the physician for clarification.

Medical and Surgical Section Guidelines (Section 0)

B2. Body System

General guidelines

B2.1a

The procedure codes in the general anatomical regions body systems can be used when the procedure is performed on an anatomical region rather than a specific body part (e.g., root operations Control and Detachment, Drainage of a body cavity) or on the rare occasion when no information is available to support assignment of a code to a specific body part.

Examples: Control of postoperative hemorrhage is coded to the root operation Control found in the general anatomical regions body systems.

Chest tube drainage of the pleural cavity is coded to the root operation Drainage found in the general anatomical regions body systems. Suture repair of the abdominal wall is coded to the root operation Repair in the general anatomical regions body system.

B2.1b

Where the general body part values "upper" and "lower" are provided as an option in the Upper Arteries, Lower Arteries, Upper Veins, Lower Veins, Muscles and Tendons body systems, "upper" or "lower "specifies body parts located above or below the diaphragm respectively.

Example: Vein body parts above the diaphragm are found in the Upper Veins body system; vein body parts below the diaphragm are found in the Lower Veins body system.

AHA Coding Clinic® Reference Notation(s) — Coding Guideline B2.1b

Upper or lower veins body system .... AHA 14:3Q:p25

B3. Root Operation

General guidelines

B3.1a

In order to determine the appropriate root operation, the full definition of the root operation as contained in the PCS Tables must be applied.

B3.1b

Components of a procedure specified in the root operation definition and explanation are not coded separately. Procedural steps necessary to reach the operative site and close the operative site, including anastomosis of a tubular body part, are also not coded separately.

Examples: Resection of a joint as part of a joint replacement procedure is included in the root operation definition of Replacement and is not coded separately. Laparotomy performed to reach the site of an open liver biopsy is not coded separately. In a resection of sigmoid colon with anastomosis of descending colon to rectum, the anastomosis is not coded separately.

AHA Coding Clinic® Reference Notation(s) — Coding Guideline B3.1b

Components in fusion procedures included in Fusion root operation .... AHA 14:3Q:p30
Coronary artery release prior to bypass .... AHA 13:2Q:p37
Debridement considered as procedure preparation .... AHA 14:3Q:p31
Decalcification of aorta in preparation for further surgery .... AHA 16:2Q:p25
FloSeal on small bleeder during cholecystectomy .... AHA 13:3Q:p22
Injection of substances with vitrectomy .... AHA 15:2Q:p24

© 2018 Channel Publishing, Ltd.

AHA Coding Clinic® Reference Notation(s) — Coding Guideline B3.1b - continued

Lysis of adhesions, integral or code separately....AHA 14:1Q:p3
Omental bleeding repair during cholecystectomy....AHA 13:3Q:p23
Orthotopic liver transplant with end-to-side cavoplasty and choledochostomy AHA 14:3Q:p13
Repositioning of aorta inherent to release of esophageal vascular ring ....AHA 15:3Q:p15

Multiple procedures

B3.2

During the same operative episode, multiple procedures are coded if:

a. The same root operation is performed on different body parts as defined by distinct values of the body part character.

Examples: Diagnostic excision of liver and pancreas are coded separately. Excision of lesion in the ascending colon and excision of lesion in the transverse colon are coded separately.

b. The same root operation is repeated in multiple body parts, and those body parts are separate and distinct body parts classified to a single ICD-10-PCS body part value.

Examples: Excision of the sartorius muscle and excision of the gracilis muscle are both included in the upper leg muscle body part value, and multiple procedures are coded.

Extraction of multiple toenails are coded separately.

AHA Coding Clinic® Reference Notation(s) — Coding Guideline B3.2b

Coil embolization of gastroduodenal artery, and chemoembolizationof hepatic artery....AHA 14:3Q:p26
Fasciotomy for compartment syndrome, foot, multiple sites ....AHA 17:2Q:p12,13
Uterine fibroids, multiple....AHA 14.4Q.p16

c. Multiple root operations with distinct objectives are performed on the same body part.

Example: Destruction of sigmoid lesion and bypass of sigmoid colon are coded separately.

AHA Coding Clinic® Reference Notation(s) — Coding Guideline B3.2c

Laminoplasty with two distinct objectives ....AHA 15:2Q:p20

d. The intended root operation is attempted using one approach, but is converted to a different approach.

Example: Laparoscopic cholecystectomy converted to an open cholecystectomy is coded as percutaneous endoscopic Inspection and open Resection.

AHA Coding Clinic® Reference Notation(s) — Coding Guideline B3.2d

Laparoscopic procedure converted to open ....AHA 15:1Q:p33

Discontinued or incomplete procedures

B3.3

If the intended procedure is discontinued or otherwise not completed, code the procedure to the root operation performed. If a procedure is discontinued before any other root operation is performed, code the root operation Inspection of the body part or anatomical region inspected.

Example: A planned aortic valve replacement procedure is discontinued after the initial thoracotomy and before any incision is made in the heart muscle, when the patient becomes hemodynamically unstable. This procedure is coded as an open Inspection of the mediastinum.

AHA Coding Clinic® Reference Notation(s) — Coding Guideline B3.3

Discontinued coronary intervention ....AHA 15:3Q:p9
Discontinued procedure after angiogram....AHA 15:3Q:p9

Biopsy procedures

B3.4a

Biopsy procedures are coded using the root operations Excision, Extraction, or Drainage and the qualifier Diagnostic.

Examples: Fine needle aspiration biopsy of fluid in the lung is coded to the root operation Drainage with the qualifier Diagnostic.

Biopsy of bone marrow is coded to the root operation Extraction with the qualifier Diagnostic.

Lymph node sampling for biopsy is coded to the root operation Excision with the qualifier Diagnostic.

AHA Coding Clinic® Reference Notation(s) — Coding Guideline B3.4a

Diagnostic and therapeutic procedures....AHA 17:3Q:p12

Biopsy followed by more definitive treatment

B3.4b

If a diagnostic Excision, Extraction, or Drainage procedure (biopsy) is followed by a more definitive procedure, such as Destruction, Excision or Resection at the same procedure site, both the biopsy and the more definitive treatment are coded.

Example: Biopsy of breast followed by partial mastectomy at the same procedure site, both the biopsy and the partial mastectomy procedure are coded.

Overlapping body layers

B3.5

If the root operations Excision, Repair or Inspection are performed on overlapping layers of the musculoskeletal system, the body part specifying the deepest layer is coded.

Example: Excisional debridement that includes skin and subcutaneous tissue and muscle is coded to the muscle body part.

AHA Coding Clinic® Reference Notation(s) — Coding Guideline B3.5

Deepest layer coded ....AHA 14:3Q:p14
Deepest layer coded - coccyx....AHA 15:3Q:p3-8
Obstetric perineal laceration repair ....AHA 16:1Q:p6-8

© 2018 Channel Publishing, Ltd.

Bypass procedures

B3.6a

Bypass procedures are coded by identifying the body part bypassed "from" and the body part bypassed "to." The fourth character body part specifies the body part bypassed from, and the qualifier specifies the body part bypassed to.

Example: Bypass from stomach to jejunum, stomach is the body part and jejunum is the qualifier.

AHA Coding Clinic® Reference Notation(s) — Coding Guideline B3.6a

Creation of percutaneous cutaneoperitoneal fistula for peritoneal dialysis ......AHA 13:4Q:p126

B3.6b

Coronary artery bypass procedures are coded differently than other bypass procedures as described in the previous guideline. Rather than identifying the body part bypassed from, the body part identifies the number of coronary arteries bypassed to, and the qualifier specifies the vessel bypassed from.

Example: Aortocoronary artery bypass of the left anterior descending coronary artery and the obtuse marginal coronary artery is classified in the body part axis of classification as two coronary arteries, and the qualifier specifies the aorta as the body part bypassed from.

AHA Coding Clinic® Reference Notation(s) — Coding Guideline B3.6b

Distinct coronary lesion sites treated ......AHA 15:2Q:p3-5

B3.6c

If multiple coronary arteries are bypassed, a separate procedure is coded for each coronary artery that uses a different device and/or qualifier.

Example: Aortocoronary artery bypass and internal mammary coronary artery bypass are coded separately.

Control vs. more definitive root operations

B3.7

The root operation Control is defined as, "Stopping, or attempting to stop, postprocedural or other acute bleeding." If an attempt to stop postprocedural or other acute bleeding is unsuccessful, and to stop the bleeding requires performing a more definitive root operation, such as Bypass, Detachment, Excision, Extraction, Reposition, Replacement, or Resection, then the more definitive root operation is coded instead of Control.

Example: Resection of spleen to stop bleeding is coded to Resection instead of Control.

AHA Coding Clinic® Reference Notation(s) — Coding Guideline B3.7

Control versus more definitive root operations......AHA 17:4Q:p106

Excision vs. Resection

B3.8

PCS contains specific body parts for anatomical subdivisions of a body part, such as lobes of the lungs or liver and regions of the intestine. Resection of the specific body part is coded whenever all of the body part is cut out or off, rather than coding Excision of a less specific body part.

Example: Left upper lung lobectomy is coded to Resection of Upper Lung Lobe, Left rather than Excision of Lung, Left.

Excision for graft

B3.9

If an autograft is obtained from a different procedure site in order to complete the objective of the procedure, a separate procedure is coded.

Example: Coronary bypass with excision of saphenous vein graft, excision of saphenous vein is coded separately.

AHA Coding Clinic® Reference Notation(s) — Coding Guideline B3.9

Autograft from same operative site ......AHA 17:3Q:p7

Excision of fat for graft to a separate site ......AHA 18:1Q:p7

Harvesting of fat graft from abdomen ......AHA 14:3Q:p22

Fusion procedures of the spine

B3.10a

The body part coded for a spinal vertebral joint(s) rendered immobile by a spinal fusion procedure is classified by the level of the spine (e.g. thoracic). There are distinct body part values for a single vertebral joint and for multiple vertebral joints at each spinal level.

Example: Body part values specify Lumbar Vertebral Joint, Lumbar Vertebral Joints, 2 or More and Lumbosacral Vertebral Joint.

AHA Coding Clinic® Reference Notation(s) — Coding Guideline B3.10a

Fusion, level of spine ......AHA 13:1Q:p29

Fusion of multiple vertebral joints......AHA 13:1Q:p21

B3.10b

If multiple vertebral joints are fused, a separate procedure is coded for each vertebral joint that uses a different device and/or qualifier.

Example: Fusion of lumbar vertebral joint, posterior approach, anterior column and fusion of lumbar vertebral joint, posterior approach, posterior column are coded separately.

B3.10c

Combinations of devices and materials are often used on a vertebral joint to render the joint immobile. When combinations of devices are used on the same vertebral joint, the device value coded for the procedure is as follows:

- If an interbody fusion device is used to render the joint immobile (alone or containing other material like bone graft), the procedure is coded with the device value Interbody Fusion Device
- If bone graft is the only device used to render the joint immobile, the procedure is coded with the device value Nonautologous Tissue Substitute or Autologous Tissue Substitute
- If a mixture of autologous and nonautologous bone graft (with or without biological or synthetic extenders or binders) is used to render the joint immobile, code the procedure with the device value Autologous Tissue Substitute

Examples: Fusion of a vertebral joint using a cage style interbody fusion device containing morsellized bone graft is coded to the device Interbody Fusion Device.

Fusion of a vertebral joint using a bone dowel interbody fusion device made of cadaver bone and packed with a mixture of local morsellized bone and demineralized bone matrix is coded to the device Interbody Fusion Device.

© 2018 Channel Publishing, Ltd.

B3.10c – *Examples:* — *continued*

Fusion of a vertebral joint using both autologous bone graft and bone bank bone graft is coded to the device Autologous Tissue Substitute.

AHA Coding Clinic® Reference Notation(s) — Coding Guideline B3.10c

Interbody fusion device .... AHA 13:1Q:p29
Bone graft with mixture of autologous and nonautologous bone .... AHA 13:3Q:p25
Fusion of multiple vertebral joints .... AHA 13:1Q:p21

Inspection procedures

B3.11a

Inspection of a body part(s) performed in order to achieve the objective of a procedure is not coded separately.

Example: Fiberoptic bronchoscopy performed for irrigation of bronchus, only the irrigation procedure is coded.

B3.11b

If multiple tubular body parts are inspected, the most distal body part (the body part furthest from the starting point of the inspection) is coded. If multiple non-tubular body parts in a region are inspected, the body part that specifies the entire area inspected is coded.

Examples: Cystoureteroscopy with inspection of bladder and ureters is coded to the ureter body part value.

Exploratory laparotomy with general inspection of abdominal contents is coded to the peritoneal cavity body part value.

B3.11c

When both an Inspection procedure and another procedure are performed on the same body part during the same episode, if the Inspection procedure is performed using a different approach than the other procedure, the Inspection procedure is coded separately.

Example: Endoscopic Inspection of the duodenum is coded separately when open Excision of the duodenum is performed during the same procedural episode.

AHA Coding Clinic® Reference Notation(s) — Coding Guideline B3.11c

Sigmoidoscopy to check anastomosis following low anterior resection .... AHA 17:2Q:p15

Occlusion vs. Restriction for vessel embolization procedures

B3.12

If the objective of an embolization procedure is to completely close a vessel, the root operation Occlusion is coded. If the objective of an embolization procedure is to narrow the lumen of a vessel, the root operation Restriction is coded.

Examples: Tumor embolization is coded to the root operation Occlusion, because the objective of the procedure is to cut off the blood supply to the vessel.

Embolization of a cerebral aneurysm is coded to the root operation Restriction, because the objective of the procedure is not to close off the vessel entirely, but to narrow the lumen of the vessel at the site of the aneurysm where it is abnormally wide.

Release procedures

B3.13

In the root operation Release, the body part value coded is the body part being freed and not the tissue being manipulated or cut to free the body part.

Example: Lysis of intestinal adhesions is coded to the specific intestine body part value.

AHA Coding Clinic® Reference Notation(s) — Coding Guideline B3.13

Lysis of adhesions, integral or code separately .... AHA 14:1Q:p3

Release vs. Division

B3.14

If the sole objective of the procedure is freeing a body part without cutting the body part, the root operation is Release. If the sole objective of the procedure is separating or transecting a body part, the root operation is Division.

Examples: Freeing a nerve root from surrounding scar tissue to relieve pain is coded to the root operation Release.

Severing a nerve root to relieve pain is coded to the root operation Division.

Reposition for fracture treatment

B3.15

Reduction of a displaced fracture is coded to the root operation Reposition and the application of a cast or splint in conjunction with the Reposition procedure is not coded separately. Treatment of a nondisplaced fracture is coded to the procedure performed.

Examples: Casting of a nondisplaced fracture is coded to the root operation Immobilization in the Placement section.

Putting a pin in a nondisplaced fracture is coded to the root operation Insertion.

Transplantation vs. Administration

B3.16

Putting in a mature and functioning living body part taken from another individual or animal is coded to the root operation Transplantation. Putting in autologous or nonautologous cells is coded to the Administration section.

Example: Putting in autologous or nonautologous bone marrow, pancreatic islet cells or stem cells is coded to the Administration section.

© 2018 Channel Publishing, Ltd.

Transfer procedures using multiple tissue layers

B3.17

The root operation Transfer contains qualifiers that can be used to specify when a transfer flap is composed of more than one tissue layer, such as a musculocutaneous flap. For procedures involving transfer of multiple tissue layers including skin, subcutaneous tissue, fascia or muscle, the procedure is coded to the body part value that describes the deepest tissue layer in the flap, and the qualifier can be used to describe the other tissue layer(s) in the transfer flap.

Example: A musculocutaneous flap transfer is coded to the appropriate body part value in the body system Muscles, and the qualifier is used to describe the additional tissue layer(s) in the transfer flap.

B4. Body Part

General guidelines

B4.1a

If a procedure is performed on a portion of a body part that does not have a separate body part value, code the body part value corresponding to the whole body part.

Example: A procedure performed on the alveolar process of the mandible is coded to the mandible body part.

B4.1b

If the prefix "peri" is combined with a body part to identify the site of the procedure, and the site of the procedure is not further specified, then the procedure is coded to the body part named. This guideline applies only when a more specific body part value is not available.

Examples: A procedure site identified as perirenal is coded to the kidney body part when the site of the procedure is not further specified.

A procedure site described in the documentation as peri-urethral, and the documentation also indicates that it is the vulvar tissue and not the urethral tissue that is the site of the procedure, then the procedure is coded to the vulva body part.

AHA Coding Clinic® Reference Notation(s) — Coding Guideline B4.1b

Catheter ablation of peripulmonary veins to target the conduction pathway of left atrium .... AHA 14:4Q:p47

Official Clarification .... AHA 16:3Q:p43

Periurethral obstetric laceration repair .... AHA 14:4Q:p18

B4.1c

If a procedure is performed on a continuous section of a tubular body part, code the body part value corresponding to the furthest anatomical site from the point of entry.

Example: A procedure performed on a continuous section of artery from the femoral artery to the external iliac artery with the point of entry at the femoral artery is coded to the external iliac body part.

Branches of body parts

B4.2

Where a specific branch of a body part does not have its own body part value in PCS, the body part is typically coded to the closest proximal branch that has a specific body part value. In the cardiovascular body systems, if a general body part is available in the correct root operation table, and coding to a proximal branch would require assigning a code in a different body system, the procedure is coded using the general body part value.

Examples: A procedure performed on the mandibular branch of the trigeminal nerve is coded to the trigeminal nerve body part value.

Occlusion of the bronchial artery is coded to the body part value Upper Artery in the body system Upper Arteries, and not to the body part value Thoracic Aorta, Descending in the body system Heart and Great Vessels.

Bilateral body part values

B4.3

Bilateral body part values are available for a limited number of body parts. If the identical procedure is performed on contralateral body parts, and a bilateral body part value exists for that body part, a single procedure is coded using the bilateral body part value. If no bilateral body part value exists, each procedure is coded separately using the appropriate body part value.

Examples: The identical procedure performed on both fallopian tubes is coded once using the body part value Fallopian Tube, Bilateral.

The identical procedure performed on both knee joints is coded twice using the body part values Knee Joint, Right and Knee Joint, Left.

AHA Coding Clinic® Reference Notation(s) — Coding Guideline B4.3

Repair of midline diaphragm (paraesophageal) hernia .... AHA 14:3Q:p28

Removal of bilateral nonviable TRAM flap .... AHA 16:2Q:p27

Coronary arteries

B4.4

The coronary arteries are classified as a single body part that is further specified by number of arteries treated. One procedure code specifying multiple arteries is used when the same procedure is performed, including the same device and qualifier values.

Examples: Angioplasty of two distinct coronary arteries with placement of two stents is coded as Dilation of Coronary Artery, Two Arteries with Two Intraluminal Devices.

Angioplasty of two distinct coronary arteries, one with stent placed and one without, is coded separately as Dilation of Coronary Artery, One Artery with Intraluminal Device, and Dilation of Coronary Artery, One Artery with no device.

© 2018 Channel Publishing, Ltd.

Tendons, ligaments, bursae and fascia near a joint

B4.5

Procedures performed on tendons, ligaments, bursae and fascia supporting a joint are coded to the body part in the respective body system that is the focus of the procedure. Procedures performed on joint structures themselves are coded to the body part in the joint body systems.

Examples: Repair of the anterior cruciate ligament of the knee is coded to the knee bursa and ligament body part in the bursae and ligaments body system.

Knee arthroscopy with shaving of articular cartilage is coded to the knee joint body part in the Lower Joints body system.

Skin, subcutaneous tissue and fascia overlying a joint

B4.6

If a procedure is performed on the skin, subcutaneous tissue or fascia overlying a joint, the procedure is coded to the following body part:

- Shoulder is coded to Upper Arm
- Elbow is coded to Lower Arm
- Wrist is coded to Lower Arm
- Hip is coded to Upper Leg
- Knee is coded to Lower Leg
- Ankle is coded to Foot

Fingers and toes

B4.7

If a body system does not contain a separate body part value for fingers, procedures performed on the fingers are coded to the body part value for the hand. If a body system does not contain a separate body part value for toes, procedures performed on the toes are coded to the body part value for the foot.

Example: Excision of finger muscle is coded to one of the hand muscle body part values in the Muscles body system.

Upper and lower intestinal tract

B4.8

In the Gastrointestinal body system, the general body part values Upper Intestinal Tract and Lower Intestinal Tract are provided as an option for the root operations Change, Inspection, Removal and Revision. Upper Intestinal Tract includes the portion of the gastrointestinal tract from the esophagus down to and including the duodenum, and Lower Intestinal Tract includes the portion of the gastrointestinal tract from the jejunum down to and including the rectum and anus.

Example: In the root operation Change table, change of a device in the jejunum is coded using the body part Lower Intestinal Tract.

B5. Approach

Open approach with percutaneous endoscopic assistance

B5.2

Procedures performed using the open approach with percutaneous endoscopic assistance are coded to the approach Open.

Example: Laparoscopic-assisted sigmoidectomy is coded to the approach Open.

External approach

B5.3a

Procedures performed within an orifice on structures that are visible without the aid of any instrumentation are coded to the approach External.

Example: Resection of tonsils is coded to the approach External.

B5.3b

Procedures performed indirectly by the application of external force through the intervening body layers are coded to the approach External.

Example: Closed reduction of fracture is coded to the approach External.

Percutaneous procedure via device

B5.4

Procedures performed percutaneously via a device placed for the procedure are coded to the approach Percutaneous.

Example: Fragmentation of kidney stone performed via percutaneous nephrostomy is coded to the approach Percutaneous.

B6. Device

General guidelines

B6.1a

A device is coded only if a device remains after the procedure is completed. If no device remains, the device value No Device is coded. In limited root operations, the classification provides the qualifier values Temporary and Intraoperative, for specific procedures involving clinically significant devices, where the purpose of the device is to be utilized for a brief duration during the procedure or current inpatient stay. If a device that is intended to remain after the procedure is completed requires removal before the end of the operative episode in which it was inserted (for example, the device size is inadequate or a complication occurs), both the insertion and removal of the device should be coded.

B6.1b

Materials such as sutures, ligatures, radiological markers and temporary post-operative wound drains are considered integral to the performance of a procedure and are not coded as devices.

AHA Coding Clinic® Reference Notation(s) — Coding Guideline B6.1b

Bronchoscopic placement of fiducial marker....AHA 14:1Q:p20
Fluoroscopic guided fiducial marker placement....AHA 14:1Q:p20

© 2018 Channel Publishing, Ltd.

B6.1c

Procedures performed on a device only and not on a body part are specified in the root operations Change, Irrigation, Removal and Revision, and are coded to the procedure performed.

Example: Irrigation of percutaneous nephrostomy tube is coded to the root operation Irrigation of indwelling device in the Administration section.

AHA Coding Clinic® Reference Notation(s) — Coding Guideline B6.1c

Replacement of arterial conduit is not coded as Removal of device ....AHA 14:3Q:p30

Drainage device

B6.2

A separate procedure to put in a drainage device is coded to the root operation Drainage with the device value Drainage Device.

Obstetric Section Guidelines (Section 1)

C. Obstetrics Section

Products of conception

C1

Procedures performed on the products of conception are coded to the Obstetrics section. Procedures performed on the pregnant female other than the products of conception are coded to the appropriate root operation in the Medical and Surgical section.

Example: Amniocentesis is coded to the products of conception body part in the Obstetrics section. Repair of obstetric urethral laceration is coded to the urethra body part in the Medical and Surgical section.

Procedures following delivery or abortion

C2

Procedures performed following a delivery or abortion for curettage of the endometrium or evacuation of retained products of conception are all coded in the Obstetrics section, to the root operation Extraction and the body part Products of Conception, Retained. Diagnostic or therapeutic dilation and curettage performed during times other than the postpartum or post-abortion period are all coded in the Medical and Surgical section, to the root operation Extraction and the body part Endometrium.

New Technology Section Guidelines (section X)

D. New Technology Section

General guidelines

D1

Section X codes are standalone codes. They are not supplemental codes. Section X codes fully represent the specific procedure described in the code title, and do not require any additional codes from other sections of ICD-10-PCS. When section X contains a code title which describes a specific new technology procedure, only that X code is reported for the procedure. There is no need to report a broader, non-specific code in another section of ICD-10-PCS.

Example: XW04321 Introduction of Ceftazidime-Avibactam Anti-infective into Central Vein, Percutaneous Approach, New Technology Group 1, can be coded to indicate that Ceftazidime-Avibactam Anti-infective was administered via a central vein. A separate code from table 3E0 in the Administration section of ICD-10-PCS is not coded in addition to this code.

Selection of Principal Procedure

The following instructions should be applied in the selection of principal procedure and clarification on the importance of the relation to the principal diagnosis when more than one procedure is performed:

1. Procedure performed for definitive treatment of both principal diagnosis and secondary diagnosis.
    a. Sequence procedure performed for definitive treatment most related to principal diagnosis as principal procedure.
2. Procedure performed for definitive treatment and diagnostic procedures performed for both principal diagnosis and secondary diagnosis.
    a. Sequence procedure performed for definitive treatment most related to principal diagnosis as principal procedure.
3. A diagnostic procedure was performed for the principal diagnosis and a procedure is performed for definitive treatment of a secondary diagnosis.
    a. Sequence diagnostic procedure as principal procedure, since the procedure most related to the principal diagnosis takes precedence.
4. No procedures performed that are related to principal diagnosis; procedures performed for definitive treatment and diagnostic procedures were performed for secondary diagnosis.
    a. Sequence procedure performed for definitive treatment of secondary diagnosis as principal procedure, since there are no procedures (definitive or nondefinitive treatment) related to principal diagnosis.

AHA Coding Clinic® Reference Notation(s) — Coding Guideline Selection of Principal Procedure

Sequencing of mechanical ventilation with other procedures ....AHA 14:4Q:p11

© 2018 Channel Publishing, Ltd.

A

3f (Aortic) Bioprosthesis valve
use Zooplastic Tissue in Heart and Great Vessels
Abdominal aortic plexus
use Nerve, Abdominal Sympathetic
Abdominal esophagus
use Esophagus, Lower
Abdominohysterectomy
see Resection, Uterus **0UT9-**
Abdominoplasty
see Alteration, Abdominal Wall **0W0F-**
see Repair, Abdominal Wall **0WQF-**
see Supplement, Abdominal Wall **0WUF-**
Abductor hallucis muscle
use Muscle, Foot, Left
use Muscle, Foot, Right
AbioCor® Total Replacement Heart
use Synthetic Substitute
Ablation *see* Destruction
Abortion
Products of Conception **10A0-**
Abortifacient **10A07ZX**
Laminaria **10A07ZW**
Vacuum **10A07Z6**
Abrasion *see* Extraction
Absolute Pro Vascular (OTW) Self-Expanding Stent System
use Intraluminal Device
Accessory cephalic vein
use Vein, Cephalic, Left
use Vein, Cephalic, Right
Accessory obturator nerve
use Nerve, Lumbar Plexus
Accessory phrenic nerve
use Nerve, Phrenic
Accessory spleen
use Spleen
Acculink (RX) Carotid Stent System
use Intraluminal Device
Acellular Hydrated Dermis
use Nonautologous Tissue Substitute
Acetabular cup
use Liner in Lower Joints
Acetabulectomy
see Excision, Lower Bones **0QB-**
see Resection, Lower Bones **0QT-**
Acetabulofemoral joint
use Joint, Hip, Left
use Joint, Hip, Right
Acetabuloplasty
see Repair, Lower Bones **0QQ-**
see Replacement, Lower Bones **0QR-**
see Supplement, Lower Bones **0QU-**
Achilles tendon
use Tendon, Lower Leg, Left
use Tendon, Lower Leg, Right
Achillorrhaphy *see* Repair, Tendons **0LQ-**
Achillotenotomy, achillotomy
see Division, Tendons **0L8-**
see Drainage, Tendons **0L9-**
Acromioclavicular ligament
use Bursa and Ligament, Shoulder, Left
use Bursa and Ligament, Shoulder, Right
Acromion (process)
use Scapula, Left
use Scapula, Right
Acromionectomy
see Excision, Upper Joints **0RB-**
see Resection, Upper Joints **0RT-**
Acromioplasty
see Repair, Upper Joints **0RQ-**
see Replacement, Upper Joints **0RR-**
see Supplement, Upper Joints **0RU-**
Activa PC neurostimulator
use Stimulator Generator, Multiple Array in **0JH-**
Activa RC neurostimulator
use Stimulator Generator, Multiple Array Rechargeable in **0JH-**
Activa SC neurostimulator
use Stimulator Generator, Single Array in **0JH-**
Activities of Daily Living Assessment F02-
Activities of Daily Living Treatment F08-
ACUITY™ Steerable Lead
use Cardiac Lead, Defibrillator in **02H-**
use Cardiac Lead, Pacemaker in **02H-**
Acupuncture
Breast
Anesthesia **8E0H300**
No Qualifier **8E0H30Z**
Integumentary System
Anesthesia **8E0H300**
No Qualifier **8E0H30Z**
Adductor brevis muscle
use Muscle, Upper Leg, Left
use Muscle, Upper Leg, Right
Adductor hallucis muscle
use Muscle, Foot, Left
use Muscle, Foot, Right
Adductor longus muscle
use Muscle, Upper Leg, Left
use Muscle, Upper Leg, Right
Adductor magnus muscle
use Muscle, Upper Leg, Left
use Muscle, Upper Leg, Right
Adenohypophysis
use Gland, Pituitary
Adenoidectomy
see Excision, Adenoids **0CBQ-**
see Resection, Adenoids **0CTQ-**
Adenoidotomy *see* Drainage, Adenoids **0C9Q-**
Adhesiolysis *see* Release
Administration
Blood products *see* Transfusion
Other substance *see* Introduction of substance in or on
Adrenalectomy
see Excision, Endocrine System **0GB-**
see Resection, Endocrine System **0GT-**
Adrenalorrhaphy *see* Repair, Endocrine System **0GQ-**
Adrenalotomy *see* Drainage, Endocrine System **0G9-**
Advancement
see Reposition
see Transfer
Advisa (MRI)
use Pacemaker, Dual Chamber in **0JH-**
AFX® Endovascular AAA System
use Intraluminal Device
AIGISRx Antibacterial Envelope
use Anti-Infective Envelope
Alar ligament of axis
use Bursa and Ligament, Head and Neck
Alfieri Stitch Valvuloplasty *see* Restriction, Valve, Mitral **02VG-**
Alimentation *see* Introduction of substance in or on
Alteration
Abdominal Wall **0W0F-**
Ankle Region
Left **0Y0L-**
Right **0Y0K-**
Arm
Lower
Left **0X0F-**
Right **0X0D-**
Upper
Left **0X09-**
Right **0X08-**
Axilla
Left **0X05-**
Right **0X04-**
Back
Lower **0W0L-**
Upper **0W0K-**
Breast
Bilateral **0H0V-**
Left **0H0U-**
Right **0H0T-**
Buttock
Left **0Y01-**
Right **0Y00-**
Chest Wall **0W08-**
Ear
Bilateral **0902-**
Left **0901-**
Right **0900-**
Elbow Region
Left **0X0C-**
Right **0X0B-**
Extremity
Lower
Left **0Y0B-**
Right **0Y09-**
Upper
Left **0X07-**
Right **0X06-**
Eyelid
Lower
Left **080R-**
Right **080Q-**
Upper
Left **080P-**
Right **080N-**
Face **0W02-**
Head **0W00-**
Jaw
Lower **0W05-**
Upper **0W04-**
Knee Region
Left **0Y0G-**
Right **0Y0F-**
Leg
Lower
Left **0Y0J-**
Right **0Y0H-**
Upper
Left **0Y0D-**
Right **0Y0C-**
Lip
Lower **0C01X-**
Upper **0C00X-**
Nasal Mucosa and Soft Tissue **090K-**
Neck **0W06-**
Perineum
Female **0W0N-**
Male **0W0M-**
Shoulder Region
Left **0X03-**
Right **0X02-**
Subcutaneous Tissue and Fascia
Abdomen **0J08-**
Back **0J07-**
Buttock **0J09-**
Chest **0J06-**
Face **0J01-**
Lower Arm
Left **0J0H-**
Right **0J0G-**
Alteration — *continued*
Subcutaneous Tissue and Fascia — *continued*
Lower Leg
Left **0J0P-**
Right **0J0N-**
Neck
Left **0J05-**
Right **0J04-**
Upper Arm
Left **0J0F-**
Right **0J0D-**
Upper Leg
Left **0J0M-**
Right **0J0L-**
Wrist Region
Left **0X0H-**
Right **0X0G-**
Alveolar process of mandible
use Mandible, Left
use Mandible, Right
Alveolar process of maxilla
use Maxilla
Alveolectomy
see Excision, Head and Facial Bones **0NB-**
see Resection, Head and Facial Bones **0NT-**
Alveoloplasty
see Repair, Head and Facial Bones **0NQ-**
see Replacement, Head and Facial Bones **0NR-**
see Supplement, Head and Facial Bones **0NU-**
Alveolotomy
see Division, Head and Facial Bones **0N8-**
see Drainage, Head and Facial Bones **0N9-**
Ambulatory cardiac monitoring 4A12X45
Amniocentesis *see* Drainage, Products of Conception **1090-**
Amnioinfusion *see* Introduction of substance in or on, Products of Conception **3E0E-**
Amnioscopy 10J08ZZ
Amniotomy *see* Drainage, Products of Conception **1090-**
AMPLATZER® Muscular VSD Occluder
use Synthetic Substitute
Amputation *see* Detachment
AMS 800® Urinary Control System
use Artificial Sphincter in Urinary System
Anal orifice
use Anus
Analog radiography *see* Plain Radiography
Analog radiology *see* Plain Radiography
Anastomosis *see* Bypass
Anatomical snuffbox
use Muscle, Lower Arm and Wrist, Left
use Muscle, Lower Arm and Wrist, Right
Andexanet Alfa, Factor Xa Inhibitor Reversal Agent XW0-
AneuRx® AAA Advantage®
use Intraluminal Device
Angiectomy
see Excision, Heart and Great Vessels **02B-**
see Excision, Lower Arteries **04B-**
see Excision, Lower Veins **06B-**
see Excision, Upper Arteries **03B-**
see Excision, Upper Veins **05B-**

© 2018 Channel Publishing, Ltd.

Angiocardiography
Combined right and left heart *see* Fluoroscopy, Heart, Right and Left **B216-**
Left Heart *see* Fluoroscopy, Heart, Left **B215-**
Right Heart *see* Fluoroscopy, Heart, Right **B214-**
SPY system intravascular fluorescence *see* Monitoring, Physiological Systems **4A1-**
Angiography
see Plain Radiography, Heart **B20-**
see Fluoroscopy, Heart **B21-**
Angioplasty
see Dilation, Heart and Great Vessels **027-**
see Dilation, Lower Arteries **047-**
see Dilation, Upper Arteries **037-**
see Repair, Heart and Great Vessels **02Q-**
see Repair, Lower Arteries **04Q-**
see Repair, Upper Arteries **03Q-**
see Replacement, Heart and Great Vessels **02R-**
see Replacement, Lower Arteries **04R-**
see Replacement, Upper Arteries **03R-**
see Supplement, Heart and Great Vessels **02U-**
see Supplement, Lower Arteries **04U-**
see Supplement, Upper Arteries **03U-**
Angiorrhaphy
see Repair, Heart and Great Vessels **02Q-**
see Repair, Lower Arteries **04Q-**
see Repair, Upper Arteries **03Q-**
Angioscopy
02JY4ZZ
03JY4ZZ
04JY4ZZ
Angiotensin II
use Synthetic Human Angiotensin II
Angiotripsy
see Occlusion, Lower Arteries **04L-**
see Occlusion, Upper Arteries **03L-**
Angular artery
use Artery, Face
Angular vein
use Vein, Face, Left
use Vein, Face, Right
Annular ligament
use Bursa and Ligament, Elbow, Left
use Bursa and Ligament, Elbow, Right
Annuloplasty
see Repair, Heart and Great Vessels **02Q-**
see Supplement, Heart and Great Vessels **02U-**
Annuloplasty ring
use Synthetic Substitute
Anoplasty
see Repair, Anus **0DQQ-**
see Supplement, Anus **0DUQ-**
Anorectal junction
use Rectum
Anoscopy 0DJD8ZZ
Ansa cervicalis
use Nerve, Cervical Plexus
Antabuse therapy HZ93ZZZ
Antebrachial fascia
use Subcutaneous Tissue and Fascia, Lower Arm, Left
use Subcutaneous Tissue and Fascia, Lower Arm, Right
Anterior (pectoral) lymph node
use Lymphatic, Axillary, Left
use Lymphatic, Axillary, Right
Anterior cerebral artery
use Artery, Intracranial
Anterior cerebral vein
use Vein, Intracranial
Anterior choroidal artery
use Artery, Intracranial
Anterior circumflex humeral artery
use Artery, Axillary, Left
use Artery, Axillary, Right
Anterior communicating artery
use Artery, Intracranial
Anterior cruciate ligament (ACL)
use Bursa and Ligament, Knee, Left
use Bursa and Ligament, Knee, Right
Anterior crural nerve
use Nerve, Femoral
Anterior facial vein
use Vein, Face, Left
use Vein, Face, Right
Anterior intercostal artery
use Artery, Internal Mammary, Left
use Artery, Internal Mammary, Right
Anterior interosseous nerve
use Nerve, Median
Anterior lateral malleolar artery
use Artery, Anterior Tibial, Left
use Artery, Anterior Tibial, Right
Anterior lingual gland
use Gland, Minor Salivary
Anterior medial malleolar artery
use Artery, Anterior Tibial, Left
use Artery, Anterior Tibial, Right
Anterior spinal artery
use Artery, Vertebral, Left
use Artery, Vertebral, Right
Anterior tibial recurrent artery
use Artery, Anterior Tibial, Left
use Artery, Anterior Tibial, Right
Anterior ulnar recurrent artery
use Artery, Ulnar, Left
use Artery, Ulnar, Right
Anterior vagal trunk
use Nerve, Vagus
Anterior vertebral muscle
use Muscle, Neck, Left
use Muscle, Neck, Right
Antigen-free air conditioning *see* Atmospheric Control, Physiological Systems **6A0-**
Antihelix
use Ear, External, Bilateral
use Ear, External, Left
use Ear, External, Right
Antimicrobial envelope
use Anti-Infective Envelope
Antitragus
use Ear, External, Bilateral
use Ear, External, Left
use Ear, External, Right
Antrostomy *see* Drainage, Ear, Nose, Sinus **099-**
Antrotomy *see* Drainage, Ear, Nose, Sinus **099-**
Antrum of Highmore
use Sinus, Maxillary, Left
use Sinus, Maxillary, Right
Aortic annulus
use Valve, Aortic
Aortic arch
use Thoracic Aorta, Ascending/Arch
Aortic intercostal artery
use Upper Artery
Aortography
see Fluoroscopy, Lower Arteries **B41-**
see Fluoroscopy, Upper Arteries **B31-**
see Plain Radiography, Lower Arteries **B40-**
see Plain Radiography, Upper Arteries **B30-**
Aortoplasty
see Repair, Aorta, Abdominal **04Q0-**
see Repair, Aorta, Thoracic, Ascending/Arch **02QX-**
see Repair, Aorta, Thoracic, Descending **02QW-**
see Replacement, Aorta, Abdominal **04R0-**
see Replacement, Aorta, Thoracic, Ascending/Arch **02RX-**
see Replacement, Aorta, Thoracic, Descending **02RW-**
see Supplement, Aorta, Abdominal **04U0-**
see Supplement, Aorta, Thoracic, Ascending/Arch **02UX-**
see Supplement, Aorta, Thoracic, Descending **02UW-**
Apical (subclavicular) lymph node
use Lymphatic, Axillary, Left
use Lymphatic, Axillary, Right
Apneustic center
use Pons
Appendectomy
see Excision, Appendix **0DBJ-**
see Resection, Appendix **0DTJ-**
Appendicolysis *see* Release, Appendix **0DNJ-**
Appendicotomy *see* Drainage, Appendix **0D9J-**
Application *see* Introduction of substance in or on
Aquablation therapy, prostate XV508A4
Aquapheresis 6A550Z3
Aqueduct of Sylvius
use Cerebral Ventricle
Aqueous humour
use Anterior Chamber, Left
use Anterior Chamber, Right
Arachnoid mater, intracranial
use Cerebral Meninges
Arachnoid mater, spinal
use Spinal Meninges
Arcuate artery
use Artery, Foot, Left
use Artery, Foot, Right
Areola
use Nipple, Left
use Nipple, Right
AROM (artificial rupture of membranes) 10907ZC
Arterial canal (duct)
use Artery, Pulmonary, Left
Arterial pulse tracing *see* Measurement, Arterial **4A03-**
Arteriectomy *see* Excision, Heart and Great Vessels **02B-**
see Excision, Lower Arteries **04B-**
see Excision, Upper Arteries **03B-**
Arteriography
see Fluoroscopy, Heart **B21-**
see Fluoroscopy, Lower Arteries **B41-**
see Fluoroscopy, Upper Arteries **B31-**
see Plain Radiography, Heart **B20-**
see Plain Radiography, Lower Arteries **B40-**
see Plain Radiography, Upper Arteries **B30-**
Arterioplasty
see Repair, Heart and Great Vessels **02Q-**
see Repair, Lower Arteries **04Q-**
see Repair, Upper Arteries **03Q-**
see Replacement, Heart and Great Vessels **02R-**
see Replacement, Lower Arteries **04R-**
see Replacement, Upper Arteries **03R-**
see Supplement, Heart and Great Vessels **02U-**
see Supplement, Lower Arteries **04U-**
see Supplement, Upper Arteries **03U-**
Arteriorrhaphy
see Repair, Heart and Great Vessels **02Q-**
see Repair, Lower Arteries **04Q-**
see Repair, Upper Arteries **03Q-**
Arterioscopy
see Inspection, Artery, Lower **04JY-**
see Inspection, Artery, Upper **03JY-**
see Inspection, Great Vessel **02JY-**
Arthrectomy
see Excision, Lower Joints **0SB-**
see Excision, Upper Joints **0RB-**
see Resection, Lower Joints **0ST-**
see Resection, Upper Joints **0RT-**
Arthrocentesis
see Drainage, Lower Joints **0S9-**
see Drainage, Upper Joints **0R9-**
Arthrodesis
see Fusion, Lower Joints **0SG-**
see Fusion, Upper Joints **0RG-**
Arthrography
see Plain Radiography, Non-Axial Lower Bones **BQ0-**
see Plain Radiography, Non-Axial Upper Bones **BP0-**
see Plain Radiography, Skull and Facial Bones **BN0-**
Arthrolysis
see Release, Lower Joints **0SN-**
see Release, Upper Joints **0RN-**
Arthropexy
see Repair, Lower Joints **0SQ-**
see Repair, Upper Joints **0RQ-**
see Reposition, Lower Joints **0SS-**
see Reposition, Upper Joints **0RS-**
Arthroplasty
see Repair, Lower Joints **0SQ-**
see Repair, Upper Joints **0RQ-**
see Replacement, Lower Joints **0SR-**
see Replacement, Upper Joints **0RR-**
see Supplement, Lower Joints **0SU-**
see Supplement, Upper Joints **0RU-**
Arthroplasty, radial head
see Replacement, Radius, Left **0PRJ-**
see Replacement, Radius, Right **0PRH-**
Arthroscopy
see Inspection, Lower Joints **0SJ-**
see Inspection, Upper Joints **0RJ-**
Arthrotomy
see Drainage, Lower Joints **0S9-**
see Drainage, Upper Joints **0R9-**
Articulating spacer (antibiotic)
use Articulating Spacer in Lower Joints
Artificial anal sphincter (AAS)
use Artificial Sphincter in Gastrointestinal System

© 2018 Channel Publishing, Ltd.

Artificial bowel sphincter (neosphincter)
use Artificial Sphincter in Gastrointestinal System
Artificial Sphincter
Insertion of device in
Anus **0DHQ-**
Bladder **0THB-**
Bladder Neck **0THC-**
Urethra **0THD-**
Removal of device from
Anus **0DPQ-**
Bladder **0TPB-**
Urethra **0TPD-**
Revision of device in
Anus **0DWQ-**
Bladder **0TWB-**
Urethra **0TWD-**
Artificial urinary sphincter (AUS)
use Artificial Sphincter in Urinary System
Aryepiglottic fold
use Larynx
Arytenoid cartilage
use Larynx
Arytenoid muscle
use Muscle, Neck, Left
use Muscle, Neck, Right
Arytenoidectomy *see* Excision, Larynx **0CBS-**
Arytenoidopexy
see Repair, Larynx **0CQS-**
Ascenda Intrathecal Catheter
use Infusion Device
Ascending aorta
use Thoracic Aorta, Ascending/Arch
Ascending palatine artery
use Artery, Face
Ascending pharyngeal artery
use Artery, External Carotid, Left
use Artery, External Carotid, Right
Aspiration, fine needle
Fluid or gas *see* Drainage
Tissue biopsy
see Excision
see Extraction
Assessment
Activities of daily living *see* Activities of Daily Living Assessment, Rehabilitation **F02-**
Hearing *see* Hearing Assessment, Diagnostic Audiology **F13-**
Hearing aid *see* Hearing Aid Assessment, Diagnostic Audiology **F14-**
Intravascular perfusion, using indocyanine green (ICG) dye *see* Monitoring, Physiological Systems **4A1-**
Motor function *see* Motor Function Assessment, Rehabilitation **F01-**
Nerve function *see* Motor Function Assessment, Rehabilitation **F01-**
Speech *see* Speech Assessment, Rehabilitation **F00-**
Vestibular *see* Vestibular Assessment, Diagnostic Audiology **F15-**
Vocational *see* Activities of Daily Living Treatment, Rehabilitation **F08-**
Assistance
Cardiac
Continuous
Balloon Pump **5A02210**
Impeller Pump **5A0221D**
Other Pump **5A02216**
Pulsatile Compression **5A02215**
Assistance — *continued*
Cardiac — *continued*
Intermittent
Balloon Pump **5A02110**
Impeller Pump **5A0211D**
Other Pump **5A02116**
Pulsatile Compression **5A02115**
Circulatory
Continuous
Hyperbaric **5A05221**
Supersaturated **5A0522C**
Intermittent
Hyperbaric **5A05121**
Supersaturated **5A0512C**
Respiratory
24-96 Consecutive Hours
Continuous Negative Airway Pressure **5A09459**
Continuous Positive Airway Pressure **5A09457**
Intermittent Negative Airway Pressure **5A0945B**
Intermittent Positive Airway Pressure **5A09458**
No Qualifier **5A0945Z**
Continuous, Filtration **5A0920Z**
Greater than 96 Consecutive Hours
Continuous Negative Airway Pressure **5A09559**
Continuous Positive Airway Pressure **5A09557**
Intermittent Negative Airway Pressure **5A0955B**
Intermittent Positive Airway Pressure **5A09558**
No Qualifier **5A0955Z**
Less than 24 Consecutive Hours
Continuous Negative Airway Pressure **5A09359**
Continuous Positive Airway Pressure **5A09357**
Intermittent Negative Airway Pressure **5A0935B**
Intermittent Positive Airway Pressure **5A09358**
No Qualifier **5A0935Z**
Assurant (Cobalt) stent
use Intraluminal Device
Atherectomy
see Extirpation, Heart and Great Vessels **02C-**
see Extirpation, Lower Arteries **04C-**
see Extirpation, Upper Arteries **03C-**
Atlantoaxial joint
use Joint, Cervical Vertebral
Atmospheric Control 6A0Z-
AtriClip LAA Exclusion System
use Extraluminal Device
Atrioseptoplasty
see Repair, Heart and Great Vessels **02Q-**
see Replacement, Heart and Great Vessels **02R-**
see Supplement, Heart and Great Vessels **02U-**
Atrioventricular node
use Conduction Mechanism
Atrium dextrum cordis
use Atrium, Right
Atrium pulmonale
use Atrium, Left
Attain Ability® lead
use Cardiac Lead, Defibrillator in **02H-**
use Cardiac Lead, Pacemaker in **02H-**
Attain StarFix® (OTW) lead
use Cardiac Lead, Defibrillator in **02H-**
use Cardiac Lead, Pacemaker in **02H-**
Audiology, diagnostic
see Hearing Aid Assessment, Diagnostic Audiology **F14-**
see Hearing Assessment, Diagnostic Audiology **F13-**
see Vestibular Assessment, Diagnostic Audiology **F15-**
Audiometry *see* Hearing Assessment, Diagnostic Audiology **F13-**
Auditory tube
use Eustachian Tube, Left
use Eustachian Tube, Right
Auerbach's (myenteric) plexus
use Nerve, Abdominal Sympathetic
Auricle
use Ear, External, Bilateral
use Ear, External, Left
use Ear, External, Right
Auricularis muscle
use Muscle, Head
Autograft
use Autologous Tissue Substitute
Autologous artery graft
use Autologous Arterial Tissue in Heart and Great Vessels
use Autologous Arterial Tissue in Lower Arteries
use Autologous Arterial Tissue in Lower Veins
use Autologous Arterial Tissue in Upper Arteries
use Autologous Arterial Tissue in Upper Veins
Autologous vein graft
use Autologous Venous Tissue in Heart and Great Vessels
use Autologous Venous Tissue in Lower Arteries
use Autologous Venous Tissue in Lower Veins
use Autologous Venous Tissue in Upper Arteries
use Autologous Venous Tissue in Upper Veins
Autotransfusion *see* Transfusion
Autotransplant
Adrenal tissue *see* Reposition, Endocrine System **0GS-**
Kidney *see* Reposition, Urinary System **0TS-**
Pancreatic tissue *see* Reposition, Pancreas **0FSG-**
Parathyroid tissue *see* Reposition, Endocrine System **0GS-**
Thyroid tissue *see* Reposition, Endocrine System **0GS-**
Tooth *see* Reattachment, Mouth and Throat **0CM-**
Avulsion *see* Extraction
Axial Lumbar Interbody Fusion System
use Interbody Fusion Device in Lower Joints
AxiaLIF® System
use Interbody Fusion Device in Lower Joints
Axicabtagene Ciloeucel
use Engineered Autologous Chimeric Antigen Receptor T-Cell Immunotherapy
Axillary fascia
use Subcutaneous Tissue and Fascia, Upper Arm, Left
use Subcutaneous Tissue and Fascia, Upper Arm, Right
Axillary nerve
use Nerve, Brachial Plexus

B

BAK/C® Interbody Cervical Fusion System
use Interbody Fusion Device in Upper Joints
BAL (bronchial alveolar lavage), diagnostic
see Drainage, Respiratory System **0B9-**
Balanoplasty
see Repair, Penis **0VQS-**
see Supplement, Penis **0VUS-**
Balloon atrial septostomy (BAS) 02163Z7
Balloon Pump
Continuous, Output **5A02210**
Intermittent, Output **5A02110**
Bandage, Elastic *see* Compression
Banding
see Occlusion
see Restriction
Banding, esophageal varices *see* Occlusion, Vein, Esophageal **06L3-**
Banding, laparoscopic (adjustable) gastric
Initial procedure **0DV64CZ**
Surgical correction *see* Revision of device in, Stomach **0DW6-**
Bard® Composix® (E/X) (LP) mesh
use Synthetic Substitute
Bard® Composix® Kugel® patch
use Synthetic Substitute
Bard® Dulex™ mesh
use Synthetic Substitute
Bard® Ventralex™ hernia patch
use Synthetic Substitute
Barium swallow *see* Fluoroscopy, Gastrointestinal System **BD1-**
Baroreflex Activation Therapy® (BAT®)
use Stimulator Generator in Subcutaneous Tissue and Fascia
use Stimulator Lead in Upper Arteries
Bartholin's (greater vestibular) gland
use Gland, Vestibular
Basal (internal) cerebral vein
use Vein, Intracranial
Basal metabolic rate (BMR) *see* Measurement, Physiological Systems **4A0Z-**
Basal nuclei
use Basal Ganglia
Base of tongue
use Pharnyx
Basilar artery
use Artery, Intracranial
Basis pontis
use Pons
Beam Radiation
Abdomen **DW03-**
Intraoperative **DW033Z0**
Adrenal Gland **DG02-**
Intraoperative **DG023Z0**
Bile Ducts **DF02-**
Intraoperative **DF023Z0**
Bladder **DT02-**
Intraoperative **DT023Z0**
Bone
Intraoperative **DP0C3Z0**
Other **DP0C-**
Bone Marrow **D700-**
Intraoperative **D7003Z0**
Brain **D000-**
Intraoperative **D0003Z0**
Brain Stem **D001-**
Intraoperative **D0013Z0**

© 2018 Channel Publishing, Ltd.

Beam Radiation — *continued*
Breast
Left **DM00-**
Intraoperative **DM003Z0**
Right **DM01-**
Intraoperative **DM013Z0**
Bronchus **DB01-**
Intraoperative **DB013Z0**
Cervix **DU01-**
Intraoperative **DU013Z0**
Chest **DW02-**
Intraoperative **DW023Z0**
Chest Wall **DB07-**
Intraoperative **DB073Z0**
Colon **DD05-**
Intraoperative **DD053Z0**
Diaphragm **DB08-**
Intraoperative **DB083Z0**
Duodenum **DD02-**
Intraoperative **DD023Z0**
Ear **D900-**
Intraoperative **D9003Z0**
Esophagus **DD00-**
Intraoperative **DD003Z0**
Eye **D800-**
Intraoperative **D8003Z0**
Femur **DP09-**
Intraoperative **DP093Z0**
Fibula **DP0B-**
Intraoperative **DP0B3Z0**
Gallbladder **DF01-**
Intraoperative **DF013Z0**
Gland
Adrenal **DG02-**
Intraoperative **DG023Z0**
Parathyroid **DG04-**
Intraoperative **DG043Z0**
Pituitary **DG00-**
Intraoperative **DG003Z0**
Thyroid **DG05-**
Intraoperative **DG053Z0**
Glands
Intraoperative **D9063Z0**
Salivary **D906-**
Head and Neck **DW01**
Intraoperative **DW013Z0**
Hemibody **DW04-**
Intraoperative **DW043Z0**
Humerus **DP06-**
Intraoperative **DP063Z0**
Hypopharynx **D903-**
Intraoperative **D9033Z0**
Ileum **DD04-**
Intraoperative **DD043Z0**
Jejunum **DD03-**
Intraoperative **DD033Z0**
Kidney **DT00-**
Intraoperative **DT003Z0**
Larynx **D90B-**
Intraoperative **D90B3Z0**
Liver **DF00-**
Intraoperative **DF003Z0**
Lung **DB02-**
Intraoperative **DB023Z0**
Lymphatics
Abdomen **D706-**
Intraoperative **D7063Z0**
Axillary **D704-**
Intraoperative **D7043Z0**
Inguinal **D708-**
Intraoperative **D7083Z0**
Neck **D703-**
Intraoperative **D7033Z0**
Pelvis **D707-**
Intraoperative **D7073Z0**
Thorax **D705-**
Intraoperative **D7053Z0**
Mandible **DP03-**
Intraoperative **DP033Z0**
Maxilla **DP02-**
Intraoperative **DP023Z0**
Mediastinum **DB06-**
Intraoperative **DB063Z0**

Beam Radiation — *continued*
Mouth **D904-**
Intraoperative **D9043Z0**
Nasopharynx **D90D-**
Intraoperative **D90D3Z0**
Neck and Head **DW01-**
Intraoperative **DW013Z0**
Nerve
Intraoperative **D0073Z0**
Peripheral **D007-**
Nose **D901-**
Intraoperative **D9013Z0**
Oropharynx **D90F-**
Intraoperative **D90F3Z0**
Ovary **DU00-**
Intraoperative **DU003Z0**
Palate
Hard **D908-**
Intraoperative **D9083Z0**
Soft **D909-**
Intraoperative **D9093Z0**
Pancreas **DF03-**
Intraoperative **DF033Z0**
Parathyroid Gland **DG04-**
Intraoperative **DG043Z0**
Pelvic Bones **DP08-**
Intraoperative **DP083Z0**
Pelvic Region **DW06-**
Intraoperative **DW063Z0**
Pineal Body **DG01-**
Intraoperative **DG013Z0**
Pituitary Gland **DG00-**
Intraoperative **DG003Z0**
Pleura **DB05-**
Intraoperative **DB053Z0**
Prostate **DV00-**
Intraoperative **DV003Z0**
Radius **DP07-**
Intraoperative **DP073Z0**
Rectum **DD07-**
Intraoperative **DD073Z0**
Rib **DP05-**
Intraoperative **DP053Z0**
Sinuses **D907-**
Intraoperative **D9073Z0**
Skin
Abdomen **DH08-**
Intraoperative **DH083Z0**
Arm **DH04-**
Intraoperative **DH043Z0**
Back **DH07-**
Intraoperative **DH073Z0**
Buttock **DH09-**
Intraoperative **DH093Z0**
Chest **DH06-**
Intraoperative **DH063Z0**
Face **DH02-**
Intraoperative **DH023Z0**
Leg **DH0B-**
Intraoperative **DH0B3Z0**
Neck **DH03-**
Intraoperative **DH033Z0**
Skull **DP00-**
Intraoperative **DP003Z0**
Spinal Cord **D006-**
Intraoperative **D0063Z0**
Spleen **D702-**
Intraoperative **D7023Z0**
Sternum **DP04-**
Intraoperative **DP043Z0**
Stomach **DD01-**
Intraoperative **DD013Z0**
Testis **DV01-**
Intraoperative **DV013Z0**
Thymus **D701-**
Intraoperative **D7013Z0**
Thyroid Gland **DG05-**
Intraoperative **DG053Z0**
Tibia **DP0B-**
Intraoperative **DP0B3Z0**
Tongue **D905-**
Intraoperative **D9053Z0**
Trachea **DB00-**
Intraoperative **DB003Z0**

Beam Radiation — *continued*
Ulna **DP07-**
Intraoperative **DP073Z0**
Ureter **DT01-**
Intraoperative **DT013Z0**
Urethra **DT03-**
Intraoperative **DT033Z0**
Uterus **DU02-**
Intraoperative **DU023Z0**
Whole Body **DW05-**
Intraoperative **DW053Z0**
Bedside swallow F00ZJWZ
Berlin Heart Ventricular Assist Device
use Implantable Heart Assist System in Heart and Great Vessels
Bezlotoxumab Monoclonal Antibody XW0-
Biceps brachii muscle
use Muscle, Upper Arm, Left
use Muscle, Upper Arm, Right
Biceps femoris muscle
use Muscle, Upper Leg, Left
use Muscle, Upper Leg, Right
Bicipital aponeurosis
use Subcutaneous Tissue and Fascia, Lower Arm, Left
use Subcutaneous Tissue and Fascia, Lower Arm, Right
Bicuspid valve
use Valve, Mitral
Bili light therapy *see* Phototherapy, Skin **6A60-**
Bioactive embolization coil(s)
use Intraluminal Device, Bioactive in Upper Arteries
Biofeedback GZC9ZZZ
Biopsy
see Drainage with qualifier Diagnostic
see Excision with qualifier Diagnostic
see Extraction with qualifier Diagnostic
BiPAP *see* Assistance, Respiratory **5A09-**
Bisection *see* Division
Biventricular external heart assist system
use Short-term External Heart Assist System in Heart and Great Vessels
Blepharectomy
see Excision, Eye **08B-**
see Resection, Eye **08T-**
Blepharoplasty
see Repair, Eye **08Q-**
see Replacement, Eye **08R-**
see Reposition, Eye **08S-**
see Supplement, Eye **08U-**
Blepharorrhaphy *see* Repair, Eye **08Q-**
Blepharotomy *see* Drainage, Eye **089-**
Blinatumomab antineoplastic immunothrerapy XW0-
Block, Nerve, anesthetic injection 3E0T3CZ
Blood glucose monitoring system
use Monitoring Device
Blood pressure *see* Measurement, Arterial 4A03-
BMR (basal metabolic rate) *see* Measurement, Physiological Systems 4A0Z-
Body of femur
use Femoral Shaft, Left
use Femoral Shaft, Right
Body of fibula
use Fibula, Left
use Fibula, Right

Bone anchored hearing device
use Hearing Device, Bone Conduction in **09H-**
use Hearing Device in Head and Facial Bones
Bone bank bone graft
use Nonautologous Tissue Substitute
Bone growth stimulator
Insertion of device in
Bone
Facial **0NHW-**
Lower **0QHY-**
Nasal **0NHB-**
Upper **0PHY-**
Skull **0NH0-**
Removal of device from
Bone
Facial **0NPW-**
Lower **0QPY-**
Nasal **0NPB-**
Upper **0PPY-**
Skull **0NP0-**
Revision of device in
Bone
Facial **0NWW-**
Lower **0QWY-**
Nasal **0NWB-**
Upper **0PWY-**
Skull **0NW0-**
Bone marrow transplant *see* Transfusion, Circulatory **302-**
Bone morphogenetic protein 2 (BMP 2)
use Recombinant Bone Morphogenetic Protein
Bone screw (interlocking) (lag) (pedicle) (recessed)
use Internal Fixation Device in Head and Facial Bones
use Internal Fixation Device in Lower Bones
use Internal Fixation Device in Upper Bones
Bony labyrinth
use Ear, Inner, Left
use Ear, Inner, Right
Bony orbit
use Orbit, Left
use Orbit, Right
Bony vestibule
use Ear, Inner, Left
use Ear, Inner, Right
Botallo's duct
use Artery, Pulmonary, Left
Bovine pericardial valve
use Zooplastic Tissue in Heart and Great Vessels
Bovine pericardium graft
use Zooplastic Tissue in Heart and Great Vessels
BP (blood pressure) *see* Measurement, Arterial **4A03-**
Brachial (lateral) lymph node
use Lymphatic, Axillary, Left
use Lymphatic, Axillary, Right
Brachialis muscle
use Muscle, Upper Arm, Left
use Muscle, Upper Arm, Right
Brachiocephalic artery
use Artery, Innominate
Brachiocephalic trunk
use Artery, Innominate
Brachiocephalic vein
use Vein, Innominate, Left
use Vein, Innominate, Right
Brachioradialis muscle
use Muscle, Lower Arm and Wrist, Left
use Muscle, Lower Arm and Wrist, Right

© 2018 Channel Publishing, Ltd.

© 2018 Channel Publishing, Ltd.

PROCEDURE INDEX

C

Caesarean section *see* Extraction, Products of Conception **10D0-**
Calcaneocuboid joint
use Joint, Tarsal, Left
use Joint, Tarsal, Right
Calcaneocuboid ligament
use Bursa and Ligament, Foot, Left
use Bursa and Ligament, Foot, Right
Calcaneofibular ligament
use Bursa and Ligament, Ankle, Left
use Bursa and Ligament, Ankle, Right
Calcaneus
use Tarsal, Left
use Tarsal, Right
Cannulation
see Bypass
see Dilation
see Drainage
see Irrigation
Canthorrhaphy *see* Repair, Eye **08Q-**
Canthotomy *see* Release, Eye **08N-**
Capitate bone
use Carpal, Left
use Carpal, Right
Capsulectomy, lens *see* Excision, Eye **08B-**
Capsulorrhaphy, joint
see Repair, Lower Joints **0SQ-**
see Repair, Upper Joints **0RQ-**
Cardia
use Esophagogastric Junction
Cardiac contractility modulation lead
use Cardiac Lead in Heart and Great Vessels
Cardiac event recorder
use Monitoring Device
Cardiac Lead
Defibrillator
Atrium
Left **02H7-**
Right **02H6-**
Pericardium **02HN-**
Vein, Coronary **02H4-**
Ventricle
Left **02HL-**
Right **02HK-**
Insertion of device in
Atrium
Left **02H7-**
Right **02H6-**
Pericardium **02HN-**
Vein, Coronary **02H4-**
Ventricle
Left **02HL-**
Right **02HK-**
Pacemaker
Atrium
Left **02H7-**
Right **02H6-**
Pericardium **02HN-**
Vein, Coronary **02H4-**
Ventricle
Left **02HL-**
Right **02HK-**
Removal of device from, Heart **02PA-**
Revision of device in, Heart **02WA-**
Cardiac plexus
use Nerve, Thoracic Sympathetic
Cardiac Resynchronization Defibrillator Pulse Generator
Abdomen **0JH8-**
Chest **0JH6-**
Cardiac Resynchronization Pacemaker Pulse Generator
Abdomen **0JH8-**
Chest **0JH6-**
Cardiac resynchronization therapy (CRT) lead
use Cardiac Lead, Defibrillator in **02H-**
use Cardiac Lead, Pacemaker in **02H-**
Cardiac Rhythm Related Device
Insertion of device in
Abdomen **0JH8-**
Chest **0JH6-**
Removal of device from, Subcutaneous Tissue and Fascia, Trunk **0JPT-**
Revision of device in, Subcutaneous Tissue and Fascia, Trunk **0JWT-**
Cardiocentesis *see* Drainage, Pericardial Cavity **0W9D-**
Cardioesophageal junction
use Esophagogastric Junction
Cardiolysis *see* Release, Heart and Great Vessels **02N-**
CardioMEMS® pressure sensor
use Monitoring Device, Pressure Sensor in **02H-**
Cardiomyotomy *see* Division, Esophagogastric Junction **0D84-**
Cardioplegia *see* Introduction of substance in or on, Heart **3E08-**
Cardiorrhaphy *see* Repair, Heart and Great Vessels **02Q-**
Cardioversion **5A2204Z**
Caregiver Training **F0FZ-**
Caroticotympanic artery
use Artery, Internal Carotid, Left
use Artery, Internal Carotid, Right
Carotid (artery) sinus (baroreceptor) lead
use Stimulator Lead in Upper Arteries
Carotid glomus
use Carotid Bodies, Bilateral
use Carotid Body, Left
use Carotid Body, Right
Carotid sinus
use Artery, Internal Carotid, Left
use Artery, Internal Carotid, Right
Carotid sinus nerve
use Nerve, Glossopharyngeal
Carotid WALLSTENT® Monorail® Endoprosthesis
use Intraluminal Device
Carpectomy
see Excision, Upper Bones **0PB-**
see Resection, Upper Bones **0PT-**
Carpometacarpal ligament
use Bursa and Ligament, Hand, Left
use Bursa and Ligament, Hand, Right
Casting *see* Immobilization
CAT scan *see* Computerized Tomography (CT Scan)
Catheterization
see Dilation
see Drainage
see Insertion of device in
see Irrigation
Heart *see* Measurement, Cardiac **4A02-**
Umbilical vein, for infusion **06H033T**
Cauda equina
use Spinal Cord, Lumbar
Cauterization
see Destruction
see Repair
Cavernous plexus
use Nerve, Head and Neck Sympathetic
CBMA (Concentrated Bone Marrow Aspirate)
use Concentrated Bone Marrow Aspirate
CBMA (Concentrated Bone Marrow Aspirate) injection, intramuscular **XK02303**
Cecectomy
see Excision, Cecum **0DBH-**
see Resection, Cecum **0DTH-**
Cecocolostomy
see Bypass, Gastrointestinal System **0D1-**
see Drainage, Gastrointestinal System **0D9-**
Cecopexy
see Repair, Cecum **0DQH-**
see Reposition, Cecum **0DSH-**
Cecoplication *see* Restriction, Cecum **0DVH-**
Cecorrhaphy *see* Repair, Cecum **0DQH-**
Cecostomy
see Bypass, Cecum **0D1H-**
see Drainage, Cecum **0D9H-**
Cecotomy *see* Drainage, Cecum **0D9H-**
Ceftazidime-avibactam anti-infective **XW0-**
Celiac (solar) plexus
use Nerve, Abdominal Sympathetic
Celiac ganglion
use Nerve, Abdominal Sympathetic
Celiac lymph node
use Lymphatic, Aortic
Celiac trunk
use Artery, Celiac
Central axillary lymph node
use Lymphatic, Axillary, Left
use Lymphatic, Axillary, Right
Central venous pressure *see* Measurement, Venous **4A04-**
Centrimag® Blood Pump
use Short-term External Heart Assist System in Heart and Great Vessels
Cephalogram **BN00ZZZ**
Ceramic on ceramic bearing surface
use Synthetic Substitute, Ceramic in **0SR-**
Cerclage *see* Restriction
Cerebral aqueduct (Sylvius)
use Cerebral Ventricle
Cerebral embolic filtration, dual filter **X2A5312**
Cerebrum
use Brain
Cervical esophagus
use Esophagus, Upper
Cervical facet joint
use Joint, Cervical Vertebral
use Joint, Cervical Vertebral, 2 or more
Cervical ganglion
use Nerve, Head and Neck Sympathetic
Cervical interspinous ligament
use Bursa and Ligament, Head and Neck
Cervical intertransverse ligament
use Bursa and Ligament, Head and Neck
Cervical ligamentum flavum
use Bursa and Ligament, Head and Neck

© 2018 Channel Publishing, Ltd.

Cervical lymph node
use Lymphatic, Neck, Left
use Lymphatic, Neck, Right
Cervicectomy
see Excision, Cervix 0UBC-
see Resection, Cervix 0UTC-
Cervicothoracic facet joint
use Joint, Cervicothoracic Vertebral
Cesarean section *see* Extraction, Products of Conception 10D0-
Cesium-131 Collagen Implant
use Radioactive Element, Cesium-131 Collagen Implant in 00H-
Change device in
Abdominal Wall 0W2FX-
Back
Lower 0W2LX-
Upper 0W2KX-
Bladder 0T2BX-
Bone
Facial 0N2WX-
Lower 0Q2YX-
Nasal 0N2BX-
Upper 0P2YX-
Bone Marrow 072TX-
Brain 0020X-
Breast
Left 0H2UX-
Right 0H2TX-
Bursa and Ligament
Lower 0M2YX-
Upper 0M2XX-
Cavity, Cranial 0W21X-
Chest Wall 0W28X-
Cisterna Chyli 072LX-
Diaphragm 0B2TX-
Duct
Hepatobiliary 0F2BX-
Pancreatic 0F2DX-
Ear
Left 092JX-
Right 092HX-
Epididymis and Spermatic Cord 0V2MX-
Extremity
Lower
Left 0Y2BX-
Right 0Y29X-
Upper
Left 0X27X-
Right 0X26X-
Eye
Left 0821X-
Right 0820X-
Face 0W22X-
Fallopian Tube 0U28X-
Gallbladder 0F24X-
Gland
Adrenal 0G25X-
Endocrine 0G2SX-
Pituitary 0G20X-
Salivary 0C2AX-
Head 0W20X-
Intestinal Tract
Lower 0D2DXUZ
Upper 0D20XUZ
Jaw
Lower 0W25X-
Upper 0W24X-
Joint
Lower 0S2YX-
Upper 0R2YX-
Kidney 0T25X-
Larynx 0C2SX-
Liver 0F20X-
Lung
Left 0B2LX-
Right 0B2KX-
Lymphatic 072NX-
Thoracic Duct 072KX-
Mediastinum 0W2CX-
Mesentery 0D2VX-
Mouth and Throat 0C2YX-
Change device in — *continued*
Muscle
Lower 0K2YX-
Upper 0K2XX-
Nasal Mucosa and Soft Tissue 092KX-
Neck 0W26X-
Nerve
Cranial 002EX-
Peripheral 012YX-
Omentum 0D2UX-
Ovary 0U23X-
Pancreas 0F2GX-
Parathyroid Gland 0G2RX-
Pelvic Cavity 0W2JX-
Penis 0V2SX-
Pericardial Cavity 0W2DX-
Perineum
Female 0W2NX-
Male 0W2MX-
Peritoneal Cavity 0W2GX-
Peritoneum 0D2WX-
Pineal Body 0G21X-
Pleura 0B2QX-
Pleural Cavity
Left 0W2BX-
Right 0W29X-
Products of Conception 10207-
Prostate and Seminal Vesicles 0V24X-
Retroperitoneum 0W2HX-
Scrotum and Tunica Vaginalis 0V28X-
Sinus 092YX-
Skin 0H2PX-
Skull 0N20X-
Spinal Canal 002UX-
Spleen 072PX-
Subcutaneous Tissue and Fascia
Head and Neck 0J2SX-
Lower Extremity 0J2WX-
Trunk 0J2TX-
Upper Extremity 0J2VX-
Tendon
Lower 0L2YX-
Upper 0L2XX-
Testis 0V2DX-
Thymus 072MX-
Thyroid Gland 0G2KX-
Trachea 0B21-
Tracheobronchial Tree 0B20X-
Ureter 0T29X-
Urethra 0T2DX-
Uterus and Cervix 0U2DXHZ
Vagina and Cul-de-sac 0U2HXGZ
Vas Deferens 0V2RX-
Vulva 0U2MX-
Change device in or on
Abdominal Wall 2W03X-
Anorectal 2Y03X5Z
Arm
Lower
Left 2W0DX-
Right 2W0CX-
Upper
Left 2W0BX-
Right 2W0AX-
Back 2W05X-
Chest Wall 2W04X-
Ear 2Y02X5Z
Extremity
Lower
Left 2W0MX-
Right 2W0LX-
Upper
Left 2W09X-
Right 2W08X-
Face 2W01X-
Finger
Left 2W0KX-
Right 2W0JX-
Foot
Left 2W0TX-
Right 2W0SX-
Genital Tract, Female 2Y04X5Z
Change device in or on — *continued*
Hand
Left 2W0FX-
Right 2W0EX-
Head 2W00X-
Inguinal Region
Left 2W07X-
Right 2W06X-
Leg
Lower
Left 2W0RX-
Right 2W0QX-
Upper
Left 2W0PX-
Right 2W0NX-
Mouth and Pharynx 2Y00X5Z
Nasal 2Y01X5Z
Neck 2W02X-
Thumb
Left 2W0HX-
Right 2W0GX-
Toe
Left 2W0VX-
Right 2W0UX-
Urethra 2Y05X5Z
Chemoembolization *see* Introduction of substance in or on
Chemosurgery, Skin 3E00XTZ
Chemothalamectomy *see* Destruction, Thalamus 0059-
Chemotherapy, Infusion for cancer *see* Introduction of substance in or on
Chest x-ray *see* Plain Radiography, Chest BW03-
Chiropractic Manipulation
Abdomen 9WB9X-
Cervical 9WB1X-
Extremities
Lower 9WB6X-
Upper 9WB7X-
Head 9WB0X-
Lumbar 9WB3X-
Pelvis 9WB5X-
Rib Cage 9WB8X-
Sacrum 9WB4X-
Thoracic 9WB2X-
Choana
use Nasopharynx
Cholangiogram
see Fluoroscopy, Hepatobiliary System and Pancreas BF1-
see Plain Radiography, Hepatobiliary System and Pancreas BF0-
Cholecystectomy
see Excision, Gallbladder 0FB4-
see Resection, Gallbladder 0FT4-
Cholecystojejunostomy
see Bypass, Hepatobiliary System and Pancreas 0F1-
see Drainage, Hepatobiliary System and Pancreas 0F9-
Cholecystopexy
see Repair, Gallbladder 0FQ4-
see Reposition, Gallbladder 0FS4-
Cholecystoscopy 0FJ44ZZ
Cholecystostomy
see Drainage, Gallbladder 0F94-
see Bypass, Gallbladder 0F14-
Cholecystotomy *see* Drainage, Gallbladder 0F94-
Choledochectomy
see Excision, Hepatobiliary System and Pancreas 0FB-
see Resection, Hepatobiliary System and Pancreas 0FT-
Choledocholithotomy *see* Extirpation, Duct, Common Bile 0FC9-
Choledochoplasty
see Repair, Hepatobiliary System and Pancreas 0FQ-
see Replacement, Hepatobiliary System and Pancreas 0FR-
see Supplement, Hepatobiliary System and Pancreas 0FU-
Choledochoscopy 0FJB8ZZ
Choledochotomy *see* Drainage, Hepatobiliary System and Pancreas 0F9-
Cholelithotomy *see* Extirpation, Hepatobiliary System and Pancreas 0FC-
Chondrectomy
see Excision, Lower Joints 0SB-
see Excision, Upper Joints 0RB-
Knee *see* Excision, Lower Joints 0SB-
Semilunar cartilage *see* Excision, Lower Joints 0SB-
Chondroglossus muscle
use Muscle, Tongue, Palate, Pharynx
Chorda tympani
use Nerve, Facial
Chordotomy *see* Division, Central Nervous System and Cranial Nerves 008-
Choroid plexus
use Cerebral Ventricle
Choroidectomy
see Excision, Eye 08B-
see Resection, Eye 08T-
Ciliary body
use Eye, Left
use Eye, Right
Ciliary ganglion
use Nerve, Head and Neck Sympathetic
Circle of Willis
use Artery, Intracranial
Circumcision 0VTTXZZ
Circumflex iliac artery
use Artery, Femoral, Left
use Artery, Femoral, Right
Clamp and rod internal fixation system (CRIF)
use Internal Fixation Device in Lower Bones
use Internal Fixation Device in Upper Bones
Clamping *see* Occlusion
Claustrum
use Basal Ganglia
Claviculectomy
see Excision, Upper Bones 0PB-
see Resection, Upper Bones 0PT-
Claviculotomy
see Division, Upper Bones 0P8-
see Drainage, Upper Bones 0P9-
Clipping, aneurysm
see Occlusion using Extraluminal Device
see Restriction using Extraluminal Device
Clitorectomy, clitoridectomy
see Excision, Clitoris 0UBJ-
see Resection, Clitoris 0UTJ-
Clolar
use Clofarabine
Closure
see Occlusion
see Repair
Clysis *see* Introduction of substance in or on
Coagulation *see* Destruction
COALESCE® radiolucent interbody fusion device
use Interbody Fusion Device, Radiolucent Porous in New Technology
CoAxia NeuroFlo catheter
use Intraluminal Device

PROCEDURE INDEX

© 2018 Channel Publishing, Ltd.

Cobalt/chromium head and polyethylene socket
use Synthetic Substitute, Metal on Polyethylene in **0SR-**
Cobalt/chromium head and socket
use Synthetic Substitute, Metal in **0SR-**
Coccygeal body
use Coccygeal Glomus
Coccygeus muscle
use Muscle, Trunk, Left
use Muscle, Trunk, Right
Cochlea
use Ear, Inner, Left
use Ear, Inner, Right
Cochlear implant (CI), multiple channel (electrode)
use Hearing Device, Multiple Channel Cochlear Prosthesis in **09H-**
Cochlear implant (CI), single channel (electrode)
use Hearing Device, Single Channel Cochlear Prosthesis in **09H-**
Cochlear Implant Treatment **F0BZ0-**
Cochlear nerve
use Nerve, Acoustic
COGNIS® CRT-D
use Cardiac Resynchronization Defibrillator Pulse Generator in **0JH-**
COHERE® radiolucent interbody fusion device
use Interbody Fusion Device, Radiolucent Porous in New Technology
Colectomy
see Excision, Gastrointestinal System **0DB-**
see Resection, Gastrointestinal System **0DT-**
Collapse *see* Occlusion
Collection from
Breast, Breast Milk **8E0HX62**
Indwelling Device
Circulatory System
Blood **8C02X6K**
Other Fluid **8C02X6L**
Nervous System
Cerebrospinal Fluid **8C01X6J**
Other Fluid **8C01X6L**
Integumentary System, Breast Milk **8E0HX62**
Reproductive System, Male, Sperm **8E0VX63**
Colocentesis *see* Drainage, Gastrointestinal System **0D9-**
Colofixation
see Repair, Gastrointestinal System **0DQ-**
see Reposition, Gastrointestinal System **0DS-**
Cololysis *see* Release, Gastrointestinal System **0DN-**
Colonic Z-Stent®
use Intraluminal Device
Colonoscopy **0DJD8ZZ**
Colopexy
see Repair, Gastrointestinal System **0DQ-**
see Reposition, Gastrointestinal System **0DS-**
Coloplication *see* Restriction, Gastrointestinal System **0DV-**
Coloproctectomy
see Excision, Gastrointestinal System **0DB-**
see Resection, Gastrointestinal System **0DT-**
Coloproctostomy
see Bypass, Gastrointestinal System **0D1-**
see Drainage, Gastrointestinal System **0D9-**
Colopuncture *see* Drainage, Gastrointestinal System **0D9-**
Colorrhaphy *see* Repair, Gastrointestinal System **0DQ-**
Colostomy
see Bypass, Gastrointestinal System **0D1-**
see Drainage, Gastrointestinal System **0D9-**
Colpectomy
see Excision, Vagina **0UBG-**
see Resection, Vagina **0UTG-**
Colpocentesis *see* Drainage, Vagina **0U9G-**
Colpopexy
see Repair, Vagina **0UQG-**
see Reposition, Vagina **0USG-**
Colpoplasty
see Repair, Vagina **0UQG-**
see Supplement, Vagina **0UUG-**
Colporrhaphy *see* Repair, Vagina **0UQG-**
Colposcopy **0UJH8ZZ**
Columella
use Nasal Mucosa and Soft Tissue
Common digital vein
use Vein, Foot, Left
use Vein, Foot, Right
Common facial vein
use Vein, Face, Left
use Vein, Face, Right
Common fibular nerve
use Nerve, Peroneal
Common hepatic artery
use Artery, Hepatic
Common iliac (subaortic) lymph node
use Lymphatic, Pelvis
Common interosseous artery
use Artery, Ulnar, Left
use Artery, Ulnar, Right
Common peroneal nerve
use Nerve, Peroneal
Complete (SE) stent
use Intraluminal Device
Compression *see* Restriction
Abdominal Wall **2W13X-**
Arm
Lower
Left **2W1DX-**
Right **2W1CX-**
Upper
Left **2W1BX-**
Right **2W1AX-**
Back **2W15X-**
Chest Wall **2W14X-**
Extremity
Lower
Left **2W1MX-**
Right **2W1LX-**
Upper
Left **2W19X-**
Right **2W18X-**
Face **2W11X-**
Finger
Left **2W1KX-**
Right **2W1JX-**
Foot
Left **2W1TX-**
Right **2W1SX-**
Hand
Left **2W1FX-**
Right **2W1EX-**
Head **2W10X-**
Inguinal Region
Left **2W17X-**
Right **2W16X-**
Compression — *continued*
Leg
Lower
Left **2W1RX-**
Right **2W1QX-**
Upper
Left **2W1PX-**
Right **2W1NX-**
Neck **2W12X-**
Thumb
Left **2W1HX-**
Right **2W1GX-**
Toe
Left **2W1VX-**
Right **2W1UX-**
Computer Assisted Procedure
Extremity
Lower
No Qualifier **8E0YXBZ**
With Computerized Tomography **8E0YXBG**
With Fluoroscopy **8E0YXBF**
With Magnetic Resonance Imaging **8E0YXBH**
Upper
No Qualifier **8E0XXBZ**
With Computerized Tomography **8E0XXBG**
With Fluoroscopy **8E0XXBF**
With Magnetic Resonance Imaging **8E0XXBH**
Head and Neck Region
No Qualifier **8E09XBZ**
With Computerized Tomography **8E09XBG**
With Fluoroscopy **8E09XBF**
With Magnetic Resonance Imaging **8E09XBH**
Trunk Region
No Qualifier **8E0WXBZ**
With Computerized Tomography **8E0WXBG**
With Fluoroscopy **8E0WXBF**
With Magnetic Resonance Imaging **8E0WXBH**
Computerized Tomography (CT Scan)
Abdomen **BW20-**
Chest and Pelvis **BW25-**
Abdomen and Chest **BW24-**
Abdomen and Pelvis **BW21-**
Airway, Trachea **BB2F-**
Ankle
Left **BQ2H-**
Right **BQ2G-**
Aorta
Abdominal **B420-**
Intravascular Optical Coherence **B420Z2Z**
Thoracic **B320-**
Intravascular Optical Coherence **B320Z2Z**
Arm
Left **BP2F-**
Right **BP2E-**
Artery
Celiac **B421-**
Intravascular Optical Coherence **B421Z2Z**
Common Carotid
Bilateral **B325-**
Intravascular Optical Coherence **B325Z2Z**
Coronary
Bypass Graft
Multiple **B223-**
Intravascular Optical Coherence **B223Z2Z**
Multiple **B221-**
Intravascular Optical Coherence **B221Z2Z**
Internal Carotid
Bilateral **B328-**
Intravascular Optical Coherence **B328Z2Z**
Computerized Tomography (CT Scan) — *continued*
Artery — *continued*
Intracranial **B32R-**
Intravascular Optical Coherence **B32RZ2Z**
Lower Extremity
Bilateral **B42H-**
Intravascular Optical Coherence **B42HZ2Z**
Left **B42G-**
Intravascular Optical Coherence **B42GZ2Z**
Right **B42F-**
Intravascular Optical Coherence **B42FZ2Z**
Pelvic **B42C-**
Intravascular Optical Coherence **B42CZ2Z**
Pulmonary
Left **B32T-**
Intravascular Optical Coherence **B32TZ2Z**
Right **B32S-**
Intravascular Optical Coherence **B32SZ2Z**
Renal
Bilateral **B428-**
Intravascular Optical Coherence **B428Z2Z**
Transplant **B42M-**
Intravascular Optical Coherence **B42MZ2Z**
Superior Mesenteric **B424-**
Intravascular Optical Coherence **B424Z2Z**
Vertebral
Bilateral **B32G-**
Intravascular Optical Coherence **B32GZ2Z**
Bladder **BT20-**
Bone
Facial **BN25-**
Temporal **BN2F-**
Brain **B020-**
Calcaneus
Left **BQ2K-**
Right **BQ2J-**
Cerebral Ventricle **B028-**
Chest, Abdomen and Pelvis **BW25-**
Chest and Abdomen **BW24-**
Cisterna **B027-**
Clavicle
Left **BP25-**
Right **BP24-**
Coccyx **BR2F-**
Colon **BD24-**
Ear **B920-**
Elbow
Left **BP2H-**
Right **BP2G-**
Extremity
Lower
Left **BQ2S-**
Right **BQ2R-**
Upper
Bilateral **BP2V-**
Left **BP2U-**
Right **BP2T-**
Eye
Bilateral **B827-**
Left **B826-**
Right **B825-**
Femur
Left **BQ24-**
Right **BQ23-**
Fibula
Left **BQ2C-**
Right **BQ2B-**
Finger
Left **BP2S-**
Right **BP2R-**

© 2018 Channel Publishing, Ltd.

Computerized Tomography (CT Scan) — *continued*
Foot
Left **BQ2M-**
Right **BQ2L-**
Forearm
Left **BP2K-**
Right **BP2J-**
Gland
Adrenal, Bilateral **BG22-**
Parathyroid **BG23-**
Parotid, Bilateral **B926-**
Salivary, Bilateral **B92D-**
Submandibular, Bilateral **B929-**
Thyroid **BG24-**
Hand
Left **BP2P-**
Right **BP2N-**
Hands and Wrists, Bilateral **BP2Q-**
Head **BW28-**
Head and Neck **BW29-**
Heart
Intravascular Optical Coherence **B226Z2Z**
Right and Left **B226-**
Hepatobiliary System, All **BF2C-**
Hip
Left **BQ21-**
Right **BQ20-**
Humerus
Left **BP2B-**
Right **BP2A-**
Intracranial Sinus **B522-**
Intravascular Optical Coherence **B522Z2Z**
Joint
Acromioclavicular, Bilateral **BP23-**
Finger
Left **BP2DZZZ**
Right **BP2CZZZ**
Foot
Left **BQ2Y-**
Right **BQ2X-**
Hand
Left **BP2DZZZ**
Right **BP2CZZZ**
Sacroiliac **BR2D-**
Sternoclavicular
Bilateral **BP22-**
Left **BP21-**
Right **BP20-**
Temporomandibular, Bilateral **BN29-**
Toe
Left **BQ2Y-**
Right **BQ2X-**
Kidney
Bilateral **BT23-**
Left **BT22-**
Right **BT21-**
Transplant **BT29-**
Knee
Left **BQ28-**
Right **BQ27-**
Larynx **B92J-**
Leg
Left **BQ2F-**
Right **BQ2D-**
Liver **BF25-**
Liver and Spleen **BF26-**
Lung, Bilateral **BB24-**
Mandible **BN26-**
Nasopharynx **B92F-**
Neck **BW2F-**
Neck and Head **BW29-**
Orbit, Bilateral **BN23-**
Oropharynx **B92F-**
Pancreas **BF27-**
Patella
Left **BQ2W-**
Right **BQ2V-**
Pelvic Region **BW2G-**

Computerized Tomography (CT Scan) — *continued*
Pelvis **BR2C-**
Chest and Abdomen **BW25-**
Pelvis and Abdomen **BW21-**
Pituitary Gland **B029-**
Prostate **BV23-**
Ribs
Left **BP2Y-**
Right **BP2X-**
Sacrum **BR2F-**
Scapula
Left **BP27-**
Right **BP26-**
Sella Turcica **B029-**
Shoulder
Left **BP29-**
Right **BP28-**
Sinus
Intracranial **B522-**
Intravascular Optical Coherence **B522Z2Z**
Paranasal **B922-**
Skull **BN20-**
Spinal Cord **B02B-**
Spine
Cervical **BR20-**
Lumbar **BR29-**
Thoracic **BR27-**
Spleen and Liver **BF26-**
Thorax **BP2W-**
Tibia
Left **BQ2C-**
Right **BQ2B-**
Toe
Left **BQ2Q-**
Right **BQ2P-**
Trachea **BB2F-**
Tracheobronchial Tree
Bilateral **BB29-**
Left **BB28-**
Right **BB27-**
Vein
Pelvic (Iliac)
Left **B52G-**
Intravascular Optical Coherence **B52GZ2Z**
Right **B52F-**
Intravascular Optical Coherence **B52FZ2Z**
Pelvic (Iliac) Bilateral **B52H-**
Intravascular Optical Coherence **B52HZ2Z**
Portal **B52T-**
Intravascular Optical Coherence **B52TZ2Z**
Pulmonary
Bilateral **B52S-**
Intravascular Optical Coherence **B52SZ2Z**
Left **B52R-**
Intravascular Optical Coherence **B52RZ2Z**
Right **B52Q-**
Intravascular Optical Coherence **B52QZ2Z**
Renal
Bilateral **B52L-**
Intravascular Optical Coherence **B52LZ2Z**
Left **B52K-**
Intravascular Optical Coherence **B52KZ2Z**
Right **B52J-**
Intravascular Optical Coherence **B52JZ2Z**
Spanchnic **B52T-**
Intravascular Optical Coherence **B52TZ2Z**

Computerized Tomography (CT Scan) — *continued*
Vena Cava
Inferior **B529-**
Intravascular Optical Coherence **B529Z2Z**
Superior **B528-**
Intravascular Optical Coherence **B528Z2Z**
Ventricle, Cerebral **B028-**
Wrist
Left **BP2M-**
Right **BP2L-**
Concentrated Bone Marrow Aspirate (CBMA) injection, intramuscular XK02303
Concerto II CRT-D
use Cardiac Resynchronization Defibrillator Pulse Generator **0JH-**
Condylectomy
see Excision, Head and Facial Bones **0NB-**
see Excision, Lower Bones **0QB-**
see Excision, Upper Bones **0PB-**
Condyloid process
use Mandible, Left
use Mandible, Right
Condylotomy
see Division, Head and Facial Bones **0N8-**
see Division, Lower Bones **0Q8-**
see Division, Upper Bones **0P8-**
see Drainage, Head and Facial Bones **0N9-**
see Drainage, Lower Bones **0Q9-**
see Drainage, Upper Bones **0P9-**
Condylysis
see Release, Head and Facial Bones **0NN-**
see Release, Lower Bones **0QN-**
see Release, Upper Bones **0PN-**
Conization, cervix *see* Excision, Cervix **0UBC-**
Conjunctivoplasty
see Repair, Eye **08Q-**
see Replacement, Eye **08R-**
CONSERVE® PLUS Total Resurfacing Hip System
use Resurfacing Device in Lower Joints
Construction
Auricle, ear *see* Replacement, Ear, Nose, Sinus **09R-**
Ileal conduit *see* Bypass, Urinary System **0T1-**
Consulta CRT-D
use Cardiac Resynchronization Defibrillator Pulse Generator in **0JH-**
Consulta CRT-P
use Cardiac Resynchronization Pacemaker Pulse Generator in **0JH-**
Contact Radiation
Abdomen **DWY37ZZ**
Adrenal Gland **DGY27ZZ**
Bile Ducts **DFY27ZZ**
Bladder **DTY27ZZ**
Bone, Other **DPYC7ZZ**
Brain **D0Y07ZZ**
Brain Stem **D0Y17ZZ**
Breast
Left **DMY07ZZ**
Right **DMY17ZZ**
Bronchus **DBY17ZZ**
Cervix **DUY17ZZ**
Chest **DWY27ZZ**
Chest Wall **DBY77ZZ**
Colon **DDY57ZZ**
Diaphragm **DBY87ZZ**
Duodenum **DDY27ZZ**
Ear **D9Y07ZZ**
Esophagus **DDY07ZZ**
Eye **D8Y07ZZ**

Contact Radiation — *continued*
Femur **DPY97ZZ**
Fibula **DPYB7ZZ**
Gallbladder **DFY17ZZ**
Gland
Adrenal **DGY27ZZ**
Parathyroid **DGY47ZZ**
Pituitary **DGY07ZZ**
Thyroid **DGY57ZZ**
Glands, Salivary **D9Y67ZZ**
Head and Neck **DWY17ZZ**
Hemibody **DWY47ZZ**
Humerus **DPY67ZZ**
Hypopharynx **D9Y37ZZ**
Ileum **DDY47ZZ**
Jejunum **DDY37ZZ**
Kidney **DTY07ZZ**
Larynx **D9YB7ZZ**
Liver **DFY07ZZ**
Lung **DBY27ZZ**
Mandible **DPY37ZZ**
Maxilla **DPY27ZZ**
Mediastinum **DBY67ZZ**
Mouth **D9Y47ZZ**
Nasopharynx **D9YD7ZZ**
Neck and Head **DWY17ZZ**
Nerve, Peripheral **D0Y77ZZ**
Nose **D9Y17ZZ**
Oropharynx **D9YF7ZZ**
Ovary **DUY07ZZ**
Palate
Hard **D9Y87ZZ**
Soft **D9Y97ZZ**
Pancreas **DFY37ZZ**
Parathyroid Gland **DGY47ZZ**
Pelvic Bones **DPY87ZZ**
Pelvic Region **DWY67ZZ**
Pineal Body **DGY17ZZ**
Pituitary Gland **DGY07ZZ**
Pleura **DBY57ZZ**
Prostate **DVY07ZZ**
Radius **DPY77ZZ**
Rectum **DDY77ZZ**
Rib **DPY57ZZ**
Sinuses **D9Y77ZZ**
Skin
Abdomen **DHY87ZZ**
Arm **DHY47ZZ**
Back **DHY77ZZ**
Buttock **DHY97ZZ**
Chest **DHY67ZZ**
Face **DHY27ZZ**
Leg **DHYB7ZZ**
Neck **DHY37ZZ**
Skull **DPY07ZZ**
Spinal Cord **D0Y67ZZ**
Sternum **DPY47ZZ**
Stomach **DDY17ZZ**
Testis **DVY17ZZ**
Thyroid Gland **DGY57ZZ**
Tibia **DPYB7ZZ**
Tongue **D9Y57ZZ**
Trachea **DBY07ZZ**
Ulna **DPY77ZZ**
Ureter **DTY17ZZ**
Urethra **DTY37ZZ**
Uterus **DUY27ZZ**
Whole Body **DWY57ZZ**
CONTAK RENEWAL® 3 RF (HE) CRT-D
use Cardiac Resynchronization Defibrillator Pulse Generator in **0JH-**
Contegra Pulmonary Valved Conduit
use Zooplastic Tissue in Heart and Great Vessels
Continuous Glucose Monitoring (CGM) device
use Monitoring Device

PROCEDURE INDEX

© 2018 Channel Publishing, Ltd.

Continuous Negative Airway Pressure
- 24-96 Consecutive Hours, Ventilation **5A09459**
- Greater than 96 Consecutive Hours, Ventilation **5A09559**
- Less than 24 Consecutive Hours, Ventilation **5A09359**

Continuous Positive Airway Pressure
- 24-96 Consecutive Hours, Ventilation **5A09457**
- Greater than 96 Consecutive Hours, Ventilation **5A09557**
- Less than 24 Consecutive Hours, Ventilation **5A09357**

Continuous renal replacement therapy (CRRT) 5A1D90Z

Contraceptive Device
- Change device in, Uterus and Cervix **0U2DXHZ**
- Insertion of device in
  - Cervix **0UHC-**
  - Subcutaneous Tissue and Fascia
    - Abdomen **0JH8-**
    - Chest **0JH6-**
    - Lower Arm
      - Left **0JHH-**
      - Right **0JHG-**
    - Lower Leg
      - Left **0JHP-**
      - Right **0JHN-**
    - Upper Arm
      - Left **0JHF-**
      - Right **0JHD-**
    - Upper Leg
      - Left **0JHM-**
      - Right **0JHL-**
  - Uterus **0UH9-**
- Removal of device from
  - Subcutaneous Tissue and Fascia
    - Lower Extremity **0JPW-**
    - Trunk **0JPT-**
    - Upper Extremity **0JPV-**
  - Uterus and Cervix **0UPD-**
- Revision of device in
  - Subcutaneous Tissue and Fascia
    - Lower Extremity **0JWW-**
    - Trunk **0JWT-**
    - Upper Extremity **0JWV-**
  - Uterus and Cervix **0UWD-**

Contractility Modulation Device
- Abdomen **0JH8-**
- Chest **0JH6-**

Control, Epistaxis *see* Control bleeding in, Nasal Mucosa and Soft Tissue **093K-**

Control bleeding in
- Abdominal Wall **0W3F-**
- Ankle Region
  - Left **0Y3L-**
  - Right **0Y3K-**
- Arm
  - Lower
    - Left **0X3F-**
    - Right **0X3D-**
  - Upper
    - Left **0X39-**
    - Right **0X38-**
- Axilla
  - Left **0X35-**
  - Right **0X34-**
- Back
  - Lower **0W3L-**
  - Upper **0W3K-**
- Buttock
  - Left **0Y31-**
  - Right **0Y30-**
- Cavity, Cranial **0W31-**
- Chest Wall **0W38-**

Control bleeding in — *continued*
- Elbow Region
  - Left **0X3C-**
  - Right **0X3B-**
- Extremity
  - Lower
    - Left **0Y3B-**
    - Right **0Y39-**
  - Upper
    - Left **0X37-**
    - Right **0X36-**
- Face **0W32-**
- Femoral Region
  - Left **0Y38-**
  - Right **0Y37-**
- Foot
  - Left **0Y3N-**
  - Right **0Y3M-**
- Gastrointestinal Tract **0W3P-**
- Genitourinary Tract **0W3R-**
- Hand
  - Left **0X3K-**
  - Right **0X3J-**
- Head **0W30-**
- Inguinal Region
  - Left **0Y36-**
  - Right **0Y35-**
- Jaw
  - Lower **0W35-**
  - Upper **0W34-**
- Knee Region
  - Left **0Y3G-**
  - Right **0Y3F-**
- Leg
  - Lower
    - Left **0Y3J-**
    - Right **0Y3H-**
  - Upper
    - Left **0Y3D-**
    - Right **0Y3C-**
- Mediastinum **0W3C-**
- Nasal Mucosa and Soft Tissue **093K-**
- Neck **0W36-**
- Oral Cavity and Throat **0W33-**
- Pelvic Cavity **0W3J-**
- Pericardial Cavity **0W3D-**
- Perineum
  - Female **0W3N-**
  - Male **0W3M-**
- Peritoneal Cavity **0W3G-**
- Pleural Cavity
  - Left **0W3B-**
  - Right **0W39-**
- Respiratory Tract **0W3Q-**
- Retroperitoneum **0W3H-**
- Shoulder Region
  - Left **0X33-**
  - Right **0X32-**
- Wrist Region
  - Left **0X3H-**
  - Right **0X3G-**

Conus arteriosus
- *use* Ventricle, Right

Conus medullaris
- *use* Spinal Cord, Lumbar

Conversion
- Cardiac rhythm **5A2204Z**
- Gastrostomy to jejunostomy feeding device *see* Insertion of device in, Jejunum **0DHA-**

Cook Biodesign® Fistula Plug(s)
- *use* Nonautologous Tissue Substitute

Cook Biodesign® Hernia Graft(s)
- *use* Nonautologous Tissue Substitute

Cook Biodesign® Layered Graft(s)
- *use* Nonautologous Tissue Substitute

Cook Zenapro™ Layered Graft(s)
- *use* Nonautologous Tissue Substitute

Cook Zenith AAA Endovascular Graft
- *use* Intraluminal Device
- *use* Intraluminal Device, Branched or Fenestrated, One or Two Arteries in **04V-**
- *use* Intraluminal Device, Branched or Fenestrated, Three or More Arteries in **04V-**

Coracoacromial ligament
- *use* Bursa and Ligament, Shoulder, Left
- *use* Bursa and Ligament, Shoulder, Right

Coracobrachialis muscle
- *use* Muscle, Upper Arm, Left
- *use* Muscle, Upper Arm, Right

Coracoclavicular ligament
- *use* Bursa and Ligament, Shoulder, Left
- *use* Bursa and Ligament, Shoulder, Right

Coracohumeral ligament
- *use* Bursa and Ligament, Shoulder, Left
- *use* Bursa and Ligament, Shoulder, Right

Coracoid process
- *use* Scapula, Left
- *use* Scapula, Right

Cordotomy *see* Division, Central Nervous System and Cranial Nerves **008-**

Core needle biopsy *see* Excision with qualifier Diagnostic

CoreValve transcatheter aortic valve
- *use* Zooplastic Tissue in Heart and Great Vessels

Cormet Hip Resurfacing System
- *use* Resurfacing Device in Lower Joints

Corniculate cartilage
- *use* Larynx

CoRoent® XL
- *use* Interbody Fusion Device in Lower Joints

Coronary arteriography
- *see* Fluoroscopy, Heart **B21-**
- *see* Plain Radiography, Heart **B20-**

Corox OTW (Bipolar) Lead
- *use* Cardiac Lead, Defibrillator in **02H-**
- *use* Cardiac Lead, Pacemaker in **02H-**

Corpus callosum
- *use* Brain

Corpus cavernosum
- *use* Penis

Corpus spongiosum
- *use* Penis

Corpus striatum
- *use* Basal Ganglia

Corrugator supercilii muscle
- *use* Muscle, Facial

Cortical strip neurostimulator lead
- *use* Neurostimulator Lead in Central Nervous System and Cranial Nerves

Costatectomy
- *see* Excision, Upper Bones **0PB-**
- *see* Resection, Upper Bones **0PT-**

Costectomy
- *see* Excision, Upper Bones **0PB-**
- *see* Resection, Upper Bones **0PT-**

Costocervical trunk
- *use* Artery, Subclavian, Left
- *use* Artery, Subclavian, Right

Costochondrectomy
- *see* Excision, Upper Bones **0PB-**
- *see* Resection, Upper Bones **0PT-**

Costoclavicular ligament
- *use* Bursa and Ligament, Shoulder, Left
- *use* Bursa and Ligament, Shoulder, Right

Costosternoplasty
- *see* Repair, Upper Bones **0PQ-**
- *see* Replacement, Upper Bones **0PR-**
- *see* Supplement, Upper Bones **0PU-**

Costotomy
- *see* Division, Upper Bones **0P8-**
- *see* Drainage, Upper Bones **0P9-**

Costotransverse joint
- *use* Joint, Thoracic Vertebral

Costotransverse ligament *use* Rib(s) Bursa and Ligament

Costovertebral joint
- *use* Joint, Thoracic Vertebral

Costoxiphoid ligament *use* Sternum Bursa and Ligament

Counseling
- Family, for substance abuse, Other Family Counseling **HZ63ZZZ**
- Group
  - 12-Step **HZ43ZZZ**
  - Behavioral **HZ41ZZZ**
  - Cognitive **HZ40ZZZ**
  - Cognitive-Behavioral **HZ42ZZZ**
  - Confrontational **HZ48ZZZ**
  - Continuing Care **HZ49ZZZ**
  - Infectious Disease
    - Post-Test **HZ4CZZZ**
    - Pre-Test **HZ4CZZZ**
  - Interpersonal **HZ44ZZZ**
  - Motivational Enhancement **HZ47ZZZ**
  - Psychoeducation **HZ46ZZZ**
  - Spiritual **HZ4BZZZ**
  - Vocational **HZ45ZZZ**
- Individual
  - 12-Step **HZ33ZZZ**
  - Behavioral **HZ31ZZZ**
  - Cognitive **HZ30ZZZ**
  - Cognitive-Behavioral **HZ32ZZZ**
  - Confrontational **HZ38ZZZ**
  - Continuing Care **HZ39ZZZ**
  - Infectious Disease
    - Post-Test **HZ3CZZZ**
    - Pre-Test **HZ3CZZZ**
  - Interpersonal **HZ34ZZZ**
  - Motivational Enhancement **HZ37ZZZ**
  - Psychoeducation **HZ36ZZZ**
  - Spiritual **HZ3BZZZ**
  - Vocational **HZ35ZZZ**
- Mental Health Services
  - Educational **GZ60ZZZ**
  - Other Counseling **GZ63ZZZ**
  - Vocational **GZ61ZZZ**

Countershock, cardiac 5A2204Z

Cowper's (bulbourethral) gland
- *use* Urethra

CPAP (continuous positive airway pressure)
- *see* Assistance, Respiratory **5A09-**

Craniectomy
- *see* Excision, Head and Facial Bones **0NB-**
- *see* Resection, Head and Facial Bones **0NT-**

Cranioplasty
- *see* Repair, Head and Facial Bones **0NQ-**
- *see* Replacement, Head and Facial Bones **0NR-**
- *see* Supplement, Head and Facial Bones **0NU-**

© 2018 Channel Publishing, Ltd.

Craniotomy
see Division, Head and Facial Bones **0N8-**
see Drainage, Central Nervous System and Cranial Nerves **009-**
see Drainage, Head and Facial Bones **0N9-**
Creation
Perineum
Female **0W4N0-**
Male **0W4M0-**
Valve
Aortic **024F0-**
Mitral **024G0-**
Tricuspid **024J0-**
Cremaster muscle
use Muscle, Perineum
Cribriform plate
use Bone, Ethmoid, Left
use Bone, Ethmoid, Right
Cricoid cartilage
use Trachea
Cricoidectomy *see* Excision, Larynx **0CBS-**
Cricothyroid artery
use Artery, Thyroid, Left
use Artery, Thyroid, Right
Cricothyroid muscle
use Muscle, Neck, Left
use Muscle, Neck, Right
Crisis Intervention GZ2ZZZZ
CRRT (Continuous renal replacement therapy) **5A1D90Z**
Crural fascia
use Subcutaneous Tissue and Fascia, Upper Leg, Left
use Subcutaneous Tissue and Fascia, Upper Leg, Right
Crushing, nerve
Cranial *see* Destruction, Central Nervous System and Cranial Nerves **005-**
Peripheral *see* Destruction, Peripheral Nervous System **015-**
Cryoablation *see* Destruction
Cryotherapy *see* Destruction
Cryptorchidectomy
see Excision, Male Reproductive System **0VB-**
see Resection, Male Reproductive System **0VT-**
Cryptorchiectomy
see Excision, Male Reproductive System **0VB-**
see Resection, Male Reproductive System **0VT-**
Cryptotomy
see Division, Gastrointestinal System **0D8-**
see Drainage, Gastrointestinal System **0D9-**
CT scan *see* Computerized Tomography (CT Scan)
CT sialogram *see* Computerized Tomography (CT Scan), Ear, Nose, Mouth and Throat **B92-**
Cubital lymph node
use Lymphatic, Upper Extremity, Left
use Lymphatic, Upper Extremity, Right
Cubital nerve
use Nerve, Ulnar
Cuboid bone
use Tarsal, Left
use Tarsal, Right
Cuboideonavicular joint
use Joint, Tarsal, Left
use Joint, Tarsal, Right
Culdocentesis *see* Drainage, Cul-de-sac **0U9F-**
Culdoplasty
see Repair, Cul-de-sac **0UQF-**
see Supplement, Cul-de-sac **0UUF-**
Culdoscopy 0UJH8ZZ
Culdotomy *see* Drainage, Cul-de-sac **0U9F-**
Culmen
use Cerebellum
Cultured epidermal cell autograft
use Autologous Tissue Substitute
Cuneiform cartilage
use Larynx
Cuneonavicular joint
use Joint, Tarsal, Left
use Joint, Tarsal, Right
Cuneonavicular ligament
use Bursa and Ligament, Foot, Left
use Bursa and Ligament, Foot, Right
Curettage
see Excision
see Extraction
Cutaneous (transverse) cervical nerve
use Nerve, Cervical Plexus
CVP (central venous pressure)
see Measurement, Venous **4A04-**
Cyclodiathermy *see* Destruction, Eye **085-**
Cyclophotocoagulation *see* Destruction, Eye **085-**
CYPHER® Stent
use Intraluminal Device, Drug-eluting in Heart and Great Vessels
Cystectomy
see Excision, Bladder **0TBB-**
see Resection, Bladder **0TTB-**
Cystocele repair *see* Repair, Subcutaneous Tissue and Fascia, Pelvic Region **0JQC-**
Cystography
see Fluoroscopy, Urinary System **BT1-**
see Plain Radiography, Urinary System **BT0-**
Cystolithotomy *see* Extirpation, Bladder **0TCB-**
Cystopexy
see Repair, Bladder **0TQB-**
see Reposition, Bladder **0TSB-**
Cystoplasty
see Repair, Bladder **0TQB-**
see Replacement, Bladder **0TRB-**
see Supplement, Bladder **0TUB-**
Cystorrhaphy *see* Repair, Bladder **0TQB-**
Cystoscopy 0TJB8ZZ
Cystostomy *see* Bypass, Bladder **0T1B-**
Cystostomy tube
use Drainage Device
Cystotomy *see* Drainage, Bladder **0T9B-**
Cystourethrography
see Fluoroscopy, Urinary System **BT1-**
see Plain Radiography, Urinary System **BT0-**
Cystourethroplasty
see Repair, Urinary System **0TQ-**
see Replacement, Urinary System **0TR-**
see Supplement, Urinary System **0TU-**
Cytarabine and Daunorubicin Liposome Antineoplastic XW0-

D

DBS lead
use Neurostimulator Lead in Central Nervous System and Cranial Nerves
DeBakey Left Ventricular Assist Device
use Implantable Heart Assist System in Heart and Great Vessels
Debridement
Excisional *see* Excision
Non-excisional *see* Extraction
Decompression, Circulatory 6A15-
Decortication, lung
see Extirpation, Respiratory System **0BC-**
see Release, Respiratory System **0BN-**
Deep brain neurostimulator lead
use Neurostimulator Lead in Central Nervous System and Cranial Nerves
Deep cervical fascia
use Subcutaneous Tissue and Fascia, Left Neck
use Subcutaneous Tissue and Fascia, Right Neck
Deep cervical vein
use Vein, Vertebral, Left
use Vein, Vertebral, Right
Deep circumflex iliac artery
use Artery, External Iliac, Left
use Artery, External Iliac, Right
Deep facial vein
use Vein, Face, Left
use Vein, Face, Right
Deep femoral (profunda femoris) vein
use Vein, Femoral, Left
use Vein, Femoral, Right
Deep femoral artery
use Artery, Femoral, Left
use Artery, Femoral, Right
Deep Inferior Epigastric Artery Perforator Flap
Replacement
Bilateral **0HRV077**
Left **0HRU077**
Right **0HRT077**
Transfer
Left **0KXG-**
Right **0KXF-**
Deep palmar arch
use Artery, Hand, Left
use Artery, Hand, Right
Deep transverse perineal muscle
use Muscle, Perineum
Deferential artery
use Artery, Internal Iliac, Left
use Artery, Internal Iliac, Right
Defibrillator Generator
Abdomen **0JH8-**
Chest **0JH6-**
Defibrotide sodium anticoagulant XW0-
Defitelio
use Defibrotide sodium anticoagulant
Delivery
Cesarean *see* Extraction, Products of Conception **10D0-**
Forceps *see* Extraction, Products of Conception **10D0-**
Manually assisted **10E0XZZ**
Products of Conception **10E0XZZ**
Vacuum assisted *see* Extraction, Products of Conception **10D0-**
Delta frame external fixator
use External Fixation Device, Hybrid in **0PH-**
use External Fixation Device, Hybrid in **0PS-**
use External Fixation Device, Hybrid in **0QH-**
use External Fixation Device, Hybrid in **0QS-**
Delta III Reverse shoulder prosthesis
use Synthetic Substitute, Reverse Ball and Socket in **0RR-**
Deltoid fascia
use Subcutaneous Tissue and Fascia, Upper Arm, Left
use Subcutaneous Tissue and Fascia, Upper Arm, Right
Deltoid ligament
use Bursa and Ligament, Ankle, Left
use Bursa and Ligament, Ankle, Right
Deltoid muscle
use Muscle, Shoulder, Left
use Muscle, Shoulder, Right
Deltopectoral (infraclavicular) lymph node
use Lymphatic, Upper Extremity, Left
use Lymphatic, Upper Extremity, Right
Denervation
Cranial nerve *see* Destruction, Central Nervous System and Cranial Nerves **005-**
Peripheral nerve *see* Destruction, Peripheral Nervous System **015-**
Dens
use Cervical Vertebra
Densitometry
Plain Radiography
Femur
Left **BQ04ZZ1**
Right **BQ03ZZ1**
Hip
Left **BQ01ZZ1**
Right **BQ00ZZ1**
Spine
Cervical **BR00ZZ1**
Lumbar **BR09ZZ1**
Thoracic **BR07ZZ1**
Whole **BR0GZZ1**
Ultrasonography
Elbow
Left **BP4HZZ1**
Right **BP4GZZ1**
Hand
Left **BP4PZZ1**
Right **BP4NZZ1**
Shoulder
Left **BP49ZZ1**
Right **BP48ZZ1**
Wrist
Left **BP4MZZ1**
Right **BP4LZZ1**
Denticulate (dentate) ligament
use Spinal Meninges
Depressor anguli oris muscle
use Muscle, Facial
Depressor labii inferioris muscle
use Muscle, Facial
Depressor septi nasi muscle
use Muscle, Facial
Depressor supercilii muscle
use Muscle, Facial
Dermabrasion *see* Extraction, Skin and Breast **0HD-**
Dermis
use Skin
Descending genicular artery
use Artery, Femoral, Left
use Artery, Femoral, Right

© 2018 Channel Publishing, Ltd.

Destruction
Acetabulum
Left **0Q55-**
Right **0Q54-**
Adenoids **0C5Q-**
Ampulla of Vater **0F5C-**
Anal Sphincter **0D5R-**
Anterior Chamber
Left **08533ZZ**
Right **08523ZZ**
Anus **0D5Q-**
Aorta
Abdominal **0450-**
Thoracic
Ascending/Arch **025X-**
Descending **025W-**
Aortic Body **0G5D-**
Appendix **0D5J-**
Artery
Anterior Tibial
Left **045Q-**
Right **045P-**
Axillary
Left **0356-**
Right **0355-**
Brachial
Left **0358-**
Right **0357-**
Celiac **0451-**
Colic
Left **0457-**
Middle **0458-**
Right **0456-**
Common Carotid
Left **035J-**
Right **035H-**
Common Iliac
Left **045D-**
Right **045C-**
External Carotid
Left **035N-**
Right **035M-**
External Iliac
Left **045J-**
Right **045H-**
Face **035R-**
Femoral
Left **045L-**
Right **045K-**
Foot
Left **045W-**
Right **045V-**
Gastric **0452-**
Hand
Left **035F-**
Right **035D-**
Hepatic **0453-**
Inferior Mesenteric **045B-**
Innominate **0352-**
Internal Carotid
Left **035L-**
Right **035K-**
Internal Iliac
Left **045F-**
Right **045E-**
Internal Mammary
Left **0351-**
Right **0350-**
Intracranial **035G-**
Lower **045Y-**
Peroneal
Left **045U-**
Right **045T-**
Popliteal
Left **045N-**
Right **045M-**
Posterior Tibial
Left **045S-**
Right **045R-**
Pulmonary
Left **025R-**
Right **025Q-**
Pulmonary Trunk **025P-**

Destruction — *continued*
Artery — *continued*
Radial
Left **035C-**
Right **035B-**
Renal
Left **045A-**
Right **0459-**
Splenic **0454-**
Subclavian
Left **0354-**
Right **0353-**
Superior Mesenteric **0455-**
Temporal
Left **035T-**
Right **035S-**
Thyroid
Left **035V-**
Right **035U-**
Ulnar
Left **035A-**
Right **0359-**
Upper **035Y-**
Vertebral
Left **035Q-**
Right **035P-**
Atrium
Left **0257-**
Right **0256-**
Auditory Ossicle
Left **095A-**
Right **0959-**
Basal Ganglia **0058-**
Bladder **0T5B-**
Bladder Neck **0T5C-**
Bone
Ethmoid
Left **0N5G-**
Right **0N5F-**
Frontal **0N51-**
Hyoid **0N5X-**
Lacrimal
Left **0N5J-**
Right **0N5H-**
Nasal **0N5B-**
Occipital **0N57-**
Palatine
Left **0N5L-**
Right **0N5K-**
Parietal
Left **0N54-**
Right **0N53-**
Pelvic
Left **0Q53-**
Right **0Q52-**
Sphenoid **0N5C-**
Temporal
Left **0N56-**
Right **0N55-**
Zygomatic
Left **0N5N-**
Right **0N5M-**
Brain **0050-**
Breast
Bilateral **0H5V-**
Left **0H5U-**
Right **0H5T-**
Bronchus
Lingula **0B59-**
Lower Lobe
Left **0B5B-**
Right **0B56-**
Main
Left **0B57-**
Right **0B53-**
Middle Lobe, Right **0B55-**
Upper Lobe
Left **0B58-**
Right **0B54-**
Buccal Mucosa **0C54-**

Destruction — *continued*
Bursa and Ligament
Abdomen
Left **0M5J-**
Right **0M5H-**
Ankle
Left **0M5R-**
Right **0M5Q-**
Elbow
Left **0M54-**
Right **0M53-**
Foot
Left **0M5T-**
Right **0M5S-**
Hand
Left **0M58-**
Right **0M57-**
Head and Neck **0M50-**
Hip
Left **0M5M-**
Right **0M5L-**
Knee
Left **0M5P-**
Right **0M5N-**
Lower Extremity
Left **0M5W-**
Right **0M5V-**
Perineum **0M5K-**
Rib(s) **0M5G-**
Shoulder
Left **0M52-**
Right **0M51-**
Spine
Lower **0M5D-**
Upper **0M5C-**
Sternum **0M5F-**
Upper Extremity
Left **0M5B-**
Right **0M59-**
Wrist
Left **0M56-**
Right **0M55-**
Carina **0B52-**
Carotid Bodies, Bilateral **0G58-**
Carotid Body
Left **0G56-**
Right **0G57-**
Carpal
Left **0P5N-**
Right **0P5M-**
Cecum **0D5H-**
Cerebellum **005C-**
Cerebral Hemisphere **0057-**
Cerebral Meninges **0051-**
Cerebral Ventricle **0056-**
Cervix **0U5C-**
Chordae Tendineae **0259-**
Choroid
Left **085B-**
Right **085A-**
Cisterna Chyli **075L-**
Clavicle
Left **0P5B-**
Right **0P59-**
Clitoris **0U5J-**
Coccygeal Glomus **0G5B-**
Coccyx **0Q5S-**
Colon
Ascending **0D5K-**
Descending **0D5M-**
Sigmoid **0D5N-**
Transverse **0D5L-**
Conduction Mechanism **0258-**
Conjunctiva
Left **085TXZZ**
Right **085SXZZ**
Cord
Bilateral **0V5H-**
Left **0V5G-**
Right **0V5F-**
Cornea
Left **0859XZZ**
Right **0858XZZ**
Cul-de-sac **0U5F-**
Diaphragm **0B5T-**

Destruction — *continued*
Disc
Cervical Vertebral **0R53-**
Cervicothoracic Vertebral **0R55-**
Lumbar Vertebral **0S52-**
Lumbosacral **0S54-**
Thoracic Vertebral **0R59-**
Thoracolumbar Vertebral **0R5B-**
Duct
Common Bile **0F59-**
Cystic **0F58-**
Hepatic
Common **0F57-**
Left **0F56-**
Right **0F55-**
Lacrimal
Left **085Y-**
Right **085X-**
Pancreatic **0F5D-**
Accessory **0F5F-**
Parotid
Left **0C5C-**
Right **0C5B-**
Duodenum **0D59-**
Dura Mater **0052-**
Ear
External
Left **0951-**
Right **0950-**
External Auditory Canal
Left **0954-**
Right **0953-**
Inner
Left **095E-**
Right **095D-**
Middle
Left **0956-**
Right **0955-**
Endometrium **0U5B-**
Epididymis
Bilateral **0V5L-**
Left **0V5K-**
Right **0V5J-**
Epiglottis **0C5R-**
Esophagogastric Junction **0D54-**
Esophagus **0D55-**
Lower **0D53-**
Middle **0D52-**
Upper **0D51-**
Eustachian Tube
Left **095G-**
Right **095F-**
Eye
Left **0851XZZ**
Right **0850XZZ**
Eyelid
Lower
Left **085R-**
Right **085Q-**
Upper
Left **085P-**
Right **085N-**
Fallopian Tube
Left **0U56-**
Right **0U55-**
Fallopian Tubes, Bilateral **0U57-**
Femoral Shaft
Left **0Q59-**
Right **0Q58-**
Femur
Lower
Left **0Q5C-**
Right **0Q5B-**
Upper
Left **0Q57-**
Right **0Q56-**
Fibula
Left **0Q5K-**
Right **0Q5J-**
Finger Nail **0H5QXZZ**
Gallbladder **0F54-**
Gingiva
Lower **0C56-**
Upper **0C55-**

© 2018 Channel Publishing, Ltd.

Destruction — *continued*
Gland
Adrenal
Bilateral **0G54-**
Left **0G52-**
Right **0G53-**
Lacrimal
Left **085W-**
Right **085V-**
Minor Salivary **0C5J-**
Parotid
Left **0C59-**
Right **0C58-**
Pituitary **0G50-**
Sublingual
Left **0C5F-**
Right **0C5D-**
Submaxillary
Left **0C5H-**
Right **0C5G-**
Vestibular **0U5L-**
Glenoid Cavity
Left **0P58-**
Right **0P57-**
Glomus Jugulare **0G5C-**
Humeral Head
Left **0P5D-**
Right **0P5C-**
Humeral Shaft
Left **0P5G-**
Right **0P5F-**
Hymen **0U5K-**
Hypothalamus **005A-**
Ileocecal Valve **0D5C-**
Ileum **0D5B-**
Intestine
Large **0D5E-**
Left **0D5G-**
Right **0D5F-**
Small **0D58-**
Iris
Left **085D3ZZ**
Right **085C3ZZ**
Jejunum **0D5A-**
Joint
Acromioclavicular
Left **0R5H-**
Right **0R5G-**
Ankle
Left **0S5G-**
Right **0S5F-**
Carpal
Left **0R5R-**
Right **0R5Q-**
Carpometacarpal
Left **0R5T-**
Right **0R5S-**
Cervical Vertebral **0R51-**
Cervicothoracic Vertebral **0R54-**
Coccygeal **0S56-**
Elbow
Left **0R5M-**
Right **0R5L-**
Finger Phalangeal
Left **0R5X-**
Right **0R5W-**
Hip
Left **0S5B-**
Right **0S59-**
Knee
Left **0S5D-**
Right **0S5C-**
Lumbar Vertebral **0S50-**
Lumbosacral **0S53-**
Metacarpophalangeal
Left **0R5V-**
Right **0R5U-**
Metatarsal-Phalangeal
Left **0S5N-**
Right **0S5M-**
Occipital-cervical **0R50-**

Destruction — *continued*
Joint — *continued*
Sacrococcygeal **0S55-**
Sacroiliac
Left **0S58-**
Right **0S57-**
Shoulder
Left **0R5K-**
Right **0R5J-**
Sternoclavicular
Left **0R5F-**
Right **0R5E-**
Tarsal
Left **0S5J-**
Right **0S5H-**
Tarsometatarsal
Left **0S5L-**
Right **0S5K-**
Temporomandibular
Left **0R5D-**
Right **0R5C-**
Thoracic Vertebral **0R56-**
Thoracolumbar Vertebral **0R5A-**
Toe Phalangeal
Left **0S5Q-**
Right **0S5P-**
Wrist
Left **0R5P-**
Right **0R5N-**
Kidney
Left **0T51-**
Right **0T50-**
Kidney Pelvis
Left **0T54-**
Right **0T53-**
Larynx **0C5S-**
Lens
Left **085K3ZZ**
Right **085J3ZZ**
Lip
Lower **0C51-**
Upper **0C50-**
Liver **0F50-**
Left Lobe **0F52-**
Right Lobe **0F51-**
Lung
Bilateral **0B5M-**
Left **0B5L-**
Lower Lobe
Left **0B5J-**
Right **0B5F-**
Middle Lobe, Right **0B5D-**
Right **0B5K-**
Upper Lobe
Left **0B5G-**
Right **0B5C-**
Lung Lingula **0B5H-**
Lymphatic
Aortic **075D-**
Axillary
Left **0756-**
Right **0755-**
Head **0750-**
Inguinal
Left **075J-**
Right **075H-**
Internal Mammary
Left **0759-**
Right **0758-**
Lower Extremity
Left **075G-**
Right **075F-**
Mesenteric **075B-**
Neck
Left **0752-**
Right **0751-**
Pelvis **075C-**
Thoracic Duct **075K-**
Thorax **0757-**
Upper Extremity
Left **0754-**
Right **0753-**

Destruction — *continued*
Mandible
Left **0N5V-**
Right **0N5T-**
Maxilla **0N5R-**
Medulla Oblongata **005D-**
Mesentery **0D5V-**
Metacarpal
Left **0P5Q-**
Right **0P5P-**
Metatarsal
Left **0Q5P-**
Right **0Q5N-**
Muscle
Abdomen
Left **0K5L-**
Right **0K5K-**
Extraocular
Left **085M-**
Right **085L-**
Facial **0K51-**
Foot
Left **0K5W-**
Right **0K5V-**
Hand
Left **0K5D-**
Right **0K5C-**
Head **0K50-**
Hip
Left **0K5P-**
Right **0K5N-**
Lower Arm and Wrist
Left **0K5B-**
Right **0K59-**
Lower Leg
Left **0K5T-**
Right **0K5S-**
Neck
Left **0K53-**
Right **0K52-**
Papillary **025D-**
Perineum **0K5M-**
Shoulder
Left **0K56-**
Right **0K55-**
Thorax
Left **0K5J-**
Right **0K5H-**
Tongue, Palate, Pharynx **0K54-**
Trunk
Left **0K5G-**
Right **0K5F-**
Upper Arm
Left **0K58-**
Right **0K57-**
Upper Leg
Left **0K5R-**
Right **0K5Q-**
Nasal Mucosa and Soft Tissue **095K-**
Nasopharynx **095N-**
Nerve
Abdominal Sympathetic **015M-**
Abducens **005L-**
Accessory **005R-**
Acoustic **005N-**
Brachial Plexus **0153-**
Cervical **0151-**
Cervical Plexus **0150-**
Facial **005M-**
Femoral **015D-**
Glossopharyngeal **005P-**
Head and Neck Sympathetic **015K-**
Hypoglossal **005S-**
Lumbar **015B-**
Lumbar Plexus **0159-**
Lumbar Sympathetic **015N-**
Lumbosacral Plexus **015A-**
Median **0155-**
Oculomotor **005H-**
Olfactory **005F-**
Optic **005G-**
Peroneal **015H-**

Destruction — *continued*
Nerve — *continued*
Phrenic **0152-**
Pudendal **015C-**
Radial **0156-**
Sacral **015R-**
Sacral Plexus **015Q-**
Sacral Sympathetic **015P-**
Sciatic **015F-**
Thoracic **0158-**
Thoracic Sympathetic **015L-**
Tibial **015G-**
Trigeminal **005K-**
Trochlear **005J-**
Ulnar **0154-**
Vagus **005Q-**
Nipple
Left **0H5X-**
Right **0H5W-**
Omentum **0D5U-**
Orbit
Left **0N5Q-**
Right **0N5P-**
Ovary
Bilateral **0U52-**
Left **0U51-**
Right **0U50-**
Palate
Hard **0C52-**
Soft **0C53-**
Pancreas **0F5G-**
Para-aortic Body **0G59-**
Paraganglion Extremity **0G5F-**
Parathyroid Gland **0G5R-**
Inferior
Left **0G5P-**
Right **0G5N-**
Multiple **0G5Q-**
Superior
Left **0G5M-**
Right **0G5L-**
Patella
Left **0Q5F-**
Right **0Q5D-**
Penis **0V5S-**
Pericardium **025N-**
Peritoneum **0D5W-**
Phalanx
Finger
Left **0P5V-**
Right **0P5T-**
Thumb
Left **0P5S-**
Right **0P5R-**
Toe
Left **0Q5R-**
Right **0Q5Q-**
Pharynx **0C5M-**
Pineal Body **0G51-**
Pleura
Left **0B5P-**
Right **0B5N-**
Pons **005B-**
Prepuce **0V5T-**
Prostate **0V50-**
Robotic Waterjet Ablation **XV508A4**
Radius
Left **0P5J-**
Right **0P5H-**
Rectum **0D5P-**
Retina
Left **085F3ZZ**
Right **085E3ZZ**
Retinal Vessel
Left **085H3ZZ**
Right **085G3ZZ**
Ribs
1 to 2 **0P51-**
3 or more **0P52-**
Sacrum **0Q51-**
Scapula
Left **0P56-**
Right **0P55-**

PROCEDURE INDEX

© 2018 Channel Publishing, Ltd.

Destruction — *continued*
Sclera
Left **0857XZZ**
Right **0856XZZ**
Scrotum **0V55-**
Septum
Atrial **0255-**
Nasal **095M-**
Ventricular **025M-**
Sinus
Accessory **095P-**
Ethmoid
Left **095V-**
Right **095U-**
Frontal
Left **095T-**
Right **095S-**
Mastoid
Left **095C-**
Right **095B-**
Maxillary
Left **095R-**
Right **095Q-**
Sphenoid
Left **095X-**
Right **095W-**
Skin
Abdomen **0H57XZ-**
Back **0H56XZ-**
Buttock **0H58XZ-**
Chest **0H55XZ-**
Ear
Left **0H53XZ-**
Right **0H52XZ-**
Face **0H51XZ-**
Foot
Left **0H5NXZ-**
Right **0H5MXZ-**
Hand
Left **0H5GXZ-**
Right **0H5FXZ-**
Inguinal **0H5AXZ-**
Lower Arm
Left **0H5EXZ-**
Right **0H5DXZ-**
Lower Leg
Left **0H5LXZ-**
Right **0H5KXZ-**
Neck **0H54XZ-**
Perineum **0H59XZ-**
Scalp **0H50XZ-**
Upper Arm
Left **0H5CXZ-**
Right **0H5BXZ-**
Upper Leg
Left **0H5JXZ-**
Right **0H5HXZ-**
Skull **0N50-**
Spinal Cord
Cervical **005W-**
Lumbar **005Y-**
Thoracic **005X-**
Spinal Meninges **005T-**
Spleen **075P-**
Sternum **0P50-**
Stomach **0D56-**
Pylorus **0D57-**
Subcutaneous Tissue and Fascia
Abdomen **0J58-**
Back **0J57-**
Buttock **0J59-**
Chest **0J56-**
Face **0J51-**
Foot
Left **0J5R-**
Right **0J5Q-**
Hand
Left **0J5K-**
Right **0J5J-**
Lower Arm
Left **0J5H-**
Right **0J5G-**

Destruction — *continued*
Subcutaneous Tissue and Fascia — *continued*
Lower Leg
Left **0J5P-**
Right **0J5N-**
Neck
Left **0J55-**
Right **0J54-**
Pelvic Region **0J5C-**
Perineum **0J5B-**
Scalp **0J50-**
Upper Arm
Left **0J5F-**
Right **0J5D-**
Upper Leg
Left **0J5M-**
Right **0J5L-**
Tarsal
Left **0Q5M-**
Right **0Q5L-**
Tendon
Abdomen
Left **0L5G-**
Right **0L5F-**
Ankle
Left **0L5T-**
Right **0L5S-**
Foot
Left **0L5W-**
Right **0L5V-**
Hand
Left **0L58-**
Right **0L57-**
Head and Neck **0L50-**
Hip
Left **0L5K-**
Right **0L5J-**
Knee
Left **0L5R-**
Right **0L5Q-**
Lower Arm and Wrist
Left **0L56-**
Right **0L55-**
Lower Leg
Left **0L5P-**
Right **0L5N-**
Perineum **0L5H-**
Shoulder
Left **0L52-**
Right **0L51-**
Thorax
Left **0L5D-**
Right **0L5C-**
Trunk
Left **0L5B-**
Right **0L59-**
Upper Arm
Left **0L54-**
Right **0L53-**
Upper Leg
Left **0L5M-**
Right **0L5L-**
Testis
Bilateral **0V5C-**
Left **0V5B-**
Right **0V59-**
Thalamus **0059-**
Thymus **075M-**
Thyroid Gland **0G5K-**
Left Lobe **0G5G-**
Right Lobe **0G5H-**
Tibia
Left **0Q5H-**
Right **0Q5G-**
Toe Nail **0H5RXZZ**
Tongue **0C57-**
Tonsils **0C5P-**
Tooth
Lower **0C5X-**
Upper **0C5W-**
Trachea **0B51-**

Destruction — *continued*
Tunica Vaginalis
Left **0V57-**
Right **0V56-**
Turbinate, Nasal **095L-**
Tympanic Membrane
Left **0958-**
Right **0957-**
Ulna
Left **0P5L-**
Right **0P5K-**
Ureter
Left **0T57-**
Right **0T56-**
Urethra **0T5D-**
Uterine Supporting Structure **0U54-**
Uterus **0U59-**
Uvula **0C5N-**
Vagina **0U5G-**
Valve
Aortic **025F-**
Mitral **025G-**
Pulmonary **025H-**
Tricuspid **025J-**
Vas Deferens
Bilateral **0V5Q-**
Left **0V5P-**
Right **0V5N-**
Vein
Axillary
Left **0558-**
Right **0557-**
Azygos **0550-**
Basilic
Left **055C-**
Right **055B-**
Brachial
Left **055A-**
Right **0559-**
Cephalic
Left **055F-**
Right **055D-**
Colic **0657-**
Common Iliac
Left **065D-**
Right **065C-**
Coronary **0254-**
Esophageal **0653-**
External Iliac
Left **065G-**
Right **065F-**
External Jugular
Left **055Q-**
Right **055P-**
Face
Left **055V-**
Right **055T-**
Femoral
Left **065N-**
Right **065M-**
Foot
Left **065V-**
Right **065T-**
Gastric **0652-**
Hand
Left **055H-**
Right **055G-**
Hemiazygos **0551-**
Hepatic **0654-**
Hypogastric
Left **065J-**
Right **065H-**
Inferior Mesenteric **0656-**
Innominate
Left **0554-**
Right **0553-**
Internal Jugular
Left **055N-**
Right **055M-**
Intracranial **055L-**
Lower **065Y-**
Portal **0658-**

Destruction — *continued*
Vein — *continued*
Pulmonary
Left **025T-**
Right **025S-**
Renal
Left **065B-**
Right **0659-**
Saphenous
Left **065Q-**
Right **065P-**
Splenic **0651-**
Subclavian
Left **0556-**
Right **0555-**
Superior Mesenteric **0655-**
Upper **055Y-**
Vertebral
Left **055S-**
Right **055R-**
Vena Cava
Inferior **0650-**
Superior **025V-**
Ventricle
Left **025L-**
Right **025K-**
Vertebra
Cervical **0P53-**
Lumbar **0Q50-**
Thoracic **0P54-**
Vesicle
Bilateral **0V53-**
Left **0V52-**
Right **0V51-**
Vitreous
Left **08553ZZ**
Right **08543ZZ**
Vocal Cord
Left **0C5V-**
Right **0C5T-**
Vulva **0U5M-**
Detachment
Arm
Lower
Left **0X6F0Z-**
Right **0X6D0Z-**
Upper
Left **0X690Z-**
Right **0X680Z-**
Elbow Region
Left **0X6C0ZZ**
Right **0X6B0ZZ**
Femoral Region
Left **0Y680ZZ**
Right **0Y670ZZ**
Finger
Index
Left **0X6P0Z-**
Right **0X6N0Z-**
Little
Left **0X6W0Z-**
Right **0X6V0Z-**
Middle
Left **0X6R0Z-**
Right **0X6Q0Z-**
Ring
Left **0X6T0Z-**
Right **0X6S0Z-**
Foot
Left **0Y6N0Z-**
Right **0Y6M0Z-**
Forequarter
Left **0X610ZZ**
Right **0X600ZZ**
Hand
Left **0X6K0Z-**
Right **0X6J0Z-**
Hindquarter
Bilateral **0Y640ZZ**
Left **0Y630ZZ**
Right **0Y620ZZ**
Knee Region
Left **0Y6G0ZZ**
Right **0Y6F0ZZ**

© 2018 Channel Publishing, Ltd.

Detachment — *continued*
Leg
Lower
Left **0Y6J0Z-**
Right **0Y6H0Z-**
Upper
Left **0Y6D0Z-**
Right **0Y6C0Z-**
Shoulder Region
Left **0X630ZZ**
Right **0X620ZZ**
Thumb
Left **0X6M0Z-**
Right **0X6L0Z-**
Toe
1st
Left **0Y6Q0Z-**
Right **0Y6P0Z-**
2nd
Left **0Y6S0Z-**
Right **0Y6R0Z-**
3rd
Left **0Y6U0Z-**
Right **0Y6T0Z-**
4th
Left **0Y6W0Z-**
Right **0Y6V0Z-**
5th
Left **0Y6Y0Z-**
Right **0Y6X0Z-**
Determination, Mental status GZ14ZZZ
Detorsion
see Release
see Reposition
Detoxification Services, for substance abuse HZ2ZZZZ
Device Fitting F0DZ-
Diagnostic Audiology *see* Audiology, Diagnostic
Diagnostic imaging *see* Imaging, Diagnostic
Diagnostic radiology *see* Imaging, Diagnostic
Dialysis
Hemodialysis *see* Performance, Urinary **5A1D-**
Peritoneal **3E1M39Z**
Diaphragma sellae
use Dura Mater
Diaphragmatic pacemaker generator
use Stimulator Generator in Subcutaneous Tissue and Fascia
Diaphragmatic Pacemaker Lead
Insertion of device in, Diaphragm **0BHT-**
Removal of device from, Diaphragm **0BPT-**
Revision of device in, Diaphragm **0BWT-**
Digital radiography, plain *see* Plain Radiography
Dilation
Ampulla of Vater **0F7C-**
Anus **0D7Q-**
Aorta
Abdominal **0470-**
Thoracic
Ascending/Arch **027X-**
Descending **027W-**
Artery
Anterior Tibial
Left **047Q-**
Right **047P-**
Axillary
Left **0376-**
Right **0375-**
Brachial
Left **0378-**
Right **0377-**
Celiac **0471-**

Dilation — *continued*
Artery — *continued*
Colic
Left **0477-**
Middle **0478-**
Right **0476-**
Common Carotid
Left **037J-**
Right **037H-**
Common Iliac
Left **047D-**
Right **047C-**
Coronary
Four or More Arteries **0273-**
One Artery **0270-**
Three Arteries **0272-**
Two Arteries **0271-**
External Carotid
Left **037N-**
Right **037M-**
External Iliac
Left **047J-**
Right **047H-**
Face **037R-**
Femoral
Left **047L-**
Right **047K-**
Foot
Left **047W-**
Right **047V-**
Gastric **0472-**
Hand
Left **037F-**
Right **037D-**
Hepatic **0473-**
Inferior Mesenteric **047B-**
Innominate **0372-**
Internal Carotid
Left **037L-**
Right **037K-**
Internal Iliac
Left **047F-**
Right **047E-**
Internal Mammary
Left **0371-**
Right **0370-**
Intracranial **037G-**
Lower **047Y-**
Peroneal
Left **047U-**
Right **047T-**
Popliteal
Left **047N-**
Right **047M-**
Posterior Tibial
Left **047S-**
Right **047R-**
Pulmonary
Left **027R-**
Right **027Q-**
Pulmonary Trunk **027P-**
Radial
Left **037C-**
Right **037B-**
Renal
Left **047A-**
Right **0479-**
Splenic **0474-**
Subclavian
Left **0374-**
Right **0373-**
Superior Mesenteric **0475-**
Temporal
Left **037T-**
Right **037S-**
Thyroid
Left **037V-**
Right **037U-**
Ulnar
Left **037A-**
Right **0379-**
Upper **037Y-**

Dilation — *continued*
Artery — *continued*
Vertebral
Left **037Q-**
Right **037P-**
Bladder **0T7B-**
Bladder Neck **0T7C-**
Bronchus
Lingula **0B79-**
Lower Lobe
Left **0B7B-**
Right **0B76-**
Main
Left **0B77-**
Right **0B73-**
Middle Lobe, Right **0B75-**
Upper Lobe
Left **0B78-**
Right **0B74-**
Carina **0B72-**
Cecum **0D7H-**
Cerebral Ventricle **0076-**
Cervix **0U7C-**
Colon
Ascending **0D7K-**
Descending **0D7M-**
Sigmoid **0D7N-**
Transverse **0D7L-**
Duct
Common Bile **0F79-**
Cystic **0F78-**
Hepatic
Common **0F77-**
Left **0F76-**
Right **0F75-**
Lacrimal
Left **087Y-**
Right **087X-**
Pancreatic **0F7D**
Accessory **0F7F-**
Parotid
Left **0C7C-**
Right **0C7B-**
Duodenum **0D79-**
Esophagogastric Junction **0D74-**
Esophagus **0D75-**
Lower **0D73-**
Middle **0D72-**
Upper **0D71-**
Eustachian Tube
Left **097G-**
Right **097F-**
Fallopian Tube
Left **0U76-**
Right **0U75-**
Fallopian Tubes, Bilateral **0U77-**
Hymen **0U7K-**
Ileocecal Valve **0D7C-**
Ileum **0D7B-**
Intestine
Large **0D7E-**
Left **0D7G-**
Right **0D7F-**
Small **0D78-**
Jejunum **0D7A-**
Kidney Pelvis
Left **0T74-**
Right **0T73-**
Larynx **0C7S-**
Pharynx **0C7M-**
Rectum **0D7P-**
Stomach **0D76-**
Pylorus **0D77-**
Trachea **0B71-**
Ureter
Left **0T77-**
Right **0T76-**
Ureters, Bilateral **0T78-**
Urethra **0T7D-**
Uterus **0U79-**
Vagina **0U7G-**

Dilation — *continued*
Valve
Aortic **027F-**
Mitral **027G-**
Pulmonary **027H-**
Tricuspid **027J-**
Vas Deferens
Bilateral **0V7Q-**
Left **0V7P-**
Right **0V7N-**
Vein
Axillary
Left **0578-**
Right **0577-**
Azygos **0570-**
Basilic
Left **057C-**
Right **057B-**
Brachial
Left **057A-**
Right **0579-**
Cephalic
Left **057F-**
Right **057D-**
Colic **0677-**
Common Iliac
Left **067D-**
Right **067C-**
Esophageal **0673-**
External Iliac
Left **067G-**
Right **067F-**
External Jugular
Left **057Q-**
Right **057P-**
Face
Left **057V-**
Right **057T-**
Femoral
Left **067N-**
Right **067M-**
Foot
Left **067V-**
Right **067T-**
Gastric **0672-**
Hand
Left **057H-**
Right **057G-**
Hemiazygos **0571**
Hepatic **0674-**
Hypogastric
Left **067J-**
Right **067H-**
Inferior Mesenteric **0676-**
Innominate
Left **0574-**
Right **0573-**
Internal Jugular
Left **057N-**
Right **057M-**
Intracranial **057L-**
Lower **067Y-**
Portal **0678-**
Pulmonary
Left **027T-**
Right **027S-**
Renal
Left **067B-**
Right **0679-**
Saphenous
Left **067Q-**
Right **067P-**
Splenic **0671-**
Subclavian
Left **0576-**
Right **0575-**
Superior Mesenteric **0675-**
Upper **057Y-**
Vertebral
Left **057S-**
Right **057R-**

© 2018 Channel Publishing, Ltd.

Dilation — *continued*
Vena Cava
Inferior **0670-**
Superior **027V-**
Ventricle
Left **027L-**
Right **027K-**
Direct Lateral Interbody Fusion (DLIF) device
use Interbody Fusion Device in Lower Joints
Disarticulation *see* Detachment
Discectomy, diskectomy
see Excision, Lower Joints **0SB-**
see Excision, Upper Joints **0RB-**
see Resection, Lower Joints **0ST-**
see Resection, Upper Joints **0RT-**
Discography
see Fluoroscopy, Axial Skeleton, Except Skull and Facial Bones **BR1-**
see Plain Radiography, Axial Skeleton, Except Skull and Facial Bones **BR0-**
Distal humerus
use Humeral Shaft, Left
use Humeral Shaft, Right
Distal humerus, involving joint
use Joint, Elbow, Left
use Joint, Elbow, Right
Distal radioulnar joint
use Joint, Wrist, Left
use Joint, Wrist, Right
Diversion *see* Bypass
Diverticulectomy *see* Excision, Gastrointestinal System **0DB-**
Division
Acetabulum
Left **0Q85-**
Right **0Q84-**
Anal Sphincter **0D8R-**
Basal Ganglia **0088-**
Bladder Neck **0T8C-**
Bone
Ethmoid
Left **0N8G-**
Right **0N8F-**
Frontal **0N81-**
Hyoid **0N8X-**
Lacrimal
Left **0N8J-**
Right **0N8H-**
Nasal **0N8B-**
Occipital **0N87-**
Palatine
Left **0N8L-**
Right **0N8K-**
Parietal
Left **0N84-**
Right **0N83-**
Pelvic
Left **0Q83-**
Right **0Q82-**
Sphenoid **0N8C-**
Temporal
Left **0N86-**
Right **0N85-**
Zygomatic
Left **0N8N-**
Right **0N8M-**
Brain **0080-**
Bursa and Ligament
Abdomen
Left **0M8J-**
Right **0M8H-**
Ankle
Left **0M8R-**
Right **0M8Q-**
Elbow
Left **0M84-**
Right **0M83-**
Foot
Left **0M8T-**
Right **0M8S-**

Division — *continued*
Bursa and Ligament — *continued*
Hand
Left **0M88-**
Right **0M87-**
Head and Neck **0M80-**
Hip
Left **0M8M-**
Right **0M8L-**
Knee
Left **0M8P-**
Right **0M8N-**
Lower Extremity
Left **0M8W-**
Right **0M8V-**
Perineum **0M8K-**
Rib(s) **0M8G-**
Shoulder
Left **0M82-**
Right **0M81-**
Spine
Lower **0M8D-**
Upper **0M8C-**
Sternum **0M8F-**
Upper Extremity
Left **0M8B-**
Right **0M89-**
Wrist
Left **0M86-**
Right **0M85-**
Carpal
Left **0P8N-**
Right **0P8M-**
Cerebral Hemisphere **0087-**
Chordae Tendineae **0289-**
Clavicle
Left **0P8B-**
Right **0P89-**
Coccyx **0Q8S-**
Conduction Mechanism **0288-**
Esophagogastric Junction **0D84-**
Femoral Shaft
Left **0Q89-**
Right **0Q88-**
Femur
Lower
Left **0Q8C-**
Right **0Q8B-**
Upper
Left **0Q87-**
Right **0Q86-**
Fibula
Left **0Q8K-**
Right **0Q8J-**
Gland, Pituitary **0G80-**
Glenoid Cavity
Left **0P88-**
Right **0P87-**
Humeral Head
Left **0P8D-**
Right **0P8C-**
Humeral Shaft
Left **0P8G-**
Right **0P8F-**
Hymen **0U8K-**
Kidneys, Bilateral **0T82-**
Mandible
Left **0N8V-**
Right **0N8T-**
Maxilla **0N8R-**
Metacarpal
Left **0P8Q-**
Right **0P8P-**
Metatarsal
Left **0Q8P-**
Right **0Q8N-**
Muscle
Abdomen
Left **0K8L-**
Right **0K8K-**
Facial **0K81-**
Foot
Left **0K8W-**
Right **0K8V-**

Division — *continued*
Muscle — *continued*
Hand
Left **0K8D-**
Right **0K8C-**
Head **0K80-**
Hip
Left **0K8P-**
Right **0K8N-**
Lower Arm and Wrist
Left **0K8B-**
Right **0K89-**
Lower Leg
Left **0K8T-**
Right **0K8S-**
Neck
Left **0K83-**
Right **0K82-**
Papillary **028D-**
Perineum **0K8M-**
Shoulder
Left **0K86-**
Right **0K85-**
Thorax
Left **0K8J-**
Right **0K8H-**
Tongue, Palate, Pharynx **0K84-**
Trunk
Left **0K8G-**
Right **0K8F-**
Upper Arm
Left **0K88-**
Right **0K87-**
Upper Leg
Left **0K8R-**
Right **0K8Q-**
Nerve
Abdominal Sympathetic **018M-**
Abducens **008L-**
Accessory **008R-**
Acoustic **008N-**
Brachial Plexus **0183-**
Cervical **0181-**
Cervical Plexus **0180-**
Facial **008M-**
Femoral **018D-**
Glossopharyngeal **008P-**
Head and Neck Sympathetic **018K-**
Hypoglossal **008S-**
Lumbar **018B-**
Lumbar Plexus **0189-**
Lumbar Sympathetic **018N-**
Lumbosacral Plexus **018A-**
Median **0185-**
Oculomotor **008H-**
Olfactory **008F-**
Optic **008G-**
Peroneal **018H-**
Phrenic **0182-**
Pudendal **018C-**
Radial **0186-**
Sacral **018R-**
Sacral Plexus **018Q-**
Sacral Sympathetic **018P-**
Sciatic **018F-**
Thoracic **0188-**
Thoracic Sympathetic **018L-**
Tibial **018G-**
Trigeminal **008K-**
Trochlear **008J-**
Ulnar **0184-**
Vagus **008Q-**
Orbit
Left **0N8Q-**
Right **0N8P-**
Ovary
Bilateral **0U82-**
Left **0U81-**
Right **0U80-**
Pancreas **0F8G-**
Patella
Left **0Q8F-**
Right **0Q8D-**

Division — *continued*
Perineum, Female **0W8NXZZ**
Phalanx
Finger
Left **0P8V-**
Right **0P8T-**
Thumb
Left **0P8S-**
Right **0P8R-**
Toe
Left **0Q8R-**
Right **0Q8Q-**
Radius
Left **0P8J-**
Right **0P8H-**
Ribs
1 to 2 **0P81-**
3 or more **0P82-**
Sacrum **0Q81-**
Scapula
Left **0P86-**
Right **0P85-**
Skin
Abdomen **0H87XZZ**
Back **0H86XZZ**
Buttock **0H88XZZ**
Chest **0H85XZZ**
Ear
Left **0H83XZZ**
Right **0H82XZZ**
Face **0H81XZZ**
Foot
Left **0H8NXZZ**
Right **0H8MXZZ**
Hand
Left **0H8GXZZ**
Right **0H8FXZZ**
Inguinal **0H8AXZZ**
Lower Arm
Left **0H8EXZZ**
Right **0H8DXZZ**
Lower Leg
Left **0H8LXZZ**
Right **0H8KXZZ**
Neck **0H84XZZ**
Perineum **0H89XZZ**
Scalp **0H80XZZ**
Upper Arm
Left **0H8CXZZ**
Right **0H8BXZZ**
Upper Leg
Left **0H8JXZZ**
Right **0H8HXZZ**
Skull **0N80-**
Spinal Cord
Cervical **008W-**
Lumbar **008Y-**
Thoracic **008X-**
Sternum **0P80-**
Stomach, Pylorus **0D87-**
Subcutaneous Tissue and Fascia
Abdomen **0J88-**
Back **0J87-**
Buttock **0J89-**
Chest **0J86-**
Face **0J81-**
Foot
Left **0J8R-**
Right **0J8Q-**
Hand
Left **0J8K-**
Right **0J8J-**
Head and Neck **0J8S-**
Lower Arm
Left **0J8H-**
Right **0J8G-**
Lower Extremity **0J8W-**
Lower Leg
Left **0J8P-**
Right **0J8N-**
Neck
Left **0J85-**
Right **0J84-**

© 2018 Channel Publishing, Ltd.

Division — *continued*
Subcutaneous Tissue and Fascia — *continued*
Pelvic Region **0J8C-**
Perineum **0J8B-**
Scalp **0J80-**
Trunk **0J8T-**
Upper Arm
Left **0J8F-**
Right **0J8D-**
Upper Extremity **0J8V-**
Upper Leg
Left **0J8M-**
Right **0J8L-**
Tarsal
Left **0Q8M-**
Right **0Q8L-**
Tendon
Abdomen
Left **0L8G-**
Right **0L8F-**
Ankle
Left **0L8T-**
Right **0L8S-**
Foot
Left **0L8W-**
Right **0L8V-**
Hand
Left **0L88-**
Right **0L87-**
Head and Neck **0L80-**
Hip
Left **0L8K-**
Right **0L8J-**
Knee
Left **0L8R-**
Right **0L8Q-**
Lower Arm and Wrist
Left **0L86-**
Right **0L85-**
Lower Leg
Left **0L8P-**
Right **0L8N-**
Perineum **0L8H-**
Shoulder
Left **0L82-**
Right **0L81-**
Thorax
Left **0L8D-**
Right **0L8C-**
Trunk
Left **0L8B-**
Right **0L89-**
Upper Arm
Left **0L84-**
Right **0L83-**
Upper Leg
Left **0L8M-**
Right **0L8L-**
Thyroid Gland Isthmus **0G8J-**
Tibia
Left **0Q8H-**
Right **0Q8G-**
Turbinate, Nasal **098L-**
Ulna
Left **0P8L-**
Right **0P8K-**
Uterine Supporting Structure **0U84-**
Vertebra
Cervical **0P83-**
Lumbar **0Q80-**
Thoracic **0P84-**
Doppler study *see* Ultrasonography
Dorsal digital nerve
use Nerve, Radial
Dorsal metacarpal vein
use Vein, Hand, Left
use Vein, Hand, Right
Dorsal metatarsal artery
use Artery, Foot, Left
use Artery, Foot, Right
Dorsal metatarsal vein
use Vein, Foot, Left
use Vein, Foot, Right
Dorsal scapular artery
use Artery, Subclavian, Left
use Artery, Subclavian, Right
Dorsal scapular nerve
use Nerve, Brachial Plexus
Dorsal venous arch
use Vein, Foot, Left
use Vein, Foot, Right
Dorsalis pedis artery
use Artery, Anterior Tibial, Left
use Artery, Anterior Tibial, Right
DownStream® System
5A0512C
5A0522C
Drainage
Abdominal Wall **0W9F-**
Acetabulum
Left **0Q95-**
Right **0Q94-**
Adenoids **0C9Q-**
Ampulla of Vater **0F9C-**
Anal Sphincter **0D9R-**
Ankle Region
Left **0Y9L-**
Right **0Y9K-**
Anterior Chamber
Left **0893-**
Right **0892-**
Anus **0D9Q-**
Aorta, Abdominal **0490-**
Aortic Body **0G9D-**
Appendix **0D9J-**
Arm
Lower
Left **0X9F-**
Right **0X9D-**
Upper
Left **0X99-**
Right **0X98-**
Artery
Anterior Tibial
Left **049Q-**
Right **049P-**
Axillary
Left **0396-**
Right **0395-**
Brachial
Left **0398-**
Right **0397-**
Celiac **0491-**
Colic
Left **0497-**
Middle **0498-**
Right **0496-**
Common Carotid
Left **039J-**
Right **039H-**
Common Iliac
Left **049D-**
Right **049C-**
External Carotid
Left **039N-**
Right **039M-**
External Iliac
Left **049J-**
Right **049H-**
Face **039R-**
Femoral
Left **049L-**
Right **049K-**
Foot
Left **049W-**
Right **049V-**
Gastric **0492-**
Hand
Left **039F-**
Right **039D-**
Hepatic **0493-**
Inferior Mesenteric **049B-**
Innominate **0392-**
Drainage — *continued*
Artery — *continued*
Internal Carotid
Left **039L-**
Right **039K-**
Internal Iliac
Left **049F-**
Right **049E-**
Internal Mammary
Left **0391-**
Right **0390-**
Intracranial **039G-**
Lower **049Y-**
Peroneal
Left **049U-**
Right **049T-**
Popliteal
Left **049N-**
Right **049M-**
Posterior Tibial
Left **049S-**
Right **049R-**
Radial
Left **039C-**
Right **039B-**
Renal
Left **049A-**
Right **0499-**
Splenic **0494-**
Subclavian
Left **0394-**
Right **0393-**
Superior Mesenteric **0495-**
Temporal
Left **039T-**
Right **039S-**
Thyroid
Left **039V-**
Right **039U-**
Ulnar
Left **039A-**
Right **0399-**
Upper **039Y-**
Vertebral
Left **039Q-**
Right **039P-**
Auditory Ossicle
Left **099A-**
Right **0999-**
Axilla
Left **0X95-**
Right **0X94-**
Back
Lower **0W9L-**
Upper **0W9K-**
Basal Ganglia **0098-**
Bladder **0T9B-**
Bladder Neck **0T9C-**
Bone
Ethmoid
Left **0N9G-**
Right **0N9F-**
Frontal **0N91-**
Hyoid **0N9X-**
Lacrimal
Left **0N9J-**
Right **0N9H-**
Nasal **0N9B-**
Occipital **0N97-**
Palatine
Left **0N9L-**
Right **0N9K-**
Parietal
Left **0N94-**
Right **0N93-**
Pelvic
Left **0Q93-**
Right **0Q92-**
Sphenoid **0N9C-**
Temporal
Left **0N96-**
Right **0N95-**
Zygomatic
Left **0N9N-**
Right **0N9M-**
Drainage — *continued*
Bone Marrow **079T-**
Brain **0090-**
Breast
Bilateral **0H9V-**
Left **0H9U-**
Right **0H9T-**
Bronchus
Lingula **0B99-**
Lower Lobe
Left **0B9B-**
Right **0B96-**
Main
Left **0B97-**
Right **0B93-**
Middle Lobe, Right **0B95-**
Upper Lobe
Left **0B98-**
Right **0B94-**
Buccal Mucosa **0C94-**
Bursa and Ligament
Abdomen
Left **0M9J-**
Right **0M9H-**
Ankle
Left **0M9R-**
Right **0M9Q-**
Elbow
Left **0M94-**
Right **0M93-**
Foot
Left **0M9T-**
Right **0M9S-**
Hand
Left **0M98-**
Right **0M97-**
Head and Neck **0M90-**
Hip
Left **0M9M-**
Right **0M9L-**
Knee
Left **0M9P-**
Right **0M9N-**
Lower Extremity
Left **0M9W-**
Right **0M9V-**
Perineum **0M9K-**
Rib(s) **0M9G-**
Shoulder
Left **0M92-**
Right **0M91-**
Spine
Lower **0M9D-**
Upper **0M9C-**
Sternum **0M9F-**
Upper Extremity
Left **0M9B-**
Right **0M99-**
Wrist
Left **0M96-**
Right **0M95-**
Buttock
Left **0Y91-**
Right **0Y90-**
Carina **0B92-**
Carotid Bodies, Bilateral **0G98-**
Carotid Body
Left **0G96-**
Right **0G97-**
Carpal
Left **0P9N-**
Right **0P9M-**
Cavity, Cranial **0W91-**
Cecum **0D9H-**
Cerebellum **009C-**
Cerebral Hemisphere **0097-**
Cerebral Meninges **0091-**
Cerebral Ventricle **0096-**
Cervix **0U9C-**
Chest Wall **0W98-**
Choroid
Left **089B-**
Right **089A-**
Cisterna Chyli **079L-**

PROCEDURE INDEX

© 2018 Channel Publishing, Ltd.

Drainage — *continued*
Clavicle
Left **0P9B-**
Right **0P99-**
Clitoris **0U9J-**
Coccygeal Glomus **0G9B-**
Coccyx **0Q9S-**
Colon
Ascending **0D9K-**
Descending **0D9M-**
Sigmoid **0D9N-**
Transverse **0D9L-**
Conjunctiva
Left **089T-**
Right **089S-**
Cord
Bilateral **0V9H-**
Left **0V9G-**
Right **0V9F-**
Cornea
Left **0899-**
Right **0898-**
Cul-de-sac **0U9F-**
Diaphragm **0B9T-**
Disc
Cervical Vertebral **0R93-**
Cervicothoracic Vertebral **0R95-**
Lumbar Vertebral **0S92-**
Lumbosacral **0S94-**
Thoracic Vertebral **0R99-**
Thoracolumbar Vertebral **0R9B-**
Duct
Common Bile **0F99-**
Cystic **0F98-**
Hepatic
Common **0F97-**
Left **0F96-**
Right **0F95-**
Lacrimal
Left **089Y-**
Right **089X-**
Pancreatic **0F9D-**
Accessory **0F9F-**
Parotid
Left **0C9C-**
Right **0C9B-**
Duodenum **0D99-**
Dura Mater **0092-**
Ear
External
Left **0991-**
Right **0990-**
External Auditory Canal
Left **0994-**
Right **0993-**
Inner
Left **099E-**
Right **099D-**
Middle
Left **0996-**
Right **0995-**
Elbow Region
Left **0X9C-**
Right **0X9B-**
Epididymis
Bilateral **0V9L-**
Left **0V9K-**
Right **0V9J-**
Epidural Space, Intracranial **0093-**
Epiglottis **0C9R-**
Esophagogastric Junction **0D94-**
Esophagus **0D95-**
Lower **0D93-**
Middle **0D92-**
Upper **0D91-**
Eustachian Tube
Left **099G-**
Right **099F-**
Extremity
Lower
Left **0Y9B-**
Right **0Y99-**

Drainage — *continued*
Extremity — *continued*
Upper
Left **0X97-**
Right **0X96-**
Eye
Left **0891-**
Right **0890-**
Eyelid
Lower
Left **089R-**
Right **089Q-**
Upper
Left **089P-**
Right **089N-**
Face **0W92-**
Fallopian Tube
Left **0U96-**
Right **0U95-**
Fallopian Tubes, Bilateral **0U97-**
Femoral Region
Left **0Y98-**
Right **0Y97-**
Femoral Shaft
Left **0Q99-**
Right **0Q98-**
Femur
Lower
Left **0Q9C-**
Right **0Q9B-**
Upper
Left **0Q97-**
Right **0Q96-**
Fibula
Left **0Q9K-**
Right **0Q9J-**
Finger Nail **0H9Q-**
Foot
Left **0Y9N-**
Right **0Y9M-**
Gallbladder **0F94-**
Gingiva
Lower **0C96-**
Upper **0C95-**
Gland
Adrenal
Bilateral **0G94-**
Left **0G92-**
Right **0G93-**
Lacrimal
Left **089W-**
Right **089V-**
Minor Salivary **0C9J-**
Parotid
Left **0C99-**
Right **0C98-**
Pituitary **0G90-**
Sublingual
Left **0C9F-**
Right **0C9D-**
Submaxillary
Left **0C9H-**
Right **0C9G-**
Vestibular **0U9L-**
Glenoid Cavity
Left **0P98-**
Right **0P97-**
Glomus Jugulare **0G9C-**
Hand
Left **0X9K-**
Right **0X9J-**
Head **0W90-**
Humeral Head
Left **0P9D-**
Right **0P9C-**
Humeral Shaft
Left **0P9G-**
Right **0P9F-**
Hymen **0U9K-**
Hypothalamus **009A-**
Ileocecal Valve **0D9C-**
Ileum **0D9B-**

Drainage — *continued*
Inguinal Region
Left **0Y96-**
Right **0Y95-**
Intestine
Large **0D9E-**
Left **0D9G-**
Right **0D9F-**
Small **0D98-**
Iris
Left **089D-**
Right **089C-**
Jaw
Lower **0W95-**
Upper **0W94-**
Jejunum **0D9A-**
Joint
Acromioclavicular
Left **0R9H-**
Right **0R9G-**
Ankle
Left **0S9G-**
Right **0S9F-**
Carpal
Left **0R9R-**
Right **0R9Q-**
Carpometacarpal
Left **0R9T-**
Right **0R9S-**
Cervical Vertebral **0R91-**
Cervicothoracic Vertebral **0R94-**
Coccygeal **0S96-**
Elbow
Left **0R9M-**
Right **0R9L-**
Finger Phalangeal
Left **0R9X-**
Right **0R9W-**
Hip
Left **0S9B-**
Right **0S99-**
Knee
Left **0S9D-**
Right **0S9C-**
Lumbar Vertebral **0S90-**
Lumbosacral **0S93-**
Metacarpophalangeal
Left **0R9V-**
Right **0R9U-**
Metatarsal-Phalangeal
Left **0S9N-**
Right **0S9M-**
Occipital-cervical **0R90-**
Sacrococcygeal **0S95-**
Sacroiliac
Left **0S98-**
Right **0S97-**
Shoulder
Left **0R9K-**
Right **0R9J-**
Sternoclavicular
Left **0R9F-**
Right **0R9E-**
Tarsal
Left **0S9J-**
Right **0S9H-**
Tarsometatarsal
Left **0S9L-**
Right **0S9K-**
Temporomandibular
Left **0R9D-**
Right **0R9C-**
Thoracic Vertebral **0R96-**
Thoracolumbar Vertebral **0R9A-**
Toe Phalangeal
Left **0S9Q-**
Right **0S9P-**
Wrist
Left **0R9P-**
Right **0R9N-**
Kidney
Left **0T91-**
Right **0T90-**

Drainage — *continued*
Kidney Pelvis
Left **0T94-**
Right **0T93-**
Knee Region
Left **0Y9G-**
Right **0Y9F-**
Larynx **0C9S-**
Leg
Lower
Left **0Y9J-**
Right **0Y9H-**
Upper
Left **0Y9D-**
Right **0Y9C-**
Lens
Left **089K-**
Right **089J-**
Lip
Lower **0C91-**
Upper **0C90-**
Liver **0F90-**
Left Lobe **0F92-**
Right Lobe **0F91-**
Lung
Bilateral **0B9M-**
Left **0B9L-**
Lower Lobe
Left **0B9J-**
Right **0B9F-**
Middle Lobe, Right **0B9D-**
Right **0B9K-**
Upper Lobe
Left **0B9G-**
Right **0B9C-**
Lung Lingula **0B9H-**
Lymphatic
Aortic **079D-**
Axillary
Left **0796-**
Right **0795-**
Head **0790-**
Inguinal
Left **079J-**
Right **079H-**
Internal Mammary
Left **0799-**
Right **0798-**
Lower Extremity
Left **079G-**
Right **079F-**
Mesenteric **079B-**
Neck
Left **0792-**
Right **0791-**
Pelvis **079C-**
Thoracic Duct **079K-**
Thorax **0797-**
Upper Extremity
Left **0794-**
Right **0793-**
Mandible
Left **0N9V-**
Right **0N9T-**
Maxilla **0N9R-**
Mediastinum **0W9C-**
Medulla Oblongata **009D-**
Mesentery **0D9V-**
Metacarpal
Left **0P9Q-**
Right **0P9P-**
Metatarsal
Left **0Q9P-**
Right **0Q9N-**
Muscle
Abdomen
Left **0K9L-**
Right **0K9K-**
Extraocular
Left **089M-**
Right **089L-**
Facial **0K91-**

© 2018 Channel Publishing, Ltd.

PROCEDURE INDEX

© 2018 Channel Publishing, Ltd.

Drainage — *continued*
Tunica Vaginalis
Left **0V97-**
Right **0V96-**
Turbinate, Nasal **099L-**
Tympanic Membrane
Left **0998-**
Right **0997-**
Ulna
Left **0P9L-**
Right **0P9K-**
Ureter
Left **0T97-**
Right **0T96-**
Ureters, Bilateral **0T98-**
Urethra **0T9D-**
Uterine Supporting Structure **0U94-**
Uterus **0U99-**
Uvula **0C9N-**
Vagina **0U9G-**
Vas Deferens
Bilateral **0V9Q-**
Left **0V9P-**
Right **0V9N-**
Vein
Axillary
Left **0598-**
Right **0597-**
Azygos **0590-**
Basilic
Left **059C-**
Right **059B-**
Brachial
Left **059A-**
Right **0599-**
Cephalic
Left **059F-**
Right **059D-**
Colic **0697-**
Common Iliac
Left **069D-**
Right **069C-**
Esophageal **0693-**
External Iliac
Left **069G-**
Right **069F-**
External Jugular
Left **059Q-**
Right **059P-**
Face
Left **059V-**
Right **059T-**
Femoral
Left **069N-**
Right **069M-**
Foot
Left **069V-**
Right **069T-**
Gastric **0692-**
Hand
Left **059H-**
Right **059G-**
Hemiazygos **0591-**
Hepatic **0694-**
Hypogastric
Left **069J-**
Right **069H-**
Inferior Mesenteric **0696-**
Innominate
Left **0594-**
Right **0593-**
Internal Jugular
Left **059N-**
Right **059M-**
Intracranial **059L-**
Lower **069Y-**
Portal **0698-**
Renal
Left **069B-**
Right **0699-**
Saphenous
Left **069Q-**
Right **069P-**

Drainage — *continued*
Vein — *continued*
Splenic **0691-**
Subclavian
Left **0596-**
Right **0595-**
Superior Mesenteric **0695-**
Upper **059Y-**
Vertebral
Left **059S-**
Right **059R-**
Vena Cava, Inferior **0690-**
Vertebra
Cervical **0P93-**
Lumbar **0Q90-**
Thoracic **0P94-**
Vesicle
Bilateral **0V93-**
Left **0V92-**
Right **0V91-**
Vitreous
Left **0895-**
Right **0894-**
Vocal Cord
Left **0C9V-**
Right **0C9T-**
Vulva **0U9M-**
Wrist Region
Left **0X9H-**
Right **0X9G-**

Dressing
Abdominal Wall **2W23X4Z**
Arm
Lower
Left **2W2DX4Z**
Right **2W2CX4Z**
Upper
Left **2W2BX4Z**
Right **2W2AX4Z**
Back **2W25X4Z**
Chest Wall **2W24X4Z**
Extremity
Lower
Left **2W2MX4Z**
Right **2W2LX4Z**
Upper
Left **2W29X4Z**
Right **2W28X4Z**
Face **2W21X4Z**
Finger
Left **2W2KX4Z**
Right **2W2JX4Z**
Foot
Left **2W2TX4Z**
Right **2W2SX4Z**
Hand
Left **2W2FX4Z**
Right **2W2EX4Z**
Head **2W20X4Z**
Inguinal Region
Left **2W27X4Z**
Right **2W26X4Z**
Leg
Lower
Left **2W2RX4Z**
Right **2W2QX4Z**
Upper
Left **2W2PX4Z**
Right **2W2NX4Z**
Neck **2W22X4Z**
Thumb
Left **2W2HX4Z**
Right **2W2GX4Z**
Toe
Left **2W2VX4Z**
Right **2W2UX4Z**

Driver stent (RX) (OTW)
use Intraluminal Device

Drotrecogin alfa, infusion *see* Introduction of Recombinant Human-activated Protein C

Duct of Santorini
use Duct, Pancreatic, Accessory

Duct of Wirsung
use Duct, Pancreatic

Ductogram, mammary *see* Plain Radiography, Skin, Subcutaneous Tissue and Breast **BH0-**

Ductography, mammary *see* Plain Radiography, Skin, Subcutaneous Tissue and Breast **BH0-**

Ductus deferens
use Vas Deferens
use Vas Deferens, Bilateral
use Vas Deferens, Left
use Vas Deferens, Right

Duodenal ampulla
use Ampulla of Vater

Duodenectomy
see Excision, Duodenum **0DB9-**
see Resection, Duodenum **0DT9-**

Duodenocholedochotomy *see* Drainage, Gallbladder **0F94-**

Duodenocystostomy
see Bypass, Gallbladder **0F14-**
see Drainage, Gallbladder **0F94-**

Duodenoenterostomy
see Bypass, Gastrointestinal System **0D1-**
see Drainage, Gastrointestinal System **0D9-**

Duodenojejunal flexure
use Jejunum

Duodenolysis *see* Release, Duodenum **0DN9-**

Duodenorrhaphy *see* Repair, Duodenum **0DQ9-**

Duodenostomy
see Bypass, Duodenum **0D19-**
see Drainage, Duodenum **0D99-**

Duodenotomy *see* Drainage, Duodenum **0D99-**

Dura mater, intracranial
use Dura Mater

Dura mater, spinal
use Spinal Meninges

DuraGraft® Endothelial Damage Inhibitor
use Endothelial Damage Inhibitor

DuraHeart Left Ventricular Assist System
use Implantable Heart Assist System in Heart and Great Vessels

Dural venous sinus
use Vein, Intracranial

Durata® Defibrillation Lead
use Cardiac Lead, Defibrillator in **02H-**

Dynesys® Dynamic Stabilization System
use Spinal Stabilization Device, Pedicle-Based in **0RH-**
use Spinal Stabilization Device, Pedicle-Based in **0SH-**

E

E-Luminexx™ (Biliary) (Vascular) Stent
use Intraluminal Device

Earlobe
use Ear, External, Bilateral
use Ear, External, Left
use Ear, External, Right

ECCO2R (Extracorporeal Carbon Dioxide Removal) **5A0920Z**

Echocardiogram *see* Ultrasonography, Heart **B24-**

Echography *see* Ultrasonography

ECMO *see* Performance, Circulatory **5A15-**

EDWARDS INTUITY Elite valve system
use Zooplastic Tissue, Rapid Deployment Technique in New Technology

EEG (electroencephalogram) *see* Measurement, Central Nervous **4A00-**

EGD (esophagogastroduodenoscopy) **0DJ08ZZ**

Eighth cranial nerve
use Nerve, Acoustic

Ejaculatory duct
use Vas Deferens
use Vas Deferens, Bilateral
use Vas Deferens, Left
use Vas Deferens, Right

EKG (electrocardiogram) *see* Measurement, Cardiac **4A02-**

Electrical bone growth stimulator (EBGS)
use Bone Growth Stimulator in Head and Facial Bones
use Bone Growth Stimulator in Lower Bones
use Bone Growth Stimulator in Upper Bones

Electrical muscle stimulation (EMS) lead
use Stimulator Lead in Muscles

Electrocautery
Destruction *see* Destruction
Repair *see* Repair

Electroconvulsive Therapy
Bilateral-Multiple Seizure **GZB3ZZZ**
Bilateral-Single Seizure **GZB2ZZZ**
Electroconvulsive Therapy, Other **GZB4ZZZ**
Unilateral-Multiple Seizure **GZB1ZZZ**
Unilateral-Single Seizure **GZB0ZZZ**

Electroencephalogram (EEG) *see* Measurement, Central Nervous **4A00-**

Electromagnetic Therapy
Central Nervous **6A22-**
Urinary **6A21-**

Electronic muscle stimulator lead
use Stimulator Lead in Muscles

Electrophysiologic stimulation (EPS) *see* Measurement, Cardiac **4A02-**

Electroshock therapy *see* Electroconvulsive Therapy

Elevation, bone fragments, skull *see* Reposition, Head and Facial Bones **0NS-**

Eleventh cranial nerve
use Nerve, Accessory

© 2018 Channel Publishing, Ltd.

E-Luminexx™ (Biliary) (Vascular) Stent
use Intraluminal Device
Embolectomy *see* Extirpation
Embolization
see Occlusion
see Restriction
Embolization coil(s)
use Intraluminal Device
EMG (electromyogram) *see* Measurement, Musculoskeletal 4A0F-
Encephalon
use Brain
Endarterectomy
see Extirpation, Lower Arteries 04C-
see Extirpation, Upper Arteries 03C-
Endeavor® (III) (IV) (Sprint) Zotarolimus-eluting Coronary Stent System
use Intraluminal Device, Drug-eluting in Heart and Great Vessels
Endologix AFX® Endovascular AAA System
use Intraluminal Device
EndoSure® sensor
use Monitoring Device, Pressure Sensor in 02H-
ENDOTAK RELIANCE® (G) Defibrillation Lead
use Cardiac Lead, Defibrillator in 02H-
Endothelial damage inhibitor, applied to vein graft XY0VX83
Endotracheal tube (cuffed) (double-lumen)
use Intraluminal Device, Endotracheal Airway in Respiratory System
Endurant® II AAA stent graft system
use Intraluminal Device
Endurant® Endovascular Stent Graft
use Intraluminal Device
Engineered Autologous Chimeric Antigen Receptor T-cell Immunotherapy XW0-
Enlargement
see Dilation
see Repair
EnRhythm
use Pacemaker, Dual Chamber 0JH-
Enterorrhaphy *see* Repair, Gastrointestinal System 0DQ-
Enterra gastric neurostimulator
use Stimulator Generator, Multiple Array in 0JH-
Enucleation
Eyeball *see* Resection, Eye 08T-
Eyeball with prosthetic implant *see* Replacement, Eye 08R-
Ependyma
use Cerebral Ventricle
Epicel® cultured epidermal autograft
use Autologous Tissue Substitute
Epic™ Stented Tissue Valve (aortic)
use Zooplastic Tissue in Heart and Great Vessels
Epidermis
use Skin
Epididymectomy
see Excision, Male Reproductive System 0VB-
see Resection, Male Reproductive System 0VT-
Epididymoplasty
see Repair, Male Reproductive System 0VQ-
see Supplement, Male Reproductive System 0VU-
Epididymorrhaphy *see* Repair, Male Reproductive System 0VQ-
Epididymotomy *see* Drainage, Male Reproductive System 0V9-
Epidural space, spinal
use Spinal Canal
Epiphysiodesis
see Insertion of device in, Lower Bones 0QH-
see Insertion of device in, Upper Bones 0PH-
see Repair, Lower Bones 0QQ-
see Repair, Upper Bones 0PQ-
Epiploic foramen
use Peritoneum
Epiretinal Visual Prosthesis
Left 08H105Z
Right 08H005Z
Episiorrhaphy *see* Repair, Perineum, Female 0WQN-
Episiotomy *see* Division, Perineum, Female 0W8N-
Epithalamus
use Thalamus
Epitrochlear lymph node
use Lymphatic, Upper Extremity, Left
use Lymphatic, Upper Extremity, Right
EPS (electrophysiologic stimulation) *see* Measurement, Cardiac 4A02-
Eptifibatide, infusion *see* Introduction of Platelet Inhibitor
ERCP (endoscopic retrograde cholangiopancreatography)
see Fluoroscopy, Hepatobiliary System and Pancreas BF1-
Erector spinae muscle
use Muscle, Trunk, Left
use Muscle, Trunk, Right
Esophageal artery
use Upper Artery
Esophageal obturator airway (EOA)
use Intraluminal Device, Airway in Gastrointestinal System
Esophageal plexus
use Nerve, Thoracic Sympathetic
Esophagectomy
see Excision, Gastrointestinal System 0DB-
see Resection, Gastrointestinal System 0DT-
Esophagocoloplasty
see Repair, Gastrointestinal System 0DQ-
see Supplement, Gastrointestinal System 0DU-
Esophagoenterostomy
see Bypass, Gastrointestinal System 0D1-
see Drainage, Gastrointestinal System 0D9-
Esophagoesophagostomy
see Bypass, Gastrointestinal System 0D1-
see Drainage, Gastrointestinal System 0D9-
Esophagogastrectomy
see Excision, Gastrointestinal System 0DB-
see Resection, Gastrointestinal System 0DT-
Esophagogastroduodenoscopy (EGD) 0DJ08ZZ
Esophagogastroplasty
see Repair, Gastrointestinal System 0DQ-
see Supplement, Gastrointestinal System 0DU-
Esophagogastroscopy 0DJ68ZZ
Esophagogastrostomy
see Bypass, Gastrointestinal System 0D1-
see Drainage, Gastrointestinal System 0D9-
Esophagojejunoplasty *see* Supplement, Gastrointestinal System 0DU-
Esophagojejunostomy
see Bypass, Gastrointestinal System 0D1-
see Drainage, Gastrointestinal System 0D9-
Esophagomyotomy *see* Division, Esophagogastric Junction 0D84-
Esophagoplasty
see Repair, Gastrointestinal System 0DQ-
see Replacement, Esophagus 0DR5-
see Supplement, Gastrointestinal System 0DU-
Esophagoplication *see* Restriction, Gastrointestinal System 0DV-
Esophagorrhaphy *see* Repair, Gastrointestinal System 0DQ-
Esophagoscopy 0DJ08ZZ
Esophagotomy *see* Drainage, Gastrointestinal System 0D9-
Esteem® implantable hearing system
use Hearing Device in Ear, Nose, Sinus
ESWL (extracorporeal shock wave lithotripsy) *see* Fragmentation
Ethmoidal air cell
use Sinus, Ethmoid, Left
use Sinus, Ethmoid, Right
Ethmoidectomy
see Excision, Ear, Nose, Sinus 09B-
see Excision, Head and Facial Bones 0NB-
see Resection, Ear, Nose, Sinus 09T-
see Resection, Head and Facial Bones 0NT-
Ethmoidotomy *see* Drainage, Ear, Nose, Sinus 099-
Evacuation
Hematoma *see* Extirpation
Other Fluid *see* Drainage
Evera (XT) (S) (DR/VR)
use Defibrillator Generator in 0JH-
Everolimus-eluting coronary stent
use Intraluminal Device, Drug-eluting in Heart and Great Vessels
Evisceration
Eyeball *see* Resection, Eye 08T-
Eyeball with prosthetic implant *see* Replacement, Eye 08R-
Ex-PRESS™ mini glaucoma shunt
use Synthetic Substitute
Examination *see* Inspection
Exchange *see* Change device in
Excision
Abdominal Wall 0WBF-
Acetabulum
Left 0QB5-
Right 0QB4-
Adenoids 0CBQ-
Ampulla of Vater 0FBC-
Excision — *continued*
Anal Sphincter 0DBR-
Ankle Region
Left 0YBL-
Right 0YBK-
Anus 0DBQ-
Aorta
Abdominal 04B0-
Thoracic
Ascending/Arch 02BX-
Descending 02BW-
Aortic Body 0GBD-
Appendix 0DBJ-
Arm
Lower
Left 0XBF-
Right 0XBD-
Upper
Left 0XB9-
Right 0XB8-
Artery
Anterior Tibial
Left 04BQ-
Right 04BP-
Axillary
Left 03B6-
Right 03B5-
Brachial
Left 03B8-
Right 03B7-
Celiac 04B1-
Colic
Left 04B7-
Middle 04B8-
Right 04B6-
Common Carotid
Left 03BJ-
Right 03BH
Common Iliac
Left 04BD-
Right 04BC-
External Carotid
Left 03BN-
Right 03BM-
External Iliac
Left 04BJ
Right 04BH-
Face 03BR-
Femoral
Left 04BL-
Right 04BK
Foot
Left 04BW-
Right 04BV-
Gastric 04B2-
Hand
Left 03BF-
Right 03BD-
Hepatic 04B3-
Inferior Mesenteric 04BB-
Innominate 03B2-
Internal Carotid
Left 03BL-
Right 03BK-
Internal Iliac
Left 04BF-
Right 04BE-
Internal Mammary
Left 03B1-
Right 03B0-
Intracranial 03BG-
Lower 04BY-
Peroneal
Left 04BU-
Right 04BT-
Popliteal
Left 04BN-
Right 04BM-
Posterior Tibial
Left 04BS-
Right 04BR-

PROCEDURE INDEX

© 2018 Channel Publishing, Ltd.

Excision — *continued*
Artery — *continued*
Pulmonary
Left **02BR**-
Right **02BQ**-
Pulmonary Trunk **02BP**-
Radial
Left **03BC**-
Right **03BB**-
Renal
Left **04BA**-
Right **04B9**-
Splenic **04B4**-
Subclavian
Left **03B4**-
Right **03B3**-
Superior Mesenteric **04B5**-
Temporal
Left **03BT**-
Right **03BS**-
Thyroid
Left **03BV**-
Right **03BU**-
Ulnar
Left **03BA**-
Right **03B9**-
Upper **03BY**-
Vertebral
Left **03BQ**-
Right **03BP**-
Atrium
Left **02B7**-
Right **02B6**-
Auditory Ossicle
Left **09BA**-
Right **09B9**-
Axilla
Left **0XB5**-
Right **0XB4**-
Back
Lower **0WBL**-
Upper **0WBK**-
Basal Ganglia **00B8**-
Bladder **0TBB**-
Bladder Neck **0TBC**-
Bone
Ethmoid
Left **0NBG**-
Right **0NBF**-
Frontal **0NB1**-
Hyoid **0NBX**-
Lacrimal
Left **0NBJ**-
Right **0NBH**-
Nasal **0NBB**-
Occipital **0NB7**-
Palatine
Left **0NBL**-
Right **0NBK**-
Parietal
Left **0NB4**-
Right **0NB3**-
Pelvic
Left **0QB3**-
Right **0QB2**-
Sphenoid **0NBC**-
Temporal
Left **0NB6**-
Right **0NB5**-
Zygomatic
Left **0NBN**-
Right **0NBM**-
Brain **00B0**-
Breast
Bilateral **0HBV**-
Left **0HBU**-
Right **0HBT**-
Supernumerary **0HBY**-
Bronchus
Lingula **0BB9**-
Lower Lobe
Left **0BBB**-
Right **0BB6**-

Excision — *continued*
Bronchus — *continued*
Main
Left **0BB7**-
Right **0BB3**-
Middle Lobe, Right **0BB5**-
Upper Lobe
Left **0BB8**-
Right **0BB4**-
Buccal Mucosa **0CB4**-
Bursa and Ligament
Abdomen
Left **0MBJ**-
Right **0MBH**-
Ankle
Left **0MBR**-
Right **0MBQ**-
Elbow
Left **0MB4**-
Right **0MB3**-
Foot
Left **0MBT**-
Right **0MBS**-
Hand
Left **0MB8**-
Right **0MB7**-
Head and Neck **0MB0**-
Hip
Left **0MBM**-
Right **0MBL**-
Knee
Left **0MBP**-
Right **0MBN**-
Lower Extremity
Left **0MBW**-
Right **0MBV**-
Perineum **0MBK**-
Rib(s) **0MBG**-
Shoulder
Left **0MB2**-
Right **0MB1**-
Spine
Lower **0MBD**-
Upper **0MBC**-
Sternum **0MBF**-
Upper Extremity
Left **0MBB**-
Right **0MB9**-
Wrist
Left **0MB6**-
Right **0MB5**-
Buttock
Left **0YB1**-
Right **0YB0**-
Carina **0BB2**-
Carotid Bodies, Bilateral **0GB8**-
Carotid Body
Left **0GB6**-
Right **0GB7**-
Carpal
Left **0PBN**-
Right **0PBM**-
Cecum **0DBH**-
Cerebellum **00BC**-
Cerebral Hemisphere **00B7**-
Cerebral Meninges **00B1**-
Cerebral Ventricle **00B6**-
Cervix **0UBC**-
Chest Wall **0WB8**-
Chordae Tendineae **02B9**-
Choroid
Left **08BB**-
Right **08BA**-
Cisterna Chyli **07BL**-
Clavicle
Left **0PBB**-
Right **0PB9**-
Clitoris **0UBJ**-
Coccygeal Glomus **0GBB**-
Coccyx **0QBS**-

Excision — *continued*
Colon
Ascending **0DBK**-
Descending **0DBM**-
Sigmoid **0DBN**-
Transverse **0DBL**-
Conduction Mechanism **02B8**-
Conjunctiva
Left **08BTXZ**-
Right **08BSXZ**-
Cord
Bilateral **0VBH**-
Left **0VBG**-
Right **0VBF**-
Cornea
Left **08B9XZ**-
Right **08B8XZ**-
Cul-de-sac **0UBF**-
Diaphragm **0BBT**-
Disc
Cervical Vertebral **0RB3**-
Cervicothoracic Vertebral **0RB5**-
Lumbar Vertebral **0SB2**-
Lumbosacral **0SB4**-
Thoracic Vertebral **0RB9**-
Thoracolumbar Vertebral **0RBB**-
Duct
Common Bile **0FB9**-
Cystic **0FB8**-
Hepatic
Common **0FB7**-
Left **0FB6**-
Right **0FB5**-
Lacrimal
Left **08BY**-
Right **08BX**-
Pancreatic **0FBD**-
Accessory **0FBF**-
Parotid
Left **0CBC**-
Right **0CBB**-
Duodenum **0DB9**-
Dura Mater **00B2**-
Ear
External
Left **09B1**-
Right **09B0**-
External Auditory Canal
Left **09B4**-
Right **09B3**-
Inner
Left **09BE**-
Right **09BD**-
Middle
Left **09B6**-
Right **09B5**-
Elbow Region
Left **0XBC**-
Right **0XBB**-
Epididymis
Bilateral **0VBL**-
Left **0VBK**-
Right **0VBJ**-
Epiglottis **0CBR**-
Esophagogastric Junction **0DB4** -
Esophagus **0DB5**-
Lower **0DB3**-
Middle **0DB2**-
Upper **0DB1**-
Eustachian Tube
Left **09BG**-
Right **09BF**-
Extremity
Lower
Left **0YBB**-
Right **0YB9**-
Upper
Left **0XB7**-
Right **0XB6**-
Eye
Left **08B1**-
Right **08B0**-

Excision — *continued*
Eyelid
Lower
Left **08BR**-
Right **08BQ**-
Upper
Left **08BP**-
Right **08BN**-
Face **0WB2**-
Fallopian Tube
Left **0UB6**-
Right **0UB5**-
Fallopian Tubes, Bilateral **0UB7**-
Femoral Region
Left **0YB8**-
Right **0YB7**-
Femoral Shaft
Left **0QB9**-
Right **0QB8**-
Femur
Lower
Left **0QBC**-
Right **0QBB**-
Upper
Left **0QB7**-
Right **0QB6**-
Fibula
Left **0QBK**-
Right **0QBJ**-
Finger Nail **0HBQXZ**-
Floor of Mouth *see* Excision, Oral Cavity and Throat **0WB3**-
Foot
Left **0YBN**-
Right **0YBM**-
Gallbladder **0FB4**-
Gingiva
Lower **0CB6**-
Upper **0CB5**-
Gland
Adrenal
Bilateral **0GB4**-
Left **0GB2**-
Right **0GB3**-
Lacrimal
Left **08BW**-
Right **08BV**-
Minor Salivary **0CBJ**-
Parotid
Left **0CB9**-
Right **0CB8**-
Pituitary **0GB0**-
Sublingual
Left **0CBF**-
Right **0CBD**-
Submaxillary
Left **0CBH**-
Right **0CBG**-
Vestibular **0UBL**-
Glenoid Cavity
Left **0PB8**-
Right **0PB7**-
Glomus Jugulare **0GBC**-
Hand
Left **0XBK**-
Right **0XBJ**-
Head **0WB0**-
Humeral Head
Left **0PBD**-
Right **0PBC**-
Humeral Shaft
Left **0PBG**-
Right **0PBF**-
Hymen **0UBK**-
Hypothalamus **00BA**-
Ileocecal Valve **0DBC**-
Ileum **0DBB**-
Inguinal Region
Left **0YB6**-
Right **0YB5**-

© 2018 Channel Publishing, Ltd.

© 2018 Channel Publishing, Ltd.

Excision — *continued*
Sinus — *continued*
Mastoid
Left **09BC-**
Right **09BB-**
Maxillary
Left **09BR-**
Right **09BQ-**
Sphenoid
Left **09BX-**
Right **09BW-**
Skin
Abdomen **0HB7XZ-**
Back **0HB6XZ-**
Buttock **0HB8XZ-**
Chest **0HB5XZ-**
Ear
Left **0HB3XZ-**
Right **0HB2XZ-**
Face **0HB1XZ-**
Foot
Left **0HBNXZ-**
Right **0HBMXZ-**
Hand
Left **0HBGXZ-**
Right **0HBFXZ-**
Inguinal **0HBAXZ-**
Lower Arm
Left **0HBEXZ-**
Right **0HBDXZ-**
Lower Leg
Left **0HBLXZ-**
Right **0HBKXZ-**
Neck **0HB4XZ-**
Perineum **0HB9XZ-**
Scalp **0HB0XZ-**
Upper Arm
Left **0HBCXZ-**
Right **0HBBXZ-**
Upper Leg
Left **0HBJXZ-**
Right **0HBHXZ-**
Skull **0NB0-**
Spinal Cord
Cervical **00BW-**
Lumbar **00BY-**
Thoracic **00BX-**
Spinal Meninges **00BT-**
Spleen **07BP-**
Sternum **0PB0-**
Stomach **0DB6-**
Pylorus **0DB7-**
Subcutaneous Tissue and Fascia
Abdomen **0JB8-**
Back **0JB7-**
Buttock **0JB9-**
Chest **0JB6-**
Face **0JB1-**
Foot
Left **0JBR-**
Right **0JBQ-**
Hand
Left **0JBK-**
Right **0JBJ-**
Lower Arm
Left **0JBH-**
Right **0JBG-**
Lower Leg
Left **0JBP-**
Right **0JBN-**
Neck
Left **0JB5-**
Right **0JB4-**
Pelvic Region **0JBC-**
Perineum **0JBB-**
Scalp **0JB0-**
Upper Arm
Left **0JBF-**
Right **0JBD-**
Upper Leg
Left **0JBM-**
Right **0JBL-**

Excision — *continued*
Tarsal
Left **0QBM-**
Right **0QBL-**
Tendon
Abdomen
Left **0LBG-**
Right **0LBF-**
Ankle
Left **0LBT-**
Right **0LBS-**
Foot
Left **0LBW-**
Right **0LBV-**
Hand
Left **0LB8-**
Right **0LB7-**
Head and Neck **0LB0-**
Hip
Left **0LBK-**
Right **0LBJ-**
Knee
Left **0LBR-**
Right **0LBQ-**
Lower Arm and Wrist
Left **0LB6-**
Right **0LB5-**
Lower Leg
Left **0LBP-**
Right **0LBN-**
Perineum **0LBH-**
Shoulder
Left **0LB2-**
Right **0LB1-**
Thorax
Left **0LBD-**
Right **0LBC-**
Trunk
Left **0LBB-**
Right **0LB9-**
Upper Arm
Left **0LB4-**
Right **0LB3-**
Upper Leg
Left **0LBM-**
Right **0LBL-**
Testis
Bilateral **0VBC-**
Left **0VBB-**
Right **0VB9-**
Thalamus **00B9-**
Thymus **07BM-**
Thyroid Gland
Left Lobe **0GBG-**
Right Lobe **0GBH-**
Thyroid Gland Isthmus **0GBJ-**
Tibia
Left **0QBH-**
Right **0QBG-**
Toe Nail **0HBRXZ -**
Tongue **0CB7-**
Tonsils **0CBP-**
Tooth
Lower **0CBX-**
Upper **0CBW-**
Trachea **0BB1-**
Tunica Vaginalis
Left **0VB7-**
Right **0VB6-**
Turbinate, Nasal **09BL-**
Tympanic Membrane
Left **09B8-**
Right **09B7-**
Ulna
Left **0PBL-**
Right **0PBK-**
Ureter
Left **0TB7-**
Right **0TB6-**
Urethra **0TBD-**
Uterine Supporting Structure **0UB4-**
Uterus **0UB9-**
Uvula **0CBN-**

Excision — *continued*
Vagina **0UBG-**
Valve
Aortic **02BF-**
Mitral **02BG-**
Pulmonary **02BH-**
Tricuspid **02BJ-**
Vas Deferens
Bilateral **0VBQ-**
Left **0VBP-**
Right **0VBN-**
Vein
Axillary
Left **05B8-**
Right **05B7-**
Azygos **05B0-**
Basilic
Left **05BC-**
Right **05BB-**
Brachial
Left **05BA-**
Right **05B9-**
Cephalic
Left **05BF-**
Right **05BD-**
Colic **06B7-**
Common Iliac
Left **06BD-**
Right **06BC-**
Coronary **02B4-**
Esophageal **06B3-**
External Iliac
Left **06BG-**
Right **06BF-**
External Jugular
Left **05BQ-**
Right **05BP-**
Face
Left **05BV-**
Right **05BT-**
Femoral
Left **06BN-**
Right **06BM-**
Foot
Left **06BV-**
Right **06BT-**
Gastric **06B2-**
Hand
Left **05BH-**
Right **05BG-**
Hemiazygos **05B1-**
Hepatic **06B4-**
Hypogastric
Left **06BJ-**
Right **06BH-**
Inferior Mesenteric **06B6-**
Innominate
Left **05B4-**
Right **05B3-**
Internal Jugular
Left **05BN-**
Right **05BM-**
Intracranial **05BL-**
Lower **06BY-**
Portal **06B8-**
Pulmonary
Left **02BT -**
Right **02BS-**
Renal
Left **06BB-**
Right **06B9-**
Saphenous
Left **06BQ-**
Right **06BP-**
Splenic **06B1-**
Subclavian
Left **05B6-**
Right **05B5-**
Superior Mesenteric **06B5-**
Upper **05BY-**
Vertebral
Left **05BS-**
Right **05BR-**

Excision — *continued*
Vena Cava
Inferior **06B0-**
Superior **02BV-**
Ventricle
Left **02BL-**
Right **02BK-**
Vertebra
Cervical **0PB3-**
Lumbar **0QB0-**
Thoracic **0PB4-**
Vesicle
Bilateral **0VB3-**
Left **0VB2-**
Right **0VB1-**
Vitreous
Left **08B53Z-**
Right **08B43Z-**
Vocal Cord
Left **0CBV-**
Right **0CBT-**
Vulva **0UBM-**
Wrist Region
Left **0XBH-**
Right **0XBG-**
EXCLUDER® AAA Endoprosthesis
use Intraluminal Device
use Intraluminal Device, Branched or Fenestrated, One or Two Arteries in **04V-**
use Intraluminal Device, Branched or Fenestrated, Three or More in Arteries **04V-**
EXCLUDER® IBE Endoprosthesis
use Intraluminal Device, Branched or Fenestrated, One or Two Arteries in **04V-**
Exclusion, Left atrial appendage (LAA) *see* Occlusion, Atrium, Left **02L7-**
Exercise, rehabilitation *see* Motor Treatment, Rehabilitation **F07-**
Exploration *see* Inspection
Express® (LD) Premounted Stent System
use Intraluminal Device
Express® Biliary SD Monorail® Premounted Stent System
use Intraluminal Device
Ex-PRESS™ mini glaucoma shunt
use Synthetic Substitute
Express® SD Renal Monorail® Premounted Stent System
use Intraluminal Device
Extensor carpi radialis muscle
use Muscle, Lower Arm and Wrist, Left
use Muscle, Lower Arm and Wrist, Right
Extensor carpi ulnaris muscle
use Muscle, Lower Arm and Wrist, Left
use Muscle, Lower Arm and Wrist, Right
Extensor digitorum brevis muscle
use Muscle, Foot, Left
use Muscle, Foot, Right
Extensor digitorum longus muscle
use Muscle, Lower Leg, Left
use Muscle, Lower Leg, Right
Extensor hallucis brevis muscle
use Muscle, Foot, Left
use Muscle, Foot, Right
Extensor hallucis longus muscle
use Muscle, Lower Leg, Left
use Muscle, Lower Leg, Right
External anal sphincter
use Anal Sphincter

© 2018 Channel Publishing, Ltd.

External auditory meatus
- *use* Ear, External Auditory Canal, Left
- *use* Ear, External Auditory Canal, Right

External fixator
- *use* External Fixation Device in Head and Facial Bones
- *use* External Fixation Device in Lower Bones
- *use* External Fixation Device in Lower Joints
- *use* External Fixation Device in Upper Bones
- *use* External Fixation Device in Upper Joints

External maxillary artery
- *use* Artery, Face

External naris
- *use* Nasal Mucosa and Soft Tissue

External oblique aponeurosis
- *use* Subcutaneous Tissue and Fascia, Trunk

External oblique muscle
- *use* Muscle, Abdomen, Left
- *use* Muscle, Abdomen, Right

External popliteal nerve
- *use* Nerve, Peroneal

External pudendal artery
- *use* Artery, Femoral, Left
- *use* Artery, Femoral, Right

External pudendal vein
- *use* Saphenous Vein, Left
- *use* Saphenous Vein, Right

External urethral sphincter
- *use* Urethra

Extirpation
- Acetabulum
  - Left **0QC5-**
  - Right **0QC4-**
- Adenoids **0CCQ-**
- Ampulla of Vater **0FCC-**
- Anal Sphincter **0DCR-**
- Anterior Chamber
  - Left **08C3-**
  - Right **08C2-**
- Anus **0DCQ-**
- Aorta
  - Abdominal **04C0-**
  - Thoracic
    - Ascending/Arch **02CX-**
    - Descending **02CW-**
- Aortic Body **0GCD-**
- Appendix **0DCJ-**
- Artery
  - Anterior Tibial
    - Left **04CQ-**
    - Right **04CP-**
  - Axillary
    - Left **03C6-**
    - Right **03C5-**
  - Brachial
    - Left **03C8-**
    - Right **03C7-**
  - Celiac **04C1-**
  - Colic
    - Left **04C7-**
    - Middle **04C8-**
    - Right **04C6-**
  - Common Carotid
    - Left **03CJ-**
    - Right **03CH-**
  - Common Iliac
    - Left **04CD-**
    - Right **04CC-**
  - Coronary
    - Four or More Arteries **02C3-**
    - One Artery **02C0-**
    - Three Arteries **02C2-**
    - Two Arteries **02C1-**
  - External Carotid
    - Left **03CN-**
    - Right **03CM-**

Extirpation — *continued*
- Artery — *continued*
  - External Iliac
    - Left **04CJ-**
    - Right **04CH-**
  - Face **03CR-**
  - Femoral
    - Left **04CL-**
    - Right **04CK-**
  - Foot
    - Left **04CW-**
    - Right **04CV-**
  - Gastric **04C2-**
  - Hand
    - Left **03CF-**
    - Right **03CD-**
  - Hepatic **04C3-**
  - Inferior Mesenteric **04CB-**
  - Innominate **03C2-**
  - Internal Carotid
    - Left **03CL-**
    - Right **03CK-**
  - Internal Iliac
    - Left **04CF-**
    - Right **04CE-**
  - Internal Mammary
    - Left **03C1-**
    - Right **03C0-**
  - Intracranial **03CG-**
  - Lower **04CY-**
  - Peroneal
    - Left **04CU-**
    - Right **04CT-**
  - Popliteal
    - Left **04CN-**
    - Right **04CM-**
  - Posterior Tibial
    - Left **04CS-**
    - Right **04CR-**
  - Pulmonary
    - Left **02CR-**
    - Right **02CQ-**
  - Pulmonary Trunk **02CP-**
  - Radial
    - Left **03CC-**
    - Right **03CB-**
  - Renal
    - Left **04CA-**
    - Right **04C9-**
  - Splenic **04C4-**
  - Subclavian
    - Left **03C4-**
    - Right **03C3-**
  - Superior Mesenteric **04C5-**
  - Temporal
    - Left **03CT-**
    - Right **03CS-**
  - Thyroid
    - Left **03CV-**
    - Right **03CU-**
  - Ulnar
    - Left **03CA-**
    - Right **03C9-**
  - Upper **03CY-**
  - Vertebral
    - Left **03CQ-**
    - Right **03CP-**
- Atrium
  - Left **02C7-**
  - Right **02C6-**
- Auditory Ossicle
  - Left **09CA-**
  - Right **09C9-**
- Basal Ganglia **00C8-**
- Bladder **0TCB-**
- Bladder Neck **0TCC-**
- Bone
  - Ethmoid
    - Left **0NCG-**
    - Right **0NCF-**
  - Frontal **0NC1-**
  - Hyoid **0NCX-**

Extirpation — *continued*
- Bone — *continued*
  - Lacrimal
    - Left **0NCJ-**
    - Right **0NCH-**
  - Nasal **0NCB-**
  - Occipital **0NC7-**
  - Palatine
    - Left **0NCL-**
    - Right **0NCK-**
  - Parietal
    - Left **0NC4-**
    - Right **0NC3-**
  - Pelvic
    - Left **0QC3-**
    - Right **0QC2-**
  - Sphenoid **0NCC-**
  - Temporal
    - Left **0NC6-**
    - Right **0NC5-**
  - Zygomatic
    - Left **0NCN-**
    - Right **0NCM-**
- Brain **00C0-**
- Breast
  - Bilateral **0HCV-**
  - Left **0HCU-**
  - Right **0HCT-**
- Bronchus
  - Lingula **0BC9-**
  - Lower Lobe
    - Left **0BCB-**
    - Right **0BC6-**
  - Main
    - Left **0BC7-**
    - Right **0BC3-**
  - Middle Lobe, Right **0BC5-**
  - Upper Lobe
    - Left **0BC8-**
    - Right **0BC4-**
- Buccal Mucosa **0CC4-**
- Bursa and Ligament
  - Abdomen
    - Left **0MCJ-**
    - Right **0MCH-**
  - Ankle
    - Left **0MCR-**
    - Right **0MCQ-**
  - Elbow
    - Left **0MC4-**
    - Right **0MC3-**
  - Foot
    - Left **0MCT-**
    - Right **0MCS-**
  - Hand
    - Left **0MC8-**
    - Right **0MC7-**
  - Head and Neck **0MC0-**
  - Hip
    - Left **0MCM-**
    - Right **0MCL-**
  - Knee
    - Left **0MCP-**
    - Right **0MCN-**
  - Lower Extremity
    - Left **0MCW-**
    - Right **0MCV-**
  - Perineum **0MCK-**
  - Rib(s) **0MCG-**
  - Shoulder
    - Left **0MC2-**
    - Right **0MC1-**
  - Spine
    - Lower **0MCD-**
    - Upper **0MCC-**
  - Sternum **0MCF-**
  - Upper Extremity
    - Left **0MCB-**
    - Right **0MC9-**
  - Wrist
    - Left **0MC6-**
    - Right **0MC5-**
- Carina **0BC2-**
- Carotid Bodies, Bilateral **0GC8-**

Extirpation — *continued*
- Carotid Body
  - Left **0GC6-**
  - Right **0GC7-**
- Carpal
  - Left **0PCN-**
  - Right **0PCM-**
- Cavity, Cranial **0WC1-**
- Cecum **0DCH-**
- Cerebellum **00CC-**
- Cerebral Hemisphere **00C7-**
- Cerebral Meninges **00C1-**
- Cerebral Ventricle **00C6-**
- Cervix **0UCC-**
- Chordae Tendineae **02C9-**
- Choroid
  - Left **08CB-**
  - Right **08CA-**
- Cisterna Chyli **07CL-**
- Clavicle
  - Left **0PCB-**
  - Right **0PC9-**
- Clitoris **0UCJ-**
- Coccygeal Glomus **0GCB-**
- Coccyx **0QCS-**
- Colon
  - Ascending **0DCK-**
  - Descending **0DCM-**
  - Sigmoid **0DCN-**
  - Transverse **0DCL-**
- Conduction Mechanism **02C8-**
- Conjunctiva
  - Left **08CTXZZ**
  - Right **08CSXZZ**
- Cord
  - Bilateral **0VCH-**
  - Left **0VCG-**
  - Right **0VCF-**
- Cornea
  - Left **08C9XZZ**
  - Right **08C8XZZ**
- Cul-de-sac **0UCF-**
- Diaphragm **0BCT-**
- Disc
  - Cervical Vertebral **0RC3-**
  - Cervicothoracic Vertebral **0RC5-**
  - Lumbar Vertebral **0SC2-**
  - Lumbosacral **0SC4-**
  - Thoracic Vertebral **0RC9-**
  - Thoracolumbar Vertebral **0RCB-**
- Duct
  - Common Bile **0FC9-**
  - Cystic **0FC8-**
  - Hepatic
    - Common **0FC7-**
    - Left **0FC6-**
    - Right **0FC5-**
  - Lacrimal
    - Left **08CY-**
    - Right **08CX-**
  - Pancreatic **0FCD-**
    - Accessory **0FCF-**
  - Parotid
    - Left **0CCC-**
    - Right **0CCB-**
- Duodenum **0DC9-**
- Dura Mater **00C2-**
- Ear
  - External
    - Left **09C1-**
    - Right **09C0-**
  - External Auditory Canal
    - Left **09C4-**
    - Right **09C3-**
  - Inner
    - Left **09CE-**
    - Right **09CD-**
  - Middle
    - Left **09C6-**
    - Right **09C5-**
- Endometrium **0UCB-**

© 2018 Channel Publishing, Ltd.

Extirpation — *continued*
- Epididymis
  - Bilateral **0VCL-**
  - Left **0VCK-**
  - Right **0VCJ-**
- Epidural Space, Intracranial **00C3-**
- Epiglottis **0CCR-**
- Esophagogastric Junction **0DC4-**
- Esophagus **0DC5-**
  - Lower **0DC3-**
  - Middle **0DC2-**
  - Upper **0DC1-**
- Eustachian Tube
  - Left **09CG-**
  - Right **09CF-**
- Eye
  - Left **08C1XZZ**
  - Right **08C0XZZ**
- Eyelid
  - Lower
    - Left **08CR-**
    - Right **08CQ-**
  - Upper
    - Left **08CP-**
    - Right **08CN-**
- Fallopian Tube
  - Left **0UC6-**
  - Right **0UC5-**
- Fallopian Tubes, Bilateral **0UC7-**
- Femoral Shaft
  - Left **0QC9-**
  - Right **0QC8-**
- Femur
  - Lower
    - Left **0QCC-**
    - Right **0QCB-**
  - Upper
    - Left **0QC7-**
    - Right **0QC6-**
- Fibula
  - Left **0QCK-**
  - Right **0QCJ-**
- Finger Nail **0HCQXZZ**
- Gallbladder **0FC4-**
- Gastrointestinal Tract **0WCP-**
- Genitourinary Tract **0WCR-**
- Gingiva
  - Lower **0CC6-**
  - Upper **0CC5-**
- Gland
  - Adrenal
    - Bilateral **0GC4-**
    - Left **0GC2-**
    - Right **0GC3-**
  - Lacrimal
    - Left **08CW-**
    - Right **08CV-**
  - Minor Salivary **0CCJ-**
  - Parotid
    - Left **0CC9-**
    - Right **0CC8-**
  - Pituitary **0GC0-**
  - Sublingual
    - Left **0CCF-**
    - Right **0CCD-**
  - Submaxillary
    - Left **0CCH-**
    - Right **0CCG-**
  - Vestibular **0UCL-**
- Glenoid Cavity
  - Left **0PC8-**
  - Right **0PC7-**
- Glomus Jugulare **0GCC-**
- Humeral Head
  - Left **0PCD-**
  - Right **0PCC-**
- Humeral Shaft
  - Left **0PCG-**
  - Right **0PCF-**
- Hymen **0UCK-**
- Hypothalamus **00CA-**
- Ileocecal Valve **0DCC-**
- Ileum **0DCB-**

Extirpation — *continued*
- Intestine
  - Large **0DCE-**
    - Left **0DCG-**
    - Right **0DCF-**
  - Small **0DC8-**
- Iris
  - Left **08CD-**
  - Right **08CC-**
- Jejunum **0DCA-**
- Joint
  - Acromioclavicular
    - Left **0RCH-**
    - Right **0RCG-**
  - Ankle
    - Left **0SCG-**
    - Right **0SCF-**
  - Carpal
    - Left **0RCR-**
    - Right **0RCQ-**
  - Carpometacarpal
    - Left **0RCT-**
    - Right **0RCS-**
  - Cervical Vertebral **0RC1-**
  - Cervicothoracic Vertebral **0RC4-**
  - Coccygeal **0SC6-**
  - Elbow
    - Left **0RCM-**
    - Right **0RCL-**
  - Finger Phalangeal
    - Left **0RCX-**
    - Right **0RCW-**
  - Hip
    - Left **0SCB-**
    - Right **0SC9-**
  - Knee
    - Left **0SCD-**
    - Right **0SCC-**
  - Lumbar Vertebral **0SC0-**
  - Lumbosacral **0SC3-**
  - Metacarpophalangeal
    - Left **0RCV-**
    - Right **0RCU-**
  - Metatarsal-Phalangeal
    - Left **0SCN-**
    - Right **0SCM-**
  - Occipital-cervical **0RC0-**
  - Sacrococcygeal **0SC5-**
  - Sacroiliac
    - Left **0SC8-**
    - Right **0SC7-**
  - Shoulder
    - Left **0RCK-**
    - Right **0RCJ-**
  - Sternoclavicular
    - Left **0RCF-**
    - Right **0RCE-**
  - Tarsal
    - Left **0SCJ-**
    - Right **0SCH-**
  - Tarsometatarsal
    - Left **0SCL-**
    - Right **0SCK-**
  - Temporomandibular
    - Left **0RCD-**
    - Right **0RCC-**
  - Thoracic Vertebral **0RC6-**
  - Thoracolumbar Vertebral **0RCA-**
  - Toe Phalangeal
    - Left **0SCQ-**
    - Right **0SCP-**
  - Wrist
    - Left **0RCP-**
    - Right **0RCN-**
- Kidney
  - Left **0TC1-**
  - Right **0TC0-**
- Kidney Pelvis
  - Left **0TC4-**
  - Right **0TC3-**
- Larynx **0CCS-**

Extirpation — *continued*
- Lens
  - Left **08CK-**
  - Right **08CJ-**
- Lip
  - Lower **0CC1-**
  - Upper **0CC0-**
- Liver **0FC0-**
  - Left Lobe **0FC2-**
  - Right Lobe **0FC1-**
- Lung
  - Bilateral **0BCM-**
  - Left **0BCL-**
  - Lower Lobe
    - Left **0BCJ-**
    - Right **0BCF-**
  - Middle Lobe, Right **0BCD-**
  - Right **0BCK-**
  - Upper Lobe
    - Left **0BCG-**
    - Right **0BCC-**
- Lung Lingula **0BCH-**
- Lymphatic
  - Aortic **07CD-**
  - Axillary
    - Left **07C6-**
    - Right **07C5-**
  - Head **07C0-**
  - Inguinal
    - Left **07CJ-**
    - Right **07CH-**
  - Internal Mammary
    - Left **07C9-**
    - Right **07C8-**
  - Lower Extremity
    - Left **07CG-**
    - Right **07CF-**
  - Mesenteric **07CB-**
  - Neck
    - Left **07C2-**
    - Right **07C1-**
  - Pelvis **07CC-**
  - Thoracic Duct **07CK-**
  - Thorax **07C7-**
  - Upper Extremity
    - Left **07C4-**
    - Right **07C3-**
- Mandible
  - Left **0NCV-**
  - Right **0NCT-**
- Maxilla **0NCR-**
- Mediastinum **0WCC-**
- Medulla Oblongata **00CD-**
- Mesentery **0DCV-**
- Metacarpal
  - Left **0PCQ-**
  - Right **0PCP-**
- Metatarsal
  - Left **0QCP-**
  - Right **0QCN-**
- Muscle
  - Abdomen
    - Left **0KCL-**
    - Right **0KCK-**
  - Extraocular
    - Left **08CM-**
    - Right **08CL-**
  - Facial **0KC1-**
  - Foot
    - Left **0KCW-**
    - Right **0KCV-**
  - Hand
    - Left **0KCD-**
    - Right **0KCC-**
  - Head **0KC0-**
  - Hip
    - Left **0KCP-**
    - Right **0KCN-**
  - Lower Arm and Wrist
    - Left **0KCB-**
    - Right **0KC9-**
  - Lower Leg
    - Left **0KCT-**
    - Right **0KCS-**

Extirpation — *continued*
- Muscle — *continued*
  - Neck
    - Left **0KC3-**
    - Right **0KC2-**
  - Papillary **02CD-**
  - Perineum **0KCM-**
  - Shoulder
    - Left **0KC6-**
    - Right **0KC5-**
  - Thorax
    - Left **0KCJ-**
    - Right **0KCH-**
  - Tongue, Palate, Pharynx **0KC4-**
  - Trunk
    - Left **0KCG-**
    - Right **0KCF-**
  - Upper Arm
    - Left **0KC8-**
    - Right **0KC7-**
  - Upper Leg
    - Left **0KCR-**
    - Right **0KCQ-**
- Nasal Mucosa and Soft Tissue **09CK-**
- Nasopharynx **09CN-**
- Nerve
  - Abdominal Sympathetic **01CM-**
  - Abducens **00CL-**
  - Accessory **00CR-**
  - Acoustic **00CN-**
  - Brachial Plexus **01C3-**
  - Cervical **01C1-**
  - Cervical Plexus **01C0-**
  - Facial **00CM-**
  - Femoral **01CD-**
  - Glossopharyngeal **00CP-**
  - Head and Neck Sympathetic **01CK-**
  - Hypoglossal **00CS-**
  - Lumbar **01CB-**
  - Lumbar Plexus **01C9-**
  - Lumbar Sympathetic **01CN-**
  - Lumbosacral Plexus **01CA-**
  - Median **01C5-**
  - Oculomotor **00CH-**
  - Olfactory **00CF-**
  - Optic **00CG-**
  - Peroneal **01CH-**
  - Phrenic **01C2-**
  - Pudendal **01CC-**
  - Radial **01C6-**
  - Sacral **01CR-**
  - Sacral Plexus **01CQ-**
  - Sacral Sympathetic **01CP-**
  - Sciatic **01CF-**
  - Thoracic **01C8-**
  - Thoracic Sympathetic **01CL-**
  - Tibial **01CG-**
  - Trigeminal **00CK-**
  - Trochlear **00CJ-**
  - Ulnar **01C4-**
  - Vagus **00CQ-**
- Nipple
  - Left **0HCX-**
  - Right **0HCW-**
- Omentum **0DCU-**
- Oral Cavity and Throat **0WC3-**
- Orbit
  - Left **0NCQ-**
  - Right **0NCP-**
- Orbital Atherectomy Technology **X2C-**
- Ovary
  - Bilateral **0UC2-**
  - Left **0UC1-**
  - Right **0UC0-**
- Palate
  - Hard **0CC2-**
  - Soft **0CC3-**
- Pancreas **0FCG-**
- Para-aortic Body **0GC9-**
- Paraganglion Extremity **0GCF-**

© 2018 Channel Publishing, Ltd.

Extirpation — *continued*
Parathyroid Gland **0GCR-**
Inferior
Left **0GCP-**
Right **0GCN-**
Multiple **0GCQ-**
Superior
Left **0GCM-**
Right **0GCL-**
Patella
Left **0QCF-**
Right **0QCD-**
Pelvic Cavity **0WCJ-**
Penis **0VCS-**
Pericardial Cavity **0WCD-**
Pericardium **02CN-**
Peritoneal Cavity **0WCG-**
Peritoneum **0DCW-**
Phalanx
Finger
Left **0PCV-**
Right **0PCT-**
Thumb
Left **0PCS-**
Right **0PCR-**
Toe
Left **0QCR-**
Right **0QCQ-**
Pharynx **0CCM-**
Pineal Body **0GC1-**
Pleura
Left **0BCP-**
Right **0BCN-**
Pleural Cavity
Left **0WCB-**
Right **0WC9-**
Pons **00CB-**
Prepuce **0VCT-**
Prostate **0VC0-**
Radius
Left **0PCJ-**
Right **0PCH-**
Rectum **0DCP-**
Respiratory Tract **0WCQ-**
Retina
Left **08CF-**
Right **08CE-**
Retinal Vessel
Left **08CH-**
Right **08CG-**
Retroperitoneum **0WCH-**
Ribs
1 to 2 **0PC1-**
3 or more **0PC2-**
Sacrum **0QC1-**
Scapula
Left **0PC6-**
Right **0PC5-**
Sclera
Left **08C7XZZ**
Right **08C6XZZ**
Scrotum **0VC5-**
Septum
Atrial **02C5-**
Nasal **09CM-**
Ventricular **02CM-**
Sinus
Accessory **09CP-**
Ethmoid
Left **09CV-**
Right **09CU-**
Frontal
Left **09CT-**
Right **09CS-**
Mastoid
Left **09CC-**
Right **09CB-**
Maxillary
Left **09CR-**
Right **09CQ-**
Sphenoid
Left **09CX-**
Right **09CW-**

Extirpation — *continued*
Skin
Abdomen **0HC7XZZ**
Back **0HC6XZZ**
Buttock **0HC8XZZ**
Chest **0HC5XZZ**
Ear
Left **0HC3XZZ**
Right **0HC2XZZ**
Face **0HC1XZZ**
Foot
Left **0HCNXZZ**
Right **0HCMXZZ**
Hand
Left **0HCGXZZ**
Right **0HCFXZZ**
Inguinal **0HCAXZZ**
Lower Arm
Left **0HCEXZZ**
Right **0HCDXZZ**
Lower Leg
Left **0HCLXZZ**
Right **0HCKXZZ**
Neck **0HC4XZZ**
Perineum **0HC9XZZ**
Scalp **0HC0XZZ**
Upper Arm
Left **0HCCXZZ**
Right **0HCBXZZ**
Upper Leg
Left **0HCJXZZ**
Right **0HCHXZZ**
Spinal Canal **00CU-**
Spinal Cord
Cervical **00CW-**
Lumbar **00CY-**
Thoracic **00CX-**
Spinal Meninges **00CT-**
Spleen **07CP-**
Sternum **0PC0-**
Stomach **0DC6-**
Pylorus **0DC7-**
Subarachnoid Space, Intracranial **00C5-**
Subcutaneous Tissue and Fascia
Abdomen **0JC8-**
Back **0JC7-**
Buttock **0JC9-**
Chest **0JC6-**
Face **0JC1-**
Foot
Left **0JCR-**
Right **0JCQ-**
Hand
Left **0JCK-**
Right **0JCJ-**
Lower Arm
Left **0JCH-**
Right **0JCG-**
Lower Leg
Left **0JCP-**
Right **0JCN-**
Neck
Left **0JC5-**
Right **0JC4-**
Pelvic Region **0JCC-**
Perineum **0JCB-**
Scalp **0JC0-**
Upper Arm
Left **0JCF-**
Right **0JCD-**
Upper Leg
Left **0JCM-**
Right **0JCL-**
Subdural Space, Intracranial **00C4-**
Tarsal
Left **0QCM-**
Right **0QCL-**
Tendon
Abdomen
Left **0LCG-**
Right **0LCF-**

Extirpation — *continued*
Tendon — *continued*
Ankle
Left **0LCT-**
Right **0LCS-**
Foot
Left **0LCW-**
Right **0LCV-**
Hand
Left **0LC8-**
Right **0LC7-**
Head and Neck **0LC0-**
Hip
Left **0LCK-**
Right **0LCJ-**
Knee
Left **0LCR-**
Right **0LCQ-**
Lower Arm and Wrist
Left **0LC6-**
Right **0LC5-**
Lower Leg
Left **0LCP-**
Right **0LCN-**
Perineum **0LCH-**
Shoulder
Left **0LC2-**
Right **0LC1-**
Thorax
Left **0LCD-**
Right **0LCC-**
Trunk
Left **0LCB-**
Right **0LC9-**
Upper Arm
Left **0LC4-**
Right **0LC3-**
Upper Leg
Left **0LCM-**
Right **0LCL-**
Testis
Bilateral **0VCC-**
Left **0VCB-**
Right **0VC9-**
Thalamus **00C9-**
Thymus **07CM-**
Thyroid Gland **0GCK-**
Left Lobe **0GCG-**
Right Lobe **0GCH-**
Tibia
Left **0QCH-**
Right **0QCG-**
Toe Nail **0HCRXZZ**
Tongue **0CC7-**
Tonsils **0CCP-**
Tooth
Lower **0CCX-**
Upper **0CCW-**
Trachea **0BC1-**
Tunica Vaginalis
Left **0VC7-**
Right **0VC6-**
Turbinate, Nasal **09CL-**
Tympanic Membrane
Left **09C8-**
Right **09C7-**
Ulna
Left **0PCL-**
Right **0PCK-**
Ureter
Left **0TC7-**
Right **0TC6-**
Urethra **0TCD-**
Uterine Supporting Structure **0UC4-**
Uterus **0UC9-**
Uvula **0CCN-**
Vagina **0UCG-**
Valve
Aortic **02CF-**
Mitral **02CG-**
Pulmonary **02CH-**
Tricuspid **02CJ-**

Extirpation — *continued*
Vas Deferens
Bilateral **0VCQ-**
Left **0VCP-**
Right **0VCN-**
Vein
Axillary
Left **05C8-**
Right **05C7-**
Azygos **05C0-**
Basilic
Left **05CC-**
Right **05CB-**
Brachial
Left **05CA-**
Right **05C9-**
Cephalic
Left **05CF-**
Right **05CD-**
Colic **06C7-**
Common Iliac
Left **06CD-**
Right **06CC-**
Coronary **02C4-**
Esophageal **06C3-**
External Iliac
Left **06CG-**
Right **06CF-**
External Jugular
Left **05CQ-**
Right **05CP-**
Face
Left **05CV-**
Right **05CT-**
Femoral
Left **06CN-**
Right **06CM-**
Foot
Left **06CV-**
Right **06CT-**
Gastric **06C2-**
Hand
Left **05CH-**
Right **05CG-**
Hemiazygos **05C1-**
Hepatic **06C4-**
Hypogastric
Left **06CJ-**
Right **06CH-**
Inferior Mesenteric **06C6-**
Innominate
Left **05C4-**
Right **05C3-**
Internal Jugular
Left **05CN-**
Right **05CM-**
Intracranial **05CL-**
Lower **06CY-**
Portal **06C8-**
Pulmonary
Left **02CT-**
Right **02CS-**
Renal
Left **06CB-**
Right **06C9-**
Saphenous
Left **06CQ-**
Right **06CP-**
Splenic **06C1-**
Subclavian
Left **05C6-**
Right **05C5-**
Superior Mesenteric **06C5-**
Upper **05CY-**
Vertebral
Left **05CS-**
Right **05CR-**
Vena Cava
Inferior **06C0-**
Superior **02CV-**
Ventricle
Left **02CL-**
Right **02CK-**

PROCEDURE INDEX

© 2018 Channel Publishing, Ltd.

Extirpation — *continued*
Vertebra
Cervical **0PC**3-
Lumbar **0QC**0-
Thoracic **0PC**4-
Vesicle
Bilateral **0VC**3-
Left **0VC**2-
Right **0VC**1-
Vitreous
Left **08C**5-
Right **08C**4-
Vocal Cord
Left **0CC**V-
Right **0CC**T-
Vulva **0UC**M-
Extracorporeal Carbon Dioxide Removal (ECCO2R) 5A0920Z
Extracorporeal shock wave lithotripsy *see* Fragmentation
Extracranial-intracranial bypass (EC-IC) *see* Bypass, Upper Arteries **031**-
Extraction
Acetabulum
Left **0QD**50ZZ
Right **0QD**40ZZ
Ampulla of Vater **0FD**C-
Anus **0DD**Q-
Appendix **0DD**J-
Auditory Ossicle
Left **09D**A0ZZ
Right **09D**90ZZ
Bone
Ethmoid
Left **0ND**G0ZZ
Right **0ND**F0ZZ
Frontal **0ND**10ZZ
Hyoid **0ND**X0ZZ
Lacrimal
Left **0ND**J0ZZ
Right **0ND**H0ZZ
Nasal **0ND**B0ZZ
Occiptal **0ND**70ZZ
Palatine
Left **0ND**L0ZZ
Right **0ND**K0ZZ
Parietal
Left **0ND**40ZZ
Right **0ND**30ZZ
Pelvic
Left **0QD**30ZZ
Right **0QD**20ZZ
Sphenoid **0ND**C0ZZ
Temporal
Left **0ND**60ZZ
Right **0ND**50ZZ
Zygomatic
Left **0ND**N0ZZ
Right **0ND**M0ZZ
Bone Marrow
Iliac **07D**R-
Sternum **07D**Q-
Vertebral **07D**S-
Bronchus
Lingula **0BD**9-
Lower Lobe
Left **0BD**B-
Right **0BD**6-
Main
Left **0BD**7-
Right **0BD**3-
Middle Lobe, Right **0BD**5-
Upper Lobe
Left **0BD**8-
Right **0BD**4-
Bursa and Ligament
Abdomen
Left **0MD**J-
Right **0MD**H-
Ankle
Left **0MD**R-
Right **0MD**Q-

Extraction — *continued*
Bursa and Ligament — *continued*
Elbow
Left **0MD**4-
Right **0MD**3-
Foot
Left **0MD**T-
Right **0MD**S-
Hand
Left **0MD**8-
Right **0MD**7-
Head and Neck **0MD**0-
Hip
Left **0MD**M-
Right **0MD**L-
Knee
Left **0MD**P-
Right **0MD**N-
Lower Extremity
Left **0MD**W-
Right **0MD**V-
Perineum **0MD**K-
Rib(s) **0MD**G-
Shoulder
Left **0MD**2-
Right **0MD**1-
Spine
Lower **0MD**D-
Upper **0MD**C-
Sternum **0MD**F-
Upper Extremity
Left **0MD**B-
Right **0MD**9-
Wrist
Left **0MD**6-
Right **0MD**5-
Carina **0BD**2-
Carpal
Left **0PD**N0ZZ
Right **0PD**M0ZZ
Cecum **0DD**H-
Cerebral Meninges **00D**1-
Cisterna Chyli **07D**L-
Clavicle
Left **0PD**B0ZZ
Right **0PD**90ZZ
Coccyx **0QD**S0ZZ
Colon
Ascending **0DD**K-
Descending **0DD**M-
Sigmoid **0DD**N-
Transverse **0DD**L-
Cornea
Left **08D**9XZ-
Right **08D**8XZ-
Duct
Common Bile **0FD**9-
Cystic **0FD**8-
Hepatic
Common **0FD**7-
Left **0FD**6-
Right **0FD**5-
Pancreatic **0FD**D-
Accessory **0FD**F-
Duodenum **0DD**9-
Dura Mater **00D**2-
Endometrium **0UD**B-
Esophagogastric Junction **0DD**4-
Esophagus **0DD**5-
Lower **0DD**3-
Middle **0DD**2-
Upper **0DD**1-
Femoral Shaft
Left **0QD**90ZZ
Right **0QD**80ZZ
Femur
Lower
Left **0QD**C0ZZ
Right **0QD**B0ZZ
Upper
Left **0QD**70ZZ
Right **0QD**60ZZ
Fibula
Left **0QD**K0ZZ
Right **0QD**J0ZZ

Extraction — *continued*
Finger Nail **0HD**QXZZ
Gallbladder **0FD**4-
Glenoid Cavity
Left **0PD**80ZZ
Right **0PD**70ZZ
Hair **0HD**SXZZ
Humeral Head
Left **0PD**D0ZZ
Right **0PD**C0ZZ
Humeral Shaft
Left **0PD**G0ZZ
Right **0PD**F0ZZ
Ileocecal Valve **0DD**C-
Ileum **0DD**B-
Intestine
Large **0DD**E-
Left **0DD**G-
Right **0DD**F-
Small **0DD**8-
Jejunum **0DD**A-
Kidney
Left **0TD**1-
Right **0TD**0-
Lens
Left **08D**K3ZZ
Right **08D**J3ZZ
Liver **0FD**0-
Left Lobe **0FD**2-
Right Lobe **0FD**1-
Lung
Bilateral **0BD**M-
Left **0BD**L-
Lower Lobe
Left **0BD**J-
Right **0BD**F-
Middle Lobe, Right **0BD**D-
Right **0BD**K-
Upper Lobe
Left **0BD**G-
Right **0BD**C-
Lung Lingula **0BD**H-
Lymphatic
Aortic **07D**D-
Axillary
Left **07D**6-
Right **07D**5-
Head **07D**0-
Inguinal
Left **07D**J-
Right **07D**H-
Internal Mammary
Left **07D**9-
Right **07D**8-
Lower Extremity
Left **07D**G-
Right **07D**F-
Mesenteric **07D**B-
Neck
Left **07D**2-
Right **07D**1-
Pelvis **07D**C-
Thoracic Duct **07D**K-
Thorax **07D**7-
Upper Extremity
Left **07D**4-
Right **07D**3-
Mandible
Left **0ND**V0ZZ
Right **0ND**T0ZZ
Maxilla **0ND**R0ZZ
Metacarpal
Left **0PD**Q0ZZ
Right **0PD**P0ZZ
Metatarsal
Left **0QD**P0ZZ
Right **0QD**N0ZZ
Muscle
Abdomen
Left **0KD**L0ZZ
Right **0KD**K0ZZ
Facial **0KD**10ZZ
Foot
Left **0KD**W0ZZ
Right **0KD**V0ZZ

Extraction — *continued*
Muscle — *continued*
Hand
Left **0KD**D0ZZ
Right **0KD**C0ZZ
Head **0KD**00ZZ
Hip
Left **0KD**P0ZZ
Right **0KD**N0ZZ
Lower Arm and Wrist
Left **0KD**B0ZZ
Right **0KD**90ZZ
Lower Leg
Left **0KD**T0ZZ
Right **0KD**S0ZZ
Neck
Left **0KD**30ZZ
Right **0KD**20ZZ
Perineum **0KD**M0ZZ
Shoulder
Left **0KD**60ZZ
Right **0KD**50ZZ
Thorax
Left **0KD**J0ZZ
Right **0KD**H0ZZ
Tongue, Palate, Pharynx **0KD**40ZZ
Trunk
Left **0KD**G0ZZ
Right **0KD**F0ZZ
Upper Arm
Left **0KD**80ZZ
Right **0KD**70ZZ
Upper Leg
Left **0KD**R0ZZ
Right **0KD**Q0ZZ
Nerve
Abdominal Sympathetic **01D**M-
Abducens **00D**L-
Accessory **00D**R-
Acoustic **00D**N-
Brachial Plexus **01D**3-
Cervical **01D**1-
Cervical Plexus **01D**0-
Facial **00D**M-
Femoral **01D**D-
Glossopharyngeal **00D**P-
Head and Neck Sympathetic **01D**K-
Hypoglossal **00D**S-
Lumbar **01D**B-
Lumbar Plexus **01D**9-
Lumbar Sympathetic **01D**N-
Lumbosacral Plexus **01D**A-
Median **01D**5-
Oculomotor **00D**H-
Olfactory **00D**F-
Optic **00D**G-
Peroneal **01D**H-
Phrenic **01D**2-
Pudendal **01D**C-
Radial **01D**6-
Sacral **01D**R-
Sacral Plexus **01D**Q-
Sacral Sympathetic **01D**P-
Sciatic **01D**F-
Thoracic **01D**8-
Thoracic Sympathetic **01D**L-
Tibial **01D**G-
Trigeminal **00D**K-
Trochlear **00D**J-
Ulnar **01D**4-
Vagus **00D**Q-
Orbit
Left **0ND**Q0ZZ
Right **0ND**P0ZZ
Ova **0UD**N-
Pancreas **0FD**G-
Patella
Left **0QD**F0ZZ
Right **0QD**D0ZZ

PROCEDURE INDEX

© 2018 Channel Publishing, Ltd.

Extraction — *continued*
- Phalanx
  - Finger
    - Left **0PD**V0ZZ
    - Right **0PD**T0ZZ
  - Thumb
    - Left **0PD**S0ZZ
    - Right **0PD**R0ZZ
  - Toe
    - Left **0QD**R0ZZ
    - Right **0QD**Q0ZZ
- Pleura
  - Left **0BD**P-
  - Right **0BD**N-
- Products of Conception
  - Ectopic **10D**2-
  - Extraperitoneal **10D**00Z2
  - High **10D**00Z0
  - High Forceps **10D**07Z5
  - Internal Version **10D**07Z7
  - Low **10D**00Z1
  - Low Forceps **10D**07Z3
  - Mid Forceps **10D**07Z4
  - Other **10D**07Z8
  - Retained **10D**1-
  - Vacuum **10D**07Z6
- Radius
  - Left **0PD**J0ZZ
  - Right **0PD**H0ZZ
- Rectum **0DD**P-
- Ribs
  - 1 to 2 **0PD**10ZZ
  - 3 or more **0PD**20ZZ
- Sacrum **0QD**10ZZ
- Scapula
  - Left **0PD**60ZZ
  - Right **0PD**50ZZ
- Septum, Nasal **09D**M-
- Sinus
  - Accessory **09D**P-
  - Ethmoid
    - Left **09D**V-
    - Right **09D**U-
  - Frontal
    - Left **09D**T-
    - Right **09D**S-
  - Mastoid
    - Left **09D**C-
    - Right **09D**B-
  - Maxillary
    - Left **09D**R-
    - Right **09D**Q-
  - Sphenoid
    - Left **09D**X-
    - Right **09D**W-
- Skin
  - Abdomen **0HD**7XZZ
  - Back **0HD**6XZZ
  - Buttock **0HD**8XZZ
  - Chest **0HD**5XZZ
  - Ear
    - Left **0HD**3XZZ
    - Right **0HD**2XZZ
  - Face **0HD**1XZZ
  - Foot
    - Left **0HD**NXZZ
    - Right **0HD**MXZZ
  - Hand
    - Left **0HD**GXZZ
    - Right **0HD**FXZZ
  - Inguinal **0HD**AXZZ
  - Lower Arm
    - Left **0HD**EXZZ
    - Right **0HD**DXZZ
  - Lower Leg
    - Left **0HD**LXZZ
    - Right **0HD**KXZZ
  - Neck **0HD**4XZZ
  - Perineum **0HD**9XZZ
  - Scalp **0HD**0XZZ
  - Upper Arm
    - Left **0HD**CXZZ
    - Right **0HD**BXZZ

Extraction — *continued*
- Skin — *continued*
  - Upper Leg
    - Left **0HD**JXZZ
    - Right **0HD**HXZZ
- Skull **0ND**00ZZ
- Spinal Meninges **00D**T-
- Spleen **07D**P-
- Sternum **0PD**00ZZ
- Stomach **0DD**6-
  - Pylorus **0DD**7-
- Subcutaneous Tissue and Fascia
  - Abdomen **0JD**8-
  - Back **0JD**7-
  - Buttock **0JD**9-
  - Chest **0JD**6-
  - Face **0JD**1-
  - Foot
    - Left **0JD**R-
    - Right **0JD**Q-
  - Hand
    - Left **0JD**K-
    - Right **0JD**J-
  - Lower Arm
    - Left **0JD**H-
    - Right **0JD**G-
  - Lower Leg
    - Left **0JD**P-
    - Right **0JD**N-
  - Neck
    - Left **0JD**5-
    - Right **0JD**4-
  - Pelvic Region **0JD**C-
  - Perineum **0JD**B-
  - Scalp **0JD**0-
  - Upper Arm
    - Left **0JD**F-
    - Right **0JD**D-
  - Upper Leg
    - Left **0JD**M-
    - Right **0JD**L-
- Tarsal
  - Left **0QD**M0ZZ
  - Right **0QD**L0ZZ
- Tendon
  - Abdomen
    - Left **0LD**G0ZZ
    - Right **0LD**F0ZZ
  - Ankle
    - Left **0LD**T0ZZ
    - Right **0LD**S0ZZ
  - Foot
    - Left **0LD**W0ZZ
    - Right **0LD**V0ZZ
  - Hand
    - Left **0LD**80ZZ
    - Right **0LD**70ZZ
  - Head and Neck **0LD**00ZZ
  - Hip
    - Left **0LD**K0ZZ
    - Right **0LD**J0ZZ
  - Knee
    - Left **0LD**R0ZZ
    - Right **0LD**Q0ZZ
  - Lower Arm and Wrist
    - Left **0LD**60ZZ
    - Right **0LD**50ZZ
  - Lower Leg
    - Left **0LD**P0ZZ
    - Right **0LD**N0ZZ
  - Perineum **0LD**H0ZZ
  - Shoulder
    - Left **0LD**20ZZ
    - Right **0LD**10ZZ
  - Thorax
    - Left **0LD**D0ZZ
    - Right **0LD**C0ZZ
  - Trunk
    - Left **0LD**B0ZZ
    - Right **0LD**90ZZ
  - Upper Arm
    - Left **0LD**40ZZ
    - Right **0LD**30ZZ

Extraction — *continued*
- Tendon — *continued*
  - Upper Leg
    - Left **0LD**M0ZZ
    - Right **0LD**L0ZZ
- Thymus **07D**M-
- Tibia
  - Left **0QD**H0ZZ
  - Right **0QD**G0ZZ
- Toe Nail **0HD**RXZZ
- Tooth
  - Lower **0CD**XXZ-
  - Upper **0CD**WXZ-
- Trachea **0BD**1-
- Turbinate, Nasal **09D**L-
- Tympanic Membrane
  - Left **09D**8-
  - Right **09D**7-
- Ulna
  - Left **0PD**L0ZZ
  - Right **0PD**K0ZZ
- Vein
  - Basilic
    - Left **05D**C-
    - Right **05D**B-
  - Brachial
    - Left **05D**A-
    - Right **05D**9-
  - Cephalic
    - Left **05D**F-
    - Right **05D**D-
  - Femoral
    - Left **06D**N-
    - Right **06D**M-
  - Foot
    - Left **06D**V-
    - Right **06D**T-
  - Hand
    - Left **05D**H-
    - Right **05D**G-
  - Lower **06D**Y-
  - Saphenous
    - Left **06D**Q-
    - Right **06D**P-
  - Upper **05D**Y-
- Vertebra
  - Cervical **0PD**30ZZ
  - Lumbar **0QD**00ZZ
  - Thoracic **0PD**40ZZ
- Vocal Cord
  - Left **0CD**V-
  - Right **0CD**T-

Extradural space, intracranial
- *use* Epidural Space, Intracranial

Extradural space, spinal
- *use* Spinal Canal

EXtreme Lateral Interbody Fusion (XLIF) device
- *use* Interbody Fusion Device in Lower Joints

F

Face lift *see* Alteration, Face **0W0**2-

Facet replacement spinal stabilization device
- *use* Spinal Stabilization Device, Facet Replacement in **0RH**-
- *use* Spinal Stabilization Device, Facet Replacement in **0SH**-

Facial artery
- *use* Artery, Face

Factor Xa Inhibitor Reversal Agent, Andexanet Alfa
- *use* Andexanet Alfa, Factor Xa Inhibitor Reversal Agent

False vocal cord
- *use* Larynx

Falx cerebri
- *use* Dura Mater

Fascia lata
- *use* Subcutaneous Tissue and Fascia, Upper Leg, Left
- *use* Subcutaneous Tissue and Fascia, Upper Leg, Right

Fasciaplasty, fascioplasty
- *see* Repair, Subcutaneous Tissue and Fascia **0JQ**-
- *see* Replacement, Subcutaneous Tissue and Fascia **0JR**-

Fasciectomy *see* Excision, Subcutaneous Tissue and Fascia **0JB**-

Fasciorrhaphy *see* Repair, Subcutaneous Tissue and Fascia **0JQ**-

Fasciotomy
- *see* Division, Subcutaneous Tissue and Fascia **0J8**-
- *see* Drainage, Subcutaneous Tissue and Fascia **0J9**-
- *see* Release

Feeding Device
- Change device in
  - Lower **0D2**DXUZ
  - Upper **0D2**0XUZ
- Insertion of device in
  - Duodenum **0DH**9-
  - Esophagus **0DH**5-
  - Ileum **0DH**B-
  - Intestine, Small **0DH**8-
  - Jejunum **0DH**A-
  - Stomach **0DH**6-
- Removal of device from
  - Esophagus **0DP**5-
  - Intestinal Tract
    - Lower **0DP**D-
    - Upper **0DP**0-
  - Stomach **0DP**6-
- Revision of device in
  - Intestinal Tract
    - Lower **0DW**D-
    - Upper **0DW**0-
  - Stomach **0DW**6-

Femoral head
- *use* Femur, Upper, Left
- *use* Femur, Upper, Right

Femoral lymph node
- *use* Lymphatic, Lower Extremity, Left
- *use* Lymphatic, Lower Extremity, Right

Femoropatellar joint
- *use* Joint, Knee, Left
- *use* Joint, Knee, Right
- *use* Joint, Knee, Left, Femoral Surface
- *use* Joint, Knee, Right, Femoral Surface

PROCEDURE INDEX

© 2018 Channel Publishing, Ltd.

Femorotibial joint
- *use* Joint, Knee, Left
- *use* Joint, Knee, Right
- *use* Joint, Knee, Left, Tibial Surface
- *use* Joint, Knee, Right, Tibial Surface

Fibular artery
- *use* Artery, Peroneal, Left
- *use* Artery, Peroneal, Right

Fibularis brevis muscle
- *use* Muscle, Lower Leg, Left
- *use* Muscle, Lower Leg, Right

Fibularis longus muscle
- *use* Muscle, Lower Leg, Left
- *use* Muscle, Lower Leg, Right

Fifth cranial nerve
- *use* Nerve, Trigeminal

Filum terminale
- *use* Spinal Meninges

Fimbriectomy
- *see* Excision, Female Reproductive System **0UB-**
- *see* Resection, Female Reproductive System **0UT-**

Fine needle aspiration
- Fluid or gas *see* Drainage
- Tissue biopsy
  - *see* Excision
  - *see* Extraction

First cranial nerve
- *use* Nerve, Olfactory

First intercostal nerve
- *use* Brachial Plexus

Fistulization
- *see* Bypass
- *see* Drainage
- *see* Repair

Fitting
- Arch bars, for fracture reduction *see* Reposition, Mouth and Throat **0CS-**
- Arch bars, for immobilization *see* Immobilization, Face **2W31-**
- Artificial limb *see* Device Fitting, Rehabilitation **F0D-**
- Hearing aid *see* Device Fitting, Rehabilitation **F0D-**
- Ocular prosthesis **F0DZ8UZ**
- Prosthesis, limb *see* Device Fitting, Rehabilitation **F0D-**
- Prosthesis, ocular **F0DZ8UZ**

Fixation, bone
- External, with fracture reduction *see* Reposition
- External, without fracture reduction *see* Insertion
- Internal, with fracture reduction *see* Reposition
- Internal, without fracture reduction *see* Insertion

FLAIR® Endovascular Stent Graft
- *use* Intraluminal Device

Flexible Composite Mesh
- *use* Synthetic Substitute

Flexor carpi radialis muscle
- *use* Muscle, Lower Arm and Wrist, Left
- *use* Muscle, Lower Arm and Wrist, Right

Flexor carpi ulnaris muscle
- *use* Muscle, Lower Arm and Wrist, Left
- *use* Muscle, Lower Arm and Wrist, Right

Flexor digitorum brevis muscle
- *use* Muscle, Foot, Left
- *use* Muscle, Foot, Right

Flexor digitorum longus muscle
- *use* Muscle, Lower Leg, Left
- *use* Muscle, Lower Leg, Right

Flexor hallucis brevis muscle
- *use* Muscle, Foot, Left
- *use* Muscle, Foot, Right

Flexor hallucis longus muscle
- *use* Muscle, Lower Leg, Left
- *use* Muscle, Lower Leg, Right

Flexor pollicis longus muscle
- *use* Muscle, Lower Arm and Wrist, Left
- *use* Muscle, Lower Arm and Wrist, Right

Fluoroscopy
- Abdomen and Pelvis **BW11-**
- Airway, Upper **BB1DZZZ**
- Ankle
  - Left **BQ1H-**
  - Right **BQ1G-**
- Aorta
  - Abdominal **B410-**
    - Laser, Intraoperative **B410-**
  - Thoracic **B310-**
    - Laser, Intraoperative **B310-**
  - Thoraco-Abdominal **B31P-**
    - Laser, Intraoperative **B31P-**
- Aorta and Bilateral Lower Extremity Arteries **B41D-**
  - Laser, Intraoperative **B41D-**
- Arm
  - Left **BP1FZZZ**
  - Right **BP1EZZZ**
- Artery
  - Brachiocephalic-Subclavian
    - Laser, Intraoperative **B311-**
    - Right **B311-**
  - Bronchial **B31L-**
    - Laser, Intraoperative **B31L-**
  - Bypass Graft, Other **B21F-**
  - Cervico-Cerebral Arch **B31Q-**
    - Laser, Intraoperative **B31Q-**
  - Common Carotid
    - Bilateral **B315-**
      - Laser, Intraoperative **B315-**
    - Left **B314-**
      - Laser, Intraoperative **B314-**
    - Right **B313-**
      - Laser, Intraoperative **B313-**
  - Coronary
    - Bypass Graft
      - Multiple **B213-**
        - Laser, Intraoperative **B213-**
      - Single **B212-**
        - Laser, Intraoperative **B212-**
    - Multiple **B211-**
      - Laser, Intraoperative **B211-**
    - Single **B210-**
      - Laser, Intraoperative **B210-**
  - External Carotid
    - Bilateral **B31C-**
      - Laser, Intraoperative **B31C-**
    - Left **B31B-**
      - Laser, Intraoperative **B31B-**
    - Right **B319-**
      - Laser, Intraoperative **B319-**
  - Hepatic **B412-**
    - Laser, Intraoperative **B412-**
  - Inferior Mesenteric **B415-**
    - Laser, Intraoperative **B415-**
  - Intercostal **B31L-**
    - Laser, Intraoperative **B31L-**
  - Internal Carotid
    - Bilateral **B318-**
      - Laser, Intraoperative **B318-**
    - Left **B317-**
      - Laser, Intraoperative **B317-**
    - Right **B316-**
      - Laser, Intraoperative **B316-**
  - Internal Mammary Bypass Graft
    - Left **B218-**
    - Right **B217-**
  - Intra-Abdominal
    - Other **B41B-**
    - Laser, Intraoperative **B41B-**
  - Intracranial **B31R-**
    - Laser, Intraoperative **B31R-**

Fluoroscopy — *continued*
- Artery — *continued*
  - Lower
    - Other **B41J-**
    - Laser, Intraoperative **B41J-**
  - Lower Extremity
    - Bilateral and Aorta **B41D-**
      - Laser, Intraoperative **B41D-**
    - Left **B41G-**
      - Laser, Intraoperative **B41G-**
    - Right **B41F-**
      - Laser, Intraoperative **B41F-**
  - Lumbar **B419-**
    - Laser, Intraoperative **B419-**
  - Pelvic **B41C-**
    - Laser, Intraoperative **B41C -**
  - Pulmonary
    - Left **B31T-**
      - Laser, Intraoperative **B31T-**
    - Right **B31S-**
      - Laser, Intraoperative **B31S-**
  - Pulmonary Trunk **B31U-**
    - Laser, Intraoperative **B31U-**
  - Renal
    - Bilateral **B418-**
      - Laser, Intraoperative **B418-**
    - Left **B417-**
      - Laser, Intraoperative **B417-**
    - Right **B416-**
      - Laser, Intraoperative **B416-**
  - Spinal **B31M-**
    - Laser, Intraoperative **B31M-**
  - Splenic **B413-**
    - Laser, Intraoperative **B413-**
  - Subclavian
    - Left **B312-**
    - Laser, Intraoperative **B312-**
  - Superior Mesenteric **B414-**
    - Laser, Intraoperative **B414-**
  - Upper
    - Laser, Intraoperative **B31N-**
    - Other **B31N-**
  - Upper Extremity
    - Bilateral **B31K-**
      - Laser, Intraoperative **B31K-**
    - Left **B31J-**
      - Laser, Intraoperative **B31J-**
    - Right **B31H-**
      - Laser, Intraoperative **B31H-**
  - Vertebral
    - Bilateral **B31G-**
      - Laser, Intraoperative **B31G-**
    - Left **B31F-**
      - Laser, Intraoperative **B31F-**
    - Right **B31D-**
      - Laser, Intraoperative **B31D-**
- Bile Duct **BF10-**
  - Pancreatic Duct and Gallbladder **BF14-**
- Bile Duct and Gallbladder **BF13-**
- Biliary Duct **BF11-**
- Bladder **BT10-**
  - Kidney and Ureter **BT14-**
    - Left **BT1F-**
    - Right **BT1D-**
- Bladder and Urethra **BT1B-**
- Bowel, Small **BD1-**
- Calcaneus
  - Left **BQ1KZZZ**
  - Right **BQ1JZZZ**
- Clavicle
  - Left **BP15ZZZ**
  - Right **BP14ZZZ**
- Coccyx **BR1F-**
- Colon **BD14-**
- Corpora Cavernosa **BV10-**
- Dialysis Fistula **B51W-**
- Dialysis Shunt **B51W-**
- Diaphragm **BB16ZZZ-**
- Disc
  - Cervical **BR11-**
  - Lumbar **BR13-**
  - Thoracic **BR12-**
- Duodenum **BD19-**

Fluoroscopy — *continued*
- Elbow
  - Left **BP1H-**
  - Right **BP1G-**
- Epiglottis **B91G-**
- Esophagus **BD11-**
- Extremity
  - Lower **BW1C-**
  - Upper **BW1J-**
- Facet Joint
  - Cervical **BR14-**
  - Lumbar **BR16-**
  - Thoracic **BR15-**
- Fallopian Tube
  - Bilateral **BU12-**
  - Left **BU11-**
  - Right **BU10-**
- Fallopian Tube and Uterus **BU18-**
- Femur
  - Left **BQ14ZZZ**
  - Right **BQ13ZZZ**
- Finger
  - Left **BP1SZZZ**
  - Right **BP1RZZZ**
- Foot
  - Left **BQ1MZZZ**
  - Right **BQ1LZZZ**
- Forearm
  - Left **BP1KZZZ**
  - Right **BP1JZZZ**
- Gallbladder **BF12-**
  - Bile Duct and Pancreatic Duct **BF14-**
- Gallbladder and Bile Duct **BF13-**
- Gastrointestinal, Upper **BD1-**
- Hand
  - Left **BP1PZZZ**
  - Right **BP1NZZZ**
- Head and Neck **BW19-**
- Heart
  - Left **B215-**
  - Right **B214-**
  - Right and Left **B216-**
- Hip
  - Left **BQ11-**
  - Right **BQ10-**
- Humerus
  - Left **BP1BZZZ**
  - Right **BP1AZZZ**
- Ileal Diversion Loop **BT1C-**
- Ileal Loop, Ureters and Kidney **BT1G-**
- Intracranial Sinus **B512-**
- Joint
  - Acromioclavicular, Bilateral **BP13ZZZ**
  - Finger
    - Left **BP1D-**
    - Right **BP1C-**
  - Foot
    - Left **BQ1Y-**
    - Right **BQ1X-**
  - Hand
    - Left **BP1D-**
    - Right **BP1C-**
  - Lumbosacral **BR1B-**
  - Sacroiliac **BR1D-**
  - Sternoclavicular
    - Bilateral **BP12ZZZ**
    - Left **BP11ZZZ**
    - Right **BP10ZZZ**
  - Temporomandibular
    - Bilateral **BN19-**
    - Left **BN18-**
    - Right **BN17-**
  - Thoracolumbar **BR18-**
  - Toe
    - Left **BQ1Y-**
    - Right **BQ1X-**

© 2018 Channel Publishing, Ltd.

Fluoroscopy — *continued*
Kidney
Bilateral **BT13-**
Ileal Loop and Ureter **BT1G-**
Left **BT12-**
Right **BT11-**
Ureter and Bladder **BT14-**
Left **BT1F-**
Right **BT1D-**
Knee
Left **BQ18-**
Right **BQ17-**
Larynx **B91J-**
Leg
Left **BQ1FZZZ**
Right **BQ1DZZZ**
Lung
Bilateral **BB14ZZZ**
Left **BB13ZZZ**
Right **BB12ZZZ**
Mediastinum **BB1CZZZ**
Mouth **BD1B-**
Neck and Head **BW19-**
Oropharynx **BD1B-**
Pancreatic Duct **BF1-**
Gallbladder and Bile Buct **BF14-**
Patella
Left **BQ1WZZZ**
Right **BQ1VZZZ**
Pelvis **BR1C-**
Pelvis and Abdomen **BW11-**
Pharynix **B91G-**
Ribs
Left **BP1YZZZ**
Right **BP1XZZZ**
Sacrum **BR1F-**
Scapula
Left **BP17ZZZ**
Right **BP16ZZZ**
Shoulder
Left **BP19-**
Right **BP18-**
Sinus, Intracranial **B512-**
Spinal Cord **B01B-**
Spine
Cervical **BR10-**
Lumbar **BR19-**
Thoracic **BR17-**
Whole **BR1G-**
Sternum **BR1H-**
Stomach **BD12-**
Toe
Left **BQ1QZZZ**
Right **BQ1PZZZ**
Tracheobronchial Tree
Bilateral **BB19YZZ**
Left **BB18YZZ**
Right **BB17YZZ**
Ureter
Ileal Loop and Kidney **BT1G-**
Kidney and Bladder **BT14-**
Left **BT1F-**
Right **BT1D-**
Left **BT17-**
Right **BT16-**
Urethra **BT15-**
Urethra and Bladder **BT1B-**
Uterus **BU16-**
Uterus and Fallopian Tube **BU18-**
Vagina **BU19-**
Vasa Vasorum **BV18-**
Vein
Cerebellar **B511-**
Cerebral **B511-**
Epidural **B510-**
Jugular
Bilateral **B515-**
Left **B514-**
Right **B513-**
Lower Extremity
Bilateral **B51D-**
Left **B51C-**
Right **B51B-**
Other **B51V-**

Fluoroscopy — *continued*
Vein — *continued*
Pelvic (Iliac)
Left **B51G-**
Right **B51F-**
Pelvic (Iliac) Bilateral **B51H-**
Portal **B51T-**
Pulmonary
Bilateral **B51S-**
Left **B51R-**
Right **B51Q-**
Renal
Bilateral **B51L-**
Left **B51K-**
Right **B51J-**
Spanchnic **B51T-**
Subclavian
Left **B517-**
Right **B516-**
Upper Extremity
Bilateral **B51P-**
Left **B51N-**
Right **B51M-**
Vena Cava
Inferior **B519-**
Superior **B518-**
Wrist
Left **BP1M-**
Right **BP1L-**
Fluoroscopy, laser intraoperative
see Fluoroscopy, Heart **B21-**
see Fluoroscopy, Lower Arteries **B41-**
see Fluoroscopy, Upper Arteries **B31-**
Flushing *see* Irrigation
Foley catheter
use Drainage Device
Fontan completion procedure Stage II *see* Bypass, Vena Cava, Inferior **0610-**
Foramen magnum
use Occipital Bone
Foramen of Monro (intraventricular)
use Cerebral Ventricle
Foreskin
use Prepuce
Formula™ Balloon-Expandable Renal Stent System
use Intraluminal Device
Fossa of Rosenmuller
use Nasopharynx
Fourth cranial nerve
use Nerve, Trochlear
Fourth ventricle
use Cerebral Ventricle
Fovea
use Retina, Left
use Retina, Right
Fragmentation
Ampulla of Vater **0FFC-**
Anus **0DFQ-**
Appendix **0DFJ-**
Bladder **0TFB-**
Bladder Neck **0TFC-**
Bronchus
Lingula **0BF9-**
Lower Lobe
Left **0BFB-**
Right **0BF6-**
Main
Left **0BF7-**
Right **0BF3-**
Middle Lobe, Right **0BF5-**
Upper Lobe
Left **0BF8-**
Right **0BF4-**
Carina **0BF2-**
Cavity, Cranial **0WF1-**
Cecum **0DFH-**
Cerebral Ventricle **00F6-**

Fragmentation — *continued*
Colon
Ascending **0DFK-**
Descending **0DFM-**
Sigmoid **0DFN-**
Transverse **0DFL-**
Duct
Common Bile **0FF9-**
Cystic **0FF8-**
Hepatic
Common **0FF7-**
Left **0FF6-**
Right **0FF5-**
Pancreatic **0FFD-**
Accessory **0FFF-**
Parotid
Left **0CFC-**
Right **0CFB-**
Duodenum **0DF9-**
Epidural Space, Intracranial **00F3-**
Esophagus **0DF5-**
Fallopian Tube
Left **0UF6-**
Right **0UF5-**
Fallopian Tubes, Bilateral **0UF7-**
Gallbladder **0FF4-**
Gastrointestinal Tract **0WFP-**
Genitourinary Tract **0WFR-**
Ileum **0DFB-**
Intestine
Large **0DFE-**
Left **0DFG-**
Right **0DFF-**
Small **0DF8-**
Jejunum **0DFA-**
Kidney Pelvis
Left **0TF4-**
Right **0TF3-**
Mediastinum **0WFC-**
Oral Cavity and Throat **0WF3-**
Pelvic Cavity **0WFJ-**
Pericardial Cavity **0WFD-**
Pericardium **02FN-**
Peritoneal Cavity **0WFG-**
Pleural Cavity
Left **0WFB-**
Right **0WF9-**
Rectum **0DFP-**
Respiratory Tract **0WFQ-**
Spinal Canal **00FU-**
Stomach **0DF6-**
Subarachnoid Space, Intracranial **00F5-**
Subdural Space, Intracranial **00F4-**
Trachea **0BF1-**
Ureter
Left **0TF7-**
Right **0TF6-**
Urethra **0TFD-**
Uterus **0UF9-**
Vitreous
Left **08F5-**
Right **08F4-**
Freestyle (Stentless) Aortic Root Bioprosthesis
use Zooplastic Tissue in Heart and Great Vessels
Frenectomy
see Excision, Mouth and Throat **0CB-**
see Resection, Mouth and Throat **0CT-**
Frenoplasty, frenuloplasty
see Repair, Mouth and Throat **0CQ-**
see Replacement, Mouth and Throat **0CR-**
see Supplement, Mouth and Throat **0CU-**

Frenotomy
see Drainage, Mouth and Throat **0C9-**
see Release, Mouth and Throat **0CN-**
Frenulotomy
see Drainage, Mouth and Throat **0C9-**
see Release, Mouth and Throat **0CN-**
Frenulum labii inferioris
use Lip, Lower
Frenulum labii superioris
use Lip, Upper
Frenulum linguae
use Tongue
Frenulumectomy
see Excision, Mouth and Throat **0CB-**
see Resection, Mouth and Throat **0CT-**
Frontal lobe
use Cerebral Hemisphere
Frontal vein
use Vein, Face, Left
use Vein, Face, Right
Fulguration *see* Destruction
Fundoplication, gastroesophageal *see* Restriction, Esophagogastric Junction **0DV4-**
Fundus uteri
use Uterus
Fusion
Acromioclavicular
Left **0RGH-**
Right **0RGG-**
Ankle
Left **0SGG-**
Right **0SGF-**
Carpal
Left **0RGR-**
Right **0RGQ-**
Carpometacarpal
Left **0RGT-**
Right **0RGS-**
Cervical Vertebral **0RG1-**
2 or more **0RG2-**
Interbody Fusion Device
Nanotextured Surface **XRG2092**
Radiolucent Porous **XRG20F3**
Interbody Fusion Device
Nanotextured Surface **XRG1092**
Radiolucent Porous **XRG10F3**
Cervicothoracic Vertebral **0RG4-**
Interbody Fusion Device
Nanotextured Surface **XRG4092**
Radiolucent Porous **XRG40F3**
Coccygeal **0SG6-**
Elbow
Left **0RGM-**
Right **0RGL-**
Finger Phalangeal
Left **0RGX-**
Right **0RGW-**
Hip
Left **0SGB-**
Right **0SG9-**
Knee
Left **0SGD-**
Right **0SGC-**
Lumbar Vertebral **0SG0-**
2 or more **0SG1-**
Interbody Fusion Device
Nanotextured Surface **XRGC092**
Radiolucent Porous **XRGC0F3**

PROCEDURE INDEX

© 2018 Channel Publishing, Ltd.

Fusion — *continued*
Lumbar Vertebral **0SG0**- — *continued*
Interbody Fusion Device
Nanotextured Surface **XRGB092**
Radiolucent Porous **XRGB0F3**
Lumbosacral **0SG3**-
Interbody Fusion Device
Nanotextured Surface **XRGD092**
Radiolucent Porous **XRGD0F3**
Metacarpophalangeal
Left **0RGV**-
Right **0RGU**-
Metatarsal-Phalangeal
Left **0SGN**-
Right **0SGM**-
Occipital-cervical **0RG0**-
Interbody Fusion Device
Nanotextured Surface **XRG0092**
Radiolucent Porous **XRG00F3**
Sacrococcygeal **0SG5**-
Sacroiliac
Left **0SG8**-
Right **0SG7**-
Shoulder
Left **0RGK**-
Right **0RGJ**-
Sternoclavicular
Left **0RGF**-
Right **0RGE**-
Tarsal
Left **0SGJ**-
Right **0SGH**-
Tarsometatarsal
Left **0SGL**-
Right **0SGK**-
Temporomandibular
Left **0RGD**-
Right **0RGC**-
Thoracic Vertebral **0RG6**-
2 to 7 **0RG7**-
Interbody Fusion Device
Nanotextured Surface **XRG7092**
Radiolucent Porous **XRG70F3**
8 or more **0RG8**-
Interbody Fusion Device
Nanotextured Surface **XRG8092**
Radiolucent Porous **XRG80F3**
Interbody Fusion Device
Nanotextured Surface **XRG6092**
Radiolucent Porous **XRG60F3**
Thoracolumbar Vertebral **0RGA**-
Interbody Fusion Device
Nanotextured Surface **XRGA092**
Radiolucent Porous **XRGA0F3**
Toe Phalangeal
Left **0SGQ**-
Right **0SGP**-
Wrist
Left **0RGP**-
Right **0RGN**-
Fusion screw (compression) (lag) (locking)
use Internal Fixation Device in Lower Joints
use Internal Fixation Device in Upper Joints

G

Gait training *see* Motor Treatment, Rehabilitation **F07**-
Galea aponeurotica
use Subcutaneous Tissue and Fascia, Scalp
GammaTile™
use Radioactive Element, Cesium-131 Collagen Implant in **00H**-
Ganglion impar (ganglion of Walther)
use Nerve, Sacral Sympathetic
Ganglionectomy
Destruction of lesion *see* Destruction
Excision of lesion *see* Excision
Gasserian ganglion
use Nerve, Trigeminal
Gastrectomy
Partial *see* Excision, Stomach **0DB6**-
Total *see* Resection, Stomach **0DT6**-
Vertical (sleeve) *see* Excision, Stomach **0DB6**-
Gastric electrical stimulation (GES) lead
use Stimulator Lead in Gastrointestinal System
Gastric lymph node
use Lymphatic, Aortic
Gastric pacemaker lead
use Stimulator Lead in Gastrointestinal System
Gastric plexus
use Nerve, Abdominal Sympathetic
Gastrocnemius muscle
use Muscle, Lower Leg, Left
use Muscle, Lower Leg, Right
Gastrocolic ligament
use Omentum
Gastrocolic omentum
use Omentum
Gastrocolostomy
see Bypass, Gastrointestinal System **0D1**-
see Drainage, Gastrointestinal System **0D9**-
Gastroduodenal artery
use Artery, Hepatic
Gastroduodenectomy
see Excision, Gastrointestinal System **0DB**-
see Resection, Gastrointestinal System **0DT**-
Gastroduodenoscopy 0DJ08ZZ
Gastroenteroplasty
see Repair, Gastrointestinal System **0DQ**-
see Supplement, Gastrointestinal System **0DU**-
Gastroenterostomy
see Bypass, Gastrointestinal System **0D1**-
see Drainage, Gastrointestinal System **0D9**-
Gastroesophageal (GE) junction
use Esophagogastric Junction
Gastrogastrostomy
see Bypass, Stomach **0D16**-
see Drainage, Stomach **0D96**-
Gastrohepatic omentum
use Omentum
Gastrojejunostomy
see Bypass, Stomach **0D16**-
see Drainage, Stomach **0D96**-
Gastrolysis *see* Release, Stomach **0DN6**-
Gastropexy
see Repair, Stomach **0DQ6**-
see Reposition, Stomach **0DS6**-
Gastrophrenic ligament
use Omentum
Gastroplasty
see Repair, Stomach **0DQ6**-
see Supplement, Stomach **0DU6**-
Gastroplication *see* Restriction, Stomach **0DV6**-
Gastropylorectomy *see* Excision, Gastrointestinal System **0DB**-
Gastrorrhaphy *see* Repair, Stomach **0DQ6**-
Gastroscopy 0DJ68ZZ
Gastrosplenic ligament
use Omentum
Gastrostomy
see Bypass, Stomach **0D16**-
see Drainage, Stomach **0D96**-
Gastrotomy *see* Drainage, Stomach **0D96**-
Gemellus muscle
use Muscle, Hip, Left
use Muscle, Hip, Right
Geniculate ganglion
use Nerve, Facial
Geniculate nucleus
use Thalamus
Genioglossus muscle
use Muscle, Tongue, Palate, Pharynx
Genioplasty *see* Alteration, Jaw, Lower **0W05**-
Genitofemoral nerve
use Nerve, Lumbar Plexus
GIAPREZA™
use Synthetic Human Angiotensin II
Gingivectomy *see* Excision, Mouth and Throat **0CB**-
Gingivoplasty
see Repair, Mouth and Throat **0CQ**-
see Replacement, Mouth and Throat **0CR**-
see Supplement, Mouth and Throat **0CU**-
Glans penis
use Prepuce
Glenohumeral joint
use Joint, Shoulder, Left
use Joint, Shoulder, Right
Glenohumeral ligament
use Bursa and Ligament, Shoulder, Left
use Bursa and Ligament, Shoulder, Right
Glenoid fossa (of scapula)
use Glenoid Cavity, Left
use Glenoid Cavity, Right
Glenoid ligament (labrum)
use Shoulder Joint, Left
use Shoulder Joint, Right
Globus pallidus
use Basal Ganglia
Glomectomy
see Excision, Endocrine System **0GB**-
see Resection, Endocrine System **0GT**-
Glossectomy
see Excision, Tongue **0CB7**-
see Resection, Tongue **0CT7**-
Glossoepiglottic fold
use Epiglottis
Glossopexy
see Repair, Tongue **0CQ7**-
see Reposition, Tongue **0CS7**-
Glossoplasty
see Repair, Tongue **0CQ7**-
see Replacement, Tongue **0CR7**-
see Supplement, Tongue **0CU7**-
Glossorrhaphy *see* Repair, Tongue **0CQ7**-
Glossotomy *see* Drainage, Tongue **0C97**-
Glottis
use Larynx
Gluteal Artery Perforator Flap
Replacement
Bilateral **0HRV079**
Left **0HRU079**
Right **0HRT079**
Transfer
Left **0KXG**-
Right **0KXF**-
Gluteal lymph node
use Lymphatic, Pelvis
Gluteal vein
use Vein, Hypogastric, Left
use Vein, Hypogastric, Right
Gluteus maximus muscle
use Muscle, Hip, Left
use Muscle, Hip, Right
Gluteus medius muscle
use Muscle, Hip, Left
use Muscle, Hip, Right
Gluteus minimus muscle
use Muscle, Hip, Left
use Muscle, Hip, Right
GORE® DUALMESH®
use Synthetic Substitute
GORE® EXCLUDER® AAA Endoprosthesis
use Intraluminal Device
use Intraluminal Device, Branched or Fenestrated, One or Two Arteries in **04V**-
use Intraluminal Device, Branched or Fenestrated, Three or More Arteries in **04V**-
GORE® EXCLUDER® IBE Endoprosthesis
use Intraluminal Device, Branched or Fenestrated, One or Two Arteries in **04V**-
GORE® TAG® Thoracic Endoprosthesis
use Intraluminal Device
Gracilis muscle
use Muscle, Upper Leg, Left
use Muscle, Upper Leg, Right
Graft
see Replacement
see Supplement
Great auricular nerve
use Cervical Plexus
Great cerebral vein
use Vein, Intracranial
Greater alar cartilage
use Nasal Mucosa and Soft Tissue
Greater occipital nerve
use Nerve, Cervical
Greater omentum
use Omentum
Great(er) saphenous vein
use Saphenous Vein, Left
use Saphenous Vein, Right
Greater splanchnic nerve
use Nerve, Thoracic Sympathetic
Greater superficial petrosal nerve
use Nerve, Facial
Greater trochanter
use Femur, Upper, Left
use Femur, Upper, Right
Greater tuberosity
use Humeral Head, Left
use Humeral Head, Right
Greater vestibular (Bartholin's) gland
use Gland, Vestibular
Greater wing *use* Sphenoid Bone
Guedel airway
use Intraluminal Device, Airway in Mouth and Throat

© 2018 Channel Publishing, Ltd.

Guidance, catheter placement
- EKG *see* Measurement, Physiological Systems **4A0-**
- Fluoroscopy *see* Fluoroscopy, Veins **B51-**
- Ultrasound *see* Ultrasonography, Veins **B54-**

H

Hallux
- *use* Toe, 1st, Left
- *use* Toe, 1st, Right

Hamate bone
- *use* Carpal, Left
- *use* Carpal, Right

Hancock Bioprosthesis (aortic) (mitral) valve
- *use* Zooplastic Tissue in Heart and Great Vessels

Hancock Bioprosthetic Valved Conduit
- *use* Zooplastic Tissue in Heart and Great Vessels

Harvesting, stem cells *see* Pheresis, Circulatory **6A55-**

Head of fibula
- *use* Fibula, Left
- *use* Fibula, Right

Hearing Aid Assessment F14Z-

Hearing Assessment F13Z-

Hearing Device
- Bone Conduction
  - Left **09HE-**
  - Right **09HD-**
- Insertion of device in
  - Left **0NH6-**
  - Right **0NH5-**
- Multiple Channel Cochlear Prosthesis
  - Left **09HE-**
  - Right **09HD-**
- Removal of device from, Skull **0NP0-**
- Revision of device in, Skull **0NW0-**
- Single Channel Cochlear Prosthesis
  - Left **09HE-**
  - Right **09HD-**

Hearing Treatment F09Z-

Heart Assist System
- Implantable
  - Insertion of device in, Heart **02HA-**
  - Removal of device from, Heart **02PA-**
  - Revision of device in, Heart **02WA-**
- Short-term External
  - Insertion of device in, Heart **02HA-**
  - Removal of device from, Heart **02PA-**
  - Revision of device in, Heart **02WA-**

HeartMate 3™ LVAS
- *use* Implantable Heart Assist System in Heart and Great Vessels

HeartMate II® Left Ventricular Assist Device (LVAD)
- *use* Implantable Heart Assist System in Heart and Great Vessels

HeartMate XVE® Left Ventricular Assist Device (LVAD)
- *use* Implantable Heart Assist System in Heart and Great Vessels

HeartMate® implantable heart assist system *see* Insertion of device in, Heart **02HA-**

Helix
- *use* Ear, External, Bilateral
- *use* Ear, External, Left
- *use* Ear, External, Right

Hematopoietic cell transplant (HCT) *see* Transfusion, Circulatory **302-**

Hemicolectomy *see* Resection, Gastrointestinal System **0DT-**

Hemicystectomy *see* Excision, Urinary System **0TB-**

Hemigastrectomy *see* Excision, Gastrointestinal System **0DB-**

Hemiglossectomy *see* Excision, Mouth and Throat **0CB-**

Hemilaminectomy
- *see* Excision, Lower Bones **0QB-**
- *see* Excision, Upper Bones **0PB-**

Hemilaminotomy
- *see* Drainage, Lower Bones **0Q9-**
- *see* Drainage, Upper Bones **0P9-**
- *see* Excision, Lower Bones **0QB-**
- *see* Excision, Upper Bones **0PB-**
- *see* Release, Central Nervous System and Cranial Nerves **00N-**
- *see* Release, Lower Bones **0QN-**
- *see* Release, Peripheral Nervous System **01N-**
- *see* Release, Upper Bones **0PN-**

Hemilaryngectomy *see* Excision, Larynx **0CBS-**

Hemimandibulectomy *see* Excision, Head and Facial Bones **0NB-**

Hemimaxillectomy *see* Excision, Head and Facial Bones **0NB-**

Hemipylorectomy *see* Excision, Gastrointestinal System **0DB-**

Hemispherectomy
- *see* Excision, Central Nervous System and Cranial Nerves **00B-**
- *see* Resection, Central Nervous System and Cranial Nerves **00T-**

Hemithyroidectomy
- *see* Excision, Endocrine System **0GB-**
- *see* Resection, Endocrine System **0GT-**

Hemodialysis *see* Performance, Urinary **5A1D-**

Hemolung® Respiratory Assist System (RAS) 5A0920Z

Hepatectomy
- *see* Excision, Hepatobiliary System and Pancreas **0FB-**
- *see* Resection, Hepatobiliary System and Pancreas **0FT-**

Hepatic artery proper
- *use* Artery, Hepatic

Hepatic flexure
- *use* Transverse Colon

Hepatic lymph node
- *use* Lymphatic, Aortic

Hepatic plexus
- *use* Nerve, Abdominal Sympathetic

Hepatic portal vein
- *use* Vein, Portal

Hepaticoduodenostomy
- *see* Bypass, Hepatobiliary System and Pancreas **0F1-**
- *see* Drainage, Hepatobiliary System and Pancreas **0F9-**

Hepaticotomy *see* Drainage, Hepatobiliary System and Pancreas **0F9-**

Hepatocholedochostomy *see* Drainage, Duct, Common Bile **0F99-**

Hepatogastric ligament
- *use* Omentum

Hepatopancreatic ampulla
- *use* Ampulla of Vater

Hepatopexy
- *see* Repair, Hepatobiliary System and Pancreas **0FQ-**
- *see* Reposition, Hepatobiliary System and Pancreas **0FS-**

Hepatorrhaphy *see* Repair, Hepatobiliary System and Pancreas **0FQ-**

Hepatotomy *see* Drainage, Hepatobiliary System and Pancreas **0F9-**

Herculink (RX) Elite Renal Stent System
- *use* Intraluminal Device

Herniorrhaphy
- *see* Repair, Anatomical Regions, General **0WQ-**
- *see* Repair, Anatomical Regions, Lower Extremities **0YQ-**
- With synthetic substitute
  - *see* Supplement, Anatomical Regions, General **0WU-**
  - *see* Supplement, Anatomical Regions, Lower Extremities **0YU-**

Hip (joint) liner
- *use* Liner in Lower Joints

Holter monitoring 4A12X45

Holter valve ventricular shunt
- *use* Synthetic Substitute

Human angiotensin II, synthetic
- *use* Synthetic Human Angiotensin II

Humeroradial joint
- *use* Joint, Elbow, Left
- *use* Joint, Elbow, Right

Humeroulnar joint
- *use* Joint, Elbow, Left
- *use* Joint, Elbow, Right

Humerus, distal
- *use* Humeral Shaft, Left
- *use* Humeral Shaft, Right

Hydrocelectomy *see* Excision, Male Reproductive System **0VB-**

Hydrotherapy
- Assisted exercise in pool *see* Motor Treatment, Rehabilitation **F07-**
- Whirlpool *see* Activities of Daily Living Treatment, Rehabilitation **F08-**

Hymenectomy
- *see* Excision, Hymen **0UBK-**
- *see* Resection, Hymen **0UTK**

Hymenoplasty
- *see* Repair, Hymen **0UQK-**
- *see* Supplement, Hymen **0UUK-**

Hymenorrhaphy *see* Repair, Hymen **0UQK-**

Hymenotomy
- *see* Division, Hymen **0U8K-**
- *see* Drainage, Hymen **0U9K-**

Hyoglossus muscle
- *use* Muscle, Tongue, Palate, Pharynx

Hyoid artery
- *use* Artery, Thyroid, Left
- *use* Artery, Thyroid, Right

Hyperalimentation *see* Introduction of substance in or on

Hyperbaric oxygenation
- Decompression sickness treatment *see* Decompression, Circulatory **6A15-**
- Wound treatment *see* Assistance, Circulatory **5A05-**

Hyperthermia
- Radiation Therapy
  - Abdomen **DWY38ZZ**
  - Adrenal Gland **DGY28ZZ**
  - Bile Ducts **DFY28ZZ**
  - Bladder **DTY28ZZ**
  - Bone, Other **DPYC8ZZ**
  - Bone Marrow **D7Y08ZZ**
  - Brain **D0Y08ZZ**

PROCEDURE INDEX

© 2018 Channel Publishing, Ltd.

Hyperthermia — *continued*
Radiation Therapy — *continued*
Brain Stem **D0Y18ZZ**
Breast
Left **DMY08ZZ**
Right **DMY18ZZ**
Bronchus **DBY18ZZ**
Cervix **DUY18ZZ**
Chest **DWY28ZZ**
Chest Wall **DBY78ZZ**
Colon **DDY58ZZ**
Diaphragm **DBY88ZZ**
Duodenum **DDY28ZZ**
Ear **D9Y08ZZ**
Esophagus **DDY08ZZ**
Eye **D8Y08ZZ**
Femur **DPY98ZZ**
Fibula **DPYB8ZZ**
Gallbladder **DFY18ZZ**
Gland
Adrenal **DGY28ZZ**
Parathyroid **DGY48ZZ**
Pituitary **DGY08ZZ**
Thyroid **DGY58ZZ**
Glands, Salivary **D9Y68ZZ**
Head and Neck **DWY18ZZ**
Hemibody **DWY48ZZ**
Humerus **DPY68ZZ**
Hypopharynx **D9Y38ZZ**
Ileum **DDY48ZZ**
Jejunum **DDY38ZZ**
Kidney **DTY08ZZ**
Larynx **D9YB8ZZ**
Liver **DFY08ZZ**
Lung **DBY28ZZ**
Lymphatics
Abdomen **D7Y68ZZ**
Axillary **D7Y48ZZ**
Inguinal **D7Y88ZZ**
Neck **D7Y38ZZ**
Pelvis **D7Y78ZZ**
Thorax **D7Y58ZZ**
Mandible **DPY38ZZ**
Maxilla **DPY28ZZ**
Mediastinum **DBY68ZZ**
Mouth **D9Y48ZZ**
Nasopharynx **D9YD8ZZ**
Neck and Head **DWY18ZZ**
Nerve, Peripheral **D0Y78ZZ**
Nose **D9Y18ZZ**
Oropharynx **D9YF8ZZ**
Ovary **DUY08ZZ**
Palate
Hard **D9Y88ZZ**
Soft **D9Y98ZZ**
Pancreas **DFY38ZZ**
Parathyroid Gland **DGY48ZZ**
Pelvic Bones **DPY88ZZ**
Pelvic Region **DWY68ZZ**
Pineal Body **DGY18ZZ**
Pituitary Gland **DGY08ZZ**
Pleura **DBY58ZZ**
Prostate **DVY08ZZ**
Radius **DPY78ZZ**
Rectum **DDY78ZZ**
Rib **DPY58ZZ**
Sinuses **D9Y78ZZ**
Skin
Abdomen **DHY88ZZ**
Arm **DHY48ZZ**
Back **DHY78ZZ**
Buttock **DHY98ZZ**
Chest **DHY68ZZ**
Face **DHY28ZZ**
Leg **DHYB8ZZ**
Neck **DHY38ZZ**
Skull **DPY08ZZ**
Spinal Cord **D0Y68ZZ**
Spleen **D7Y28ZZ**
Sternum **DPY48ZZ**
Stomach **DDY18ZZ**
Testis **DVY18ZZ**
Thymus **D7Y18ZZ**
Thyroid Gland **DGY58ZZ**

Hyperthermia — *continued*
Radiation Therapy — *continued*
Tibia **DPYB8ZZ**
Tongue **D9Y58ZZ**
Trachea **DBY08ZZ**
Ulna **DPY78ZZ**
Ureter **DTY18ZZ**
Urethra **DTY38ZZ**
Uterus **DUY28ZZ**
Whole Body **DWY58ZZ**
Whole Body **6A3Z-**
Hypnosis GZFZZZZ
Hypogastric artery
use Artery, Internal Iliac, Left
use Artery, Internal Iliac, Right
Hypopharynx
use Pharynx
Hypophysectomy
see Excision, Gland, Pituitary **0GB0-**
see Resection, Gland, Pituitary **0GT0-**
Hypophysis
use Gland, Pituitary
Hypothalamotomy *see* Destruction, Thalamus **0059-**
Hypothenar muscle
use Muscle, Hand, Left
use Muscle, Hand, Right
Hypothermia, Whole Body 6A4Z-
Hysterectomy
Supracervical
see Resection, Uterus **0UT9-**
Total *see* Resection, Uterus **0UT9-**
Hysterolysis *see* Release, Uterus **0UN9-**
Hysteropexy
see Repair, Uterus **0UQ9-**
see Reposition, Uterus **0US9-**
Hysteroplasty *see* Repair, Uterus **0UQ9-**
Hysterorrhaphy *see* Repair, Uterus **0UQ9-**
Hysteroscopy 0UJD8ZZ
Hysterotomy *see* Drainage, Uterus **0U99-**
Hysterotrachelectomy
see Resection, Cervix **0UTC-**
see Resection, Uterus **0UT9-**
Hysterotracheloplasty *see* Repair, Uterus **0UQ9-**
Hysterotrachelorrhaphy *see* Repair, Uterus **0UQ9-**

I

IABP (Intra-aortic balloon pump)
see Assistance, Cardiac **5A02-**
IAEMT (Intraoperative anesthetic effect monitoring and titration) *see* Monitoring, Central Nervous **4A10-**
Idarucizumab, Dabigatran reversal agent XW0-
IHD (Intermittent hemodialysis) 5A1D70Z
Ileal artery
use Artery, Superior Mesenteric
Ileectomy
see Excision, Ileum **0DBB-**
see Resection, Ileum **0DTB-**
Ileocolic artery
use Artery, Superior Mesenteric
Ileocolic vein
use Vein, Colic
Ileopexy
see Repair, Ileum **0DQB-**
see Reposition, Ileum **0DSB-**
Ileorrhaphy *see* Repair, Ileum **0DQB-**
Ileoscopy 0DJD8ZZ
Ileostomy
see Bypass, Ileum **0D1B-**
see Drainage, Ileum **0D9B-**
Ileotomy *see* Drainage, Ileum **0D9B-**
Ileoureterostomy *see* Bypass, Urinary System **0T1-**
Iliac crest
use Bone, Pelvic, Left
use Bone, Pelvic, Right
Iliac fascia
use Subcutaneous Tissue and Fascia, Upper Leg, Left
use Subcutaneous Tissue and Fascia, Upper Leg, Right
Iliac lymph node
use Lymphatic, Pelvis
Iliacus muscle
use Muscle, Hip, Left
use Muscle, Hip, Right
Iliofemoral ligament
use Bursa and Ligament, Hip, Left
use Bursa and Ligament, Hip, Right
Iliohypogastric nerve
use Nerve, Lumbar Plexus
Ilioinguinal nerve
use Nerve, Lumbar Plexus
Iliolumbar artery
use Artery, Internal Iliac, Left
use Artery, Internal Iliac, Right
Iliolumbar ligament *use* Lower Spine Bursa and Ligament
Iliotibial tract (band)
use Subcutaneous Tissue and Fascia, Upper Leg, Left
use Subcutaneous Tissue and Fascia, Upper Leg, Right
Ilium
use Bone, Pelvic, Left
use Bone, Pelvic, Right
Ilizarov external fixator
use External Fixation Device, Ring in **0PH-**
use External Fixation Device, Ring in **0PS-**
use External Fixation Device, Ring in **0QH-**
use External Fixation Device, Ring in **0QS-**
Ilizarov-Vecklich device
use External Fixation Device, Limb Lengthening in **0PH-**
use External Fixation Device, Limb Lengthening in **0QH-**
Imaging, diagnostic
see Computerized Tomography (CT Scan)
see Fluoroscopy
see Magnetic Resonance Imaging (MRI)
see Plain Radiography
see Ultrasonography
Immobilization
Abdominal Wall **2W33X-**
Arm
Lower
Left **2W3DX-**
Right **2W3CX-**
Upper
Left **2W3BX-**
Right **2W3AX-**
Back **2W35X-**
Chest Wall **2W34X-**
Extremity
Lower
Left **2W3MX-**
Right **2W3LX-**
Upper
Left **2W39X-**
Right **2W38X-**
Face **2W31X-**
Finger
Left **2W3KX-**
Right **2W3JX-**
Foot
Left **2W3TX-**
Right **2W3SX-**
Hand
Left **2W3FX-**
Right **2W3EX-**
Head **2W30X-**
Inguinal Region
Left **2W37X-**
Right **2W36X-**
Leg
Lower
Left **2W3RX-**
Right **2W3QX-**
Upper
Left **2W3PX-**
Right **2W3NX-**
Neck **2W32X-**
Thumb
Left **2W3HX-**
Right **2W3GX-**
Toe
Left **2W3VX-**
Right **2W3UX-**
Immunization *see* Introduction of Serum, Toxoid, and Vaccine
Immunotherapy *see* Introduction of Immunotherapeutic Substance
Immunotherapy, antineoplastic
Interferon *see* Introduction of Low-dose Interleukin-2
Interleukin-2, high-dose *see* Introduction of High-dose Interleukin-2
Interleukin-2, low-dose *see* Introduction of Low-dose Interleukin-2
Monoclonal antibody *see* Introduction of Monoclonal Antibody
Proleukin, high-dose *see* Introduction of High-dose Interleukin-2
Proleukin, low-dose *see* Introduction of Low-dose Interleukin-2

© 2018 Channel Publishing, Ltd.

Impella® heart pump
use Short-term External Heart Assist System in Heart and Great Vessels
Impeller Pump
Continuous, Output **5A0221D**
Intermittent, Output **5A0211D**
Implantable cardioverter-defibrillator (ICD)
use Defibrillator Generator in **0JH-**
Implantable drug infusion pump (anti-spasmodic) (chemotherapy) (pain)
use Infusion Device, Pump in Subcutaneous Tissue and Fascia
Implantable gastric pacemaker generator
use Stimulator Generator in Subcutaneous Tissue and Fascia
Implantable glucose monitoring device
use Monitoring Device
Implantable hemodynamic monitor (IHM)
use Monitoring Device, Hemodynamic in **0JH-**
Implantable hemodynamic monitoring system (IHMS)
use Monitoring Device, Hemodynamic in **0JH-**
Implantable Miniature Telescope™ (IMT)
use Synthetic Substitute, Intraocular Telescope in **08R-**
Implantation
see Insertion
see Replacement
Implanted (venous) (access) port
use Vascular Access Device, Totally Implantable in Subcutaneous Tissue and Fascia
IMV (intermittent mandatory ventilation) *see* Assistance, Respiratory **5A09-**
In Vitro Fertilization 8E0ZXY1
Incision, abscess *see* Drainage
Incudectomy
see Excision, Ear, Nose, Sinus **09B-**
see Resection, Ear, Nose, Sinus **09T-**
Incudopexy
see Repair, Ear, Nose, Sinus **09Q-**
see Reposition, Ear, Nose, Sinus **09S-**
Incus
use Auditory Ossicle, Left
use Auditory Ossicle, Right
Induction of labor
Artificial rupture of membranes *see* Drainage, Pregnancy **109-**
Oxytocin *see* Introduction of Hormone
InDura, intrathecal catheter (1P) (spinal)
use Infusion Device
Inferior cardiac nerve
use Nerve, Thoracic Sympathetic
Inferior cerebellar vein
use Vein, Intracranial
Inferior cerebral vein
use Vein, Intracranial
Inferior epigastric artery
use Artery, External Iliac, Left
use Artery, External Iliac, Right
Inferior epigastric lymph node
use Lymphatic, Pelvis
Inferior genicular artery
use Artery, Popliteal, Left
use Artery, Popliteal, Right
Inferior gluteal artery
use Artery, Internal Iliac, Left
use Artery, Internal Iliac, Right
Inferior gluteal nerve
use Nerve, Sacral Plexus
Inferior hypogastric plexus
use Nerve, Abdominal Sympathetic
Inferior labial artery
use Artery, Face
Inferior longitudinal muscle
use Muscle, Tongue, Palate, Pharynx
Inferior mesenteric ganglion
use Nerve, Abdominal Sympathetic
Inferior mesenteric lymph node
use Lymphatic, Mesenteric
Inferior mesenteric plexus
use Nerve, Abdominal Sympathetic
Inferior oblique muscle
use Muscle, Extraocular, Left
use Muscle, Extraocular, Right
Inferior pancreaticoduodenal artery
use Artery, Superior Mesenteric
Inferior phrenic artery
use Aorta, Abdominal
Inferior rectus muscle
use Muscle, Extraocular, Left
use Muscle, Extraocular, Right
Inferior suprarenal artery
use Artery, Renal, Left
use Artery, Renal, Right
Inferior tarsal plate
use Eyelid, Lower, Left
use Eyelid, Lower, Right
Inferior thyroid vein
use Vein, Innominate, Left
use Vein, Innominate, Right
Inferior tibiofibular joint
use Joint, Ankle, Left
use Joint, Ankle, Right
Inferior turbinate
use Turbinate, Nasal
Inferior ulnar collateral artery
use Artery, Brachial, Left
use Artery, Brachial, Right
Inferior vesical artery
use Artery, Internal Iliac, Left
use Artery, Internal Iliac, Right
Infraauricular lymph node
use Lymphatic, Head
Infraclavicular (deltopectoral) lymph node
use Lymphatic, Upper Extremity, Left
use Lymphatic, Upper Extremity, Right
Infrahyoid muscle
use Muscle, Neck, Left
use Muscle, Neck, Right
Infraparotid lymph node
use Lymphatic, Head
Infraspinatus fascia
use Subcutaneous Tissue and Fascia, Upper Arm, Left
use Subcutaneous Tissue and Fascia, Upper Arm, Right
Infraspinatus muscle
use Muscle, Shoulder, Left
use Muscle, Shoulder, Right
Infundibulopelvic ligament
use Uterine Supporting Structure
Infusion *see* Introduction of substance in or on
Infusion Device, Pump
Insertion of device in
Abdomen **0JH8-**
Back **0JH7-**
Chest **0JH6-**
Lower Arm
Left **0JHH-**
Right **0JHG-**
Lower Leg
Left **0JHP-**
Right **0JHN-**
Trunk **0JHT-**
Upper Arm
Left **0JHF-**
Right **0JHD-**
Upper Leg
Left **0JHM-**
Right **0JHL-**
Removal of device from
Lower Extremity **0JPW-**
Trunk **0JPT-**
Upper Extremity **0JPV-**
Revision of device in
Lower Extremity **0JWW-**
Trunk **0JWT-**
Upper Extremity **0JWV-**
Infusion, glucarpidase
Central vein **3E043GQ**
Peripheral vein **3E033GQ**
Inguinal canal
use Inguinal Region, Bilateral
use Inguinal Region, Left
use Inguinal Region, Right
Inguinal triangle
use Inguinal Region, Bilateral
use Inguinal Region, Left
use Inguinal Region, Right
Injection *see* Introduction of substance in or on
Injection, Concentrated Bone Marrow Aspirate (CBMA), intramuscular XK02303
Injection reservoir, port
use Vascular Access Device, Totally Implantable in Subcutaneous Tissue and Fascia
Injection reservoir, pump
use Infusion Device, Pump in Subcutaneous Tissue and Fascia
Insemination, artificial 3E0P7LZ
Insertion
Antimicrobial envelope *see* Introduction of Anti-infective
Aqueous drainage shunt
see Bypass, Eye **081-**
see Drainage, Eye **089-**
Products of Conception **10H0-**
Spinal Stabilization Device
see Insertion of device in, Lower Joints **0SH-**
see Insertion of device in, Upper Joints **0RH-**
Insertion of device in
Abdominal Wall **0WHF-**
Acetabulum
Left **0QH5-**
Right **0QH4-**
Anal Sphincter **0DHR-**
Ankle Region
Left **0YHL-**
Right **0YHK-**
Anus **0DHQ-**
Aorta
Abdominal **04H0-**
Thoracic
Ascending/Arch **02HX-**
Descending **02HW-**
Insertion of device in — *continued*
Arm
Lower
Left **0XHF-**
Right **0XHD-**
Upper
Left **0XH9-**
Right **0XH8-**
Artery
Anterior Tibial
Left **04HQ-**
Right **04HP-**
Axillary
Left **03H6-**
Right **03H5-**
Brachial
Left **03H8-**
Right **03H7-**
Celiac **04H1-**
Colic
Left **04H7-**
Middle **04H8-**
Right **04H6-**
Common Carotid
Left **03HJ-**
Right **03HH-**
Common Iliac
Left **04HD-**
Right **04HC-**
External Carotid
Left **03HN-**
Right **03HM-**
External Iliac
Left **04HJ-**
Right **04HH-**
Face **03HR-**
Femoral
Left **04HL-**
Right **04HK-**
Foot
Left **04HW-**
Right **04HV-**
Gastric **04H2-**
Hand
Left **03HF-**
Right **03HD-**
Hepatic **04H3-**
Inferior Mesenteric **04HB**
Innominate **03H2-**
Internal Carotid
Left **03HL-**
Right **03HK-**
Internal Iliac
Left **04HF-**
Right **04HE-**
Internal Mammary
Left **03H1-**
Right **03H0-**
Intracranial **03HG-**
Lower **04HY-**
Peroneal
Left **04HU-**
Right **04HT-**
Popliteal
Left **04HN-**
Right **04HM-**
Posterior Tibial
Left **04HS-**
Right **04HR-**
Pulmonary
Left **02HR-**
Right **02HQ-**
Pulmonary Trunk **02HP-**
Radial
Left **03HC-**
Right **03HB-**
Renal
Left **04HA-**
Right **04H9-**
Splenic **04H4-**
Subclavian
Left **03H4-**
Right **03H3-**

PROCEDURE INDEX

© 2018 Channel Publishing, Ltd.

Insertion of device in — *continued*
Artery — *continued*
Superior Mesenteric **04H5-**
Temporal
Left **03HT-**
Right **03HS-**
Thyroid
Left **03HV-**
Right **03HU-**
Ulnar
Left **03HA-**
Right **03H9-**
Upper **03HY-**
Vertebral
Left **03HQ-**
Right **03HP-**
Atrium
Left **02H7-**
Right **02H6-**
Axilla
Left **0XH5-**
Right **0XH4-**
Back
Lower **0WHL-**
Upper **0WHK-**
Bladder **0THB-**
Bladder Neck **0THC-**
Bone
Ethmoid
Left **0NHG-**
Right **0NHF-**
Facial **0NHW-**
Frontal **0NH1-**
Hyoid **0NHX-**
Lacrimal
Left **0NHJ-**
Right **0NHH-**
Lower **0QHY-**
Nasal **0NHB-**
Occipital **0NH7-**
Palatine
Left **0NHL-**
Right **0NHK-**
Parietal
Left **0NH4-**
Right **0NH3-**
Pelvic
Left **0QH3-**
Right **0QH2-**
Sphenoid **0NHC-**
Temporal
Left **0NH6-**
Right **0NH5-**
Upper **0PHY-**
Zygomatic
Left **0NHN-**
Right **0NHM-**
Brain **00H0-**
Breast
Bilateral **0HHV-**
Left **0HHU-**
Right **0HHT-**
Bronchus
Lingula **0BH9-**
Lower Lobe
Left **0BHB-**
Right **0BH6-**
Main
Left **0BH7-**
Right **0BH3-**
Middle Lobe, Right **0BH5-**
Upper Lobe
Left **0BH8-**
Right **0BH4-**
Bursa and Ligament
Lower **0MHY-**
Upper **0MHX-**
Buttock
Left **0YH1-**
Right **0YH0-**
Carpal
Left **0PHN-**
Right **0PHM-**

Insertion of device in — *continued*
Cavity, Cranial **0WH1-**
Cerebral Ventricle **00H6-**
Cervix **0UHC-**
Chest Wall **0WH8-**
Cisterna Chyli **07HL-**
Clavicle
Left **0PHB-**
Right **0PH9-**
Coccyx **0QHS-**
Cul-de-sac **0UHF-**
Diaphragm **0BHT-**
Disc
Cervical Vertebral **0RH3-**
Cervicothoracic Vertebral **0RH5-**
Lumbar Vertebral **0SH2-**
Lumbosacral **0SH4-**
Thoracic Vertebral **0RH9-**
Thoracolumbar Vertebral **0RHB-**
Duct
Hepatobiliary **0FHB-**
Pancreatic **0FHD-**
Duodenum **0DH9-**
Ear
Inner
Left **09HE-**
Right **09HD-**
Left **09HJ-**
Right **09HH-**
Elbow Region
Left **0XHC-**
Right **0XHB-**
Epididymis and Spermatic Cord **0VHM-**
Esophagus **0DH5-**
Extremity
Lower
Left **0YHB-**
Right **0YH9-**
Upper
Left **0XH7-**
Right **0XH6-**
Eye
Left **08H1-**
Right **08H0-**
Face **0WH2-**
Fallopian Tube **0UH8-**
Femoral Region
Left **0YH8-**
Right **0YH7-**
Femoral Shaft
Left **0QH9-**
Right **0QH8-**
Femur
Lower
Left **0QHC-**
Right **0QHB-**
Upper
Left **0QH7-**
Right **0QH6-**
Fibula
Left **0QHK-**
Right **0QHJ-**
Foot
Left **0YHN-**
Right **0YHM-**
Gallbladder **0FH4-**
Gastrointestinal Tract **0WHP-**
Genitourinary Tract **0WHR-**
Gland
Endocrine **0GHS-**
Salivary **0CHA-**
Glenoid Cavity
Left **0PH8-**
Right **0PH7-**
Hand
Left **0XHK-**
Right **0XHJ-**
Head **0WH0-**
Heart **02HA-**

Insertion of device in — *continued*
Humeral Head
Left **0PHD-**
Right **0PHC-**
Humeral Shaft
Left **0PHG-**
Right **0PHF-**
Ileum **0DHB-**
Inguinal Region
Left **0YH6-**
Right **0YH5-**
Intestinal Tract
Lower **0DHD-**
Upper **0DH0-**
Intestine
Large **0DHE-**
Small **0DH8-**
Jaw
Lower **0WH5-**
Upper **0WH4-**
Jejunum **0DHA-**
Joint
Acromioclavicular
Left **0RHH-**
Right **0RHG-**
Ankle
Left **0SHG-**
Right **0SHF-**
Carpal
Left **0RHR-**
Right **0RHQ-**
Carpometacarpal
Left **0RHT-**
Right **0RHS-**
Cervical Vertebral **0RH1-**
Cervicothoracic Vertebral **0RH4-**
Coccygeal **0SH6-**
Elbow
Left **0RHM-**
Right **0RHL-**
Finger Phalangeal
Left **0RHX-**
Right **0RHW-**
Hip
Left **0SHB-**
Right **0SH9-**
Knee
Left **0SHD-**
Right **0SHC-**
Lumbar Vertebral **0SH0-**
Lumbosacral **0SH3-**
Metacarpophalangeal
Left **0RHV-**
Right **0RHU-**
Metatarsal-Phalangeal
Left **0SHN-**
Right **0SHM-**
Occipital-cervical **0RH0-**
Sacrococcygeal **0SH5-**
Sacroiliac
Left **0SH8-**
Right **0SH7-**
Shoulder
Left **0RHK-**
Right **0RHJ-**
Sternoclavicular
Left **0RHF-**
Right **0RHE-**
Tarsal
Left **0SHJ-**
Right **0SHH-**
Tarsometatarsal
Left **0SHL-**
Right **0SHK-**
Temporomandibular
Left **0RHD-**
Right **0RHC-**
Thoracic Vertebral **0RH6-**
Thoracolumbar Vertebral **0RHA-**

Insertion of device in — *continued*
Joint — *continued*
Toe Phalangeal
Left **0SHQ-**
Right **0SHP-**
Wrist
Left **0RHP-**
Right **0RHN-**
Kidney **0TH5-**
Knee Region
Left **0YHG-**
Right **0YHF-**
Larynx **0CHS-**
Leg
Lower
Left **0YHJ-**
Right **0YHH-**
Upper
Left **0YHD-**
Right **0YHC-**
Liver **0FH0-**
Left Lobe **0FH2-**
Right Lobe **0FH1-**
Lung
Left **0BHL-**
Right **0BHK-**
Lymphatic **07HN-**
Thoracic Duct **07HK-**
Mandible
Left **0NHV-**
Right **0NHT**
Maxilla **0NHR-**
Mediastinum **0WHC-**
Metacarpal
Left **0PHQ-**
Right **0PHP-**
Metatarsal
Left **0QHP-**
Right **0QHN-**
Mouth and Throat **0CHY-**
Muscle
Lower **0KHY-**
Upper **0KHX-**
Nasal Mucosa and Soft Tissue **09HK-**
Nasopharynx **09HN-**
Neck **0WH6-**
Nerve
Cranial **00HE-**
Peripheral **01HY-**
Nipple
Left **0HHX-**
Right **0HHW-**
Oral Cavity and Throat **0WH3-**
Orbit
Left **0NHQ-**
Right **0NHP-**
Ovary **0UH3-**
Pancreas **0FHG-**
Patella
Left **0QHF-**
Right **0QHD-**
Pelvic Cavity **0WHJ-**
Penis **0VHS-**
Pericardial Cavity **0WHD-**
Pericardium **02HN-**
Perineum
Female **0WHN-**
Male **0WHM-**
Peritoneal Cavity **0WHG-**
Phalanx
Finger
Left **0PHV-**
Right **0PHT-**
Thumb
Left **0PHS-**
Right **0PHR-**
Toe
Left **0QHR-**
Right **0QHQ-**
Pleura **0BHQ-**

© 2018 Channel Publishing, Ltd.

Insertion of device in — *continued*
Pleural Cavity
Left **0WHB-**
Right **0WH9-**
Prostate **0VH0-**
Prostate and Seminal Vesicles **0VH4-**
Radius
Left **0PHJ-**
Right **0PHH-**
Rectum **0DHP-**
Respiratory Tract **0WHQ-**
Retroperitoneum **0WHH-**
Ribs
1 to 2 **0PH1-**
3 or more **0PH2-**
Sacrum **0QH1-**
Scapula
Left **0PH6-**
Right **0PH5-**
Scrotum and Tunica Vaginalis **0VH8-**
Shoulder Region
Left **0XH3-**
Right **0XH2-**
Sinus **09HY-**
Skin **0HHPXYZ**
Skull **0NH0-**
Spinal Canal **00HU-**
Spinal Cord **00HV-**
Spleen **07HP-**
Sternum **0PH0-**
Stomach **0DH6-**
Subcutaneous Tissue and Fascia
Abdomen **0JH8-**
Back **0JH7-**
Buttock **0JH9-**
Chest **0JH6-**
Face **0JH1-**
Foot
Left **0JHR-**
Right **0JHQ-**
Hand
Left **0JHK-**
Right **0JHJ-**
Head and Neck **0JHS-**
Lower Arm
Left **0JHH-**
Right **0JHG-**
Lower Extremity **0JHW-**
Lower Leg
Left **0JHP-**
Right **0JHN-**
Neck
Left **0JH5-**
Right **0JH4-**
Pelvic Region **0JHC-**
Perineum **0JHB-**
Scalp **0JH0-**
Trunk **0JHT-**
Upper Arm
Left **0JHF-**
Right **0JHD-**
Upper Extremity **0JHV-**
Upper Leg
Left **0JHM-**
Right **0JHL-**
Tarsal
Left **0QHM-**
Right **0QHL-**
Tendon
Lower **0LHY-**
Upper **0LHX-**
Testis **0VHD-**
Thymus **07HM-**
Tibia
Left **0QHH-**
Right **0QHG-**
Tongue **0CH7-**
Trachea **0BH1-**
Tracheobronchial Tree **0BH0-**

Insertion of device in — *continued*
Ulna
Left **0PHL-**
Right **0PHK-**
Ureter **0TH9-**
Urethra **0THD-**
Uterus **0UH9-**
Uterus and Cervix **0UHD-**
Vagina **0UHG-**
Vagina and Cul-de-sac **0UHH-**
Vas Deferens **0VHR-**
Vein
Axillary
Left **05H8-**
Right **05H7-**
Azygos **05H0-**
Basilic
Left **05HC-**
Right **05HB-**
Brachial
Left **05HA-**
Right **05H9-**
Cephalic
Left **05HF-**
Right **05HD-**
Colic **06H7-**
Common Iliac
Left **06HD-**
Right **06HC-**
Coronary **02H4-**
Esophageal **06H3-**
External Iliac
Left **06HG-**
Right **06HF-**
External Jugular
Left **05HQ-**
Right **05HP-**
Face
Left **05HV-**
Right **05HT-**
Femoral
Left **06HN-**
Right **06HM-**
Foot
Left **06HV-**
Right **06HT-**
Gastric **06H2-**
Hand
Left **05HH-**
Right **05HG-**
Hemiazygos **05H1-**
Hepatic **06H4-**
Hypogastric
Left **06HJ-**
Right **06HH-**
Inferior Mesenteric **06H6-**
Innominate
Left **05H4-**
Right **05H3-**
Internal Jugular
Left **05HN-**
Right **05HM-**
Intracranial **05HL-**
Lower **06HY-**
Portal **06H8-**
Pulmonary
Left **02HT-**
Right **02HS-**
Renal
Left **06HB-**
Right **06H9-**
Saphenous
Left **06HQ-**
Right **06HP-**
Splenic **06H1-**
Subclavian
Left **05H6-**
Right **05H5-**
Superior Mesenteric **06H5-**
Upper **05HY-**
Vertebral
Left **05HS-**
Right **05HR-**

Insertion of device in — *continued*
Vena Cava
Inferior **06H0-**
Superior **02HV-**
Ventricle
Left **02HL-**
Right **02HK-**
Vertebra
Cervical **0PH3-**
Lumbar **0QH0-**
Thoracic **0PH4-**
Wrist Region
Left **0XHH-**
Right **0XHG-**

Inspection
Abdominal Wall **0WJF-**
Ankle Region
Left **0YJL-**
Right **0YJK-**
Arm
Lower
Left **0XJF-**
Right **0XJD-**
Upper
Left **0XJ9-**
Right **0XJ8-**
Artery
Lower **04JY-**
Upper **03JY-**
Axilla
Left **0XJ5-**
Right **0XJ4-**
Back
Lower **0WJL-**
Upper **0WJK-**
Bladder **0TJB-**
Bone
Facial **0NJW**
Lower **0QJY-**
Nasal **0NJB-**
Upper **0PJY-**
Bone Marrow **07JT-**
Brain **00J0-**
Breast
Left **0HJU-**
Right **0HJT-**
Bursa and Ligament
Lower **0MJY-**
Upper **0MJX-**
Buttock
Left **0YJ1-**
Right **0YJ0-**
Cavity, Cranial **0WJ1-**
Chest Wall **0WJ8-**
Cisterna Chyli **07JL-**
Diaphragm **0BJT-**
Disc
Cervical Vertebral **0RJ3-**
Cervicothoracic Vertebral **0RJ5-**
Lumbar Vertebral **0SJ2-**
Lumbosacral **0SJ4-**
Thoracic Vertebral **0RJ9-**
Thoracolumbar Vertebral **0RJB-**
Duct
Hepatobiliary **0FJB-**
Pancreatic **0FJD-**
Ear
Inner
Left **09JE-**
Right **09JD-**
Left **09JJ-**
Right **09JH-**
Elbow Region
Left **0XJC-**
Right **0XJB-**
Epididymis and Spermatic Cord **0VJM-**
Extremity
Lower
Left **0YJB-**
Right **0YJ9-**

Inspection — *continued*
Extremity — *continued*
Upper
Left **0XJ7-**
Right **0XJ6-**
Eye
Left **08J1XZZ**
Right **08J0XZZ**
Face **0WJ2-**
Fallopian Tube **0UJ8-**
Femoral Region
Bilateral **0YJE-**
Left **0YJ8-**
Right **0YJ7-**
Finger Nail **0HJQXZZ**
Foot
Left **0YJN-**
Right **0YJM-**
Gallbladder **0FJ4-**
Gastrointestinal Tract **0WJP**
Genitourinary Tract **0WJR**
Gland
Adrenal **0GJ5-**
Endocrine **0GJS-**
Pituitary **0GJ0-**
Salivary **0CJA-**
Great Vessel **02JY-**
Hand
Left **0XJK-**
Right **0XJJ-**
Head **0WJ0-**
Heart **02JA-**
Inguinal Region
Bilateral **0YJA-**
Left **0YJ6-**
Right **0YJ5-**
Intestinal Tract
Lower **0DJD-**
Upper **0DJ0-**
Jaw
Lower **0WJ5-**
Upper **0WJ4-**
Joint
Acromioclavicular
Left **0RJH-**
Right **0RJG-**
Ankle
Left **0SJG-**
Right **0SJF-**
Carpal
Left **0RJR-**
Right **0RJQ-**
Carpometacarpal
Left **0RJT-**
Right **0RJS-**
Cervical Vertebral **0RJ1-**
Cervicothoracic Vertebral **0RJ4-**
Coccygeal **0SJ6-**
Elbow
Left **0RJM-**
Right **0RJL-**
Finger Phalangeal
Left **0RJX-**
Right **0RJW-**
Hip
Left **0SJB-**
Right **0SJ9-**
Knee
Left **0SJD-**
Right **0SJC-**
Lumbar Vertebral **0SJ0-**
Lumbosacral **0SJ3-**
Metacarpophalangeal
Left **0RJV-**
Right **0RJU-**
Metatarsal-Phalangeal
Left **0SJN-**
Right **0SJM-**
Occipital-cervical **0RJ0-**
Sacrococcygeal **0SJ5-**
Sacroiliac
Left **0SJ8-**
Right **0SJ7-**

PROCEDURE INDEX

© 2018 Channel Publishing, Ltd.

Inspection — *continued*
Joint — *continued*
Shoulder
Left **0RJK-**
Right **0RJJ-**
Sternoclavicular
Left **0RJF-**
Right **0RJE-**
Tarsal
Left **0SJJ-**
Right **0SJH-**
Tarsometatarsal
Left **0SJL-**
Right **0SJK-**
Temporomandibular
Left **0RJD-**
Right **0RJC-**
Thoracic Vertebral **0RJ6-**
Thoracolumbar Vertebral **0RJA-**
Toe Phalangeal
Left **0SJQ-**
Right **0SJP-**
Wrist
Left **0RJP-**
Right **0RJN-**
Kidney **0TJ5-**
Knee Region
Left **0YJG-**
Right **0YJF-**
Larynx **0CJS-**
Leg
Lower
Left **0YJJ-**
Right **0YJH-**
Upper
Left **0YJD-**
Right **0YJC-**
Lens
Left **08JKXZZ**
Right **08JJXZZ**
Liver **0FJ0-**
Lung
Left **0BJL-**
Right **0BJK-**
Lymphatic **07JN-**
Thoracic Duct **07JK-**
Mediastinum **0WJC-**
Mesentery **0DJV-**
Mouth and Throat **0CJY-**
Muscle
Extraocular
Left **08JM-**
Right **08JL-**
Lower **0KJY-**
Upper **0KJX-**
Nasal Mucosa and Soft Tissue **09JK-**
Neck **0WJ6-**
Nerve
Cranial **00JE-**
Peripheral **01JY-**
Omentum **0DJU-**
Oral Cavity and Throat **0WJ3-**
Ovary **0UJ3-**
Pancreas **0FJG-**
Parathyroid Gland **0GJR-**
Pelvic Cavity **0WJJ-**
Penis **0VJS-**
Pericardial Cavity **0WJD-**
Perineum
Female **0WJN-**
Male **0WJM-**
Peritoneal Cavity **0WJG-**
Peritoneum **0DJW-**
Pineal Body **0GJ1-**
Pleura **0BJQ-**
Pleural Cavity
Left **0WJB-**
Right **0WJ9-**
Products of Conception **10J0-**
Ectopic **10J2-**
Retained **10J1-**
Prostate and Seminal Vesicles **0VJ4-**

Inspection — *continued*
Respiratory Tract **0WJQ-**
Retroperitoneum **0WJH-**
Scrotum and Tunica Vaginalis **0VJ8-**
Shoulder Region
Left **0XJ3-**
Right **0XJ2-**
Sinus **09JY-**
Skin **0HJPXZZ**
Skull **0NJ0-**
Spinal Canal **00JU-**
Spinal Cord **00JV-**
Spleen **07JP-**
Stomach **0DJ6-**
Subcutaneous Tissue and Fascia
Head and Neck **0JJS-**
Lower Extremity **0JJW-**
Trunk **0JJT-**
Upper Extremity **0JJV-**
Tendon
Lower **0LJY-**
Upper **0LJX-**
Testis **0VJD-**
Thymus **07JM-**
Thyroid Gland **0GJK-**
Toe Nail **0HJRXZZ**
Trachea **0BJ1-**
Tracheobronchial Tree **0BJ0-**
Tympanic Membrane
Left **09J8-**
Right **09J7-**
Ureter **0TJ9-**
Urethra **0TJD-**
Uterus and Cervix **0UJD-**
Vagina and Cul-de-sac **0UJH-**
Vas Deferens **0VJR-**
Vein
Lower **06JY-**
Upper **05JY-**
Vulva **0UJM-**
Wrist Region
Left **0XJH-**
Right **0XJG-**
Instillation *see* Introduction of substance in or on
Insufflation *see* Introduction of substance in or on
Interatrial septum
use Septum, Atrial
Interbody fusion (spine) cage
use Interbody Fusion Device in Lower Joints
use Interbody Fusion Device in Upper Joints
Interbody fusion device
Nanotextured Surface
Cervical Vertebral **XRG**1092
2 or more **XRG**2092
Cervicothoracic Vertebral **XRG**4092
Lumbar Vertebral **XRG**B092
2 or more **XRG**C092
Lumbosacral **XRG**D092
Occipital-cervical **XRG**0092
Thoracic Vertebral **XRG**6092
2 to 7 **XRG**7092
8 or more **XRG**8092
Thoracolumbar Vertebral **XRG**A092
Radiolucent Porous
Cervical Vertebral **XRG**10F3
2 or more **XRG**20F3
Cervicothoracic Vertebral **XRG**40F3
Lumbar Vertebral **XRG**B0F3
2 or more **XRG**C0F3
Lumbosacral **XRG**D0F3
Occipital-cervical **XRG**00F3
Thoracic Vertebral **XRG**60F3
2 to 7 **XRG**70F3
8 or more **XRG**80F3
Thoracolumbar Vertebral **XRG**A0F3

Intercarpal joint
use Joint, Carpal, Left
use Joint, Carpal, Right
Intercarpal ligament
use Bursa and Ligament, Hand, Left
use Bursa and Ligament, Hand, Right
Interclavicular ligament
use Bursa and Ligament, Shoulder, Left
use Bursa and Ligament, Shoulder, Right
Intercostal lymph node
use Lymphatic, Thorax
Intercostal muscle
use Muscle, Thorax, Left
use Muscle, Thorax, Right
Intercostal nerve
use Nerve, Thoracic
Intercostobrachial nerve
use Nerve, Thoracic
Intercuneiform joint
use Joint, Tarsal, Left
use Joint, Tarsal, Right
Intercuneiform ligament
use Bursa and Ligament, Foot, Left
use Bursa and Ligament, Foot, Right
Intermediate bronchus
use Main Bronchus, Right
Intermediate cuneiform bone
use Tarsal, Left
use Tarsal, Right
Intermittent hemodialysis (IHD) 5A1D70Z
Intermittent mandatory ventilation *see* Assistance, Respiratory **5A09-**
Intermittent Negative Airway Pressure
24-96 Consecutive Hours, Ventilation **5A0945B**
Greater than 96 Consecutive Hours, Ventilation **5A0955B**
Less than 24 Consecutive Hours, Ventilation **5A0935B**
Intermittent Positive Airway Pressure
24-96 Consecutive Hours, Ventilation **5A09458**
Greater than 96 Consecutive Hours, Ventilation **5A09558**
Less than 24 Consecutive Hours, Ventilation **5A09358**
Intermittent positive pressure breathing *see* Assistance, Respiratory **5A09-**
Internal (basal) cerebral vein
use Vein, Intracranial
Internal anal sphincter
use Anal Sphincter
Internal carotid artery, intracranial portion
use Intracranial Artery
Internal carotid plexus
use Nerve, Head and Neck Sympathetic
Internal iliac vein
use Vein, Hypogastric, Left
use Vein, Hypogastric, Right
Internal maxillary artery
use Artery, External Carotid, Left
use Artery, External Carotid, Right
Internal naris
use Nasal Mucosa and Soft Tissue
Internal oblique muscle
use Muscle, Abdomen, Left
use Muscle, Abdomen, Right
Internal pudendal artery
use Artery, Internal Iliac, Left
use Artery, Internal Iliac, Right

Internal pudendal vein
use Vein, Hypogastric, Left
use Vein, Hypogastric, Right
Internal thoracic artery
use Artery, Internal Mammary, Left
use Artery, Internal Mammary, Right
use Artery, Subclavian, Left
use Artery, Subclavian, Right
Internal urethral sphincter
use Urethra
Interphalangeal (IP) joint
use Joint, Finger Phalangeal, Left
use Joint, Finger Phalangeal, Right
use Joint, Toe Phalangeal, Left
use Joint, Toe Phalangeal, Right
Interphalangeal ligament
use Bursa and Ligament, Foot, Left
use Bursa and Ligament, Foot, Right
use Bursa and Ligament, Hand, Left
use Bursa and Ligament, Hand, Right
Interrogation, cardiac rhythm related device
Interrogation only *see* Measurement, Cardiac **4B02-**
With cardiac function testing *see* Measurement, Cardiac **4A02-**
Interruption *see* Occlusion
Interspinalis muscle
use Muscle, Trunk, Left
use Muscle, Trunk, Right
Interspinous ligament, cervical
use Head and Neck Bursa and Ligament
Interspinous ligament, lumbar
use Lower Spine Bursa and Ligament
Interspinous ligament, thoracic
use Upper Spine Bursa and Ligament
Interspinous process spinal stabilization device
use Spinal Stabilization Device, Interspinous Process in **0RH-**
use Spinal Stabilization Device, Interspinous Process in **0SH-**
InterStim® Therapy lead
use Neurostimulator Lead in Peripheral Nervous System
InterStim® Therapy neurostimulator
use Stimulator Generator, Single Array in **0JH-**
Intertransversarius muscle
use Muscle, Trunk, Left
use Muscle, Trunk, Right
Intertransverse ligament, cervical
use Head and Neck Bursa and Ligament
Intertransverse ligament, lumbar
use Lower Spine Bursa and Ligament
Intertransverse ligament, thoracic
use Upper Spine Bursa and Ligament
Interventricular foramen (Monro)
use Cerebral Ventricle
Interventricular septum
use Septum, Ventricular
Intestinal lymphatic trunk
use Cisterna Chyli

PROCEDURE INDEX

© 2018 Channel Publishing, Ltd.

Intraluminal Device
Airway
Esophagus **0DH5-**
Mouth and Throat **0CHY-**
Nasopharynx **09HN-**
Bioactive
Occlusion
Common Carotid
Left **03LJ-**
Right **03LH-**
External Carotid
Left **03LN-**
Right **03LM-**
Internal Carotid
Left **03LL-**
Right **03LK-**
Intracranial **03LG-**
Vertebral
Left **03LQ-**
Right **03LP-**
Restriction
Common Carotid
Left **03VJ-**
Right **03VH-**
External Carotid
Left **03VN-**
Right **03VM-**
Internal Carotid
Left **03VL-**
Right **03VK-**
Intracranial **03VG-**
Vertebral
Left **03VQ-**
Right **03VP-**
Endobronchial Valve
Lingula **0BH9-**
Lower Lobe
Left **0BHB-**
Right **0BH6-**
Main
Left **0BH7**
Right **0BH3-**
Middle Lobe, Right **0BH5-**
Upper Lobe
Left **0BH8-**
Right **0BH4-**
Endotracheal Airway
Change device in, Trachea **0B21XEZ**
Insertion of device in, Trachea **0BH1-**
Pessary
Change device in, Vagina and Cul-de-sac **0U2HXGZ**
Insertion of device in
Cul-de-sac **0UHF-**
Vagina **0UHG-**
Intramedullary (IM) rod (nail)
use Internal Fixation Device, Intramedullary in Lower Bones
use Internal Fixation Device, Intramedullary in Upper Bones
Intramedullary skeletal kinetic distractor (ISKD)
use Internal Fixation Device, Intramedullary in Lower Bones
use Internal Fixation Device, Intramedullary in Upper Bones
Intraocular Telescope
Left **08RK30Z**
Right **08RJ30Z**
Intraoperative knee replacement sensor XR2-
Intraoperative Radiation Therapy (IORT)
Anus **DDY8CZZ**
Bile Ducts **DFY2CZZ**
Bladder **DTY2CZZ**
Cervix **DUY1CZZ**
Colon **DDY5CZZ**
Duodenum **DDY2CZZ**
Intraoperative Radiation Therapy (IORT) — *continued*
Gallbladder **DFY1CZZ**
Ileum **DDY4CZZ**
Jejunum **DDY3CZZ**
Kidney **DTY0CZZ**
Larynx **D9YBCZZ**
Liver **DFY0CZZ**
Mouth **D9Y4CZZ**
Nasopharynx **D9YDCZZ**
Ovary **DUY0CZZ**
Pancreas **DFY3CZZ**
Pharynx **D9YCCZZ**
Prostate **DVY0CZZ**
Rectum **DDY7CZZ**
Stomach **DDY1CZZ**
Ureter **DTY1CZZ**
Urethra **DTY3CZZ**
Uterus **DUY2CZZ**
Intrauterine device (IUD)
use Contraceptive Device in Female Reproductive System
Intravascular fluorescence angiography (IFA) *see* Monitoring, Physiological Systems **4A1-**
Introduction of substance in or on
Artery
Central **3E06-**
Analgesics **3E06-**
Anesthetic, Intracirculatory **3E06-**
Antiarrhythmic **3E06-**
Anti-infective **3E06-**
Anti-inflammatory **3E06-**
Antineoplastic **3E06-**
Destructive Agent **3E06-**
Diagnostic Substance, Other **3E06-**
Electrolytic Substance **3E06-**
Hormone **3E06-**
Hypnotics **3E06-**
Immunotherapeutic **3E06-**
Nutritional Substance **3E06-**
Platelet Inhibitor **3E06-**
Radioactive Substance **3E06-**
Sedatives **3E06-**
Serum **3E06-**
Thrombolytic **3E06-**
Toxoid **3E06-**
Vaccine **3E06-**
Vasopressor **3E06-**
Water Balance Substance **3E06-**
Coronary **3E07-**
Diagnostic Substance, Other **3E07-**
Platelet Inhibitor **3E07-**
Thrombolytic **3E07-**
Peripheral **3E05-**
Analgesics **3E05-**
Anesthetic, Intracirculatory **3E05-**
Antiarrhythmic **3E05-**
Anti-infective **3E05-**
Anti-inflammatory **3E05-**
Antineoplastic **3E05-**
Destructive Agent **3E05-**
Diagnostic Substance, Other **3E05-**
Electrolytic Substance **3E05-**
Hormone **3E05-**
Hypnotics **3E05-**
Immunotherapeutic **3E05-**
Nutritional Substance **3E05-**
Platelet Inhibitor **3E05-**
Radioactive Substance **3E05-**
Sedatives **3E05-**
Serum **3E05-**
Thrombolytic **3E05-**
Toxoid **3E05-**
Vaccine **3E05-**
Vasopressor **3E05-**
Water Balance Substance **3E05-**
Introduction of substance in or on — *continued*
Biliary Tract **3E0J-**
Analgesics **3E0J-**
Anesthetic Agent **3E0J-**
Anti-infective **3E0J**
Anti-inflammatory **3E0J**
Antineoplastic **3E0J-**
Destructive Agent **3E0J-**
Diagnostic Substance, Other **3E0J-**
Electrolytic Substance **3E0J-**
Gas **3E0J-**
Hypnotics **3E0J-**
Islet Cells, Pancreatic **3E0J-**
Nutritional Substance **3E0J-**
Radioactive Substance **3E0J-**
Sedatives **3E0J-**
Water Balance Substance **3E0J-**
Bone **3E0V-**
Analgesics **3E0V3NZ**
Anesthetic Agent **3E0V3BZ**
Anti-infective **3E0V32-**
Anti-inflammatory **3E0V33Z**
Antineoplastic **3E0V30-**
Destructive Agent **3E0V3TZ**
Diagnostic Substance, Other **3E0V3KZ**
Electrolytic Substance **3E0V37Z**
Hypnotics **3E0V3NZ**
Nutritional Substance **3E0V36Z**
Radioactive Substance **3E0V3HZ**
Sedatives **3E0V3NZ**
Water Balance Substance **3E0V37Z**
Bone Marrow **3E0A3GC**
Antineoplastic **3E0A30-**
Brain **3E0Q**
Analgesics **3E0Q-**
Anesthetic Agent **3E0Q-**
Anti-infective **3E0Q-**
Anti-inflammatory **3E0Q-**
Antineoplastic **3E0Q-**
Destructive Agent **3E0Q-**
Diagnostic Substance, Other **3E0Q-**
Electrolytic Substance **3E0Q-**
Gas **3E0Q-**
Hypnotics **3E0Q-**
Nutritional Substance **3E0Q-**
Radioactive Substance **3E0Q-**
Sedatives **3E0Q-**
Stem Cells
Embryonic **3E0Q-**
Somatic **3E0Q-**
Water Balance Substance **3E0Q-**
Cranial Cavity **3E0Q-**
Analgesics **3E0Q-**
Anesthetic Agent **3E0Q-**
Anti-infective **3E0Q-**
Anti-inflammatory **3E0Q-**
Antineoplastic **3E0Q-**
Destructive Agent **3E0Q-**
Diagnostic Substance, Other **3E0Q-**
Electrolytic Substance **3E0Q-**
Gas **3E0Q-**
Hypnotics **3E0Q-**
Nutritional Substance **3E0Q-**
Radioactive Substance **3E0Q-**
Sedatives **3E0Q-**
Stem Cells
Embryonic **3E0Q-**
Somatic **3E0Q-**
Water Balance Substance **3E0Q-**
Introduction of substance in or on — *continued*
Ear **3E0B**
Analgesics **3E0B-**
Anesthetic Agent **3E0B-**
Anti-infective **3E0B-**
Anti-inflammatory **3E0B-**
Antineoplastic **3E0B-**
Destructive Agent **3E0B-**
Diagnostic Substance, Other **3E0B-**
Hypnotics **3E0B-**
Radioactive Substance **3E0B-**
Sedatives **3E0B-**
Epidural Space **3E0S3GC**
Analgesics **3E0S3NZ**
Anesthetic Agent **3E0S3BZ**
Anti-infective **3E0S32-**
Anti-inflammatory **3E0S33Z**
Antineoplastic **3E0S30-**
Destructive Agent **3E0S3TZ**
Diagnostic Substance, Other **3E0S3KZ**
Electrolytic Substance **3E0S37Z**
Gas **3E0S-**
Hypnotics **3E0S3NZ**
Nutritional Substance **3E0S36Z**
Radioactive Substance **3E0S3HZ**
Sedatives **3E0S3NZ**
Water Balance Substance **3E0S37Z**
Eye **3E0C-**
Analgesics **3E0C-**
Anesthetic Agent **3E0C-**
Anti-infective **3E0C-**
Anti-inflammatory **3E0C-**
Antineoplastic **3E0C-**
Destructive Agent **3E0C-**
Diagnostic Substance, Other **3E0C-**
Gas **3E0C-**
Hypnotics **3E0C-**
Pigment **3E0C-**
Radioactive Substance **3E0C-**
Sedatives **3E0C-**
Gastrointestinal Tract
Lower **3E0H-**
Analgesics **3E0H-**
Anesthetic Agent **3E0H-**
Anti-infective **3E0H-**
Anti-inflammatory **3E0H-**
Antineoplastic **3E0H-**
Destructive Agent **3E0H-**
Diagnostic Substance, Other **3E0H-**
Electrolytic Substance **3E0H-**
Gas **3E0H-**
Hypnotics **3E0H-**
Nutritional Substance **3E0H-**
Radioactive Substance **3E0H-**
Sedatives **3E0H-**
Water Balance Substance **3E0H-**
Upper **3E0G-**
Analgesics **3E0G-**
Anesthetic Agent **3E0G-**
Anti-infective **3E0G-**
Anti-inflammatory **3E0G-**
Antineoplastic **3E0G-**
Destructive Agent **3E0G-**
Diagnostic Substance, Other **3E0G-**
Electrolytic Substance **3E0G-**
Gas **3E0G-**
Hypnotics **3E0G-**
Nutritional Substance **3E0G-**
Radioactive Substance **3E0G-**
Sedatives **3E0G-**
Water Balance Substance **3E0G-**

© 2018 Channel Publishing, Ltd.

- **Introduction of substance in or on** — *continued*
  - Genitourinary Tract **3E0K-**
    - Analgesics **3E0K-**
    - Anesthetic Agent **3E0K-**
    - Anti-infective **3E0K-**
    - Anti-inflammatory **3E0K-**
    - Antineoplastic **3E0K-**
    - Destructive Agent **3E0K-**
    - Diagnostic Substance, Other **3E0K-**
    - Electrolytic Substance **3E0K-**
    - Gas **3E0K-**
    - Hypnotics **3E0K-**
    - Nutritional Substance **3E0K-**
    - Radioactive Substance **3E0K-**
    - Sedatives **3E0K-**
    - Water Balance Substance **3E0K-**
  - Heart **3E08-**
    - Diagnostic Substance, Other **3E08-**
    - Platelet Inhibitor **3E08-**
    - Thrombolytic **3E08-**
  - Joint **3E0U-**
    - Analgesics **3E0U3NZ**
    - Anesthetic Agent **3E0U3BZ**
    - Anti-infective **3E0U-**
    - Anti-inflammatory **3E0U33Z**
    - Antineoplastic **3E0U30-**
    - Destructive Agent **3E0U3TZ**
    - Diagnostic Substance, Other **3E0U3KZ**
    - Electrolytic Substance **3E0U37Z**
    - Gas **3E0U3SF**
    - Hypnotics **3E0U3NZ**
    - Nutritional Substance **3E0U36Z**
    - Radioactive Substance **3E0U3HZ**
    - Sedatives **3E0U3NZ**
    - Water Balance Substance **3E0U37Z**
  - Lymphatic **3E0W3GC**
    - Analgesics **3E0W3NZ**
    - Anesthetic Agent **3E0W3BZ**
    - Anti-infective **3E0W32-**
    - Anti-inflammatory **3E0W33Z**
    - Antineoplastic **3E0W30-**
    - Destructive Agent **3E0W3TZ**
    - Diagnostic Substance, Other **3E0W3KZ**
    - Electrolytic Substance **3E0W37Z**
    - Hypnotics **3E0W3NZ**
    - Nutritional Substance **3E0W36Z**
    - Radioactive Substance **3E0W3HZ**
    - Sedatives **3E0W3NZ**
    - Water Balance Substance **3E0W37Z**
  - Mouth **3E0D-**
    - Analgesics **3E0D-**
    - Anesthetic Agent **3E0D-**
    - Antiarrhythmic **3E0D-**
    - Anti-infective **3E0D-**
    - Anti-inflammatory **3E0D-**
    - Antineoplastic **3E0D-**
    - Destructive Agent **3E0D-**
    - Diagnostic Substance, Other **3E0D-**
    - Electrolytic Substance **3E0D-**
    - Hypnotics **3E0D-**
    - Nutritional Substance **3E0D-**
    - Radioactive Substance **3E0D-**
    - Sedatives **3E0D-**
    - Serum **3E0D-**
    - Toxoid **3E0D-**
    - Vaccine **3E0D-**
    - Water Balance Substance **3E0D-**
  - Mucous Membrane **3E00XGC**
    - Analgesics **3E00XNZ**
    - Anesthetic Agent **3E00XBZ**
    - Anti-infective **3E00X2-**
    - Anti-inflammatory **3E00X3Z**
    - Antineoplastic **3E00X0-**
    - Destructive Agent **3E00XTZ**
    - Diagnostic Substance, Other **3E00XKZ**
    - Hypnotics **3E00XNZ**
    - Pigment **3E00XMZ**
    - Sedatives **3E00XNZ**
    - Serum **3E00X4Z**
    - Toxoid **3E00X4Z**
    - Vaccine **3E00X4Z**
  - Muscle **3E023GC**
    - Analgesics **3E023NZ**
    - Anesthetic Agent **3E023BZ**
    - Anti-infective **3E0232-**
    - Anti-inflammatory **3E0233Z**
    - Antineoplastic **3E0230-**
    - Destructive Agent **3E023TZ**
    - Diagnostic Substance, Other **3E023KZ**
    - Electrolytic Substance **3E0237Z**
    - Hypnotics **3E023NZ**
    - Nutritional Substance **3E0236Z**
    - Radioactive Substance **3E023HZ**
    - Sedatives **3E023NZ**
    - Serum **3E0234Z**
    - Toxoid **3E0234Z**
    - Vaccine **3E0234Z**
    - Water Balance Substance **3E0237Z**
  - Nerve
    - Cranial **3E0X3GC**
      - Anesthetic Agent **3E0X3BZ**
      - Anti-inflammatory **3E0X33Z**
      - Destructive Agent **3E0X3TZ**
    - Peripheral **3E0T3GC**
      - Anesthetic Agent **3E0T3BZ**
      - Anti-inflammatory **3E0T33Z**
      - Destructive Agent **3E0T3TZ**
    - Plexus **3E0T3GC**
      - Anesthetic Agent **3E0T3BZ**
      - Anti-inflammatory **3E0T33Z**
      - Destructive Agent **3E0T3TZ**
  - Nose **3E09-**
    - Analgesics **3E09-**
    - Anesthetic Agent **3E09-**
    - Anti-infective **3E09-**
    - Anti-inflammatory **3E09-**
    - Antineoplastic **3E09-**
    - Destructive Agent **3E09-**
    - Diagnostic Substance, Other **3E09-**
    - Hypnotics **3E09-**
    - Radioactive Substance **3E09-**
    - Sedatives **3E09-**
    - Serum **3E09-**
    - Toxoid **3E09-**
    - Vaccine **3E09-**
  - Pancreatic Tract **3E0J-**
    - Analgesics **3E0J-**
    - Anesthetic Agent **3E0J-**
    - Anti-infective **3E0J-**
    - Anti-inflammatory **3E0J-**
    - Antineoplastic **3E0J-**
    - Destructive Agent **3E0J-**
    - Diagnostic Substance, Other **3E0J-**
    - Electrolytic Substance **3E0J-**
    - Gas **3E0J-**
    - Hypnotics **3E0J-**
    - Islet Cells, Pancreatic **3E0J-**
    - Nutritional Substance **3E0J-**
    - Radioactive Substance **3E0J-**
    - Sedatives **3E0J-**
    - Water Balance Substance **3E0J-**
  - Pericardial Cavity **3E0Y-**
    - Analgesics **3E0Y3NZ**
    - Anesthetic Agent **3E0Y3BZ**
    - Anti-infective **3E0Y32-**
    - Anti-inflammatory **3E0Y33Z**
    - Antineoplastic **3E0Y-**
    - Destructive Agent **3E0Y3TZ**
    - Diagnostic Substance, Other **3E0Y3KZ**
    - Electrolytic Substance **3E0Y37Z**
    - Gas **3E0Y-**
    - Hypnotics **3E0Y3NZ**
    - Nutritional Substance **3E0Y36Z**
    - Radioactive Substance **3E0Y3HZ**
    - Sedatives **3E0Y3NZ**
    - Water Balance Substance **3E0Y37Z**
  - Peritoneal Cavity **3E0M-**
    - Adhesion Barrier **3E0M-**
    - Analgesics **3E0M3NZ**
    - Anesthetic Agent **3E0M3BZ**
    - Anti-infective **3E0M32-**
    - Anti-inflammatory **3E0M33Z**
    - Antineoplastic **3E0M-**
    - Destructive Agent **3E0M3TZ**
    - Diagnostic Substance, Other **3E0M3KZ**
    - Electrolytic Substance **3E0M37Z**
    - Gas **3E0M-**
    - Hypnotics **3E0M3NZ**
    - Nutritional Substance **3E0M36Z**
    - Radioactive Substance **3E0M3HZ**
    - Sedatives **3E0M3NZ**
    - Water Balance Substance **3E0M37Z**
  - Pharynx **3E0D-**
    - Analgesics **3E0D-**
    - Anesthetic Agent **3E0D-**
    - Antiarrhythmic **3E0D-**
    - Anti-infective **3E0D-**
    - Anti-inflammatory **3E0D-**
    - Antineoplastic **3E0D-**
    - Destructive Agent **3E0D-**
    - Diagnostic Substance, Other **3E0D-**
    - Electrolytic Substance **3E0D-**
    - Hypnotics **3E0D-**
    - Nutritional Substance **3E0D-**
    - Radioactive Substance **3E0D-**
    - Sedatives **3E0D-**
    - Serum **3E0D-**
    - Toxoid **3E0D-**
    - Vaccine **3E0D-**
    - Water Balance Substance **3E0D-**
  - Pleural Cavity **3E0L-**
    - Adhesion Barrier **3E0L-**
    - Analgesics **3E0L3NZ**
    - Anesthetic Agent **3E0L3BZ**
    - Anti-infective **3E0L32-**
    - Anti-inflammatory **3E0L33Z**
    - Antineoplastic **3E0L-**
    - Destructive Agent **3E0L3TZ**
    - Diagnostic Substance, Other **3E0L3KZ**
    - Electrolytic Substance **3E0L37Z**
    - Gas **3E0L-**
    - Hypnotics **3E0L3NZ**
    - Nutritional Substance **3E0L36Z**
    - Radioactive Substance **3E0L3HZ**
    - Sedatives **3E0L3NZ**
    - Water Balance Substance **3E0L37Z**
  - Products of Conception **3E0E-**
    - Analgesics **3E0E-**
    - Anesthetic Agent **3E0E-**
    - Anti-infective **3E0E-**
    - Anti-inflammatory **3E0E-**
    - Antineoplastic **3E0E-**
    - Destructive Agent **3E0E-**
    - Diagnostic Substance, Other **3E0E-**
    - Electrolytic Substance **3E0E-**
    - Gas **3E0E-**
    - Hypnotics **3E0E-**
    - Nutritional Substance **3E0E-**
    - Radioactive Substance **3E0E-**
    - Sedatives **3E0E-**
    - Water Balance Substance **3E0E-**
  - Reproductive
    - Female **3E0P-**
      - Adhesion Barrier **3E0P-**
      - Analgesics **3E0P-**
      - Anesthetic Agent **3E0P-**
      - Anti-infective **3E0P-**
      - Anti-inflammatory **3E0P-**
      - Antineoplastic **3E0P-**
      - Destructive Agent **3E0P-**
      - Diagnostic Substance, Other **3E0P-**
      - Electrolytic Substance **3E0P-**
      - Gas **3E0P-**
      - Hormone **3E0P-**
      - Hypnotics **3E0P-**
      - Nutritional Substance **3E0P-**
      - Ovum, Fertilized **3E0P-**
      - Radioactive Substance **3E0P-**
      - Sedatives **3E0P-**
      - Sperm **3E0P-**
      - Water Balance Substance **3E0P-**
    - Male **3E0N-**
      - Analgesics **3E0N-**
      - Anesthetic Agent **3E0N-**
      - Anti-infective **3E0N-**
      - Anti-inflammatory **3E0N-**
      - Antineoplastic **3E0N-**
      - Destructive Agent **3E0N-**
      - Diagnostic Substance, Other **3E0N-**
      - Electrolytic Substance **3E0N-**
      - Gas **3E0N-**
      - Hypnotics **3E0N-**
      - Nutritional Substance **3E0N-**
      - Radioactive Substance **3E0N-**
      - Sedatives **3E0N-**
      - Water Balance Substance **3E0N-**
  - Respiratory Tract **3E0F-**
    - Analgesics **3E0F-**
    - Anesthetic Agent **3E0F-**
    - Anti-infective **3E0F-**
    - Anti-inflammatory **3E0F-**
    - Antineoplastic **3E0F-**
    - Destructive Agent **3E0F-**
    - Diagnostic Substance, Other **3E0F-**
    - Electrolytic Substance **3E0F-**
    - Gas **3E0F-**
    - Hypnotics **3E0F-**
    - Nutritional Substance **3E0F-**
    - Radioactive Substance **3E0F-**
    - Sedatives **3E0F-**
    - Water Balance Substance **3E0F-**
  - Skin **3E00XGC**
    - Analgesics **3E00XNZ**
    - Anesthetic Agent **3E00XBZ**
    - Anti-infective **3E00X2-**
    - Anti-inflammatory **3E00X3Z**
    - Antineoplastic **3E00X0-**
    - Destructive Agent **3E00XTZ**
    - Diagnostic Substance, Other **3E00XKZ**
    - Hypnotics **3E00XNZ**
    - Pigment **3E00XMZ**

© 2018 Channel Publishing, Ltd.

Introduction of substance in or on — *continued*
Skin 3E00XGC — *continued*
Sedatives 3E00XNZ
Serum 3E00X4Z
Toxoid 3E00X4Z
Vaccine 3E00X4Z
Spinal Canal 3E0R3GC
Analgesics 3E0R3NZ
Anesthetic Agent 3E0R3BZ
Anti-infective 3E0R32-
Anti-inflammatory 3E0R33Z
Antineoplastic 3E0R30-
Destructive Agent 3E0R3TZ
Diagnostic Substance, Other 3E0R3KZ
Electrolytic Substance 3E0R37Z
Gas 3E0R-
Hypnotics 3E0R3NZ
Nutritional Substance 3E0R36Z
Radioactive Substance 3E0R3HZ
Sedatives 3E0R3NZ
Stem Cells
Embryonic 3E0R-
Somatic 3E0R-
Water Balance Substance 3E0R37Z
Subcutaneous Tissue 3E013GC
Analgesics 3E013NZ
Anesthetic Agent 3E013BZ
Anti-infective 3E01-
Anti-inflammatory 3E0133Z
Antineoplastic 3E0130-
Destructive Agent 3E013TZ
Diagnostic Substance, Other 3E013KZ
Electrolytic Substance 3E0137Z
Hormone 3E013V-
Hypnotics 3E013NZ
Nutritional Substance 3E0136Z
Radioactive Substance 3E013HZ
Sedatives 3E013NZ
Serum 3E0134Z
Toxoid 3E0134Z
Vaccine 3E0134Z
Water Balance Substance 3E0137Z
Vein
Central 3E04-
Analgesics 3E04-
Anesthetic, Intracirculatory 3E04-
Antiarrhythmic 3E04-
Anti-infective 3E04-
Anti-inflammatory 3E04-
Antineoplastic 3E04-
Destructive Agent 3E04-
Diagnostic Substance, Other 3E04-
Electrolytic Substance 3E04-
Hormone 3E04-
Hypnotics 3E04-
Immunotherapeutic 3E04-
Nutritional Substance 3E04-
Platelet Inhibitor 3E04-
Radioactive Substance 3E04-
Sedatives 3E04-
Serum 3E04-
Thrombolytic 3E04-
Toxoid 3E04-
Vaccine 3E04-
Vasopressor 3E04-
Water Balance Substance 3E04-

Introduction of substance in or on — *continued*
Vein — *continued*
Peripheral 3E03-
Analgesics 3E03-
Anesthetic, Intracirculatory 3E03-
Antiarrhythmic 3E03-
Anti-infective 3E03-
Anti-inflammatory 3E03-
Antineoplastic 3E03-
Destructive Agent 3E03-
Diagnostic Substance, Other 3E03-
Electrolytic Substance 3E03-
Hormone 3E03-
Hypnotics 3E03-
Immunotherapeutic 3E03-
Islet Cells, Pancreatic 3E03-
Nutritional Substance 3E03-
Platelet Inhibitor 3E03-
Radioactive Substance 3E03-
Sedatives 3E03-
Serum 3E03-
Thrombolytic 3E03-
Toxoid 3E03-
Vaccine 3E03-
Vasopressor 3E03-
Water Balance Substance 3E03-
Intubation
Airway
see Insertion of device in, Esophagus 0DH5-
see Insertion of device in, Mouth and Throat 0CHY-
see Insertion of device in, Trachea 0BH1-
Drainage device *see* Drainage
Feeding Device *see* Insertion of device in, Gastrointestinal System 0DH-
INTUITY Elite valve system, EDWARDS
use Zooplastic Tissue, Rapid Deployment Technique in New Technology
IPPB (intermittent positive pressure breathing) *see* Assistance, Respiratory 5A09-
IRE (irreversible electroporation)
see Destruction, Hepatobiliary System and Pancreas 0F5-
Iridectomy
see Excision, Eye 08B-
see Resection, Eye 08T-
Iridoplasty
see Repair, Eye 08Q-
see Replacement, Eye 08R-
see Supplement, Eye 08U-
Iridotomy *see* Drainage, Eye 089-
Irreversible Electroporation (IRE)
see Destruction, Hepatobiliary System and Pancreas 0F5-
Irrigation
Biliary Tract, Irrigating Substance 3E1J-
Brain, Irrigating Substance 3E1Q38Z
Cranial Cavity, Irrigating Substance 3E1Q38Z
Ear, Irrigating Substance 3E1B-
Epidural Space, Irrigating Substance 3E1S38Z
Eye, Irrigating Substance 3E1C-
Gastrointestinal Tract
Lower, Irrigating Substance 3E1H-
Upper, Irrigating Substance 3E1G-
Genitourinary Tract, Irrigating Substance 3E1K-
Irrigating Substance 3C1ZX8Z
Joint, Irrigating Substance 3E1U38Z

Irrigation — *continued*
Mucous Membrane, Irrigating Substance 3E10-
Nose, Irrigating Substance 3E19-
Pancreatic Tract, Irrigating Substance 3E1J-
Pericardial Cavity, Irrigating Substance 3E1Y38Z
Peritoneal Cavity
Dialysate 3E1M39Z
Irrigating Substance 3E1M38Z
Pleural Cavity, Irrigating Substance 3E1L38Z
Reproductive
Female, Irrigating Substance 3E1P-
Male, Irrigating Substance 3E1N-
Respiratory Tract, Irrigating Substance 3E1F-
Skin, Irrigating Substance 3E10-
Spinal Canal, Irrigating Substance 3E1R38Z
Isavuconazole anti-infective XW0-
Ischiatic nerve
use Nerve, Sciatic
Ischiocavernosus muscle
use Muscle, Perineum
Ischiofemoral ligament
use Bursa and Ligament, Hip, Left
use Bursa and Ligament, Hip, Right
Ischium
use Bone, Pelvic, Left
use Bone, Pelvic, Right
Isolation 8E0ZXY6
Isotope Administration, Whole Body DWY5G-
Itrel (3) (4) neurostimulator
use Stimulator Generator, Single Array in 0JH-

J

PROCEDURE INDEX

© 2018 Channel Publishing, Ltd.

PROCEDURE INDEX

K

Kappa
use Pacemaker, Dual Chamber in 0JH-
Kcentra
use 4-Factor Prothrombin Complex Concentrate
Keratectomy, kerectomy
see Excision, Eye **08B-**
see Resection, Eye **08T-**
Keratocentesis *see* Drainage, Eye **089-**
Keratoplasty
see Repair, Eye **08Q-**
see Replacement, Eye **08R-**
see Supplement, Eye **08U-**
Keratotomy
see Drainage, Eye **089-**
see Repair, Eye **08Q-**
Kirschner wire (K-wire)
use Internal Fixation Device in Head and Facial Bones
use Internal Fixation Device in Lower Bones
use Internal Fixation Device in Lower Joints
use Internal Fixation Device in Upper Bones
use Internal Fixation Device in Upper Joints
Knee (implant) insert
use Liner in Lower Joints
KUB x-ray *see* Plain Radiography, Kidney, Ureter and Bladder **BT04-**
Kuntscher nail
use Internal Fixation Device, Intramedullary in Lower Bones
use Internal Fixation Device, Intramedullary in Upper Bones
KYMRIAH
use Engineered Autologous Chimeric Antigen Receptor T-cell Immunotherapy

L

Labia majora
use Vulva
Labia minora
use Vulva
Labial gland
use Lip, Lower
use Lip, Upper
Labiectomy
see Excision, Female Reproductive System **0UB-**
see Resection, Female Reproductive System **0UT-**
Lacrimal canaliculus
use Duct, Lacrimal, Left
use Duct, Lacrimal, Right
Lacrimal punctum
use Duct, Lacrimal, Left
use Duct, Lacrimal, Right
Lacrimal sac
use Duct, Lacrimal, Left
use Duct, Lacrimal, Right
LAGB (laparoscopic adjustable gastric banding)
Initial procedure **0DV64CZ**
Surgical correction *see* Revision of device in, Stomach **0DW6-**
Laminectomy
see Excision, Lower Bones **0QB-**
see Excision, Upper Bones **0PB-**
see Release, Central Nervous System and Cranial Nerves **00N-**
see Release, Peripheral Nervous System **01N-**
Laminotomy
see Drainage, Lower Bones **0Q9-**
see Drainage, Upper Bones **0P9-**
see Excision, Lower Bones **0QB-**
see Excision, Upper Bones **0PB-**
see Release, Central Nervous System and Cranial Nerves **00N-**
see Release, Lower Bones **0QN-**
see Release, Peripheral Nervous System **01N-**
see Release, Upper Bones **0PN-**
LAP-BAND® adjustable gastric banding system
use Extraluminal Device
Laparoscopic-assisted transanal pull-through
see Excision, Gastrointestinal System **0DB-**
see Resection, Gastrointestinal System **0DT-**
Laparoscopy *see* Inspection
Laparotomy
Drainage *see* Drainage, Peritoneal Cavity **0W9G-**
Exploratory *see* Inspection, Peritoneal Cavity **0WJG-**
Laryngectomy
see Excision, Larynx **0CBS-**
see Resection, Larynx **0CTS-**
Laryngocentesis *see* Drainage, Larynx **0C9S-**
Laryngogram *see* Fluoroscopy, Larynx **B91J-**
Laryngopexy *see* Repair, Larynx **0CQS-**
Laryngopharynx
use Pharynx
Laryngoplasty
see Repair, Larynx **0CQS-**
see Replacement, Larynx **0CRS-**
see Supplement, Larynx **0CUS-**
Laryngorrhaphy *see* Repair, Larynx **0CQS-**
Laryngoscopy **0CJS8ZZ**
Laryngotomy *see* Drainage, Larynx **0C9S-**
Laser Interstitial Thermal Therapy
Adrenal Gland **DGY2KZZ**
Anus **DDY8KZZ**
Bile Ducts **DFY2KZZ**
Brain **D0Y0KZZ**
Brain Stem **D0Y1KZZ**
Breast
Left **DMY0KZZ**
Right **DMY1KZZ**
Bronchus **DBY1KZZ**
Chest Wall **DBY7KZZ**
Colon **DDY5KZZ**
Diaphragm **DBY8KZZ**
Duodenum **DDY2KZZ**
Esophagus **DDY0KZZ**
Gallbladder **DFY1KZZ**
Gland
Adrenal **DGY2KZZ**
Parathyroid **DGY4KZZ**
Pituitary **DGY0KZZ**
Thyroid **DGY5KZZ**
Ileum **DDY4KZZ**
Jejunum **DDY3KZZ**
Liver **DFY0KZZ**
Lung **DBY2KZZ**
Mediastinum **DBY6KZZ**
Nerve, Peripheral **D0Y7KZZ**
Pancreas **DFY3KZZ**
Parathyroid Gland **DGY4KZZ**
Pineal Body **DGY1KZZ**
Pituitary Gland **DGY0KZZ**
Pleura **DBY5KZZ**
Prostate **DVY0KZZ**
Rectum **DDY7KZZ**
Spinal Cord **D0Y6KZZ**
Stomach **DDY1KZZ**
Thyroid Gland **DGY5KZZ**
Trachea **DBY0KZZ**
Lateral (brachial) lymph node
use Lymphatic, Axillary, Left
use Lymphatic, Axillary, Right
Lateral canthus
use Eyelid, Upper, Left
use Eyelid, Upper, Right
Lateral collateral ligament (LCL)
use Bursa and Ligament, Knee, Left
use Bursa and Ligament, Knee, Right
Lateral condyle of femur
use Femur, Lower, Left
use Femur, Lower, Right
Lateral condyle of tibia
use Tibia, Left
use Tibia, Right
Lateral cuneiform bone
use Tarsal, Left
use Tarsal, Right
Lateral epicondyle of femur
use Femur, Lower, Left
use Femur, Lower, Right
Lateral epicondyle of humerus
use Humeral Shaft, Left
use Humeral Shaft, Right
Lateral femoral cutaneous nerve
use Nerve, Lumbar Plexus
Lateral malleolus
use Fibula, Left
use Fibula, Right
Lateral meniscus
use Joint, Knee, Left
use Joint, Knee, Right
Lateral nasal cartilage
use Nasal Mucosa and Soft Tissue
Lateral plantar artery
use Artery, Foot, Left
use Artery, Foot, Right
Lateral plantar nerve
use Nerve, Tibial
Lateral rectus muscle
use Muscle, Extraocular, Left
use Muscle, Extraocular, Right
Lateral sacral artery
use Artery, Internal Iliac, Left
use Artery, Internal Iliac, Right
Lateral sacral vein
use Vein, Hypogastric, Left
use Vein, Hypogastric, Right
Lateral sural cutaneous nerve
use Nerve, Peroneal
Lateral tarsal artery
use Artery, Foot, Left
use Artery, Foot, Right
Lateral temporomandibular ligament
use Bursa and Ligament, Head and Neck
Lateral thoracic artery
use Artery, Axillary, Left
use Artery, Axillary, Right
Latissimus dorsi muscle
use Muscle, Trunk, Left
use Muscle, Trunk, Right
Latissimus Dorsi Myocutaneous Flap
Replacement
Bilateral **0HRV075**
Left **0HRU075**
Right **0HRT075**
Transfer
Left **0KXG-**
Right **0KXF-**
Lavage
see Irrigation
Bronchial alveolar, diagnostic *see* Drainage, Respiratory System **0B9-**
Least splanchnic nerve
use Nerve, Thoracic Sympathetic
Left ascending lumbar vein
use Vein, Hemiazygos
Left atrioventricular valve
use Valve, Mitral
Left auricular appendix
use Atrium, Left
Left colic vein
use Vein, Colic
Left coronary sulcus
use Heart, Left
Left gastric artery
use Artery, Gastric
Left gastroepiploic artery
use Artery, Splenic
Left gastroepiploic vein
use Vein, Splenic
Left inferior phrenic vein
use Vein, Renal, Left
Left inferior pulmonary vein
use Vein, Pulmonary, Left
Left jugular trunk
use Lymphatic, Thoracic Duct
Left lateral ventricle
use Cerebral Ventricle
Left ovarian vein
use Vein, Renal, Left
Left second lumbar vein
use Vein, Renal, Left
Left subclavian trunk
use Lymphatic, Thoracic Duct
Left subcostal vein
use Vein, Hemiazygos
Left superior pulmonary vein
use Vein, Pulmonary, Left
Left suprarenal vein
use Vein, Renal, Left
Left testicular vein
use Vein, Renal, Left
Lengthening
Bone, with device *see* Insertion of Limb Lengthening Device
Muscle, by incision *see* Division, Muscles **0K8-**
Tendon, by incision *see* Division, Tendons **0L8-**
Leptomeninges, intracranial
use Cerebral Meninges

© 2018 Channel Publishing, Ltd.

Leptomeninges, spinal
use Spinal Meninges
Lesser alar cartilage
use Nasal Mucosa and Soft Tissue
Lesser occipital nerve
use Nerve, Cervical Plexus
Lesser omentum
use Omentum
Lesser saphenous vein
use Saphenous Vein, Left
use Saphenous Vein, Right
Lesser splanchnic nerve
use Nerve, Thoracic Sympathetic
Lesser trochanter
use Femur, Upper, Left
use Femur, Upper, Right
Lesser tuberosity
use Humeral Head, Left
use Humeral Head, Right
Lesser wing *use* Sphenoid Bone
Leukopheresis, therapeutic *see* Pheresis, Circulatory **6A55-**
Levator anguli oris muscle
use Muscle, Facial
Levator ani muscle
use Perineum Muscle
Levator labii superioris alaeque nasi muscle
use Muscle, Facial
Levator labii superioris muscle
use Muscle, Facial
Levator palpebrae superioris muscle
use Eyelid, Upper, Left
use Eyelid, Upper, Right
Levator scapulae muscle
use Muscle, Neck, Left
use Muscle, Neck, Right
Levator veli palatini muscle
use Muscle, Tongue, Palate, Pharynx
Levatores costarum muscle
use Muscle, Thorax, Left
use Muscle, Thorax, Right
LifeStent® (Flexstar) (XL) Vascular Stent System
use Intraluminal Device
Ligament of head of fibula
use Bursa and Ligament, Knee, Left
use Bursa and Ligament, Knee, Right
Ligament of the lateral malleolus
use Bursa and Ligament, Ankle, Left
use Bursa and Ligament, Ankle, Right
Ligamentum flavum, cervical
use Head and Neck Bursa and Ligament
Ligamentum flavum, lumbar
use Lower Spine Bursa and Ligament
Ligamentum flavum, thoracic
use Upper Spine Bursa and Ligament
Ligation *see* Occlusion
Ligation, hemorrhoid *see* Occlusion, Lower Veins, Hemorrhoidal Plexus
Light Therapy GZJZZZZ
Liner
Removal of device from
Hip
Left **0SPB09Z**
Right **0SP909Z**
Knee
Left **0SPD09Z**
Right **0SPC09Z**
Liner — *continued*
Revision of device in
Hip
Left **0SWB09Z**
Right **0SW909Z**
Knee
Left **0SWD09Z**
Right **0SWC09Z**
Supplement
Hip
Left **0SUB09Z**
Acetabular Surface **0SUE09Z**
Femoral Surface **0SUS09Z**
Right **0SU909Z**
Acetabular Surface **0SUA09Z**
Femoral Surface **0SUR09Z**
Knee
Left **0SUD09-**
Femoral Surface **0SUU09Z**
Tibial Surface **0SUW09Z**
Right **0SUC09-**
Femoral Surface **0SUT09Z**
Tibial Surface **0SUV09Z**
Lingual artery
use Artery, External Carotid, Left
use Artery, External Carotid, Right
Lingual tonsil
use Pharynx
Lingulectomy, lung
see Excision, Lung Lingula **0BBH-**
see Resection, Lung Lingula **0BTH-**
Lithotripsy
see Fragmentation
With removal of fragments *see* Extirpation
LITT (laser interstitial thermal therapy)
see Laser Interstitial Thermal Therapy
LIVIAN™ CRT-D
use Cardiac Resynchronization Defibrillator Pulse Generator in **0JH-**
Lobectomy
see Excision, Central Nervous System and Cranial Nerves **00B-**
see Excision, Endocrine System **0GB-**
see Excision, Hepatobiliary System and Pancreas **0FB-**
see Excision, Respiratory System **0BB-**
see Resection, Endocrine System **0GT-**
see Resection, Hepatobiliary System and Pancreas **0FT-**
see Resection, Respiratory System **0BT-**
Lobotomy *see* Division, Brain **0080-**
Localization
see Imaging
see Map
Locus ceruleus
use Pons
Long thoracic nerve
use Nerve, Brachial Plexus
Loop ileostomy *see* Bypass, Ileum **0D1B-**
Loop recorder, implantable
use Monitoring Device
Lower GI series *see* Fluoroscopy, Colon **BD14-**
Lumbar artery
use Aorta, Abdominal
Lumbar facet joint
use Joint, Lumbar Vertebral
Lumbar ganglion
use Nerve, Lumbar Sympathetic
Lumbar lymph node
use Lymphatic, Aortic
Lumbar lymphatic trunk
use Cisterna Chyli
Lumbar splanchnic nerve
use Nerve, Lumbar Sympathetic
Lumbosacral facet joint
use Joint, Lumbosacral
Lumbosacral trunk
use Nerve, Lumbar
Lumpectomy *see* Excision
Lunate bone
use Carpal, Left
use Carpal, Right
Lunotriquetral ligament
use Bursa and Ligament, Hand, Left
use Bursa and Ligament, Hand, Right
Lymphadenectomy
see Excision, Lymphatic and Hemic Systems **07B-**
see Resection, Lymphatic and Hemic Systems **07T-**
Lymphadenotomy *see* Drainage, Lymphatic and Hemic Systems **079-**
Lymphangiectomy
see Excision, Lymphatic and Hemic Systems **07B-**
see Resection, Lymphatic and Hemic Systems **07T-**
Lymphangiogram *see* Plain Radiography, Lymphatic System **B70-**
Lymphangioplasty
see Repair, Lymphatic and Hemic Systems **07Q-**
see Supplement, Lymphatic and Hemic Systems **07U-**
Lymphangiorrhaphy *see* Repair, Lymphatic and Hemic Systems **07Q-**
Lymphangiotomy *see* Drainage, Lymphatic and Hemic Systems **079-**
Lysis *see* Release

M

Macula
use Retina, Left
use Retina, Right
MAGEC® Spinal Bracing and Distraction System
use Magnetically Controlled Growth Rod(s) in New Technology
Magnet extraction, ocular foreign body *see* Extirpation, Eye **08C-**
Magnetically controlled growth rod(s)
Cervical **XNS3-**
Lumbar **XNS0-**
Thoracic **XNS4-**
Magnetic Resonance Imaging (MRI)
Abdomen **BW30-**
Ankle
Left **BQ3H-**
Right **BQ3G-**
Aorta
Abdominal **B430-**
Thoracic **B330-**
Arm
Left **BP3F-**
Right **BP3E-**
Artery
Celiac **B431-**
Cervico-Cerebral Arch **B33Q-**
Common Carotid, Bilateral **B335-**
Coronary
Bypass Graft, Multiple **B233-**
Multiple **B231-**
Internal Carotid, Bilateral **B338-**
Intracranial **B33R-**
Lower Extremity
Bilateral **B43H-**
Left **B43G-**
Right **B43F-**
Pelvic **B43C-**
Renal, Bilateral **B438-**
Spinal **B33M-**
Superior Mesenteric **B434-**
Upper Extremity
Bilateral **B33K-**
Left **B33J-**
Right **B33H-**
Vertebral, Bilateral **B33G-**
Bladder **BT30-**
Brachial Plexus **BW3P-**
Brain **B030-**
Breast
Bilateral **BH32-**
Left **BH31-**
Right **BH30-**
Calcaneus
Left **BQ3K-**
Right **BQ3J-**
Chest **BW33Y-**
Coccyx **BR3F-**
Connective Tissue
Lower Extremity **BL31-**
Upper Extremity **BL30-**
Corpora Cavernosa **BV30-**
Disc
Cervical **BR31-**
Lumbar **BR33-**
Thoracic **BR32-**
Ear **B930-**
Elbow
Left **BP3H-**
Right **BP3G-**
Eye
Bilateral **B837-**
Left **B836-**
Right **B835-**

© 2018 Channel Publishing, Ltd.

Magnetic Resonance Imaging (MRI) — *continued*
Femur
Left **BQ34-**
Right **BQ33-**
Fetal Abdomen **BY33-**
Fetal Extremity **BY35-**
Fetal Head **BY30-**
Fetal Heart **BY31-**
Fetal Spine **BY34-**
Fetal Thorax **BY32-**
Fetus, Whole **BY36-**
Foot
Left **BQ3M-**
Right **BQ3L-**
Forearm
Left **BP3K-**
Right **BP3J-**
Gland
Adrenal, Bilateral **BG32-**
Parathyroid **BG33-**
Parotid, Bilateral **B936-**
Salivary, Bilateral **B93D-**
Submandibular, Bilateral **B939-**
Thyroid **BG34-**
Head **BW38-**
Heart, Right and Left **B236-**
Hip
Left **BQ31-**
Right **BQ30-**
Intracranial Sinus **B532-**
Joint
Finger
Left **BP3D-**
Right **BP3C-**
Hand
Left **BP3D-**
Right **BP3C-**
Temporomandibular, Bilateral **BN39-**
Kidney
Bilateral **BT33-**
Left **BT32-**
Right **BT31-**
Transplant **BT39-**
Knee
Left **BQ38-**
Right **BQ37-**
Larynx **B93J-**
Leg
Left **BQ3F-**
Right **BQ3D-**
Liver **BF35-**
Liver and Spleen **BF36-**
Lung Apices **BB3G-**
Nasopharynx **B93F-**
Neck **BW3F-**
Nerve
Acoustic **B03C-**
Brachial Plexus **BW3P-**
Oropharynx **B93F-**
Ovary
Bilateral **BU35-**
Left **BU34-**
Right **BU33-**
Ovary and Uterus **BU3C-**
Pancreas **BF37-**
Patella
Left **BQ3W-**
Right **BQ3V-**
Pelvic Region **BW3G-**
Pelvis **BR3C-**
Pituitary Gland **B039-**
Plexus, Brachial **BW3P-**
Prostate **BV33-**
Retroperitoneum **BW3H-**
Sacrum **BR3F-**
Scrotum **BV34-**
Sella Turcica **B039-**

Magnetic Resonance Imaging (MRI) — *continued*
Shoulder
Left **BP39-**
Right **BP38-**
Sinus
Intracranial **B532-**
Paranasal **B932-**
Spinal Cord **B03B-**
Spine
Cervical **BR30-**
Lumbar **BR39-**
Thoracic **BR37-**
Spleen and Liver **BF36-**
Subcutaneous Tissue
Abdomen **BH3H-**
Extremity
Lower **BH3J-**
Upper **BH3F-**
Head **BH3D-**
Neck **BH3D-**
Pelvis **BH3H-**
Thorax **BH3G-**
Tendon
Lower Extremity **BL33-**
Upper Extremity **BL32-**
Testicle
Bilateral **BV37-**
Left **BV36-**
Right **BV35-**
Toe
Left **BQ3Q-**
Right **BQ3P-**
Uterus **BU36-**
Pregnant **BU3B-**
Uterus and Ovary **BU3C-**
Vagina **BU39-**
Vein
Cerebellar **B531-**
Cerebral **B531-**
Jugular, Bilateral **B535-**
Lower Extremity
Bilateral **B53D-**
Left **B53C-**
Right **B53B-**
Other **B53V-**
Pelvic (Iliac) Bilateral **B53H-**
Portal **B53T-**
Pulmonary, Bilateral **B53S-**
Renal, Bilateral **B53L-**
Spanchnic **B53T-**
Upper Extremity
Bilateral **B53P-**
Left **B53N-**
Right **B53M-**
Vena Cava
Inferior **B539-**
Superior **B538-**
Wrist
Left **BP3M-**
Right **BP3L-**
Malleotomy *see* Drainage, Ear, Nose, Sinus **099-**
Malleus
use Auditory Ossicle, Left
use Auditory Ossicle, Right
Mammaplasty, mammoplasty
see Alteration, Skin and Breast **0H0-**
see Repair, Skin and Breast **0HQ-**
see Replacement, Skin and Breast **0HR-**
see Supplement, Skin and Breast **0HU-**
Mammary duct
use Breast, Bilateral
use Breast, Left
use Breast, Right
Mammary gland
use Breast, Bilateral
use Breast, Left
use Breast, Right

Mammectomy
see Excision, Skin and Breast **0HB-**
see Resection, Skin and Breast **0HT-**
Mammillary body
use Hypothalamus
Mammography *see* Plain Radiography, Skin, Subcutaneous Tissue and Breast **BH0-**
Mammotomy *see* Drainage, Skin and Breast **0H9-**
Mandibular nerve
use Nerve, Trigeminal
Mandibular notch
use Mandible, Left
use Mandible, Right
Mandibulectomy
see Excision, Head and Facial Bones **0NB-**
see Resection, Head and Facial Bones **0NT-**
Manipulation
Adhesions *see* Release
Chiropractic *see* Chiropractic Manipulation
Manual removal, retained placenta
see Extraction, Products of Conception, Retained **10D1-**
Manubrium
use Sternum
Map
Basal Ganglia **00K8-**
Brain **00K0-**
Cerebellum **00KC-**
Cerebral Hemisphere **00K7-**
Conduction Mechanism **02K8-**
Hypothalamus **00KA-**
Medulla Oblongata **00KD-**
Pons **00KB-**
Thalamus **00K9-**
Mapping
Doppler ultrasound *see* Ultrasonography
Electrocardiogram only *see* Measurement, Cardiac **4A02-**
Mark IV Breathing Pacemaker System
use Stimulator Generator in Subcutaneous Tissue and Fascia
Marsupialization
see Drainage
see Excision
Massage, cardiac
External **5A12012**
Open **02QA0ZZ**
Masseter muscle
use Muscle, Head
Masseteric fascia
use Subcutaneous Tissue and Fascia, Face
Mastectomy
see Excision, Skin and Breast **0HB-**
see Resection, Skin and Breast **0HT-**
Mastoid (postauricular) lymph node
use Lymphatic, Neck, Left
use Lymphatic, Neck, Right
Mastoid air cells
use Sinus, Mastoid, Left
use Sinus, Mastoid, Right
Mastoid process
use Bone, Temporal, Left
use Bone, Temporal, Right
Mastoidectomy
see Excision, Ear, Nose, Sinus **09B-**
see Resection, Ear, Nose, Sinus **09T-**

Mastoidotomy *see* Drainage, Ear, Nose, Sinus **099-**
Mastopexy
see Reposition, Skin and Breast **0HS-**
see Repair, Skin and Breast **0HQ-**
Mastorrhaphy *see* Repair, Skin and Breast **0HQ-**
Mastotomy *see* Drainage, Skin and Breast **0H9-**
Maxillary artery
use Artery, External Carotid, Left
use Artery, External Carotid, Right
Maxillary nerve
use Nerve, Trigeminal
Maximo II DR (VR)
use Defibrillator, Generator in **0JH-**
Maximo II DR CRT-D
use Cardiac Resynchronization Defibrillator Pulse Generator in **0JH-**
Measurement
Arterial
Flow
Coronary **4A03-**
Peripheral **4A03-**
Pulmonary **4A03-**
Pressure
Coronary **4A03-**
Peripheral **4A03-**
Pulmonary **4A03-**
Thoracic, Other **4A03-**
Pulse
Coronary **4A03-**
Peripheral **4A03-**
Pulmonary **4A03-**
Saturation, Peripheral **4A03-**
Sound, Peripheral **4A03-**
Biliary
Flow **4A0C-**
Pressure **4A0C-**
Cardiac
Action Currents **4A02-**
Defibrillator **4B02XTZ**
Electrical Activity **4A02-**
Guidance **4A02X4A**
No Qualifier **4A02X4Z**
Output **4A02-**
Pacemaker **4B02XSZ**
Rate **4A02-**
Rhythm **4A02-**
Sampling and Pressure
Bilateral **4A02-**
Left Heart **4A02-**
Right Heart **4A02-**
Sound **4A02-**
Total Activity, Stress **4A02XM4**
Central Nervous
Conductivity **4A00-**
Electrical Activity **4A00-**
Pressure **4A000BZ**
Intracranial **4A00-**
Saturation, Intracranial **4A00-**
Stimulator **4B00XVZ**
Temperature, Intracranial **4A00-**
Circulatory, Volume **4A05XLZ**
Gastrointestinal
Motility **4A0B-**
Pressure **4A0B-**
Secretion **4A0B-**
Lymphatic
Flow **4A06-**
Pressure **4A06-**
Metabolism **4A0Z-**
Musculoskeletal
Contractility **4A0F-**
Stimulator **4B0FXVZ**
Olfactory, Acuity **4A08X0Z**

© 2018 Channel Publishing, Ltd.

Measurement — *continued*
Peripheral Nervous
Conductivity
Motor **4A01**-
Sensory **4A01**-
Electrical Activity **4A01**-
Stimulator **4B01**XVZ
Products of Conception
Cardiac
Electrical Activity **4A0H**-
Rate **4A0H**-
Rhythm **4A0H**-
Sound **4A0H**-
Nervous
Conductivity **4A0J**-
Electrical Activity **4A0J**-
Pressure **4A0J**-
Respiratory
Capacity **4A09**-
Flow **4A09**-
Pacemaker **4B09**XSZ
Rate **4A09**-
Resistance **4A09**-
Total Activity **4A09**-
Volume **4A09**-
Sleep **4A0Z**XQZ
Temperature **4A0Z**-
Urinary
Contractility **4A0D**-
Flow **4A0D**-
Pressure **4A0D**-
Resistance **4A0D**-
Volume **4A0D**-
Venous
Flow
Central **4A04**-
Peripheral **4A04**-
Portal **4A04**-
Pulmonary **4A04**-
Pressure
Central **4A04**-
Peripheral **4A04**-
Portal **4A04**-
Pulmonary **4A04**-
Pulse
Central **4A04**-
Peripheral **4A04**-
Portal **4A04**-
Pulmonary **4A04**-
Saturation, Peripheral **4A04**-
Visual
Acuity **4A07**X0Z
Mobility **4A07**X7Z
Pressure **4A07**XBZ
Meatoplasty, urethra *see* Repair, Urethra **0TQD**-
Meatotomy *see* Drainage, Urinary System **0T9**-
Mechanical ventilation *see* Performance, Respiratory **5A19**-
Medial canthus
use Eyelid, Lower, Left
use Eyelid, Lower, Right
Medial collateral ligament (MCL)
use Bursa and Ligament, Knee, Left
use Bursa and Ligament, Knee, Right
Medial condyle of femur
use Femur, Lower, Left
use Femur, Lower, Right
Medial condyle of tibia
use Tibia, Left
use Tibia, Right
Medial cuneiform bone
use Tarsal, Left
use Tarsal, Right
Medial epicondyle of femur
use Femur, Lower, Left
use Femur, Lower, Right
Medial epicondyle of humerus
use Humeral Shaft, Left
use Humeral Shaft, Right
Medial malleolus
use Tibia, Left
use Tibia, Right
Medial meniscus
use Joint, Knee, Left
use Joint, Knee, Right
Medial plantar artery
use Artery, Foot, Left
use Artery, Foot, Right
Medial plantar nerve
use Nerve, Tibial
Medial popliteal nerve
use Nerve, Tibial
Medial rectus muscle
use Muscle, Extraocular, Left
use Muscle, Extraocular, Right
Medial sural cutaneous nerve
use Nerve, Tibial
Median antebrachial vein
use Vein, Basilic, Left
use Vein, Basilic, Right
Median cubital vein
use Vein, Basilic, Left
use Vein, Basilic, Right
Median sacral artery
use Aorta, Abdominal
Mediastinal cavity
use Mediastinum
Mediastinal lymph node
use Lymphatic, Thorax
Mediastinal space
use Mediastinum
Mediastinoscopy **0WJC**4ZZ
Medication Management **GZ3**ZZZZ
For substance abuse
Antabuse **HZ83**ZZZ
Bupropion **HZ87**ZZZ
Clonidine **HZ86**ZZZ
Levo-alpha-acetyl-methadol (LAAM) **HZ82**ZZZ
Methadone Maintenance **HZ81**ZZZ
Naloxone **HZ85**ZZZ
Naltrexone **HZ84**ZZZ
Nicotine Replacement **HZ80**ZZZ
Other Replacement Medication **HZ89**ZZZ
Psychiatric Medication **HZ88**ZZZ
Meditation **8E0**ZXY5
Medtronic Endurant® II AAA stent graft system
use Intraluminal Device
Meissner's (submucous) plexus
use Nerve, Abdominal Sympathetic
Melody® transcatheter pulmonary valve
use Zooplastic Tissue in Heart and Great Vessels
Membranous urethra
use Urethra
Meningeorrhaphy
see Repair, Cerebral Meninges **00Q1**-
see Repair, Spinal Meninges **00QT**-
Meniscectomy, knee
see Excision, Joint, Knee, Left **0SBD**-
see Excision, Joint, Knee, Right **0SBC**-
Mental foramen
use Mandible, Left
use Mandible, Right
Mentalis muscle
use Muscle, Facial
Mentoplasty *see* Alteration, Jaw, Lower **0W05**-
Mesenterectomy *see* Excision, Mesentery **0DBV**-
Mesenteriorrhaphy, mesenterorrhaphy *see* Repair, Mesentery **0DQV**-
Mesenteriplication *see* Repair, Mesentery **0DQV**-
Mesoappendix
use Mesentery
Mesocolon
use Mesentery
Metacarpal ligament
use Bursa and Ligament, Hand, Left
use Bursa and Ligament, Hand, Right
Metacarpophalangeal ligament
use Bursa and Ligament, Hand, Left
use Bursa and Ligament, Hand, Right
Metal on metal bearing surface
use Synthetic Substitute, Metal in **0SR**-
Metatarsal ligament
use Bursa and Ligament, Foot, Left
use Bursa and Ligament, Foot, Right
Metatarsectomy
see Excision, Lower Bones **0QB**-
see Resection, Lower Bones **0QT**-
Metatarsophalangeal (MTP) joint
use Joint, Metatarsal-Phalangeal, Left
use Joint, Metatarsal-Phalangeal, Right
Metatarsophalangeal ligament
use Bursa and Ligament, Foot, Left
use Bursa and Ligament, Foot, Right
Metathalamus
use Thalamus
Micro-Driver stent (RX) (OTW)
use Intraluminal Device
MicroMed HeartAssist
use Implantable Heart Assist System in Heart and Great Vessels
Micrus CERECYTE microcoil
use Intraluminal Device, Bioactive in Upper Arteries
Midcarpal joint
use Joint, Carpal, Left
use Joint, Carpal, Right
Middle cardiac nerve
use Nerve, Thoracic Sympathetic
Middle cerebral artery
use Artery, Intracranial
Middle cerebral vein
use Vein, Intracranial
Middle colic vein
use Vein, Colic
Middle genicular artery
use Artery, Popliteal, Left
use Artery, Popliteal, Right
Middle hemorrhoidal vein
use Vein, Hypogastric, Left
use Vein, Hypogastric, Right
Middle rectal artery
use Artery, Internal Iliac, Left
use Artery, Internal Iliac, Right
Middle suprarenal artery
use Aorta, Abdominal
Middle temporal artery
use Artery, Temporal, Left
use Artery, Temporal, Right
Middle turbinate
use Turbinate, Nasal
MIRODERM™ Biologic Wound Matrix
use Skin Substitute, Porcine Liver Derived in New Technology
MitraClip valve repair system
use Synthetic Substitute
Mitral annulus
use Valve, Mitral
Mitroflow® Aortic Pericardial Heart Valve
use Zooplastic Tissue in Heart and Great Vessels
Mobilization, adhesions *see* Release
Molar gland
use Buccal Mucosa
Monitoring
Arterial
Flow
Coronary **4A13**-
Peripheral **4A13**-
Pulmonary **4A13**-
Pressure
Coronary **4A13**-
Peripheral **4A13**-
Pulmonary **4A13**-
Pulse
Coronary **4A13**-
Peripheral **4A13**-
Pulmonary **4A13**-
Saturation, Peripheral **4A13**-
Sound, Peripheral **4A13**-
Cardiac
Electrical Activity **4A12**-
Ambulatory **4A12**X45
No Qualifier **4A12**X4Z
Output **4A12**-
Rate **4A12**-
Rhythm **4A12**-
Sound **4A12**-
Total Activity, Stress **4A12**XM4
Vascular Perfusion, Indocyanine Green Dye **4A12**XSH
Central Nervous
Conductivity **4A10**-
Electrical Activity
Intraoperative **4A10**-
No Qualifier **4A10**-
Pressure **4A10**0BZ
Intracranial **4A10**-
Saturation, Intracranial **4A10**-
Temperature, Intracranial **4A10**-
Gastrointestinal
Motility **4A1B**
Pressure **4A1B**-
Secretion **4A1B**-
Vascular Perfusion, Indocyanine Green Dye **4A1B**XSH
Intraoperative Knee Replacement Sensor **XR2**-
Lymphatic
Flow **4A16**-
Pressure **4A16**-
Peripheral Nervous
Conductivity
Motor **4A11**-
Sensory **4A11**-
Electrical Activity
Intraoperative **4A11**-
No Qualifier **4A11**-
Products of Conception
Cardiac
Electrical Activity **4A1H**-
Rate **4A1H**-
Rhythm **4A1H**-
Sound **4A1H**-
Nervous
Conductivity **4A1J**-
Electrical Activity **4A1J**-
Pressure **4A1J**-
Respiratory
Capacity **4A19**-
Flow **4A19**-
Rate **4A19**-
Resistance **4A19**-
Volume **4A19**-
Skin and Breast
Vascular Perfusion, Indocyanine Green Dye **4A1G**XSH
Sleep **4A1Z**XQZ

PROCEDURE INDEX

© 2018 Channel Publishing, Ltd.

Monitoring — *continued*
Temperature **4A1Z-**
Urinary
Contractility **4A1D-**
Flow **4A1D-**
Pressure **4A1D-**
Resistance **4A1D-**
Volume **4A1D-**
Venous
Flow
Central **4A14-**
Peripheral **4A14-**
Portal **4A14-**
Pulmonary **4A14-**
Pressure
Central **4A14-**
Peripheral **4A14-**
Portal **4A14-**
Pulmonary **4A14-**
Pulse
Central **4A14-**
Peripheral **4A14-**
Portal **4A14-**
Pulmonary **4A14-**
Saturation
Central **4A14-**
Portal **4A14-**
Pulmonary **4A14-**
Monitoring Device, Hemodynamic
Abdomen **0JH8-**
Chest **0JH6-**
Mosaic Bioprosthesis (aortic) (mitral) valve
use Zooplastic Tissue in Heart and Great Vessels
Motor Function Assessment F01-
Motor Treatment F07-
MR Angiography
see Magnetic Resonance Imaging (MRI), Heart **B23-**
see Magnetic Resonance Imaging (MRI), Lower Arteries **B43-**
see Magnetic Resonance Imaging (MRI), Upper Arteries **B33-**
MULTI-LINK (VISION) (MINI-VISION) (ULTRA) Coronary Stent System
use Intraluminal Device
Multiple sleep latency test 4A0ZXQZ
Musculocutaneous nerve
use Nerve, Brachial Plexus
Musculopexy
see Repair, Muscles **0KQ-**
see Reposition, Muscles **0KS-**
Musculophrenic artery
use Artery, Internal Mammary, Left
use Artery, Internal Mammary, Right
Musculoplasty
see Repair, Muscles **0KQ-**
see Supplement, Muscles **0KU-**
Musculorrhaphy *see* Repair, Muscles **0KQ-**
Musculospiral nerve
use Nerve, Radial
Myectomy
see Excision, Muscles **0KB-**
see Resection, Muscles **0KT-**
Myelencephalon
use Medulla Oblongata
Myelogram
CT *see* Computerized Tomography (CT Scan), Central Nervous System **B02-**
MRI *see* Magnetic Resonance Imaging (MRI), Central Nervous System **B03-**
Myenteric (Auerbach's) plexus
use Nerve, Abdominal Sympathetic
Myocardial Bridge Release
see Release, Artery, Coronary
Myomectomy *see* Excision, Female Reproductive System **0UB-**
Myometrium
use Uterus
Myopexy
see Repair, Muscles **0KQ-**
see Reposition, Muscles **0KS-**
Myoplasty
see Repair, Muscles **0KQ-**
see Supplement, Muscles **0KU-**
Myorrhaphy *see* Repair, Muscles **0KQ-**
Myoscopy *see* Inspection, Muscles **0KJ-**
Myotomy
see Division, Muscles **0K8-**
see Drainage, Muscles **0K9-**
Myringectomy
see Excision, Ear, Nose, Sinus **09B-**
see Resection, Ear, Nose, Sinus **09T-**
Myringoplasty
see Repair, Ear, Nose, Sinus **09Q-**
see Replacement, Ear, Nose, Sinus **09R-**
see Supplement, Ear, Nose, Sinus **09U-**
Myringostomy *see* Drainage, Ear, Nose, Sinus **099-**
Myringotomy *see* Drainage, Ear, Nose, Sinus **099-**

N

Nail bed
use Finger Nail
use Toe Nail
Nail plate
use Finger Nail
use Toe Nail
nanoLOCK™ interbody fusion device
use Interbody Fusion Device, Nanotextured Surface in New Technology
Narcosynthesis GZGZZZZ
Nasal cavity
use Nasal Mucosa and Soft Tissue
Nasal concha
use Turbinate, Nasal
Nasalis muscle
use Muscle, Facial
Nasolacrimal duct
use Duct, Lacrimal, Left
use Duct, Lacrimal, Right
Nasopharyngeal airway (NPA)
use Intraluminal Device, Airway in Ear, Nose, Sinus
Navicular bone
use Tarsal, Left
use Tarsal, Right
Near Infrared Spectroscopy, Circulatory System 8E023DZ
Neck of femur
use Femur, Upper, Left
use Femur, Upper, Right
Neck of humerus (anatomical) (surgical)
use Humeral Head, Left
use Humeral Head, Right
Nephrectomy
see Excision, Urinary System **0TB-**
see Resection, Urinary System **0TT-**
Nephrolithotomy *see* Extirpation, Urinary System **0TC-**
Nephrolysis *see* Release, Urinary System **0TN-**
Nephropexy
see Repair, Urinary System **0TQ-**
see Reposition, Urinary System **0TS-**
Nephroplasty
see Repair, Urinary System **0TQ-**
see Supplement, Urinary System **0TU-**
Nephropyeloureterostomy
see Bypass, Urinary System **0T1-**
see Drainage, Urinary System **0T9-**
Nephrorrhaphy *see* Repair, Urinary System **0TQ-**
Nephroscopy, transurethral 0TJ58ZZ
Nephrostomy
see Bypass, Urinary System **0T1-**
see Drainage, Urinary System **0T9-**
Nephrotomography
see Fluoroscopy, Urinary System **BT1-**
see Plain Radiography, Urinary System **BT0-**
Nephrotomy
see Drainage, Urinary System **0T9-**
see Division, Urinary System **0T8-**
Nerve conduction study
see Measurement, Central Nervous **4A00-**
see Measurement, Peripheral Nervous **4A01-**
Nerve Function Assessment F01-
Nerve to the stapedius
use Nerve, Facial
Nesiritide
use Human B-type Natriuretic Peptide
Neurectomy
see Excision, Central Nervous System and Cranial Nerves **00B-**
see Excision, Peripheral Nervous System **01B-**
Neurexeresis
see Extraction, Central Nervous System and Cranial Nerves **00D-**
see Extraction, Peripheral Nervous System **01D-**
Neurohypophysis
use Gland, Pituitary
Neurolysis
see Release, Central Nervous System and Cranial Nerves **00N-**
see Release, Peripheral Nervous System **01N-**
Neuromuscular electrical stimulation (NEMS) lead
use Stimulator Lead in Muscles
Neurophysiologic monitoring
see Monitoring, Central Nervous **4A10-**
Neuroplasty
see Repair, Central Nervous System and Cranial Nerves **00Q-**
see Repair, Peripheral Nervous System **01Q-**
see Supplement, Central Nervous System and Cranial Nerves **00U-**
see Supplement, Peripheral Nervous System **01U-**
Neurorrhaphy
see Repair, Central Nervous System and Cranial Nerves **00Q-**
see Repair, Peripheral Nervous System **01Q-**
Neurostimulator Generator
Insertion of device in, Skull **0NH00NZ**
Removal of device from, Skull **0NP00NZ**
Revision of device in, Skull **0NW00NZ**
Neurostimulator generator, multiple channel
use Stimulator Generator, Multiple Array in **0JH-**
Neurostimulator generator, multiple channel rechargeable
use Stimulator Generator, Multiple Array Rechargeable in **0JH-**
Neurostimulator generator, single channel
use Stimulator Generator, Single Array in **0JH-**
Neurostimulator generator, single channel rechargeable
use Stimulator Generator, Single Array Rechargeable in **0JH-**
Neurostimulator Lead
Insertion of device in
Brain **00H0-**
Cerebral Ventricle **00H6-**
Nerve
Cranial **00HE-**
Peripheral **01HY-**
Spinal Canal **00HU-**
Spinal Cord **00HV-**
Vein
Azygos **05H0-**
Innominate
Left **05H4-**
Right **05H3-**

© 2018 Channel Publishing, Ltd.

Neurostimulator Lead — *continued*
Removal of device from
Brain **00P0-**
Cerebral Ventricle **00P6-**
Nerve
Cranial **00PE-**
Peripheral **01PY-**
Spinal Canal **00PU-**
Spinal Cord **00PV-**
Vein
Azygos **05P0-**
Innominate
Left **05P4-**
Right **05P3-**
Revision of device in
Brain **00W0-**
Cerebral Ventricle **00W6-**
Nerve
Cranial **00WE-**
Peripheral **01WY-**
Spinal Canal **00WU-**
Spinal Cord **00WV-**
Vein
Azygos **05W0-**
Innominate
Left **05W4-**
Right **05W3-**
Neurotomy
see Division, Central Nervous System and Cranial Nerves **008-**
see Division, Peripheral Nervous System **018-**
Neurotripsy
see Destruction, Central Nervous System and Cranial Nerves **005-**
see Destruction, Peripheral Nervous System **015-**
Neutralization plate
use Internal Fixation Device in Head and Facial Bones
use Internal Fixation Device in Lower Bones
use Internal Fixation Device in Upper Bones
New Technology
Andexanet Alfa, Factor Xa Inhibitor Reversal Agent **XW0-**
Bezlotoxumab Monoclonal Antibody **XW0-**
Blinatumomab antineoplastic immunotherapy **XW0-**
Ceftazidime-avibactam anti-infective **XW0-**
Cerebral Embolic Filtration, Dual Filter **X2A5312**
Concentrated Bone Marrow Aspirate **XK02303**
Cytarabine and Daunorubicin Liposome Antineoplastic **XW0-**
Defibrotide Sodium Anticoagulant **XW0-**
Destruction, Prostate, Robotic Waterjet Ablation **XV508A4**
Endothelial Damage Inhibitor **XY0VX83**
Engineered Autologous Chimeric Antigen Receptor T-cell Immunotherapy **XW0-**
Fusion
Cervical Vertebral
2 or more
Nanotextured Surface **XRG2092**
Radiolucent Porous **XRG20F3**
Interbody Fusion Device
Nanotextured Surface **XRG1092**
Radiolucent Porous **XRG10F3**

New Technology — *continued*
Fusion — *continued*
Cervicothoracic Vertebral
Nanotextured Surface **XRG4092**
Radiolucent Porous **XRG40F3**
Lumbar Vertebral
2 or more
Nanotextured Surface **XRGC092**
Radiolucent Porous **XRGC0F3**
Interbody Fusion Device
Nanotextured Surface **XRGB092**
Radiolucent Porous **XRGB0F3**
Lumbosacral
Nanotextured Surface **XRGD092**
Radiolucent Porous **XRGD0F3**
Occipital-cervical
Nanotextured Surface **XRG0092**
Radiolucent Porous **XRG00F3**
Thoracic Vertebral
2 to 7
Nanotextured Surface **XRG7092**
Radiolucent Porous **XRG70F3**
8 or more
Nanotextured Surface **XRG8092**
Radiolucent Porous **XRG80F3**
Interbody Fusion Device
Nanotextured Surface **XRG6092**
Radiolucent Porous **XRG60F3**
Thoracolumbar Vertebral
Nanotextured Surface **XRGA092**
Radiolucent Porous **XRGA0F3**
Idarucizumab, Dabigatran reversal agent **XW0-**
Intraoperative knee replacement sensor **XR2-**
Isavuconazole anti-infective **XW0-**
Orbital atherectomy technology **X2C-**
Other New Technology Therapeutic Substance **XW0-**
Plazomicin Anti-infective **XW0-**
Replacement
Skin Substitute, Porcine Liver Derived **XHRPXL2**
Zooplastic Tissue, Rapid Deployment Technique **X2RF-**
Reposition
Cervical, Magnetically Controlled Growth Rod(s) **XNS3-**
Lumbar, Magnetically Controlled Growth Rod(s) **XNS0-**
Thoracic, Magnetically Controlled Growth Rod(s) **XNS4-**
Synthetic Human Angiotensin II **XW0-**
Uridine Triacetate **XW0DX82**
Ninth cranial nerve
use Nerve, Glossopharyngeal
Nitinol framed polymer mesh
use Synthetic Substitute
Non-tunneled central venous catheter
use Infusion Device

Nonimaging Nuclear Medicine Assay
Bladder, Kidneys and Ureters **CT63-**
Blood **C763-**
Kidneys, Ureters and Bladder **CT63-**
Lymphatics and Hematologic System **C76YYZZ**
Ureters, Kidneys and Bladder **CT63-**
Urinary System **CT6YYZZ**
Nonimaging Nuclear Medicine Probe
Abdomen **CW50-**
Abdomen and Chest **CW54-**
Abdomen and Pelvis **CW51-**
Brain **C050-**
Central Nervous System **C05YYZZ**
Chest **CW53-**
Chest and Abdomen **CW54-**
Chest and Neck **CW56-**
Extremity
Lower **CP5PZZZ**
Upper **CP5NZZZ**
Head and Neck **CW5B-**
Heart **C25YYZZ**
Right and Left **C256-**
Lymphatics
Head **C75J-**
Head and Neck **C755-**
Lower Extremity **C75P-**
Neck **C75K-**
Pelvic **C75D-**
Trunk **C75M-**
Upper Chest **C75L-**
Upper Extremity **C75N**
Lymphatics and Hematologic System **C76YYZZ**
Musculoskeletal System, Other **CP5YYZZ**
Neck and Chest **CW56-**
Neck and Head **CW5B-**
Pelvic Region **CW5J-**
Pelvis and Abdomen **CW51-**
Spine **CP55ZZZ**
Nonimaging Nuclear Medicine Uptake
Endocrine System **CG4YYZZ**
Gland, Thyroid **CG42-**
Nostril
use Nasal Mucosa and Soft Tissue
Novacor Left Ventricular Assist Device
use Implantable Heart Assist System in Heart and Great Vessels
Novation® Ceramic AHS® (Articulation Hip System)
use Synthetic Substitute, Ceramic in **0SR-**
Nuclear medicine
see Nonimaging Nuclear Medicine Assay
see Nonimaging Nuclear Medicine Probe
see Nonimaging Nuclear Medicine Uptake
see Planar Nuclear Medicine Imaging
see Positron Emission Tomographic (PET) Imaging
see Systemic Nuclear Medicine Therapy
see Tomographic (Tomo) Nuclear Medicine Imaging
Nuclear scintigraphy *see* Nuclear Medicine
Nutrition, concentrated substances
Enteral infusion **3E0G36Z**
Parenteral (peripheral) infusion
see Introduction of Nutritional Substance

O

Obliteration *see* Destruction
Obturator artery
use Artery, Internal Iliac, Left
use Artery, Internal Iliac, Right
Obturator lymph node
use Lymphatic, Pelvis
Obturator muscle
use Muscle, Hip, Left
use Muscle, Hip, Right
Obturator nerve
use Nerve, Lumbar Plexus
Obturator vein
use Vein, Hypogastric, Left
use Vein, Hypogastric, Right
Obtuse margin
use Heart, Left
Occipital artery
use Artery, External Carotid, Left
use Artery, External Carotid, Right
Occipital lobe
use Cerebral Hemisphere
Occipital lymph node
use Lymphatic, Neck, Left
use Lymphatic, Neck, Right
Occipitofrontalis muscle
use Muscle, Facial
Occlusion
Ampulla of Vater **0FLC-**
Anus **0DLQ-**
Aorta
Abdominal **04L0-**
Thoracic, Descending **02LW3DJ**
Artery
Anterior Tibial
Left **04LQ-**
Right **04LP-**
Axillary
Left **03L6-**
Right **03L5**
Brachial
Left **03L8-**
Right **03L7-**
Celiac **04L1-**
Colic
Left **04L7-**
Middle **04L8-**
Right **04L6-**
Common Carotid
Left **03LJ-**
Right **03LH-**
Common Iliac
Left **04LD-**
Right **04LC-**
External Carotid
Left **03LN-**
Right **03LM-**
External Iliac
Left **04LJ-**
Right **04LH-**
Face **03LR-**
Femoral
Left **04LL-**
Right **04LK-**
Foot
Left **04LW-**
Right **04LV-**
Gastric **04L2-**
Hand
Left **03LF-**
Right **03LD-**
Hepatic **04L3-**
Inferior Mesenteric **04LB-**
Innominate **03L2-**
Internal Carotid
Left **03LL-**
Right **03LK-**
Internal Iliac
Left, **04LF-**
Right, **04LE-**

PROCEDURE INDEX

© 2018 Channel Publishing, Ltd.

Occlusion — *continued*
Artery — *continued*
Internal Mammary
Left **03L1**-
Right **03L0**-
Intracranial **03LG**-
Lower **04LY**-
Peroneal
Left **04LU**-
Right **04LT**-
Popliteal
Left **04LN**-
Right **04LM**-
Posterior Tibial
Left **04LS**-
Right **04LR**-
Pulmonary
Left **02LR**-
Right **02LQ**-
Pulmonary Trunk **02LP**-
Radial
Left **03LC**-
Right **03LB**-
Renal
Left **04LA**-
Right **04L9**-
Splenic **04L4**-
Subclavian
Left **03L4**-
Right **03L3**-
Superior Mesenteric **04L5**-
Temporal
Left **03LT**-
Right **03LS**-
Thyroid
Left **03LV**-
Right **03LU**-
Ulnar
Left **03LA**-
Right **03L9**-
Upper **03LY**-
Vertebral
Left **03LQ**-
Right **03LP**-
Atrium, Left **02L7**-
Bladder **0TLB**-
Bladder Neck **0TLC**-
Bronchus
Lingula **0BL9**-
Lower Lobe
Left **0BLB**-
Right **0BL6**-
Main
Left **0BL7**-
Right **0BL3**-
Middle Lobe, Right **0BL5**-
Upper Lobe
Left **0BL8**-
Right **0BL4**-
Carina **0BL2**-
Cecum **0DLH**-
Cisterna Chyli **07LL**-
Colon
Ascending **0DLK**-
Descending **0DLM**-
Sigmoid **0DLN**-
Transverse **0DLL**-
Cord
Bilateral **0VLH**-
Left **0VLG**-
Right **0VLF**-
Cul-de-sac **0ULF**-
Duct
Common Bile **0FL9**-
Cystic **0FL8**-
Hepatic
Common **0FL7**-
Left **0FL6**-
Right **0FL5**-
Lacrimal
Left **08LY**-
Right **08LX**-
Pancreatic **0FLD**-
Accessory **0FLF**-

Occlusion — *continued*
Duct — *continued*
Parotid
Left **0CLC**-
Right **0CLB**-
Duodenum **0DL9**-
Esophagogastric Junction **0DL4**-
Esophagus **0DL5**-
Lower **0DL3**-
Middle **0DL2**-
Upper **0DL1**-
Fallopian Tube
Left **0UL6**-
Right **0UL5**-
Fallopian Tubes, Bilateral **0UL7**-
Ileocecal Valve **0DLC**-
Ileum **0DLB**-
Intestine
Large **0DLE**-
Left **0DLG**-
Right **0DLF**-
Small **0DL8**-
Jejunum **0DLA**-
Kidney Pelvis
Left **0TL4**-
Right **0TL3**-
Left atrial appendage (LAA) *see* Occlusion, Atrium, Left **02L7**-
Lymphatic
Aortic **07LD**-
Axillary
Left **07L6**-
Right **07L5**-
Head **07L0**-
Inguinal
Left **07LJ**-
Right **07LH**-
Internal Mammary
Left **07L9**-
Right **07L8**-
Lower Extremity
Left **07LG**-
Right **07LF**-
Mesenteric **07LB**-
Neck
Left **07L2**-
Right **07L1**-
Pelvis **07LC**-
Thoracic Duct **07LK**-
Thorax **07L7**-
Upper Extremity
Left **07L4**-
Right **07L3**-
Rectum **0DLP**-
Stomach **0DL6**-
Pylorus **0DL7**-
Trachea **0BL1**-
Ureter
Left **0TL7**-
Right **0TL6**-
Urethra **0TLD**-
Vagina **0ULG**-
Valve, Pulmonary **02LH**-
Vas Deferens
Bilateral **0VLQ**-
Left **0VLP**-
Right **0VLN**-
Vein
Axillary
Left **05L8**-
Right **05L7**-
Azygos **05L0**-
Basilic
Left **05LC**-
Right **05LB**-
Brachial
Left **05LA**-
Right **05L9**-
Cephalic
Left **05LF**-
Right **05LD**-
Colic **06L7**-

Occlusion — *continued*
Vein — *continued*
Common Iliac
Left **06LD**-
Right **06LC**-
Esophageal **06L3**-
External Iliac
Left **06LG**-
Right **06LF**-
External Jugular
Left **05LQ**-
Right **05LP**-
Face
Left **05LV**-
Right **05LT**-
Femoral
Left **06LN**-
Right **06LM**-
Foot
Left **06LV**-
Right **06LT**-
Gastric **06L2**-
Hand
Left **05LH**-
Right **05LG**-
Hemiazygos **05L1**-
Hepatic **06L4**-
Hypogastric
Left **06LJ**-
Right **06LH**-
Inferior Mesenteric **06L6**-
Innominate
Left **05L4**-
Right **05L3**-
Internal Jugular
Left **05LN**-
Right **05LM**-
Intracranial **05LL**-
Lower **06LY**-
Portal **06L8**-
Pulmonary
Left **02LT**-
Right **02LS**-
Renal
Left **06LB**-
Right **06L9**-
Saphenous
Left **06LQ**-
Right **06LP**-
Splenic **06L1**-
Subclavian
Left **05L6**-
Right **05L5**-
Superior Mesenteric **06L5**-
Upper **05LY**-
Vertebral
Left **05LS**-
Right **05LR**-
Vena Cava
Inferior **06L0**-
Superior **02LV**-
Occlusion, REBOA (resuscitative endovascular balloon occlusion of the aorta)
Abdominal Aorta **04L03DJ**
Thoracic Aorta, Descending **02LW3DJ**
Occupational therapy *see* Activities of Daily Living Treatment, Rehabilitation **F08**-
Odentectomy
see Excision, Mouth and Throat **0CB**-
see Resection, Mouth and Throat **0CT**-
Odontoid process
use Cervical Vertebra
Olecranon bursa
use Bursa and Ligament, Elbow, Left
use Bursa and Ligament, Elbow, Right

Olecranon process
use Ulna, Left
use Ulna, Right
Olfactory bulb
use Nerve, Olfactory
Omentectomy, omentumectomy
see Excision, Gastrointestinal System **0DB**-
see Resection, Gastrointestinal System **0DT**-
Omentofixation *see* Repair, Gastrointestinal System **0DQ**-
Omentoplasty
see Repair, Gastrointestinal System **0DQ**-
see Replacement, Gastrointestinal System **0DR**-
see Supplement, Gastrointestinal System **0DU**-
Omentorrhaphy *see* Repair, Gastrointestinal System **0DQ**-
Omentotomy *see* Drainage, Gastrointestinal System **0D9**-
Omnilink Elite Vascular Balloon Expandable Stent System
use Intraluminal Device
Onychectomy
see Excision, Skin and Breast **0HB**-
see Resection, Skin and Breast **0HT**-
Onychoplasty
see Repair, Skin and Breast **0HQ**-
see Replacement, Skin and Breast **0HR**-
Onychotomy *see* Drainage, Skin and Breast **0H9**-
Oophorectomy
see Excision, Female Reproductive System **0UB**-
see Resection, Female Reproductive System **0UT**-
Oophoropexy
see Repair, Female Reproductive System **0UQ**-
see Reposition, Female Reproductive System **0US**-
Oophoroplasty
see Repair, Female Reproductive System **0UQ**-
see Supplement, Female Reproductive System **0UU**-
Oophororrhaphy *see* Repair, Female Reproductive System **0UQ**-
Oophorostomy *see* Drainage, Female Reproductive System **0U9**-
Oophorotomy
see Drainage, Female Reproductive System **0U9**-
see Division, Female Reproductive System **0U8**-
Oophorrhaphy *see* Repair, Female Reproductive System **0UQ**-
Open Pivot Aortic Valve Graft (AVG)
use Synthetic Substitute
Open Pivot (mechanical) valve
use Synthetic Substitute
Ophthalmic artery
use Intracranial Artery
Ophthalmic nerve
use Nerve, Trigeminal
Ophthalmic vein
use Vein, Intracranial
Opponensplasty
Tendon replacement *see* Replacement, Tendons **0LR**-
Tendon transfer *see* Transfer, Tendons **0LX**-
Optic chiasma
use Nerve, Optic

© 2018 Channel Publishing, Ltd.

Optic disc
use Retina, Left
use Retina, Right
Optic foramen *use* Sphenoid Bone
Optical coherence tomography, intravascular *see* Computerized Tomography (CT Scan)
Optimizer™ III implantable pulse generator
use Contractility Modulation Device in **0JH-**
Orbicularis oculi muscle
use Eyelid, Upper, Left
use Eyelid, Upper, Right
Orbicularis oris muscle
use Muscle, Facial
Orbital atherectomy technology X2C-
Orbital fascia
use Subcutaneous Tissue and Fascia, Face
Orbital portion of ethmoid bone
use Orbit, Left
use Orbit, Right
Orbital portion of frontal bone
use Orbit, Left
use Orbit, Right
Orbital portion of lacrimal bone
use Orbit, Left
use Orbit, Right
Orbital portion of maxilla
use Orbit, Left
use Orbit, Right
Orbital portion of palatine bone
use Orbit, Left
use Orbit, Right
Orbital portion of sphenoid bone
use Orbit, Left
use Orbit, Right
Orbital portion of zygomatic bone
use Orbit, Left
use Orbit, Right
Orchectomy, orchidectomy, orchiectomy
see Excision, Male Reproductive System **0VB-**
see Resection, Male Reproductive System **0VT-**
Orchidoplasty, orchioplasty
see Repair, Male Reproductive System **0VQ-**
see Replacement, Male Reproductive System **0VR-**
see Supplement, Male Reproductive System **0VU-**
Orchidorrhaphy, orchiorrhaphy
see Repair, Male Reproductive System **0VQ-**
Orchidotomy, orchiotomy, orchotomy *see* Drainage, Male Reproductive System **0V9-**
Orchiopexy
see Repair, Male Reproductive System **0VQ-**
see Reposition, Male Reproductive System **0VS-**
Oropharyngeal airway (OPA)
use Intraluminal Device, Airway in Mouth and Throat
Oropharynx
use Pharynx
Ossiculectomy
see Excision, Ear, Nose, Sinus **09B-**
see Resection, Ear, Nose, Sinus **09T-**
Ossiculotomy *see* Drainage, Ear, Nose, Sinus **099-**
Ostectomy
see Excision, Head and Facial Bones **0NB-**
see Excision, Lower Bones **0QB-**
see Excision, Upper Bones **0PB-**
see Resection, Head and Facial Bones **0NT-**
see Resection, Lower Bones **0QT-**
see Resection, Upper Bones **0PT-**
Osteoclasis
see Division, Head and Facial Bones **0N8-**
see Division, Lower Bones **0Q8-**
see Division, Upper Bones **0P8-**
Osteolysis
see Release, Head and Facial Bones **0NN-**
see Release, Lower Bones **0QN-**
see Release, Upper Bones **0PN-**
Osteopathic Treatment
Abdomen **7W09X-**
Cervical **7W01X-**
Extremity
Lower **7W06X-**
Upper **7W07X-**
Head **7W00X-**
Lumbar **7W03X-**
Pelvis **7W05X-**
Rib Cage **7W08X-**
Sacrum **7W04X-**
Thoracic **7W02X-**
Osteopexy
see Repair, Head and Facial Bones **0NQ-**
see Repair, Lower Bones **0QQ-**
see Repair, Upper Bones **0PQ-**
see Reposition, Head and Facial Bones **0NS-**
see Reposition, Lower Bones **0QS-**
see Reposition, Upper Bones **0PS-**
Osteoplasty
see Repair, Head and Facial Bones **0NQ**
see Repair, Lower Bones **0QQ-**
see Repair, Upper Bones **0PQ-**
see Replacement, Head and Facial Bones **0NR-**
see Replacement, Lower Bones **0QR-**
see Replacement, Upper Bones **0PR-**
see Supplement, Head and Facial Bones **0NU-**
see Supplement, Lower Bones **0QU-**
see Supplement, Upper Bones **0PU-**
Osteorrhaphy
see Repair, Head and Facial Bones **0NQ-**
see Repair, Lower Bones **0QQ-**
see Repair, Upper Bones **0PQ-**
Osteotomy, ostotomy
see Division, Head and Facial Bones **0N8-**
see Division, Lower Bones **0Q8-**
see Division, Upper Bones **0P8-**
see Drainage, Head and Facial Bones **0N9-**
see Drainage, Lower Bones **0Q9-**
see Drainage, Upper Bones **0P9-**
Otic ganglion
use Nerve, Head and Neck Sympathetic
Otoplasty
see Repair, Ear, Nose, Sinus **09Q-**
see Replacement, Ear, Nose, Sinus **09R-**
see Supplement, Ear, Nose, Sinus **09U-**
Otoscopy *see* Inspection, Ear, Nose, Sinus **09J-**
Oval window
use Ear, Middle, Left
use Ear, Middle, Right
Ovarian artery
use Aorta, Abdominal
Ovarian ligament
use Uterine Supporting Structure
Ovariectomy
see Excision, Female Reproductive System **0UB-**
see Resection, Female Reproductive System **0UT-**
Ovariocentesis *see* Drainage, Female Reproductive System **0U9-**
Ovariopexy
see Repair, Female Reproductive System **0UQ-**
see Reposition, Female Reproductive System **0US-**
Ovariotomy
see Drainage, Female Reproductive System **0U9-**
see Division, Female Reproductive System **0U8-**
Ovatio™ CRT-D
use Cardiac Resynchronization Defibrillator Pulse Generator in **0JH-**
Oversewing
Gastrointestinal ulcer *see* Repair, Gastrointestinal System **0DQ-**
Pleural bleb *see* Repair, Respiratory System **0BQ-**
Oviduct
use Fallopian Tube, Left
use Fallopian Tube, Right
Oximetry, Fetal pulse 10H073Z
OXINIUM
use Synthetic Substitute, Oxidized Zirconium on Polyethylene in **0SR-**
Oxygenation
Extracorporeal membrane (ECMO) *see* Performance, Circulatory **5A15-**
Hyperbaric *see* Assistance, Circulatory **5A05-**
Supersaturated *see* Assistance, Circulatory **5A05-**

P

Pacemaker
Dual Chamber
Abdomen **0JH8-**
Chest **0JH6-**
Intracardiac
Insertion of device in
Atrium
Left **02H7-**
Right **02H6-**
Vein, Coronary **02H4-**
Ventricle
Left **02HL-**
Right **02HK-**
Removal of device from, Heart **02PA-**
Revision of device in, Heart **02WA-**
Single Chamber
Abdomen **0JH8-**
Chest **0JH6-**
Single Chamber Rate Responsive
Abdomen **0JH8-**
Chest **0JH6-**
Packing
Abdominal Wall **2W43X5Z**
Anorectal **2Y43X5Z**
Arm
Lower
Left **2W4DX5Z**
Right **2W4CX5Z**
Upper
Left **2W4BX5Z**
Right **2W4AX5Z**
Back **2W45X5Z**
Chest Wall **2W44X5Z**
Ear **2Y42X5Z**
Extremity
Lower
Left **2W4MX5Z**
Right **2W4LX5Z**
Upper
Left **2W49X5Z**
Right **2W48X5Z**
Face **2W41X5Z**
Finger
Left **2W4KX5Z**
Right **2W4JX5Z**
Foot
Left **2W4TX5Z**
Right **2W4SX5Z**
Genital Tract, Female **2Y44X5Z**
Hand
Left **2W4FX5Z**
Right **2W4EX5Z**
Head **2W40X5Z**
Inguinal Region
Left **2W47X5Z**
Right **2W46X5Z**
Leg
Lower
Left **2W4RX5Z**
Right **2W4QX5Z**
Upper
Left **2W4PX5Z**
Right **2W4NX5Z**
Mouth and Pharynx **2Y40X5Z**
Nasal **2Y41X5Z**
Neck **2W42X5Z**
Thumb
Left **2W4HX5Z**
Right **2W4GX5Z**
Toe
Left **2W4VX5Z**
Right **2W4UX5Z**
Urethra **2Y45X5Z**

PROCEDURE INDEX

© 2018 Channel Publishing, Ltd.

Paclitaxel-eluting coronary stent
use Intraluminal Device, Drug-eluting in Heart and Great Vessels
Paclitaxel-eluting peripheral stent
use Intraluminal Device, Drug-eluting in Lower Arteries
use Intraluminal Device, Drug-eluting in Upper Arteries
Palatine gland
use Buccal Mucosa
Palatine tonsil
use Tonsils
Palatine uvula
use Uvula
Palatoglossal muscle
use Muscle, Tongue, Palate, Pharynx
Palatopharyngeal muscle
use Muscle, Tongue, Palate, Pharynx
Palatoplasty
see Repair, Mouth and Throat **0CQ-**
see Replacement, Mouth and Throat **0CR-**
see Supplement, Mouth and Throat **0CU-**
Palatorrhaphy *see* Repair, Mouth and Throat **0CQ-**
Palmar (volar) digital vein
use Vein, Hand, Left
use Vein, Hand, Right
Palmar (volar) metacarpal vein
use Vein, Hand, Left
use Vein, Hand, Right
Palmar cutaneous nerve
use Nerve, Median
use Nerve, Radial
Palmar fascia (aponeurosis)
use Subcutaneous Tissue and Fascia, Hand, Left
use Subcutaneous Tissue and Fascia, Hand, Right
Palmar interosseous muscle
use Muscle, Hand, Left
use Muscle, Hand, Right
Palmar ulnocarpal ligament
use Bursa and Ligament, Wrist, Left
use Bursa and Ligament, Wrist, Right
Palmaris longus muscle
use Muscle, Lower Arm and Wrist, Left
use Muscle, Lower Arm and Wrist, Right
Pancreatectomy
see Excision, Pancreas **0FBG-**
see Resection, Pancreas **0FTG-**
Pancreatic artery
use Artery, Splenic
Pancreatic plexus
use Nerve, Abdominal Sympathetic
Pancreatic vein
use Vein, Splenic
Pancreaticoduodenostomy *see* Bypass, Hepatobiliary System and Pancreas **0F1-**
Pancreaticosplenic lymph node
use Lymphatic, Aortic
Pancreatogram, endoscopic retrograde *see* Fluoroscopy, Pancreatic Duct **BF18-**
Pancreatolithotomy *see* Extirpation, Pancreas **0FCG-**
Pancreatotomy
see Drainage, Pancreas **0F9G-**
see Division, Pancreas **0F8G-**
Panniculectomy
see Excision, Abdominal Wall **0WBF-**
see Excision, Skin, Abdomen **0HB7-**
Paraaortic lymph node
use Lymphatic, Aortic
Paracentesis
Eye *see* Drainage, Eye **089-**
Peritoneal Cavity *see* Drainage, Peritoneal Cavity **0W9G-**
Tympanum *see* Drainage, Ear, Nose, Sinus **099-**
Pararectal lymph node
use Lymphatic, Mesenteric
Parasternal lymph node
use Lymphatic, Thorax
Parathyroidectomy
see Excision, Endocrine System **0GB-**
see Resection, Endocrine System **0GT-**
Paratracheal lymph node
use Lymphatic, Thorax
Paraurethral (Skene's) gland
use Gland, Vestibular
Parenteral nutrition, total *see* Introduction of Nutritional Substance
Parietal lobe
use Cerebral Hemisphere
Parotid lymph node
use Lymphatic, Head
Parotid plexus
use Nerve, Facial
Parotidectomy
see Excision, Mouth and Throat **0CB-**
see Resection, Mouth and Throat **0CT-**
Pars flaccida
use Tympanic Membrane, Left
use Tympanic Membrane, Right
Partial joint replacement
Hip *see* Replacement, Lower Joints **0SR-**
Knee *see* Replacement, Lower Joints **0SR-**
Shoulder *see* Replacement, Upper Joints **0RR-**
Partially absorbable mesh
use Synthetic Substitute
Patch, blood, spinal 3E0R3GC
Patellapexy
see Repair, Lower Bones **0QQ-**
see Reposition, Lower Bones **0QS-**
Patellaplasty
see Repair, Lower Bones **0QQ-**
see Replacement, Lower Bones **0QR-**
see Supplement, Lower Bones **0QU-**
Patellar ligament
use Bursa and Ligament, Knee, Left
use Bursa and Ligament, Knee, Right
Patellar tendon
use Tendon, Knee, Left
use Tendon, Knee, Right
Patellectomy
see Excision, Lower Bones **0QB-**
see Resection, Lower Bones **0QT-**
Patellofemoral joint
use Joint, Knee, Left
use Joint, Knee, Right
use Joint, Knee, Left, Femoral Surface
use Joint, Knee, Right, Femoral Surface
Pectineus muscle
use Muscle, Upper Leg, Left
use Muscle, Upper Leg, Right
Pectoral (anterior) lymph node
use Lymphatic, Axillary, Left
use Lymphatic, Axillary, Right
Pectoral fascia
use Subcutaneous Tissue and Fascia, Chest
Pectoralis major muscle
use Muscle, Thorax, Left
use Muscle, Thorax, Right
Pectoralis minor muscle
use Muscle, Thorax, Left
use Muscle, Thorax, Right
Pedicle-based dynamic stabilization device
use Spinal Stabilization Device, Pedicle-Based in **0RH-**
use Spinal Stabilization Device, Pedicle-Based in **0SH-**
PEEP (positive end expiratory pressure) *see* Assistance, Respiratory **5A09-**
PEG (percutaneous endoscopic gastrostomy) 0DH63UZ
PEJ (percutaneous endoscopic jejunostomy) 0DHA3UZ
Pelvic splanchnic nerve
use Nerve, Abdominal Sympathetic
use Nerve, Sacral Sympathetic
Penectomy
see Excision, Male Reproductive System **0VB-**
see Resection, Male Reproductive System **0VT-**
Penile urethra
use Urethra
Perceval sutureless valve
use Zooplastic Tissue, Rapid Deployment Technique in New Technology
Percutaneous endoscopic gastrojejunostomy (PEG/J) tube
use Feeding Device in Gastrointestinal System
Percutaneous endoscopic gastrostomy (PEG) tube
use Feeding Device in Gastrointestinal System
Percutaneous nephrostomy catheter
use Drainage Device
Percutaneous transluminal coronary angioplasty (PTCA)
see Dilation, Heart and Great Vessels **027-**
Performance
Biliary
Multiple, Filtration **5A1C60Z**
Single, Filtration **5A1C00Z**
Cardiac
Continuous
Output **5A1221Z**
Pacing **5A1223Z**
Intermittent, Pacing **5A1213Z**
Single, Output, Manual **5A12012**
Circulatory
Central Membrane **5A1522F**
Peripheral Veno-arterial Membrane **5A1522G**
Peripheral Veno-venous Membrane **5A1522H**
Respiratory
24-96 Consecutive Hours, Ventilation **5A1945Z**
Greater than 96 Consecutive Hours, Ventilation **5A1955Z**
Less than 24 Consecutive Hours, Ventilation **5A1935Z**
Single, Ventilation, Nonmechanical **5A19054**
Performance — *continued*
Urinary
Continuous, Greater than 18 hours per day, Filtration **5A1D90Z**
Intermittent, Less than 6 hours per day, Filtration **5A1D70Z**
Prolonged Intermittent, 6-18 hours per day, Filtration **5A1D80Z**
Perfusion *see* Introduction of substance in or on
Perfusion, donor organ
Heart **6AB50BZ**
Kidney(s) **6ABT0BZ**
Liver **6ABF0BZ**
Lung(s) **6ABB0BZ**
Pericardiectomy
see Excision, Pericardium **02BN-**
see Resection, Pericardium **02TN-**
Pericardiocentesis *see* Drainage, Pericardial Cavity **0W9D-**
Pericardiolysis *see* Release, Pericardium **02NN-**
Pericardiophrenic artery
use Artery, Internal Mammary, Left
use Artery, Internal Mammary, Right
Pericardioplasty
see Repair, Pericardium **02QN-**
see Replacement, Pericardium **02RN-**
see Supplement, Pericardium **02UN-**
Pericardiorrhaphy *see* Repair, Pericardium **02QN-**
Pericardiostomy *see* Drainage, Pericardial Cavity **0W9D-**
Pericardiotomy *see* Drainage, Pericardial Cavity **0W9D-**
Perimetrium
use Uterus
Peripheral parenteral nutrition
see Introduction of Nutritional Substance
Peripherally inserted central catheter (PICC)
use Infusion Device
Peritoneal dialysis 3E1M39Z
Peritoneocentesis
see Drainage, Peritoneal Cavity **0W9G-**
see Drainage, Peritoneum **0D9W-**
Peritoneoplasty
see Repair, Peritoneum **0DQW-**
see Replacement, Peritoneum **0DRW-**
see Supplement, Peritoneum **0DUW-**
Peritoneoscopy 0DJW4ZZ
Peritoneotomy *see* Drainage, Peritoneum **0D9W-**
Peritoneumectomy *see* Excision, Peritoneum **0DBW-**
Peroneus brevis muscle
use Muscle, Lower Leg, Left
use Muscle, Lower Leg, Right
Peroneus longus muscle
use Muscle, Lower Leg, Left
use Muscle, Lower Leg, Right
Pessary ring
use Intraluminal Device, Pessary in Female Reproductive System
PET scan *see* Positron Emission Tomographic (PET) Imaging
Petrous part of temporal bone
use Bone, Temporal, Left
use Bone, Temporal, Right

© 2018 Channel Publishing, Ltd.

Phacoemulsification, lens
With IOL implant *see* Replacement, Eye **08R-**
Without IOL implant *see* Extraction, Eye **08D-**
Phalangectomy
see Excision, Lower Bones **0QB-**
see Excision, Upper Bones **0PB-**
see Resection, Lower Bones **0QT-**
see Resection, Upper Bones **0PT-**
Phallectomy
see Excision, Penis **0VBS-**
see Resection, Penis **0VTS-**
Phalloplasty
see Repair, Penis **0VQS-**
see Supplement, Penis **0VUS-**
Phallotomy *see* Drainage, Penis **0V9S-**
Pharmacotherapy, for substance abuse
Antabuse **HZ93ZZZ**
Bupropion **HZ97ZZZ**
Clonidine **HZ96ZZZ**
Levo-alpha-acetyl-methadol (LAAM) **HZ92ZZZ**
Methadone Maintenance **HZ91ZZZ**
Naloxone **HZ95ZZZ**
Naltrexone **HZ94ZZZ**
Nicotine Replacement **HZ90ZZZ**
Psychiatric Medication **HZ98ZZZ**
Replacement Medication, Other **HZ99ZZZ**
Pharyngeal constrictor muscle
use Muscle, Tongue, Palate, Pharynx
Pharyngeal plexus
use Nerve, Vagus
Pharyngeal recess
use Nasopharynx
Pharyngeal tonsil
use Adenoids
Pharyngogram *see* Fluoroscopy, Pharynix **B91G-**
Pharyngoplasty
see Repair, Mouth and Throat **0CQ-**
see Replacement, Mouth and Throat **0CR-**
see Supplement, Mouth and Throat **0CU-**
Pharyngorrhaphy *see* Repair, Mouth and Throat **0CQ-**
Pharyngotomy *see* Drainage, Mouth and Throat **0C9**
Pharyngotympanic tube
use Eustachian Tube, Left
use Eustachian Tube, Right
Pheresis
Erythrocytes **6A55-**
Leukocytes **6A55-**
Plasma **6A55-**
Platelets **6A55-**
Stem Cells
Cord Blood **6A55-**
Hematopoietic **6A55-**
Phlebectomy
see Excision, Lower Veins **06B-**
see Excision, Upper Veins **05B-**
see Extraction, Lower Veins **06D-**
see Extraction, Upper Veins **05D-**
Phlebography
see Plain Radiography, Veins **B50-**
Impedance **4A04X51**
Phleborrhaphy
see Repair, Lower Veins **06Q-**
see Repair, Upper Veins **05Q-**
Phlebotomy
see Drainage, Lower Veins **069-**
see Drainage, Upper Veins **059-**
Photocoagulation
For Destruction *see* Destruction
For Repair *see* Repair
Photopheresis, therapeutic *see* Phototherapy, Circulatory **6A65-**
Phototherapy
Circulatory **6A65-**
Skin **6A60-**
Ultraviolet light *see* Ultraviolet Light Therapy, Physiological Systems **6A8-**
Phrenectomy, phrenoneurectomy
see Excision, Nerve, Phrenic **01B2-**
Phrenemphraxis *see* Destruction, Nerve, Phrenic **0152-**
Phrenic nerve stimulator generator
use Stimulator Generator in Subcutaneous Tissue and Fascia
Phrenic nerve stimulator lead
use Diaphragmatic Pacemaker Lead in Respiratory System
Phreniclasis *see* Destruction, Nerve, Phrenic **0152-**
Phrenicoexeresis *see* Extraction, Nerve, Phrenic **01D2-**
Phrenicotomy *see* Division, Nerve, Phrenic **0182-**
Phrenicotripsy *see* Destruction, Nerve, Phrenic **0152-**
Phrenoplasty
see Repair, Respiratory System **0BQ-**
see Supplement, Respiratory System **0BU-**
Phrenotomy *see* Drainage, Respiratory System **0B9-**
Physiatry *see* Motor Treatment, Rehabilitation **F07-**
Physical medicine *see* Motor Treatment, Rehabilitation **F07-**
Physical therapy *see* Motor Treatment, Rehabilitation **F07-**
PHYSIOMESH™ Flexible Composite Mesh
use Synthetic Substitute
Pia mater, intracranial
use Cerebral Meninges
Pia mater, spinal
use Spinal Meninges
Pinealectomy
see Excision, Pineal Body **0GB1-**
see Resection, Pineal Body **0GT1-**
Pinealoscopy **0GJ14ZZ**
Pinealotomy *see* Drainage, Pineal Body **0G91-**
Pinna
use Ear, External, Bilateral
use Ear, External, Left
use Ear, External, Right
Pipeline™ Embolization device (PED)
use Intraluminal Device
Piriform recess (sinus)
use Pharynx
Piriformis muscle
use Muscle, Hip, Left
use Muscle, Hip, Right
PIRRT (prolonged intermittent renal replacement therapy) **5A1D80Z**
Pisiform bone
use Carpal, Left
use Carpal, Right
Pisohamate ligament
use Bursa and Ligament, Hand, Left
use Bursa and Ligament, Hand, Right
Pisometacarpal ligament
use Bursa and Ligament, Hand, Left
use Bursa and Ligament, Hand, Right
Pituitectomy
see Excision, Gland, Pituitary **0GB0-**
see Resection, Gland, Pituitary **0GT0-**
Plain film radiology *see* Plain Radiography
Plain Radiography
Abdomen **BW00ZZZ**
Abdomen and Pelvis **BW01ZZZ**
Abdominal Lymphatic
Bilateral **B701-**
Unilateral **B700-**
Airway, Upper **BB0DZZZ**
Ankle
Left **BQ0H-**
Right **BQ0G-**
Aorta
Abdominal **B400-**
Thoracic **B300-**
Thoraco-Abdominal **B30P-**
Aorta and Bilateral Lower Extremity Arteries **B40D-**
Arch
Bilateral **BN0DZZZ**
Left **BN0CZZZ**
Right **BN0BZZZ**
Arm
Left **BP0FZZZ**
Right **BP0EZZZ**
Artery
Brachiocephalic-Subclavian, Right **B301-**
Bronchial **B30L-**
Bypass Graft, Other **B20F-**
Cervico-Cerebral Arch **B30Q-**
Common Carotid
Bilateral **B305-**
Left **B304-**
Right **B303-**
Coronary
Bypass Graft
Multiple **B203-**
Single **B202-**
Multiple **B201-**
Single **B200-**
External Carotid
Bilateral **B30C-**
Left **B30B-**
Right **B309-**
Hepatic **B402-**
Inferior Mesenteric **B405-**
Intercostal **B30L-**
Internal Carotid
Bilateral **B308-**
Left **B307-**
Right **B306-**
Internal Mammary Bypass Graft
Left **B208-**
Right **B207-**
Intra-Abdominal, Other **B40B-**
Intracranial **B30R-**
Lower, Other **B40J-**
Lower Extremity
Bilateral and Aorta **B40D-**
Left **B40G-**
Right **B40F-**
Lumbar **B409-**
Pelvic **B40C-**
Pulmonary
Left **B30T-**
Right **B30S-**
Renal
Bilateral **B408-**
Left **B407-**
Right **B406-**
Transplant **B40M-**
Spinal **B30M-**
Splenic **B403-**
Plain Radiography — *continued*
Artery — *continued*
Subclavian, Left **B302-**
Superior Mesenteric **B404-**
Upper, Other **B30N-**
Upper Extremity
Bilateral **B30K-**
Left **B30J-**
Right **B30H-**
Vertebral
Bilateral **B30G-**
Left **B30F-**
Right **B30D-**
Bile Duct **BF00-**
Bile Duct and Gallbladder **BF03-**
Bladder **BT00-**
Kidney and Ureter **BT04-**
Bladder and Urethra **BT0B-**
Bone
Facial **BN05ZZZ**
Nasal **BN04ZZZ**
Bones, Long, All **BW0BZZZ**
Breast
Bilateral **BH02ZZZ**
Left **BH01ZZZ**
Right **BH00ZZZ**
Calcaneus
Left **BQ0KZZZ**
Right **BQ0JZZZ**
Chest **BW03ZZZ**
Clavicle
Left **BP05ZZZ**
Right **BP04ZZZ**
Coccyx **BR0FZZZ**
Corpora Cavernosa **BV00-**
Dialysis Fistula **B50W-**
Dialysis Shunt **B50W-**
Disc
Cervical **BR01-**
Lumbar **BR03-**
Thoracic **BR02-**
Duct
Lacrimal
Bilateral **B802-**
Left **B801-**
Right **B800-**
Mammary
Multiple
Left **BH06**
Right **BH05-**
Single
Left **BH04-**
Right **BH03-**
Elbow
Left **BP0H-**
Right **BP0G-**
Epididymis
Left **BV02-**
Right **BV01-**
Extremity
Lower **BW0CZZZ**
Upper **BW0JZZZ**
Eye
Bilateral **B807ZZZ**
Left **B806ZZZ**
Right **B805ZZZ**
Facet Joint
Cervical **BR04-**
Lumbar **BR06-**
Thoracic **BR05-**
Fallopian Tube
Bilateral **BU02-**
Left **BU01-**
Right **BU00-**
Fallopian Tube and Uterus **BU08-**
Femur
Left, Densitometry **BQ04ZZ1**
Right, Densitometry **BQ03ZZ1**
Finger
Left **BP0SZZZ**
Right **BP0RZZZ**
Foot
Left **BQ0MZZZ**
Right **BQ0LZZZ**

PROCEDURE INDEX

© 2018 Channel Publishing, Ltd.

Plain Radiography — *continued*
Forearm
Left **BP0K**ZZZ
Right **BP0J**ZZZ
Gallbladder and Bile Duct **BF03**-
Gland
Parotid
Bilateral **B906**-
Left **B905**-
Right **B904**-
Salivary
Bilateral **B90D**-
Left **B90C**-
Right **B90B**-
Submandibular
Bilateral **B909**-
Left **B908**-
Right **B907**-
Hand
Left **BP0P**ZZZ
Right **BP0N**ZZZ
Heart
Left **B205**-
Right **B204**-
Right and Left **B206**-
Hepatobiliary System, All **BF0C**-
Hip
Left **BQ01**-
Densitometry **BQ01**ZZ1
Right **BQ00**-
Densitometry **BQ00**ZZ1
Humerus
Left **BP0B**ZZZ
Right **BP0A**ZZZ
Ileal Diversion Loop **BT0C**-
Intracranial Sinus **B502**-
Joint
Acromioclavicular, Bilateral **BP03**ZZZ
Finger
Left **BP0D**-
Right **BP0C**-
Foot
Left **BQ0Y**-
Right **BQ0X**-
Hand
Left **BP0D**-
Right **BP0C**-
Lumbosacral **BR0B**ZZZ
Sacroiliac **BR0D**-
Sternoclavicular
Bilateral **BP02**ZZZ
Left **BP01**ZZZ
Right **BP00**ZZZ
Temporomandibular
Bilateral **BN09**-
Left **BN08**-
Right **BN07**-
Thoracolumbar **BR08**ZZZ
Toe
Left **BQ0Y**-
Right **BQ0X**-
Kidney
Bilateral **BT03**-
Left **BT02**-
Right **BT01**-
Ureter and Bladder **BT04**-
Knee
Left **BQ08**-
Right **BQ07**-
Leg
Left **BQ0F**ZZZ
Right **BQ0D**ZZZ
Lymphatic
Head **B704**-
Lower Extremity
Bilateral **B70B**-
Left **B709**-
Right **B708**-
Neck **B704**-
Pelvic **B70C**-

Plain Radiography — *continued*
Lymphatic — *continued*
Upper Extremity
Bilateral **B707**-
Left **B706**-
Right **B705**-
Mandible **BN06**ZZZ
Mastoid **B90H**ZZZ
Nasopharynx **B90F**ZZZ
Optic Foramina
Left **B804**ZZZ
Right **B803**ZZZ
Orbit
Bilateral **BN03**ZZZ
Left **BN02**ZZZ
Right **BN01**ZZZ
Oropharynx **B90F**ZZZ
Patella
Left **BQ0W**ZZZ
Right **BQ0V**ZZZ
Pelvis **BR0C**ZZZ
Pelvis and Abdomen **BW01**ZZZ
Prostate **BV03**-
Retroperitoneal Lymphatic
Bilateral **B701**-
Unilateral **B700**-
Ribs
Left **BP0Y**ZZZ
Right **BP0X**ZZZ
Sacrum **BR0F**ZZZ
Scapula
Left **BP07**ZZZ
Right **BP06**ZZZ
Shoulder
Left **BP09**-
Right **BP08**-
Sinus
Intracranial **B502**-
Paranasal **B902**ZZZ
Skull **BN00**ZZZ
Spinal Cord **B00B**-
Spine
Cervical, Densitometry **BR00**ZZ1
Lumbar, Densitometry **BR09**ZZ1
Thoracic, Densitometry **BR07**ZZ1
Whole, Densitometry **BR0G**ZZ1
Sternum **BR0H**ZZZ
Teeth
All **BN0J**ZZZ
Multiple **BN0H**ZZZ
Testicle
Left **BV06**-
Right **BV05**-
Toe
Left **BQ0Q**ZZZ
Right **BQ0P**ZZZ
Tooth, Single **BN0G**ZZZ
Tracheobronchial Tree
Bilateral **BB09**YZZ
Left **BB08**YZZ
Right **BB07**YZZ
Ureter
Bilateral **BT08**-
Kidney and Bladder **BT04**-
Left **BT07**-
Right **BT06**-
Urethra **BT05**-
Urethra and Bladder **BT0B**-
Uterus **BU06**-
Uterus and Fallopian Tube **BU08**-
Vagina **BU09**-
Vasa Vasorum **BV08**-
Vein
Cerebellar **B501**-
Cerebral **B501**-
Epidural **B500**-
Jugular
Bilateral **B505**-
Left **B504**-
Right **B503**-

Plain Radiography — *continued*
Vein — *continued*
Lower Extremity
Bilateral **B50D**-
Left **B50C**-
Right **B50B**-
Other **B50V**-
Pelvic (Iliac)
Bilateral **B50H**-
Left **B50G**-
Right **B50F**-
Portal **B50T**-
Pulmonary
Bilateral **B50S**-
Left **B50R**-
Right **B50Q**-
Renal
Bilateral **B50L**-
Left **B50K**-
Right **B50J**-
Spanchnic **B50T**-
Subclavian
Left **B507**-
Right **B506**-
Upper Extremity
Bilateral **B50P**-
Left **B50N**-
Right **B50M**-
Vena Cava
Inferior **B509**-
Superior **B508**-
Whole Body **BW0K**ZZZ
Infant **BW0M**ZZZ
Whole Skeleton **BW0L**ZZZ
Wrist
Left **BP0M**-
Right **BP0L**-

Planar Nuclear Medicine Imaging
Abdomen **CW10**-
Abdomen and Chest **CW14**-
Abdomen and Pelvis **CW11**-
Anatomical Region, Other **CW1Z**ZZZ
Anatomical Regions, Multiple **CW1Y**YZZ
Bladder and Ureters **CT1H**-
Bladder, Kidneys and Ureters **CT13**-
Blood **C713**-
Bone Marrow **C710**-
Brain **C010**-
Breast **CH1Y**YZZ
Bilateral **CH12**-
Left **CH11**-
Right **CH10**-
Bronchi and Lungs **CB12**-
Central Nervous System **C01Y**YZZ
Cerebrospinal Fluid **C015**-
Chest **CW13**-
Chest and Abdomen **CW14**-
Chest and Neck **CW16**-
Digestive System **CD1Y**YZZ
Ducts, Lacrimal, Bilateral **C819**-
Ear, Nose, Mouth and Throat **C91Y**YZZ
Endocrine System **CG1Y**YZZ
Extremity
Lower **CW1D**-
Bilateral **CP1F**-
Left **CP1D**-
Right **CP1C**-
Upper **CW1M**-
Bilateral **CP1B**-
Left **CP19**-
Right **CP18**-
Eye **C81Y**YZZ
Gallbladder **CF14**-
Gastrointestinal Tract **CD17**-
Upper **CD15**-
Gland
Adrenal, Bilateral **CG14**-
Parathyroid **CG11**-
Thyroid **CG12**-

Planar Nuclear Medicine Imaging — *continued*
Glands, Salivary, Bilateral **C91B**-
Head and Neck **CW1B**-
Heart **C21Y**YZZ
Right and Left **C216**-
Hepatobiliary System, All **CF1C**-
Hepatobiliary System and Pancreas **CF1Y**YZZ
Kidneys, Ureters and Bladder **CT13**-
Liver **CF15**-
Liver and Spleen **CF16**-
Lungs and Bronchi **CB12**-
Lymphatics
Head **C71J**-
Head and Neck **C715**-
Lower Extremity **C71P**-
Neck **C71K**-
Pelvic **C71D**-
Trunk **C71M** -
Upper Chest **C71L**-
Upper Extremity **C71N**-
Lymphatics and Hematologic System **C71Y**YZZ
Musculoskeletal System
All **CP1Z**-
Other **CP1Y**YZZ-
Myocardium **C21G**-
Neck and Chest **CW16**-
Neck and Head **CW1B**-
Pancreas and Hepatobiliary System **CF1Y**YZZ
Pelvic Region **CW1J**-
Pelvis **CP16**-
Pelvis and Abdomen **CW11**-
Pelvis and Spine **CP17**-
Reproductive System, Male **CV1Y**YZZ
Respiratory System **CB1Y**YZZ
Skin **CH1Y**YZZ
Skull **CP11**-
Spine **CP15**-
Spine and Pelvis **CP17**-
Spleen **C712**-
Spleen and Liver **CF16**-
Subcutaneous Tissue **CH1Y**YZZ
Testicles, Bilateral **CV19**-
Thorax **CP14**-
Ureters, Kidneys and Bladder **CT13**-
Ureters and Bladder **CT1H**-
Urinary System **CT1Y**YZZ
Veins **C51Y**YZZ
Central **C51R**-
Lower Extremity
Bilateral **C51D**-
Left **C51C**-
Right **C51B**-
Upper Extremity
Bilateral **C51Q**-
Left **C51P**-
Right **C51N**-
Whole Body **CW1N**-

Plantar digital vein
use Vein, Foot, Left
use Vein, Foot, Right

Plantar fascia (aponeurosis)
use Subcutaneous Tissue and Fascia, Foot, Left
use Subcutaneous Tissue and Fascia, Foot, Right

Plantar metatarsal vein
use Vein, Foot, Left
use Vein, Foot, Right

Plantar venous arch
use Vein, Foot, Left
use Vein, Foot, Right

Plaque Radiation
Abdomen **DWY3**FZZ
Adrenal Gland **DGY2**FZZ
Anus **DDY8**FZZ
Bile Ducts **DFY2**FZZ
Bladder **DTY2**FZZ

PROCEDURE INDEX

© 2018 Channel Publishing, Ltd.

Plaque Radiation — *continued*
Bone, Other **DPY**CFZZ
Bone Marrow **D7Y**0FZZ
Brain **D0Y**0FZZ
Brain Stem **D0Y**1FZZ
Breast
Left **DMY**0FZZ
Right **DMY**1FZZ
Bronchus **DBY**1FZZ
Cervix **DUY**1FZZ
Chest **DWY**2FZZ
Chest Wall **DBY**7FZZ
Colon **DDY**5FZZ
Diaphragm **DBY**8FZZ
Duodenum **DDY**2FZZ
Ear **D9Y**0FZZ
Esophagus **DDY**0FZZ
Eye **D8Y**0FZZ
Femur **DPY**9FZZ
Fibula **DPY**BFZZ
Gallbladder **DFY**1FZZ
Gland
Adrenal **DGY**2FZZ
Parathyroid **DGY**4FZZ
Pituitary **DGY**0FZZ
Thyroid **DGY**5FZZ
Glands, Salivary **D9Y**6FZZ
Head and Neck **DWY**1FZZ
Hemibody **DWY**4FZZ
Humerus **DPY**6FZZ
Ileum **DDY**4FZZ
Jejunum **DDY**3FZZ
Kidney **DTY**0FZZ
Larynx **D9Y**BFZZ
Liver **DFY**0FZZ
Lung **DBY**2FZZ
Lymphatics
Abdomen **D7Y**6FZZ
Axillary **D7Y**4FZZ
Inguinal **D7Y**8FZZ
Neck **D7Y**3FZZ
Pelvis **D7Y**7FZZ
Thorax **D7Y**5FZZ
Mandible **DPY**3FZZ
Maxilla **DPY**2FZZ
Mediastinum **DBY**6FZZ
Mouth **D9Y**4FZZ
Nasopharynx **D9Y**DFZZ
Neck and Head **DWY**1FZZ
Nerve, Peripheral **D0Y**7FZZ
Nose **D9Y**1FZZ
Ovary **DUY**0FZZ
Palate
Hard **D9Y**8FZZ
Soft **D9Y**9FZZ
Pancreas **DFY**3FZZ
Parathyroid Gland **DGY**4FZZ
Pelvic Bones **DPY**8FZZ
Pelvic Region **DWY**6FZZ
Pharynx **D9Y**CFZZ
Pineal Body **DGY**1FZZ
Pituitary Gland **DGY**0FZZ
Pleura **DBY**5FZZ
Prostate **DVY**0FZZ
Radius **DPY**7FZZ
Rectum **DDY**7FZZ
Rib **DPY**5FZZ
Sinuses **D9Y**7FZZ
Skin
Abdomen **DHY**8FZZ
Arm **DHY**4FZZ
Back **DHY**7FZZ
Buttock **DHY**9FZZ
Chest **DHY**6FZZ
Face **DHY**2FZZ
Foot **DHY**CFZZ
Hand **DHY**5FZZ
Leg **DHY**BFZZ
Neck **DHY**3FZZ
Skull **DPY**0FZZ
Spinal Cord **D0Y**6FZZ
Spleen **D7Y**2FZZ
Sternum **DPY**4FZZ
Stomach **DDY**1FZZ

Plaque Radiation — *continued*
Testis **DVY**1FZZ
Thymus **D7Y**1FZZ
Thyroid Gland **DGY**5FZZ
Tibia **DPY**BFZZ
Tongue **D9Y**5FZZ
Trachea **DBY**0FZZ
Ulna **DPY**7FZZ
Ureter **DTY**1FZZ
Urethra **DTY**3FZZ
Uterus **DUY**2FZZ
Whole Body **DWY**5FZZ
Plasmapheresis, therapeutic
see Pheresis, Physiological Systems **6A5-**
Plateletpheresis, therapeutic
see Pheresis, Physiological Systems **6A5-**
Platysma muscle
use Muscle, Neck, Left
use Muscle, Neck, Right
Plazomicin Anti-infective XW0-
Pleurectomy
see Excision, Respiratory System **0BB-**
see Resection, Respiratory System **0BT-**
Pleurocentesis *see* Drainage, Anatomical Regions, General **0W9-**
Pleurodesis, pleurosclerosis
Chemical injection *see* Introduction of substance in or on, Pleural Cavity **3E0L-**
Surgical *see* Destruction, Respiratory System **0B5-**
Pleurolysis *see* Release, Respiratory System **0BN-**
Pleuroscopy 0BJQ4ZZ
Pleurotomy *see* Drainage, Respiratory System **0B9-**
Plica semilunaris
use Conjunctiva, Left
use Conjunctiva, Right
Plication *see* Restriction
Pneumectomy
see Excision, Respiratory System **0BB-**
see Resection, Respiratory System **0BT-**
Pneumocentesis *see* Drainage, Respiratory System **0B9-**
Pneumogastric nerve
use Nerve, Vagus
Pneumolysis *see* Release, Respiratory System **0BN-**
Pneumonectomy
see Resection, Respiratory System **0BT-**
Pneumonolysis *see* Release, Respiratory System **0BN-**
Pneumonopexy
see Repair, Respiratory System **0BQ-**
see Reposition, Respiratory System **0BS-**
Pneumonorrhaphy *see* Repair, Respiratory System **0BQ-**
Pneumonotomy *see* Drainage, Respiratory System **0B9-**
Pneumotaxic center
use Pons
Pneumotomy *see* Drainage, Respiratory System **0B9-**
Pollicization *see* Transfer, Anatomical Regions, Upper Extremities **0XX-**
Polyethylene socket
use Synthetic Substitute, Polyethylene in **0SR-**
Polymethylmethacrylate (PMMA)
use Synthetic Substitute
Polypectomy, gastrointestinal *see* Excision, Gastrointestinal System **0DB-**

Polypropylene mesh
use Synthetic Substitute
Polysomnogram 4A1ZXQZ
Pontine tegmentum
use Pons
Popliteal ligament
use Bursa and Ligament, Knee, Left
use Bursa and Ligament, Knee, Right
Popliteal lymph node
use Lymphatic, Lower Extremity, Left
use Lymphatic, Lower Extremity, Right
Popliteal vein
use Vein, Femoral, Left
use Vein, Femoral, Right
Popliteus muscle
use Muscle, Lower Leg, Left
use Muscle, Lower Leg, Right
Porcine (bioprosthetic) valve
use Zooplastic Tissue in Heart and Great Vessels
Positive end expiratory pressure
see Performance, Respiratory **5A19-**
Positron Emission Tomographic (PET) Imaging
Brain **C030-**
Bronchi and Lungs **CB32-**
Central Nervous System **C03**YYZZ
Heart **C23**YYZZ
Lungs and Bronchi **CB32-**
Myocardium **C23G-**
Respiratory System **CB3**YYZZ
Whole Body **CW3**NYZZ
Positron emission tomography
see Positron Emission Tomographic (PET) Imaging
Postauricular (mastoid) lymph node
use Lymphatic, Neck, Left
use Lymphatic, Neck, Right
Postcava
use Vena Cava, Inferior
Posterior (subscapular) lymph node
use Lymphatic, Axillary, Left
use Lymphatic, Axillary, Right
Posterior auricular artery
use Artery, External Carotid, Left
use Artery, External Carotid, Right
Posterior auricular nerve
use Nerve, Facial
Posterior auricular vein
use Vein, External Jugular, Left
use Vein, External Jugular, Right
Posterior cerebral artery
use Artery, Intracranial
Posterior chamber
use Eye, Left
use Eye, Right
Posterior circumflex humeral artery
use Artery, Axillary, Left
use Artery, Axillary, Right
Posterior communicating artery
use Artery, Intracranial
Posterior cruciate ligament (PCL)
use Bursa and Ligament, Knee, Left
use Bursa and Ligament, Knee, Right
Posterior facial (retromandibular) vein
use Vein, Face, Left
use Vein, Face, Right
Posterior femoral cutaneous nerve
use Nerve, Sacral Plexus
Posterior inferior cerebellar artery (PICA)
use Artery, Intracranial

Posterior interosseous nerve
use Nerve, Radial
Posterior labial nerve
use Nerve, Pudendal
Posterior scrotal nerve
use Nerve, Pudendal
Posterior spinal artery
use Artery, Vertebral, Left
use Artery, Vertebral, Right
Posterior tibial recurrent artery
use Artery, Anterior Tibial, Left
use Artery, Anterior Tibial, Right
Posterior ulnar recurrent artery
use Artery, Ulnar, Left
use Artery, Ulnar, Right
Posterior vagal trunk
use Nerve, Vagus
PPN (peripheral parenteral nutrition) *see* Introduction of Nutritional Substance
Preauricular lymph node
use Lymphatic, Head
Precava
use Vena Cava, Superior
Prepatellar bursa
use Bursa and Ligament, Knee, Left
use Bursa and Ligament, Knee, Right
Preputiotomy *see* Drainage, Male Reproductive System **0V9-**
Pressure support ventilation *see* Performance, Respiratory **5A19-**
PRESTIGE® Cervical Disc
use Synthetic Substitute
Pretracheal fascia
use Subcutaneous Tissue and Fascia, Left Neck
use Subcutaneous Tissue and Fascia, Right Neck
Prevertebral fascia
use Subcutaneous Tissue and Fascia, Left Neck
use Subcutaneous Tissue and Fascia, Right Neck
PrimeAdvanced neurostimulator (SureScan) (MRI Safe)
use Stimulator Generator, Multiple Array in **0JH-**
Princeps pollicis artery
use Artery, Hand, Left
use Artery, Hand, Right
Probing, duct
Diagnostic *see* Inspection
Dilation *see* Dilation
PROCEED™ Ventral Patch
use Synthetic Substitute
Procerus muscle
use Muscle, Facial
Proctectomy
see Excision, Rectum **0DBP-**
see Resection, Rectum **0DTP-**
Proctoclysis *see* Introduction of substance in or on, Gastrointestinal Tract, Lower **3E0H-**
Proctocolectomy
see Excision, Gastrointestinal System **0DB-**
see Resection, Gastrointestinal System **0DT-**
Proctocolpoplasty
see Repair, Gastrointestinal System **0DQ-**
see Supplement, Gastrointestinal System **0DU-**
Proctoperineoplasty
see Repair, Gastrointestinal System **0DQ-**
see Supplement, Gastrointestinal System **0DU-**
Proctoperineorrhaphy *see* Repair, Gastrointestinal System **0DQ-**

© 2018 Channel Publishing, Ltd.

Proctopexy
see Repair, Rectum **0DQP-**
see Reposition, Rectum **0DSP-**
Proctoplasty
see Repair, Rectum **0DQP-**
see Supplement, Rectum **0DUP-**
Proctorrhaphy *see* Repair, Rectum **0DQP-**
Proctoscopy 0DJD8ZZ
Proctosigmoidectomy
see Excision, Gastrointestinal System **0DB-**
see Resection, Gastrointestinal System **0DT-**
Proctosigmoidoscopy 0DJD8ZZ
Proctostomy *see* Drainage, Rectum **0D9P-**
Proctotomy *see* Drainage, Rectum **0D9P-**
Prodisc-C
use Synthetic Substitute
Prodisc-L
use Synthetic Substitute
Production, atrial septal defect
see Excision, Septum, Atrial **02B5-**
Profunda brachii
use Artery, Brachial, Left
use Artery, Brachial, Right
Profunda femoris (deep femoral) vein
use Vein, Femoral, Left
use Vein, Femoral, Right
PROLENE Polypropylene Hernia System (PHS)
use Synthetic Substitute
Prolonged intermittent renal replacement therapy (PIRRT) 5A1D80Z
Pronator quadratus muscle
use Muscle, Lower Arm and Wrist, Left
use Muscle, Lower Arm and Wrist, Right
Pronator teres muscle
use Muscle, Lower Arm and Wrist, Left
use Muscle, Lower Arm and Wrist, Right
Prostatectomy
see Excision, Prostate **0VB0-**
see Resection, Prostate **0VT0-**
Prostatic urethra
use Urethra
Prostatomy, prostatotomy *see* Drainage, Prostate **0V90-**
Protecta XT CRT-D
use Cardiac Resynchronization Defibrillator Pulse Generator in **0JH-**
Protecta XT DR (XT VR)
use Defibrillator Generator in **0JH-**
Protégé® RX Carotid Stent System
use Intraluminal Device
Proximal radioulnar joint
use Joint, Elbow, Left
use Joint, Elbow, Right
Psoas muscle
use Muscle, Hip, Left
use Muscle, Hip, Right
PSV (pressure support ventilation) *see* Performance, Respiratory **5A19-**
Psychoanalysis GZ54ZZZ
Psychological Tests
Cognitive Status **GZ14ZZZ**
Developmental **GZ10ZZZ**
Intellectual and Psychoeducational **GZ12ZZZ**
Neurobehavioral Status **GZ14ZZZ**
Neuropsychological **GZ13ZZZ**
Personality and Behavioral **GZ11ZZZ**
Psychotherapy
Family, Mental Health Services **GZ72ZZZ**
Group **GZHZZZZ**
Mental Health Services **GZHZZZZ**
Individual
see Psychotherapy, Individual, Mental Health Services
For substance abuse
12-Step **HZ53ZZZ**
Behavioral **HZ51ZZZ**
Cognitive **HZ50ZZZ**
Cognitive-Behavioral **HZ52ZZZ**
Confrontational **HZ58ZZZ**
Interactive **HZ55ZZZ**
Interpersonal **HZ54ZZZ**
Motivational Enhancement **HZ57ZZZ**
Psychoanalysis **HZ5BZZZ**
Psychodynamic **HZ5CZZZ**
Psychoeducation **HZ56ZZZ**
Psychophysiological **HZ5DZZZ**
Supportive **HZ59ZZZ**
Mental Health Services
Behavioral **GZ51ZZZ**
Cognitive **GZ52ZZZ**
Cognitive-Behavioral **GZ58ZZZ**
Interactive **GZ50ZZZ**
Interpersonal **GZ53ZZZ**
Psychoanalysis **GZ54ZZZ**
Psychodynamic **GZ55ZZZ**
Psychophysiological **GZ59ZZZ**
Supportive **GZ56ZZZ**
PTCA (percutaneous transluminal coronary angioplasty) *see* Dilation, Heart and Great Vessels **027-**
Pterygoid muscle
use Muscle, Head
Pterygoid process *use* Sphenoid Bone
Pterygopalatine (sphenopalatine) ganglion
use Nerve, Head and Neck Sympathetic
Pubis
use Bone, Pelvic, Left
use Bone, Pelvic, Right
Pubofemoral ligament
use Bursa and Ligament, Hip, Left
use Bursa and Ligament, Hip, Right
Pudendal nerve
use Nerve, Sacral Plexus
Pull-through, laparoscopic-assisted transanal
see Excision, Gastrointestinal System **0DB-**
see Resection, Gastrointestinal System **0DT-**
Pull-through, rectal
see Resection, Rectum **0DTP-**
Pulmoaortic canal
use Artery, Pulmonary, Left
Pulmonary annulus
use Valve, Pulmonary
Pulmonary artery wedge monitoring *see* Monitoring, Arterial **4A13-**
Pulmonary plexus
use Nerve, Thoracic Sympathetic
use Nerve, Vagus
Pulmonic valve
use Valve, Pulmonary
Pulpectomy *see* Excision, Mouth and Throat **0CB-**
Pulverization *see* Fragmentation
Pulvinar
use Thalamus
Pump reservoir
use Infusion Device, Pump in Subcutaneous Tissue and Fascia
Punch biopsy *see* Excision with qualifier Diagnostic
Puncture *see* Drainage
Puncture, lumbar *see* Drainage, Spinal Canal **009U-**
Pyelography
see Fluoroscopy, Urinary System **BT1-**
see Plain Radiography, Urinary System **BT0-**
Pyeloileostomy, urinary diversion
see Bypass, Urinary System **0T1-**
Pyeloplasty
see Repair, Urinary System **0TQ-**
see Replacement, Urinary System **0TR-**
see Supplement, Urinary System **0TU-**
Pyelorrhaphy *see* Repair, Urinary System **0TQ-**
Pyeloscopy 0TJ58ZZ
Pyelostomy
see Drainage, Urinary System **0T9-**
see Bypass, Urinary System **0T1-**
Pyelotomy *see* Drainage, Urinary System **0T9-**
Pylorectomy
see Excision, Stomach, Pylorus **0DB7-**
see Resection, Stomach, Pylorus **0DT7-**
Pyloric antrum
use Stomach, Pylorus
Pyloric canal
use Stomach, Pylorus
Pyloric sphincter
use Stomach, Pylorus
Pylorodiosis *see* Dilation, Stomach, Pylorus **0D77-**
Pylorogastrectomy
see Excision, Gastrointestinal System **0DB-**
see Resection, Gastrointestinal System **0DT-**
Pyloroplasty
see Repair, Stomach, Pylorus **0DQ7-**
see Supplement, Stomach, Pylorus **0DU7-**
Pyloroscopy 0DJ68ZZ
Pylorotomy *see* Drainage, Stomach, Pylorus **0D97-**
Pyramidalis muscle
use Muscle, Abdomen, Left
use Muscle, Abdomen, Right

Q

Quadrangular cartilage
use Septum, Nasal
Quadrant resection of breast *see* Excision, Skin and Breast **0HB-**
Quadrate lobe
use Liver
Quadratus femoris muscle
use Muscle, Hip, Left
use Muscle, Hip, Right
Quadratus lumborum muscle
use Muscle, Trunk, Left
use Muscle, Trunk, Right
Quadratus plantae muscle
use Muscle, Foot, Left
use Muscle, Foot, Right
Quadriceps (femoris)
use Muscle, Upper Leg, Left
use Muscle, Upper Leg, Right
Quarantine 8E0ZXY6

© 2018 Channel Publishing, Ltd.

R

Radial collateral carpal ligament
use Bursa and Ligament, Wrist, Left
use Bursa and Ligament, Wrist, Right
Radial collateral ligament
use Bursa and Ligament, Elbow, Left
use Bursa and Ligament, Elbow, Right
Radial notch
use Ulna, Left
use Ulna, Right
Radial recurrent artery
use Artery, Radial, Left
use Artery, Radial, Right
Radial vein
use Vein, Brachial, Left
use Vein, Brachial, Right
Radialis indicis
use Artery, Hand, Left
use Artery, Hand, Right
Radiation Therapy
see Beam Radiation
see Brachytherapy
see Stereotactic Radiosurgery
Radiation treatment *see* Radiation Therapy
Radiocarpal joint
use Joint, Wrist, Left
use Joint, Wrist, Right
Radiocarpal ligament
use Bursa and Ligament, Wrist, Left
use Bursa and Ligament, Wrist, Right
Radiography *see* Plain Radiography
Radiology, analog *see* Plain Radiography
Radiology, diagnostic *see* Imaging, Diagnostic
Radioulnar ligament
use Bursa and Ligament, Wrist, Left
use Bursa and Ligament, Wrist, Right
Range of motion testing *see* Motor Function Assessment, Rehabilitation **F01-**
REALIZE® Adjustable Gastric Band
use Extraluminal Device
Reattachment
Abdominal Wall **0WMF0ZZ**
Ampulla of Vater **0FMC-**
Ankle Region
Left **0YML0ZZ**
Right **0YMK0ZZ**
Arm
Lower
Left **0XMF0ZZ**
Right **0XMD0ZZ**
Upper
Left **0XM90ZZ**
Right **0XM80ZZ**
Axilla
Left **0XM50ZZ**
Right **0XM40ZZ**
Back
Lower **0WML0ZZ**
Upper **0WMK0ZZ**
Bladder **0TMB-**
Bladder Neck **0TMC-**
Breast
Bilateral **0HMVXZZ**
Left **0HMUXZZ**
Right **0HMTXZZ**

Reattachment — *continued*
Bronchus
Lingula **0BM90ZZ**
Lower Lobe
Left **0BMB0ZZ**
Right **0BM60ZZ**
Main
Left **0BM70ZZ**
Right **0BM30ZZ**
Middle Lobe, Right **0BM50ZZ**
Upper Lobe
Left **0BM80ZZ**
Right **0BM40ZZ**
Bursa and Ligament
Abdomen
Left **0MMJ-**
Right **0MMH-**
Ankle
Left **0MMR-**
Right **0MMQ-**
Elbow
Left **0MM4-**
Right **0MM3-**
Foot
Left **0MMT-**
Right **0MMS-**
Hand
Left **0MM8-**
Right **0MM7-**
Head and Neck **0MM0-**
Hip
Left **0MMM-**
Right **0MML-**
Knee
Left **0MMP-**
Right **0MMN-**
Lower Extremity
Left **0MMW-**
Right **0MMV-**
Perineum **0MMK-**
Rib(s) **0MMG-**
Shoulder
Left **0MM2-**
Right **0MM1-**
Spine
Lower **0MMD-**
Upper **0MMC-**
Sternum **0MMF-**
Upper Extremity
Left **0MMB-**
Right **0MM9-**
Wrist
Left **0MM6-**
Right **0MM5-**
Buttock
Left **0YM10ZZ**
Right **0YM00ZZ**
Carina **0BM20ZZ**
Cecum **0DMH-**
Cervix **0UMC-**
Chest Wall **0WM80ZZ**
Clitoris **0UMJXZZ**
Colon
Ascending **0DMK-**
Descending **0DMM-**
Sigmoid **0DMN-**
Transverse **0DML-**
Cord
Bilateral **0VMH-**
Left **0VMG-**
Right **0VMF-**
Cul-de-sac **0UMF-**
Diaphragm **0BMT0ZZ**
Duct
Common Bile **0FM9-**
Cystic **0FM8-**
Hepatic
Common **0FM7-**
Left **0FM6-**
Right **0FM5-**
Pancreatic **0FMD-**
Accessory **0FMF-**
Duodenum **0DM9-**

Reattachment — *continued*
Ear
Left **09M1XZZ**
Right **09M0XZZ**
Elbow Region
Left **0XMC0ZZ**
Right **0XMB0ZZ**
Esophagus **0DM5-**
Extremity
Lower
Left **0YMB0ZZ**
Right **0YM90ZZ**
Upper
Left **0XM70ZZ**
Right **0XM60ZZ**
Eyelid
Lower
Left **08MRXZZ**
Right **08MQXZZ**
Upper
Left **08MPXZZ**
Right **08MNXZZ**
Face **0WM20ZZ**
Fallopian Tube
Left **0UM6-**
Right **0UM5-**
Fallopian Tubes, Bilateral **0UM7-**
Femoral Region
Left **0YM80ZZ**
Right **0YM70ZZ**
Finger
Index
Left **0XMP0ZZ**
Right **0XMN0ZZ**
Little
Left **0XMW0ZZ**
Right **0XMV0ZZ**
Middle
Left **0XMR0ZZ**
Right **0XMQ0ZZ**
Ring
Left **0XMT0ZZ**
Right **0XMS0ZZ**
Foot
Left **0YMN0ZZ**
Right **0YMM0ZZ**
Forequarter
Left **0XM10ZZ**
Right **0XM00ZZ**
Gallbladder **0FM4**
Gland
Left **0GM2-**
Right **0GM3-**
Hand
Left **0XMK0ZZ**
Right **0XMJ0ZZ**
Hindquarter
Bilateral **0YM40ZZ**
Left **0YM30ZZ**
Right **0YM20ZZ**
Hymen **0UMK-**
Ileum **0DMB-**
Inguinal Region
Left **0YM60ZZ**
Right **0YM50ZZ**
Intestine
Large **0DME-**
Left **0DMG-**
Right **0DMF-**
Small **0DM8-**
Jaw
Lower **0WM50ZZ**
Upper **0WM40ZZ**
Jejunum **0DMA-**
Kidney
Left **0TM1-**
Right **0TM0-**
Kidney Pelvis
Left **0TM4-**
Right **0TM3-**
Kidneys, Bilateral **0TM2-**
Knee Region
Left **0YMG0ZZ**
Right **0YMF0ZZ**

Reattachment — *continued*
Leg
Lower
Left **0YMJ0ZZ**
Right **0YMH0ZZ**
Upper
Left **0YMD0ZZ**
Right **0YMC0ZZ**
Lip
Lower **0CM10ZZ**
Upper **0CM00ZZ**
Liver **0FM0-**
Left Lobe **0FM2-**
Right Lobe **0FM1-**
Lung
Left **0BML0ZZ**
Lower Lobe
Left **0BMJ0ZZ**
Right **0BMF0ZZ**
Middle Lobe, Right **0BMD0ZZ**
Right **0BMK0ZZ**
Upper Lobe
Left **0BMG0ZZ**
Right **0BMC0ZZ**
Lung Lingula **0BMH0ZZ**
Muscle
Abdomen
Left **0KML-**
Right **0KMK-**
Facial **0KM1-**
Foot
Left **0KMW-**
Right **0KMV-**
Hand
Left **0KMD-**
Right **0KMC-**
Head **0KM0**
Hip
Left **0KMP-**
Right **0KMN-**
Lower Arm and Wrist
Left **0KMB-**
Right **0KM9-**
Lower Leg
Left **0KMT-**
Right **0KMS**
Neck
Left **0KM3-**
Right **0KM2**
Perineum **0KMM-**
Shoulder
Left **0KM6-**
Right **0KM5-**
Thorax
Left **0KMJ-**
Right **0KMH-**
Tongue, Palate, Pharynx **0KM4-**
Trunk
Left **0KMG-**
Right **0KMF-**
Upper Arm
Left **0KM8-**
Right **0KM7-**
Upper Leg
Left **0KMR-**
Right **0KMQ-**
Nasal Mucosa and Soft Tissue **09MKXZZ**
Neck **0WM60ZZ**
Nipple
Left **0HMXXZZ**
Right **0HMWXZZ**
Ovary
Bilateral **0UM2-**
Left **0UM1-**
Right **0UM0-**
Palate, Soft **0CM30ZZ**
Pancreas **0FMG-**

© 2018 Channel Publishing, Ltd.

Reattachment — *continued*
Parathyroid Gland **0GMR-**
Inferior
Left **0GMP-**
Right **0GMN-**
Multiple **0GMQ-**
Superior
Left **0GMM-**
Right **0GML-**
Penis **0VMSXZZ**
Perineum
Female **0WMN0ZZ**
Male **0WMM0ZZ**
Rectum **0DMP-**
Scrotum **0VM5XZZ**
Shoulder Region
Left **0XM30ZZ**
Right **0XM20ZZ**
Skin
Abdomen **0HM7XZZ**
Back **0HM6XZZ**
Buttock **0HM8XZZ**
Chest **0HM5XZZ**
Ear
Left **0HM3XZZ**
Right **0HM2XZZ**
Face **0HM1XZZ**
Foot
Left **0HMNXZZ**
Right **0HMMXZZ**
Hand
Left **0HMGXZZ**
Right **0HMFXZZ**
Inguinal **0HMAXZZ**
Lower Arm
Left **0HMEXZZ**
Right **0HMDXZZ**
Lower Leg
Left **0HMLXZZ**
Right **0HMKXZZ**
Neck **0HM4XZZ**
Perineum **0HM9XZZ**
Scalp **0HM0XZZ**
Upper Arm
Left **0HMCXZZ**
Right **0HMBXZZ**
Upper Leg
Left **0HMJXZZ**
Right **0HMHXZZ**
Stomach **0DM6-**
Tendon
Abdomen
Left **0LMG-**
Right **0LMF-**
Ankle
Left **0LMT-**
Right **0LMS-**
Foot
Left **0LMW-**
Right **0LMV-**
Hand
Left **0LM8-**
Right **0LM7-**
Head and Neck **0LM0-**
Hip
Left **0LMK-**
Right **0LMJ-**
Knee
Left **0LMR-**
Right **0LMQ-**
Lower Arm and Wrist
Left **0LM6-**
Right **0LM5-**
Lower Leg
Left **0LMP-**
Right **0LMN-**
Perineum **0LMH-**
Shoulder
Left **0LM2-**
Right **0LM1-**
Thorax
Left **0LMD-**
Right **0LMC-**

Reattachment — *continued*
Tendon — *continued*
Trunk
Left **0LMB-**
Right **0LM9-**
Upper Arm
Left **0LM4-**
Right **0LM3-**
Upper Leg
Left **0LMM-**
Right **0LML-**
Testis
Bilateral **0VMC-**
Left **0VMB-**
Right **0VM9-**
Thumb
Left **0XMM0ZZ**
Right **0XML0ZZ**
Thyroid Gland
Left Lobe **0GMG-**
Right Lobe **0GMH-**
Toe
1st
Left **0YMQ0ZZ**
Right **0YMP0ZZ**
2nd
Left **0YMS0ZZ**
Right **0YMR0ZZ**
3rd
Left **0YMU0ZZ**
Right **0YMT0ZZ**
4th
Left **0YMW0ZZ**
Right **0YMV0ZZ**
5th
Left **0YMY0ZZ**
Right **0YMX0ZZ**
Tongue **0CM70ZZ**
Tooth
Lower **0CMX-**
Upper **0CMW-**
Trachea **0BM10ZZ**
Tunica Vaginalis
Left **0VM7-**
Right **0VM6-**
Ureter
Left **0TM7-**
Right **0TM6-**
Ureters, Bilateral **0TM8-**
Urethra **0TMD-**
Uterine Supporting Structure **0UM4-**
Uterus **0UM9-**
Uvula **0CMN0ZZ**
Vagina **0UMG-**
Vulva **0UMMXZZ**
Wrist Region
Left **0XMH0ZZ**
Right **0XMG0ZZ**
REBOA (resuscitative endovascular balloon occlusion of the aorta)
Abdominal Aorta **04L03DJ**
Thoracic Aorta, Descending **02LW3DJ**
Rebound HRD® (Hernia Repair Device)
use Synthetic Substitute
Recession
see Repair
see Reposition
Reclosure, disrupted abdominal wall 0WQFXZZ
Reconstruction
see Repair
see Replacement
see Supplement
Rectectomy
see Excision, Rectum **0DBP-**
see Resection, Rectum **0DTP-**
Rectocele repair
see Repair, Subcutaneous Tissue and Fascia, Pelvic Region **0JQC-**

Rectopexy
see Repair, Gastrointestinal System **0DQ-**
see Reposition, Gastrointestinal System **0DS-**
Rectoplasty
see Repair, Gastrointestinal System **0DQ-**
see Supplement, Gastrointestinal System **0DU-**
Rectorrhaphy *see* Repair, Gastrointestinal System **0DQ-**
Rectoscopy 0DJD8ZZ
Rectosigmoid junction
use Colon, Sigmoid
Rectosigmoidectomy
see Excision, Gastrointestinal System **0DB-**
see Resection, Gastrointestinal System **0DT-**
Rectostomy *see* Drainage, Rectum **0D9P-**
Rectotomy *see* Drainage, Rectum **0D9P-**
Rectus abdominis muscle
use Muscle, Abdomen, Left
use Muscle, Abdomen, Right
Rectus femoris muscle
use Muscle, Upper Leg, Left
use Muscle, Upper Leg, Right
Recurrent laryngeal nerve
use Nerve, Vagus
Reduction
Dislocation *see* Reposition
Fracture *see* Reposition
Intussusception, intestinal *see* Reposition, Gastrointestinal System **0DS-**
Mammoplasty *see* Excision, Skin and Breast **0HB-**
Prolapse *see* Reposition
Torsion *see* Reposition
Volvulus, gastrointestinal *see* Reposition, Gastrointestinal System **0DS-**
Refusion *see* Fusion
Rehabilitation
see Activities of Daily Living Assessment, Rehabilitation **F02-**
see Activities of Daily Living Treatment, Rehabilitation **F08-**
see Caregiver Training, Rehabilitation **F0F-**
see Cochlear Implant Treatment, Rehabilitation **F0B-**
see Device Fitting, Rehabilitation **F0D-**
see Hearing Treatment, Rehabilitation **F09-**
see Motor Function Assessment, Rehabilitation **F01-**
see Motor Treatment, Rehabilitation **F07-**
see Speech Assessment, Rehabilitation **F00-**
see Speech Treatment, Rehabilitation **F06-**
see Vestibular Treatment, Rehabilitation **F0C-**
Reimplantation
see Reattachment
see Reposition
see Transfer
Reinforcement
see Repair
see Supplement
Relaxation, scar tissue *see* Release
Release
Acetabulum
Left **0QN5-**
Right **0QN4-**

Release — *continued*
Adenoids **0CNQ-**
Ampulla of Vater **0FNC-**
Anal Sphincter **0DNR-**
Anterior Chamber
Left **08N33ZZ**
Right **08N23ZZ**
Anus **0DNQ-**
Aorta
Abdominal **04N0-**
Thoracic
Ascending/Arch **02NX-**
Descending **02NW-**
Aortic Body **0GND-**
Appendix **0DNJ-**
Artery
Anterior Tibial
Left **04NQ-**
Right **04NP-**
Axillary
Left **03N6-**
Right **03N5-**
Brachial
Left **03N8-**
Right **03N7-**
Celiac **04N1-**
Colic
Left **04N7-**
Middle **04N8-**
Right **04N6-**
Common Carotid
Left **03NJ-**
Right **03NH-**
Common Iliac
Left **04ND-**
Right **04NC-**
Coronary
Four or More Arteries **02N3-**
One Artery **02N0-**
Three Arteries **02N2-**
Two Arteries **02N1-**
External Carotid
Left **03NN-**
Right **03NM-**
External Iliac
Left **04NJ-**
Right **04NH-**
Face **03NR-**
Femoral
Left **04NL-**
Right **04NK-**
Foot
Left **04NW-**
Right **04NV-**
Gastric **04N2-**
Hand
Left **03NF-**
Right **03ND-**
Hepatic **04N3-**
Inferior Mesenteric **04NB-**
Innominate **03N2-**
Internal Carotid
Left **03NL-**
Right **03NK-**
Internal Iliac
Left **04NF-**
Right **04NE-**
Internal Mammary
Left **03N1-**
Right **03N0-**
Intracranial **03NG-**
Lower **04NY-**
Peroneal
Left **04NU-**
Right **04NT-**
Popliteal
Left **04NN-**
Right **04NM-**
Posterior Tibial
Left **04NS-**
Right **04NR-**

© 2018 Channel Publishing, Ltd.

Release — *continued*
- Artery — *continued*
  - Pulmonary
    - Left **02NR-**
    - Right **02NQ-**
  - Pulmonary Trunk **02NP-**
  - Radial
    - Left **03NC-**
    - Right **03NB-**
  - Renal
    - Left **04NA-**
    - Right **04N9-**
  - Splenic **04N4-**
  - Subclavian
    - Left **03N4-**
    - Right **03N3-**
  - Superior Mesenteric **04N5-**
  - Temporal
    - Left **03NT-**
    - Right **03NS-**
  - Thyroid
    - Left **03NV-**
    - Right **03NU-**
  - Ulnar
    - Left **03NA-**
    - Right **03N9-**
  - Upper **03NY-**
  - Vertebral
    - Left **03NQ-**
    - Right **03NP-**
- Atrium
  - Left **02N7-**
  - Right **02N6-**
- Auditory Ossicle
  - Left **09NA-**
  - Right **09N9-**
- Basal Ganglia **00N8-**
- Bladder **0TNB-**
- Bladder Neck **0TNC-**
- Bone
  - Ethmoid
    - Left **0NNG-**
    - Right **0NNF-**
  - Frontal **0NN1-**
  - Hyoid **0NNX-**
  - Lacrimal
    - Left **0NNJ-**
    - Right **0NNH-**
  - Nasal **0NNB-**
  - Occipital **0NN7-**
  - Palatine
    - Left **0NNL-**
    - Right **0NNK-**
  - Parietal
    - Left **0NN4-**
    - Right **0NN3-**
  - Pelvic
    - Left **0QN3-**
    - Right **0QN2-**
  - Sphenoid **0NNC-**
  - Temporal
    - Left **0NN6-**
    - Right **0NN5-**
  - Zygomatic
    - Left **0NNN-**
    - Right **0NNM-**
- Brain **00N0-**
- Breast
  - Bilateral **0HNV-**
  - Left **0HNU-**
  - Right **0HNT-**
- Bronchus
  - Lingula **0BN9-**
  - Lower Lobe
    - Left **0BNB-**
    - Right **0BN6-**
  - Main
    - Left **0BN7-**
    - Right **0BN3-**
  - Middle Lobe, Right **0BN5-**
  - Upper Lobe
    - Left **0BN8-**
    - Right **0BN4-**
- Buccal Mucosa **0CN4-**

Release — *continued*
- Bursa and Ligament
  - Abdomen
    - Left **0MNJ-**
    - Right **0MNH-**
  - Ankle
    - Left **0MNR-**
    - Right **0MNQ-**
  - Elbow
    - Left **0MN4-**
    - Right **0MN3-**
  - Foot
    - Left **0MNT-**
    - Right **0MNS-**
  - Hand
    - Left **0MN8-**
    - Right **0MN7-**
  - Head and Neck **0MN0-**
  - Hip
    - Left **0MNM-**
    - Right **0MNL-**
  - Knee
    - Left **0MNP-**
    - Right **0MNN-**
  - Lower Extremity
    - Left **0MNW-**
    - Right **0MNV-**
  - Perineum **0MNK-**
  - Rib(s) **0MNG-**
  - Shoulder
    - Left **0MN2-**
    - Right **0MN1-**
  - Spine
    - Lower **0MND-**
    - Upper **0MNC-**
  - Sternum **0MNF-**
  - Upper Extremity
    - Left **0MNB-**
    - Right **0MN9-**
  - Wrist
    - Left **0MN6-**
    - Right **0MN5-**
- Carina **0BN2-**
- Carotid Bodies, Bilateral **0GN8-**
- Carotid Body
  - Left **0GN6-**
  - Right **0GN7**
- Carpal
  - Left **0PNN-**
  - Right **0PNM-**
- Cecum **0DNH-**
- Cerebellum **00NC-**
- Cerebral Hemisphere **00N7-**
- Cerebral Meninges **00N1-**
- Cerebral Ventricle **00N6-**
- Cervix **0UNC-**
- Chordae Tendineae **02N9-**
- Choroid
  - Left **08NB-**
  - Right **08NA-**
- Cisterna Chyli **07NL-**
- Clavicle
  - Left **0PNB-**
  - Right **0PN9-**
- Clitoris **0UNJ-**
- Coccygeal Glomus **0GNB-**
- Coccyx **0QNS-**
- Colon
  - Ascending **0DNK-**
  - Descending **0DNM-**
  - Sigmoid **0DNN-**
  - Transverse **0DNL-**
- Conduction Mechanism **02N8-**
- Conjunctiva
  - Left **08NTXZZ**
  - Right **08NSXZZ**
- Cord
  - Bilateral **0VNH-**
  - Left **0VNG-**
  - Right **0VNF-**
- Cornea
  - Left **08N9XZZ**
  - Right **08N8XZZ**
- Cul-de-sac **0UNF-**

Release — *continued*
- Diaphragm **0BNT-**
- Disc
  - Cervical Vertebral **0RN3-**
  - Cervicothoracic Vertebral **0RN5-**
  - Lumbar Vertebral **0SN2-**
  - Lumbosacral **0SN4-**
  - Thoracic Vertebral **0RN9-**
  - Thoracolumbar Vertebral **0RNB-**
- Duct
  - Common Bile **0FN9-**
  - Cystic **0FN8-**
  - Hepatic
    - Common **0FN7-**
    - Left **0FN6-**
    - Right **0FN5-**
  - Lacrimal
    - Left **08NY-**
    - Right **08NX-**
  - Pancreatic **0FND-**
    - Accessory **0FNF-**
  - Parotid
    - Left **0CNC-**
    - Right **0CNB-**
- Duodenum **0DN9-**
- Dura Mater **00N2-**
- Ear
  - External
    - Left **09N1-**
    - Right **09N0-**
  - External Auditory Canal
    - Left **09N4-**
    - Right **09N3-**
  - Inner
    - Left **09NE-**
    - Right **09ND-**
  - Middle
    - Left **09N6-**
    - Right **09N5-**
- Epididymis
  - Bilateral **0VNL-**
  - Left **0VNK-**
  - Right **0VNJ-**
- Epiglottis **0CNR-**
- Esophagogastric Junction **0DN4-**
- Esophagus **0DN5-**
  - Lower **0DN3-**
  - Middle **0DN2-**
  - Upper **0DN1-**
- Eustachian Tube
  - Left **09NG-**
  - Right **09NF-**
- Eye
  - Left **08N1XZZ**
  - Right **08N0XZZ**
- Eyelid
  - Lower
    - Left **08NR-**
    - Right **08NQ-**
  - Upper
    - Left **08NP-**
    - Right **08NN-**
- Fallopian Tube
  - Left **0UN6-**
  - Right **0UN5-**
- Fallopian Tubes, Bilateral **0UN7-**
- Femoral Shaft
  - Left **0QN9-**
  - Right **0QN8-**
- Femur
  - Lower
    - Left **0QNC-**
    - Right **0QNB-**
  - Upper
    - Left **0QN7-**
    - Right **0QN6-**
- Fibula
  - Left **0QNK-**
  - Right **0QNJ-**
- Finger Nail **0HNQXZZ**
- Gallbladder **0FN4-**

Release — *continued*
- Gingiva
  - Lower **0CN6-**
  - Upper **0CN5-**
- Gland
  - Adrenal
    - Bilateral **0GN4-**
    - Left **0GN2-**
    - Right **0GN3-**
  - Lacrimal
    - Left **08NW-**
    - Right **08NV-**
  - Minor Salivary **0CNJ-**
  - Parotid
    - Left **0CN9-**
    - Right **0CN8-**
  - Pituitary **0GN0-**
  - Sublingual
    - Left **0CNF-**
    - Right **0CND-**
  - Submaxillary
    - Left **0CNH-**
    - Right **0CNG-**
  - Vestibular **0UNL-**
- Glenoid Cavity
  - Left **0PN8-**
  - Right **0PN7-**
- Glomus Jugulare **0GNC-**
- Humeral Head
  - Left **0PND-**
  - Right **0PNC-**
- Humeral Shaft
  - Left **0PNG-**
  - Right **0PNF-**
- Hymen **0UNK-**
- Hypothalamus **00NA-**
- Ileocecal Valve **0DNC-**
- Ileum **0DNB-**
- Intestine
  - Large **0DNE-**
    - Left **0DNG-**
    - Right **0DNF-**
  - Small **0DN8-**
- Iris
  - Left **08ND3ZZ**
  - Right **08NC3ZZ**
- Jejunum **0DNA-**
- Joint
  - Acromioclavicular
    - Left **0RNH-**
    - Right **0RNG-**
  - Ankle
    - Left **0SNG-**
    - Right **0SNF-**
  - Carpal
    - Left **0RNR-**
    - Right **0RNQ-**
  - Carpometacarpal
    - Left **0RNT-**
    - Right **0RNS-**
  - Cervical Vertebral **0RN1-**
  - Cervicothoracic Vertebral **0RN4-**
  - Coccygeal **0SN6-**
  - Elbow
    - Left **0RNM-**
    - Right **0RNL-**
  - Finger Phalangeal
    - Left **0RNX-**
    - Right **0RNW-**
  - Hip
    - Left **0SNB-**
    - Right **0SN9-**
  - Knee
    - Left **0SND-**
    - Right **0SNC-**
  - Lumbar Vertebral **0SN0-**
  - Lumbosacral **0SN3-**
  - Metacarpophalangeal
    - Left **0RNV-**
    - Right **0RNU-**
  - Metatarsal-Phalangeal
    - Left **0SNN-**
    - Right **0SNM-**

© 2018 Channel Publishing, Ltd.

Release — *continued*
Joint — *continued*
Occipital-cervical **0RN0-**
Sacrococcygeal **0SN5-**
Sacroiliac
Left **0SN8-**
Right **0SN7-**
Shoulder
Left **0RNK-**
Right **0RNJ-**
Sternoclavicular
Left **0RNF-**
Right **0RNE-**
Tarsal
Left **0SNJ-**
Right **0SNH-**
Tarsometatarsal
Left **0SNL-**
Right **0SNK-**
Temporomandibular
Left **0RND-**
Right **0RNC-**
Thoracic Vertebral **0RN6-**
Thoracolumbar Vertebral **0RNA-**
Toe Phalangeal
Left **0SNQ-**
Right **0SNP-**
Wrist
Left **0RNP-**
Right **0RNN-**
Kidney
Left **0TN1-**
Right **0TN0-**
Kidney Pelvis
Left **0TN4-**
Right **0TN3-**
Larynx **0CNS-**
Lens
Left **08NK3ZZ**
Right **08NJ3ZZ**
Lip
Lower **0CN1-**
Upper **0CN0-**
Liver **0FN0-**
Left Lobe **0FN2-**
Right Lobe **0FN1-**
Lung
Bilateral **0BNM-**
Left **0BNL-**
Lower Lobe
Left **0BNJ-**
Right **0BNF-**
Middle Lobe, Right **0BND-**
Right **0BNK-**
Upper Lobe
Left **0BNG-**
Right **0BNC-**
Lung Lingula **0BNH-**
Lymphatic
Aortic **07ND-**
Axillary
Left **07N6-**
Right **07N5-**
Head **07N0-**
Inguinal
Left **07NJ-**
Right **07NH-**
Internal Mammary
Left **07N9-**
Right **07N8-**
Lower Extremity
Left **07NG-**
Right **07NF-**
Mesenteric **07NB-**
Neck
Left **07N2-**
Right **07N1-**
Pelvis **07NC-**
Thoracic Duct **07NK-**
Thorax **07N7-**
Upper Extremity
Left **07N4-**
Right **07N3-**

Release — *continued*
Mandible
Left **0NNV-**
Right **0NNT-**
Maxilla **0NNR-**
Medulla Oblongata **00ND-**
Mesentery **0DNV-**
Metacarpal
Left **0PNQ-**
Right **0PNP-**
Metatarsal
Left **0QNP-**
Right **0QNN-**
Muscle
Abdomen
Left **0KNL-**
Right **0KNK-**
Extraocular
Left **08NM-**
Right **08NL-**
Facial **0KN1-**
Foot
Left **0KNW-**
Right **0KNV-**
Hand
Left **0KND-**
Right **0KNC-**
Head **0KN0-**
Hip
Left **0KNP-**
Right **0KNN-**
Lower Arm and Wrist
Left **0KNB-**
Right **0KN9-**
Lower Leg
Left **0KNT-**
Right **0KNS-**
Neck
Left **0KN3-**
Right **0KN2-**
Papillary **02ND-**
Perineum **0KNM-**
Shoulder
Left **0KN6-**
Right **0KN5-**
Thorax
Left **0KNJ-**
Right **0KNH-**
Tongue, Palate, Pharynx **0KN4-**
Trunk
Left **0KNG-**
Right **0KNF-**
Upper Arm
Left **0KN8-**
Right **0KN7-**
Upper Leg
Left **0KNR-**
Right **0KNQ-**
Myocardial Bridge *see* Release, Artery, Coronary
Nasal Mucosa and Soft Tissue **09NK-**
Nasopharynx **09NN-**
Nerve
Abdominal Sympathetic **01NM-**
Abducens **00NL-**
Accessory **00NR-**
Acoustic **00NN-**
Brachial Plexus **01N3-**
Cervical **01N1-**
Cervical Plexus **01N0-**
Facial **00NM-**
Femoral **01ND-**
Glossopharyngeal **00NP-**
Head and Neck Sympathetic **01NK-**
Hypoglossal **00NS-**
Lumbar **01NB-**
Lumbar Plexus **01N9-**
Lumbar Sympathetic **01NN-**
Lumbosacral Plexus **01NA-**
Median **01N5-**
Oculomotor **00NH-**
Olfactory **00NF-**

Release — *continued*
Nerve — *continued*
Optic **00NG-**
Peroneal **01NH-**
Phrenic **01N2-**
Pudendal **01NC-**
Radial **01N6-**
Sacral **01NR-**
Sacral Plexus **01NQ-**
Sacral Sympathetic **01NP-**
Sciatic **01NF-**
Thoracic **01N8-**
Thoracic Sympathetic **01NL -**
Tibial **01NG-**
Trigeminal **00NK-**
Trochlear **00NJ-**
Ulnar **01N4-**
Vagus **00NQ-**
Nipple
Left **0HNX-**
Right **0HNW-**
Omentum **0DNU-**
Orbit
Left **0NNQ-**
Right **0NNP-**
Ovary
Bilateral **0UN2-**
Left **0UN1-**
Right **0UN0-**
Palate
Hard **0CN2-**
Soft **0CN3-**
Pancreas **0FNG-**
Para-aortic Body **0GN9-**
Paraganglion Extremity **0GNF-**
Parathyroid Gland **0GNR-**
Inferior
Left **0GNP-**
Right **0GNN-**
Multiple **0GNQ-**
Superior
Left **0GNM-**
Right **0GNL-**
Patella
Left **0QNF-**
Right **0QND-**
Penis **0VNS-**
Pericardium **02NN-**
Peritoneum **0DNW-**
Phalanx
Finger
Left **0PNV-**
Right **0PNT-**
Thumb
Left **0PNS-**
Right **0PNR-**
Toe
Left **0QNR-**
Right **0QNQ-**
Pharynx **0CNM-**
Pineal Body **0GN1-**
Pleura
Left **0BNP-**
Right **0BNN-**
Pons **00NB-**
Prepuce **0VNT-**
Prostate **0VN0-**
Radius
Left **0PNJ-**
Right **0PNH-**
Rectum **0DNP-**
Retina
Left **08NF3ZZ**
Right **08NE3ZZ**
Retinal Vessel
Left **08NH3ZZ**
Right **08NG3ZZ**
Ribs
1 to 2 **0PN1-**
3 or more **0PN2-**
Sacrum **0QN1-**
Scapula
Left **0PN6-**
Right **0PN5-**

Release — *continued*
Sclera
Left **08N7XZZ**
Right **08N6XZZ**
Scrotum **0VN5-**
Septum
Atrial **02N5-**
Nasal **09NM-**
Ventricular **02NM-**
Sinus
Accessory **09NP-**
Ethmoid
Left **09NV-**
Right **09NU-**
Frontal
Left **09NT-**
Right **09NS-**
Mastoid
Left **09NC-**
Right **09NB-**
Maxillary
Left **09NR-**
Right **09NQ-**
Sphenoid
Left **09NX-**
Right **09NW-**
Skin
Abdomen **0HN7XZZ**
Back **0HN6XZZ**
Buttock **0HN8XZZ**
Chest **0HN5XZZ**
Ear
Left **0HN3XZZ**
Right **0HN2XZZ**
Face **0HN1XZZ**
Foot
Left **0HNNXZZ**
Right **0HNMXZZ**
Hand
Left **0HNGXZZ**
Right **0HNFXZZ**
Inguinal **0HNAXZZ**
Lower Arm
Left **0HNEXZZ**
Right **0HNDXZZ**
Lower Leg
Left **0HNLXZZ**
Right **0HNKXZZ**
Neck **0HN4XZZ**
Perineum **0HN9XZZ**
Scalp **0HN0XZZ**
Upper Arm
Left **0HNCXZZ**
Right **0HNBXZZ**
Upper Leg
Left **0HNJXZZ**
Right **0HNHXZZ**
Spinal Cord
Cervical **00NW-**
Lumbar **00NY-**
Thoracic **00NX-**
Spinal Meninges **00NT-**
Spleen **07NP-**
Sternum **0PN0-**
Stomach **0DN6-**
Pylorus **0DN7-**
Subcutaneous Tissue and Fascia
Abdomen **0JN8-**
Back **0JN7-**
Buttock **0JN9-**
Chest **0JN6-**
Face **0JN1-**
Foot
Left **0JNR-**
Right **0JNQ-**
Hand
Left **0JNK-**
Right **0JNJ-**
Lower Arm
Left **0JNH-**
Right **0JNG-**
Lower Leg
Left **0JNP-**
Right **0JNN-**

PROCEDURE INDEX

© 2018 Channel Publishing, Ltd.

© 2018 Channel Publishing, Ltd.

- **Removal of device from** — *continued*
  - Femur
    - Lower
      - Left **0QPC**-
      - Right **0QPB**-
    - Upper
      - Left **0QP7**-
      - Right **0QP6**-
  - Fibula
    - Left **0QPK**-
    - Right **0QPJ**
  - Finger Nail **0HPQX**-
  - Gallbladder **0FP4**-
  - Gastrointestinal Tract **0WPP**-
  - Genitourinary Tract **0WPR**-
  - Gland
    - Adrenal **0GP5**-
    - Endocrine **0GPS**-
    - Pituitary **0GP0**-
    - Salivary **0CPA**-
  - Glenoid Cavity
    - Left **0PP8**-
    - Right **0PP7**-
  - Great Vessel **02PY**-
  - Hair **0HPSX**-
  - Head **0WP0**-
  - Heart **02PA**-
  - Humeral Head
    - Left **0PPD**-
    - Right **0PPC**-
  - Humeral Shaft
    - Left **0PPG**-
    - Right **0PPF**-
  - Intestinal Tract
    - Lower **0DPD**-
    - Upper **0DP0**-
  - Jaw
    - Lower **0WP5**-
    - Upper **0WP4**-
  - Joint
    - Acromioclavicular
      - Left **0RPH**-
      - Right **0RPG**-
    - Ankle
      - Left **0SPG**-
      - Right **0SPF**-
    - Carpal
      - Left **0RPR**-
      - Right **0RPQ**-
    - Carpometacarpal
      - Left **0RPT**-
      - Right **0RPS**-
    - Cervical Vertebral **0RP1**-
    - Cervicothoracic Vertebral **0RP4**-
    - Coccygeal **0SP6**-
    - Elbow
      - Left **0RPM**-
      - Right **0RPL**-
    - Finger Phalangeal
      - Left **0RPX**-
      - Right **0RPW**-
    - Hip
      - Left **0SPB**-
        - Acetabular Surface **0SPE**-
        - Femoral Surface **0SPS**-
      - Right **0SP9**-
        - Acetabular Surface **0SPA**-
        - Femoral Surface **0SPR**-
    - Knee
      - Left **0SPD**-
        - Femoral Surface **0SPU**-
        - Tibial Surface **0SPW**-
      - Right **0SPC**-
        - Femoral Surface **0SPT**-
        - Tibial Surface **0SPV**-
    - Lumbar Vertebral **0SP0**-
    - Lumbosacral **0SP3**-
    - Metacarpophalangeal
      - Left **0RPV**-
      - Right **0RPU**-
    - Metatarsal-Phalangeal
      - Left **0SPN**-
      - Right **0SPM**-

- **Removal of device from** — *continued*
  - Joint — *continued*
    - Occipital-cervical **0RP0**-
    - Sacrococcygeal **0SP5**-
    - Sacroiliac
      - Left **0SP8**-
      - Right **0SP7**-
    - Shoulder
      - Left **0RPK**-
      - Right **0RPJ**-
    - Sternoclavicular
      - Left **0RPF**-
      - Right **0RPE**-
    - Tarsal
      - Left **0SPJ**-
      - Right **0SPH**-
    - Tarsometatarsal
      - Left **0SPL**-
      - Right **0SPK**-
    - Temporomandibular
      - Left **0RPD**-
      - Right **0RPC**-
    - Thoracic Vertebral **0RP6**-
    - Thoracolumbar Vertebral **0RPA**-
    - Toe Phalangeal
      - Left **0SPQ**-
      - Right **0SPP**-
    - Wrist
      - Left **0RPP**-
      - Right **0RPN**-
  - Kidney **0TP5**-
  - Larynx **0CPS**-
  - Lens
    - Left **08PK3**-
    - Right **08PJ3**-
  - Liver **0FP0**-
  - Lung
    - Left **0BPL**-
    - Right **0BPK**-
  - Lymphatic **07PN**-
    - Thoracic Duct **07PK**-
  - Mediastinum **0WPC**-
  - Mesentery **0DPV**-
  - Metacarpal
    - Left **0PPQ**-
    - Right **0PPP**-
  - Metatarsal
    - Left **0QPP**-
    - Right **0QPN**-
  - Mouth and Throat **0CPY**-
  - Muscle
    - Extraocular
      - Left **08PM**-
      - Right **08PL**-
    - Lower **0KPY**-
    - Upper **0KPX**-
  - Nasal Mucosa and Soft Tissue **09PK**-
  - Neck **0WP6**-
  - Nerve
    - Cranial **00PE**-
    - Peripheral **01PY**-
  - Omentum **0DPU**-
  - Ovary **0UP3**-
  - Pancreas **0FPG**-
  - Parathyroid Gland **0GPR**-
  - Patella
    - Left **0QPF**-
    - Right **0QPD**-
  - Pelvic Cavity **0WPJ**-
  - Penis **0VPS**-
  - Pericardial Cavity **0WPD**-
  - Perineum
    - Female **0WPN**-
    - Male **0WPM**-
  - Peritoneal Cavity **0WPG**-
  - Peritoneum **0DPW**-

- **Removal of device from** — *continued*
  - Phalanx
    - Finger
      - Left **0PPV**-
      - Right **0PPT**-
    - Thumb
      - Left **0PPS**-
      - Right **0PPR**-
    - Toe
      - Left **0QPR**-
      - Right **0QPQ**-
  - Pineal Body **0GP1**-
  - Pleura **0BPQ**-
  - Pleural Cavity
    - Left **0WPB**-
    - Right **0WP9**-
  - Products of Conception **10P0**-
  - Prostate and Seminal Vesicles **0VP4**-
  - Radius
    - Left **0PPJ**-
    - Right **0PPH**-
  - Rectum **0DPP**-
  - Respiratory Tract **0WPQ**-
  - Retroperitoneum **0WPH**-
  - Ribs
    - 1 to 2 **0PP1**-
    - 3 or more **0PP2**-
  - Sacrum **0QP1**-
  - Scapula
    - Left **0PP6**-
    - Right **0PP5**-
  - Scrotum and Tunica Vaginalis **0VP8**-
  - Sinus **09PY**-
  - Skin **0HPPX**-
  - Skull **0NP0**-
  - Spinal Canal **00PU**-
  - Spinal Cord **00PV**-
  - Spleen **07PP**-
  - Sternum **0PP0**-
  - Stomach **0DP6**-
  - Subcutaneous Tissue and Fascia
    - Head and Neck **0JPS**-
    - Lower Extremity **0JPW**-
    - Trunk **0JPT**-
    - Upper Extremity **0JPV**-
  - Tarsal
    - Left **0QPM**-
    - Right **0QPL**-
  - Tendon
    - Lower **0LPY**-
    - Upper **0LPX**-
  - Testis **0VPD**-
  - Thymus **07PM**-
  - Thyroid Gland **0GPK**-
  - Tibia
    - Left **0QPH**-
    - Right **0QPG**-
  - Toe Nail **0HPRX**-
  - Trachea **0BP1**-
  - Tracheobronchial Tree **0BP0**-
  - Tympanic Membrane
    - Left **09P8**-
    - Right **09P7**-
  - Ulna
    - Left **0PPL**-
    - Right **0PPK**-
  - Ureter **0TP9**-
  - Urethra **0TPD**-
  - Uterus and Cervix **0UPD**-
  - Vagina and Cul-de-sac **0UPH**-
  - Vas Deferens **0VPR**-
  - Vein
    - Azygos **05P0**-
    - Innominate
      - Left **05P4**-
      - Right **05P3**-
    - Lower **06PY**-
    - Upper **05PY**-

- **Removal of device from** — *continued*
  - Vertebra
    - Cervical **0PP3**-
    - Lumbar **0QP0**-
    - Thoracic **0PP4**-
  - Vulva **0UPM**-
- **Renal calyx**
  - *use* Kidney
  - *use* Kidneys, Bilateral
  - *use* Kidney, Left
  - *use* Kidney, Right
- **Renal capsule**
  - *use* Kidney
  - *use* Kidneys, Bilateral
  - *use* Kidney, Left
  - *use* Kidney, Right
- **Renal cortex**
  - *use* Kidney
  - *use* Kidneys, Bilateral
  - *use* Kidney, Left
  - *use* Kidney, Right
- **Renal dialysis** *see* Performance, Urinary **5A1D**-
- **Renal plexus**
  - *use* Nerve, Abdominal Sympathetic
- **Renal segment**
  - *use* Kidney
  - *use* Kidney, Left
  - *use* Kidney, Right
  - *use* Kidneys, Bilateral
- **Renal segmental artery**
  - *use* Artery, Renal, Left
  - *use* Artery, Renal, Right
- **Reopening, operative site**
  - Control of bleeding *see* Control bleeding in
  - Inspection only *see* Inspection
- **Repair**
  - Abdominal Wall **0WQF**-
  - Acetabulum
    - Left **0QQ5**-
    - Right **0QQ4**-
  - Adenoids **0CQQ**-
  - Ampulla of Vater **0FQC**-
  - Anal Sphincter **0DQR**-
  - Ankle Region
    - Left **0YQL**-
    - Right **0YQK**-
  - Anterior Chamber
    - Left **08Q33ZZ**
    - Right **08Q23ZZ**
  - Anus **0DQQ**-
  - Aorta
    - Abdominal **04Q0**-
    - Thoracic
      - Ascending/Arch **02QX**-
      - Descending **02QW**-
  - Aortic Body **0GQD**-
  - Appendix **0DQJ**-
  - Arm
    - Lower
      - Left **0XQF**-
      - Right **0XQD**-
    - Upper
      - Left **0XQ9**-
      - Right **0XQ8**-
  - Artery
    - Anterior Tibial
      - Left **04QQ**-
      - Right **04QP**-
    - Axillary
      - Left **03Q6**-
      - Right **03Q5**-
    - Brachial
      - Left **03Q8**-
      - Right **03Q7**-
    - Celiac **04Q1**-
    - Colic
      - Left **04Q7**-
      - Middle **04Q8**-
      - Right **04Q6**-

© 2018 Channel Publishing, Ltd.

- **Repair** — *continued*
  - Artery — *continued*
    - Common Carotid
      - Left **03QJ**-
      - Right **03QH**-
    - Common Iliac
      - Left **04QD**-
      - Right **04QC**-
    - Coronary
      - Four or More Arteries **02Q3**-
      - One Artery **02Q0**-
      - Three Arteries **02Q2**-
      - Two Arteries **02Q1**-
    - External Carotid
      - Left **03QN**-
      - Right **03QM**-
    - External Iliac
      - Left **04QJ**-
      - Right **04QH**-
    - Face **03QR**-
    - Femoral
      - Left **04QL**-
      - Right **04QK**-
    - Foot
      - Left **04QW**-
      - Right **04QV**-
    - Gastric **04Q2**-
    - Hand
      - Left **03QF**-
      - Right **03QD**-
    - Hepatic **04Q3**-
    - Inferior Mesenteric **04QB**-
    - Innominate **03Q2**-
    - Internal Carotid
      - Left **03QL**-
      - Right **03QK**-
    - Internal Iliac
      - Left **04QF**-
      - Right **04QE**-
    - Internal Mammary
      - Left **03Q1**-
      - Right **03Q0**-
    - Intracranial **03QG**-
    - Lower **04QY**-
    - Peroneal
      - Left **04QU**-
      - Right **04QT**-
    - Popliteal
      - Left **04QN**-
      - Right **04QM**-
    - Posterior Tibial
      - Left **04QS**-
      - Right **04QR**-
    - Pulmonary
      - Left **02QR**-
      - Right **02QQ**-
    - Pulmonary Trunk **02QP**-
    - Radial
      - Left **03QC**-
      - Right **03QB**-
    - Renal
      - Left **04QA**-
      - Right **04Q9**-
    - Splenic **04Q4**-
    - Subclavian
      - Left **03Q4**-
      - Right **03Q3**-
    - Superior Mesenteric **04Q5**-
    - Temporal
      - Left **03QT**-
      - Right **03QS**-
    - Thyroid
      - Left **03QV**-
      - Right **03QU**-
    - Ulnar
      - Left **03QA**-
      - Right **03Q9**-
    - Upper **03QY**-
    - Vertebral
      - Left **03QQ**-
      - Right **03QP**-

- **Repair** — *continued*
  - Atrium
    - Left **02Q7**-
    - Right **02Q6**-
  - Auditory Ossicle
    - Left **09QA**-
    - Right **09Q9**-
  - Axilla
    - Left **0XQ5**-
    - Right **0XQ4**-
  - Back
    - Lower **0WQL**-
    - Upper **0WQK**-
  - Basal Ganglia **00Q8**-
  - Bladder **0TQB**-
  - Bladder Neck **0TQC**-
  - Bone
    - Ethmoid
      - Left **0NQG**-
      - Right **0NQF**-
    - Frontal **0NQ1**-
    - Hyoid **0NQX**-
    - Lacrimal
      - Left **0NQJ**-
      - Right **0NQH**-
    - Nasal **0NQB**-
    - Occipital **0NQ7**-
    - Palatine
      - Left **0NQL**-
      - Right **0NQK**-
    - Parietal
      - Left **0NQ4**-
      - Right **0NQ3**-
    - Pelvic
      - Left **0QQ3**-
      - Right **0QQ2**-
    - Sphenoid **0NQC**-
    - Temporal
      - Left **0NQ6**-
      - Right **0NQ5**-
    - Zygomatic
      - Left **0NQN**-
      - Right **0NQM**-
  - Brain **00Q0**-
  - Breast
    - Bilateral **0HQV**-
    - Left **0HQU**-
    - Right **0HQT**-
    - Supernumerary **0HQY**-
  - Bronchus
    - Lingula **0BQ9**-
    - Lower Lobe
      - Left **0BQB**-
      - Right **0BQ6**-
    - Main
      - Left **0BQ7**-
      - Right **0BQ3**-
    - Middle Lobe, Right **0BQ5**-
    - Upper Lobe
      - Left **0BQ8**-
      - Right **0BQ4**-
  - Buccal Mucosa **0CQ4**-
  - Bursa and Ligament
    - Abdomen
      - Left **0MQJ**-
      - Right **0MQH**-
    - Ankle
      - Left **0MQR**-
      - Right **0MQQ**-
    - Elbow
      - Left **0MQ4**-
      - Right **0MQ3**-
    - Foot
      - Left **0MQT**-
      - Right **0MQS**-
    - Hand
      - Left **0MQ8**-
      - Right **0MQ7**-
    - Head and Neck **0MQ0**-
    - Hip
      - Left **0MQM**-
      - Right **0MQL**-

- **Repair** — *continued*
  - Bursa and Ligament — *continued*
    - Knee
      - Left **0MQP**-
      - Right **0MQN**-
    - Lower Extremity
      - Left **0MQW**-
      - Right **0MQV**-
    - Perineum **0MQK**-
    - Rib(s) **0MQG**-
    - Shoulder
      - Left **0MQ2**-
      - Right **0MQ1**-
    - Spine
      - Lower **0MQD**-
      - Upper **0MQC**-
    - Sternum **0MQF**-
    - Upper Extremity
      - Left **0MQB**-
      - Right **0MQ9**-
    - Wrist
      - Left **0MQ6**-
      - Right **0MQ5**-
  - Buttock
    - Left **0YQ1**-
    - Right **0YQ0**-
  - Carina **0BQ2**
  - Carotid Bodies, Bilateral **0GQ8**-
  - Carotid Body
    - Left **0GQ6**-
    - Right **0GQ7**-
  - Carpal
    - Left **0PQN**-
    - Right **0PQM**-
  - Cecum **0DQH**-
  - Cerebellum **00QC**-
  - Cerebral Hemisphere **00Q7**-
  - Cerebral Meninges **00Q1**-
  - Cerebral Ventricle **00Q6**-
  - Cervix **0UQC**-
  - Chest Wall **0WQ8**-
  - Chordae Tendineae **02Q9**-
  - Choroid
    - Left **08QB**-
    - Right **08QA**-
  - Cisterna Chyli **07QL**-
  - Clavicle
    - Left **0PQB**-
    - Right **0PQ9**-
  - Clitoris **0UQJ**-
  - Coccygeal Glomus **0GQB**-
  - Coccyx **0QQS**-
  - Colon
    - Ascending **0DQK**-
    - Descending **0DQM**-
    - Sigmoid **0DQN**-
    - Transverse **0DQL**-
  - Conduction Mechanism **02Q8**-
  - Conjunctiva
    - Left **08QTXZZ**
    - Right **08QSXZZ**
  - Cord
    - Bilateral **0VQH**-
    - Left **0VQG**-
    - Right **0VQF**-
  - Cornea
    - Left **08Q9XZZ**
    - Right **08Q8XZZ**
  - Cul-de-sac **0UQF**-
  - Diaphragm **0BQT**-
  - Disc
    - Cervical Vertebral **0RQ3**-
    - Cervicothoracic Vertebral **0RQ5**-
    - Lumbar Vertebral **0SQ2**-
    - Lumbosacral **0SQ4**-
    - Thoracic Vertebral **0RQ9**-
    - Thoracolumbar Vertebral **0RQB**-

- **Repair** — *continued*
  - Duct
    - Common Bile **0FQ9**-
    - Cystic **0FQ8**-
    - Hepatic
      - Common **0FQ7**-
      - Left **0FQ6**-
      - Right **0FQ5**-
    - Lacrimal
      - Left **08QY**-
      - Right **08QX**-
    - Pancreatic **0FQD**-
      - Accessory **0FQF**-
    - Parotid
      - Left **0CQC**-
      - Right **0CQB**-
  - Duodenum **0DQ9**-
  - Dura Mater **00Q2**-
  - Ear
    - External
      - Bilateral **09Q2**-
      - Left **09Q1**-
      - Right **09Q0**-
    - External Auditory Canal
      - Left **09Q4**-
      - Right **09Q3**-
    - Inner
      - Left **09QE**-
      - Right **09QD**-
    - Middle
      - Left **09Q6**-
      - Right **09Q5**-
  - Elbow Region
    - Left **0XQC**-
    - Right **0XQB**-
  - Epididymis
    - Bilateral **0VQL**-
    - Left **0VQK**-
    - Right **0VQJ**-
  - Epiglottis **0CQR**-
  - Esophagogastric Junction **0DQ4**-
  - Esophagus **0DQ5**-
    - Lower **0DQ3**-
    - Middle **0DQ2**-
    - Upper **0DQ1**-
  - Eustachian Tube
    - Left **09QG**-
    - Right **09QF**-
  - Extremity
    - Lower
      - Left **0YQB**-
      - Right **0YQ9**-
    - Upper
      - Left **0XQ7**-
      - Right **0XQ6**-
  - Eye
    - Left **08Q1XZZ**
    - Right **08Q0XZZ**
  - Eyelid
    - Lower
      - Left **08QR**-
      - Right **08QQ**-
    - Upper
      - Left **08QP**-
      - Right **08QN**-
  - Face **0WQ2**-
  - Fallopian Tube
    - Left **0UQ6**-
    - Right **0UQ5**-
  - Fallopian Tubes, Bilateral **0UQ7**-
  - Femoral Region
    - Bilateral **0YQE**-
    - Left **0YQ8**-
    - Right **0YQ7**-
  - Femoral Shaft
    - Left **0QQ9**-
    - Right **0QQ8**-
  - Femur
    - Lower
      - Left **0QQC**-
      - Right **0QQB**-
    - Upper
      - Left **0QQ7**-
      - Right **0QQ6**-

© 2018 Channel Publishing, Ltd.

- **Repair** — *continued*
  - Fibula
    - Left **0QQK**-
    - Right **0QQJ**-
  - Finger
    - Index
      - Left **0XQP**-
      - Right **0XQN**-
    - Little
      - Left **0XQW**-
      - Right **0XQV**-
    - Middle
      - Left **0XQR**-
      - Right **0XQQ**-
    - Ring
      - Left **0XQT**-
      - Right **0XQS**-
  - Finger Nail **0HQQXZZ**
  - Floor of mouth *see* Repair, Oral Cavity and Throat **0WQ3**-
  - Foot
    - Left **0YQN**-
    - Right **0YQM**-
  - Gallbladder **0FQ4**-
  - Gingiva
    - Lower **0CQ6**-
    - Upper **0CQ5**-
  - Gland
    - Adrenal
      - Bilateral **0GQ4**-
      - Left **0GQ2**-
      - Right **0GQ3**-
    - Lacrimal
      - Left **08QW**-
      - Right **08QV**-
    - Minor Salivary **0CQJ**-
    - Parotid
      - Left **0CQ9**-
      - Right **0CQ8**-
    - Pituitary **0GQ0**-
    - Sublingual
      - Left **0CQF**-
      - Right **0CQD**-
    - Submaxillary
      - Left **0CQH**-
      - Right **0CQG**-
    - Vestibular **0UQL**-
  - Glenoid Cavity
    - Left **0PQ8**-
    - Right **0PQ7**-
  - Glomus Jugulare **0GQC**-
  - Hand
    - Left **0XQK**-
    - Right **0XQJ**-
  - Head **0WQ0**-
  - Heart **02QA**-
    - Left **02QC**-
    - Right **02QB**-
  - Humeral Head
    - Left **0PQD**-
    - Right **0PQC**-
  - Humeral Shaft
    - Left **0PQG**-
    - Right **0PQF**-
  - Hymen **0UQK**-
  - Hypothalamus **00QA**-
  - Ileocecal Valve **0DQC**-
  - Ileum **0DQB**-
  - Inguinal Region
    - Bilateral **0YQA**-
    - Left **0YQ6**-
    - Right **0YQ5**-
  - Intestine
    - Large **0DQE**-
      - Left **0DQG**-
      - Right **0DQF**-
    - Small **0DQ8**-
  - Iris
    - Left **08QD3ZZ**
    - Right **08QC3ZZ**
  - Jaw
    - Lower **0WQ5**-
    - Upper **0WQ4**-
- **Repair** — *continued*
  - Jejunum **0DQA**-
  - Joint
    - Acromioclavicular
      - Left **0RQH**-
      - Right **0RQG**-
    - Ankle
      - Left **0SQG**-
      - Right **0SQF**-
    - Carpal
      - Left **0RQR**-
      - Right **0RQQ**-
    - Carpometacarpal
      - Left **0RQT**-
      - Right **0RQS**-
    - Cervical Vertebral **0RQ1**-
    - Cervicothoracic Vertebral **0RQ4**-
    - Coccygeal **0SQ6**-
    - Elbow
      - Left **0RQM**-
      - Right **0RQL**-
    - Finger Phalangeal
      - Left **0RQX**-
      - Right **0RQW**-
    - Hip
      - Left **0SQB**-
      - Right **0SQ9**-
    - Knee
      - Left **0SQD**-
      - Right **0SQC**-
    - Lumbar Vertebral **0SQ0**-
    - Lumbosacral **0SQ3**-
    - Metacarpophalangeal
      - Left **0RQV**-
      - Right **0RQU**-
    - Metatarsal-Phalangeal
      - Left **0SQN**-
      - Right **0SQM**-
    - Occipital-cervical **0RQ0**-
    - Sacrococcygeal **0SQ5**-
    - Sacroiliac
      - Left **0SQ8**-
      - Right **0SQ7**-
    - Shoulder
      - Left **0RQK**-
      - Right **0RQJ**-
    - Sternoclavicular
      - Left **0RQF**-
      - Right **0RQE**-
    - Tarsal
      - Left **0SQJ**-
      - Right **0SQH**-
    - Tarsometatarsal
      - Left **0SQL**-
      - Right **0SQK**-
    - Temporomandibular
      - Left **0RQD**-
      - Right **0RQC**-
    - Thoracic Vertebral **0RQ6**-
    - Thoracolumbar Vertebral **0RQA**-
    - Toe Phalangeal
      - Left **0SQQ**-
      - Right **0SQP**
    - Wrist
      - Left **0RQP**-
      - Right **0RQN**-
  - Kidney
    - Left **0TQ1**-
    - Right **0TQ0**-
  - Kidney Pelvis
    - Left **0TQ4**-
    - Right **0TQ3**-
  - Knee Region
    - Left **0YQG**-
    - Right **0YQF**-
  - Larynx **0CQS**-
  - Leg
    - Lower
      - Left **0YQJ**-
      - Right **0YQH**-
- **Repair** — *continued*
  - Leg — *continued*
    - Upper
      - Left **0YQD**-
      - Right **0YQC**-
  - Lens
    - Left **08QK3ZZ**
    - Right **08QJ3ZZ**
  - Lip
    - Lower **0CQ1**-
    - Upper **0CQ0**-
  - Liver **0FQ0**-
    - Left Lobe **0FQ2**-
    - Right Lobe **0FQ1**-
  - Lung
    - Bilateral **0BQM**-
    - Left **0BQL**-
    - Lower Lobe
      - Left **0BQJ**-
      - Right **0BQF**-
    - Middle Lobe, Right **0BQD**-
    - Right **0BQK**-
    - Upper Lobe
      - Left **0BQG**-
      - Right **0BQC**-
  - Lung Lingula **0BQH**-
  - Lymphatic
    - Aortic **07QD**-
    - Axillary
      - Left **07Q6**-
      - Right **07Q5**-
    - Head **07Q0**-
    - Inguinal
      - Left **07QJ**-
      - Right **07QH**-
    - Internal Mammary
      - Left **07Q9**-
      - Right **07Q8**-
    - Lower Extremity
      - Left **07QG**-
      - Right **07QF**-
    - Mesenteric **07QB**-
    - Neck
      - Left **07Q2**-
      - Right **07Q1**-
    - Pelvis **07QC**-
    - Thoracic Duct **07QK**-
    - Thorax **07Q7**-
    - Upper Extremity
      - Left **07Q4**-
      - Right **07Q3**-
  - Mandible
    - Left **0NQV**-
    - Right **0NQT**-
  - Maxilla **0NQR**-
  - Mediastinum **0WQC**-
  - Medulla Oblongata **00QD**-
  - Mesentery **0DQV**-
  - Metacarpal
    - Left **0PQQ**-
    - Right **0PQP**-
  - Metatarsal
    - Left **0QQP**-
    - Right **0QQN**-
  - Muscle
    - Abdomen
      - Left **0KQL**-
      - Right **0KQK**-
    - Extraocular
      - Left **08QM**-
      - Right **08QL**-
    - Facial **0KQ1**-
    - Foot
      - Left **0KQW**-
      - Right **0KQV**-
    - Hand
      - Left **0KQD**-
      - Right **0KQC**-
    - Head **0KQ0**-
    - Hip
      - Left **0KQP**-
      - Right **0KQN**-
- **Repair** — *continued*
  - Muscle — *continued*
    - Lower Arm and Wrist
      - Left **0KQB**-
      - Right **0KQ9**-
    - Lower Leg
      - Left **0KQT**-
      - Right **0KQS**-
    - Neck
      - Left **0KQ3**-
      - Right **0KQ2**-
    - Papillary **02QD**-
    - Perineum **0KQM**-
    - Shoulder
      - Left **0KQ6**-
      - Right **0KQ5**-
    - Thorax
      - Left **0KQJ**-
      - Right **0KQH**-
    - Tongue, Palate, Pharynx **0KQ4**-
    - Trunk
      - Left **0KQG**-
      - Right **0KQF**-
    - Upper Arm
      - Left **0KQ8**-
      - Right **0KQ7**-
    - Upper Leg
      - Left **0KQR**-
      - Right **0KQQ**-
  - Nasal Mucosa and Soft Tissue **09QK**-
  - Nasopharynx **09QN**-
  - Neck **0WQ6**-
  - Nerve
    - Abdominal Sympathetic **01QM**-
    - Abducens **00QL**-
    - Accessory **00QR**-
    - Acoustic **00QN**-
    - Brachial Plexus **01Q3**-
    - Cervical **01Q1**-
    - Cervical Plexus **01Q0**-
    - Facial **00QM**-
    - Femoral **01QD**-
    - Glossopharyngeal **00QP**-
    - Head and Neck Sympathetic **01QK**-
    - Hypoglossal **00QS**-
    - Lumbar **01QB**-
    - Lumbar Plexus **01Q9**-
    - Lumbar Sympathetic **01QN**-
    - Lumbosacral Plexus **01QA**-
    - Median **01Q5**-
    - Oculomotor **00QH**-
    - Olfactory **00QF**-
    - Optic **00QG**-
    - Peroneal **01QH**-
    - Phrenic **01Q2**-
    - Pudendal **01QC**-
    - Radial **01Q6**-
    - Sacral **01QR**-
    - Sacral Plexus **01QQ**-
    - Sacral Sympathetic **01QP**-
    - Sciatic **01QF**-
    - Thoracic **01Q8**-
    - Thoracic Sympathetic **01QL**-
    - Tibial **01QG**-
    - Trigeminal **00QK**-
    - Trochlear **00QJ**-
    - Ulnar **01Q4**-
    - Vagus **00QQ**-
  - Nipple
    - Left **0HQX**-
    - Right **0HQW**-
  - Omentum **0DQU**-
  - Oral Cavity and Throat **0WQ3**-
  - Orbit
    - Left **0NQQ**-
    - Right **0NQP**-
  - Ovary
    - Bilateral **0UQ2**-
    - Left **0UQ1**-
    - Right **0UQ0**-

© 2018 Channel Publishing, Ltd.

Repair — *continued*
- Palate
  - Hard **0CQ2**-
  - Soft **0CQ3**-
- Pancreas **0FQG**-
- Para-aortic Body **0GQ9**-
- Paraganglion Extremity **0GQF**-
- Parathyroid Gland **0GQR**-
  - Inferior
    - Left **0GQP**-
    - Right **0GQN**-
  - Multiple **0GQQ**-
  - Superior
    - Left **0GQM**-
    - Right **0GQL**-
- Patella
  - Left **0QQF**-
  - Right **0QQD**-
- Penis **0VQS**-
- Pericardium **02QN**-
- Perineum
  - Female **0WQN**-
  - Male **0WQM**-
- Peritoneum **0DQW**-
- Phalanx
  - Finger
    - Left **0PQV**-
    - Right **0PQT**-
  - Thumb
    - Left **0PQS**-
    - Right **0PQR**-
  - Toe
    - Left **0QQR**-
    - Right **0QQQ**-
- Pharynx **0CQM**-
- Pineal Body **0GQ1**-
- Pleura
  - Left **0BQP**-
  - Right **0BQN**-
- Pons **00QB**-
- Prepuce **0VQT**-
- Products of Conception **10Q0**-
- Prostate **0VQ0**-
- Radius
  - Left **0PQJ**-
  - Right **0PQH**-
- Rectum **0DQP**-
- Retina
  - Left **08QF**3ZZ
  - Right **08QE**3ZZ
- Retinal Vessel
  - Left **08QH**3ZZ
  - Right **08QG**3ZZ
- Ribs
  - 1 to 2 **0PQ1**-
  - 3 or more **0PQ2**-
- Sacrum **0QQ1**-
- Scapula
  - Left **0PQ6**-
  - Right **0PQ5**-
- Sclera
  - Left **08Q7**XZZ
  - Right **08Q6**XZZ
- Scrotum **0VQ5**-
- Septum
  - Atrial **02Q5**-
  - Nasal **09QM**-
  - Ventricular **02QM**-
- Shoulder Region
  - Left **0XQ3**-
  - Right **0XQ2**-
- Sinus
  - Accessory **09QP**-
  - Ethmoid
    - Left **09QV**-
    - Right **09QU**-
  - Frontal
    - Left **09QT**-
    - Right **09QS**-
  - Mastoid
    - Left **09QC**-
    - Right **09QB**-

Repair — *continued*
- Sinus — *continued*
  - Maxillary
    - Left **09QR**-
    - Right **09QQ**-
  - Sphenoid
    - Left **09QX**-
    - Right **09QW**-
- Skin
  - Abdomen **0HQ7**XZZ
  - Back **0HQ6**XZZ
  - Buttock **0HQ8**XZZ
  - Chest **0HQ5**XZZ
  - Ear
    - Left **0HQ3**XZZ
    - Right **0HQ2**XZZ
  - Face **0HQ1**XZZ
  - Foot
    - Left **0HQN**XZZ
    - Right **0HQM**XZZ
  - Hand
    - Left **0HQG**XZZ
    - Right **0HQF**XZZ
  - Inguinal **0HQA**XZZ
  - Lower Arm
    - Left **0HQE**XZZ
    - Right **0HQD**XZZ
  - Lower Leg
    - Left **0HQL**XZZ
    - Right **0HQK**XZZ
  - Neck **0HQ4**XZZ
  - Perineum **0HQ9**XZZ
  - Scalp **0HQ0**XZZ
  - Upper Arm
    - Left **0HQC**XZZ
    - Right **0HQB**XZZ
  - Upper Leg
    - Left **0HQJ**XZZ
    - Right **0HQH**XZZ
- Skull **0NQ0**-
- Spinal Cord
  - Cervical **00QW**-
  - Lumbar **00QY**-
  - Thoracic **00QX**-
- Spinal Meninges **00QT**-
- Spleen **07QP**-
- Sternum **0PQ0**-
- Stomach **0DQ6**-
  - Pylorus **0DQ7**-
- Subcutaneous Tissue and Fascia
  - Abdomen **0JQ8**-
  - Back **0JQ7**-
  - Buttock **0JQ9**-
  - Chest **0JQ6**-
  - Face **0JQ1**-
  - Foot
    - Left **0JQR**-
    - Right **0JQQ**-
  - Hand
    - Left **0JQK**-
    - Right **0JQJ**-
  - Lower Arm
    - Left **0JQH**-
    - Right **0JQG**-
  - Lower Leg
    - Left **0JQP**-
    - Right **0JQN**-
  - Neck
    - Left **0JQ5**-
    - Right **0JQ4**-
  - Pelvic Region **0JQC**-
  - Perineum **0JQB**-
  - Scalp **0JQ0**-
  - Upper Arm
    - Left **0JQF**-
    - Right **0JQD**-
  - Upper Leg
    - Left **0JQM**-
    - Right **0JQL**-
- Tarsal
  - Left **0QQM**-
  - Right **0QQL**-

Repair — *continued*
- Tendon
  - Abdomen
    - Left **0LQG**-
    - Right **0LQF**-
  - Ankle
    - Left **0LQT**-
    - Right **0LQS**-
  - Foot
    - Left **0LQW**-
    - Right **0LQV**-
  - Hand
    - Left **0LQ8**-
    - Right **0LQ7**-
  - Head and Neck **0LQ0**-
  - Hip
    - Left **0LQK**-
    - Right **0LQJ**-
  - Knee
    - Left **0LQR**-
    - Right **0LQQ**-
  - Lower Arm and Wrist
    - Left **0LQ6**-
    - Right **0LQ5**-
  - Lower Leg
    - Left **0LQP**-
    - Right **0LQN**-
  - Perineum **0LQH**-
  - Shoulder
    - Left **0LQ2**-
    - Right **0LQ1**-
  - Thorax
    - Left **0LQD**-
    - Right **0LQC**-
  - Trunk
    - Left **0LQB**-
    - Right **0LQ9**-
  - Upper Arm
    - Left **0LQ4**-
    - Right **0LQ3**-
  - Upper Leg
    - Left **0LQM**-
    - Right **0LQL**-
- Testis
  - Bilateral **0VQC**-
  - Left **0VQB**-
  - Right **0VQ9**-
- Thalamus **00Q9**-
- Thumb
  - Left **0XQM**-
  - Right **0XQL**-
- Thymus **07QM**-
- Thyroid Gland **0GQK**-
  - Left Lobe **0GQG**-
  - Right Lobe **0GQH**-
- Thyroid Gland Isthmus **0GQJ**-
- Tibia
  - Left **0QQH**-
  - Right **0QQG**-
- Toe
  - 1st
    - Left **0YQQ**-
    - Right **0YQP**-
  - 2nd
    - Left **0YQS**-
    - Right **0YQR**-
  - 3rd
    - Left **0YQU**-
    - Right **0YQT**-
  - 4th
    - Left **0YQW**-
    - Right **0YQV**-
  - 5th
    - Left **0YQY**-
    - Right **0YQX**-
- Toe Nail **0HQR**XZZ
- Tongue **0CQ7**-
- Tonsils **0CQP**-
- Tooth
  - Lower **0CQX**-
  - Upper **0CQW**-
- Trachea **0BQ1**-

Repair — *continued*
- Tunica Vaginalis
  - Left **0VQ7**-
  - Right **0VQ6**-
- Turbinate, Nasal **09QL**-
- Tympanic Membrane
  - Left **09Q8**-
  - Right **09Q7**-
- Ulna
  - Left **0PQL**-
  - Right **0PQK**-
- Ureter
  - Left **0TQ7**-
  - Right **0TQ6**-
- Urethra **0TQD**-
- Uterine Supporting Structure **0UQ4**-
- Uterus **0UQ9**-
- Uvula **0CQN**-
- Vagina **0UQG**-
- Valve
  - Aortic **02QF**-
  - Mitral **02QG**-
  - Pulmonary **02QH**-
  - Tricuspid **02QJ**-
- Vas Deferens
  - Bilateral **0VQQ**-
  - Left **0VQP**-
  - Right **0VQN**-
- Vein
  - Axillary
    - Left **05Q8**-
    - Right **05Q7**-
  - Azygos **05Q0**-
  - Basilic
    - Left **05QC**-
    - Right **05QB**
  - Brachial
    - Left **05QA**-
    - Right **05Q9**-
  - Cephalic
    - Left **05QF**-
    - Right **05QD**-
  - Colic **06Q7**-
  - Common Iliac
    - Left **06QD**
    - Right **06QC**-
  - Coronary **02Q4**-
  - Esophageal **06Q3**-
  - External Iliac
    - Left **06QG**-
    - Right **06QF**-
  - External Jugular
    - Left **05QQ**-
    - Right **05QP**-
  - Face
    - Left **05QV**-
    - Right **05QT**-
  - Femoral
    - Left **06QN**-
    - Right **06QM**-
  - Foot
    - Left **06QV**-
    - Right **06QT**-
  - Gastric **06Q2**-
  - Hand
    - Left **05QH**-
    - Right **05QG**-
  - Hemiazygos **05Q1**-
  - Hepatic **06Q4**-
  - Hypogastric
    - Left **06QJ**-
    - Right **06QH**-
  - Inferior Mesenteric **06Q6**-
  - Innominate
    - Left **05Q4**-
    - Right **05Q3**-
  - Internal Jugular
    - Left **05QN**-
    - Right **05QM**-
  - Intracranial **05QL**-
  - Lower **06QY**-
  - Portal **06Q8**-

PROCEDURE INDEX

© 2018 Channel Publishing, Ltd.

- **Repair** — *continued*
  - Vein — *continued*
    - Pulmonary
      - Left 02QT-
      - Right 02QS-
    - Renal
      - Left 06QB-
      - Right 06Q9-
    - Saphenous
      - Left 06QQ-
      - Right 06QP-
    - Splenic 06Q1-
    - Subclavian
      - Left 05Q6-
      - Right 05Q5-
    - Superior Mesenteric 06Q5-
    - Upper 05QY-
    - Vertebral
      - Left 05QS-
      - Right 05QR-
  - Vena Cava
    - Inferior 06Q0-
    - Superior 02QV-
  - Ventricle
    - Left 02QL-
    - Right 02QK-
  - Vertebra
    - Cervical 0PQ3-
    - Lumbar 0QQ0-
    - Thoracic 0PQ4-
  - Vesicle
    - Bilateral 0VQ3-
    - Left 0VQ2-
    - Right 0VQ1-
  - Vitreous
    - Left 08Q53ZZ
    - Right 08Q43ZZ
  - Vocal Cord
    - Left 0CQV-
    - Right 0CQT-
  - Vulva 0UQM-
  - Wrist Region
    - Left 0XQH-
    - Right 0XQG-
- **Repair, obstetric laceration, periurethral** 0UQMXZZ
- **Replacement**
  - Acetabulum
    - Left 0QR5-
    - Right 0QR4
  - Ampulla of Vater 0FRC-
  - Anal Sphincter 0DRR-
  - Aorta
    - Abdominal 04R0-
    - Thoracic
      - Ascending/Arch 02RX-
      - Descending 02RW-
  - Artery
    - Anterior Tibial
      - Left 04RQ-
      - Right 04RP-
    - Axillary
      - Left 03R6-
      - Right 03R5-
    - Brachial
      - Left 03R8-
      - Right 03R7-
    - Celiac 04R1-
    - Colic
      - Left 04R7-
      - Middle 04R8-
      - Right 04R6-
    - Common Carotid
      - Left 03RJ-
      - Right 03RH-
    - Common Iliac
      - Left 04RD-
      - Right 04RC-
    - External Carotid
      - Left 03RN-
      - Right 03RM-
    - External Iliac
      - Left 04RJ-
      - Right 04RH-

- **Replacement** — *continued*
  - Artery — *continued*
    - Face 03RR-
    - Femoral
      - Left 04RL-
      - Right 04RK-
    - Foot
      - Left 04RW-
      - Right 04RV-
    - Gastric 04R2-
    - Hand
      - Left 03RF-
      - Right 03RD-
    - Hepatic 04R3-
    - Inferior Mesenteric 04RB-
    - Innominate 03R2-
    - Internal Carotid
      - Left 03RL-
      - Right 03RK-
    - Internal Iliac
      - Left 04RF-
      - Right 04RE-
    - Internal Mammary
      - Left 03R1-
      - Right 03R0-
    - Intracranial 03RG-
    - Lower 04RY-
    - Peroneal
      - Left 04RU-
      - Right 04RT-
    - Popliteal
      - Left 04RN-
      - Right 04RM-
    - Posterior Tibial
      - Left 04RS-
      - Right 04RR-
    - Pulmonary
      - Left 02RR-
      - Right 02RQ-
    - Pulmonary Trunk 02RP-
    - Radial
      - Left 03RC-
      - Right 03RB-
    - Renal
      - Left 04RA-
      - Right 04R9-
    - Splenic 04R4-
    - Subclavian
      - Left 03R4-
      - Right 03R3-
    - Superior Mesenteric 04R5-
    - Temporal
      - Left 03RT-
      - Right 03RS-
    - Thyroid
      - Left 03RV-
      - Right 03RU-
    - Ulnar
      - Left 03RA-
      - Right 03R9-
    - Upper 03RY-
    - Vertebral
      - Left 03RQ-
      - Right 03RP-
  - Atrium
    - Left 02R7-
    - Right 02R6-
  - Auditory Ossicle
    - Left 09RA0-
    - Right 09R90-
  - Bladder 0TRB-
  - Bladder Neck 0TRC-
  - Bone
    - Ethmoid
      - Left 0NRG-
      - Right 0NRF-
    - Frontal 0NR1-
    - Hyoid 0NRX-
    - Lacrimal
      - Left 0NRJ-
      - Right 0NRH-
    - Nasal 0NRB-
    - Occipital 0NR7-

- **Replacement** — *continued*
  - Bone — *continued*
    - Palatine
      - Left 0NRL-
      - Right 0NRK-
    - Parietal
      - Left 0NR4-
      - Right 0NR3-
    - Pelvic
      - Left 0QR3-
      - Right 0QR2-
    - Sphenoid 0NRC-
    - Temporal
      - Left 0NR6-
      - Right 0NR5-
    - Zygomatic
      - Left 0NRN-
      - Right 0NRM-
  - Breast
    - Bilateral 0HRV-
    - Left 0HRU-
    - Right 0HRT-
  - Bronchus
    - Lingula 0BR9-
    - Lower Lobe
      - Left 0BRB-
      - Right 0BR6-
    - Main
      - Left 0BR7-
      - Right 0BR3-
    - Middle Lobe, Right 0BR5-
    - Upper Lobe
      - Left 0BR8-
      - Right 0BR4-
  - Buccal Mucosa 0CR4-
  - Bursa and Ligament
    - Abdomen
      - Left 0MRJ-
      - Right 0MRH-
    - Ankle
      - Left 0MRR-
      - Right 0MRQ-
    - Elbow
      - Left 0MR4-
      - Right 0MR3-
    - Foot
      - Left 0MRT-
      - Right 0MRS-
    - Hand
      - Left 0MR8-
      - Right 0MR7-
    - Head and Neck 0MR0-
    - Hip
      - Left 0MRM-
      - Right 0MRL-
    - Knee
      - Left 0MRP-
      - Right 0MRN-
    - Lower Extremity
      - Left 0MRW-
      - Right 0MRV-
    - Perineum 0MRK-
    - Rib(s) 0MRG-
    - Shoulder
      - Left 0MR2-
      - Right 0MR1-
    - Spine
      - Lower 0MRD-
      - Upper 0MRC-
    - Sternum 0MRF-
    - Upper Extremity
      - Left 0MRB-
      - Right 0MR9-
    - Wrist
      - Left 0MR6-
      - Right 0MR5-
  - Carina 0BR2-
  - Carpal
    - Left 0PRN-
    - Right 0PRM-
  - Cerebral Meninges 00R1-
  - Cerebral Ventricle 00R6-
  - Chordae Tendineae 02R9-

- **Replacement** — *continued*
  - Choroid
    - Left 08RB-
    - Right 08RA-
  - Clavicle
    - Left 0PRB-
    - Right 0PR9-
  - Coccyx 0QRS-
  - Conjunctiva
    - Left 08RTX-
    - Right 08RSX-
  - Cornea
    - Left 08R9-
    - Right 08R8-
  - Diaphragm 0BRT-
  - Disc
    - Cervical Vertebral 0RR30-
    - Cervicothoracic Vertebral 0RR50-
    - Lumbar Vertebral 0SR20-
    - Lumbosacral 0SR40-
    - Thoracic Vertebral 0RR90-
    - Thoracolumbar Vertebral 0RRB0-
  - Duct
    - Common Bile 0FR9-
    - Cystic 0FR8-
    - Hepatic
      - Common 0FR7-
      - Left 0FR6-
      - Right 0FR5-
    - Lacrimal
      - Left 08RY-
      - Right 08RX-
    - Pancreatic 0FRD-
      - Accessory 0FRF-
    - Parotid
      - Left 0CRC-
      - Right 0CRB-
  - Dura Mater 00R2-
  - Ear
    - External
      - Bilateral 09R2-
      - Left 09R1-
      - Right 09R0-
    - Inner
      - Left 09RE0-
      - Right 09RD0-
    - Middle
      - Left 09R60-
      - Right 09R50-
  - Epiglottis 0CRR-
  - Esophagus 0DR5-
  - Eye
    - Left 08R1-
    - Right 08R0-
  - Eyelid
    - Lower
      - Left 08RR-
      - Right 08RQ-
    - Upper
      - Left 08RP-
      - Right 08RN-
  - Femoral Shaft
    - Left 0QR9-
    - Right 0QR8-
  - Femur
    - Lower
      - Left 0QRC-
      - Right 0QRB-
    - Upper
      - Left 0QR7-
      - Right 0QR6-
  - Fibula
    - Left 0QRK-
    - Right 0QRJ-
  - Finger Nail 0HRQX-
  - Gingiva
    - Lower 0CR6-
    - Upper 0CR5-
  - Glenoid Cavity
    - Left 0PR8-
    - Right 0PR7-
  - Hair 0HRSX-

© 2018 Channel Publishing, Ltd.

Replacement — *continued*
Humeral Head
Left **0PRD**-
Right **0PRC**-
Humeral Shaft
Left **0PRG**-
Right **0PRF**
Iris
Left **08RD3**-
Right **08RC3**-
Joint
Acromioclavicular
Left **0RRH0**-
Right **0RRG0**-
Ankle
Left **0SRG**-
Right **0SRF**-
Carpal
Left **0RRR0**-
Right **0RRQ0**-
Carpometacarpal
Left **0RRT0**-
Right **0RRS0**-
Cervical Vertebral **0RR10**-
Cervicothoracic Vertebral **0RR40**-
Coccygeal **0SR60**-
Elbow
Left **0RRM0**-
Right **0RRL0**-
Finger Phalangeal
Left **0RRX0**-
Right **0RRW0**-
Hip
Left **0SRB**-
Acetabular Surface **0SRE**-
Femoral Surface **0SRS**-
Right **0SR9**-
Acetabular Surface **0SRA**-
Femoral Surface **0SRR**-
Knee
Left **0SRD**-
Femoral Surface **0SRU**-
Tibial Surface **0SRW**-
Right **0SRC**-
Femoral Surface **0SRT**-
Tibial Surface **0SRV**-
Lumbar Vertebral **0SR00**-
Lumbosacral **0SR30**-
Metacarpophalangeal
Left **0RRV0**-
Right **0RRU0**-
Metatarsal-Phalangeal
Left **0SRN0**-
Right **0SRM0**-
Occipital-cervical **0RR00**-
Sacrococcygeal **0SR50**-
Sacroiliac
Left **0SR80**-
Right **0SR70**-
Shoulder
Left **0RRK**-
Right **0RRJ**-
Sternoclavicular
Left **0RRF0**-
Right **0RRE0**-
Tarsal
Left **0SRJ0**-
Right **0SRH0**-
Tarsometatarsal
Left **0SRL0**-
Right **0SRK0**-
Temporomandibular
Left **0RRD0**-
Right **0RRC0**-
Thoracic Vertebral **0RR60**-
Thoracolumbar Vertebral **0RRA0**-
Toe Phalangeal
Left **0SRQ0**-
Right **0SRP0**-
Wrist
Left **0RRP0**-
Right **0RRN0**-

Replacement — *continued*
Kidney Pelvis
Left **0TR4**-
Right **0TR3**-
Larynx **0CRS**-
Lens
Left **08RK30Z**
Right **08RJ30Z**
Lip
Lower **0CR1**-
Upper **0CR0**-
Mandible
Left **0NRV**-
Right **0NRT**-
Maxilla **0NRR**-
Mesentery **0DRV**-
Metacarpal
Left **0PRQ**-
Right **0PRP**-
Metatarsal
Left **0QRP**-
Right **0QRN**-
Muscle
Abdomen
Left **0KRL**-
Right **0KRK**-
Facial **0KR1**-
Foot
Left **0KRW**-
Right **0KRV**-
Hand
Left **0KRD**-
Right **0KRC**-
Head **0KR0**-
Hip
Left **0KRP**-
Right **0KRN**-
Lower Arm and Wrist
Left **0KRB**-
Right **0KR9**-
Lower Leg
Left **0KRT**-
Right **0KRS**-
Neck
Left **0KR3**-
Right **0KR2**-
Papillary **02RD**-
Perineum **0KRM**-
Shoulder
Left **0KR6**-
Right **0KR5**-
Thorax
Left **0KRJ**-
Right **0KRH**-
Tongue, Palate, Pharynx **0KR4**-
Trunk
Left **0KRG**-
Right **0KRF**-
Upper Arm
Left **0KR8**-
Right **0KR7**-
Upper Leg
Left **0KRR**-
Right **0KRQ**-
Nasal Mucosa and Soft Tissue **09RK**-
Nasopharynx **09RN**-
Nerve
Abducens **00RL**-
Accessory **00RR**-
Acoustic **00RN**-
Cervical **01R1**-
Facial **00RM**-
Femoral **01RD**-
Glossopharyngeal **00RP**-
Hypoglossal **00RS**-
Lumbar **01RB**-
Median **01R5**-
Oculomotor **00RH**-
Olfactory **00RF**-
Optic **00RG**-
Peroneal **01RH**-
Phrenic **01R2**-
Pudendal **01RC**-

Replacement — *continued*
Nerve — *continued*
Radial **01R6**-
Sacral **01RR**-
Sciatic **01RF**-
Thoracic **01R8**-
Tibial **01RG**-
Trigeminal **00RK**-
Trochlear **00RJ**-
Ulnar **01R4**-
Vagus **00RQ**-
Nipple
Left **0HRX**-
Right **0HRW**-
Omentum **0DRU**-
Orbit
Left **0NRQ**-
Right **0NRP**-
Palate
Hard **0CR2**-
Soft **0CR3**-
Patella
Left **0QRF**-
Right **0QRD**-
Pericardium **02RN**-
Peritoneum **0DRW**-
Phalanx
Finger
Left **0PRV**-
Right **0PRT**-
Thumb
Left **0PRS**-
Right **0PRR**-
Toe
Left **0QRR**-
Right **0QRQ**-
Pharynx **0CRM**-
Radius
Left **0PRJ**-
Right **0PRH**-
Retinal Vessel
Left **08RH3**-
Right **08RG3**-
Ribs
1 to 2 **0PR1**-
3 or more **0PR2**-
Sacrum **0QR1**-
Scapula
Left **0PR6**-
Right **0PR5**-
Sclera
Left **08R7X**-
Right **08R6X**-
Septum
Atrial **02R5**-
Nasal **09RM**-
Ventricular **02RM**-
Skin
Abdomen **0HR7**-
Back **0HR6**-
Buttock **0HR8**-
Chest **0HR5**-
Ear
Left **0HR3**-
Right **0HR2**-
Face **0HR1**-
Foot
Left **0HRN**-
Right **0HRM**-
Hand
Left **0HRG**-
Right **0HRF**-
Inguinal **0HRA**-
Lower Arm
Left **0HRE**-
Right **0HRD**-
Lower Leg
Left **0HRL**-
Right **0HRK**-
Neck **0HR4**-
Perineum **0HR9**-
Scalp **0HR0**-

Replacement — *continued*
Skin — *continued*
Upper Arm
Left **0HRC**-
Right **0HRB**-
Upper Leg
Left **0HRJ**-
Right **0HRH**-
Skin Substitute, Porcine Liver Derived **XHRPXL2**
Skull **0NR0**-
Spinal Meninges **00RT**-
Sternum **0PR0**-
Subcutaneous Tissue and Fascia
Abdomen **0JR8**-
Back **0JR7**-
Buttock **0JR9**-
Chest **0JR6**-
Face **0JR1**-
Foot
Left **0JRR**-
Right **0JRQ**-
Hand
Left **0JRK**-
Right **0JRJ**-
Lower Arm
Left **0JRH**-
Right **0JRG**-
Lower Leg
Left **0JRP**-
Right **0JRN**-
Neck
Left **0JR5**-
Right **0JR4**-
Pelvic Region **0JRC**-
Perineum **0JRB**-
Scalp **0JR0**-
Upper Arm
Left **0JRF**-
Right **0JRD**-
Upper Leg
Left **0JRM**-
Right **0JRL**-
Tarsal
Left **0QRM**-
Right **0QRL**-
Tendon
Abdomen
Left **0LRG**-
Right **0LRF**-
Ankle
Left **0LRT**-
Right **0LRS**-
Foot
Left **0LRW**-
Right **0LRV**-
Hand
Left **0LR8**-
Right **0LR7**-
Head and Neck **0LR0**-
Hip
Left **0LRK**-
Right **0LRJ**-
Knee
Left **0LRR**-
Right **0LRQ**-
Lower Arm and Wrist
Left **0LR6**-
Right **0LR5**-
Lower Leg
Left **0LRP**-
Right **0LRN**-
Perineum **0LRH**-
Shoulder
Left **0LR2**-
Right **0LR1**-
Thorax
Left **0LRD**-
Right **0LRC**-
Trunk
Left **0LRB**-
Right **0LR9**-

© 2018 Channel Publishing, Ltd.

PROCEDURE INDEX

© 2018 Channel Publishing, Ltd.

Reposition — *continued*
Bursa and Ligament — *continued*
Wrist
Left **0MS6-**
Right **0MS5-**
Carina **0BS20ZZ**
Carpal
Left **0PSN-**
Right **0PSM-**
Cecum **0DSH-**
Cervix **0USC-**
Clavicle
Left **0PSB-**
Right **0PS9-**
Coccyx **0QSS-**
Colon
Ascending **0DSK-**
Descending **0DSM-**
Sigmoid **0DSN-**
Transverse **0DSL-**
Cord
Bilateral **0VSH-**
Left **0VSG-**
Right **0VSF-**
Cul-de-sac **0USF-**
Diaphragm **0BST0ZZ**
Duct
Common Bile **0FS9-**
Cystic **0FS8-**
Hepatic
Common **0FS7-**
Left **0FS6-**
Right **0FS5-**
Lacrimal
Left **08SY-**
Right **08SX-**
Pancreatic **0FSD-**
Accessory **0FSF-**
Parotid
Left **0CSC-**
Right **0CSB-**
Duodenum **0DS9-**
Ear
Bilateral **09S2-**
Left **09S1-**
Right **09S0-**
Epiglottis **0CSR-**
Esophagus **0DS5-**
Eustachian Tube
Left **09SG-**
Right **09SF-**
Eyelid
Lower
Left **08SR-**
Right **08SQ-**
Upper
Left **08SP-**
Right **08SN-**
Fallopian Tube
Left **0US6-**
Right **0US5-**
Fallopian Tubes, Bilateral **0US7-**
Femoral Shaft
Left **0QS9-**
Right **0QS8-**
Femur
Lower
Left **0QSC-**
Right **0QSB-**
Upper
Left **0QS7-**
Right **0QS6-**
Fibula
Left **0QSK-**
Right **0QSJ-**
Gallbladder **0FS4-**
Gland
Adrenal
Left **0GS2-**
Right **0GS3-**
Lacrimal
Left **08SW-**
Right **08SV-**

Reposition — *continued*
Glenoid Cavity
Left **0PS8-**
Right **0PS7-**
Hair **0HSSXZZ**
Humeral Head
Left **0PSD-**
Right **0PSC-**
Humeral Shaft
Left **0PSG-**
Right **0PSF-**
Ileum **0DSB-**
Intestine
Large **0DSE-**
Small **0DS8-**
Iris
Left **08SD3ZZ**
Right **08SC3ZZ**
Jejunum **0DSA-**
Joint
Acromioclavicular
Left **0RSH-**
Right **0RSG-**
Ankle
Left **0SSG-**
Right **0SSF-**
Carpal
Left **0RSR-**
Right **0RSQ-**
Carpometacarpal
Left **0RST-**
Right **0RSS-**
Cervical Vertebral **0RS1-**
Cervicothoracic Vertebral **0RS4-**
Coccygeal **0SS6-**
Elbow
Left **0RSM-**
Right **0RSL-**
Finger Phalangeal
Left **0RSX-**
Right **0RSW-**
Hip
Left **0SSB-**
Right **0SS9-**
Knee
Left **0SSD-**
Right **0SSC-**
Lumbar Vertebral **0SS0-**
Lumbosacral **0SS3-**
Metacarpophalangeal
Left **0RSV-**
Right **0RSU-**
Metatarsal-Phalangeal
Left **0SSN-**
Right **0SSM-**
Occipital-cervical **0RS0-**
Sacrococcygeal **0SS5-**
Sacroiliac
Left **0SS8-**
Right **0SS7-**
Shoulder
Left **0RSK-**
Right **0RSJ-**
Sternoclavicular
Left **0RSF-**
Right **0RSE-**
Tarsal
Left **0SSJ-**
Right **0SSH-**
Tarsometatarsal
Left **0SSL-**
Right **0SSK-**
Temporomandibular
Left **0RSD-**
Right **0RSC-**
Thoracic Vertebral **0RS6-**
Thoracolumbar Vertebral **0RSA-**
Toe Phalangeal
Left **0SSQ-**
Right **0SSP-**
Wrist
Left **0RSP-**
Right **0RSN-**

Reposition — *continued*
Kidney
Left **0TS1-**
Right **0TS0-**
Kidney Pelvis
Left **0TS4-**
Right **0TS3-**
Kidneys, Bilateral **0TS2-**
Lens
Left **08SK3ZZ**
Right **08SJ3ZZ**
Lip
Lower **0CS1-**
Upper **0CS0-**
Liver **0FS0-**
Lung
Left **0BSL0ZZ**
Lower Lobe
Left **0BSJ0ZZ**
Right **0BSF0ZZ**
Middle Lobe, Right **0BSD0ZZ**
Right **0BSK0ZZ**
Upper Lobe
Left **0BSG0ZZ**
Right **0BSC0ZZ**
Lung Lingula **0BSH0ZZ**
Mandible
Left **0NSV-**
Right **0NST-**
Maxilla **0NSR-**
Metacarpal
Left **0PSQ-**
Right **0PSP-**
Metatarsal
Left **0QSP-**
Right **0QSN-**
Muscle
Abdomen
Left **0KSL-**
Right **0KSK-**
Extraocular
Left **08SM-**
Right **08SL-**
Facial **0KS1-**
Foot
Left **0KSW-**
Right **0KSV-**
Hand
Left **0KSD-**
Right **0KSC-**
Head **0KS0-**
Hip
Left **0KSP-**
Right **0KSN-**
Lower Arm and Wrist
Left **0KSB-**
Right **0KS9-**
Lower Leg
Left **0KST-**
Right **0KSS-**
Neck
Left **0KS3-**
Right **0KS2-**
Perineum **0KSM-**
Shoulder
Left **0KS6-**
Right **0KS5-**
Thorax
Left **0KSJ-**
Right **0KSH-**
Tongue, Palate, Pharynx **0KS4-**
Trunk
Left **0KSG-**
Right **0KSF-**
Upper Arm
Left **0KS8-**
Right **0KS7-**
Upper Leg
Left **0KSR-**
Right **0KSQ-**
Nasal Mucosa and Soft Tissue **09SK-**

Reposition — *continued*
Nerve
Abducens **00SL-**
Accessory **00SR-**
Acoustic **00SN-**
Brachial Plexus **01S3-**
Cervical **01S1-**
Cervical Plexus **01S0-**
Facial **00SM-**
Femoral **01SD-**
Glossopharyngeal **00SP-**
Hypoglossal **00SS-**
Lumbar **01SB-**
Lumbar Plexus **01S9-**
Lumbosacral Plexus **01SA-**
Median **01S5-**
Oculomotor **00SH-**
Olfactory **00SF-**
Optic **00SG-**
Peroneal **01SH-**
Phrenic **01S2-**
Pudendal **01SC-**
Radial **01S6-**
Sacral **01SR-**
Sacral Plexus **01SQ-**
Sciatic **01SF-**
Thoracic **01S8-**
Tibial **01SG-**
Trigeminal **00SK-**
Trochlear **00SJ-**
Ulnar **01S4-**
Vagus **00SQ-**
Nipple
Left **0HSXXZZ**
Right **0HSWXZZ**
Orbit
Left **0NSQ-**
Right **0NSP-**
Ovary
Bilateral **0US2-**
Left **0US1-**
Right **0US0-**
Palate
Hard **0CS2-**
Soft **0CS3-**
Pancreas **0FSG-**
Parathyroid Gland **0GSR-**
Inferior
Left **0GSP-**
Right **0GSN-**
Multiple **0GSQ-**
Superior
Left **0GSM-**
Right **0GSL-**
Patella
Left **0QSF-**
Right **0QSD-**
Phalanx
Finger
Left **0PSV-**
Right **0PST-**
Thumb
Left **0PSS-**
Right **0PSR-**
Toe
Left **0QSR-**
Right **0QSQ-**
Products of Conception **10S0-**
Ectopic **10S2-**
Radius
Left **0PSJ-**
Right **0PSH-**
Rectum **0DSP-**
Retinal Vessel
Left **08SH3ZZ**
Right **08SG3ZZ**
Ribs
1 to 2 **0PS1-**
3 or more **0PS2-**
Sacrum **0QS1-**
Scapula
Left **0PS6-**
Right **0PS5-**

PROCEDURE INDEX

© 2018 Channel Publishing, Ltd.

Reposition — *continued*
Septum, Nasal **09SM-**
Sesamoid Bone(s) 1st Toe
see Reposition, Metatarsal, Left **0QSP-**
see Reposition, Metatarsal, Right **0QSN-**
Skull **0NS0-**
Spinal Cord
Cervical **00SW-**
Lumbar **00SY-**
Thoracic **00SX-**
Spleen **07SP0ZZ**
Sternum **0PS0-**
Stomach **0DS6-**
Tarsal
Left **0QSM-**
Right **0QSL-**
Tendon
Abdomen
Left **0LSG-**
Right **0LSF-**
Ankle
Left **0LST-**
Right **0LSS-**
Foot
Left **0LSW-**
Right **0LSV-**
Hand
Left **0LS8-**
Right **0LS7-**
Head and Neck **0LS0-**
Hip
Left **0LSK-**
Right **0LSJ-**
Knee
Left **0LSR-**
Right **0LSQ-**
Lower Arm and Wrist
Left **0LS6-**
Right **0LS5-**
Lower Leg
Left **0LSP-**
Right **0LSN-**
Perineum **0LSH-**
Shoulder
Left **0LS2-**
Right **0LS1-**
Thorax
Left **0LSD-**
Right **0LSC-**
Trunk
Left **0LSB-**
Right **0LS9-**
Upper Arm
Left **0LS4-**
Right **0LS3-**
Upper Leg
Left **0LSM-**
Right **0LSL-**
Testis
Bilateral **0VSC-**
Left **0VSB-**
Right **0VS9-**
Thymus **07SM0ZZ**
Thyroid Gland
Left Lobe **0GSG-**
Right Lobe **0GSH-**
Tibia
Left **0QSH-**
Right **0QSG-**
Tongue **0CS7-**
Tooth
Lower **0CSX-**
Upper **0CSW-**
Trachea **0BS10ZZ**
Turbinate, Nasal **09SL-**
Tympanic Membrane
Left **09S8-**
Right **09S7-**
Ulna
Left **0PSL-**
Right **0PSK-**

Reposition — *continued*
Ureter
Left **0TS7-**
Right **0TS6-**
Ureters, Bilateral **0TS8-**
Urethra **0TSD-**
Uterine Supporting Structure **0US4-**
Uterus **0US9-**
Uvula **0CSN-**
Vagina **0USG-**
Vein
Axillary
Left **05S8-**
Right **05S7-**
Azygos **05S0-**
Basilic
Left **05SC-**
Right **05SB-**
Brachial
Left **05SA-**
Right **05S9-**
Cephalic
Left **05SF-**
Right **05SD-**
Colic **06S7-**
Common Iliac
Left **06SD-**
Right **06SC-**
Esophageal **06S3-**
External Iliac
Left **06SG-**
Right **06SF-**
External Jugular
Left **05SQ-**
Right **05SP-**
Face
Left **05SV-**
Right **05ST-**
Femoral
Left **06SN-**
Right **06SM-**
Foot
Left **06SV-**
Right **06ST-**
Gastric **06S2-**
Hand
Left **05SH-**
Right **05SG-**
Hemiazygos **05S1-**
Hepatic **06S4-**
Hypogastric
Left **06SJ-**
Right **06SH-**
Inferior Mesenteric **06S6-**
Innominate
Left **05S4-**
Right **05S3-**
Internal Jugular
Left **05SN-**
Right **05SM-**
Intracranial **05SL-**
Lower **06SY-**
Portal **06S8-**
Pulmonary
Left **02ST0ZZ**
Right **02SS0ZZ**
Renal
Left **06SB-**
Right **06S9-**
Saphenous
Left **06SQ-**
Right **06SP-**
Splenic **06S1-**
Subclavian
Left **05S6-**
Right **05S5-**
Superior Mesenteric **06S5-**
Upper **05SY-**
Vertebral
Left **05SS-**
Right **05SR-**

Reposition — *continued*
Vena Cava
Inferior **06S0-**
Superior **02SV0ZZ**
Vertebra
Cervical **0PS3-**
Magnetically Controlled Growth Rod(s) **XNS3-**
Lumbar **0QS0-**
Magnetically Controlled Growth Rod(s) **XNS0-**
Thoracic **0PS4-**
Magnetically Controlled Growth Rod(s) **XNS4-**
Vocal Cord
Left **0CSV-**
Right **0CST-**

Resection
Acetabulum
Left **0QT50ZZ**
Right **0QT40ZZ**
Adenoids **0CTQ-**
Ampulla of Vater **0FTC-**
Anal Sphincter **0DTR-**
Anus **0DTQ-**
Aortic Body **0GTD-**
Appendix **0DTJ-**
Auditory Ossicle
Left **09TA-**
Right **09T9-**
Bladder **0TTB-**
Bladder Neck **0TTC-**
Bone
Ethmoid
Left **0NTG0ZZ**
Right **0NTF0ZZ**
Frontal **0NT10ZZ**
Hyoid **0NTX0ZZ**
Lacrimal
Left **0NTJ0ZZ**
Right **0NTH0ZZ**
Nasal **0NTB0ZZ**
Occipital **0NT70ZZ**
Palatine
Left **0NTL0ZZ**
Right **0NTK0ZZ**
Parietal
Left **0NT40ZZ**
Right **0NT30ZZ**
Pelvic
Left **0QT30ZZ**
Right **0QT20ZZ**
Sphenoid **0NTC0ZZ**
Temporal
Left **0NT60ZZ**
Right **0NT50ZZ**
Zygomatic
Left **0NTN0ZZ**
Right **0NTM0ZZ**
Breast
Bilateral **0HTV0ZZ**
Left **0HTU0ZZ**
Right **0HTT0ZZ**
Supernumerary **0HTY0ZZ**
Bronchus
Lingula **0BT9-**
Lower Lobe
Left **0BTB-**
Right **0BT6-**
Main
Left **0BT7-**
Right **0BT3-**
Middle Lobe, Right **0BT5-**
Upper Lobe
Left **0BT8-**
Right **0BT4-**
Bursa and Ligament
Abdomen
Left **0MTJ-**
Right **0MTH-**
Ankle
Left **0MTR-**
Right **0MTQ-**

Resection — *continued*
Bursa and Ligament — *continued*
Elbow
Left **0MT4-**
Right **0MT3-**
Foot
Left **0MTT-**
Right **0MTS-**
Hand
Left **0MT8-**
Right **0MT7-**
Head and Neck **0MT0-**
Hip
Left **0MTM-**
Right **0MTL-**
Knee
Left **0MTP-**
Right **0MTN-**
Lower Extremity
Left **0MTW-**
Right **0MTV-**
Perineum **0MTK-**
Rib(s) **0MTG-**
Shoulder
Left **0MT2-**
Right **0MT1-**
Spine
Lower **0MTD-**
Upper **0MTC-**
Sternum **0MTF-**
Upper Extremity
Left **0MTB-**
Right **0MT9-**
Wrist
Left **0MT6-**
Right **0MT5-**
Carina **0BT2-**
Carotid Bodies, Bilateral **0GT8-**
Carotid Body
Left **0GT6-**
Right **0GT7-**
Carpal
Left **0PTN0ZZ**
Right **0PTM0ZZ**
Cecum **0DTH-**
Cerebral Hemisphere **00T7-**
Cervix **0UTC-**
Chordae Tendineae **02T9-**
Cisterna Chyli **07TL-**
Clavicle
Left **0PTB0ZZ**
Right **0PT90ZZ**
Clitoris **0UTJ-**
Coccygeal Glomus **0GTB-**
Coccyx **0QTS0ZZ**
Colon
Ascending **0DTK-**
Descending **0DTM-**
Sigmoid **0DTN-**
Transverse **0DTL-**
Conduction Mechanism **02T8-**
Cord
Bilateral **0VTH-**
Left **0VTG-**
Right **0VTF-**
Cornea
Left **08T9XZZ**
Right **08T8XZZ**
Cul-de-sac **0UTF-**
Diaphragm **0BTT-**
Disc
Cervical Vertebral **0RT30ZZ**
Cervicothoracic Vertebral **0RT50ZZ**
Lumbar Vertebral **0ST20ZZ**
Lumbosacral **0ST40ZZ**
Thoracic Vertebral **0RT90ZZ**
Thoracolumbar Vertebral **0RTB0ZZ**
Duct
Common Bile **0FT9-**
Cystic **0FT8-**

© 2018 Channel Publishing, Ltd.

- **Resection** — *continued*
  - Duct — *continued*
    - Hepatic
      - Common **0FT7-**
      - Left **0FT6-**
      - Right **0FT5-**
    - Lacrimal
      - Left **08TY-**
      - Right **08TX-**
    - Pancreatic **0FTD-**
      - Accessory **0FTF-**
    - Parotid
      - Left **0CTC0ZZ**
      - Right **0CTB0ZZ**
  - Duodenum **0DT9-**
  - Ear
    - External
      - Left **09T1-**
      - Right **09T0-**
    - Inner
      - Left **09TE-**
      - Right **09TD-**
    - Middle
      - Left **09T6-**
      - Right **09T5-**
  - Epididymis
    - Bilateral **0VTL-**
    - Left **0VTK-**
    - Right **0VTJ-**
  - Epiglottis **0CTR-**
  - Esophagogastric Junction **0DT4-**
  - Esophagus **0DT5-**
    - Lower **0DT3-**
    - Middle **0DT2-**
    - Upper **0DT1-**
  - Eustachian Tube
    - Left **09TG-**
    - Right **09TF-**
  - Eye
    - Left **08T1XZZ**
    - Right **08T0XZZ**
  - Eyelid
    - Lower
      - Left **08TR-**
      - Right **08TQ**
    - Upper
      - Left **08TP-**
      - Right **08TN-**
  - Fallopian Tube
    - Left **0UT6-**
    - Right **0UT5-**
  - Fallopian Tubes, Bilateral **0UT7-**
  - Femoral Shaft
    - Left **0QT90ZZ**
    - Right **0QT80ZZ**
  - Femur
    - Lower
      - Left **0QTC0ZZ**
      - Right **0QTB0ZZ**
    - Upper
      - Left **0QT70ZZ**
      - Right **0QT60ZZ**
  - Fibula
    - Left **0QTK0ZZ**
    - Right **0QTJ0ZZ**
  - Finger Nail **0HTQXZZ**
  - Gallbladder **0FT4-**
  - Gland
    - Adrenal
      - Bilateral **0GT4-**
      - Left **0GT2-**
      - Right **0GT3-**
    - Lacrimal
      - Left **08TW-**
      - Right **08TV-**
    - Minor Salivary **0CTJ0ZZ**
    - Parotid
      - Left **0CT90ZZ**
      - Right **0CT80ZZ**
    - Pituitary **0GT0-**
    - Sublingual
      - Left **0CTF0ZZ**
      - Right **0CTD0ZZ**
- **Resection** — *continued*
  - Gland — *continued*
    - Submaxillary
      - Left **0CTH0ZZ**
      - Right **0CTG0ZZ**
    - Vestibular **0UTL-**
  - Glenoid Cavity
    - Left **0PT80ZZ**
    - Right **0PT70ZZ**
  - Glomus Jugulare **0GTC-**
  - Humeral Head
    - Left **0PTD0ZZ**
    - Right **0PTC0ZZ**
  - Humeral Shaft
    - Left **0PTG0ZZ**
    - Right **0PTF0ZZ**
  - Hymen **0UTK-**
  - Ileocecal Valve **0DTC-**
  - Ileum **0DTB-**
  - Intestine
    - Large **0DTE-**
      - Left **0DTG-**
      - Right **0DTF-**
    - Small **0DT8-**
  - Iris
    - Left **08TD3ZZ**
    - Right **08TC3ZZ**
  - Jejunum **0DTA-**
  - Joint
    - Acromioclavicular
      - Left **0RTH0ZZ**
      - Right **0RTG0ZZ**
    - Ankle
      - Left **0STG0ZZ**
      - Right **0STF0ZZ**
    - Carpal
      - Left **0RTR0ZZ**
      - Right **0RTQ0ZZ**
    - Carpometacarpal
      - Left **0RTT0ZZ**
      - Right **0RTS0ZZ**
    - Cervicothoracic Vertebral **0RT40ZZ**
    - Coccygeal **0ST60ZZ**
    - Elbow
      - Left **0RTM0ZZ**
      - Right **0RTL0ZZ**
    - Finger Phalangeal
      - Left **0RTX0ZZ**
      - Right **0RTW0ZZ**
    - Hip
      - Left **0STB0ZZ**
      - Right **0ST90ZZ**
    - Knee
      - Left **0STD0ZZ**
      - Right **0STC0ZZ**
    - Metacarpophalangeal
      - Left **0RTV0ZZ**
      - Right **0RTU0ZZ**
    - Metatarsal-Phalangeal
      - Left **0STN0ZZ**
      - Right **0STM0ZZ**
    - Sacrococcygeal **0ST50ZZ**
    - Sacroiliac
      - Left **0ST80ZZ**
      - Right **0ST70ZZ**
    - Shoulder
      - Left **0RTK0ZZ**
      - Right **0RTJ0ZZ**
    - Sternoclavicular
      - Left **0RTF0ZZ**
      - Right **0RTE0ZZ**
    - Tarsal
      - Left **0STJ0ZZ**
      - Right **0STH0ZZ**
    - Tarsometatarsal
      - Left **0STL0ZZ**
      - Right **0STK0ZZ**
    - Temporomandibular
      - Left **0RTD0ZZ**
      - Right **0RTC0ZZ**
    - Toe Phalangeal
      - Left **0STQ0ZZ**
      - Right **0STP0ZZ**
- **Resection** — *continued*
  - Joint — *continued*
    - Wrist
      - Left **0RTP0ZZ**
      - Right **0RTN0ZZ**
  - Kidney
    - Left **0TT1-**
    - Right **0TT0-**
  - Kidney Pelvis
    - Left **0TT4-**
    - Right **0TT3-**
  - Kidneys, Bilateral **0TT2-**
  - Larynx **0CTS-**
  - Lens
    - Left **08TK3ZZ**
    - Right **08TJ3ZZ**
  - Lip
    - Lower **0CT1-**
    - Upper **0CT0-**
  - Liver **0FT0-**
    - Left Lobe **0FT2-**
    - Right Lobe **0FT1-**
  - Lung
    - Bilateral **0BTM-**
    - Left **0BTL-**
    - Lower Lobe
      - Left **0BTJ-**
      - Right **0BTF-**
    - Middle Lobe, Right **0BTD-**
    - Right **0BTK-**
    - Upper Lobe
      - Left **0BTG-**
      - Right **0BTC-**
  - Lung Lingula **0BTH-**
  - Lymphatic
    - Aortic **07TD-**
    - Axillary
      - Left **07T6-**
      - Right **07T5-**
    - Head **07T0-**
    - Inguinal
      - Left **07TJ-**
      - Right **07TH-**
    - Internal Mammary
      - Left **07T9-**
      - Right **07T8-**
    - Lower Extremity
      - Left **07TG-**
      - Right **07TF-**
    - Mesenteric **07TB-**
    - Neck
      - Left **07T2-**
      - Right **07T1-**
    - Pelvis **07TC-**
    - Thoracic Duct **07TK-**
    - Thorax **07T7-**
    - Upper Extremity
      - Left **07T4-**
      - Right **07T3-**
  - Mandible
    - Left **0NTV0ZZ**
    - Right **0NTT0ZZ**
  - Maxilla **0NTR0ZZ**
  - Metacarpal
    - Left **0PTQ0ZZ**
    - Right **0PTP0ZZ**
  - Metatarsal
    - Left **0QTP0ZZ**
    - Right **0QTN0ZZ**
  - Muscle
    - Abdomen
      - Left **0KTL-**
      - Right **0KTK-**
    - Extraocular
      - Left **08TM-**
      - Right **08TL-**
    - Facial **0KT1-**
    - Foot
      - Left **0KTW-**
      - Right **0KTV-**
    - Hand
      - Left **0KTD-**
      - Right **0KTC-**
- **Resection** — *continued*
  - Muscle — *continued*
    - Head **0KT0-**
    - Hip
      - Left **0KTP-**
      - Right **0KTN-**
    - Lower Arm and Wrist
      - Left **0KTB-**
      - Right **0KT9-**
    - Lower Leg
      - Left **0KTT-**
      - Right **0KTS-**
    - Neck
      - Left **0KT3-**
      - Right **0KT2-**
    - Papillary **02TD-**
    - Perineum **0KTM-**
    - Shoulder
      - Left **0KT6-**
      - Right **0KT5-**
    - Thorax
      - Left **0KTJ-**
      - Right **0KTH-**
    - Tongue, Palate, Pharynx **0KT4-**
    - Trunk
      - Left **0KTG-**
      - Right **0KTF-**
    - Upper Arm
      - Left **0KT8-**
      - Right **0KT7-**
    - Upper Leg
      - Left **0KTR-**
      - Right **0KTQ-**
  - Nasal Mucosa and Soft Tissue **09TK-**
  - Nasopharynx **09TN-**
  - Nipple
    - Left **0HTXXZZ**
    - Right **0HTWXZZ**
  - Omentum **0DTU-**
  - Orbit
    - Left **0NTQ0ZZ**
    - Right **0NTP0ZZ**
  - Ovary
    - Bilateral **0UT2-**
    - Left **0UT1-**
    - Right **0UT0-**
  - Palate
    - Hard **0CT2-**
    - Soft **0CT3-**
  - Pancreas **0FTG-**
  - Para-aortic Body **0GT9-**
  - Paraganglion Extremity **0GTF-**
  - Parathyroid Gland **0GTR-**
    - Inferior
      - Left **0GTP-**
      - Right **0GTN-**
    - Multiple **0GTQ-**
    - Superior
      - Left **0GTM-**
      - Right **0GTL-**
  - Patella
    - Left **0QTF0ZZ**
    - Right **0QTD0ZZ**
  - Penis **0VTS-**
  - Pericardium **02TN-**
  - Phalanx
    - Finger
      - Left **0PTV0ZZ**
      - Right **0PTT0ZZ**
    - Thumb
      - Left **0PTS0ZZ**
      - Right **0PTR0ZZ**
    - Toe
      - Left **0QTR0ZZ**
      - Right **0QTQ0ZZ**
  - Pharynx **0CTM-**
  - Pineal Body **0GT1-**
  - Prepuce **0VTT-**
  - Products of Conception, Ectopic **10T2-**
  - Prostate **0VT0-**

PROCEDURE INDEX

© 2018 Channel Publishing, Ltd.

Resection — *continued*
Radius
Left **0PTJ**0ZZ
Right **0PTH**0ZZ
Rectum **0DTP**-
Ribs
1 or 2 **0PT1**0ZZ
3 or more **0PT2**0ZZ
Scapula
Left **0PT6**0ZZ
Right **0PT5**0ZZ
Scrotum **0VT5**-
Septum
Atrial **02T5**-
Nasal **09TM**-
Ventricular **02TM**-
Sinus
Accessory **09TP**-
Ethmoid
Left **09TV**-
Right **09TU**-
Frontal
Left **09TT**-
Right **09TS**-
Mastoid
Left **09TC**-
Right **09TB**-
Maxillary
Left **09TR**-
Right **09TQ**-
Sphenoid
Left **09TX**-
Right **09TW**-
Spleen **07TP**-
Sternum **0PT0**0ZZ
Stomach **0DT6**-
Pylorus **0DT7**-
Tarsal
Left **0QTM**0ZZ
Right **0QTL**0ZZ
Tendon
Abdomen
Left **0LTG**-
Right **0LTF**-
Ankle
Left **0LTT**-
Right **0LTS**-
Foot
Left **0LTW**-
Right **0LTV**-
Hand
Left **0LT8**-
Right **0LT7**-
Head and Neck **0LT0**-
Hip
Left **0LTK**-
Right **0LTJ**-
Knee
Left **0LTR**-
Right **0LTQ**-
Lower Arm and Wrist
Left **0LT6**-
Right **0LT5**-
Lower Leg
Left **0LTP**-
Right **0LTN**-
Perineum **0LTH**-
Shoulder
Left **0LT2**-
Right **0LT1**-
Thorax
Left **0LTD**-
Right **0LTC**-
Trunk
Left **0LTB**-
Right **0LT9**-
Upper Arm
Left **0LT4**-
Right **0LT3**-
Upper Leg
Left **0LTM**-
Right **0LTL**-

Resection — *continued*
Testis
Bilateral **0VTC**-
Left **0VTB**-
Right **0VT9**-
Thymus **07TM**-
Thyroid Gland **0GTK**-
Left Lobe **0GTG**-
Right Lobe **0GTH**-
Thyroid Gland Isthmus **0GTJ**-
Tibia
Left **0QTH**0ZZ
Right **0QTG**0ZZ
Toe Nail **0HTR**XZZ
Tongue **0CT7**-
Tonsils **0CTP**-
Tooth
Lower **0CTX**0Z-
Upper **0CTW**0Z-
Trachea **0BT1**-
Tunica Vaginalis
Left **0VT7**-
Right **0VT6**-
Turbinate, Nasal **09TL**-
Tympanic Membrane
Left **09T8**-
Right **09T7**-
Ulna
Left **0PTL**0ZZ
Right **0PTK**0ZZ
Ureter
Left **0TT7**-
Right **0TT6**-
Urethra **0TTD**-
Uterine Supporting Structure **0UT4**-
Uterus **0UT9**-
Uvula **0CTN**-
Vagina **0UTG**-
Valve, Pulmonary **02TH**-
Vas Deferens
Bilateral **0VTQ**-
Left **0VTP**-
Right **0VTN**-
Vesicle
Bilateral **0VT3**-
Left **0VT2**-
Right **0VT1**-
Vitreous
Left **08T5**3ZZ
Right **08T4**3ZZ
Vocal Cord
Left **0CTV**-
Right **0CTT**-
Vulva **0UTM**-
Resection, Left ventricular outflow tract obstruction (LVOT)
see Dilation, Ventricle, Left **027L**-
Resection, Subaortic membrane (Left ventricular outflow tract obstruction)
see Dilation, Ventricle, Left **027L**-
Restoration, Cardiac, Single, Rhythm 5A2204Z
RestoreAdvanced neurostimulator (SureScan) (MRI Safe)
use Stimulator Generator, Multiple Array Rechargeable in **0JH**-
RestoreSensor neurostimulator (SureScan) (MRI Safe)
use Stimulator Generator, Multiple Array Rechargeable in **0JH**-
RestoreUltra neurostimulator (SureScan) (MRI Safe)
use Stimulator Generator, Multiple Array Rechargeable in **0JH**-

Restriction
Ampulla of Vater **0FVC**-
Anus **0DVQ**-
Aorta
Abdominal **04V0**-
Intraluminal Device, Branched or Fenestrated **04V0**-
Thoracic
Ascending/Arch, Intraluminal Device, Branched or Fenestrated **02VX**-
Descending, Intraluminal Device, Branched or Fenestrated **02VW**-
Artery
Anterior Tibial
Left **04VQ**-
Right **04VP**-
Axillary
Left **03V6**-
Right **03V5**-
Brachial
Left **03V8**-
Right **03V7**-
Celiac **04V1**-
Colic
Left **04V7**-
Middle **04V8**-
Right **04V6**-
Common Carotid
Left **03VJ**-
Right **03VH**-
Common Iliac
Left **04VD**-
Right **04VC**-
External Carotid
Left **03VN**-
Right **03VM**-
External Iliac
Left **04VJ**-
Right **04VH**-
Face **03VR**-
Femoral
Left **04VL**-
Right **04VK**-
Foot
Left **04VW**-
Right **04VV**-
Gastric **04V2**-
Hand
Left **03VF**-
Right **03VD**-
Hepatic **04V3**-
Inferior Mesenteric **04VB**-
Innominate **03V2**-
Internal Carotid
Left **03VL**-
Right **03VK**-
Internal Iliac
Left **04VF**-
Right **04VE**-
Internal Mammary
Left **03V1**-
Right **03V0**-
Intracranial **03VG**-
Lower **04VY**-
Peroneal
Left **04VU**-
Right **04VT**-
Popliteal
Left **04VN**-
Right **04VM**-
Posterior Tibial
Left **04VS**-
Right **04VR**-
Pulmonary
Left **02VR**-
Right **02VQ**-
Pulmonary Trunk **02VP**-
Radial
Left **03VC**-
Right **03VB**-

Restriction — *continued*
Artery — *continued*
Renal
Left **04VA**-
Right **04V9**-
Splenic **04V4**-
Subclavian
Left **03V4**-
Right **03V3**-
Superior Mesenteric **04V5**-
Temporal
Left **03VT**-
Right **03VS**-
Thyroid
Left **03VV**-
Right **03VU**-
Ulnar
Left **03VA**-
Right **03V9**-
Upper **03VY**-
Vertebral
Left **03VQ**-
Right **03VP**-
Bladder **0TVB**-
Bladder Neck **0TVC**-
Bronchus
Lingula **0BV9**-
Lower Lobe
Left **0BVB**-
Right **0BV6**-
Main
Left **0BV7**-
Right **0BV3**-
Middle Lobe, Right **0BV5**-
Upper Lobe
Left **0BV8**-
Right **0BV4**-
Carina **0BV2**-
Cecum **0DVH**-
Cervix **0UVC**-
Cisterna Chyli **07VL**-
Colon
Ascending **0DVK**-
Descending **0DVM**-
Sigmoid **0DVN**-
Transverse **0DVL**-
Duct
Common Bile **0FV9**-
Cystic **0FV8**-
Hepatic
Common **0FV7**-
Left **0FV6**-
Right **0FV5**-
Lacrimal
Left **08VY**-
Right **08VX**-
Pancreatic **0FVD**-
Accessory **0FVF**-
Parotid
Left **0CVC**-
Right **0CVB**-
Duodenum **0DV9**-
Esophagogastric Junction **0DV4**-
Esophagus **0DV5**-
Lower **0DV3**-
Middle **0DV2**-
Upper **0DV1**-
Heart **02VA**-
Ileocecal Valve **0DVC**-
Ileum **0DVB**-
Intestine
Large **0DVE**-
Left **0DVG**-
Right **0DVF**-
Small **0DV8**-
Jejunum **0DVA**-
Kidney Pelvis
Left **0TV4**-
Right **0TV3**-
Lymphatic
Aortic **07VD**-
Axillary
Left **07V6**-
Right **07V5**-

© 2018 Channel Publishing, Ltd.

Restriction — *continued*
Lymphatic — *continued*
Head **07V0-**
Inguinal
Left **07VJ-**
Right **07VH-**
Internal Mammary
Left **07V9-**
Right **07V8-**
Lower Extremity
Left **07VG-**
Right **07VF-**
Mesenteric **07VB-**
Neck
Left **07V2-**
Right **07V1-**
Pelvis **07VC-**
Thoracic Duct **07VK-**
Thorax **07V7-**
Upper Extremity
Left **07V4-**
Right **07V3-**
Rectum **0DVP-**
Stomach **0DV6-**
Pylorus **0DV7-**
Trachea **0BV1-**
Ureter
Left **0TV7-**
Right **0TV6-**
Urethra **0TVD-**
Valve, Mitral **02VG-**
Vein
Axillary
Left **05V8-**
Right **05V7-**
Azygos **05V0-**
Basilic
Left **05VC-**
Right **05VB-**
Brachial
Left **05VA-**
Right **05V9-**
Cephalic
Left **05VF-**
Right **05VD-**
Colic **06V7-**
Common Iliac
Left **06VD-**
Right **06VC-**
Esophageal **06V3-**
External Iliac
Left **06VG-**
Right **06VF-**
External Jugular
Left **05VQ-**
Right **05VP-**
Face
Left **05VV-**
Right **05VT-**
Femoral
Left **06VN-**
Right **06VM-**
Foot
Left **06VV-**
Right **06VT-**
Gastric **06V2-**
Hand
Left **05VH-**
Right **05VG-**
Hemiazygos **05V1-**
Hepatic **06V4-**
Hypogastric
Left **06VJ-**
Right **06VH-**
Inferior Mesenteric **06V6-**
Innominate
Left **05V4-**
Right **05V3-**
Internal Jugular
Left **05VN-**
Right **05VM-**
Intracranial **05VL-**
Lower **06VY-**
Portal **06V8-**

Restriction — *continued*
Vein — *continued*
Pulmonary
Left **02VT-**
Right **02VS-**
Renal
Left **06VB-**
Right **06V9-**
Saphenous
Left **06VQ-**
Right **06VP-**
Splenic **06V1-**
Subclavian
Left **05V6-**
Right **05V5-**
Superior Mesenteric **06V5-**
Upper **05VY-**
Vertebral
Left **05VS-**
Right **05VR-**
Vena Cava
Inferior **06V0-**
Superior **02VV-**
Resurfacing Device
Removal of device from
Hip joint
Left **0SPB0BZ**
Right **0SP90BZ**
Revision of device in
Hip joint
Left **0SWB0BZ**
Right **0SW90BZ**
Supplement
Hip joint
Left **0SUB0BZ**
Acetabular Surface **0SUE0BZ**
Femoral Surface **0SUS0BZ**
Right **0SU90BZ**
Acetabular Surface **0SUA0BZ**
Femoral Surface **0SUR0BZ**
Resuscitation
Cardiopulmonary *see* Assistance, Cardiac **5A02-**
Cardioversion **5A2204Z**
Defibrillation **5A2204Z**
Endotracheal intubation *see* Insertion of device in, Trachea **0BH1-**
External chest compression **5A12012**
Pulmonary **5A19054**
Resuscitative endovascular balloon occlusion of the aorta (REBOA)
Abdomial Aorta **04L03DJ**
Thoracic Aorta, Descending **02LW3DJ**
Resuture, Heart valve prosthesis *see* Revision of device in, Heart and Great Vessels **02W-**
Retained placenta, manual removal
see Extraction, Products of Conception, Retained **10D1-**
Retraining
Cardiac *see* Motor Treatment, Rehabilitation **F07-**
Vocational *see* Activities of Daily Living Treatment, Rehabilitation **F08-**
Retrogasserian rhizotomy *see* Division, Nerve, Trigeminal **008K-**
Retroperitoneal cavity
use Retroperitoneum
Retroperitoneal lymph node
use Lymphatic, Aortic
Retroperitoneal space
use Retroperitoneum
Retropharyngeal lymph node
use Lymphatic, Neck, Left
use Lymphatic, Neck, Right

Retropubic space
use Pelvic Cavity
Reveal (DX) (XT)
use Monitoring Device
Reverse total shoulder replacement *see* Replacement, Upper Joints **0RR-**
Reverse® Shoulder Prosthesis
use Synthetic Substitute, Reverse Ball and Socket in **0RR-**
Revision
Correcting a portion of existing device *see* Revision of device in
Removal of device without replacement *see* Removal of device from
Replacement of existing device
see Removal of device from
see Root operation to place new device, e.g., Insertion, Replacement, Supplement
Revision of device in
Abdominal Wall **0WWF-**
Acetabulum
Left **0QW5-**
Right **0QW4-**
Anal Sphincter **0DWR-**
Anus **0DWQ-**
Artery
Lower **04WY-**
Upper **03WY-**
Auditory Ossicle
Left **09WA-**
Right **09W9-**
Back
Lower **0WWL-**
Upper **0WWK-**
Bladder **0TWB-**
Bone
Facial **0NWW-**
Lower **0QWY-**
Nasal **0NWB-**
Pelvic
Left **0QW3-**
Right **0QW2-**
Upper **0PWY-**
Bone Marrow **07WT-**
Brain **00W0-**
Breast
Left **0HWU-**
Right **0HWT-**
Bursa and Ligament
Lower **0MWY-**
Upper **0MWX-**
Carpal
Left **0PWN-**
Right **0PWM-**
Cavity, Cranial **0WW1-**
Cerebral Ventricle **00W6-**
Chest Wall **0WW8-**
Cisterna Chyli **07WL-**
Clavicle
Left **0PWB-**
Right **0PW9-**
Coccyx **0QWS-**
Diaphragm **0BWT-**
Disc
Cervical Vertebral **0RW3-**
Cervicothoracic Vertebral **0RW5-**
Lumbar Vertebral **0SW2-**
Lumbosacral **0SW4-**
Thoracic Vertebral **0RW9-**
Thoracolumbar Vertebral **0RWB-**
Duct
Hepatobiliary **0FWB-**
Pancreatic **0FWD-**
Ear
Inner
Left **09WE-**
Right **09WD-**
Left **09WJ-**
Right **09WH-**

Revision of device in — *continued*
Epididymis and Spermatic Cord **0VWM-**
Esophagus **0DW5-**
Extremity
Lower
Left **0YWB-**
Right **0YW9-**
Upper
Left **0XW7-**
Right **0XW6-**
Eye
Left **08W1-**
Right **08W0-**
Face **0WW2-**
Fallopian Tube **0UW8-**
Femoral Shaft
Left **0QW9-**
Right **0QW8-**
Femur
Lower
Left **0QWC-**
Right **0QWB-**
Upper
Left **0QW7-**
Right **0QW6-**
Fibula
Left **0QWK-**
Right **0QWJ-**
Finger Nail **0HWQX-**
Gallbladder **0FW4-**
Gastrointestinal Tract **0WWP-**
Genitourinary Tract **0WWR-**
Gland
Adrenal **0GW5-**
Endocrine **0GWS-**
Pituitary **0GW0-**
Salivary **0CWA-**
Glenoid Cavity
Left **0PW8-**
Right **0PW7-**
Great Vessel **02WY-**
Hair **0HWSX-**
Head **0WW0-**
Heart **02WA-**
Humeral Head
Left **0PWD-**
Right **0PWC-**
Humeral Shaft
Left **0PWG-**
Right **0PWF-**
Intestinal Tract
Lower **0DWD-**
Upper **0DW0-**
Intestine
Large **0DWE-**
Small **0DW8-**
Jaw
Lower **0WW5-**
Upper **0WW4-**
Joint
Acromioclavicular
Left **0RWH-**
Right **0RWG-**
Ankle
Left **0SWG-**
Right **0SWF-**
Carpal
Left **0RWR-**
Right **0RWQ-**
Carpometacarpal
Left **0RWT-**
Right **0RWS-**
Cervical Vertebral **0RW1-**
Cervicothoracic Vertebral **0RW4-**
Coccygeal **0SW6-**
Elbow
Left **0RWM-**
Right **0RWL-**
Finger Phalangeal
Left **0RWX-**
Right **0RWW-**

PROCEDURE INDEX

© 2018 Channel Publishing, Ltd.

Revision of device in — *continued*
Joint — *continued*
Hip
Left **0SWB-**
Acetabular Surface **0SWE-**
Femoral Surface **0SWS-**
Right **0SW9-**
Acetabular Surface **0SWA-**
Femoral Surface **0SWR-**
Knee
Left **0SWD-**
Femoral Surface **0SWU-**
Tibial Surface **0SWW-**
Right **0SWC-**
Femoral Surface **0SWT-**
Tibial Surface **0SWV-**
Lumbar Vertebral **0SW0-**
Lumbosacral **0SW3-**
Metacarpophalangeal
Left **0RWV-**
Right **0RWU-**
Metatarsal-Phalangeal
Left **0SWN-**
Right **0SWM-**
Occipital-cervical **0RW0-**
Sacrococcygeal **0SW5-**
Sacroiliac
Left **0SW8-**
Right **0SW7-**
Shoulder
Left **0RWK-**
Right **0RWJ-**
Sternoclavicular
Left **0RWF-**
Right **0RWE-**
Tarsal
Left **0SWJ-**
Right **0SWH-**
Tarsometatarsal
Left **0SWL-**
Right **0SWK-**
Temporomandibular
Left **0RWD-**
Right **0RWC-**
Thoracic Vertebral **0RW6-**
Thoracolumbar Vertebral **0RWA-**
Toe Phalangeal
Left **0SWQ-**
Right **0SWP-**
Wrist
Left **0RWP-**
Right **0RWN-**
Kidney **0TW5-**
Larynx **0CWS-**
Lens
Left **08WK-**
Right **08WJ-**
Liver **0FW0-**
Lung
Left **0BWL-**
Right **0BWK-**
Lymphatic **07WN-**
Thoracic Duct **07WK-**
Mediastinum **0WWC-**
Mesentery **0DWV-**
Metacarpal
Left **0PWQ-**
Right **0PWP-**
Metatarsal
Left **0QWP-**
Right **0QWN-**
Mouth and Throat **0CWY-**
Muscle
Extraocular
Left **08WM-**
Right **08WL-**
Lower **0KWY-**
Upper **0KWX-**
Nasal Mucosa and Soft Tissue **09WK-**
Neck **0WW6-**

Revision of device in — *continued*
Nerve
Cranial **00WE-**
Peripheral **01WY-**
Omentum **0DWU-**
Ovary **0UW3-**
Pancreas **0FWG-**
Parathyroid Gland **0GWR-**
Patella
Left **0QWF-**
Right **0QWD-**
Pelvic Cavity **0WWJ-**
Penis **0VWS-**
Pericardial Cavity **0WWD-**
Perineum
Female **0WWN-**
Male **0WWM-**
Peritoneal Cavity **0WWG-**
Peritoneum **0DWW-**
Phalanx
Finger
Left **0PWV-**
Right **0PWT-**
Thumb
Left **0PWS-**
Right **0PWR-**
Toe
Left **0QWR-**
Right **0QWQ-**
Pineal Body **0GW1-**
Pleura **0BWQ -**
Pleural Cavity-
Left **0WWB-**
Right **0WW9-**
Prostate and Seminal Vesicles **0VW4-**
Radius
Left **0PWJ-**
Right **0PWH-**
Respiratory Tract **0WWQ-**
Retroperitoneum **0WWH-**
Ribs
1 to 2 **0PW1-**
3 or more **0PW2-**
Sacrum **0QW1-**
Scapula
Left **0PW6-**
Right **0PW5-**
Scrotum and Tunica Vaginalis **0VW8-**
Septum
Atrial **02W5-**
Ventricular **02WM-**
Sinus **09WY-**
Skin **0HWPX-**
Skull **0NW0-**
Spinal Canal **00WU-**
Spinal Cord **00WV-**
Spleen **07WP-**
Sternum **0PW0-**
Stomach **0DW6-**
Subcutaneous Tissue and Fascia
Head and Neck **0JWS-**
Lower Extremity **0JWW-**
Trunk **0JWT-**
Upper Extremity **0JWV-**
Tarsal
Left **0QWM-**
Right **0QWL-**
Tendon
Lower **0LWY-**
Upper **0LWX-**
Testis **0VWD-**
Thymus **07WM-**
Thyroid Gland **0GWK-**
Tibia
Left **0QWH-**
Right **0QWG-**
Toe Nail **0HWRX-**
Trachea **0BW1-**
Tracheobronchial Tree **0BW0-**

Revision of device in — *continued*
Tympanic Membrane
Left **09W8-**
Right **09W7-**
Ulna
Left **0PWL-**
Right **0PWK-**
Ureter **0TW9-**
Urethra **0TWD-**
Uterus and Cervix **0UWD-**
Vagina and Cul-de-sac **0UWH-**
Valve
Aortic **02WF-**
Mitral **02WG-**
Pulmonary **02WH-**
Tricuspid **02WJ-**
Vas Deferens **0VWR-**
Vein
Azygos **05W0-**
Innominate
Left **05W4-**
Right **05W3-**
Lower **06WY-**
Upper **05WY-**
Vertebra
Cervical **0PW3-**
Lumbar **0QW0-**
Thoracic **0PW4-**
Vulva **0UWM-**
Revo MRI™ SureScan® pacemaker
use Pacemaker, Dual Chamber in **0JH-**
rhBMP-2
use Recombinant Bone Morphogenetic Protein
Rheos® System device
use Stimulator Generator in Subcutaneous Tissue and Fascia
Rheos® System lead
use Stimulator Lead in Upper Arteries
Rhinopharynx
use Nasopharynx
Rhinoplasty
see Alteration, Nasal Mucosa and Soft Tissue **090K-**
see Repair, Nasal Mucosa and Soft Tissue **09QK-**
see Replacement, Nasal Mucosa and Soft Tissue **09RK-**
see Supplement, Nasal Mucosa and Soft Tissue **09UK-**
Rhinorrhaphy *see* Repair, Nasal Mucosa and Soft Tissue **09QK-**
Rhinoscopy 09JKXZZ
Rhizotomy
see Division, Central Nervous System and Cranial Nerves **008-**
see Division, Peripheral Nervous System **018-**
Rhomboid major muscle
use Muscle, Trunk, Left
use Muscle, Trunk, Right
Rhomboid minor muscle
use Muscle, Trunk, Left
use Muscle, Trunk, Right
Rhythm electrocardiogram *see* Measurement, Cardiac **4A02-**
Rhytidectomy *see* Alteration, Face **0W02-**
Right ascending lumbar vein
use Vein, Azygos
Right atrioventricular valve
use Valve, Tricuspid
Right auricular appendix
use Atrium, Right
Right colic vein
use Vein, Colic
Right coronary sulcus
use Heart, Right

Right gastric artery
use Artery, Gastric
Right gastroepiploic vein
use Vein, Superior Mesenteric
Right inferior phrenic vein
use Vena Cava, Inferior
Right inferior pulmonary vein
use Vein, Pulmonary, Right
Right jugular trunk
use Lymphatic, Neck, Right
Right lateral ventricle
use Cerebral Ventricle
Right lymphatic duct
use Lymphatic, Neck, Right
Right ovarian vein
use Vena Cava, Inferior
Right second lumbar vein
use Vena Cava, Inferior
Right subclavian trunk
use Lymphatic, Neck, Right
Right subcostal vein
use Vein, Azygos
Right superior pulmonary vein
use Vein, Pulmonary, Right
Right suprarenal vein
use Vena Cava, Inferior
Right testicular vein
use Vena Cava, Inferior
Rima glottidis
use Larynx
Risorius muscle
use Muscle, Facial
RNS system lead
use Neurostimulator Lead in Central Nervous System and Cranial Nerves
RNS system neurostimulator generator
use Neurostimulator Generator in Head and Facial Bones
Robotic Assisted Procedure
Extremity
Lower **8E0Y-**
Upper **8E0X-**
Head and Neck Region **8E09-**
Trunk Region **8E0W-**
Robotic Waterjet Ablation, Destruction, Prostate XV508A4
Rotation of fetal head
Forceps **10S07ZZ**
Manual **10S0XZZ**
Round ligament of uterus
use Uterine Supporting Structure
Round window
use Ear, Inner, Left
use Ear, Inner, Right
Roux-en-Y operation
see Bypass, Gastrointestinal System **0D1-**
see Bypass, Hepatobiliary System and Pancreas **0F1-**
Rupture
Adhesions *see* Release
Fluid collection *see* Drainage

© 2018 Channel Publishing, Ltd.

S

Sacral ganglion
use Nerve, Sacral Sympathetic
Sacral lymph node
use Lymphatic, Pelvis
Sacral nerve modulation (SNM) lead
use Stimulator Lead in Urinary System
Sacral neuromodulation lead
use Stimulator Lead in Urinary System
Sacral splanchnic nerve
use Nerve, Sacral Sympathetic
Sacrectomy *see* Excision, Lower Bones **0QB-**
Sacrococcygeal ligament
use Lower Spine Bursa and Ligament
Sacrococcygeal symphysis
use Joint, Sacrococcygeal
Sacroiliac ligament
use Lower Spine Bursa and Ligament
Sacrospinous ligament
use Lower Spine Bursa and Ligament
Sacrotuberous ligament
use Lower Spine Bursa and Ligament
Salpingectomy
see Excision, Female Reproductive System **0UB-**
see Resection, Female Reproductive System **0UT-**
Salpingolysis *see* Release, Female Reproductive System **0UN-**
Salpingopexy
see Repair, Female Reproductive System **0UQ-**
see Reposition, Female Reproductive System **0US-**
Salpingopharyngeus muscle
use Muscle, Tongue, Palate, Pharynx
Salpingoplasty
see Repair, Female Reproductive System **0UQ-**
see Supplement, Female Reproductive System **0UU-**
Salpingorrhaphy *see* Repair, Female Reproductive System **0UQ-**
Salpingoscopy 0UJ88ZZ
Salpingostomy *see* Drainage, Female Reproductive System **0U9-**
Salpingotomy *see* Drainage, Female Reproductive System **0U9-**
Salpinx
use Fallopian Tube, Left
use Fallopian Tube, Right
Saphenous nerve
use Nerve, Femoral
SAPIEN transcatheter aortic valve
use Zooplastic Tissue in Heart and Great Vessels
Sartorius muscle
use Muscle, Upper Leg, Left
use Muscle, Upper Leg, Right
Scalene muscle
use Muscle, Neck, Left
use Muscle, Neck, Right
Scan
Computerized Tomography (CT) *see* Computerized Tomography (CT Scan)
Radioisotope *see* Planar Nuclear Medicine Imaging
Scaphoid bone
use Carpal, Left
use Carpal, Right
Scapholunate ligament
use Bursa and Ligament, Hand, Left
use Bursa and Ligament, Hand, Right
Scaphotrapezium ligament
use Bursa and Ligament, Hand, Left
use Bursa and Ligament, Hand, Right
Scapulectomy
see Excision, Upper Bones **0PB-**
see Resection, Upper Bones **0PT-**
Scapulopexy
see Repair, Upper Bones **0PQ-**
see Reposition, Upper Bones **0PS-**
Scarpa's (vestibular) ganglion
use Nerve, Acoustic
Sclerectomy *see* Excision, Eye **08B-**
Sclerotherapy, mechanical *see* Destruction
Sclerotherapy, via injection of sclerosing agent *see* Introduction, Destructive Agent
Sclerotomy *see* Drainage, Eye **089-**
Scrotectomy
see Excision, Male Reproductive System **0VB-**
see Resection, Male Reproductive System **0VT-**
Scrotoplasty
see Repair, Male Reproductive System **0VQ-**
see Supplement, Male Reproductive System **0VU-**
Scrotorrhaphy *see* Repair, Male Reproductive System **0VQ-**
Scrototomy *see* Drainage, Male Reproductive System **0V9**
Sebaceous gland
use Skin
Second cranial nerve
use Nerve, Optic
Section, cesarean *see* Extraction, Pregnancy **10D-**
Secura (DR) (VR)
use Defibrillator Generator in **0JH-**
Sella Turcica
use Sphenoid Bone
Semicircular canal
use Ear, Inner, Left
use Ear, Inner, Right
Semimembranosus muscle
use Muscle, Upper Leg, Left
use Muscle, Upper Leg, Right
Semitendinosus muscle
use Muscle, Upper Leg, Left
use Muscle, Upper Leg, Right
Seprafilm
use Adhesion Barrier
Septal cartilage
use Septum, Nasal
Septectomy
see Excision, Ear, Nose, Sinus **09B-**
see Excision, Heart and Great Vessels **02B-**
see Resection, Ear, Nose, Sinus **09T-**
see Resection, Heart and Great Vessels **02T-**
Septoplasty
see Repair, Ear, Nose, Sinus **09Q-**
see Repair, Heart and Great Vessels **02Q-**
see Replacement, Ear, Nose, Sinus **09R-**
see Replacement, Heart and Great Vessels **02R-**
Septoplasty — *continued*
see Reposition, Ear, Nose, Sinus **09S-**
see Supplement, Ear, Nose, Sinus **09U-**
see Supplement, Heart and Great Vessels **02U-**
Septostomy, balloon atrial 02163Z7
Septotomy *see* Drainage, Ear, Nose, Sinus **099-**
Sequestrectomy, bone *see* Extirpation
Serratus anterior muscle
use Muscle, Thorax, Left
use Muscle, Thorax, Right
Serratus posterior muscle
use Muscle, Trunk, Left
use Muscle, Trunk, Right
Seventh cranial nerve
use Nerve, Facial
Sheffield hybrid external fixator
use External Fixation Device, Hybrid in **0PH-**
use External Fixation Device, Hybrid in **0PS-**
use External Fixation Device, Hybrid in **0QH-**
use External Fixation Device, Hybrid in **0QS-**
Sheffield ring external fixator
use External Fixation Device, Ring in **0PH-**
use External Fixation Device, Ring in **0PS-**
use External Fixation Device, Ring in **0QH-**
use External Fixation Device, Ring in **0QS-**
Shirodkar cervical cerclage 0UVC7ZZ
Shock Wave Therapy, Musculoskeletal 6A93-
Short gastric artery
use Artery, Splenic
Shortening
see Excision
see Repair
see Reposition
Shunt creation *see* Bypass
Sialoadenectomy
Complete *see* Resection, Mouth and Throat **0CT-**
Partial *see* Excision, Mouth and Throat **0CB-**
Sialodochoplasty
see Repair, Mouth and Throat **0CQ-**
see Replacement, Mouth and Throat **0CR-**
see Supplement, Mouth and Throat **0CU-**
Sialoectomy
see Excision, Mouth and Throat **0CB-**
see Resection, Mouth and Throat **0CT-**
Sialography *see* Plain Radiography, Ear, Nose, Mouth and Throat **B90-**
Sialolithotomy *see* Extirpation, Mouth and Throat **0CC-**
Sigmoid artery
use Artery, Inferior Mesenteric
Sigmoid flexure
use Colon, Sigmoid
Sigmoid vein
use Vein, Inferior Mesenteric
Sigmoidectomy
see Excision, Gastrointestinal System **0DB-**
see Resection, Gastrointestinal System **0DT-**
Sigmoidorrhaphy *see* Repair, Gastrointestinal System **0DQ-**
Sigmoidoscopy 0DJD8ZZ
Sigmoidotomy *see* Drainage, Gastrointestinal System **0D9-**
Single lead pacemaker (atrium) (ventricle)
use Pacemaker, Single Chamber in **0JH-**
Single lead rate responsive pacemaker (atrium) (ventricle)
use Pacemaker, Single Chamber Rate Responsive in **0JH-**
Sinoatrial node
use Conduction Mechanism
Sinogram
Abdominal Wall *see* Fluoroscopy, Abdomen and Pelvis **BW11-**
Chest Wall *see* Plain Radiography, Chest **BW03-**
Retroperitoneum *see* Fluoroscopy, Abdomen and Pelvis **BW11-**
Sinus venosus
use Atrium, Right
Sinusectomy
see Excision, Ear, Nose, Sinus **09B-**
see Resection, Ear, Nose, Sinus **09T-**
Sinusoscopy 09JY4ZZ
Sinusotomy *see* Drainage, Ear, Nose, Sinus **099-**
Sirolimus-eluting coronary stent
use Intraluminal Device, Drug-eluting in Heart and Great Vessels
Sixth cranial nerve
use Nerve, Abducens
Size reduction, breast *see* Excision, Skin and Breast **0HB-**
SJM Biocor® Stented Valve System
use Zooplastic Tissue in Heart and Great Vessels
Skene's (paraurethral) gland
use Gland, Vestibular
Skin substitute, porcine liver derived, replacement XHRPXL2
Sling
Fascial, orbicularis muscle (mouth) *see* Supplement, Muscle, Facial **0KU1-**
Levator muscle, for urethral suspension *see* Reposition, Bladder Neck **0TSC-**
Pubococcygeal, for urethral suspension *see* Reposition, Bladder Neck **0TSC-**
Rectum *see* Reposition, Rectum **0DSP-**
Small bowel series *see* Fluoroscopy, Bowel, Small **BD13-**
Small saphenous vein
use Saphenous Vein, Left
use Saphenous Vein, Right
Snaring, polyp, colon *see* Excision, Gastrointestinal System **0DB-**
Solar (celiac) plexus
use Nerve, Abdominal Sympathetic
Soleus muscle
use Muscle, Lower Leg, Left
use Muscle, Lower Leg, Right
Spacer
Insertion of device in
Disc
Lumbar Vertebral **0SH2-**
Lumbosacral **0SH4-**
Joint
Acromioclavicular
Left **0RHH-**
Right **0RHG-**

PROCEDURE IN

© 2018 Channel Publishing, Ltd.

- **Spacer** — *continued*
  - Insertion of device in — *continued*
    - Joint — *continued*
      - Ankle
        - Left **0SHG-**
        - Right **0SHF-**
      - Carpal
        - Left **0RHR-**
        - Right **0RHQ-**
      - Carpometacarpal
        - Left **0RHT-**
        - Right **0RHS-**
      - Cervical Vertebral **0RH1-**
      - Cervicothoracic Vertebral **0RH4-**
      - Coccygeal **0SH6-**
      - Elbow
        - Left **0RHM-**
        - Right **0RHL-**
      - Finger Phalangeal
        - Left **0RHX-**
        - Right **0RHW-**
      - Hip
        - Left **0SHB-**
        - Right **0SH9-**
      - Knee
        - Left **0SHD-**
        - Right **0SHC-**
      - Lumbar Vertebral **0SH0-**
      - Lumbosacral **0SH3-**
      - Metacarpophalangeal
        - Left **0RHV-**
        - Right **0RHU-**
      - Metatarsal-Phalangeal
        - Left **0SHN-**
        - Right **0SHM-**
      - Occipital-cervical **0RH0-**
      - Sacrococcygeal **0SH5-**
      - Sacroiliac
        - Left **0SH8-**
        - Right **0SH7-**
      - Shoulder
        - Left **0RHK-**
        - Right **0RHJ-**
      - Sternoclavicular
        - Left **0RHF-**
        - Right **0RHE-**
      - Tarsal
        - Left **0SHJ-**
        - Right **0SHH-**
      - Tarsometatarsal
        - Left **0SHL-**
        - Right **0SHK-**
      - Temporomandibular
        - Left **0RHD-**
        - Right **0RHC-**
      - Thoracic Vertebral **0RH6-**
      - Thoracolumbar Vertebral **0RHA-**
      - Toe Phalangeal
        - Left **0SHQ-**
        - Right **0SHP-**
      - Wrist
        - Left **0RHP-**
        - Right **0RHN-**
  - Removal of device from
    - Acromioclavicular
      - Left **0RPH-**
      - Right **0RPG-**
    - Ankle
      - Left **0SPG-**
      - Right **0SPF-**
    - Carpal
      - Left **0RPR-**
      - Right **0RPQ-**
    - Carpometacarpal
      - Left **0RPT-**
      - Right **0RPS-**
    - Cervical Vertebral **0RP1-**
    - Cervicothoracic Vertebral **0RP4-**
    - Coccygeal **0SP6-**
    - Elbow
      - Left **0RPM -**
      - Right **0RPL-**
    - Finger Phalangeal
      - Left **0RPX-**
      - Right **0RPW-**
    - Hip
      - Left **0SPB-**
      - Right **0SP9-**
    - Knee
      - Left **0SPD-**
      - Right **0SPC-**
    - Lumbar Vertebral **0SP0-**
    - Lumbosacral **0SP3-**
    - Metacarpophalangeal
      - Left **0RPV-**
      - Right **0RPU-**
    - Metatarsal-Phalangeal
      - Left **0SPN-**
      - Right **0SPM-**
    - Occipital-cervical **0RP0-**
    - Sacrococcygeal **0SP5-**
    - Sacroiliac
      - Left **0SP8-**
      - Right **0SP7-**
    - Shoulder
      - Left **0RPK-**
      - Right **0RPJ-**
    - Sternoclavicular
      - Left **0RPF-**
      - Right **0RPE-**
    - Tarsal
      - Left **0SPJ-**
      - Right **0SPH-**
    - Tarsometatarsal
      - Left **0SPL-**
      - Right **0SPK-**
    - Temporomandibular
      - Left **0RPD-**
      - Right **0RPC-**
    - Thoracic Vertebral **0RP6-**
    - Thoracolumbar Vertebral **0RPA-**
    - Toe Phalangeal
      - Left **0SPQ-**
      - Right **0SPP-**
    - Wrist
      - Left **0RPP-**
      - Right **0RPN-**
  - Revision of device in
    - Acromioclavicular
      - Left **0RWH-**
      - Right **0RWG-**
    - Ankle
      - Left **0SWG-**
      - Right **0SWF-**
    - Carpal
      - Left **0RWR-**
      - Right **0RWQ-**
    - Carpometacarpal
      - Left **0RWT-**
      - Right **0RWS-**
    - Cervical Vertebral **0RW1-**
    - Cervicothoracic Vertebral **0RW4-**
    - Coccygeal **0SW6-**
    - Elbow
      - Left **0RWM-**
      - Right **0RWL-**
    - Finger Phalangeal
      - Left **0RWX-**
      - Right **0RWW-**
    - Hip
      - Left **0SWB-**
      - Right **0SW9-**
    - Knee
      - Left **0SWD-**
      - Right **0SWC-**
    - Lumbar Vertebral **0SW0-**
    - Lumbosacral **0SW3-**
    - Metacarpophalangeal
      - Left **0RWV-**
      - Right **0RWU-**
    - Metatarsal-Phalangeal
      - Left **0SWN-**
      - Right **0SWM-**
    - Occipital-cervical **0RW0-**
    - Sacrococcygeal **0SW5-**
    - Sacroiliac
      - Left **0SW8-**
      - Right **0SW7-**
    - Shoulder
      - Left **0RWK-**
      - Right **0RWJ-**
    - Sternoclavicular
      - Left **0RWF-**
      - Right **0RWE-**
    - Tarsal
      - Left **0SWJ-**
      - Right **0SWH-**
    - Tarsometatarsal
      - Left **0SWL-**
      - Right **0SWK-**
    - Temporomandibular
      - Left **0RWD-**
      - Right **0RWC-**
    - Thoracic Vertebral **0RW6-**
    - Thoracolumbar Vertebral **0RWA-**
    - Toe Phalangeal
      - Left **0SWQ-**
      - Right **0SWP-**
    - Wrist
      - Left **0RWP-**
      - Right **0RWN-**
- **Spacer, articulating (antibiotic)**
  - *use* Articulating Spacer in Lower Joints
- **Spacer, static (antibiotic)**
  - *use* Spacer in Lower Joints
- **Spectroscopy**
  - Intravascular **8E023DZ**
  - Near infrared **8E023DZ**
- **Speech Assessment F00-**
- **Speech therapy** *see* Speech Treatment, Rehabilitation **F06-**
- **Speech Treatment F06-**
- **Sphenoidectomy**
  - *see* Excision, Ear, Nose, Sinus **09B-**
  - *see* Excision, Head and Facial Bones **0NB-**
  - *see* Resection, Ear, Nose, Sinus **09T-**
  - *see* Resection, Head and Facial Bones **0NT-**
- **Sphenoidotomy** *see* Drainage, Ear, Nose, Sinus **099-**
- **Sphenomandibular ligament**
  - *use* Bursa and Ligament, Head and Neck
- **Sphenopalatine (pterygopalatine) ganglion**
  - *use* Nerve, Head and Neck Sympathetic
- **Sphincterorrhaphy, anal** *see* Repair, Anal Sphincter **0DQR-**
- **Sphincterotomy, anal**
  - *see* Division, Anal Sphincter **0D8R-**
  - *see* Drainage, Anal Sphincter **0D9R-**
- **Spinal cord neurostimulator lead**
  - *use* Neurostimulator Lead in Central Nervous System and Cranial Nerves
- **Spinal growth rods, magnetically controlled**
  - *use* Magnetically Controlled Growth Rod(s) in New Technology
- **Spinal nerve, cervical**
  - *use* Nerve, Cervical
- **Spinal nerve, lumbar**
  - *use* Nerve, Lumbar
- **Spinal nerve, sacral**
  - *use* Nerve, Sacral
- **Spinal nerve, thoracic**
  - *use* Nerve, Thoracic
- **Spinal Stabilization Device**
  - Facet Replacement
    - Cervical Vertebral **0RH1-**
    - Cervicothoracic Vertebral **0RH4-**
    - Lumbar Vertebral **0SH0-**
    - Lumbosacral **0SH3-**
    - Occipital-cervical **0RH0-**
    - Thoracic Vertebral **0RH6-**
    - Thoracolumbar Vertebral **0RHA-**
  - Interspinous Process
    - Cervical Vertebral **0RH1-**
    - Cervicothoracic Vertebral **0RH4-**
    - Lumbar Vertebral **0SH0-**
    - Lumbosacral **0SH3-**
    - Occipital-cervical **0RH0-**
    - Thoracic Vertebral **0RH6-**
    - Thoracolumbar Vertebral **0RHA-**
  - Pedicle-Based
    - Cervical Vertebral **0RH1-**
    - Cervicothoracic Vertebral **0RH4-**
    - Lumbar Vertebral **0SH0-**
    - Lumbosacral **0SH3-**
    - Occipital-cervical **0RH0-**
    - Thoracic Vertebral **0RH6-**
    - Thoracolumbar Vertebral **0RHA-**
- **Spinous process**
  - *use* Vertebra, Cervical
  - *use* Vertebra, Lumbar
  - *use* Vertebra, Thoracic
- **Spiral ganglion**
  - *use* Nerve, Acoustic
- **Spiration IBV™ Valve System**
  - *use* Intraluminal Device, Endobronchial Valve in Respiratory System
- **Splenectomy**
  - *see* Excision, Lymphatic and Hemic Systems **07B-**
  - *see* Resection, Lymphatic and Hemic Systems **07T-**
- **Splenic flexure**
  - *use* Colon, Transverse
- **Splenic plexus**
  - *use* Nerve, Abdominal Sympathetic
- **Splenius capitis muscle**
  - *use* Muscle, Head
- **Splenius cervicis muscle**
  - *use* Muscle, Neck, Left
  - *use* Muscle, Neck, Right
- **Splenolysis** *see* Release, Lymphatic and Hemic Systems **07N-**
- **Splenopexy**
  - *see* Repair, Lymphatic and Hemic Systems **07Q-**
  - *see* Reposition, Lymphatic and Hemic Systems **07S-**
- **Splenoplasty** *see* Repair, Lymphatic and Hemic Systems **07Q-**
- **Splenorrhaphy** *see* Repair, Lymphatic and Hemic Systems **07Q-**
- **Splenotomy** *see* Drainage, Lymphatic and Hemic Systems **079-**
- **Splinting, musculoskeletal** *see* Immobilization, Anatomical Regions **2W3-**

© 2018 Channel Publishing, Ltd.

SPY system intravascular fluorescence angiography
see Monitoring, Physiological Systems **4A1-**
Stapedectomy
see Excision, Ear, Nose, Sinus **09B-**
see Resection, Ear, Nose, Sinus **09T-**
Stapediolysis *see* Release, Ear, Nose, Sinus **09N-**
Stapedioplasty
see Repair, Ear, Nose, Sinus **09Q-**
see Replacement, Ear, Nose, Sinus **09R-**
see Supplement, Ear, Nose, Sinus **09U-**
Stapedotomy *see* Drainage, Ear, Nose, Sinus **099-**
Stapes
use Auditory Ossicle, Left
use Auditory Ossicle, Right
Static, spacer (antibiotic)
use Spacer in Lower Joints
STELARA®
use Other New Technology Therapeutic Substance
Stellate ganglion
use Nerve, Head and Neck Sympathetic
Stem cell transplant *see* Transfusion, Circulatory **302-**
Stensen's duct
use Duct, Parotid, Left
use Duct, Parotid, Right
Stent, intraluminal (cardiovascular) (gastrointestinal) (hepatobiliary) (urinary)
use Intraluminal Device
Stent retriever thrombectomy *see* Extirpation, Upper Arteries **03C-**
Stented tissue valve
use Zooplastic Tissue in Heart and Great Vessels
Stereotactic Radiosurgery
Abdomen **DW23-**
Adrenal Gland **DG22-**
Bile Ducts **DF22-**
Bladder **DT22-**
Bone Marrow **D720-**
Brain **D020-**
Brain Stem **D021-**
Breast
Left **DM20-**
Right **DM21-**
Bronchus **DB21-**
Cervix **DU21-**
Chest **DW22-**
Chest Wall **DB27-**
Colon **DD25-**
Diaphragm **DB28-**
Duodenum **DD22-**
Ear **D920-**
Esophagus **DD20-**
Eye **D820-**
Gallbladder **DF21-**
Gamma Beam
Abdomen **DW23JZZ**
Adrenal Gland **DG22JZZ**
Bile Ducts **DF22JZZ**
Bladder **DT22JZZ**
Bone Marrow **D720JZZ**
Brain **D020JZZ**
Brain Stem **D021JZZ**
Breast
Left **DM20JZZ**
Right **DM21JZZ**
Bronchus **DB21JZZ**
Cervix **DU21JZZ**
Chest **DW22JZZ**
Chest Wall **DB27JZZ**
Colon **DD25JZZ**
Diaphragm **DB28JZZ**

Stereotactic Radiosurgery — *continued*
Gamma Beam — *continued*
Duodenum **DD22JZZ**
Ear **D920JZZ**
Esophagus **DD20JZZ**
Eye **D820JZZ**
Gallbladder **DF21JZZ**
Gland
Adrenal **DG22JZZ**
Parathyroid **DG24JZZ**
Pituitary **DG20JZZ**
Thyroid **DG25JZZ**
Glands, Salivary **D926JZZ**
Head and Neck **DW21JZZ**
Ileum **DD24JZZ**
Jejunum **DD23JZZ**
Kidney **DT20JZZ**
Larynx **D92BJZZ**
Liver **DF20JZZ**
Lung **DB22JZZ**
Lymphatics
Abdomen **D726JZZ**
Axillary **D724JZZ**
Inguinal **D728JZZ**
Neck **D723JZZ**
Pelvis **D727JZZ**
Thorax **D725JZZ**
Mediastinum **DB26JZZ**
Mouth **D924JZZ**
Nasopharynx **D92DJZZ**
Neck and Head **DW21JZZ**
Nerve, Peripheral **D027JZZ**
Nose **D921JZZ**
Ovary **DU20JZZ**
Palate
Hard **D928JZZ**
Soft **D929JZZ**
Pancreas **DF23JZZ**
Parathyroid Gland **DG24JZZ**
Pelvic Region **DW26JZZ**
Pharynx **D92CJZZ**
Pineal Body **DG21JZZ**
Pituitary Gland **DG20JZZ**
Pleura **DB25JZZ**
Prostate **DV20JZZ**
Rectum **DD27JZZ**
Sinuses **D927JZZ**
Spinal Cord **D026JZZ**
Spleen **D722JZZ**
Stomach **DD21JZZ**
Testis **DV21JZZ**
Thymus **D721JZZ**
Thyroid Gland **DG25JZZ**
Tongue **D925JZZ**
Trachea **DB20JZZ**
Ureter **DT21JZZ**
Urethra **DT23JZZ**
Uterus **DU22JZZ**
Gland
Adrenal **DG22-**
Parathyroid **DG24-**
Pituitary **DG20-**
Thyroid **DG25-**
Glands, Salivary **D926-**
Head and Neck **DW21-**
Ileum **DD24-**
Jejunum **DD23-**
Kidney **DT20-**
Larnyx **D92B-**
Liver **DF20-**
Lung **DB22-**
Lymphatics
Abdomen **D726-**
Axillary **D724-**
Inguinal **D728-**
Neck **D723-**
Pelvis **D727-**
Thorax **D725-**
Mediastinum **DB26-**
Mouth **D924-**
Nasopharynx **D92D-**
Neck and Head **DW21-**
Nerve, Peripheral **D027-**
Nose **D921-**

Stereotactic Radiosurgery — *continued*
Other Photon
Abdomen **DW23DZZ**
Adrenal Gland **DG22DZZ**
Bile Ducts **DF22DZZ**
Bladder **DT22DZZ**
Bone Marrow **D720DZZ**
Brain **D020DZZ**
Brain Stem **D021DZZ**
Breast
Left **DM20DZZ**
Right **DM21DZZ**
Bronchus **DB21DZZ**
Cervix **DU21DZZ**
Chest **DW22DZZ**
Chest Wall **DB27DZZ**
Colon **DD25DZZ**
Diaphragm **DB28DZZ**
Duodenum **DD22DZZ**
Ear **D920DZZ**
Esophagus **DD20DZZ**
Eye **D820DZZ**
Gallbladder **DF21DZZ**
Gland
Adrenal **DG22DZZ**
Parathyroid **DG24DZZ**
Pituitary **DG20DZZ**
Thyroid **DG25DZZ**
Glands, Salivary **D926DZZ**
Head and Neck **DW21DZZ**
Ileum **DD24DZZ**
Jejunum **DD23DZZ**
Kidney **DT20DZZ**
Larynx **D92BDZZ**
Liver **DF20DZZ**
Lung **DB22DZZ**
Lymphatics
Abdomen **D726DZZ**
Axillary **D724DZZ**
Inguinal **D728DZZ**
Neck **D723DZZ**
Pelvis **D727DZZ**
Thorax **D725DZZ**
Mediastinum **DB26DZZ**
Mouth **D924DZZ**
Nasopharynx **D92DDZZ**
Neck and Head **DW21DZZ**
Nerve, Peripheral **D027DZZ**
Nose **D921DZZ**
Ovary **DU20DZZ**
Palate
Hard **D928DZZ**
Soft **D929DZZ**
Pancreas **DF23DZZ**
Parathyroid Gland **DG24DZZ**
Pelvic Region **DW26DZZ**
Pharynx **D92CDZZ**
Pineal Body **DG21DZZ**
Pituitary Gland **DG20DZZ**
Pleura **DB25DZZ**
Prostate **DV20DZZ**
Rectum **DD27DZZ**
Sinuses **D927DZZ**
Spinal Cord **D026DZZ**
Spleen **D722DZZ**
Stomach **DD21DZZ**
Testis **DV21DZZ**
Thymus **D721DZZ**
Thyroid Gland **DG25DZZ**
Tongue **D925DZZ**
Trachea **DB20DZZ**
Ureter **DT21DZZ**
Urethra **DT23DZZ**
Uterus **DU22DZZ**
Ovary **DU20-**
Palate
Hard **D928-**
Soft **D929-**
Pancreas **DF23-**
Parathyroid Gland **DG24-**
Particulate
Abdomen **DW23HZZ**
Adrenal Gland **DG22HZZ**
Bile Ducts **DF22HZZ**

Stereotactic Radiosurgery — *continued*
Particulate — *continued*
Bladder **DT22HZZ**
Bone Marrow **D720HZZ**
Brain **D020HZZ**
Brain Stem **D021HZZ**
Breast
Left **DM20HZZ**
Right **DM21HZZ**
Bronchus **DB21HZZ**
Cervix **DU21HZZ**
Chest **DW22HZZ**
Chest Wall **DB27HZZ**
Colon **DD25HZZ**
Diaphragm **DB28HZZ**
Duodenum **DD22HZZ**
Ear **D920HZZ**
Esophagus **DD20HZZ**
Eye **D820HZZ**
Gallbladder **DF21HZZ**
Gland
Adrenal **DG22HZZ**
Parathyroid **DG24HZZ**
Pituitary **DG20HZZ**
Thyroid **DG25HZZ**
Glands, Salivary **D926HZZ**
Head and Neck **DW21HZZ**
Ileum **DD24HZZ**
Jejunum **DD23HZZ**
Kidney **DT20HZZ**
Larynx **D92BHZZ**
Liver **DF20HZZ**
Lung **DB22HZZ**
Lymphatics
Abdomen **D726HZZ**
Axillary **D724HZZ**
Inguinal **D728HZZ**
Neck **D723HZZ**
Pelvis **D727HZZ**
Thorax **D725HZZ**
Mediastinum **DB26HZZ**
Mouth **D924HZZ**
Nasopharynx **D92DHZZ**
Neck and Head **DW21HZZ**
Nerve, Peripheral **D027HZZ**
Nose **D921HZZ**
Ovary **DU20HZZ**
Palate
Hard **D928HZZ**
Soft **D929HZZ**
Pancreas **DF23HZZ**
Parathyroid Gland **DG24HZZ**
Pelvic Region **DW26HZZ**
Pharynx **D92CHZZ**
Pineal Body **DG21HZZ**
Pituitary Gland **DG20HZZ**
Pleura **DB25HZZ**
Prostate **DV20HZZ**
Rectum **DD27HZZ**
Sinuses **D927HZZ**
Spinal Cord **D026HZZ**
Spleen **D722HZZ**
Stomach **DD21HZZ**
Testis **DV21HZZ**
Thymus **D721HZZ**
Thyroid Gland **DG25HZZ**
Tongue **D925HZZ**
Trachea **DB20HZZ**
Ureter **DT21HZZ**
Urethra **DT23HZZ**
Uterus **DU22HZZ**
Pelvic Region **DW26-**
Pharynx **D92C-**
Pineal Body **DG21-**
Pituitary Gland **DG20-**
Pleura **DB25-**
Prostate **DV20-**
Rectum **DD27-**
Sinuses **D927-**
Spinal Cord **D026-**
Spleen **D722-**
Stomach **DD21-**
Testis **DV21-**
Thymus **D721-**

© 2018 Channel Publishing, Ltd.

PROCEDURE INDEX

© 2018 Channel Publishing, Ltd.

Superficial palmar arch
use Artery, Hand, Left
use Artery, Hand, Right
Superficial palmar venous arch
use Vein, Hand, Left
use Vein, Hand, Right
Superficial temporal artery
use Artery, Temporal, Left
use Artery, Temporal, Right
Superficial transverse perineal muscle
use Muscle, Perineum
Superior cardiac nerve
use Nerve, Thoracic Sympathetic
Superior cerebellar vein
use Vein, Intracranial
Superior cerebral vein
use Vein, Intracranial
Superior clunic (cluneal) nerve
use Nerve, Lumbar
Superior epigastric artery
use Artery, Internal Mammary, Left
use Artery, Internal Mammary, Right
Superior genicular artery
use Artery, Popliteal, Left
use Artery, Popliteal, Right
Superior gluteal artery
use Artery, Internal Iliac, Left
use Artery, Internal Iliac, Right
Superior gluteal nerve
use Nerve, Lumbar Plexus
Superior hypogastric plexus
use Nerve, Abdominal Sympathetic
Superior labial artery
use Artery, Face
Superior laryngeal artery
use Artery, Thyroid, Left
use Artery, Thyroid, Right
Superior laryngeal nerve
use Nerve, Vagus
Superior longitudinal muscle
use Muscle, Tongue, Palate, Pharynx
Superior mesenteric ganglion
use Nerve, Abdominal Sympathetic
Superior mesenteric lymph node
use Lymphatic, Mesenteric
Superior mesenteric plexus
use Nerve, Abdominal Sympathetic
Superior oblique muscle
use Muscle, Extraocular, Left
use Muscle, Extraocular, Right
Superior olivary nucleus
use Pons
Superior rectal artery
use Artery, Inferior Mesenteric
Superior rectal vein
use Vein, Inferior Mesenteric
Superior rectus muscle
use Muscle, Extraocular, Left
use Muscle, Extraocular, Right
Superior tarsal plate
use Eyelid, Upper, Left
use Eyelid, Upper, Right
Superior thoracic artery
use Artery, Axillary, Left
use Artery, Axillary, Right
Superior thyroid artery
use Artery, External Carotid, Left
use Artery, External Carotid, Right
use Artery, Thyroid, Left
use Artery, Thyroid, Right
Superior turbinate
use Turbinate, Nasal
Superior ulnar collateral artery
use Artery, Brachial, Left
use Artery, Brachial, Right

Supersaturated Oxygen Therapy
5A0512C
5A0522C

Supplement
Abdominal Wall **0WUF-**
Acetabulum
Left **0QU5-**
Right **0QU4-**
Ampulla of Vater **0FUC-**
Anal Sphincter **0DUR-**
Ankle Region
Left **0YUL-**
Right **0YUK-**
Anus **0DUQ-**
Aorta
Abdominal **04U0-**
Thoracic
Ascending/Arch **02UX-**
Descending **02UW-**
Arm
Lower
Left **0XUF-**
Right **0XUD-**
Upper
Left **0XU9-**
Right **0XU8-**
Artery
Anterior Tibial
Left **04UQ-**
Right **04UP-**
Axillary
Left **03U6-**
Right **03U5-**
Brachial
Left **03U8-**
Right **03U7-**
Celiac **04U1-**
Colic
Left **04U7-**
Middle **04U8-**
Right **04U6-**
Common Carotid
Left **03UJ-**
Right **03UH-**
Common Iliac
Left **04UD-**
Right **04UC-**
External Carotid
Left **03UN-**
Right **03UM-**
External Iliac
Left **04UJ-**
Right **04UH-**
Face **03UR-**
Femoral
Left **04UL-**
Right **04UK-**
Foot
Left **04UW-**
Right **04UV-**
Gastric **04U2-**
Hand
Left **03UF-**
Right **03UD-**
Hepatic **04U3-**
Inferior Mesenteric **04UB-**
Innominate **03U2-**
Internal Carotid
Left **03UL-**
Right **03UK-**
Internal Iliac
Left **04UF-**
Right **04UE-**
Internal Mammary
Left **03U1-**
Right **03U0-**
Intracranial **03UG-**
Lower **04UY-**
Peroneal
Left **04UU-**
Right **04UT-**
Popliteal
Left **04UN-**
Right **04UM-**

Supplement — *continued*
Artery — *continued*
Posterior Tibial
Left **04US-**
Right **04UR-**
Pulmonary
Left **02UR-**
Right **02UQ-**
Pulmonary Trunk **02UP-**
Radial
Left **03UC-**
Right **03UB-**
Renal
Left **04UA-**
Right **04U9-**
Splenic **04U4-**
Subclavian
Left **03U4-**
Right **03U3-**
Superior Mesenteric **04U5-**
Temporal
Left **03UT-**
Right **03US-**
Thyroid
Left **03UV-**
Right **03UU-**
Ulnar
Left **03UA-**
Right **03U9-**
Upper **03UY-**
Vertebral
Left **03UQ-**
Right **03UP-**
Atrium
Left **02U7-**
Right **02U6-**
Auditory Ossicle
Left **09UA-**
Right **09U9-**
Axilla
Left **0XU5-**
Right **0XU4-**
Back
Lower **0WUL-**
Upper **0WUK-**
Bladder **0TUB-**
Bladder Neck **0TUC-**
Bone
Ethmoid
Left **0NUG-**
Right **0NUF-**
Frontal **0NU1-**
Hyoid **0NUX-**
Lacrimal
Left **0NUJ-**
Right **0NUH-**
Nasal **0NUB-**
Occipital **0NU7-**
Palatine
Left **0NUL-**
Right **0NUK-**
Parietal
Left **0NU4-**
Right **0NU3-**
Pelvic
Left **0QU3-**
Right **0QU2-**
Sphenoid **0NUC-**
Temporal
Left **0NU6-**
Right **0NU5-**
Zygomatic
Left **0NUN-**
Right **0NUM-**
Breast
Bilateral **0HUV-**
Left **0HUU-**
Right **0HUT-**
Bronchus
Lingula **0BU9-**
Lower Lobe
Left **0BUB-**
Right **0BU6-**

Supplement — *continued*
Bronchus — *continued*
Main
Left **0BU7-**
Right **0BU3-**
Middle Lobe, Right **0BU5-**
Upper Lobe
Left **0BU8-**
Right **0BU4-**
Buccal Mucosa **0CU4-**
Bursa and Ligament
Abdomen
Left **0MUJ-**
Right **0MUH-**
Ankle
Left **0MUR-**
Right **0MUQ-**
Elbow
Left **0MU4-**
Right **0MU3-**
Foot
Left **0MUT-**
Right **0MUS-**
Hand
Left **0MU8-**
Right **0MU7-**
Head and Neck **0MU0-**
Hip
Left **0MUM-**
Right **0MUL-**
Knee
Left **0MUP-**
Right **0MUN-**
Lower Extremity
Left **0MUW-**
Right **0MUV-**
Perineum **0MUK-**
Rib(s) **0MUG-**
Shoulder
Left **0MU2-**
Right **0MU1-**
Spine
Lower **0MUD-**
Upper **0MUC-**
Sternum **0MUF-**
Upper Extremity
Left **0MUB-**
Right **0MU9-**
Wrist
Left **0MU6-**
Right **0MU5-**
Buttock
Left **0YU1-**
Right **0YU0-**
Carina **0BU2-**
Carpal
Left **0PUN-**
Right **0PUM-**
Cecum **0DUH-**
Cerebral Meninges **00U1-**
Cerebral Ventricle **00U6-**
Chest Wall **0WU8-**
Chordae Tendineae **02U9-**
Cisterna Chyli **07UL-**
Clavicle
Left **0PUB-**
Right **0PU9-**
Clitoris **0UUJ-**
Coccyx **0QUS-**
Colon
Ascending **0DUK-**
Descending **0DUM-**
Sigmoid **0DUN-**
Transverse **0DUL-**
Cord
Bilateral **0VUH-**
Left **0VUG-**
Right **0VUF-**
Cornea
Left **08U9-**
Right **08U8-**
Cul-de-sac **0UUF-**
Diaphragm **0BUT-**

© 2018 Channel Publishing, Ltd.

- **Supplement** — *continued*
  - Disc
    - Cervical Vertebral **0RU3**-
    - Cervicothoracic Vertebral **0RU5**-
    - Lumbar Vertebral **0SU2**-
    - Lumbosacral **0SU4**-
    - Thoracic Vertebral **0RU9**-
    - Thoracolumbar Vertebral **0RUB**-
  - Duct
    - Common Bile **0FU9**-
    - Cystic **0FU8**-
    - Hepatic
      - Common **0FU7**-
      - Left **0FU6**-
      - Right **0FU5**-
    - Lacrimal
      - Left **08UY**-
      - Right **08UX**-
    - Pancreatic **0FUD**-
      - Accessory **0FUF**-
  - Duodenum **0DU9**-
  - Dura Mater **00U2**-
  - Ear
    - External
      - Bilateral **09U2**-
      - Left **09U1**-
      - Right **09U0**-
    - Inner
      - Left **09UE**-
      - Right **09UD**-
    - Middle
      - Left **09U6**-
      - Right **09U5**-
  - Elbow Region
    - Left **0XUC**-
    - Right **0XUB**-
  - Epididymis
    - Bilateral **0VUL**-
    - Left **0VUK**-
    - Right **0VUJ**-
  - Epiglottis **0CUR**-
  - Esophagogastric Junction **0DU4**-
  - Esophagus **0DU5**-
    - Lower **0DU3**-
    - Middle **0DU2**-
    - Upper **0DU1**-
  - Extremity
    - Lower
      - Left **0YUB**-
      - Right **0YU9**-
    - Upper
      - Left **0XU7**-
      - Right **0XU6**-
  - Eye
    - Left **08U1**-
    - Right **08U0**-
  - Eyelid
    - Lower
      - Left **08UR**-
      - Right **08UQ**-
    - Upper
      - Left **08UP**-
      - Right **08UN**-
  - Face **0WU2**-
  - Fallopian Tube
    - Left **0UU6**-
    - Right **0UU5**-
  - Fallopian Tubes, Bilateral **0UU7**-
  - Femoral Region
    - Bilateral **0YUE**-
    - Left **0YU8**-
    - Right **0YU7**-
  - Femoral Shaft
    - Left **0QU9**-
    - Right **0QU8**-
  - Femur
    - Lower
      - Left **0QUC**-
      - Right **0QUB**-
    - Upper
      - Left **0QU7**-
      - Right **0QU6**-

- **Supplement** — *continued*
  - Fibula
    - Left **0QUK**-
    - Right **0QUJ**-
  - Finger
    - Index
      - Left **0XUP**-
      - Right **0XUN**-
    - Little
      - Left **0XUW**-
      - Right **0XUV**-
    - Middle
      - Left **0XUR**-
      - Right **0XUQ**-
    - Ring
      - Left **0XUT**-
      - Right **0XUS**-
  - Foot
    - Left **0YUN**-
    - Right **0YUM**-
  - Gingiva
    - Lower **0CU6**-
    - Upper **0CU5**-
  - Glenoid Cavity
    - Left **0PU8**-
    - Right **0PU7**-
  - Hand
    - Left **0XUK**-
    - Right **0XUJ**-
  - Head **0WU0**-
  - Heart **02UA**-
  - Humeral Head
    - Left **0PUD**-
    - Right **0PUC**-
  - Humeral Shaft
    - Left **0PUG**-
    - Right **0PUF**-
  - Hymen **0UUK**-
  - Ileocecal Valve **0DUC**-
  - Ileum **0DUB**-
  - Inguinal Region
    - Bilateral **0YUA**-
    - Left **0YU6**-
    - Right **0YU5**-
  - Intestine
    - Large **0DUE**-
      - Left **0DUG**-
      - Right **0DUF**-
    - Small **0DU8**-
  - Iris
    - Left **08UD**-
    - Right **08UC**-
  - Jaw
    - Lower **0WU5**-
    - Upper **0WU4**-
  - Jejunum **0DUA**-
  - Joint
    - Acromioclavicular
      - Left **0RUH**-
      - Right **0RUG**-
    - Ankle
      - Left **0SUG**-
      - Right **0SUF**-
    - Carpal
      - Left **0RUR**-
      - Right **0RUQ**-
    - Carpometacarpal
      - Left **0RUT**-
      - Right **0RUS**-
    - Cervical Vertebral **0RU1**-
    - Cervicothoracic Vertebral **0RU4**-
    - Coccygeal **0SU6**-
    - Elbow
      - Left **0RUM**-
      - Right **0RUL**-
    - Finger Phalangeal
      - Left **0RUX**-
      - Right **0RUW**-
    - Hip
      - Left **0SUB**-
        - Acetabular Surface **0SUE**-
        - Femoral Surface **0SUS**-
      - Right **0SU9**-
        - Acetabular Surface **0SUA**-
        - Femoral Surface **0SUR**-

- **Supplement** — *continued*
  - Joint — *continued*
    - Knee
      - Left **0SUD**-
        - Femoral Surface **0SUU09Z**
        - Tibial Surface **0SUW09Z**
      - Right **0SUC**-
        - Femoral Surface **0SUT09Z**
        - Tibial Surface **0SUV09Z**
    - Lumbar Vertebral **0SU0**-
    - Lumbosacral **0SU3**-
    - Metacarpophalangeal
      - Left **0RUV**-
      - Right **0RUU**-
    - Metatarsal-Phalangeal
      - Left **0SUN**-
      - Right **0SUM**-
    - Occipital-cervical **0RU0**-
    - Sacrococcygeal **0SU5**-
    - Sacroiliac
      - Left **0SU8**-
      - Right **0SU7**-
    - Shoulder
      - Left **0RUK**-
      - Right **0RUJ**-
    - Sternoclavicular
      - Left **0RUF**-
      - Right **0RUE**-
    - Tarsal
      - Left **0SUJ**-
      - Right **0SUH**-
    - Tarsometatarsal
      - Left **0SUL**-
      - Right **0SUK**-
    - Temporomandibular
      - Left **0RUD**-
      - Right **0RUC**-
    - Thoracic Vertebral **0RU6**-
    - Thoracolumbar Vertebral **0RUA**-
    - Toe Phalangeal
      - Left **0SUQ**-
      - Right **0SUP**-
    - Wrist
      - Left **0RUP**-
      - Right **0RUN**-
  - Kidney Pelvis
    - Left **0TU4**-
    - Right **0TU3**-
  - Knee Region
    - Left **0YUG**-
    - Right **0YUF**-
  - Larynx **0CUS**-
  - Leg
    - Lower
      - Left **0YUJ**-
      - Right **0YUH**-
    - Upper
      - Left **0YUD**-
      - Right **0YUC**-
  - Lip
    - Lower **0CU1**-
    - Upper **0CU0**-
  - Lymphatic
    - Aortic **07UD**-
    - Axillary
      - Left **07U6**-
      - Right **07U5**-
    - Head **07U0**-
    - Inguinal
      - Left **07UJ**-
      - Right **07UH**-
    - Internal Mammary
      - Left **07U9**-
      - Right **07U8**-
    - Lower Extremity
      - Left **07UG**-
      - Right **07UF**-
    - Mesenteric **07UB**-
    - Neck
      - Left **07U2**-
      - Right **07U1**-
    - Pelvis **07UC**-
    - Thoracic Duct **07UK**-

- **Supplement** — *continued*
  - Lymphatic — *continued*
    - Thorax **07U7**-
    - Upper Extremity
      - Left **07U4**-
      - Right **07U3**-
  - Mandible
    - Left **0NUV**-
    - Right **0NUT**-
  - Maxilla **0NUR**-
  - Mediastinum **0WUC**-
  - Mesentery **0DUV**-
  - Metacarpal
    - Left **0PUQ**-
    - Right **0PUP**-
  - Metatarsal
    - Left **0QUP**-
    - Right **0QUN**-
  - Muscle
    - Abdomen
      - Left **0KUL**-
      - Right **0KUK**-
    - Extraocular
      - Left **08UM**-
      - Right **08UL**-
    - Facial **0KU1**-
    - Foot
      - Left **0KUW**-
      - Right **0KUV**-
    - Hand
      - Left **0KUD**-
      - Right **0KUC**-
    - Head **0KU0**-
    - Hip
      - Left **0KUP**-
      - Right **0KUN**-
    - Lower Arm and Wrist
      - Left **0KUB**-
      - Right **0KU9**-
    - Lower Leg
      - Left **0KUT**-
      - Right **0KUS**-
    - Neck
      - Left **0KU3**-
      - Right **0KU2**-
    - Papillary **02UD**-
    - Perineum **0KUM**-
    - Shoulder
      - Left **0KU6**-
      - Right **0KU5**-
    - Thorax
      - Left **0KUJ**-
      - Right **0KUH**-
    - Tongue, Palate, Pharynx **0KU4**-
    - Trunk
      - Left **0KUG**-
      - Right **0KUF**-
    - Upper Arm
      - Left **0KU8**-
      - Right **0KU7**-
    - Upper Leg
      - Left **0KUR**-
      - Right **0KUQ**-
  - Nasal Mucosa and Soft Tissue **09UK**-
  - Nasopharynx **09UN**-
  - Neck **0WU6**-
  - Nerve
    - Abducens **00UL**-
    - Accessory **00UR**-
    - Acoustic **00UN**-
    - Cervical **01U1**-
    - Facial **00UM**-
    - Femoral **01UD**-
    - Glossopharyngeal **00UP**-
    - Hypoglossal **00US**-
    - Lumbar **01UB**-
    - Median **01U5**-
    - Oculomotor **00UH**-
    - Olfactory **00UF**-
    - Optic **00UG**-
    - Peroneal **01UH**-
    - Phrenic **01U2**-
    - Pudendal **01UC**-
    - Radial **01U6**-

© 2018 Channel Publishing, Ltd.

- **Supplement** — *continued*
  - Nerve — *continued*
    - Sacral **01UR**-
    - Sciatic **01UF**-
    - Thoracic **01U8**-
    - Tibial **01UG**-
    - Trigeminal **00UK**-
    - Trochlear **00UJ**-
    - Ulnar **01U4**-
    - Vagus **00UQ**-
  - Nipple
    - Left **0HUX**-
    - Right **0HUW**-
  - Omentum **0DUU**-
  - Orbit
    - Left **0NUQ**-
    - Right **0NUP**-
  - Palate
    - Hard **0CU2**-
    - Soft **0CU3**-
  - Patella
    - Left **0QUF**-
    - Right **0QUD**-
  - Penis **0VUS**-
  - Pericardium **02UN**-
  - Perineum
    - Female **0WUN**-
    - Male **0WUM**-
  - Peritoneum **0DUW**-
  - Phalanx
    - Finger
      - Left **0PUV**-
      - Right **0PUT**-
    - Thumb
      - Left **0PUS**-
      - Right **0PUR**-
    - Toe
      - Left **0QUR**-
      - Right **0QUQ**-
  - Pharynx **0CUM**-
  - Prepuce **0VUT**-
  - Radius
    - Left **0PUJ**-
    - Right **0PUH**-
  - Rectum **0DUP**-
  - Retina
    - Left **08UF**-
    - Right **08UE**-
  - Retinal Vessel
    - Left **08UH**-
    - Right **08UG**-
  - Ribs
    - 1 to 2 **0PU1**-
    - 3 or more **0PU2**-
  - Sacrum **0QU1**-
  - Scapula
    - Left **0PU6**-
    - Right **0PU5**-
  - Scrotum **0VU5**-
  - Septum
    - Atrial **02U5**-
    - Nasal **09UM**-
    - Ventricular **02UM**-
  - Shoulder Region
    - Left **0XU3**-
    - Right **0XU2**-
  - Skull **0NU0**-
  - Spinal Meninges **00UT**-
  - Sternum **0PU0**-
  - Stomach **0DU6**-
    - Pylorus **0DU7**-
  - Subcutaneous Tissue and Fascia
    - Abdomen **0JU8**-
    - Back **0JU7**-
    - Buttock **0JU9**-
    - Chest **0JU6**-
    - Face **0JU1**-
    - Foot
      - Left **0JUR**-
      - Right **0JUQ**-
    - Hand
      - Left **0JUK**-
      - Right **0JUJ**-

- **Supplement** — *continued*
  - Subcutaneous Tissue and Fascia — *continued*
    - Lower Arm
      - Left **0JUH**-
      - Right **0JUG**-
    - Lower Leg
      - Left **0JUP**-
      - Right **0JUN**-
    - Neck
      - Left **0JU5**-
      - Right **0JU4**-
    - Pelvic Region **0JUC**-
    - Perineum **0JUB**-
    - Scalp **0JU0**-
    - Upper Arm
      - Left **0JUF**-
      - Right **0JUD**-
    - Upper Leg
      - Left **0JUM**-
      - Right **0JUL**-
  - Tarsal
    - Left **0QUM**-
    - Right **0QUL**-
  - Tendon
    - Abdomen
      - Left **0LUG**-
      - Right **0LUF**-
    - Ankle
      - Left **0LUT**-
      - Right **0LUS**-
    - Foot
      - Left **0LUW**-
      - Right **0LUV**-
    - Hand
      - Left **0LU8**-
      - Right **0LU7**-
    - Head and Neck **0LU0**-
    - Hip
      - Left **0LUK**-
      - Right **0LUJ**-
    - Knee
      - Left **0LUR**-
      - Right **0LUQ**-
    - Lower Arm and Wrist
      - Left **0LU6**-
      - Right **0LU5**-
    - Lower Leg
      - Left **0LUP**-
      - Right **0LUN**-
    - Perineum **0LUH**-
    - Shoulder
      - Left **0LU2**-
      - Right **0LU1**-
    - Thorax
      - Left **0LUD**-
      - Right **0LUC**-
    - Trunk
      - Left **0LUB**-
      - Right **0LU9**-
    - Upper Arm
      - Left **0LU4**-
      - Right **0LU3**-
    - Upper Leg
      - Left **0LUM**-
      - Right **0LUL**-
  - Testis
    - Bilateral **0VUC0**-
    - Left **0VUB0**-
    - Right **0VU90**-
  - Thumb
    - Left **0XUM**-
    - Right **0XUL**-
  - Tibia
    - Left **0QUH**-
    - Right **0QUG**-
  - Toe
    - 1st
      - Left **0YUQ**-
      - Right **0YUP**-
    - 2nd
      - Left **0YUS**-
      - Right **0YUR**-

- **Supplement** — *continued*
  - Toe — *continued*
    - 3rd
      - Left **0YUU**-
      - Right **0YUT**-
    - 4th
      - Left **0YUW**-
      - Right **0YUV**-
    - 5th
      - Left **0YUY**-
      - Right **0YUX**-
  - Tongue **0CU7**-
  - Trachea **0BU1**-
  - Tunica Vaginalis
    - Left **0VU7**-
    - Right **0VU6**-
  - Turbinate, Nasal **09UL**-
  - Tympanic Membrane
    - Left **09U8**-
    - Right **09U7**-
  - Ulna
    - Left **0PUL**-
    - Right **0PUK**-
  - Ureter
    - Left **0TU7**-
    - Right **0TU6**-
  - Urethra **0TUD**-
  - Uterine Supporting Structure **0UU4**-
  - Uvula **0CUN**-
  - Vagina **0UUG**-
  - Valve
    - Aortic **02UF**-
    - Mitral **02UG**-
    - Pulmonary **02UH**-
    - Tricuspid **02UJ**-
  - Vas Deferens
    - Bilateral **0VUQ**-
    - Left **0VUP**-
    - Right **0VUN**-
  - Vein
    - Axillary
      - Left **05U8**-
      - Right **05U7**-
    - Azygos **05U0**-
    - Basilic
      - Left **05UC**-
      - Right **05UB**-
    - Brachial
      - Left **05UA**-
      - Right **05U9**-
    - Cephalic
      - Left **05UF**-
      - Right **05UD**-
    - Colic **06U7**-
    - Common Iliac
      - Left **06UD**-
      - Right **06UC**-
    - Esophageal **06U3**-
    - External Iliac
      - Left **06UG**-
      - Right **06UF**-
    - External Jugular
      - Left **05UQ**-
      - Right **05UP**-
    - Face
      - Left **05UV**-
      - Right **05UT**-
    - Femoral
      - Left **06UN**-
      - Right **06UM**-
    - Foot
      - Left **06UV**-
      - Right **06UT**-
    - Gastric **06U2**-
    - Hand
      - Left **05UH**-
      - Right **05UG**-
    - Hemiazygos **05U1**-
    - Hepatic **06U4**-
    - Hypogastric
      - Left **06UJ**-
      - Right **06UH**-
    - Inferior Mesenteric **06U6**-

- **Supplement** — *continued*
  - Vein — *continued*
    - Innominate
      - Left **05U4**-
      - Right **05U3**-
    - Internal Jugular
      - Left **05UN**-
      - Right **05UM**-
    - Intracranial **05UL**-
    - Lower **06UY**-
    - Portal **06U8**-
    - Pulmonary
      - Left **02UT**-
      - Right **02US**-
    - Renal
      - Left **06UB**-
      - Right **06U9**-
    - Saphenous
      - Left **06UQ**-
      - Right **06UP**-
    - Splenic **06U1**-
    - Subclavian
      - Left **05U6**-
      - Right **05U5**-
    - Superior Mesenteric **06U5**-
    - Upper **05UY**-
    - Vertebral
      - Left **05US**-
      - Right **05UR**-
  - Vena Cava
    - Inferior **06U0**-
    - Superior **02UV**-
  - Ventricle
    - Left **02UL**-
    - Right **02UK**-
  - Vertebra
    - Cervical **0PU3**-
    - Lumbar **0QU0**-
    - Thoracic **0PU4**-
  - Vesicle
    - Bilateral **0VU3**-
    - Left **0VU2**-
    - Right **0VU1**-
  - Vocal Cord
    - Left **0CUV**-
    - Right **0CUT**-
  - Vulva **0UUM**-
  - Wrist Region
    - Left **0XUH**-
    - Right **0XUG**-
- **Supraclavicular (Virchow's) lymph node**
  - *use* Lymphatic, Neck, Left
  - *use* Lymphatic, Neck, Right
- **Supraclavicular nerve**
  - *use* Nerve, Cervical Plexus
- **Suprahyoid lymph node**
  - *use* Lymphatic, Head
- **Suprahyoid muscle**
  - *use* Muscle, Neck, Left
  - *use* Muscle, Neck, Right
- **Suprainguinal lymph node**
  - *use* Lymphatic, Pelvis
- **Supraorbital vein**
  - *use* Vein, Face, Left
  - *use* Vein, Face, Right
- **Suprarenal gland**
  - *use* Gland, Adrenal
  - *use* Gland, Adrenal, Bilateral
  - *use* Gland, Adrenal, Left
  - *use* Gland, Adrenal, Right
- **Suprarenal plexus**
  - *use* Nerve, Abdominal Sympathetic
- **Suprascapular nerve**
  - *use* Nerve, Brachial Plexus
- **Supraspinatus fascia**
  - *use* Subcutaneous Tissue and Fascia, Upper Arm, Left
  - *use* Subcutaneous Tissue and Fascia, Upper Arm, Right
- **Supraspinatus muscle**
  - *use* Muscle, Shoulder, Left
  - *use* Muscle, Shoulder, Right

© 2018 Channel Publishing, Ltd.

Supraspinous ligament
- *use* Lower Spine Bursa and Ligament
- *use* Upper Spine Bursa and Ligament

Suprasternal notch
- *use* Sternum

Supratrochlear lymph node
- *use* Lymphatic, Upper Extremity, Left
- *use* Lymphatic, Upper Extremity, Right

Sural artery
- *use* Artery, Popliteal, Left
- *use* Artery, Popliteal, Right

Suspension
- Bladder Neck *see* Reposition, Bladder Neck **0TSC-**
- Kidney *see* Reposition, Urinary System **0TS-**
- Urethra *see* Reposition, Urinary System **0TS-**
- Urethrovesical *see* Reposition, Bladder Neck **0TSC-**
- Uterus *see* Reposition, Uterus **0US9-**
- Vagina *see* Reposition, Vagina **0USG-**

Suture
- Laceration repair *see* Repair
- Ligation *see* Occlusion

Suture Removal
- Extremity
  - Lower **8E0YXY8**
  - Upper **8E0XXY8**
- Head and Neck Region **8E09XY8**
- Trunk Region **8E0WXY8**

Sutureless valve, Perceval
- *use* Zooplastic Tissue, Rapid Deployment Technique in New Technology

Sweat gland
- *use* Skin

Sympathectomy *see* Excision, Peripheral Nervous System **01B-**

SynCardia Total Artificial Heart
- *use* Synthetic Substitute

Synchra CRT-P
- *use* Cardiac Resynchronization Pacemaker Pulse Generator in **0JH-**

SynchroMed pump
- *use* Infusion Device, Pump in Subcutaneous Tissue and Fascia

Synechiotomy, iris *see* Release, Eye **08N-**

Synovectomy
- Lower joint *see* Excision, Lower Joints **0SB-**
- Upper joint *see* Excision, Upper Joints **0RB-**

Synthetic Human Angiotensin II XW0-

Systemic Nuclear Medicine Therapy
- Abdomen **CW70-**
- Anatomical Regions, Multiple **CW7YYZZ**
- Chest **CW73-**
- Thyroid **CW7G-**
- Whole Body **CW7N-**

T

Takedown
- Arteriovenous shunt *see* Removal of device from, Upper Arteries **03P-**
- Arteriovenous shunt, with creation of new shunt *see* Bypass, Upper Arteries **031-**
- Stoma
  - *see* Excision
  - *see* Reposition

Talent® Converter
- *use* Intraluminal Device

Talent® Occluder
- *use* Intraluminal Device

Talent® Stent Graft (abdominal) (thoracic)
- *use* Intraluminal Device

Talocalcaneal (subtalar) joint
- *use* Joint, Tarsal, Left
- *use* Joint, Tarsal, Right

Talocalcaneal ligament
- *use* Bursa and Ligament, Foot, Left
- *use* Bursa and Ligament, Foot, Right

Talocalcaneonavicular joint
- *use* Joint, Tarsal, Left
- *use* Joint, Tarsal, Right

Talocalcaneonavicular ligament
- *use* Bursa and Ligament, Foot, Left
- *use* Bursa and Ligament, Foot, Right

Talocrural joint
- *use* Joint, Ankle, Left
- *use* Joint, Ankle, Right

Talofibular ligament
- *use* Bursa and Ligament, Ankle, Left
- *use* Bursa and Ligament, Ankle, Right

Talus bone
- *use* Tarsal, Left
- *use* Tarsal, Right

TandemHeart® System
- *use* Short-term External Heart Assist System in Heart and Great Vessels

Tarsectomy
- *see* Excision, Lower Bones **0QB-**
- *see* Resection, Lower Bones **0QT-**

Tarsometatarsal ligament
- *use* Bursa and Ligament, Foot, Left
- *use* Bursa and Ligament, Foot, Right

Tarsorrhaphy *see* Repair, Eye **08Q-**

Tattooing
- Cornea **3E0CXMZ**
- Skin *see* Introduction of substance in or on, Skin **3E00-**

TAXUS® Liberté® Paclitaxel-eluting Coronary Stent System
- *use* Intraluminal Device, Drug-eluting in Heart and Great Vessels

TBNA (transbronchial needle aspiration)
- Fluid or gas *see* Drainage, Respiratory System **0B9-**
- Tissue biopsy *see* Extraction, Respiratory System **0BD-**

Telemetry 4A12X4Z
- Ambulatory **4A12X45**

Temperature gradient study 4A0ZXKZ

Temporal lobe
- *use* Cerebral Hemisphere

Temporalis muscle
- *use* Muscle, Head

Temporoparietalis muscle
- *use* Muscle, Head

Tendolysis *see* Release, Tendons **0LN-**

Tendonectomy
- *see* Excision, Tendons **0LB-**
- *see* Resection, Tendons **0LT-**

Tendonoplasty, tenoplasty
- *see* Repair, Tendons **0LQ-**
- *see* Replacement, Tendons **0LR-**
- *see* Supplement, Tendons **0LU-**

Tendorrhaphy *see* Repair, Tendons **0LQ-**

Tendototomy
- *see* Division, Tendons **0L8-**
- *see* Drainage, Tendons **0L9-**

Tenectomy, tenonectomy
- *see* Excision, Tendons **0LB-**
- *see* Resection, Tendons **0LT-**

Tenolysis *see* Release, Tendons **0LN-**

Tenontorrhaphy *see* Repair, Tendons **0LQ-**

Tenontotomy
- *see* Division, Tendons **0L8-**
- *see* Drainage, Tendons **0L9-**

Tenorrhaphy *see* Repair, Tendons **0LQ-**

Tenosynovectomy
- *see* Excision, Tendons **0LB-**
- *see* Resection, Tendons **0LT-**

Tenotomy
- *see* Division, Tendons **0L8-**
- *see* Drainage, Tendons **0L9-**

Tensor fasciae latae muscle
- *use* Muscle, Hip, Left
- *use* Muscle, Hip, Right

Tensor veli palatini muscle
- *use* Muscle, Tongue, Palate, Pharynx

Tenth cranial nerve
- *use* Nerve, Vagus

Tentorium cerebelli
- *use* Dura Mater

Teres major muscle
- *use* Muscle, Shoulder, Left
- *use* Muscle, Shoulder, Right

Teres minor muscle
- *use* Muscle, Shoulder, Left
- *use* Muscle, Shoulder, Right

Termination of pregnancy
- Aspiration curettage **10A07ZZ**
- Dilation and curettage **10A07ZZ**
- Hysterotomy **10A00ZZ**
- Intra-amniotic injection **10A03ZZ**
- Laminaria **10A07ZW**
- Vacuum **10A07Z6**

Testectomy
- *see* Excision, Male Reproductive System **0VB-**
- *see* Resection, Male Reproductive System **0VT-**

Testicular artery
- *use* Aorta, Abdominal

Testing
- Glaucoma **4A07XBZ**
- Hearing *see* Hearing Assessment, Diagnostic Audiology **F13-**
- Mental health *see* Psychological Tests
- Muscle function, electromyography (EMG) *see* Measurement, Musculoskeletal **4A0F-**
- Muscle function, manual *see* Motor Function Assessment, Rehabilitation **F01-**
- Neurophysiologic monitoring, intra-operative *see* Monitoring, Physiological Systems **4A1-**
- Range of motion *see* Motor Function Assessment, Rehabilitation **F01-**

Testing — *continued*
- Vestibular function *see* Vestibular Assessment, Diagnostic Audiology **F15-**

Thalamectomy *see* Excision, Thalamus **00B9-**

Thalamotomy *see* Drainage, Thalamus **0099-**

Thenar muscle
- *use* Muscle, Hand, Left
- *use* Muscle, Hand, Right

Therapeutic Massage
- Musculoskeletal System **8E0KX1Z**
- Reproductive System
  - Prostate **8E0VX1C**
  - Rectum **8E0VX1D**

Therapeutic occlusion coil(s)
- *use* Intraluminal Device

Thermography 4A0ZXKZ

Thermotherapy, prostate *see* Destruction, Prostate **0V50-**

Third cranial nerve
- *use* Nerve, Oculomotor

Third occipital nerve
- *use* Nerve, Cervical

Third ventricle
- *use* Cerebral Ventricle

Thoracectomy *see* Excision, Anatomical Regions, General **0WB-**

Thoracentesis *see* Drainage, Anatomical Regions, General **0W9-**

Thoracic aortic plexus
- *use* Nerve, Thoracic Sympathetic

Thoracic esophagus
- *use* Esophagus, Middle

Thoracic facet joint
- *use* Joint, Thoracic Vertebral

Thoracic ganglion
- *use* Nerve, Thoracic Sympathetic

Thoracoacromial artery
- *use* Artery, Axillary, Left
- *use* Artery, Axillary, Right

Thoracocentesis *see* Drainage, Anatomical Regions, General **0W9-**

Thoracolumbar facet joint
- *use* Joint, Thoracolumbar Vertebral

Thoracoplasty
- *see* Repair, Anatomical Regions, General **0WQ-**
- *see* Supplement, Anatomical Regions, General **0WU-**

Thoracostomy tube
- *use* Drainage Device

Thoracostomy, for lung collapse
- *see* Drainage, Respiratory System **0B9-**

Thoracotomy *see* Drainage, Anatomical Regions, General **0W9-**

Thoratec IVAD (Implantable Ventricular Assist Device)
- *use* Implantable Heart Assist System in Heart and Great Vessels

Thoratec Paracorporeal Ventricular Assist Device
- *use* Short-term External Heart Assist System in Heart and Great Vessels

Thrombectomy *see* Extirpation

Thymectomy
- *see* Excision, Lymphatic and Hemic Systems **07B-**
- *see* Resection, Lymphatic and Hemic Systems **07T-**

Thymopexy
- *see* Repair, Lymphatic and Hemic Systems **07Q-**
- *see* Reposition, Lymphatic and Hemic Systems **07S-**

© 2018 Channel Publishing, Ltd.

Thymus gland
use Thymus
Thyroarytenoid muscle
use Muscle, Neck, Left
use Muscle, Neck, Right
Thyrocervical trunk
use Artery, Thyroid, Left
use Artery, Thyroid, Right
Thyroid cartilage
use Larynx
Thyroidectomy
see Excision, Endocrine System **0GB-**
see Resection, Endocrine System **0GT-**
Thyroidorrhaphy *see* Repair, Endocrine System **0GQ-**
Thyroidoscopy 0GJK4ZZ
Thyroidotomy *see* Drainage, Endocrine System **0G9-**
Tibial insert
use Liner in Lower Joints
Tibialis anterior muscle
use Muscle, Lower Leg, Left
use Muscle, Lower Leg, Right
Tibialis posterior muscle
use Muscle, Lower Leg, Left
use Muscle, Lower Leg, Right
Tibiofemoral joint
use Joint, Knee, Left
use Joint, Knee, Right
use Joint, Knee, Left, Tibial Surface
use Joint, Knee, Right, Tibial Surface
Tisagenlecleucel
use Engineered Autologous Chimeric Antigen Receptor T-cell Immunotherapy
Tissue bank graft
use Nonautologous Tissue Substitute
Tissue Expander
Insertion of device in
Breast
Bilateral **0HHV-**
Left **0HHU-**
Right **0HHT-**
Nipple
Left **0HHX-**
Right **0HHW-**
Subcutaneous Tissue and Fascia
Abdomen **0JH8-**
Back **0JH7-**
Buttock **0JH9-**
Chest **0JH6-**
Face **0JH1-**
Foot
Left **0JHR-**
Right **0JHQ-**
Hand
Left **0JHK-**
Right **0JHJ-**
Lower Arm
Left **0JHH-**
Right **0JHG-**
Lower Leg
Left **0JHP-**
Right **0JHN-**
Neck
Left **0JH5-**
Right **0JH4-**
Pelvic Region **0JHC-**
Perineum **0JHB-**
Scalp **0JH0-**
Upper Arm
Left **0JHF-**
Right **0JHD-**
Upper Leg
Left **0JHM-**
Right **0JHL-**
Removal of device from
Breast
Left **0HPU-**
Right **0HPT-**

Tissue Expander — *continued*
Removal of device from — *continued*
Subcutaneous Tissue and Fascia
Head and Neck **0JPS-**
Lower Extremity **0JPW-**
Trunk **0JPT-**
Upper Extremity **0JPV-**
Revision of device in
Breast
Left **0HWU-**
Right **0HWT-**
Subcutaneous Tissue and Fascia
Head and Neck **0JWS-**
Lower Extremity **0JWW-**
Trunk **0JWT-**
Upper Extremity **0JWV-**
Tissue expander (inflatable) (injectable)
use Tissue Expander in Skin and Breast
use Tissue Expander in Subcutaneous Tissue and Fascia
Tissue Plasminogen Activator (tPA) (r-tPA)
use Thrombolytic, Other
Titanium Sternal Fixation System (TSFS)
use Internal Fixation Device, Rigid Plate in **0PS-**
use Internal Fixation Device, Rigid Plate in **0PH-**
Tomographic (Tomo) Nuclear Medicine Imaging
Abdomen **CW20-**
Abdomen and Chest **CW24-**
Abdomen and Pelvis **CW21-**
Anatomical Regions, Multiple **CW2YYZZ**
Bladder, Kidneys and Ureters **CT23-**
Brain **C020-**
Breast **CH2YYZZ**
Bilateral **CH22-**
Left **CH21-**
Right **CH20-**
Bronchi and Lungs **CB22-**
Central Nervous System **C02YYZZ**
Cerebrospinal Fluid **C025-**
Chest **CW23-**
Chest and Abdomen **CW24-**
Chest and Neck **CW26-**
Digestive System **CD2YYZZ**
Endocrine System **CG2YYZZ**
Extremity
Lower **CW2D-**
Bilateral **CP2F-**
Left **CP2D-**
Right **CP2C-**
Upper **CW2M-**
Bilateral **CP2B-**
Left **CP29-**
Right **CP28-**
Gallbladder **CF24-**
Gastrointestinal Tract **CD27-**
Gland, Parathyroid **CG21-**
Head and Neck **CW2B-**
Heart **C22YYZZ**
Right and Left **C226-**
Hepatobiliary System and Pancreas **CF2YYZZ**
Kidneys, Ureters and Bladder **CT23-**
Liver **CF25-**
Liver and Spleen **CF26-**
Lungs and Bronchi **CB22-**
Lymphatics and Hematologic System **C72YYZZ**
Musculoskeletal System, Other **CP2YYZZ**
Myocardium **C22G-**
Neck and Chest **CW26-**
Neck and Head **CW2B-**

Tomographic (Tomo) Nuclear Medicine Imaging — *continued*
Pancreas and Hepatobiliary System **CF2YYZZ**
Pelvic Region **CW2J-**
Pelvis **CP26-**
Pelvis and Abdomen **CW21-**
Pelvis and Spine **CP27-**
Respiratory System **CB2YYZZ**
Skin **CH2YYZZ**
Skull **CP21-**
Skull and Cervical Spine **CP23-**
Spine
Cervical **CP22-**
Cervical and Skull **CP23-**
Lumbar **CP2H-**
Thoracic **CP2G-**
Thoracolumbar **CP2J-**
Spine and Pelvis **CP27-**
Spleen **C722-**
Spleen and Liver **CF26-**
Subcutaneous Tissue **CH2YYZZ**
Thorax **CP24-**
Ureters, Kidneys and Bladder **CT23-**
Urinary System **CT2YYZZ**
Tomography, computerized *see* Computerized Tomography (CT Scan)
Tongue, base of
use Pharynx
Tonometry 4A07XBZ
Tonsillectomy
see Excision, Mouth and Throat **0CB-**
see Resection, Mouth and Throat **0CT-**
Tonsillotomy *see* Drainage, Mouth and Throat **0C9-**
Total anomalous pulmonary venous return (TAPVR) repair
see Bypass, Atrium **0217-**
see Bypass, Vena Cava, Superior **021V-**
Total artificial (replacement) heart
use Synthetic Substitute
Total parenteral nutrition (TPN)
see Introduction of Nutritional Substance
Trachectomy
see Excision, Trachea **0BB1-**
see Resection, Trachea **0BT1-**
Trachelectomy
see Excision, Cervix **0UBC-**
see Resection, Cervix **0UTC-**
Trachelopexy
see Repair, Cervix **0UQC-**
see Reposition, Cervix **0USC-**
Tracheloplasty *see* Repair, Cervix **0UQC-**
Trachelorrhaphy *see* Repair, Cervix **0UQC-**
Trachelotomy *see* Drainage, Cervix **0U9C-**
Tracheobronchial lymph node
use Lymphatic, Thorax
Tracheoesophageal fistulization 0B110D6
Tracheolysis *see* Release, Respiratory System **0BN-**
Tracheoplasty
see Repair, Respiratory System **0BQ-**
see Supplement, Respiratory System **0BU-**
Tracheorrhaphy *see* Repair, Respiratory System **0BQ-**
Tracheoscopy 0BJ18ZZ
Tracheostomy *see* Bypass, Respiratory System **0B1-**

Tracheostomy Device
Bypass, Trachea **0B11-**
Change device in, Trachea **0B21XFZ**
Removal of device from, Trachea **0BP1-**
Revision of device in, Trachea **0BW1-**
Tracheostomy tube
use Tracheostomy Device in Respiratory System
Tracheotomy *see* Drainage, Respiratory System **0B9-**
Traction
Abdominal Wall **2W63X-**
Arm
Lower
Left **2W6DX-**
Right **2W6CX-**
Upper
Left **2W6BX-**
Right **2W6AX-**
Back **2W65X-**
Chest Wall **2W64X-**
Extremity
Lower
Left **2W6MX-**
Right **2W6LX-**
Upper
Left **2W69X-**
Right **2W68X-**
Face **2W61X-**
Finger
Left **2W6KX-**
Right **2W6JX-**
Foot
Left **2W6TX-**
Right **2W6SX-**
Hand
Left **2W6FX-**
Right **2W6EX-**
Head **2W60X-**
Inguinal Region
Left **2W67X-**
Right **2W66X-**
Leg
Lower
Left **2W6RX-**
Right **2W6QX-**
Upper
Left **2W6PX-**
Right **2W6NX-**
Neck **2W62X-**
Thumb
Left **2W6HX-**
Right **2W6GX-**
Toe
Left **2W6VX-**
Right **2W6UX-**
Tractotomy *see* Division, Central Nervous System and Cranial Nerves **008-**
Tragus
use Ear, External, Bilateral
use Ear, External, Left
use Ear, External, Right
Training, caregiver *see* Caregiver Training
TRAM (transverse rectus abdominis myocutaneous) flap reconstruction
Free *see* Replacement, Skin and Breast **0HR-**
Pedicled *see* Transfer, Muscles **0KX-**
Transection *see* Division
Transfer
Buccal Mucosa **0CX4-**
Bursa and Ligament
Abdomen
Left **0MXJ-**
Right **0MXH-**
Ankle
Left **0MXR-**
Right **0MXQ-**

© 2018 Channel Publishing, Ltd.

© 2018 Channel Publishing, Ltd.

Transplantation
Bone marrow *see* Transfusion, Circulatory **302**-
Esophagus **0DY**50Z-
Face **0WY**20Z-
Hand
Left **0XY**K0Z-
Right **0XY**J0Z-
Heart **02Y**A0Z-
Hematopoietic cell *see* Transfusion, Circulatory **302**-
Intestine
Large **0DY**E0Z-
Small **0DY**80Z-
Kidney
Left **0TY**10Z-
Right **0TY**00Z-
Liver **0FY**00Z-
Lung
Bilateral **0BY**M0Z-
Left **0BY**L0Z-
Lower Lobe
Left **0BY**J0Z-
Right **0BY**F0Z-
Middle Lobe, Right **0BY**D0Z-
Right **0BY**K0Z-
Upper Lobe
Left **0BY**G0Z-
Right **0BY**C0Z-
Lung Lingula **0BY**H0Z-
Ovary
Left **0UY**10Z-
Right **0UY**00Z-
Pancreas **0FY**G0Z-
Products of Conception **10Y0**-
Spleen **07Y**P0Z-
Stem cell *see* Transfusion, Circulatory **302**-
Stomach **0DY**60Z-
Thymus **07Y**M0Z-
Uterus **0UY**90Z-
Transposition
see Bypass
see Reposition
see Transfer
Transversalis fascia
use Subcutaneous Tissue and Fascia, Trunk
Transverse (cutaneous) cervical nerve
use Nerve, Cervical Plexus
Transverse acetabular ligament
use Bursa and Ligament, Hip, Left
use Bursa and Ligament, Hip, Right
Transverse facial artery
use Artery, Temporal, Left
use Artery, Temporal, Right
Transverse foramen
use Cervical Vertebra
Transverse humeral ligament
use Bursa and Ligament, Shoulder, Left
use Bursa and Ligament, Shoulder, Right
Transverse ligament of atlas
use Bursa and Ligament, Head and Neck
Transverse process
use Cervical Vertebra
use Lumbar Vertebra
use Thoracic Vertebra
Transverse Rectus Abdominis Myocutaneous Flap
Replacement
Bilateral **0HR**V076
Left **0HR**U076
Right **0HR**T076
Transfer
Left **0KX**L-
Right **0KX**K-
Transverse scapular ligament
use Bursa and Ligament, Shoulder, Left
use Bursa and Ligament, Shoulder, Right
Transverse thoracis muscle
use Muscle, Thorax, Left
use Muscle, Thorax, Right
Transversospinalis muscle
use Muscle, Trunk, Left
use Muscle, Trunk, Right
Transversus abdominis muscle
use Muscle, Abdomen, Left
use Muscle, Abdomen, Right
Trapezium bone
use Carpal, Left
use Carpal, Right
Trapezius muscle
use Muscle, Trunk, Left
use Muscle, Trunk, Right
Trapezoid bone
use Carpal, Left
use Carpal, Right
Triceps brachii muscle
use Muscle, Upper Arm, Left
use Muscle, Upper Arm, Right
Tricuspid annulus
use Valve, Tricuspid
Trifacial nerve
use Nerve, Trigeminal
Trifecta™ Valve (aortic)
use Zooplastic Tissue in Heart and Great Vessels
Trigone of bladder
use Bladder
Trimming, excisional *see* Excision
Triquetral bone
use Carpal, Left
use Carpal, Right
Trochanteric bursa
use Bursa and Ligament, Hip, Left
use Bursa and Ligament, Hip, Right
TUMT (Transurethral microwave thermotherapy of prostate)
0V507ZZ
TUNA (transurethral needle ablation of prostate)
0V507ZZ
Tunneled central venous catheter
use Vascular Access Device, Tunneled in Subcutaneous Tissue and Fascia
Tunneled spinal (intrathecal) catheter
use Infusion Device
Turbinectomy
see Excision, Ear, Nose, Sinus **09B**-
see Resection, Ear, Nose, Sinus **09T**-
Turbinoplasty
see Repair, Ear, Nose, Sinus **09Q**-
see Replacement, Ear, Nose, Sinus **09R**-
see Supplement, Ear, Nose, Sinus **09U**-
Turbinotomy
see Drainage, Ear, Nose, Sinus **099**-
see Division, Ear, Nose, Sinus **098**-
TURP (transurethral resection of prostate)
see Excision, Prostate **0VB0**-
see Resection, Prostate **0VT0**-
Twelfth cranial nerve
use Nerve, Hypoglossal
Two lead pacemaker
use Pacemaker, Dual Chamber in **0JH**-
Tympanic cavity
use Ear, Middle, Left
use Ear, Middle, Right
Tympanic nerve
use Nerve, Glossopharyngeal
Tympanic part of temporal bone
use Bone, Temporal, Left
use Bone, Temporal, Right
Tympanogram *see* Hearing Assessment, Diagnostic Audiology **F13**-
Tympanoplasty
see Repair, Ear, Nose, Sinus **09Q**-
see Replacement, Ear, Nose, Sinus **09R**-
see Supplement, Ear, Nose, Sinus **09U**-
Tympanosympathectomy *see* Excision, Nerve, Head and Neck Sympathetic **01B**K-
Tympanotomy *see* Drainage, Ear, Nose, Sinus **099**-

U

Ulnar collateral carpal ligament
use Bursa and Ligament, Wrist, Left
use Bursa and Ligament, Wrist, Right
Ulnar collateral ligament
use Bursa and Ligament, Elbow, Left
use Bursa and Ligament, Elbow, Right
Ulnar notch
use Radius, Left
use Radius, Right
Ulnar vein
use Vein, Brachial, Left
use Vein, Brachial, Right
Ultrafiltration
Hemodialysis *see* Performance, Urinary **5A1D**-
Therapeutic plasmapheresis *see* Pheresis, Circulatory **6A55**-
Ultraflex™ Precision Colonic Stent System
use Intraluminal Device
ULTRAPRO Hernia System (UHS)
use Synthetic Substitute
ULTRAPRO Partially Absorbable Lightweight Mesh
use Synthetic Substitute
ULTRAPRO Plug
use Synthetic Substitute
Ultrasonic osteogenic stimulator
use Bone Growth Stimulator in Head and Facial Bones
use Bone Growth Stimulator in Lower Bones
use Bone Growth Stimulator in Upper Bones
Ultrasonography
Abdomen **BW40ZZZ**
Abdomen and Pelvis **BW41ZZZ**
Abdominal Wall **BH49ZZZ**
Aorta
Abdominal, Intravascular **B440ZZ3**
Thoracic, Intravascular **B340ZZ3**
Appendix **BD48ZZZ**
Artery
Brachiocephalic-Subclavian, Right, Intravascular **B341ZZ3**
Celiac and Mesenteric, Intravascular **B44KZZ3**
Common Carotid
Bilateral, Intravascular **B345ZZ3**
Left, Intravascular **B344ZZ3**
Right, Intravascular **B343ZZ3**
Coronary
Multiple **B241YZZ**
Intravascular **B241ZZ3**
Transesophageal **B241ZZ4**
Single **B240YZZ**
Intravascular **B240ZZ3**
Transesophageal **B240ZZ4**
Femoral, Intravascular **B44LZZ3**
Inferior Mesenteric, Intravascular **B445ZZ3**
Internal Carotid
Bilateral, Intravascular **B348ZZ3**
Left, Intravascular **B347ZZ3**
Right, Intravascular **B346ZZ3**
Intra-Abdominal, Other, Intravascular **B44BZZ3**
Intracranial, Intravascular **B34RZZ3**

© 2018 Channel Publishing, Ltd.

Ultrasonography — *continued*
Artery — *continued*
Lower Extremity
Bilateral, Intravascular **B44HZZ3**
Left, Intravascular **B44GZZ3**
Right, Intravascular **B44FZZ3**
Mesenteric and Celiac, Intravascular **B44KZZ3**
Ophthalmic, Intravascular **B34VZZ3**
Penile, Intravascular **B44NZZ3**
Pulmonary
Left, Intravascular **B34TZZ3**
Right, Intravascular **B34SZZ3**
Renal
Bilateral, Intravascular **B448ZZ3**
Left, Intravascular **B447ZZ3**
Right, Intravascular **B446ZZ3**
Subclavian, Left, Intravascular **B342ZZ3**
Superior Mesenteric, Intravascular **B444ZZ3**
Upper Extremity
Bilateral, Intravascular **B34KZZ3**
Left, Intravascular **B34JZZ3**
Right, Intravascular **B34HZZ3**
Bile Duct **BF40ZZZ**
Bile Duct and Gallbladder **BF43ZZZ**
Bladder **BT40ZZZ**
and Kidney **BT4JZZZ**
Brain **B040ZZZ**
Breast
Bilateral **BH42ZZZ**
Left **BH41ZZZ**
Right **BH40ZZZ**
Chest Wall **BH4BZZZ**
Coccyx **BR4FZZZ**
Connective Tissue
Lower Extremity **BL41ZZZ**
Upper Extremity **BL40ZZZ**
Duodenum **BD49ZZZ**
Elbow
Left, Densitometry **BP4HZZ1**
Right, Densitometry **BP4GZZ1**
Esophagus **BD41ZZZ**
Extremity
Lower **BH48ZZZ**
Upper **BH47ZZZ**
Eye
Bilateral **B847ZZZ**
Left **B846ZZZ**
Right **B845ZZZ**
Fallopian Tube
Bilateral **BU42-**
Left **BU41-**
Right **BU40-**
Fetal Umbilical Cord **BY47ZZZ**
Fetus
First Trimester, Multiple Gestation **BY4BZZZ**
Second Trimester, Multiple Gestation **BY4DZZZ**
Single
First Trimester **BY49ZZZ**
Second Trimester **BY4CZZZ**
Third Trimester **BY4FZZZ**
Third Trimester, Multiple Gestation **BY4GZZZ**
Gallbladder **BF42ZZZ**
Gallbladder and Bile Duct **BF43ZZZ**
Gastrointestinal Tract **BD47ZZZ**
Gland
Adrenal
Bilateral **BG42ZZZ**
Left **BG41ZZZ**
Right **BG40ZZZ**
Parathyroid **BG43ZZZ**
Thyroid **BG44ZZZ**

Ultrasonography — *continued*
Hand
Left, Densitometry **BP4PZZ1**
Right, Densitometry **BP4NZZ1**
Head and Neck **BH4CZZZ**
Heart
Left **B245YZZ**
Intravascular **B245ZZ3**
Transesophageal **B245ZZ4**
Pediatric **B24DYZZ**
Intravascular **B24DZZ3**
Transesophageal **B24DZZ4**
Right **B244YZZ**
Intravascular **B244ZZ3**
Transesophageal **B244ZZ4**
Right and Left **B246YZZ**
Intravascular **B246ZZ3**
Transesophageal **B246ZZ4**
Heart with Aorta **B24BYZZ**
Intravascular **B24BZZ3**
Transesophageal **B24BZZ4**
Hepatobiliary System, All **BF4CZZZ**
Hip
Bilateral **BQ42ZZZ**
Left **BQ41ZZZ**
Right **BQ40ZZZ**
Kidney
and Bladder **BT4JZZZ**
Bilateral **BT43ZZZ**
Left **BT42ZZZ**
Right **BT41ZZZ**
Transplant **BT49ZZZ**
Knee
Bilateral **BQ49ZZZ**
Left **BQ48ZZZ**
Right **BQ47ZZZ**
Liver **BF45ZZZ**
Liver and Spleen **BF46ZZZ**
Mediastinum **BB4CZZZ**
Neck **BW4FZZZ**
Ovary
Bilateral **BU45-**
Left **BU44-**
Right **BU43-**
Ovary and Uterus **BU4C-**
Pancreas **BF47ZZZ**
Pelvic Region **BW4GZZZ**
Pelvis and Abdomen **BW41ZZZ**
Penis **BV4BZZZ**
Pericardium **B24CYZZ**
Intravascular **B24CZZ3**
Transesophageal **B24CZZ4**
Placenta **BY48ZZZ**
Pleura **BB4BZZZ**
Prostate and Seminal Vesicle **BV49ZZZ**
Rectum **BD4CZZZ**
Sacrum **BR4FZZZ**
Scrotum **BV44ZZZ**
Seminal Vesicle and Prostate **BV49ZZZ**
Shoulder
Left, Densitometry **BP49ZZ1**
Right, Densitometry **BP48ZZ1**
Spinal Cord **B04BZZZ**
Spine
Cervical **BR40ZZZ**
Lumbar **BR49ZZZ**
Thoracic **BR47ZZZ**
Spleen and Liver **BF46ZZZ**
Stomach **BD42ZZZ**
Tendon
Lower Extremity **BL43ZZZ**
Upper Extremity **BL42ZZZ**
Ureter
Bilateral **BT48ZZZ**
Left **BT47ZZZ**
Right **BT46ZZZ**
Urethra **BT45ZZZ**
Uterus **BU46-**
Uterus and Ovary **BU4C-**

Ultrasonography — *continued*
Vein
Jugular
Left, Intravascular **B544ZZ3**
Right, Intravascular **B543ZZ3**
Lower Extremity
Bilateral, Intravascular **B54DZZ3**
Left, Intravascular **B54CZZ3**
Right, Intravascular **B54BZZ3**
Portal, Intravascular **B54TZZ3**
Renal
Bilateral, Intravascular **B54LZZ3**
Left, Intravascular **B54KZZ3**
Right, Intravascular **B54JZZ3**
Spanchnic, Intravascular **B54TZZ3**
Subclavian
Left, Intravascular **B547ZZ3**
Right, Intravascular **B546ZZ3**
Upper Extremity
Bilateral, Intravascular **B54PZZ3**
Left, Intravascular **B54NZZ3**
Right, Intravascular **B54MZZ3**
Vena Cava
Inferior, Intravascular **B549ZZ3**
Superior, Intravascular **B548ZZ3**
Wrist
Left, Densitometry **BP4MZZ1**
Right, Densitometry **BP4LZZ1**
Ultrasound bone healing system
use Bone Growth Stimulator in Head and Facial Bones
use Bone Growth Stimulator in Lower Bones
use Bone Growth Stimulator in Upper Bones
Ultrasound Therapy
Heart **6A75-**
No Qualifier **6A75-**
Vessels
Head and Neck **6A75-**
Other **6A75-**
Peripheral **6A75-**
Ultraviolet Light Therapy, Skin 6A80-
Umbilical artery
use Artery, Internal Iliac, Left
use Artery, Internal Iliac, Right
use Lower Artery
Uniplanar external fixator
use External Fixation Device, Monoplanar in **0PH-**
use External Fixation Device, Monoplanar in **0PS-**
use External Fixation Device, Monoplanar in **0QH-**
use External Fixation Device, Monoplanar in **0QS-**
Upper GI series *see* Fluoroscopy, Gastrointestinal, Upper **BD15-**
Ureteral orifice
use Ureter
use Ureter, Left
use Ureter, Right
use Ureters, Bilateral
Ureterectomy
see Excision, Urinary System **0TB-**
see Resection, Urinary System **0TT-**
Ureterocolostomy *see* Bypass, Urinary System **0T1-**
Ureterocystostomy *see* Bypass, Urinary System **0T1-**
Ureteroenterostomy *see* Bypass, Urinary System **0T1-**
Ureteroileostomy *see* Bypass, Urinary System **0T1-**
Ureterolithotomy *see* Extirpation, Urinary System **0TC-**
Ureterolysis *see* Release, Urinary System **0TN-**

Ureteroneocystostomy
see Bypass, Urinary System **0T1-**
see Reposition, Urinary System **0TS-**
Ureteropelvic junction (UPJ)
use Kidney Pelvis, Left
use Kidney Pelvis, Right
Ureteropexy
see Repair, Urinary System **0TQ-**
see Reposition, Urinary System **0TS-**
Ureteroplasty
see Repair, Urinary System **0TQ-**
see Replacement, Urinary System **0TR-**
see Supplement, Urinary System **0TU-**
Ureteroplication *see* Restriction, Urinary System **0TV-**
Ureteropyelography *see* Fluoroscopy, Urinary System **BT1-**
Ureterorrhaphy *see* Repair, Urinary System **0TQ-**
Ureteroscopy 0TJ98ZZ
Ureterostomy
see Bypass, Urinary System **0T1-**
see Drainage, Urinary System **0T9-**
Ureterotomy *see* Drainage, Urinary System **0T9-**
Ureteroureterostomy *see* Bypass, Urinary System **0T1-**
Ureterovesical orifice
use Ureter
use Ureter, Left
use Ureter, Right
use Ureters, Bilateral
Urethral catheterization, indwelling 0T9B70Z
Urethrectomy
see Excision, Urethra **0TBD-**
see Resection, Urethra **0TTD-**
Urethrolithotomy *see* Extirpation, Urethra **0TCD-**
Urethrolysis *see* Release, Urethra **0TND-**
Urethropexy
see Repair, Urethra **0TQD-**
see Reposition, Urethra **0TSD-**
Urethroplasty
see Repair, Urethra **0TQD-**
see Replacement, Urethra **0TRD-**
see Supplement, Urethra **0TUD-**
Urethrorrhaphy *see* Repair, Urethra **0TQD-**
Urethroscopy 0TJD8ZZ
Urethrotomy *see* Drainage, Urethra **0T9D-**
Uridine triacetate XW0DX82
Urinary incontinence stimulator lead
use Stimulator Lead in Urinary System
Urography *see* Fluoroscopy, Urinary System **BT1-**
Ustekinumab
use Other New Technology Therapeutic Substance
Uterine Artery
use Artery, Internal Iliac, Left
use Artery, Internal Iliac, Right
Uterine artery embolization (UAE)
see Occlusion, Lower Arteries **04L-**
Uterine cornu
use Uterus
Uterine tube
use Fallopian Tube, Left
use Fallopian Tube, Right
Uterine vein
use Vein, Hypogastric, Left
use Vein, Hypogastric, Right

© 2018 Channel Publishing, Ltd.

Uvulectomy
see Excision, Uvula **0CBN-**
see Resection, Uvula **0CTN-**
Uvulorrhaphy *see* Repair, Uvula **0CQN-**
Uvulotomy *see* Drainage, Uvula **0C9N-**

V

Vaccination *see* Introduction of Serum, Toxoid, and Vaccine
Vacuum extraction, obstetric 10D07Z6
Vaginal artery
use Artery, Internal Iliac, Left
use Artery, Internal Iliac, Right
Vaginal pessary
use Intraluminal Device, Pessary in Female Reproductive System
Vaginal vein
use Vein, Hypogastric, Left
use Vein, Hypogastric, Right
Vaginectomy
see Excision, Vagina **0UBG-**
see Resection, Vagina **0UTG-**
Vaginofixation
see Repair, Vagina **0UQG-**
see Reposition, Vagina **0USG-**
Vaginoplasty
see Repair, Vagina **0UQG-**
see Supplement, Vagina **0UUG-**
Vaginorrhaphy *see* Repair, Vagina **0UQG-**
Vaginoscopy 0UJH8ZZ
Vaginotomy *see* Drainage, Female Reproductive System **0U9-**
Vagotomy *see* Division, Nerve, Vagus **008Q-**
Valiant Thoracic Stent Graft
use Intraluminal Device
Valvotomy, valvulotomy
see Division, Heart and Great Vessels **028-**
see Release, Heart and Great Vessels **02N-**
Valvuloplasty
see Repair, Heart and Great Vessels **02Q-**
see Replacement, Heart and Great Vessels **02R-**
see Supplement, Heart and Great Vessels **02U-**
Valvuloplasty, Alfieri Stitch
see Restriction, Valve, Mitral **02VG-**
Vascular Access Device
Totally Implantable
Insertion of device in
Abdomen **0JH8-**
Chest **0JH6-**
Lower Arm
Left **0JHH-**
Right **0JHG-**
Lower Leg
Left **0JHP-**
Right **0JHN-**
Upper Arm
Left **0JHF-**
Right **0JHD-**
Upper Leg
Left **0JHM-**
Right **0JHL-**
Removal of device from
Lower Extremity **0JPW-**
Trunk **0JPT-**
Upper Extremity **0JPV-**
Revision of device in
Lower Extremity **0JWW-**
Trunk **0JWT-**
Upper Extremity **0JWV**
Tunneled
Insertion of device in
Abdomen **0JH8-**
Chest **0JH6-**
Lower Arm
Left **0JHH-**
Right **0JHG-**
Vascular Access Device — *continued*
Tunneled — *continued*
Insertion of device in — *continued*
Lower Leg
Left **0JHP-**
Right **0JHN-**
Upper Arm
Left **0JHF-**
Right **0JHD-**
Upper Leg
Left **0JHM-**
Right **0JHL-**
Removal of device from
Lower Extremity **0JPW-**
Trunk **0JPT-**
Upper Extremity **0JPV-**
Revision of device in
Lower Extremity **0JWW-**
Trunk **0JWT-**
Upper Extremity **0JWV-**
Vasectomy *see* Excision, Male Reproductive System **0VB-**
Vasography
see Fluoroscopy, Male Reproductive System **BV1-**
see Plain Radiography, Male Reproductive System **BV0-**
Vasoligation *see* Occlusion, Male Reproductive System **0VL-**
Vasorrhaphy *see* Repair, Male Reproductive System **0VQ-**
Vasostomy *see* Bypass, Male Reproductive System **0V1-**
Vasotomy
Drainage *see* Drainage, Male Reproductive System **0V9-**
With ligation *see* Occlusion, Male Reproductive System **0VL-**
Vasovasostomy *see* Repair, Male Reproductive System **0VQ-**
Vastus intermedius muscle
use Muscle, Upper Leg, Left
use Muscle, Upper Leg, Right
Vastus lateralis muscle
use Muscle, Upper Leg, Left
use Muscle, Upper Leg, Right
Vastus medialis muscle
use Muscle, Upper Leg, Left
use Muscle, Upper Leg, Right
VCG (vectorcardiogram) *see* Measurement, Cardiac **4A02-**
Vectra® Vascular Access Graft
use Vascular Access Device Tunneled in Subcutaneous Tissue and Fascia
Venectomy
see Excision, Lower Veins **06B-**
see Excision, Upper Veins **05B-**
Venography
see Fluoroscopy, Veins **B51-**
see Plain Radiography, Veins **B50-**
Venorrhaphy
see Repair, Lower Veins **06Q-**
see Repair, Upper Veins **05Q-**
Venotripsy
see Occlusion, Lower Veins **06L-**
see Occlusion, Upper Veins **05L-**
Ventricular fold
use Larynx
Ventriculoatriostomy *see* Bypass, Central Nervous System and Cranial Nerves **001-**
Ventriculocisternostomy *see* Bypass, Central Nervous System and Cranial Nerves **001-**
Ventriculogram, cardiac
Combined left and right heart *see* Fluoroscopy, Heart, Right and Left **B216-**
Left ventricle *see* Fluoroscopy, Heart, Left **B215-**
Right ventricle *see* Fluoroscopy, Heart, Right **B214-**
Ventriculopuncture, through previously implanted catheter 8C01X6J
Ventriculoscopy 00J04ZZ
Ventriculostomy
External drainage *see* Drainage, Cerebral Ventricle **0096-**
Internal shunt *see* Bypass, Cerebral Ventricle **0016-**
Ventriculovenostomy *see* Bypass, Cerebral Ventricle **0016-**
Ventrio™ Hernia Patch
use Synthetic Substitute
VEP (visual evoked potential) 4A07X0Z
Vermiform appendix
use Appendix
Vermilion border
use Lip, Lower
use Lip, Upper
Versa
use Pacemaker, Dual chamber in **0JH-**
Version, obstetric
External **10S0XZZ**
Internal **10S07ZZ**
Vertebral arch
use Vertebra, Cervical
use Vertebra, Lumbar
use Vertebra, Thoracic
Vertebral body
use Cervical Vertebra
use Lumbar Vertebra
use Thoracic Vertebra
Vertebral canal
use Spinal Canal
Vertebral foramen
use Vertebra, Cervical
use Vertebra, Lumbar
use Vertebra, Thoracic
Vertebral lamina
use Vertebra, Cervical
use Vertebra, Lumbar
use Vertebra, Thoracic
Vertebral pedicle
use Vertebra, Cervical
use Vertebra, Lumbar
use Vertebra, Thoracic
Vesical vein
use Vein, Hypogastric, Left
use Vein, Hypogastric, Right
Vesicotomy *see* Drainage, Urinary System **0T9-**
Vesiculectomy
see Excision, Male Reproductive System **0VB-**
see Resection, Male Reproductive System **0VT-**
Vesiculogram, seminal *see* Plain Radiography, Male Reproductive System **BV0-**
Vesiculotomy *see* Drainage, Male Reproductive System **0V9-**
Vestibular (Scarpa's) ganglion
use Nerve, Acoustic
Vestibular Assessment F15Z-
Vestibular nerve
use Nerve, Acoustic
Vestibular Treatment F0C-
Vestibulocochlear nerve
use Nerve, Acoustic
VH-IVUS (virtual histology intravascular ultrasound)
see Ultrasonography, Heart **B24-**
Virchow's (supraclavicular) lymph node
use Lymphatic, Neck, Left
use Lymphatic, Neck, Right
Virtuoso (II) (DR) (VR)
use Defibrillator Generator in **0JH-**
Vistogard®
use Uridine Triacetate

PROCEDURE INDEX

© 2018 Channel Publishing, Ltd.

Vitrectomy
see Excision, Eye **08B-**
see Resection, Eye **08T-**
Vitreous body
use Vitreous, Left
use Vitreous, Right
Viva (XT) (S)
use Cardiac Resynchronization Defibrillator Pulse Generator in **0JH-**
Vocal fold
use Vocal Cord, Left
use Vocal Cord, Right
Vocational
Assessment *see* Activities of Daily Living Assessment, Rehabilitation **F02-**
Retraining *see* Activities of Daily Living Treatment, Rehabilitation **F08-**
Volar (palmar) digital vein
use Vein, Hand, Left
use Vein, Hand, Right
Volar (palmar) metacarpal vein
use Vein, Hand, Left
use Vein, Hand, Right
Vomer bone
use Septum, Nasal
Vomer of nasal septum
use Bone, Nasal
Voraxaze
use Glucarpidase
Vulvectomy
see Excision, Female Reproductive System **0UB-**
see Resection, Female Reproductive System **0UT-**
VYXEOS™
use Cytarabine and Daunorubicin Liposome Antineoplastic

W

WALLSTENT® Endoprosthesis
use Intraluminal Device
Washing *see* Irrigation
Wedge resection, pulmonary *see* Excision, Respiratory System **0BB-**
Window *see* Drainage
Wiring, dental **2W3**1X9Z

X

Xact Carotid Stent System
use Intraluminal Device
X-ray *see* Plain Radiography
X-STOP® Spacer
use Spinal Stabilization Device, Interspinous Process in **0RH-**
use Spinal Stabilization Device, Interspinous Process in **0SH-**
Xenograft
use Zooplastic Tissue in Heart and Great Vessels
XIENCE Everolimus Eluting Coronary Stent System
use Intraluminal Device, Drug-eluting in Heart and Great Vessels
Xiphoid process
use Sternum
XLIF® System
use Interbody Fusion Device in Lower Joints

Y

Z

Z-plasty, skin for scar contracture
see Release, Skin and Breast **0HN-**
Zenith AAA Endovascular Graft
use Intraluminal Device
use Intraluminal Device, Branched or Fenestrated, One or Two Arteries **04V-**
use Intraluminal Device, Branched or Fenestrated, Three or More Arteries **04V-**
Zenith Flex® AAA Endovascular Graft
use Intraluminal Device
Zenith TX2® TAA Endovascular Graft
use Intraluminal Device
Zenith® Renu™ AAA Ancillary Graft
use Intraluminal Device
Zilver® PTX® (paclitaxel) Drug-Eluting Peripheral Stent
use Intraluminal Device, Drug-eluting in Lower Arteries
use Intraluminal Device, Drug-eluting in Upper Arteries
Zimmer® NexGen® LPS Mobile Bearing Knee
use Synthetic Substitute
Zimmer® NexGen® LPS-Flex Mobile Knee
use Synthetic Substitute
ZINPLAVA™
use Bezlotoxumab Monoclonal Antibody
Zonule of Zinn
use Lens, Left
use Lens, Right
Zooplastic tissue, rapid deployment technique, replacement **X2R**F-
Zotarolimus-eluting coronary stent
use Intraluminal Device, Drug-eluting in Heart and Great Vessels
Zygomatic process of frontal bone
use Frontal Bone
Zygomatic process of temporal bone
use Bone, Temporal, Left
use Bone, Temporal, Right
Zygomaticus muscle
use Muscle, Facial
Zyvox
use Oxazolidinones

© 2018 Channel Publishing, Ltd.

Educational Annotations | 0 – Central Nervous System and Cranial Nerves

Body System Specific Educational Annotations for the Central Nervous System and Cranial Nerves include:

- Anatomy and Physiology Review
- Anatomical Illustrations
- Definitions of Common Procedures
- AHA Coding Clinic® Reference Notations
- Body Part Key Listings
- Device Key Listings
- Device Aggregation Table Listings
- Coding Notes

Anatomy and Physiology Review of Central Nervous System and Cranial Nerves

BODY PART VALUES – 0 - CENTRAL NERVOUS SYSTEM AND CRANIAL NERVES

Abducens Nerve – The sixth (VI) cranial nerve that innervates the lateral rectus muscles of the eye.

Accessory Nerve – The eleventh (XI) cranial nerve that innervates the sternocleidomastoideus and trapezius muscles.

Acoustic Nerve – The cochlear (hearing) portion of the eighth (VIII) cranial nerve (also known as the vestibulocochlear or auditory nerve).

Basal Ganglia – ANATOMY – The basal ganglia are masses of gray matter located deep within the cerebral hemispheres, including the globus pallidus. The corpus striatum consists of 2 of the basal ganglia, the caudate and lentiform nuclei. PHYSIOLOGY – The basal ganglia function as relay stations for motor impulses.

Brain – ANATOMY – The brain is the largest and most complex part of the nervous system, and is located in the cranial cavity. The cerebrum is the largest part of the brain, and is divided sagittally (front and back through the center) into 2 hemispheres. The corpus callosum lies below and connects the 2 hemispheres. The frontal lobe forms the anterior portion of each cerebral hemisphere. The temporal lobes lie below the frontal lobe on the lateral side of each cerebral hemisphere. The parietal lobe forms the superior portion of the cerebrum, lying posterior to the frontal lobe. The occipital lobe forms the posterior portion of each cerebral hemisphere. The brain stem connects the upper end of the spinal cord with the cerebrum. It contains the pons, cerebral peduncle, medulla oblongata, and midbrain. The tapetum is a layer of fibers from the corpus callosum forming the roof and lateral walls of the lateral ventricles. PHYSIOLOGY – The cerebrum, including its lobes and cerebral cortex, is concerned with the higher brain functions, such as memory, learning, thought, reasoning, hearing, vision, speech, language, and voluntary muscle control.

Cerebellum – ANATOMY – The cerebellum is the second largest portion of the brain, located below the occipital lobe and behind the brain stem. PHYSIOLOGY – The cerebellum functions primarily as a reflex center in the coordination of skeletal muscle movements and the maintenance of equilibrium.

Cerebral Hemisphere – ANATOMY – The cerebrum is the largest portion of the brain and is symmetrically divided into left and right cerebral hemispheres that are linked by the corpus callosum. PHYSIOLOGY – Although both hemispheres are involved in most brain functions, the left hemisphere generally controls the right half of the body, and the right hemisphere generally controls the left half of the body.

Cerebral Meninges – ANATOMY – The cerebral meninges are continuous with the spinal meninges, completely enclosing the brain (and spinal cord), and consist of three layers: Dura mater, arachnoid mater, and pia mater. The dura mater is the outermost tough, fibroelastic tissue layer. The arachnoid mater is the thin, transparent middle layer. The pia mater is the thin, delicate layer that adheres to the brain and spinal cord tissues.
PHYSIOLOGY – The spinal meninges function to protect the spinal cord and contain the cerebrospinal fluid. The subarachnoid space is the cerebrospinal fluid-filled space between the arachnoid and the pia mater.

Cerebral Ventricle – ANATOMY – The ventricles are a series of four interconnected cavities of the brain and are continuous with the central canal of the spinal cord, which are filled with the cerebrospinal fluid. The tapetum is a layer of fibers from the corpus callosum forming the roof and lateral walls of the lateral ventricles.
PHYSIOLOGY – The ventricles produce and are filled by continuously replaced cerebrospinal fluid which serves to protect the brain by absorbing shocks and removing any waste substances. It also provides a stable ionic concentration in the central nervous system, which is important for maximum nerve impulse transfers.

Cervical Spinal Cord – That portion within the cervical vertebral column.

Cranial Nerve – ANATOMY – The 12 pairs of nerves arising from the brain stem and cerebrum.
PHYSIOLOGY – The cranial nerves serve the various specific organs of the head and neck, with some being mostly sensory (olfactory, optic), others being mostly motor (abducens), and most being of mixed sensory and motor nerve fibers and function.

Dura Mater – ANATOMY – The dura mater is the outermost cerebral and spinal cord layer comprised of tough, fibroelastic tissue. PHYSIOLOGY – The dura mater protects the brain and spinal cord from injury, pathogens, and any contaminates.

Epidural Space – The space inside the vertebral column and outside of the dura mater spinal meninges layer.

Facial Nerve – The seventh (VII) cranial nerve that innervates a significant number of structures both motor and sensory including facial expression and sensation, salivary glands, taste sense from the anterior portion of the tongue, and the oral and nasal cavities.

Glossopharyngeal Nerve – The ninth (IX) cranial nerve that innervates most of the motor and sensory structures of the tongue and pharynx.

Hypoglossal Nerve – The twelfth (XII) cranial nerve that innervates the musculature of the tongue and pharynx.

Hypothalamus – ANATOMY – The hypothalamus lies above the brain stem and forms the floor of the third ventricle. PHYSIOLOGY – The hypothalamus functions to control homeostasis by regulation of the heart rate, arterial blood pressure, body temperature, body weight, and sleep, and controls the anterior pituitary gland.

Lumbar Spinal Cord – That portion within the lumbar vertebral column.

Medulla Oblongata – ANATOMY – The cone-shaped part of the brainstem that is situated between the pons and the spinal cord. PHYSIOLOGY – The medulla oblongata connects the higher levels of the cerebrum to the spinal cord and transmits ascending and descending impulses. The medulla oblongata helps regulate breathing, heart rate, blood pressure, digestion, sneezing, and swallowing.

Oculomotor Nerve – The third (III) cranial nerve that innervates most of the motor function of the eye, both somatic and autonomic.

Olfactory Nerve – The first (I) cranial nerve that innervates the olfactory epithelium (sense of smell).

Optic Nerve – The second (II) cranial nerve that innervates the retina.

Pons – ANATOMY – The pons is part of the brainstem that is situated between the midbrain and above the medulla oblongata. PHYSIOLOGY – The pons transmits impulses between the cerebrum and cerebellum and other parts of the nervous system.

Spinal Canal – The spinal canal is the round space in the vertebrae through which the spinal cord passes.

Continued on next page

© 2018 Channel Publishing, Ltd.

Educational Annotations | 0 – Central Nervous System and Cranial Nerves

Anatomy and Physiology Review of Central Nervous System and Cranial Nerves

BODY PART VALUES – 0 - CENTRAL NERVOUS SYSTEM AND CRANIAL NERVES

Continued from previous page

Spinal Cord – ANATOMY – The spinal cord is a long cylindrical structure of nervous tissue that runs the length of the vertebral column from the medulla oblongata to the lumbar vertebral column. There are two consecutive rows of nerve roots that form 31 pairs of spinal nerves that emerge on each side. PHYSIOLOGY – The spinal cord is the nervous system link between the brain and most of the body through sensory, autonomic, and motor pathways.

Spinal Meninges – ANATOMY – The spinal meninges are continuous with the cerebral meninges, completely enclosing the spinal cord (and brain), and consist of three layers: Dura mater, arachnoid mater, and pia mater. The dura mater is the outermost tough, fibroelastic tissue layer. The arachnoid mater is the thin, transparent middle layer. The pia mater is the thin, delicate layer that adheres to the brain and spinal cord tissues.
PHYSIOLOGY – The spinal meninges function to protect the spinal cord and contain the cerebrospinal fluid. The subarachnoid space is the cerebrospinal fluid-filled space between the arachnoid and the pia mater.

Subarachnoid Space – The subarachnoid space is the cerebrospinal fluid-filled space between the arachnoid and the pia mater.

Subdural Space – The potential space between the dura mater and the subarachnoid mater. Any actual space may develop due to illness or trauma.

Thalamus – ANATOMY – The thalamus lies below the corpus callosum on either side of the third ventricle. PHYSIOLOGY – The thalamus functions as a central relay station for sensory impulses and regulation of motor functions. It also functions to regulate the states of sleep and consciousness.

Thoracic Spinal Cord – That portion within the thoracic vertebral column.

Trigeminal Nerve – The fifth (V) cranial nerve that innervates a large number of structures, both motor and sensory, including touch, pain, and temperature of the face, nose, and mouth.

Trochlear Nerve – The fourth (IV) cranial nerve that innervates the superior oblique muscle of the orbit.

Vagus Nerve – The tenth (X) cranial nerve that innervates a large number of parasympathetic nerves of the heart, lungs, and digestive tract and controls the muscles of swallowing.

Anatomical Illustrations of Central Nervous System and Cranial Nerves

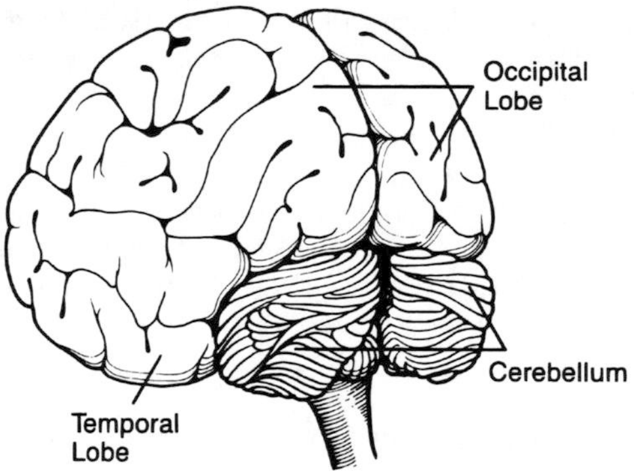

BRAIN — POSTERIOR VIEW

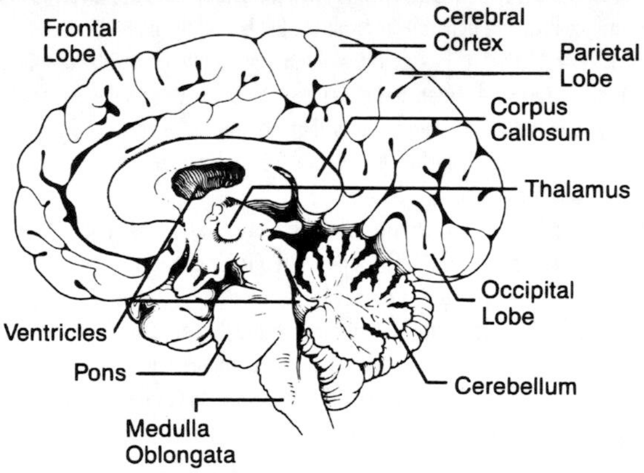

BRAIN — SAGITTAL VIEW

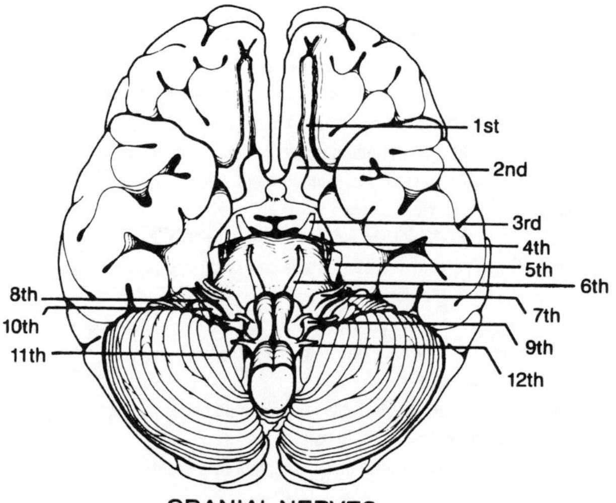

CRANIAL NERVES

Continued on next page

CENTRAL NERVOUS 0 0

© 2018 Channel Publishing, Ltd.

Educational Annotations | 0 – Central Nervous System and Cranial Nerves

Anatomical Illustrations of Central Nervous System and Cranial Nerves

Continued from previous page

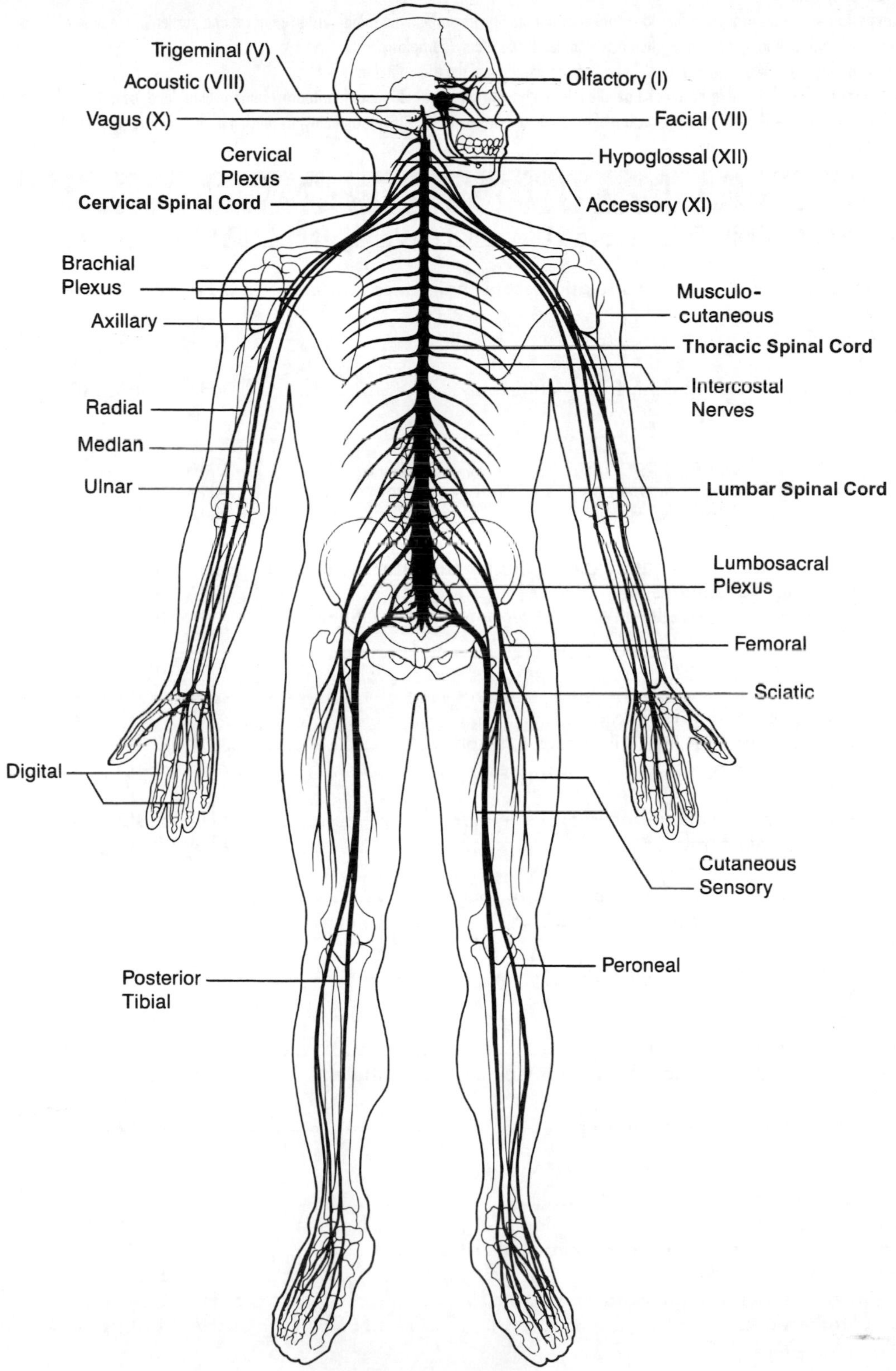

NERVOUS SYSTEM

© 2018 Channel Publishing, Ltd.

Educational Annotations | 0 – Central Nervous System and Cranial Nerves

Definitions of Common Procedures of Central Nervous System and Cranial Nerves

Anterior temporal lobectomy – The surgical removal of a portion of the temporal lobe of the brain to treat medically intractable temporal lobe epilepsy.
Brain biopsy – The removal of brain tissue for microscopic examination that is performed through a small hole (burr hole) drilled into the skull, often using the stereotactic navigation system.
Chiari decompression – The surgical procedure to reduce or eliminate the pressure on the spinal cord by removal of a portion of the base of the skull that creates space at the level of the foramen magnum and is often accompanied by durotomy/duraplasty.
Gasserian ganglionectomy – The surgical removal of gasserian ganglion of the trigeminal nerve.
Lumbar puncture (spinal tap) – The insertion of a needle into the lumbar subarachnoid space to withdraw cerebrospinal fluid, usually for diagnostic reasons.
Ventriculoperitoneal shunt – The shunting redirection of excessive cerebrospinal fluid (hydrocephalus) by placing a catheter into a cerebral ventricle and tunneling it under the skin and into the peritoneal cavity.

AHA Coding Clinic® Reference Notations of Central Nervous System and Cranial Nerves

ROOT OPERATION SPECIFIC - 0 - CENTRAL NERVOUS SYSTEM AND CRANIAL NERVES

BYPASS - 1
- Ventriculoperitoneal shunt (VP) with laparoscopic assistance ....AHA 13:2Q:p36

CHANGE - 2

DESTRUCTION - 5

DILATION - 7
- Reopening of the endoscopic third ventriculostomy ....AHA 17:4Q:p39

DIVISION - 8

DRAINAGE - 9
- Aspiration via a lumbar drain port ....AHA 14:1Q:p8
- Burr hole drainage of hydrocephalus with catheter placement ....AHA 15:3Q:p12
- Drainage of (fluid) subdural hematoma ....AHA 15:3Q:p10
- Diagnostic lumbar tap ....AHA 14:1Q:p8
- Percutaneous burr hole drainage of (fluid) chronic subdural hematoma ....AHA 15:3Q:p11
- Shunting (drainage) of spinal syrinx ....AHA 15:2Q:p30
- Subdural drainage using subdural evacuation portal system (SEPS) ....AHA 15:3Q:p12

EXCISION - B
- Amygdalohippocampectomy ....AHA 16:2Q:p18
- Brain biopsy....AHA 15:1Q:p12
- Excision of spinal cord lipoma ....AHA 14:3Q:p24
- Infratemporal fossa malignancy with nerve excision ....AHA 16:2Q:p12
- Resection of brain tumor ....AHA 14:4Q:p34

EXTIRPATION - C
- Burr hole evacuation of solid intracerebral hematoma ....AHA 15:3Q:p13
- Decompressive craniectomy ....AHA 16:2Q:p29
- Evacuation of brain hematoma....AHA 15:1Q:p12
- Evacuation of solid hematoma of the epidural space ....AHA 17:4Q:p48
- Extirpation of (solid) subdural hematoma ....AHA 15:3Q:p10

EXTRACTION - D
- Nonexcisional debridement of dura mater ....AHA 15:3Q:p13

FRAGMENTATION - F

INSERTION - H
- Cesium-131 collagen brain implant ....AHA 17:4Q:p30
- Replacement of Baclofen medication pump/spinal canal catheter ....AHA 14:3Q:p19

INSPECTION - J
- Lumbar puncture with no fluid removed ....AHA 17:1Q:p50

MAP - K

RELEASE - N
- Chiari decompression ....AHA 17:3Q:p10
- Decompression of spinal cord without fusion ....AHA 17:2Q:p23
- Decompressive cervical laminectomy at multiple sites ....AHA 15:2Q:p21
- Decompressive craniectomy ....AHA 16:2Q:p29
- Laminoplasty to expand spinal canal space....AHA 15:2Q:p20
- Release of tethered spinal cord ....AHA 14:3Q:p24

Continued on next page

© 2018 Channel Publishing, Ltd.

Educational Annotations | 0 – Central Nervous System and Cranial Nerves

AHA Coding Clinic® Reference Notations of Central Nervous System and Cranial Nerves

Continued from previous page

REMOVAL - P
- Replacement of Baclofen medication pump/spinal canal catheter .... AHA 14:3Q:p19

REPAIR - Q
- Dural rent repair .... AHA 13:3Q:p25
- .... AHA 14:3Q:p7

REPOSITION - S
- Reimplantation of transected facial nerve into muscle .... AHA 14:4Q:p35

RESECTION - T

SUPPLEMENT - U
- AlloDerm dural graft .... AHA 17:3Q:p10
- Dural patch graft with Durepair® .... AHA 14:3Q:p24
- Dural patch graft with Durepair® Official Clarification .... AHA 15:4Q:p39
- Placement of DuraGuard barrier patch .... AHA 18:1Q:p9

REVISION - W

TRANSFER - X

Body Part Key Listings of Central Nervous System and Cranial Nerves

See also Body Part Key in Appendix C

Anterior vagal trunk .... use Vagus Nerve
Apneustic center .... use Pons
Aqueduct of Sylvius .... use Cerebral Ventricle
Arachnoid mater, intracranial .... use Cerebral Meninges
Arachnoid mater, spinal .... use Spinal Meninges
Basal nuclei .... use Basal Ganglia
Basis pontis .... use Pons
Carotid sinus nerve .... use Glossopharyngeal Nerve
Cauda equina .... use Lumbar Spinal Cord
Cerebral aqueduct (Sylvius) .... use Cerebral Ventricle
Cerebrum .... use Brain
Chorda tympani .... use Facial Nerve
Choroid plexus .... use Cerebral Ventricle
Claustrum .... use Basal Ganglia
Cochlear nerve .... use Acoustic Nerve
Conus medullaris .... use Lumbar Spinal Cord
Corpus callosum .... use Brain
Corpus striatum .... use Basal Ganglia
Culmen .... use Cerebellum
Denticulate (dentate) ligament .... use Spinal Meninges
Diaphragma sellae .... use Dura Mater
Dura mater, intracranial .... use Dura Mater
Dura mater, spinal .... use Spinal Meninges
Eighth cranial nerve .... use Acoustic Nerve
Eleventh cranial nerve .... use Accessory Nerve
Encephalon .... use Brain
Ependyma .... use Cerebral Ventricle
Epidural space, spinal .... use Spinal Canal
Epithalamus .... use Thalamus
Extradural space, intracranial .... use Epidural Space, Intracranial
Extradural space, spinal .... use Spinal Canal
Extradural space .... use Epidural Space
Falx cerebri .... use Dura Mater
Fifth cranial nerve .... use Trigeminal Nerve
Filum terminale .... use Spinal Meninges
First cranial nerve .... use Olfactory Nerve
Foramen of Monro (intraventricular) .... use Cerebral Ventricle
Fourth cranial nerve .... use Trochlear Nerve
Fourth ventricle .... use Cerebral Ventricle
Frontal lobe .... use Cerebral Hemisphere
Gasserian ganglion .... use Trigeminal Nerve
Geniculate ganglion .... use Facial Nerve
Geniculate nucleus .... use Thalamus
Globus pallidus .... use Basal Ganglia
Greater superficial petrosal nerve .... use Facial Nerve
Interventricular foramen (Monro) .... use Cerebral Ventricle
Left lateral ventricle .... use Cerebral Ventricle
Leptomeninges, intracranial .... use Cerebral Meninges
Leptomeninges, spinal .... use Spinal Meninges
Locus ceruleus .... use Pons
Mammillary body .... use Hypothalamus
Mandibular nerve .... use Trigeminal Nerve
Maxillary nerve .... use Trigeminal Nerve
Metathalamus .... use Thalamus
Myelencephalon .... use Medulla Oblongata
Nerve to the stapedius .... use Facial Nerve
Ninth cranial nerve .... use Glossopharyngeal Nerve
Occipital lobe .... use Cerebral Hemisphere
Olfactory bulb .... use Olfactory Nerve
Ophthalmic nerve .... use Trigeminal Nerve
Optic chiasma .... use Optic Nerve
Parietal lobe .... use Cerebral Hemisphere
Parotid plexus .... use Facial Nerve
Pharyngeal plexus .... use Vagus Nerve
Pia mater, intracranial .... use Cerebral Meninges
Pia mater, spinal .... use Spinal Meninges
Pneumogastric nerve .... use Vagus Nerve
Pneumotaxic center .... use Pons
Pontine tegmentum .... use Pons
Posterior auricular nerve .... use Facial Nerve
Posterior vagal trunk .... use Vagus Nerve
Pulmonary plexus .... use Vagus Nerve/Thoracic Sympathetic Nerve
Pulvinar .... use Thalamus
Recurrent laryngeal nerve .... use Vagus Nerve
Right lateral ventricle .... use Cerebral Ventricle

Continued on next page

CENTRAL NERVOUS 0 0

© 2018 Channel Publishing, Ltd.

Educational Annotations | 0 – Central Nervous System and Cranial Nerves

Body Part Key Listings of Central Nervous System and Cranial Nerves

Continued from previous page

Scarpa's (vestibular) ganglion ....use Acoustic Nerve
Second cranial nerve ....use Optic Nerve
Seventh cranial nerve ....use Facial Nerve
Sixth cranial nerve............use Abducens Nerve
Spiral ganglion ....use Acoustic Nerve
Subarachnoid space, spinal ....use Spinal Canal
Subdural space, spinal............use Spinal Canal
Submandibular ganglion............use Facial Nerve
Substantia nigra ....use Basal Ganglia
Subthalamic nucleus ....use Basal Ganglia
Superior laryngeal nerve............use Vagus Nerve
Superior olivary nucleus ....use Pons
Temporal lobe ....use Cerebral Hemisphere
Tenth cranial nerve ....use Vagus Nerve
Tentorium cerebelli ....use Dura Mater
Third cranial nerve ....use Oculomotor Nerve
Third ventricle ....use Cerebral Ventricle
Trifacial nerve ....use Trigeminal Nerve
Twelfth cranial nerve ....use Hypoglossal Nerve
Tympanic nerve ....use Glossopharyngeal Nerve
Vertebral canal ....use Spinal Canal
Vestibular (Scarpa's) ganglion ....use Acoustic Nerve
Vestibular nerve............use Acoustic Nerve
Vestibulocochlear nerve............use Acoustic Nerve

Device Key Listings of Central Nervous System and Cranial Nerves

See also Device Key in Appendix D

Ascenda Intrathecal Catheter............use Infusion Device
Autograft ....use Autologous Tissue Substitute
Cesium-131 Collagen Implant ....use Radioactive Element, Cesium-131 Collagen Implant for Insertion in Central Nervous System and Cranial Nerves
Cortical strip neurostimulator lead ....use Neurostimulator Lead in Central Nervous System and Cranial Nerves
DBS lead ....use Neurostimulator Lead in Central Nervous System and Cranial Nerves
Deep brain neurostimulator lead ....use Neurostimulator Lead in Central Nervous System and Cranial Nerves
GammaTile™ ....use Radioactive Element, Cesium-131 Collagen Implant for Insertion in Central Nervous System and Cranial Nerves
Holter valve ventricular shunt ....use Synthetic Substitute
InDura, intrathecal catheter (1P) (spinal)............use Infusion Device
RNS System lead ....use Neurostimulator Lead in Central Nervous System and Cranial Nerves
Spinal cord neurostimulator lead ....use Neurostimulator Lead in Central Nervous System and Cranial Nerves
Tissue bank graft............use Nonautologous Tissue Substitute
Tunneled spinal (intrathecal) catheter............use Infusion Device

Device Aggregation Table Listings of Central Nervous System and Cranial Nerves

See also Device Aggregation Table in Appendix E

Specific Device	For Operation	In Body System	General Device
None Listed in Device Aggregation Table for this Body System			

Coding Notes of Central Nervous System and Cranial Nerves

CENTRAL NERVOUS 0 0

© 2018 Channel Publishing, Ltd.

1ST - 0 Medical and Surgical
2ND - 0 Central Nervous System & Cranial Nerves
3RD - 1 BYPASS

TUBULAR GROUP: Bypass, Dilation, (Occlusion), (Restriction)
Root Operations that alter the diameter/route of a tubular body part.

BYPASS: Altering the route of passage of the contents of a tubular body part.

Explanation: Rerouting contents to a downstream part ... with or without the use of a device ...
Examples: Ventriculoperitoneal shunt – CMS Ex: Coronary artery bypass

Body Part – 4TH	Approach – 5TH	Device – 6TH	Qualifier – 7TH
6 Cerebral Ventricle	0 Open 3 Percutaneous 4 Percutaneous endoscopic	7 Autologous tissue substitute J Synthetic substitute K Nonautologous tissue substitute	0 Nasopharynx 1 Mastoid sinus 2 Atrium 3 Blood vessel 4 Pleural cavity 5 Intestine 6 Peritoneal cavity 7 Urinary tract 8 Bone marrow B Cerebral cisterns
6 Cerebral Ventricle	0 Open 3 Percutaneous 4 Percutaneous endoscopic	Z No device	B Cerebral cisterns
U Spinal Canal	0 Open 3 Percutaneous 4 Percutaneous endoscopic	7 Autologous tissue substitute J Synthetic substitute K Nonautologous tissue substitute	2 Atrium 4 Pleural cavity 6 Peritoneal cavity 7 Urinary tract 9 Fallopian tube

1ST - 0 Medical and Surgical
2ND - 0 Central Nervous System & Cranial Nerves
3RD - 2 CHANGE

DEVICE GROUP: Change, Insertion, Removal, Replacement, Revision, Supplement
Root Operations that always involve a device.

CHANGE: Taking out or off a device from a body part and putting back an identical or similar device in or on the same body part without cutting or puncturing the skin or a mucous membrane.

Explanation: All CHANGE procedures are coded using the approach External
Examples: Exchange ventriculostomy tube – CMS Ex: Urinary catheter change

Body Part – 4TH	Approach – 5TH	Device – 6TH	Qualifier – 7TH
0 Brain E Cranial Nerve U Spinal Canal	X External	0 Drainage device Y Other device	Z No qualifier

1ST - 0 Medical and Surgical
2ND - 0 Central Nervous System & Cranial Nerves
3RD - 5 DESTRUCTION

EXCISION GROUP: Excision, Resection, Destruction, Extraction, (Detachment)
Root Operations that take out some or all of a body part.

DESTRUCTION: Physical eradication of all or a portion of a body part by the direct use of energy, force, or a destructive agent.

Explanation: None of the body part is physically taken out
Examples: Ablation trigeminal nerve – CMS Ex: Fulguration of rectal polyp

Body Part – 4TH			Approach – 5TH	Device – 6TH	Qualifier – 7TH
0 Brain 1 Cerebral Meninges 2 Dura Mater 6 Cerebral Ventricle 7 Cerebral Hemisphere 8 Basal Ganglia 9 Thalamus A Hypothalamus B Pons	C Cerebellum D Medulla Oblongata F Olfactory Nerve G Optic Nerve H Oculomotor Nerve J Trochlear Nerve K Trigeminal Nerve L Abducens Nerve M Facial Nerve	N Acoustic Nerve P Glossopharyngeal Nerve Q Vagus Nerve R Accessory Nerve S Hypoglossal Nerve T Spinal Meninges W Cervical Spinal Cord X Thoracic Spinal Cord Y Lumbar Spinal Cord	0 Open 3 Percutaneous 4 Percutaneous endoscopic	Z No device	Z No qualifier

CENTRAL NERVOUS 005

© 2018 Channel Publishing, Ltd.

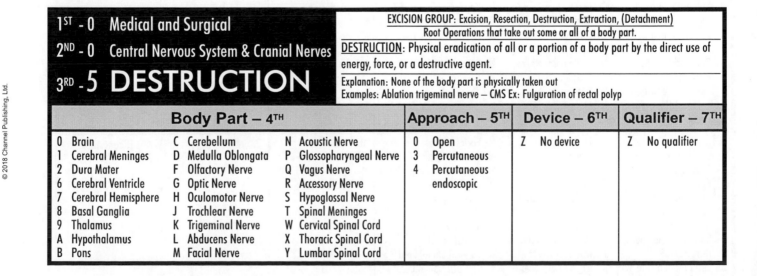

1ST - 0 Medical and Surgical
2ND - 0 Central Nervous System & Cranial Nerves
3RD - 7 DILATION

TUBULAR GROUP: Bypass, Dilation, (Occlusion), (Restriction)
Root Operations that alter the diameter/route of a tubular body part.

DILATION: Expanding an orifice or the lumen of a tubular body part.

Explanation: Accomplished by stretching or cutting ... tubular body part or orifice ...
Examples: Dilation cerebral ventricle – CMS Ex: Percutaneous transluminal angioplasty

Body Part – 4TH	Approach – 5TH	Device – 6TH	Qualifier – 7TH
6 Cerebral Ventricle	0 Open 3 Percutaneous 4 Percutaneous endoscopic	Z No device	Z No qualifier

1ST - 0 Medical and Surgical
2ND - 0 Central Nervous System & Cranial Nerves
3RD - 8 DIVISION

DIVISION GROUP: Division, Release
Root Operations involving cutting or separation only.

DIVISION: Cutting into a body part, without draining fluids and/or gases from the body part, in order to separate or transect a body part.

Explanation: All or a portion of the body part is separated into two or more portions
Examples: Bisection facial nerve – CMS Ex: Spinal cordotomy

Body Part – 4TH	Approach – 5TH	Device – 6TH	Qualifier – 7TH
0 Brain 7 Cerebral Hemisphere 8 Basal Ganglia F Olfactory Nerve G Optic Nerve H Oculomotor Nerve J Trochlear Nerve K Trigeminal Nerve L Abducens Nerve M Facial Nerve N Acoustic Nerve P Glossopharyngeal Nerve Q Vagus Nerve R Accessory Nerve S Hypoglossal Nerve W Cervical Spinal Cord X Thoracic Spinal Cord Y Lumbar Spinal Cord	0 Open 3 Percutaneous 4 Percutaneous endoscopic	Z No device	Z No qualifier

1ST - 0 Medical and Surgical
2ND - 0 Central Nervous System & Cranial Nerves
3RD - 9 DRAINAGE

DRAINAGE GROUP: Drainage, Extirpation, Fragmentation
Root Operations that take out solids/fluids/gases from a body part.

DRAINAGE: Taking or letting out fluids and/or gases from a body part.

Explanation: Qualifier "X Diagnostic" indicates drainage procedures that are biopsies
Examples: Lumbar puncture – CMS Ex: Thoracentesis

Body Part – 4TH	Approach – 5TH	Device – 6TH	Qualifier – 7TH
0 Brain 1 Cerebral Meninges 2 Dura Mater 3 Epidural Space, Intracranial 4 Subdural Space, Intracranial 5 Subarachnoid Space, Intracranial 6 Cerebral Ventricle 7 Cerebral Hemisphere 8 Basal Ganglia 9 Thalamus A Hypothalamus B Pons C Cerebellum D Medulla Oblongata F Olfactory Nerve G Optic Nerve H Oculomotor Nerve J Trochlear Nerve K Trigeminal Nerve L Abducens Nerve M Facial Nerve N Acoustic Nerve P Glossopharyngeal Nerve Q Vagus Nerve R Accessory Nerve S Hypoglossal Nerve T Spinal Meninges U Spinal Canal W Cervical Spinal Cord X Thoracic Spinal Cord Y Lumbar Spinal Cord	0 Open 3 Percutaneous 4 Percutaneous endoscopic	0 Drainage device	Z No qualifier
0 Brain 1 Cerebral Meninges 2 Dura Mater 3 Epidural Space, Intracranial 4 Subdural Space, Intracranial 5 Subarachnoid Space, Intracranial 6 Cerebral Ventricle 7 Cerebral Hemisphere 8 Basal Ganglia 9 Thalamus A Hypothalamus B Pons C Cerebellum D Medulla Oblongata F Olfactory Nerve G Optic Nerve H Oculomotor Nerve J Trochlear Nerve K Trigeminal Nerve L Abducens Nerve M Facial Nerve N Acoustic Nerve P Glossopharyngeal Nerve Q Vagus Nerve R Accessory Nerve S Hypoglossal Nerve T Spinal Meninges U Spinal Canal W Cervical Spinal Cord X Thoracic Spinal Cord Y Lumbar Spinal Cord	0 Open 3 Percutaneous 4 Percutaneous endoscopic	Z No device	X Diagnostic Z No qualifier

© 2018 Channel Publishing, Ltd.

1ST - 0 Medical and Surgical
2ND - 0 Central Nervous System & Cranial Nerves
3RD - B EXCISION

EXCISION GROUP: Excision, Resection, Destruction, Extraction, (Detachment)
Root Operations that take out some or all of a body part.

EXCISION: Cutting out or off, without replacement, a portion of a body part.

Explanation: Qualifier "X Diagnostic" indicates excision procedures that are biopsies
Examples: Stereotactic thalamic biopsy – CMS Ex: Liver biopsy

Body Part – 4TH			Approach – 5TH	Device – 6TH	Qualifier – 7TH
0 Brain	C Cerebellum	N Acoustic Nerve	0 Open	Z No device	X Diagnostic
1 Cerebral Meninges	D Medulla Oblongata	P Glossopharyngeal Nerve	3 Percutaneous		Z No qualifier
2 Dura Mater	F Olfactory Nerve	Q Vagus Nerve	4 Percutaneous endoscopic		
6 Cerebral Ventricle	G Optic Nerve	R Accessory Nerve			
7 Cerebral Hemisphere	H Oculomotor Nerve	S Hypoglossal Nerve			
8 Basal Ganglia	J Trochlear Nerve	T Spinal Meninges			
9 Thalamus	K Trigeminal Nerve	W Cervical Spinal Cord			
A Hypothalamus	L Abducens Nerve	X Thoracic Spinal Cord			
B Pons	M Facial Nerve	Y Lumbar Spinal Cord			

1ST - 0 Medical and Surgical
2ND - 0 Central Nervous System & Cranial Nerves
3RD - C EXTIRPATION

DRAINAGE GROUP: Drainage, Extirpation, Fragmentation
Root Operations that take out solids/fluids/gases from a body part.

EXTIRPATION: Taking or cutting out solid matter from a body part.

Explanation: Abnormal byproduct or foreign body ...
Examples: Removal foreign body lumbar spinal cord – CMS Ex: Thrombectomy

Body Part – 4TH			Approach – 5TH	Device – 6TH	Qualifier – 7TH
0 Brain	9 Thalamus	M Facial Nerve	0 Open	Z No device	Z No qualifier
1 Cerebral Meninges	A Hypothalamus	N Acoustic Nerve	3 Percutaneous		
2 Dura Mater	B Pons	P Glossopharyngeal Nerve	4 Percutaneous endoscopic		
3 Epidural Space, Intracranial	C Cerebellum	Q Vagus Nerve			
4 Subdural Space, Intracranial	D Medulla Oblongata	R Accessory Nerve			
5 Subarachnoid Space, Intracranial	F Olfactory Nerve	S Hypoglossal Nerve			
6 Cerebral Ventricle	G Optic Nerve	T Spinal Meninges			
7 Cerebral Hemisphere	H Oculomotor Nerve	U Spinal Canal			
8 Basal Ganglia	J Trochlear Nerve	W Cervical Spinal Cord			
	K Trigeminal Nerve	X Thoracic Spinal Cord			
	L Abducens Nerve	Y Lumbar Spinal Cord			

1ST - 0 Medical and Surgical
2ND - 0 Central Nervous System & Cranial Nerves
3RD - D EXTRACTION

EXCISION GROUP: Excision, Resection, Destruction, Extraction, (Detachment)
Root Operations that take out some or all of a body part.

EXTRACTION: Pulling or stripping out or off all or a portion of a body part by the use of force.

Explanation: None for this Body System
Examples: Extraction vagus nerve segment – CMS Ex: Dilation and curettage

Body Part – 4TH			Approach – 5TH	Device – 6TH	Qualifier – 7TH
1 Cerebral Meninges	J Trochlear Nerve	P Glossopharyngeal Nerve	0 Open	Z No device	Z No qualifier
2 Dura Mater	K Trigeminal Nerve	Q Vagus Nerve	3 Percutaneous		
F Olfactory Nerve	L Abducens Nerve	R Accessory Nerve	4 Percutaneous endoscopic		
G Optic Nerve	M Facial Nerve	S Hypoglossal Nerve			
H Oculomotor Nerve	N Acoustic Nerve	T Spinal Meninges			

© 2018 Channel Publishing, Ltd.

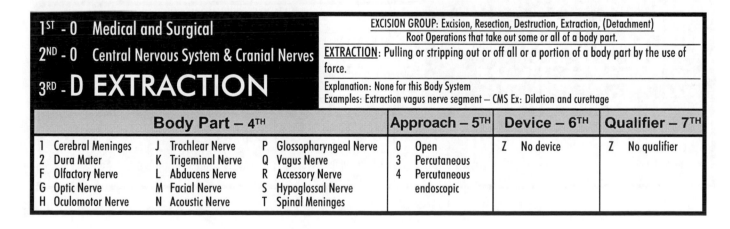

1ST - 0 Medical and Surgical
2ND - 0 Central Nervous System & Cranial Nerves
3RD - F FRAGMENTATION

DRAINAGE GROUP: Drainage, Extirpation, Fragmentation
Root Operations that take out solids/fluids/gases from a body part.

FRAGMENTATION: Breaking solid matter in a body part into pieces.

Explanation: Pieces are not taken out during the procedure ...
Examples: Fragmentation foreign body spinal canal – CMS Ex: Extracorporeal shockwave lithotripsy

Body Part – 4TH	Approach – 5TH	Device – 6TH	Qualifier – 7TH
3 Epidural Space, Intracranial 4 Subdural Space, Intracranial 5 Subarachnoid Space, Intracranial 6 Cerebral Ventricle U Spinal Canal	0 Open 3 Percutaneous 4 Percutaneous endoscopic X External NC*	Z No device	Z No qualifier

NC* – Some procedures are considered non-covered by Medicare. See current Medicare Code Editor for details.

1ST - 0 Medical and Surgical
2ND - 0 Central Nervous System & Cranial Nerves
3RD - H INSERTION

DEVICE GROUP: Change, Insertion, Removal, Replacement, Revision, Supplement
Root Operations that always involve a device.

INSERTION: Putting in a nonbiological appliance that monitors, assists, performs, or prevents a physiological function but does not physically take the place of a body part.

Explanation: None
Examples: Intrathecal spinal cord catheter – CMS Ex: Insertion of central venous catheter

Body Part – 4TH	Approach – 5TH	Device – 6TH	Qualifier – 7TH
0 Brain	0 Open	2 Monitoring device 3 Infusion device 4 Radioactive Element, Cesium-131 Collagen Implant M Neurostimulator lead Y Other device	Z No qualifier
0 Brain	3 Percutaneous 4 Percutaneous endoscopic	2 Monitoring device 3 Infusion device M Neurostimulator lead Y Other device	Z No qualifier
6 Cerebral Ventricle E Cranial Nerve U Spinal Canal V Spinal Cord	0 Open 3 Percutaneous 4 Percutaneous endoscopic	2 Monitoring device 3 Infusion device M Neurostimulator lead Y Other device	Z No qualifier

1ST - 0 Medical and Surgical
2ND - 0 Central Nervous System & Cranial Nerves
3RD - J INSPECTION

EXAMINATION GROUP: Inspection, (Map)
Root Operations involving examination only.

INSPECTION: Visually and/or manually exploring a body part.

Explanation: Direct or instrumental visualization ...
Examples: Examination cranial nerve – CMS Ex: Exploratory laparotomy

Body Part – 4TH	Approach – 5TH	Device – 6TH	Qualifier – 7TH
0 Brain E Cranial Nerve U Spinal Canal V Spinal Cord	0 Open 3 Percutaneous 4 Percutaneous endoscopic	Z No device	Z No qualifier

© 2018 Channel Publishing, Ltd.

1ST - 0 Medical and Surgical
2ND - 0 Central Nervous System & Cranial Nerves
3RD - K MAP

EXAMINATION GROUP: Inspection, Map
Root Operations involving examination only.

MAP: Locating the route of passage of electrical impulses and/or locating functional areas in a body part.

Explanation: Applicable only to the cardiac conduction mechanism and the central nervous system
Examples: Mapping basal ganglia – CMS Ex: Cardiac mapping

Body Part – 4TH		Approach – 5TH	Device – 6TH	Qualifier – 7TH
0 Brain 7 Cerebral Hemisphere 8 Basal Ganglia 9 Thalamus	A Hypothalamus B Pons C Cerebellum D Medulla Oblongata	0 Open 3 Percutaneous 4 Percutaneous endoscopic	Z No device	Z No qualifier

1ST - 0 Medical and Surgical
2ND - 0 Central Nervous System & Cranial Nerves
3RD - N RELEASE

DIVISION GROUP: Division, Release
Root Operations involving cutting or separation only.

RELEASE: Freeing a body part from an abnormal physical constraint by cutting or by the use of force.

Explanation: Some of the restraining tissue may be taken out but none of the body part is taken out
Examples: Lysis acoustic nerve scar tissue – CMS Ex: Carpal tunnel release

Body Part – 4TH			Approach – 5TH	Device – 6TH	Qualifier – 7TH
0 Brain 1 Cerebral Meninges 2 Dura Mater 6 Cerebral Ventricle 7 Cerebral Hemisphere 8 Basal Ganglia 9 Thalamus A Hypothalamus B Pons	C Cerebellum D Medulla Oblongata F Olfactory Nerve G Optic Nerve H Oculomotor Nerve J Trochlear Nerve K Trigeminal Nerve L Abducens Nerve M Facial Nerve	N Acoustic Nerve P Glossopharyngeal Nerve Q Vagus Nerve R Accessory Nerve S Hypoglossal Nerve T Spinal Meninges W Cervical Spinal Cord X Thoracic Spinal Cord Y Lumbar Spinal Cord	0 Open 3 Percutaneous 4 Percutaneous endoscopic	Z No device	Z No qualifier

© 2018 Channel Publishing, Ltd.

1ST - 0 Medical and Surgical
2ND - 0 Central Nervous System & Cranial Nerves
3RD - P REMOVAL

DEVICE GROUP: Change, Insertion, Removal, Replacement, Revision, Supplement
Root Operations that always involve a device.

REMOVAL: Taking out or off a device from a body part.

Explanation: Removal device without reinsertion ...
Examples: Removal neurostimulator lead – CMS Ex: Cardiac pacemaker removal

Body Part – 4TH	Approach – 5TH	Device – 6TH	Qualifier – 7TH
0 Brain V Spinal Cord	0 Open 3 Percutaneous 4 Percutaneous endoscopic	0 Drainage device 2 Monitoring device 3 Infusion device 7 Autologous tissue substitute J Synthetic substitute K Nonautologous tissue substitute M Neurostimulator lead Y Other device	Z No qualifier
0 Brain V Spinal Cord	X External	0 Drainage device 2 Monitoring device 3 Infusion device M Neurostimulator lead	Z No qualifier
6 Cerebral Ventricle U Spinal Canal	0 Open 3 Percutaneous 4 Percutaneous endoscopic	0 Drainage device 2 Monitoring device 3 Infusion device J Synthetic substitute M Neurostimulator lead Y Other device	Z No qualifier
6 Cerebral Ventricle U Spinal Canal	X External	0 Drainage device 2 Monitoring device 3 Infusion device M Neurostimulator lead	Z No qualifier
E Cranial Nerve	0 Open 3 Percutaneous 4 Percutaneous endoscopic	0 Drainage device 2 Monitoring device 3 Infusion device 7 Autologous tissue substitute M Neurostimulator lead Y Other device	Z No qualifier
E Cranial Nerve	X External	0 Drainage device 2 Monitoring device 3 Infusion device M Neurostimulator lead	Z No qualifier

1ST - 0 Medical and Surgical
2ND - 0 Central Nervous System & Cranial Nerves
3RD - Q REPAIR

OTHER REPAIRS GROUP: (Control), Repair
Root Operations that define other repairs.

REPAIR: Restoring, to the extent possible, a body part to its normal anatomic structure and function.

Explanation: Used only when the method to accomplish the repair is not one of the other root operations
Examples: Cerebral meningeorrhaphy – CMS Ex: Suture of laceration

Body Part – 4TH			Approach – 5TH	Device – 6TH	Qualifier – 7TH
0 Brain 1 Cerebral Meninges 2 Dura Mater 6 Cerebral Ventricle 7 Cerebral Hemisphere 8 Basal Ganglia 9 Thalamus A Hypothalamus B Pons	C Cerebellum D Medulla Oblongata F Olfactory Nerve G Optic Nerve H Oculomotor Nerve J Trochlear Nerve K Trigeminal Nerve L Abducens Nerve M Facial Nerve	N Acoustic Nerve P Glossopharyngeal Nerve Q Vagus Nerve R Accessory Nerve S Hypoglossal Nerve T Spinal Meninges W Cervical Spinal Cord X Thoracic Spinal Cord Y Lumbar Spinal Cord	0 Open 3 Percutaneous 4 Percutaneous endoscopic	Z No device	Z No qualifier

CENTRAL NERVOUS 0 0 P

© 2018 Channel Publishing, Ltd.

1ST - 0 Medical and Surgical
2ND - 0 Central Nervous System & Cranial Nerves
3RD - R REPLACEMENT

DEVICE GROUP: Change, Insertion, Removal, Replacement, Revision, Supplement
Root Operations that always involve a device.

REPLACEMENT: Putting in or on biological or synthetic material that physically takes the place and/or function of all or a portion of a body part.

Explanation: Includes taking out or eradicating, or rendering non-functional, the body part ...
Examples: Dural graft implant – CMS Ex: Total hip replacement

Body Part – 4TH			Approach – 5TH	Device – 6TH	Qualifier – 7TH
1 Cerebral Meninges 2 Dura Mater 6 Cerebral Ventricle F Olfactory Nerve G Optic Nerve H Oculomotor Nerve	J Trochlear Nerve K Trigeminal Nerve L Abducens Nerve M Facial Nerve N Acoustic Nerve	P Glossopharyngeal Nerve Q Vagus Nerve R Accessory Nerve S Hypoglossal Nerve T Spinal Meninges	0 Open 4 Percutaneous endoscopic	7 Autologous tissue substitute J Synthetic substitute K Nonautologous tissue substitute	Z No qualifier

1ST - 0 Medical and Surgical
2ND - 0 Central Nervous System & Cranial Nerves
3RD - S REPOSITION

MOVE GROUP: (Reattachment), Reposition, Transfer, (Transplantation)
Root Operations that put in/put back or move some/all of a body part.

REPOSITION: Moving to its normal location, or other suitable location, all or a portion of a body part.

Explanation: The body part may or may not be cut out or off to be moved to the new location ...
Examples: Relocation hypoglossal nerve – CMS Ex: Fracture reduction

Body Part – 4TH			Approach – 5TH	Device – 6TH	Qualifier – 7TH
F Olfactory Nerve G Optic Nerve H Oculomotor Nerve J Trochlear Nerve K Trigeminal Nerve	L Abducens Nerve M Facial Nerve N Acoustic Nerve P Glossopharyngeal Nerve Q Vagus Nerve	R Accessory Nerve S Hypoglossal Nerve W Cervical Spinal Cord X Thoracic Spinal Cord Y Lumbar Spinal Cord	0 Open 3 Percutaneous 4 Percutaneous endoscopic	Z No device	Z No qualifier

1ST - 0 Medical and Surgical
2ND - 0 Central Nervous System & Cranial Nerves
3RD T RESECTION

EXCISION GROUP: Excision, Resection, Destruction, Extraction, (Detachment)
Root Operations that take out some or all of a body part.

RESECTION: Cutting out or off, without replacement, all of a body part.

Explanation: None
Examples: Cerebral hemispherectomy – CMS Ex: Total lobectomy of lung

Body Part – 4TH	Approach – 5TH	Device – 6TH	Qualifier – 7TH
7 Cerebral Hemisphere	0 Open 3 Percutaneous 4 Percutaneous endoscopic	Z No device	Z No qualifier

1ST - 0 Medical and Surgical
2ND - 0 Central Nervous System & Cranial Nerves
3RD - U SUPPLEMENT

DEVICE GROUP: Change, Insertion, Removal, Replacement, Revision, Supplement
Root Operations that always involve a device.

SUPPLEMENT: Putting in or on biological or synthetic material that physically reinforces and/or augments the function of a portion of a body part.

Explanation: Biological material is non-living, or is living and from the same individual ...
Examples: Dural patch graft – CMS Ex: Herniorrhaphy using mesh

Body Part – 4TH			Approach – 5TH	Device – 6TH	Qualifier – 7TH
1 Cerebral Meninges 2 Dura Mater 6 Cerebral Ventricle F Olfactory Nerve G Optic Nerve H Oculomotor Nerve	J Trochlear Nerve K Trigeminal Nerve L Abducens Nerve M Facial Nerve N Acoustic Nerve	P Glossopharyngeal Nerve Q Vagus Nerve R Accessory Nerve S Hypoglossal Nerve T Spinal Meninges	0 Open 3 Percutaneous 4 Percutaneous endoscopic	7 Autologous tissue substitute J Synthetic substitute K Nonautologous tissue substitute	Z No qualifier

© 2018 Channel Publishing, Ltd.

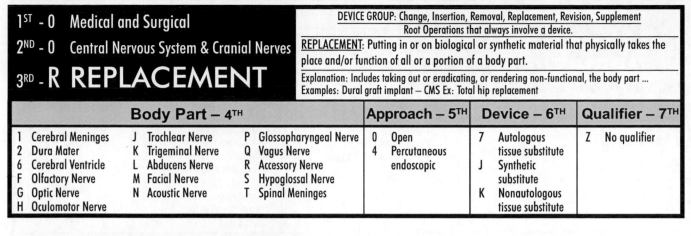

1ST - 0 Medical and Surgical
2ND - 0 Central Nervous System & Cranial Nerves
3RD - W REVISION

DEVICE GROUP: Change, Insertion, Removal, Replacement, Revision, Supplement
Root Operations that always involve a device.

REVISION: Correcting, to the extent possible, a portion of a malfunctioning device or the position of a displaced device.

Explanation: Correcting by taking out or putting in components of a device such as a screw or pin ...
Examples: Reposition neurostimulator lead – CMS Ex: Recementing of hip prosthesis

Body Part – 4TH	Approach – 5TH	Device – 6TH	Qualifier – 7TH
0 Brain V Spinal Cord	0 Open 3 Percutaneous 4 Percutaneous endoscopic	0 Drainage device 2 Monitoring device 3 Infusion device 7 Autologous tissue substitute J Synthetic substitute K Nonautologous tissue substitute M Neurostimulator lead Y Other device	Z No qualifier
0 Brain V Spinal Cord	X External	0 Drainage device 2 Monitoring device 3 Infusion device 7 Autologous tissue substitute J Synthetic substitute K Nonautologous tissue substitute M Neurostimulator lead	Z No qualifier
6 Cerebral Ventricle U Spinal Canal	0 Open 3 Percutaneous 4 Percutaneous endoscopic	0 Drainage device 2 Monitoring device 3 Infusion device J Synthetic substitute M Neurostimulator lead Y Other device	Z No qualifier
6 Cerebral Ventricle U Spinal Canal	X External	0 Drainage device 2 Monitoring device 3 Infusion device J Synthetic substitute M Neurostimulator lead	Z No qualifier
E Cranial Nerve	0 Open 3 Percutaneous 4 Percutaneous endoscopic	0 Drainage device 2 Monitoring device 3 Infusion device 7 Autologous tissue substitute M Neurostimulator lead Y Other device	Z No qualifier
E Cranial Nerve	X External	0 Drainage device 2 Monitoring device 3 Infusion device 7 Autologous tissue substitute M Neurostimulator lead	Z No qualifier

1ST - 0 Medical and Surgical
2ND - 0 Central Nervous System & Cranial Nerves
3RD - X TRANSFER

MOVE GROUP: (Reattachment), Reposition, Transfer, (Transplantation)
Root Operations that put in/put back or move some/all of a body part.

TRANSFER: Moving, without taking out, all or a portion of a body part to another location to take over the function of all or a portion of a body part.

Explanation: The body part transferred remains connected to its vascular and nervous supply
Examples: Transfer trigeminal nerve to facial nerve – CMS Ex: Tendon transfer

Body Part – 4TH		Approach – 5TH	Device – 6TH	Qualifier – 7TH
F Olfactory Nerve G Optic Nerve H Oculomotor Nerve J Trochlear Nerve K Trigeminal Nerve L Abducens Nerve	M Facial Nerve N Acoustic Nerve P Glossopharyngeal Nerve Q Vagus Nerve R Accessory Nerve S Hypoglossal Nerve	0 Open 4 Percutaneous endoscopic	Z No device	F Olfactory Nerve G Optic Nerve H Oculomotor Nerve J Trochlear Nerve K Trigeminal Nerve L Abducens Nerve M Facial Nerve N Acoustic Nerve P Glossopharyngeal Nerve Q Vagus Nerve R Accessory Nerve S Hypoglossal Nerve

© 2018 Channel Publishing, Ltd.

Educational Annotations | 1 – Peripheral Nervous System

Body System Specific Educational Annotations for the Peripheral Nervous System include:

- Anatomy and Physiology Review
- Anatomical Illustrations
- Definitions of Common Procedures
- AHA Coding Clinic® Reference Notations
- Body Part Key Listings
- Device Key Listings
- Device Aggregation Table Listings
- Coding Notes

Anatomy and Physiology Review of Peripheral Nervous System

BODY PART VALUES – 1 - PERIPHERAL NERVOUS SYSTEM

Abdominal Sympathetic Nerve – The autonomic nervous system sympathetic nerve trunk portion that innervates the smooth muscles, glands, and organs of the abdominal region.

Brachial Plexus – A branching network of the last four cervical spinal nerves and the first thoracic spinal nerve (C5-C8, T1) that primarily innervates the skin and muscles of the upper limbs.

Cervical Nerve – One of eight pairs of spinal nerves emerging from the cervical vertebrae.

Cervical Plexus – A branching network of the first four cervical spinal nerves (C1-C4) that primarily innervates the skin and muscles of the head and neck.

Femoral Nerve – The femoral nerve is the major nerve that innervates the muscles and skin of the thigh and leg.

Head and Neck Sympathetic Nerve – The autonomic nervous system sympathetic nerve trunk portion that innervates the smooth muscles, glands, and organs of the head and neck region.

Lumbar Nerve – One of five pairs of spinal nerves emerging from the lumbar vertebrae.

Lumbar Plexus – A branching network of the first four lumbar spinal nerves and the last thoracic spinal nerve (L1-L4, T12) that primarily innervates the skin and muscles of the lower abdomen and upper legs.

Lumbar Sympathetic Nerve – The autonomic nervous system sympathetic nerve trunk portion that innervates the smooth muscles, glands, and organs of the lower abdominal and pelvic regions.

Lumbosacral Plexus – A branching network of the lumbar spinal nerves, the last thoracic spinal nerve (L1-L5, T12), the sacral plexus (S1-S3), and pudondal plexus (S4-S5 and coccygeal nerve) that primarily innervates the skin and muscles of the lower abdomen and legs.

Median Nerve – The median nerve is one of the three major upper limb nerves that innervates the muscles and skin of the forearm and hand.

Peripheral Nerve – ANATOMY – A nerve outside of the brain and spinal cord. PHYSIOLOGY – The peripheral nervous system consists of a network of nerves that coordinates its voluntary and involuntary actions and communication among its parts.

Peroneal Nerve – The peroneal nerve is a division of the sciatic nerve that innervates the muscles and skin of the lower leg.

Phrenic Nerve – The phrenic nerve is the major nerve that innervates the muscles of the diaphragm and is the nerve responsible for the hiccough reflex.

Pudendal Nerve – The pudendal nerve is the major nerve that innervates the perineum, external genitalia, and anus.

Radial Nerve – The radial nerve is one of the three major upper limb nerves that innervates the muscles and skin of the arm (specifically the triceps muscle), wrist, and hand.

Sacral Nerve – One of five pairs of spinal nerves emerging from the sacrum.

Sacral Plexus – A branching network of the sacral nerves (S1-S5) and coccygeal nerve that primarily innervates the skin and muscles of the legs.

Sacral Sympathetic Nerve – The autonomic nervous system sympathetic nerve trunk portion that innervates the smooth muscles, glands, and organs of the pelvic region.

Sciatic Nerve – The sciatic nerve is the major nerve that innervates the muscles and skin of the thighs, lower legs, and feet.

Thoracic Nerve – One of twelve pairs of spinal nerves emerging from the thoracic vertebrae.

Thoracic Sympathetic Nerve – The autonomic nervous system sympathetic nerve trunk portion that innervates the smooth muscles, glands, and organs of the thoracic region.

Tibial Nerve – The tibial nerve is a division of the sciatic nerve that innervates the muscles and skin of the lower legs and feet.

Ulnar Nerve – The ulnar nerve is one of the three major upper limb nerves that innervates the muscles and skin of the arm, hand, little finger, and half of the ring finger.

© 2018 Channel Publishing, Ltd.

Educational Annotations | 1 – Peripheral Nervous System

Anatomical Illustrations of Peripheral Nervous System

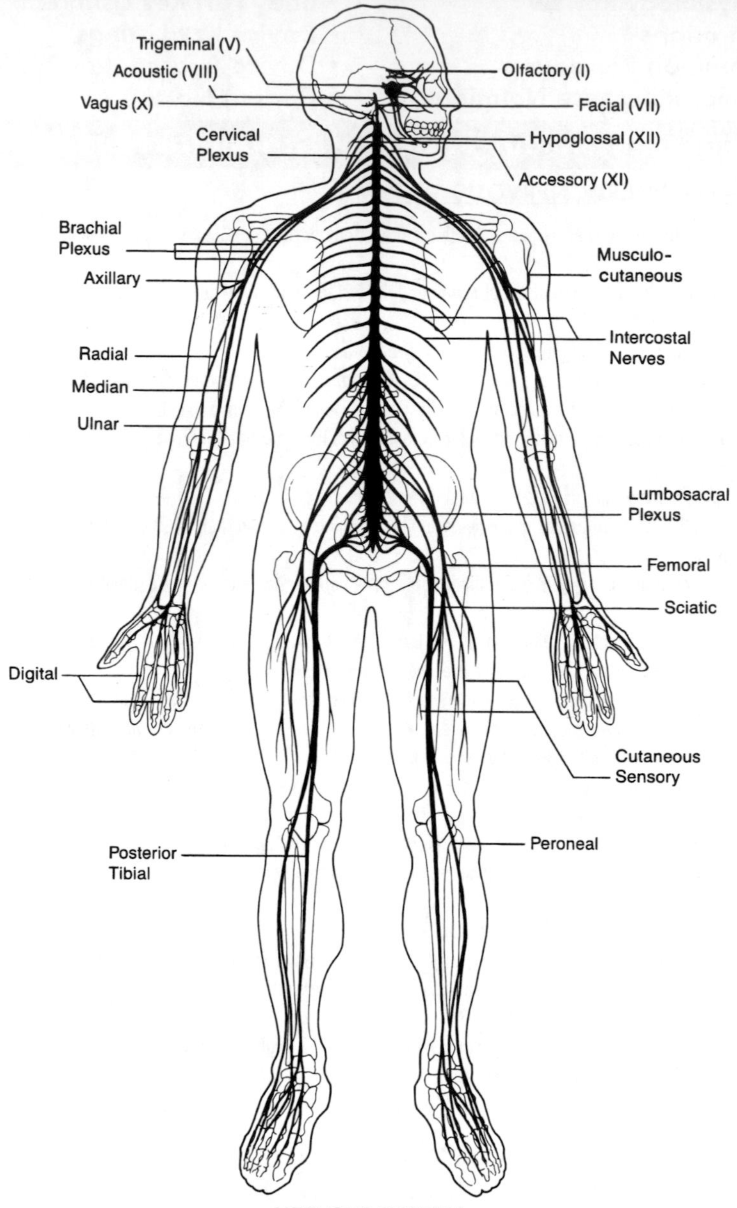

NERVOUS SYSTEM

Definitions of Common Procedures of Peripheral Nervous System

Carpal tunnel release – The surgical relief from pain and weakness of the hand due to compression of the median nerve at the wrist by dividing the transverse carpal ligament causing the compression.

Free nerve graft – The surgical repair of a damaged nerve to restore nerve function using a harvested nerve section to connect both ends of the damaged nerve.

Nerve transfer – The surgical dissection to free a viable redundant nerve branch to connect to the damaged nerve in order to restore movement or sensory function.

Thoracic sympathectomy – The surgical excision or destruction of the thoracic sympathetic nerve chain ganglia to alleviate the symptoms of hyperhidrosis, sweaty palms, or Raynaud's disease.

PERIPHERAL NERVOUS 0 1

© 2018 Channel Publishing, Ltd.

Educational Annotations | 1 – Peripheral Nervous System

AHA Coding Clinic® Reference Notations of Peripheral Nervous System

ROOT OPERATION SPECIFIC - 1 - PERIPHERAL NERVOUS SYSTEM

CHANGE - 2
DESTRUCTION - 5
DIVISION - 8
DRAINAGE - 9
EXCISION - B
Sympathectomy with thoracic outlet decompression ....AHA 17:2Q:p19
EXTIRPATION - C
EXTRACTION - D
INSERTION - H
INSPECTION - J
RELEASE - N
Carpal tunnel release ....AHA 14:3Q:p33
Cervical neural foraminal decompression ....AHA 16:2Q:p17
Complete release of brachial plexus ....AHA 16:2Q:p23
Discectomy with decompressive foraminotomy/laminectomy ....AHA 16:2Q:p16
Dissection of synovial lumbar facet cyst ....AHA 18:2Q:p22
REMOVAL - P
REPAIR - Q
REPOSITION - S
SUPPLEMENT - U
Nerve repair with neurogen tube graft ....AHA 17:4Q:p62
REVISION - W
TRANSFER - X

Body Part Key Listings of Peripheral Nervous System

See also Body Part Key in Appendix C

Abdominal aortic plexus ....use Abdominal Sympathetic Nerve
Accessory obturator nerve ....use Lumbar Plexus
Accessory phrenic nerve ....use Phrenic Nerve
Ansa cervicalis ....use Cervical Plexus
Anterior crural nerve ....use Femoral Nerve
Anterior interosseous nerve ....use Median Nerve
Auerbach's (myenteric) plexus ....use Abdominal Sympathetic Nerve
Axillary nerve ....use Brachial Plexus
Cardiac plexus ....use Thoracic Sympathetic Nerve
Cavernous plexus ....use Head and Neck Sympathetic Nerve
Celiac ganglion ....use Abdominal Sympathetic Nerve
Celiac (solar) plexus ....use Abdominal Sympathetic Nerve
Cervical ganglion ....use Head and Neck Sympathetic Nerve
Ciliary ganglion ....use Head and Neck Sympathetic Nerve
Common fibular nerve ....use Peroneal Nerve
Common peroneal nerve ....use Peroneal Nerve
Cubital nerve ....use Ulnar Nerve
Cutaneous (transverse) cervical nerve ..use Cervical Plexus
Dorsal digital nerve ....use Radial Nerve
Dorsal scapular nerve ....use Brachial Plexus
Esophageal plexus ....use Thoracic Sympathetic Nerve
External popliteal nerve ....use Peroneal Nerve
First intercostal nerve ....use Brachial Plexus
Ganglion impar (ganglion of Walther) use Sacral Sympathetic Nerve
Gastric plexus ....use Abdominal Sympathetic Nerve
Genitofemoral nerve ....use Lumbar Plexus
Great auricular nerve ....use Cervical Plexus
Greater occipital nerve ....use Cervical Nerve
Greater splanchnic nerve ....use Thoracic Sympathetic Nerve
Hepatic plexus ....use Abdominal Sympathetic Nerve
Iliohypogastric nerve ....use Lumbar Plexus
Ilioinguinal nerve ....use Lumbar Plexus
Inferior cardiac nerve ....use Thoracic Sympathetic Nerve
Inferior gluteal nerve ....use Sacral Plexus
Inferior hypogastric plexus ....use Abdominal Sympathetic Nerve
Inferior mesenteric ganglion ....use Abdominal Sympathetic Nerve
Inferior mesenteric plexus ....use Abdominal Sympathetic Nerve
Intercostal nerve ....use Thoracic Nerve
Intercostobrachial nerve ....use Thoracic Nerve
Internal carotid plexus ....use Head and Neck Sympathetic Nerve
Ischiatic nerve ....use Sciatic Nerve
Lateral femoral cutaneous nerve ....use Lumbar Plexus
Lateral plantar nerve ....use Tibial Nerve
Lateral sural cutaneous nerve ....use Peroneal Nerve
Least splanchnic nerve ....use Thoracic Sympathetic Nerve
Lesser occipital nerve ....use Cervical Plexus
Lesser splanchnic nerve ....use Thoracic Sympathetic Nerve
Long thoracic nerve ....use Brachial Plexus
Lumbar ganglion ....use Lumbar Sympathetic Nerve
Lumbar splanchnic nerve ....use Lumbar Sympathetic Nerve
Lumbosacral trunk ....use Lumbar Nerve
Medial plantar nerve ....use Tibial Nerve
Medial popliteal nerve ....use Tibial Nerve
Medial sural cutaneous nerve ....use Tibial Nerve
Meissner's (submucous) plexus ....use Abdominal Sympathetic Nerve
Middle cardiac nerve ....use Thoracic Sympathetic Nerve
Musculocutaneous nerve ....use Brachial Plexus

Continued on next page

© 2018 Channel Publishing, Ltd.

Educational Annotations | 1 – Peripheral Nervous System

Body Part Key Listings of Peripheral Nervous System

Continued from previous page

Musculospiral nerve	use Radial Nerve
Myenteric (Auerbach's) plexus	use Abdominal Sympathetic Nerve
Obturator nerve	use Lumbar Plexus
Otic ganglion	use Head and Neck Sympathetic Nerve
Palmar cutaneous nerve	use Median Nerve, Radial Nerve
Pancreatic plexus	use Abdominal Sympathetic Nerve
Pelvic splanchnic nerve	use Abdominal Sympathetic Nerve
	use Sacral Sympathetic Nerve
Posterior femoral cutaneous nerve	use Sacral Plexus
Posterior interosseous nerve	use Radial Nerve
Posterior labial nerve	use Pudendal Nerve
Posterior scrotal nerve	use Pudendal Nerve
Pterygopalatine (sphenopalatine) ganglion	use Head and Neck Sympathetic Nerve
Pudendal nerve	use Sacral Plexus
Pulmonary plexus	use Vagus Nerve/Thoracic Sympathetic Nerve
Renal plexus	use Abdominal Sympathetic Nerve
Sacral ganglion	use Sacral Sympathetic Nerve
Sacral splanchnic nerve	use Sacral Sympathetic Nerve
Saphenous nerve	use Femoral Nerve
Solar (celiac) plexus	use Abdominal Sympathetic Nerve
Sphenopalatine (pterygopalatine) ganglion	use Head and Neck Sympathetic Nerve
Spinal nerve, cervical	use Cervical Nerve
Spinal nerve, lumbar	use Lumbar Nerve
Spinal nerve, sacral	use Sacral Nerve
Spinal nerve, thoracic	use Thoracic Nerve
Splenic plexus	use Abdominal Sympathetic Nerve
Stellate ganglion	use Head and Neck Sympathetic Nerve
Subclavius nerve	use Brachial Plexus
Subcostal nerve	use Thoracic Nerve
Submandibular ganglion	use Head and Neck Sympathetic Nerve
Submaxillary ganglion	use Head and Neck Sympathetic Nerve
Submucous (Meissner's) plexus	use Abdominal Sympathetic Nerve
Suboccipital nerve	use Cervical Nerve
Superior cardiac nerve	use Thoracic Sympathetic Nerve
Superior clunic (cluneal) nerve	use Lumbar Nerve
Superior gluteal nerve	use Lumbar Plexus
Superior hypogastric plexus	use Abdominal Sympathetic Nerve
Superior mesenteric ganglion	use Abdominal Sympathetic Nerve
Superior mesenteric plexus	use Abdominal Sympathetic Nerve
Supraclavicular nerve	use Cervical Plexus
Suprascapular nerve	use Brachial Plexus
Suprarenal plexus	use Abdominal Sympathetic Nerve
Third occipital nerve	use Cervical Nerve
Thoracic aortic plexus	use Thoracic Sympathetic Nerve
Thoracic ganglion	use Thoracic Sympathetic Nerve
Transverse (cutaneous) cervical nerve	use Cervical Plexus

Device Key Listings of Peripheral Nervous System

See also Device Key in Appendix D

Autograft	use Autologous Tissue Substitute
InterStim® Therapy lead	use Neurostimulator Lead in Peripheral Nervous System

Device Aggregation Table Listings of Peripheral Nervous System

See also Device Aggregation Table in Appendix E

Specific Device	For Operation	In Body System	General Device
None Listed in Device Aggregation Table for this Body System			

Coding Notes of Peripheral Nervous System

Body System Relevant Coding Guidelines

Branches of body parts

B4.2

Where a specific branch of a body part does not have its own body part value in PCS, the body part is typically coded to the closest proximal branch that has a specific body part value. In the cardiovascular body systems, if a general body part is available in the correct root operation table, and coding to a proximal branch would require assigning a code in a different body system, the procedure is coded using the general body part value.

Examples: A procedure performed on the mandibular branch of the trigeminal nerve is coded to the trigeminal nerve body part value.

Occlusion of the bronchial artery is coded to the body part value Upper Artery in the body system Upper Arteries, and not to the body part value Thoracic Aorta, Descending in the body system Heart and Great Vessels.

PERIPHERAL NERVOUS 0 1

© 2018 Channel Publishing, Ltd.

1ST - 0 Medical and Surgical
2ND - 1 Peripheral Nervous System
3RD - 2 CHANGE

DEVICE GROUP: Change, Insertion, Removal, (Replacement), Revision, Supplement
Root Operations that always involve a device.

CHANGE: Taking out or off a device from a body part and putting back an identical or similar device in or on the same body part without cutting or puncturing the skin or a mucous membrane.

Explanation: All CHANGE procedures are coded using the approach External
Examples: Exchange ulnar nerve drain tube – CMS Ex: Urinary catheter change

Body Part – 4TH	Approach – 5TH	Device – 6TH	Qualifier – 7TH
Y Peripheral Nerve	X External	0 Drainage device Y Other device	Z No qualifier

1ST - 0 Medical and Surgical
2ND - 1 Peripheral Nervous System
3RD - 5 DESTRUCTION

EXCISION GROUP: Excision, Resection, Destruction, Extraction, (Detachment)
Root Operations that take out some or all of a body part.

DESTRUCTION: Physical eradication of all or a portion of a body part by the direct use of energy, force, or a destructive agent.

Explanation: None of the body part is physically taken out
Examples: Cryoablation nerve lesion – CMS Ex: Fulguration of rectal polyp

Body Part – 4TH			Approach – 5TH	Device – 6TH	Qualifier – 7TH
0 Cervical Plexus 1 Cervical Nerve 2 Phrenic Nerve 3 Brachial Plexus 4 Ulnar Nerve 5 Median Nerve 6 Radial Nerve 8 Thoracic Nerve	9 Lumbar Plexus A Lumbosacral Plexus B Lumbar Nerve C Pudendal Nerve D Femoral Nerve F Sciatic Nerve G Tibial Nerve H Peroneal Nerve	K Head and Neck Sympathetic Nerve L Thoracic Sympathetic Nerve M Abdominal Sympathetic Nerve N Lumbar Sympathetic Nerve P Sacral Sympathetic Nerve Q Sacral Plexus R Sacral Nerve	0 Open 3 Percutaneous 4 Percutaneous endoscopic	Z No device	Z No qualifier

1ST - 0 Medical and Surgical
2ND - 1 Peripheral Nervous System
3RD - 8 DIVISION

DIVISION GROUP: Division, Release
Root Operations involving cutting or separation only.

DIVISION: Cutting into a body part, without draining fluids and/or gases from the body part, in order to separate or transect a body part.

Explanation: All or a portion of the body part is separated into two or more portions
Examples: Sacral nerve rhizotomy – CMS Ex: Spinal cordotomy

Body Part – 4TH			Approach – 5TH	Device – 6TH	Qualifier – 7TH
0 Cervical Plexus 1 Cervical Nerve 2 Phrenic Nerve 3 Brachial Plexus 4 Ulnar Nerve 5 Median Nerve 6 Radial Nerve 8 Thoracic Nerve	9 Lumbar Plexus A Lumbosacral Plexus B Lumbar Nerve C Pudendal Nerve D Femoral Nerve F Sciatic Nerve G Tibial Nerve H Peroneal Nerve	K Head and Neck Sympathetic Nerve L Thoracic Sympathetic Nerve M Abdominal Sympathetic Nerve N Lumbar Sympathetic Nerve P Sacral Sympathetic Nerve Q Sacral Plexus R Sacral Nerve	0 Open 3 Percutaneous 4 Percutaneous endoscopic	Z No device	Z No qualifier

© 2018 Channel Publishing, Ltd.

1ST - 0 Medical and Surgical
2ND - 1 Peripheral Nervous System
3RD - 9 DRAINAGE

DRAINAGE GROUP: Drainage, Extirpation, (Fragmentation)
Root Operations that take out solids/fluids/gases from a body part.

DRAINAGE: Taking or letting out fluids and/or gases from a body part.

Explanation: Qualifier "X Diagnostic" indicates drainage procedures that are biopsies
Examples: Aspiration nerve abscess – CMS Ex: Thoracentesis

Body Part – 4TH			Approach – 5TH	Device – 6TH	Qualifier – 7TH
0 Cervical Plexus 1 Cervical Nerve 2 Phrenic Nerve 3 Brachial Plexus 4 Ulnar Nerve 5 Median Nerve 6 Radial Nerve 8 Thoracic Nerve	9 Lumbar Plexus A Lumbosacral Plexus B Lumbar Nerve C Pudendal Nerve D Femoral Nerve F Sciatic Nerve G Tibial Nerve H Peroneal Nerve	K Head and Neck Sympathetic Nerve L Thoracic Sympathetic Nerve M Abdominal Sympathetic Nerve N Lumbar Sympathetic Nerve P Sacral Sympathetic Nerve Q Sacral Plexus R Sacral Nerve	0 Open 3 Percutaneous 4 Percutaneous endoscopic	0 Drainage device	Z No qualifier
0 Cervical Plexus 1 Cervical Nerve 2 Phrenic Nerve 3 Brachial Plexus 4 Ulnar Nerve 5 Median Nerve 6 Radial Nerve 8 Thoracic Nerve	9 Lumbar Plexus A Lumbosacral Plexus B Lumbar Nerve C Pudendal Nerve D Femoral Nerve F Sciatic Nerve G Tibial Nerve H Peroneal Nerve	K Head and Neck Sympathetic Nerve L Thoracic Sympathetic Nerve M Abdominal Sympathetic Nerve N Lumbar Sympathetic Nerve P Sacral Sympathetic Nerve Q Sacral Plexus R Sacral Nerve	0 Open 3 Percutaneous 4 Percutaneous endoscopic	Z No device	X Diagnostic Z No qualifier

1ST - 0 Medical and Surgical
2ND - 1 Peripheral Nervous System
3RD - B EXCISION

EXCISION GROUP: Excision, Resection, Destruction, Extraction, (Detachment)
Root Operations that take out some or all of a body part.

EXCISION: Cutting out or off, without replacement, a portion of a body part.

Explanation: Qualifier "X Diagnostic" indicates excision procedures that are biopsies
Examples: Biopsy lumbosacral plexus – CMS Ex: Liver biopsy

Body Part – 4TH			Approach – 5TH	Device – 6TH	Qualifier – 7TH
0 Cervical Plexus 1 Cervical Nerve 2 Phrenic Nerve 3 Brachial Plexus 4 Ulnar Nerve 5 Median Nerve 6 Radial Nerve 8 Thoracic Nerve	9 Lumbar Plexus A Lumbosacral Plexus B Lumbar Nerve C Pudendal Nerve D Femoral Nerve F Sciatic Nerve G Tibial Nerve H Peroneal Nerve	K Head and Neck Sympathetic Nerve L Thoracic Sympathetic Nerve M Abdominal Sympathetic Nerve N Lumbar Sympathetic Nerve P Sacral Sympathetic Nerve Q Sacral Plexus R Sacral Nerve	0 Open 3 Percutaneous 4 Percutaneous endoscopic	Z No device	X Diagnostic Z No qualifier

1ST - 0 Medical and Surgical
2ND - 1 Peripheral Nervous System
3RD - C EXTIRPATION

DRAINAGE GROUP: Drainage, Extirpation, (Fragmentation)
Root Operations that take out solids/fluids/gases from a body part.

EXTIRPATION: Taking or cutting out solid matter from a body part.

Explanation: Abnormal byproduct or foreign body ...
Examples: Removal foreign body cervical plexus – CMS Ex: Thrombectomy

Body Part – 4TH			Approach – 5TH	Device – 6TH	Qualifier – 7TH
0 Cervical Plexus 1 Cervical Nerve 2 Phrenic Nerve 3 Brachial Plexus 4 Ulnar Nerve 5 Median Nerve 6 Radial Nerve 8 Thoracic Nerve	9 Lumbar Plexus A Lumbosacral Plexus B Lumbar Nerve C Pudendal Nerve D Femoral Nerve F Sciatic Nerve G Tibial Nerve H Peroneal Nerve	K Head and Neck Sympathetic Nerve L Thoracic Sympathetic Nerve M Abdominal Sympathetic Nerve N Lumbar Sympathetic Nerve P Sacral Sympathetic Nerve Q Sacral Plexus R Sacral Nerve	0 Open 3 Percutaneous 4 Percutaneous endoscopic	Z No device	Z No qualifier

© 2018 Channel Publishing, Ltd.

1ST - 0 Medical and Surgical
2ND - 1 Peripheral Nervous System
3RD - D EXTRACTION

EXCISION GROUP: Excision, Resection, Destruction, Extraction, (Detachment)
Root Operations that take out some or all of a body part.

EXTRACTION: Pulling or stripping out or off all or a portion of a body part by the use of force.

Explanation: None for this Body System
Examples: Neurexeresis radial nerve – CMS Ex: Dilation and curettage

Body Part – 4TH			Approach – 5TH	Device – 6TH	Qualifier – 7TH
0 Cervical Plexus	9 Lumbar Plexus	K Head and Neck Sympathetic Nerve	0 Open	Z No device	Z No qualifier
1 Cervical Nerve	A Lumbosacral Plexus	L Thoracic Sympathetic Nerve	3 Percutaneous		
2 Phrenic Nerve	B Lumbar Nerve	M Abdominal Sympathetic Nerve	4 Percutaneous endoscopic		
3 Brachial Plexus	C Pudendal Nerve	N Lumbar Sympathetic Nerve			
4 Ulnar Nerve	D Femoral Nerve	P Sacral Sympathetic Nerve			
5 Median Nerve	F Sciatic Nerve	Q Sacral Plexus			
6 Radial Nerve	G Tibial Nerve	R Sacral Nerve			
8 Thoracic Nerve	H Peroneal Nerve				

1ST - 0 Medical and Surgical
2ND - 1 Peripheral Nervous System
3RD - H INSERTION

DEVICE GROUP: Change, Insertion, Removal, Replacement, Revision, Supplement
Root Operations that always involve a device.

INSERTION: Putting in a nonbiological appliance that monitors, assists, performs, or prevents a physiological function but does not physically take the place of a body part.

Explanation: None
Examples: Insertion neurostimulator lead – CMS Ex: Insertion of central venous catheter

Body Part – 4TH	Approach – 5TH	Device – 6TH	Qualifier – 7TH
Y Peripheral Nerve	0 Open	2 Monitoring device	Z No qualifier
	3 Percutaneous	M Neurostimulator lead	
	4 Percutaneous endoscopic	Y Other device	

1ST - 0 Medical and Surgical
2ND - 1 Peripheral Nervous System
3RD - J INSPECTION

EXAMINATION GROUP: Inspection, (Map)
Root Operations involving examination only.

INSPECTION: Visually and/or manually exploring a body part.

Explanation: Direct or instrumental visualization ...
Examples: Examination injured nerve – CMS Ex: Exploratory laparotomy

Body Part – 4TH	Approach – 5TH	Device – 6TH	Qualifier – 7TH
Y Peripheral Nerve	0 Open	Z No device	Z No qualifier
	3 Percutaneous		
	4 Percutaneous endoscopic		

1ST - 0 Medical and Surgical
2ND - 1 Peripheral Nervous System
3RD - N RELEASE

DIVISION GROUP: Division, Release
Root Operations involving cutting or separation only.

RELEASE: Freeing a body part from an abnormal physical constraint by cutting or by the use of force.

Explanation: Some of the restraining tissue may be taken out but none of the body part is taken out
Examples: Carpal tunnel release – CMS Ex: Carpal tunnel release

Body Part – 4TH			Approach – 5TH	Device – 6TH	Qualifier – 7TH
0 Cervical Plexus	9 Lumbar Plexus	K Head and Neck Sympathetic Nerve	0 Open	Z No device	Z No qualifier
1 Cervical Nerve	A Lumbosacral Plexus	L Thoracic Sympathetic Nerve	3 Percutaneous		
2 Phrenic Nerve	B Lumbar Nerve	M Abdominal Sympathetic Nerve	4 Percutaneous endoscopic		
3 Brachial Plexus	C Pudendal Nerve	N Lumbar Sympathetic Nerve			
4 Ulnar Nerve	D Femoral Nerve	P Sacral Sympathetic Nerve			
5 Median Nerve	F Sciatic Nerve	Q Sacral Plexus			
6 Radial Nerve	G Tibial Nerve	R Sacral Nerve			
8 Thoracic Nerve	H Peroneal Nerve				

© 2018 Channel Publishing, Ltd.

1ST - 0 Medical and Surgical
2ND - 1 Peripheral Nervous System
3RD - P REMOVAL

DEVICE GROUP: Change, Insertion, Removal, Replacement, Revision, Supplement
Root Operations that always involve a device.

REMOVAL: Taking out or off a device from a body part.

Explanation: Removal device without reinsertion ...
Examples: Removal neurostimulator lead – CMS Ex: Cardiac pacemaker removal

Body Part – 4TH	Approach – 5TH	Device – 6TH	Qualifier – 7TH
Y Peripheral Nerve	0 Open 3 Percutaneous 4 Percutaneous endoscopic	0 Drainage device 2 Monitoring device 7 Autologous tissue substitute M Neurostimulator lead Y Other device	Z No qualifier
Y Peripheral Nerve	X External	0 Drainage device 2 Monitoring device M Neurostimulator lead	Z No qualifier

1ST - 0 Medical and Surgical
2ND - 1 Peripheral Nervous System
3RD - Q REPAIR

OTHER REPAIRS GROUP: (Control), Repair
Root Operations that define other repairs.

REPAIR: Restoring, to the extent possible, a body part to its normal anatomic structure and function.

Explanation: Used only when the method to accomplish the repair is not one of the other root operations
Examples: Microsurgical repair nerve – CMS Ex: Suture of laceration

Body Part – 4TH			Approach – 5TH	Device – 6TH	Qualifier – 7TH
0 Cervical Plexus 1 Cervical Nerve 2 Phrenic Nerve 3 Brachial Plexus 4 Ulnar Nerve 5 Median Nerve 6 Radial Nerve 8 Thoracic Nerve	9 Lumbar Plexus A Lumbosacral Plexus B Lumbar Nerve C Pudendal Nerve D Femoral Nerve F Sciatic Nerve G Tibial Nerve H Peroneal Nerve	K Head and Neck Sympathetic Nerve L Thoracic Sympathetic Nerve M Abdominal Sympathetic Nerve N Lumbar Sympathetic Nerve P Sacral Sympathetic Nerve Q Sacral Plexus R Sacral Nerve	0 Open 3 Percutaneous 4 Percutaneous endoscopic	Z No device	Z No qualifier

1ST - 0 Medical and Surgical
2ND - 1 Peripheral Nervous System
3RD - R REPLACEMENT

DEVICE GROUP: Change, Insertion, Removal, Replacement, Revision, Supplement
Root Operations that always involve a device.

REPLACEMENT: Putting in or on biological or synthetic material that physically takes the place and/or function of all or a portion of a body part.

Explanation: Includes taking out or eradicating, or rendering non-functional, the body part ...
Examples: Peroneal nerve replacement – CMS Ex: Total hip replacement

Body Part – 4TH		Approach – 5TH	Device – 6TH	Qualifier – 7TH
1 Cervical Nerve 2 Phrenic Nerve 4 Ulnar Nerve 5 Median Nerve 6 Radial Nerve 8 Thoracic Nerve B Lumbar Nerve	C Pudendal Nerve D Femoral Nerve F Sciatic Nerve G Tibial Nerve H Peroneal Nerve R Sacral Nerve	0 Open 4 Percutaneous endoscopic	7 Autologous tissue substitute J Synthetic substitute K Nonautologous tissue substitute	Z No qualifier

© 2018 Channel Publishing, Ltd.

1ST - 0 Medical and Surgical
2ND - 1 Peripheral Nervous System
3RD - S REPOSITION

MOVE GROUP: (Reattachment), Reposition, Transfer, (Transplantation)
Root Operations that put in/put back or move some/all of a body part.

REPOSITION: Moving to its normal location, or other suitable location, all or a portion of a body part.

Explanation: The body part may or may not be cut out or off to be moved to the new location ...
Examples: Relocation femoral nerve – CMS Ex: Fracture reduction

Body Part – 4TH			Approach – 5TH	Device – 6TH	Qualifier – 7TH
0 Cervical Plexus 1 Cervical Nerve 2 Phrenic Nerve 3 Brachial Plexus 4 Ulnar Nerve 5 Median Nerve	6 Radial Nerve 8 Thoracic Nerve 9 Lumbar Plexus A Lumbosacral Plexus B Lumbar Nerve C Pudendal Nerve	D Femoral Nerve F Sciatic Nerve G Tibial Nerve H Peroneal Nerve Q Sacral Plexus R Sacral Nerve	0 Open 3 Percutaneous 4 Percutaneous endoscopic	Z No device	Z No qualifier

1ST - 0 Medical and Surgical
2ND - 1 Peripheral Nervous System
3RD - U SUPPLEMENT

DEVICE GROUP: Change, Insertion, Removal, Replacement, Revision, Supplement
Root Operations that always involve a device.

SUPPLEMENT: Putting in or on biological or synthetic material that physically reinforces and/or augments the function of a portion of a body part.

Explanation: Biological material is non-living, or is living and from the same individual ...
Examples: Free nerve autograft – CMS Ex: Herniorrhaphy using mesh

Body Part – 4TH		Approach – 5TH	Device – 6TH	Qualifier – 7TH
1 Cervical Nerve 2 Phrenic Nerve 4 Ulnar Nerve 5 Median Nerve 6 Radial Nerve 8 Thoracic Nerve B Lumbar Nerve	C Pudendal Nerve D Femoral Nerve F Sciatic Nerve G Tibial Nerve H Peroneal Nerve R Sacral Nerve	0 Open 3 Percutaneous 4 Percutaneous endoscopic	7 Autologous tissue substitute J Synthetic substitute K Nonautologous tissue substitute	Z No qualifier

1ST - 0 Medical and Surgical
2ND - 1 Peripheral Nervous System
3RD - W REVISION

DEVICE GROUP: Change, Insertion, Removal, Replacement, Revision, Supplement
Root Operations that always involve a device.

REVISION: Correcting, to the extent possible, a portion of a malfunctioning device or the position of a displaced device.

Explanation: Correcting by taking out or putting in components of a device such as a screw or pin ...
Examples: Reposition neurostimulator lead – CMS Ex: Recementing of hip prosthesis

Body Part – 4TH	Approach – 5TH	Device – 6TH	Qualifier – 7TH
Y Peripheral Nerve	0 Open 3 Percutaneous 4 Percutaneous endoscopic	0 Drainage device 2 Monitoring device 7 Autologous tissue substitute M Neurostimulator lead Y Other device	Z No qualifier
Y Peripheral Nerve	X External	0 Drainage device 2 Monitoring device 7 Autologous tissue substitute M Neurostimulator lead	Z No qualifier

© 2018 Channel Publishing, Ltd.

1ST - 0 Medical and Surgical
2ND - 1 Peripheral Nervous System
3RD - X TRANSFER

MOVE GROUP: (Reattachment), Reposition, Transfer, (Transplantation)
Root Operations that put in/put back or move some/all of a body part.

TRANSFER: Moving, without taking out, all or a portion of a body part to another location to take over the function of all or a portion of a body part.

Explanation: The body part transferred remains connected to its vascular and nervous supply
Examples: Radial to median nerve transfer – CMS Ex: Tendon transfer

Body Part – 4TH	Approach – 5TH	Device – 6TH	Qualifier – 7TH
1 Cervical Nerve 2 Phrenic Nerve	0 Open 4 Percutaneous endoscopic	Z No device	1 Cervical Nerve 2 Phrenic Nerve
4 Ulnar Nerve 5 Median Nerve 6 Radial Nerve	0 Open 4 Percutaneous endoscopic	Z No device	4 Ulnar Nerve 5 Median Nerve 6 Radial Nerve
8 Thoracic Nerve	0 Open 4 Percutaneous endoscopic	Z No device	8 Thoracic Nerve
B Lumbar Nerve C Pudendal Nerve	0 Open 4 Percutaneous endoscopic	Z No device	B Lumbar Nerve C Perineal Nerve
D Femoral Nerve F Sciatic Nerve G Tibial Nerve H Peroneal Nerve	0 Open 4 Percutaneous endoscopic	Z No device	D Femoral Nerve F Sciatic Nerve G Tibial Nerve H Peroneal Nerve

© 2018 Channel Publishing, Ltd.

Educational Annotations | 2 – Heart and Great Vessels

Body System Specific Educational Annotations for the Heart and Great Vessels include:

- Anatomy and Physiology Review
- Anatomical Illustrations
- Definitions of Common Procedures
- AHA Coding Clinic® Reference Notations
- Body Part Key Listings
- Device Key Listings
- Device Aggregation Table Listings
- Coding Notes

Anatomy and Physiology Review of Heart and Great Vessels

BODY PART VALUES – 2 - HEART AND GREAT VESSELS

Aortic Valve – ANATOMY – The aortic valve has three cusps and is located between the outlet of the left ventricle and the base of the aorta. PHYSIOLOGY – The aortic valve prevents backflow of blood into the left ventricle from the aorta via its one-way valve function.

Atrial Septum – The strong tissue wall that separates the left and right atria.

Atrium, Left – ANATOMY – One of the two smaller chambers of the heart's four chambers. PHYSIOLOGY – The left atrium receives and pools the oxygenated blood from the lungs briefly before the tricuspid valve opens and the blood flows into the left ventricle.

Atrium, Right – ANATOMY – One of the two smaller chambers of the heart's four chambers. PHYSIOLOGY – The right atrium receives and pools the deoxygenated blood from the inferior vena cava and the superior vena cava briefly before the pulmonary valve opens and the blood flows into the right ventricle.

Chordae Tendineae – The very strong tendinous cord attaching a papillary muscle to a valve leaflet.

Conduction Mechanism – The electrical signal transmission system that controls the rhythmical heart beat through various structures and fibers including the sinoatrial node (the heart's pacemaker), the atrioventricular node, and the Bundle of HIS.

Coronary Artery – Coronary arteries supply oxygenated blood to the heart.

Coronary Vein – Coronary veins remove the deoxygenated blood from the heart muscle and return it to the right atrium.

Great Vessel – The major vessels associated with the heart that lie within the thoracic cavity including: Thoracic aorta, pulmonary arteries, pulmonary veins, and the superior vena cava and thoracic portion of the inferior vena cava.

Heart – ANATOMY – The heart is the 4 chambered, muscular, blood pumping organ behind the mediastinum in the thorax, and is approximately 5.5 inches (14 cm) long and 3.5 inches (9 cm) wide. The heart has 3 layers: The endocardium, myocardium, and pericardium. The endocardium is the interior lining of endothelium. The myocardium is the thick muscular layer. The pericardium is the double-layered serous membrane protecting the heart from friction as it beats. The heart has 4 valves and 4 chambers: The tricuspid valve, mitral valve, aortic valve, the pulmonary valve, right and left atria, and right and left ventricles. The mediastinum is the mass of tissue between the sternum and vertebral column which divides the thoracic cavity. PHYSIOLOGY – The heart functions to pump and maintain sufficient pressure of the blood to constantly meet the needs of the body cells. The venous blood is returned from the body via the inferior and superior vena cava to the right atrium where it is pooled momentarily before the tricuspid valve opens and allows the venous blood to enter the right ventricle. The right ventricle then contracts forcing the blood through the pulmonary valve to the lungs. The lungs return the reoxygenated blood to the left atrium where it is pooled momentarily before the mitral valve opens and allows the venous blood to enter the left ventricle. The left ventricle then contracts, forcing the blood through the aortic valve to all the tissues of the body.

Heart, Left – ANATOMY – The portion of the heart that includes the left atria and left ventricle.
PHYSIOLOGY – The left heart receives the reoxygenated blood from the lungs and pumps it out to the body.

Heart, Right – ANATOMY – The portion of the heart that includes the right atria and right ventricle.
PHYSIOLOGY – The right heart receives the venous blood and pumps it to the lungs for reoxygenation.

Mitral Valve – ANATOMY – The mitral valve (also known as the bicuspid valve) has two cusps and is located between the left atrium and the left ventricle.
PHYSIOLOGY – The mitral valve prevents backflow of blood from the left ventricle back into the left atrium via its one-way valve function. The mitral valve's closure is strengthened by the papillary muscles and their chordae tendineae during the left ventricle's forceful contraction.

Papillary Muscle – ANATOMY – The intraventricular muscles that connect with the mitral and tricuspid valves via a chordae tendineae. PHYSIOLOGY – The papillary muscles contract at the same time as the ventricle, thus reinforcing the closure of the atrial inlet valve.

Pericardium – The pericardium is the double-layered serous membrane protecting the heart from friction as it beats.

Pulmonary Artery, Left – The major blood vessel transporting deoxygenated blood from the right ventricle to the left lobes of the lungs. Blood vessels with blood flow going away from the heart are termed arteries. Pulmonary arteries carry venous blood, the opposite of the rest of the arteries.

Pulmonary Artery, Right – The major blood vessel transporting deoxygenated blood from the right ventricle to the right lobes of the lungs. Blood vessels with blood flow going away from the heart are termed arteries. Pulmonary arteries carry venous blood, the opposite of the rest of the arteries.

Pulmonary Trunk – The short, large blood vessel connecting the right ventricle to the right and left pulmonary arteries.

Pulmonary Valve – ANATOMY – The pulmonary valve has three cusps and is located between the outlet of the right ventricle and the base of the pulmonary artery.
PHYSIOLOGY – The pulmonary valve prevents backflow of blood into the right ventricle from the pulmonary artery via its one-way valve function.

Pulmonary Vein, Left – The major blood vessel transporting oxygenated blood from the left lobes of the lungs to the left atrium. Blood vessels with blood flow going to the heart are termed veins. Pulmonary veins carry arterial blood, the opposite of the rest of the veins.

Pulmonary Vein, Right – The major blood vessel transporting oxygenated blood from the right lobes of the lungs to the left atrium. Blood vessels with blood flow going to the heart are termed veins. Pulmonary veins carry arterial blood, the opposite of the rest of the veins.

Superior Vena Cava – The major vein transporting deoxygenated blood from the upper body and head that empties into the right atrium.

Thoracic Aorta – The uppermost portion of the aorta that lies within the thoracic cavity.

Tricuspid Valve – ANATOMY – The tricuspid valve has three cusps and is located between the right atrium and the right ventricle. PHYSIOLOGY – The tricuspid valve prevents backflow of blood from the right ventricle back into the right atrium via its one-way valve function. The tricuspid valve's closure is strengthened by the papillary muscles and their chordae tendineae during the right ventricle's forceful contraction.

Continued on next page

© 2018 Channel Publishing, Ltd.

Educational Annotations | 2 – Heart and Great Vessels

Anatomy and Physiology Review of Heart and Great Vessels

BODY PART VALUES – 2 - HEART AND GREAT VESSELS

Continued from previous page

Ventricle, Left – ANATOMY – One of the two large chambers of the heart's four chambers. PHYSIOLOGY – The left ventricle pumps oxygenated blood from the heart into the aorta to be carried throughout the body.

Ventricle, Right – ANATOMY – One of the two large chambers of the heart's four chambers. PHYSIOLOGY – The right ventricle pumps deoxygenated blood from the heart to the lungs through the pulmonary arteries.

Ventricular Septum – The strong tissue wall that separates the left and right ventricles.

Anatomical Illustrations of Heart and Great Vessels

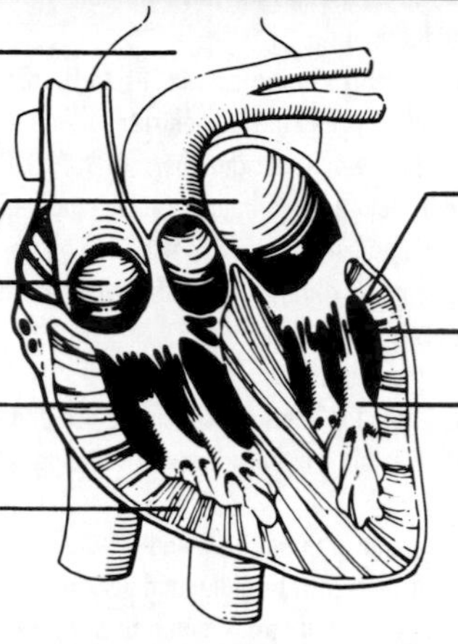

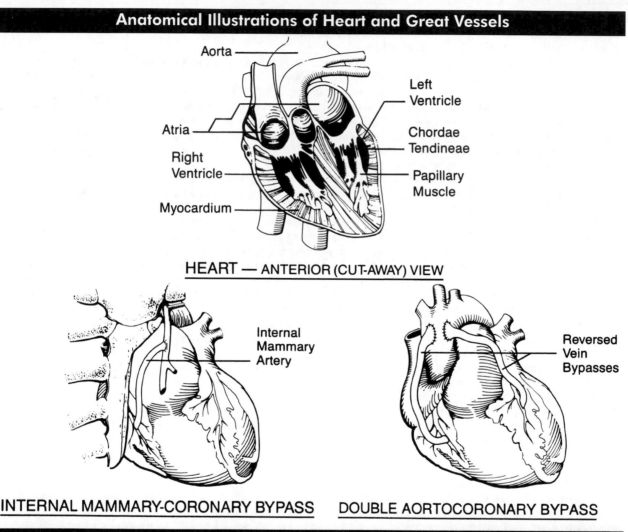

HEART — ANTERIOR (CUT-AWAY) VIEW

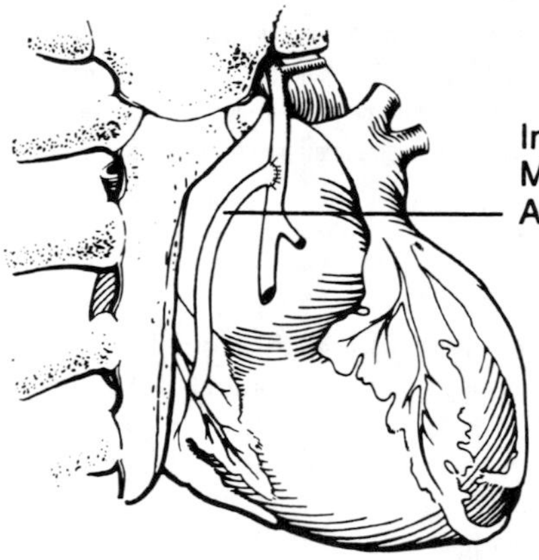

INTERNAL MAMMARY-CORONARY BYPASS

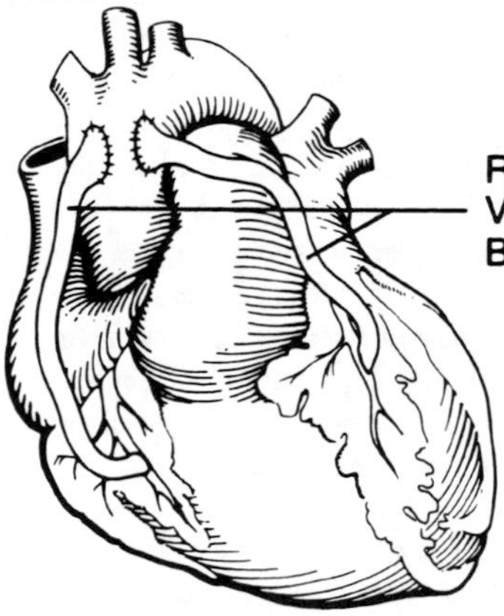

DOUBLE AORTOCORONARY BYPASS

Definitions of Common Procedures of Heart and Great Vessels

Aortocoronary artery bypass – The restoration of coronary artery blood flow by using a tubular graft (usually a saphenous vein) to bring blood from the aorta to the coronary artery that is distal to the blocked site.

Coronary artery stent – The widening of the coronary artery lumen by placing a stent (tubular supporting device) in the narrowed arterial site. The stent may or may not be coated in a drug-eluting substance.

Heart transplant – The removal of the end-staged diseased heart and replacement with a donor heart.

Internal mammary artery coronary artery bypass – The restoration of coronary artery blood flow by using the direct connection of an internal mammary artery to the coronary artery that is distal to the blocked site.

Intra-aortic balloon pump (IABP) – The computer-controlled inflatable circulatory assist device that is placed in the descending thoracic aorta. The balloon is inflated during diastole (heart not contracting and filling with blood) to increase cardiac output pressure and increase coronary blood flow.

MAZE procedure (Cox-MAZE) – The surgical cutting or destruction of atrial tissue to disrupt the electrical pathways and re-direct them through a maze-like pattern that creates only one path that the electrical impulse can take from the SA node to the AV node, which prevents the irregular electrical impulses of atrial fibrillation.

Continued on next page

© 2018 Channel Publishing, Ltd.

Educational Annotations | 2 – Heart and Great Vessels

Definitions of Common Procedures of Heart and Great Vessels

Continued from previous page

Occlusion of left atrial appendage – The surgical closure or blockage of the left atrial appendage (small pouch in muscle wall of the left atrium) to prevent blood clot formation in patients with atrial fibrillation.

Valve replacement – The replacement of a heart valve (aortic, mitral, pulmonary, or tricuspid) using a mechanical or bioprosthetic valve that replaces the entire valve.

Valvuloplasty – The restoration of the heart valve (aortic, mitral, pulmonary, or tricuspid) anatomy and/or function using a tissue graft or synthetic material, or using a balloon catheter.

AHA Coding Clinic® Reference Notations of Heart and Great Vessels

ROOT OPERATION SPECIFIC - 2 - HEART AND GREAT VESSELS

BYPASS - 1

Atrial balloon septostomy....AHA 17:4Q:p56
Bypass with pericardial patch of the pulmonary artery....AHA 16:4Q:p144
Coronary artery bypass graft, using greater saphenous vein ....AHA 14:3Q:p20
....AHA 14:1Q:p10
Coronary artery bypass graft, using internal mammary artery ....AHA 14:3Q:p8,20
Coronary artery bypass graft, using radial artery ....AHA 16:4Q:p82
Coronary bypass from internal mammary and aorta ....AHA 16:1Q:p27
Fontan completion stage II procedure....AHA 14:3Q:p29
Modified Blalock-Taussig shunt procedure....AHA 14:3Q:p3
....AHA 16:4Q:p102
Modified Warden procedure....AHA 16:4Q:p145
Norwood procedure with Sano shunt ....AHA 17:1Q:p19
Rastelli operation ....AHA 15:4Q:p22
Repair of anomalous pulmonary venous return....AHA 16:4Q:p108
Repair of truncus arteriosus ....AHA 15:4Q:p24
Replacement of pulmonary artery conduit....AHA 15:3Q:p16
Replacement of right ventricle (RV) to pulmonary artery conduit ....AHA 14:3Q:p30

CREATION - 4

Creation of a functional heart valve ....AHA 16:4Q:p101,104,106

DESTRUCTION - 5

Catheter ablation of peripulmonary veins to target the conduction pathway of left atrium ....AHA 14:4Q:p47
Catheter ablation of peripulmonary veins to target the conduction pathway of left atrium - Official Clarification ....AHA 16:3Q:p43
Modified left atrial MAZE procedure using ablation and AtrioClip® ....AHA 14:3Q:p20
Modified left atrial MAZE procedure using ablation and AtrioClip® - Official Clarification....AHA 16:3Q:p44
Photodynamic therapy of pericardium ....AHA 16:2Q:p17
Ventricular tachycardia ablation ....AHA 14:3Q:p19

DILATION - 7

Coronary angioplasty with unsuccessful stent placement....AHA 15:3Q:p10
Coronary artery bifurcation ....AHA 16:4Q:p86
Coronary artery bifurcation - Official Clarification ....AHA 18:2Q:p24
Corrective surgery for left ventricular outflow tract obstruction ....AHA 17:4Q:p32
Distinct coronary lesion sites treated....AHA 15:2Q:p3-5
Number of coronary artery stents ....AHA 16:4Q:p84
Orbital atherectomy and drug-eluting balloon angioplasty of coronary artery ....AHA 15:4Q:p13
Placement of pulmonary artery stent ....AHA 15:3Q:p16
Pulmonary valvotomy with commisurotomies ....AHA 16:1Q:p16
Restenosis of saphenous vein coronary artery bypass graft using a stent ....AHA 14:2Q:p4

DIVISION - 8

EXCISION - B

Resection of mitral valve leaflet with chordae tendineae transfer....AHA 17:1Q:p38
Wedge resection of mitral valve leaflet ....AHA 15:2Q:p.23

Continued on next page

© 2018 Channel Publishing, Ltd.

Educational Annotations | 2 – Heart and Great Vessels

AHA Coding Clinic® Reference Notations of Heart and Great Vessels

Continued from previous page

EXTIRPATION - C

Decalcification of mitral valve....AHA 16:2Q:p24

FRAGMENTATION - F

INSERTION - H

Exchange of tunneled hemodialysis catheter with chest port....AHA 15:4Q:p31
Insertion and removal of left atrial appendage device....AHA 17:4Q:p104
Insertion of CapSureFix Novus right atrial lead....AHA 18:2Q:p19
Insertion of central venous catheter though jugular vein into superior vena cava....AHA 15:4Q:p28
Insertion of central venous line ending in the cavoatrial junction....AHA 15:4Q:p28
Insertion of dialysis catheter ending in the cavoatrial junction....AHA 15:4Q:p29
Insertion of dual-lumen PICC line ending in the right atrial junction....AHA 15:4Q:p29
Insertion of heart assist device systems....AHA 16:4Q:p137
Insertion of heart assist systems....AHA 17:1Q:p10-12
Insertion of Impella® external heart assist device....AHA 17:4Q:p43,44
Insertion of infusion device into right atrium....AHA 17:2Q:p24
Insertion of infusion device into superior vena cava....AHA 15:2Q:p.33
Insertion of infusion device into superior vena cava....AHA 15:4Q:p14
Insertion of intracardiac pacemakers....AHA 16:4Q:p95
Insertion of leadless pacemaker....AHA 15:2Q:p.31
Insertion of Swan Ganz catheter for pressure monitoring....AHA 15:3Q:p35
Insertion of tunneled hemodialysis catheter into superior vena cava with port chest pocket....AHA 15:4Q:p30
Insertion of vascular access device in superior vena cava....AHA 17:4Q:p63
Placement of peripherally inserted central catheter (PICC line) into superior vena cava....AHA 13:3Q:p18
Removal with new insertion of jugular tunneled catheter in right atrium....AHA 16:2Q:p15

INSPECTION - J

MAP - K

OCCLUSION - L

Closure of patent ductus arteriosus....AHA 15:4Q:p23
Modified left atrial MAZE procedure using ablation and AtrioClip®....AHA 14:3Q:p20
Occlusion/ligation of pulmonary trunk and right pulmonary artery....AHA 17:4Q:p33
Occlusion of right pulmonary artery....AHA 16:2Q:p26
Rastelli procedure....AHA 16:4Q:p104
Resuscitative endovascular balloon occlusion of the aorta....AHA 17:4Q:p31

RELEASE - N

Release of myocardial bridge....AHA 17:4Q:p35
Widening of right ventricular outflow tract....AHA 14:3Q:p16

REMOVAL - P

Exchange of tunneled hemodialysis catheter with chest port....AHA 15:4Q:p31
Nonoperative removal of PICC line....AHA 16:3Q:p19
Removal of cardiac lead....AHA 15:3Q:p33
Removal of heart assist device systems....AHA 16:4Q:p137
Removal of heart assist systems....AHA 17:1Q:p10-12
Removal of intracardiac pacemakers....AHA 16:4Q:p95
Removal with new insertion of jugular tunneled catheter in right atrium....AHA 16:2Q:p15

REPAIR - Q

Division (repair) of double aortic arch....AHA 15:3Q:p16
Repair of atrial septal defect....AHA 15:4Q:p23
Sutureless repair of pulmonary vein stenosis....AHA 17:1Q:p18
Thoracic aortic valve repair (TAVR)....AHA 13:3Q:p26

Continued on next page

© 2018 Channel Publishing, Ltd.

Educational Annotations | 2 – Heart and Great Vessels

AHA Coding Clinic® Reference Notations of Heart and Great Vessels

Continued from previous page

REPLACEMENT - R

- Graft repair of thoracic aortic arch aneurysm ....AHA 14:1Q:p10
- Implantation of SynCardia total artificial heart ....AHA 17:1Q:p13
- Percutaneous transcatheter tricuspid valve replacement (see also new 2018 table approach value for Percutaneous) ....AHA 16:3Q:p32
- Percutaneous tricuspid valve implantation ....AHA 17:4Q:p56

REPOSITION - S

- Arterial switch procedure ....AHA 16:4Q:p103
- Correction surgery for transposition of great arteries ....AHA 15:4Q:p23

RESECTION - T

SUPPLEMENT - U

- Aortic root enlargement ....AHA 16:2Q:p26
- Closure of ventricular septal defect with Goretex® patch ....AHA 14:3Q:p16
- Enlargement of pulmonary artery and trunk ....AHA 16:2Q:p23
- Mitral valve ring annuloplasty ....AHA 15:2Q:p.23
- Pulmonary artery patch allograft ....AHA 15:3Q:p16
- Pulmonary homograft to the aortic arch ....AHA 17:1Q:p19
- Rastelli operation ....AHA 15:4Q:p22
- Repair of truncal valve ....AHA 15:4Q:p24
- Repair of ventricular septal defect....AHA 15:4Q:p24
- Right and left atrium patches using pericardial tissue ....AHA 17:3Q:p7

RESTRICTION - V

- Alfieri stitch procedure ....AHA 17:4Q:p35
- Branched/fenestrated endograft repair of aneurysms ....AHA 16:4Q:p89

REVISION - W

- Closure of paravalvular leak ....AHA 14:3Q:p31
- Repositioning of Impella short-term external heart assist device ....AHA 18:1Q:p17
- Reposition of dislocated pacemaker lead ....AHA 15:3Q:p32
- Revision of intracardiac pacemakers....AHA 16:4Q:p95

TRANSPLANTATION - Y

- Heart transplant....AHA 13:3Q:p18

© 2018 Channel Publishing, Ltd.

Educational Annotations | 2 – Heart and Great Vessels

Body Part Key Listings of Heart and Great Vessels

See also Body Part Key in Appendix C

Aortic annulus .... use Aortic Valve
Aortic arch .... use Thoracic Aorta, Ascending/Arch
Arterial canal (duct) .... use Pulmonary Artery, Left
Ascending aorta .... use Thoracic Aorta, Ascending/Arch
Atrioventricular node .... use Conduction Mechanism
Atrium dextrum cordis .... use Atrium, Right
Atrium pulmonale .... use Atrium, Left
Bicuspid valve .... use Mitral Valve
Botallo's duct .... use Pulmonary Artery, Left
Bundle of His .... use Conduction Mechanism
Bundle of Kent .... use Conduction Mechanism
Conus arteriosus .... use Ventricle, Right
Interatrial septum .... use Atrial Septum
Interventricular septum .... use Ventricular Septum
Left atrioventricular valve .... use Mitral Valve
Left auricular appendix .... use Atrium, Left
Left coronary sulcus .... use Heart, Left
Left inferior pulmonary vein .... use Pulmonary Vein, Left
Left superior pulmonary vein .... use Pulmonary Vein, Left
Mitral annulus .... use Mitral Valve
Obtuse margin .... use Heart, Left
Precava .... use Superior Vena Cava
Pulmoaortic canal .... use Pulmonary Artery, Left
Pulmonary annulus .... use Pulmonary Valve
Pulmonic valve .... use Pulmonary Valve
Right atrioventricular valve .... use Tricuspid Valve
Right auricular appendix .... use Atrium, Right
Right coronary sulcus .... use Heart, Right
Right inferior pulmonary vein .... use Pulmonary Vein, Right
Right superior pulmonary vein .... use Pulmonary Vein, Right
Sinoatrial node .... use Conduction Mechanism
Sinus venosus .... use Atrium, Right
Tricuspid annulus .... use Tricuspid Valve

Device Key Listings of Heart and Great Vessels

See also Device Key in Appendix D

3f (Aortic) Bioprosthesis valve .... use Zooplastic Tissue in Heart and Great Vessels
AbioCor® Total Replacement Heart .... use Synthetic Substitute
ACUITY™ Steerable Lead .... use Cardiac Lead, Pacemaker for Insertion in Heart and Great Vessels
.... use Cardiac Lead, Defibrillator for Insertion in Heart and Great Vessels
AMPLATZER® Muscular VSD Occluder .... use Synthetic Substitute
Annuloplasty ring .... use Synthetic Substitute
AtriClip LAA Exclusion System .... use Extraluminal Device
Attain Ability® lead .... use Cardiac Lead, Pacemaker for Insertion in Heart and Great Vessels
.... use Cardiac Lead, Defibrillator for Insertion in Heart and Great Vessels
Attain StarFix® (OTW) lead .... use Cardiac Lead, Pacemaker for Insertion in Heart and Great Vessels
.... use Cardiac Lead, Defibrillator for Insertion in Heart and Great Vessels
Autograft .... use Autologous Tissue Substitute
Autologous artery graft .... use Autologous Arterial Tissue in Heart and Great Vessels
Autologous vein graft .... use Autologous Venous Tissue in Heart and Great Vessels
Berlin Heart Ventricular Assist Device .... use Implantable Heart Assist System in Heart and Great Vessels
Biventricular external heart assist system .... use Short-term External Heart Assist System in Heart and Great Vessels
Bovine pericardial valve .... use Zooplastic Tissue in Heart and Great Vessels
Bovine pericardium graft .... use Zooplastic Tissue in Heart and Great Vessels
BVS 5000 Ventricular Assist Device .... use Short-term External Heart Assist System in Heart and Great Vessels
Cardiac contractility modulation lead .... use Cardiac Lead in Heart and Great Vessels
Cardiac event recorder .... use Monitoring Device
Cardiac resynchronization therapy (CRT) lead .... use Cardiac Lead, Pacemaker for Insertion in Heart and Great Vessels
.... use Cardiac Lead, Defibrillator for Insertion in Heart and Great Vessels
CardioMEMS® pressure sensor .... use Monitoring Device, Pressure Sensor for Insertion in Heart and Great Vessels
Centrimag® Blood Pump .... use Short-term External Heart Assist System in Heart and Great Vessels
CoAxia NeuroFlo catheter .... use Intraluminal Device
Contegra Pulmonary Valved Conduit .... use Zooplastic Tissue in Heart and Great Vessels
CoreValve transcatheter aortic valve .... use Zooplastic Tissue in Heart and Great Vessels
Corox (OTW) Bipolar Lead .... use Cardiac Lead, Pacemaker for Insertion in Heart and Great Vessels
.... use Cardiac Lead, Defibrillator for Insertion in Heart and Great Vessels
CYPHER® Stent .... use Intraluminal Device, Drug-eluting in Heart and Great Vessels
DeBakey Left Ventricular Assist Device .... use Implantable Heart Assist System in Heart and Great Vessels
Driver stent (RX) (OTW) .... use Intraluminal Device
DuraHeart Left Ventricular Assist System .... use Implantable Heart Assist System in Heart and Great Vessels
Durata® Defibrillation Lead .... use Cardiac Lead, Defibrillator for Insertion in Heart and Great Vessels
Endeavor® (III) (IV) (Sprint) Zotarolimus-eluting Coronary Stent System .... use Intraluminal Device, Drug-eluting in Heart and Great Vessels
EndoSure® sensor .... use Monitoring Device, Pressure Sensor for Insertion in Heart and Great Vessels

Continued on next page

© 2018 Channel Publishing, Ltd.

Educational Annotations | 2 – Heart and Great Vessels

Device Key Listings of Heart and Great Vessels

Continued from previous page

ENDOTAK RELIANCE® (G) Defibrillation Lead ....use Cardiac Lead, Defibrillator for Insertion in Heart and Great Vessels
Epic™ Stented Tissue Valve (aortic) ....use Zooplastic Tissue in Heart and Great Vessels
Everolimus-eluting coronary stent ....use Intraluminal Device, Drug-eluting in Heart and Great Vessels
Freestyle (Stentless) Aortic Root Bioprosthesis ....use Zooplastic Tissue in Heart and Great Vessels
Hancock Bioprosthesis (aortic) (mitral) valve ....use Zooplastic Tissue in Heart and Great Vessels
Hancock Bioprosthetic Valved Conduit ....use Zooplastic Tissue in Heart and Great Vessels
HeartMate 3™ Left Ventricular Assist Device (LVAD) ....use Implantable Heart Assist System in Heart and Great Vessels
HeartMate II® Left Ventricular Assist Device (LVAD) ....use Implantable Heart Assist System in Heart and Great Vessels
HeartMate XVE® Left Ventricular Assist Device (LVAD) ....use Implantable Heart Assist System in Heart and Great Vessels
Impella® Heart Pump ....use Short-term External Heart Assist System in Heart and Great Vessels
Melody® transcatheter pulmonary valve ....use Zooplastic Tissue in Heart and Great Vessels
Micro-Driver stent (RX) (OTW) ....use Intraluminal Device
MicroMed HeartAssist ....use Implantable Heart Assist System in Heart and Great Vessels
MitraClip valve repair system ....use Synthetic Substitute
Mitroflow® Aortic Pericardial Heart Valve ....use Zooplastic Tissue in Heart and Great Vessels
Mosaic Bioprosthesis (aortic) (mitral) valve ....use Zooplastic Tissue in Heart and Great Vessels
MULTI-LINK (VISION) (MINI-VISION) (ULTRA) Coronary Stent System ....use Intraluminal Device
Novacor Left Ventricular Assist Device ....use Implantable Heart Assist System in Heart and Great Vessels
Open Pivot Aortic Valve Graft (AVG) ....use Synthetic Substitute
Open Pivot (mechanical) valve ....use Synthetic Substitute
Paclitaxel-eluting coronary stent ....use Intraluminal Device, Drug-eluting in Heart and Great Vessels
Peripherally inserted central catheter (PICC) ....use Infusion Device
Porcine (bioprosthetic) valve ....use Zooplastic Tissue in Heart and Great Vessels
SAPIEN transcatheter aortic valve ....use Zooplastic Tissue in Heart and Great Vessels
Sirolimus-eluting coronary stent ....use Intraluminal Device, Drug-eluting in Heart and Great Vessels
SJM Biocor® Stented Valve System ....use Zooplastic Tissue in Heart and Great Vessels
Stent, intraluminal (cardiovascular) (gastrointestinal) (hepatobiliary) (urinary) ....use Intraluminal Device
Stented tissue valve ....use Zooplastic Tissue in Heart and Great Vessels
SynCardia Total Artificial Heart ....use Synthetic Substitute
TandemHeart® System ....use Short-term External Heart Assist System in Heart and Great Vessels
TAXUS® Liberté® Paclitaxel-eluting Coronary Stent System ....use Intraluminal Device, Drug-eluting in Heart and Great Vessels
Thoratec IVAD (Implantable Ventricular Assist Device) ....use Implantable Heart Assist System in Heart and Great Vessels
Thoratec Paracorporeal Ventricular Assist Device ....use Short-term External Heart Assist System in Heart and Great Vessels
Tissue bank graft ....use Nonautologous Tissue Substitute
Total artificial (replacement) heart ....use Synthetic Substitute
Trifecta™ Valve (aortic) ....use Zooplastic Tissue in Heart and Great Vessels
Valiant Thoracic Stent Graft ....use Intraluminal Device
Xenograft ....use Zooplastic Tissue in Heart and Great Vessels
XIENCE Everolimus Eluting Coronary Stent System ....use Intraluminal Device, Drug-eluting in Heart and Great Vessels
Zenith TX2® TAA Endovascular Graft ....use Intraluminal Device
Zotarolimus-eluting coronary stent ....use Intraluminal Device, Drug-eluting in Heart and Great Vessels

© 2018 Channel Publishing, Ltd.

Educational Annotations | 2 – Heart and Great Vessels

Device Aggregation Table Listings of Heart and Great Vessels

See also Device Aggregation Table in Appendix E

Specific Device	For Operation	In Body System	General Device
Autologous Arterial Tissue	All applicable	Heart and Great Vessels	Autologous Tissue Substitute
Autologous Venous Tissue	All applicable	Heart and Great Vessels	Autologous Tissue Substitute
Cardiac Lead, Defibrillator	Insertion	Heart and Great Vessels	Cardiac Lead
Cardiac Lead, Pacemaker	Insertion	Heart and Great Vessels	Cardiac Lead
Intraluminal Device, Branched or Fenestrated, One or Two Arteries	All applicable	Heart and Great Vessels	Intraluminal Device
Intraluminal Device, Branched or Fenestrated, Three or More Arteries	All applicable	Heart and Great Vessels	Intraluminal Device
Intraluminal Device, Drug-eluting	All applicable	Heart and Great Vessels	Intraluminal Device
Intraluminal Device, Drug-eluting, Four or More	All applicable	Heart and Great Vessels	Intraluminal Device
Intraluminal Device, Drug-eluting, Three	All applicable	Heart and Great Vessels	Intraluminal Device
Intraluminal Device, Drug-eluting, Two	All applicable	Heart and Great Vessels	Intraluminal Device
Intraluminal Device, Four or More	All applicable	Heart and Great Vessels	Intraluminal Device
Intraluminal Device, Radioactive	All applicable	Heart and Great Vessels	Intraluminal Device
Intraluminal Device, Three	All applicable	Heart and Great Vessels	Intraluminal Device
Intraluminal Device, Two	All applicable	Heart and Great Vessels	Intraluminal Device
Monitoring Device, Pressure Sensor	Insertion	Heart and Great Vessels	Monitoring Device

© 2018 Channel Publishing, Ltd.

Educational Annotations | 2 – Heart and Great Vessels

Coding Notes of Heart and Great Vessels

Body System Relevant Coding Guidelines

Bypass procedures

B3.6b

Coronary artery bypass procedures are coded differently than other bypass procedures as described in the previous guideline. Rather than identifying the body part bypassed from, the body part identifies the number of coronary arteries bypassed to, and the qualifier specifies the vessel bypassed from.

Example: Aortocoronary artery bypass of the left anterior descending coronary artery and the obtuse marginal coronary artery is classified in the body part axis of classification as two coronary arteries, and the qualifier specifies the aorta as the body part bypassed from.

B3.6c

If multiple coronary arteries are bypassed, a separate procedure is coded for each coronary artery that uses a different device and/or qualifier.

Example: Aortocoronary artery bypass and internal mammary coronary artery bypass are coded separately.

Coronary arteries

B4.4

The coronary arteries are classified as a single body part that is further specified by number of arteries treated. One procedure code specifying multiple arteries is used when the same procedure is performed, including the same device and qualifier values.

Examples: Angioplasty of two distinct coronary arteries with placement of two stents is coded as Dilation of Coronary Artery, Two Arteries with Two Intraluminal Devices.

Angioplasty of two distinct coronary arteries, one with stent placed and one without, is coded separately as Dilation of Coronary Artery, One Artery with Intraluminal Device, and Dilation of Coronary Artery, One Artery with no device.

Device, General Guidelines

B6.1a

A device is coded only if a device remains after the procedure is completed. If no device remains, the device value No Device is coded. In limited root operations, the classification provides the qualifier values Temporary and Intraoperative, for specific procedures involving clinically significant devices, where the purpose of the device is to be utilized for a brief duration during the procedure or current inpatient stay. If a device that is intended to remain after the procedure is completed requires removal before the end of the operative episode in which it was inserted (for example, the device size is inadequate or a complication occurs), both the insertion and removal of the device should be coded.

© 2018 Channel Publishing, Ltd.

1ST - 0 Medical and Surgical
2ND - 2 Heart and Great Vessels
3RD - 1 BYPASS

TUBULAR GROUP: Bypass, Dilation, Occlusion, Restriction
Root Operations that alter the diameter/route of a tubular body part.
BYPASS: Altering the route of passage of the contents of a tubular body part.

Explanation: Rerouting contents to a downstream part ... with or without the use of a device ...
Examples: Coronary artery bypass – CMS Ex: Coronary artery bypass

Body Part – 4TH	Approach – 5TH	Device – 6TH	Qualifier – 7TH
0 Coronary Artery, One Artery 1 Coronary Artery, Two Arteries 2 Coronary Artery, Three Arteries 3 Coronary Artery, Four or More Arteries	0 Open	8 Zooplastic tissue 9 Autologous venous tissue A Autologous arterial tissue J Synthetic substitute K Nonautologous tissue substitute	3 Coronary Artery 8 Internal Mammary, Right 9 Internal Mammary, Left C Thoracic Artery F Abdominal Artery W Aorta
0 Coronary Artery, One Artery 1 Coronary Artery, Two Arteries 2 Coronary Artery, Three Arteries 3 Coronary Artery, Four or More Arteries	0 Open	Z No device	3 Coronary Artery 8 Internal Mammary, Right 9 Internal Mammary, Left C Thoracic Artery F Abdominal Artery
0 Coronary Artery, One Artery 1 Coronary Artery, Two Arteries 2 Coronary Artery, Three Arteries 3 Coronary Artery, Four or More Arteries	3 Percutaneous	4 Drug-eluting intraluminal device D Intraluminal device	4 Coronary Vein
0 Coronary Artery, One Artery 1 Coronary Artery, Two Arteries 2 Coronary Artery, Three Arteries 3 Coronary Artery, Four or More Arteries	4 Percutaneous endoscopic	4 Drug-eluting intraluminal device D Intraluminal device	4 Coronary Vein
0 Coronary Artery, One Artery 1 Coronary Artery, Two Arteries 2 Coronary Artery, Three Arteries 3 Coronary Artery, Four or More Arteries	4 Percutaneous endoscopic	8 Zooplastic tissue 9 Autologous venous tissue A Autologous arterial tissue J Synthetic substitute K Nonautologous tissue substitute	3 Coronary Artery 8 Internal Mammary, Right 9 Internal Mammary, Left C Thoracic Artery F Abdominal Artery W Aorta
0 Coronary Artery, One Artery 1 Coronary Artery, Two Arteries 2 Coronary Artery, Three Arteries 3 Coronary Artery, Four or More Arteries	4 Percutaneous endoscopic	Z No device	3 Coronary Artery 8 Internal Mammary, Right 9 Internal Mammary, Left C Thoracic Artery F Abdominal Artery
6 Atrium, Right	0 Open 4 Percutaneous endoscopic	8 Zooplastic tissue 9 Autologous venous tissue A Autologous arterial tissue J Synthetic substitute K Nonautologous tissue substitute	P Pulmonary Trunk Q Pulmonary Artery, Right R Pulmonary Artery, Left
6 Atrium, Right	0 Open 4 Percutaneous endoscopic	Z No device	7 Atrium, Left P Pulmonary Trunk Q Pulmonary Artery, Right R Pulmonary Artery, Left
6 Atrium, Right	3 Percutaneous	Z No device	7 Atrium, Left
7 Atrium, Left V Superior Vena Cava	0 Open 4 Percutaneous endoscopic	8 Zooplastic tissue 9 Autologous venous tissue A Autologous arterial tissue J Synthetic substitute K Nonautologous tissue substitute Z No device	P Pulmonary Trunk Q Pulmonary Artery, Right R Pulmonary Artery, Left S Pulmonary Vein, Right T Pulmonary Vein, Left U Pulmonary Vein, Confluence

continued ⇨

© 2018 Channel Publishing, Ltd.

0 2 1 BYPASS – *continued*

Body Part – 4TH	Approach – 5TH	Device – 6TH	Qualifier – 7TH
K Ventricle, Right L Ventricle, Left	0 Open 4 Percutaneous endoscopic	8 Zooplastic tissue 9 Autologous venous tissue A Autologous arterial tissue J Synthetic substitute K Nonautologous tissue substitute	P Pulmonary Trunk Q Pulmonary Artery, Right R Pulmonary Artery, Left
K Ventricle, Right L Ventricle, Left	0 Open 4 Percutaneous endoscopic	Z No device	5 Coronary Circulation 8 Internal Mammary, Right 9 Internal Mammary, Left C Thoracic Artery F Abdominal Artery P Pulmonary Trunk Q Pulmonary Artery, Right R Pulmonary Artery, Left W Aorta
P Pulmonary Trunk Q Pulmonary Artery, Right R Pulmonary Artery, Left	0 Open 4 Percutaneous endoscopic	8 Zooplastic tissue 9 Autologous venous tissue A Autologous arterial tissue J Synthetic substitute K Nonautologous tissue substitute Z No device	A Innominate Artery B Subclavian D Carotid
W Thoracic Aorta, Descending	0 Open	8 Zooplastic tissue 9 Autologous venous tissue A Autologous arterial tissue J Synthetic substitute K Nonautologous tissue substitute	B Subclavian D Carotid F Abdominal Artery G Axillary Artery H Brachial Artery P Pulmonary Trunk Q Pulmonary Artery, Right R Pulmonary Artery, Left V Lower Extremity Artery
W Thoracic Aorta, Descending	0 Open	Z No device	B Subclavian D Carotid P Pulmonary Trunk Q Pulmonary Artery, Right R Pulmonary Artery, Left
W Thoracic Aorta, Descending	4 Percutaneous endoscopic	8 Zooplastic tissue 9 Autologous venous tissue A Autologous arterial tissue J Synthetic substitute K Nonautologous tissue substitute Z No device	B Subclavian D Carotid P Pulmonary Trunk Q Pulmonary Artery, Right R Pulmonary Artery, Left
X Thoracic Aorta, Ascending/Arch	0 Open 4 Percutaneous endoscopic	8 Zooplastic tissue 9 Autologous venous tissue A Autologous arterial tissue J Synthetic substitute K Nonautologous tissue substitute Z No device	B Subclavian D Carotid P Pulmonary Trunk Q Pulmonary Artery, Right R Pulmonary Artery, Left

© 2018 Channel Publishing, Ltd.

1ST - 0 Medical and Surgical
2ND - 2 Heart and Great Vessels
3RD - 4 CREATION

OTHER OBJECTIVES GROUP: (Alteration), Creation, (Fusion)
Root Operations that define other objectives.

CREATION: Putting in or on biological or synthetic material to form a new body part that to the extent possible replicates the anatomic structure or function of an absent body part.

Explanation: Gender reassignment surgery and corrective procedures for congenital anomalies
Examples: Creation aortic valve – CMS Ex: Creation of vagina in male

Body Part – 4TH	Approach – 5TH	Device – 6TH	Qualifier – 7TH
F Aortic Valve	0 Open	7 Autologous tissue substitute 8 Zooplastic tissue J Synthetic substitute K Nonautologous tissue substitute	J Truncal Valve
G Mitral Valve J Tricuspid Valve	0 Open	7 Autologous tissue substitute 8 Zooplastic tissue J Synthetic substitute K Nonautologous tissue substitute	2 Common Atrioventricular Valve

1ST - 0 Medical and Surgical
2ND - 2 Heart and Great Vessels
3RD - 5 DESTRUCTION

EXCISION GROUP: Excision, Resection, Destruction, (Extraction), (Detachment)
Root Operations that take out some or all of a body part.

DESTRUCTION: Physical eradication of all or a portion of a body part by the direct use of energy, force, or a destructive agent.

Explanation: None of the body part is physically taken out
Examples: Atrioventricular node ablation – CMS Ex: Fulguration of rectal polyp

Body Part – 4TH			Approach – 5TH	Device – 6TH	Qualifier – 7TH
4 Coronary Vein 5 Atrial Septum 6 Atrium, Right 8 Conduction Mechanism 9 Chordae Tendineae D Papillary Muscle F Aortic Valve G Mitral Valve H Pulmonary Valve	J Tricuspid Valve K Ventricle, Right L Ventricle, Left M Ventricular Septum N Pericardium P Pulmonary Trunk Q Pulmonary Artery, Right	R Pulmonary Artery, Left S Pulmonary Vein, Right T Pulmonary Vein, Left V Superior Vena Cava W Thoracic Aorta, Descending X Thoracic Aorta, Ascending/Arch	0 Open 3 Percutaneous 4 Percutaneous endoscopic	Z No device	Z No qualifier
7 Atrium, Left			0 Open 3 Percutaneous 4 Percutaneous endoscopic	Z No device	K Left Atrial Appendage Z No qualifier

© 2018 Channel Publishing, Ltd.

1ST - 0 Medical and Surgical
2ND - 2 Heart and Great Vessels
3RD - 7 DILATION

TUBULAR GROUP: Bypass, Dilation, Occlusion, Restriction
Root Operations that alter the diameter/route of a tubular body part.
DILATION: Expanding an orifice or the lumen of a tubular body part.

Explanation: Accomplished by stretching or cutting ... tubular body part or orifice ...
Examples: PTCA coronary artery – CMS Ex: Percutaneous transluminal angioplasty

Body Part – 4TH	Approach – 5TH	Device – 6TH	Qualifier – 7TH
0 Coronary Artery, One Artery 1 Coronary Artery, Two Arteries 2 Coronary Artery, Three Arteries 3 Coronary Artery, Four or More Arteries	0 Open 3 Percutaneous 4 Percutaneous endoscopic	4 Drug-eluting intraluminal device 5 Drug-eluting intraluminal device, two 6 Drug-eluting intraluminal device, three 7 Drug-eluting intraluminal device, four or more D Intraluminal device E Intraluminal device, two F Intraluminal device, three G Intraluminal device, four or more T Intraluminal device, radioactive Z No device	6 Bifurcation Z No qualifier
F Aortic Valve G Mitral Valve H Pulmonary Valve J Tricuspid Valve K Ventricle, Right L Ventricle, Left P Pulmonary Trunk Q Pulmonary Artery, Right S Pulmonary Vein, Right T Pulmonary Vein, Left V Superior Vena Cava W Thoracic Aorta, Descending X Thoracic Aorta, Ascending/Arch	0 Open 3 Percutaneous 4 Percutaneous endoscopic	4 Drug-eluting intraluminal device D Intraluminal device Z No device	Z No qualifier
R Pulmonary Artery, Left	0 Open 3 Percutaneous 4 Percutaneous endoscopic	4 Drug-eluting intraluminal device D Intraluminal device Z No device	T Ductus Arteriosus Z No qualifier

1ST - 0 Medical and Surgical
2ND - 2 Heart and Great Vessels
3RD - 8 DIVISION

DIVISION GROUP: Division, Release
Root Operations involving cutting or separation only.
DIVISION: Cutting into a body part, without draining fluids and/or gases from the body part, in order to separate or transect a body part.

Explanation: All or a portion of the body part is separated into two or more portions
Examples: Division bundle of HIS – CMS Ex: Spinal cordotomy

Body Part – 4TH	Approach – 5TH	Device – 6TH	Qualifier – 7TH
8 Conduction Mechanism 9 Chordae Tendineae D Papillary Muscle	0 Open 3 Percutaneous 4 Percutaneous endoscopic	Z No device	Z No qualifier

© 2018 Channel Publishing, Ltd.

1ST - 0 Medical and Surgical
2ND - 2 Heart and Great Vessels
3RD - B **EXCISION**

EXCISION GROUP: Excision, Resection, Destruction, (Extraction), (Detachment)
Root Operations that take out some or all of a body part.
EXCISION: Cutting out or off, without replacement, a portion of a body part.

Explanation: Qualifier "X Diagnostic" indicates excision procedures that are biopsies
Examples: Pericardial biopsy – CMS Ex: Liver biopsy

Body Part – 4TH	Approach – 5TH	Device – 6TH	Qualifier – 7TH
4 Coronary Vein 5 Atrial Septum 6 Atrium, Right 8 Conduction Mechanism 9 Chordae Tendineae D Papillary Muscle F Aortic Valve G Mitral Valve H Pulmonary Valve J Tricuspid Valve K Ventricle, Right NC* L Ventricle, Left NC* M Ventricular Septum N Pericardium P Pulmonary Trunk Q Pulmonary Artery, Right R Pulmonary Artery, Left S Pulmonary Vein, Right T Pulmonary Vein, Left V Superior Vena Cava W Thoracic Aorta, Descending X Thoracic Aorta, Ascending/Arch	0 Open 3 Percutaneous 4 Percutaneous endoscopic	Z No device	X Diagnostic Z No qualifier
7 Atrium, Left	0 Open 3 Percutaneous 4 Percutaneous endoscopic	Z No device	K Left Atrial Appendage X Diagnostic Z No qualifier

NC* – Some procedures are considered non-covered by Medicare. See current Medicare Code Editor for details.

1ST - 0 Medical and Surgical
2ND - 2 Heart and Great Vessels
3RD - C **EXTIRPATION**

DRAINAGE GROUP: (Drainage), Extirpation, Fragmentation
Root Operations that take out solids/fluids/gases from a body part.
EXTIRPATION: Taking or cutting out solid matter from a body part.

Explanation: Abnormal byproduct or foreign body ...
Examples: Pulmonary artery thrombectomy – CMS Ex: Thrombectomy

Body Part – 4TH	Approach – 5TH	Device – 6TH	Qualifier – 7TH
0 Coronary Artery, One Artery 1 Coronary Artery, Two Arteries 2 Coronary Artery, Three Arteries 3 Coronary Artery, Four or More Arteries	0 Open 3 Percutaneous 4 Percutaneous endoscopic	Z No device	6 Bifurcation Z No qualifier
4 Coronary Vein 5 Atrial Septum 6 Atrium, Right 7 Atrium, Left 8 Conduction Mechanism 9 Chordae Tendineae D Papillary Muscle F Aortic Valve G Mitral Valve H Pulmonary Valve J Tricuspid Valve K Ventricle, Right L Ventricle, Left M Ventricular Septum N Pericardium P Pulmonary Trunk Q Pulmonary Artery, Right R Pulmonary Artery, Left S Pulmonary Vein, Right T Pulmonary Vein, Left V Superior Vena Cava W Thoracic Aorta, Descending X Thoracic Aorta, Ascending/Arch	0 Open 3 Percutaneous 4 Percutaneous endoscopic	Z No device	Z No qualifier

1ST - 0 Medical and Surgical
2ND - 2 Heart and Great Vessels
3RD - F **FRAGMENTATION**

DRAINAGE GROUP: (Drainage), Extirpation, Fragmentation
Root Operations that take out solids/fluids/gases from a body part.
FRAGMENTATION: Breaking solid matter in a body part into pieces.

Explanation: Pieces are not taken out during the procedure ...
Examples: Pulverization pericardial calcifications – CMS Ex: Extracorporeal shockwave lithotripsy

Body Part – 4TH	Approach – 5TH	Device – 6TH	Qualifier – 7TH
N Pericardium	0 Open 3 Percutaneous 4 Percutaneous endoscopic X External NC*	Z No device	Z No qualifier

NC* – Non-covered by Medicare. See current Medicare Code Editor for details.

© 2018 Channel Publishing, Ltd.

1ST - 0 Medical and Surgical
2ND - 2 Heart and Great Vessels
3RD - H INSERTION

DEVICE GROUP: (Change), Insertion, Removal, Replacement, Revision, Supplement
Root Operations that always involve a device.

INSERTION: Putting in a nonbiological appliance that monitors, assists, performs, or prevents a physiological function but does not physically take the place of a body part.

Explanation: None
Examples: Insertion pacemaker lead – CMS Ex: Insertion of central venous catheter

Body Part – 4TH	Approach – 5TH	Device – 6TH	Qualifier – 7TH
4 Coronary Vein 6 Atrium, Right 7 Atrium, Left K Ventricle, Right L Ventricle, Left	0 Open 3 Percutaneous 4 Percutaneous endoscopic	0 Monitoring device, pressure sensor 2 Monitoring device 3 Infusion device D Intraluminal device J Cardiac lead, pacemaker K Cardiac lead, defibrillator M Cardiac lead N Intracardiac pacemaker Y Other device	Z No qualifier
A Heart NC*LC*	0 Open 3 Percutaneous 4 Percutaneous endoscopic	Q Implantable heart assist system Y Other device	Z No qualifier
A Heart	0 Open 3 Percutaneous 4 Percutaneous endoscopic	R Short-term external heart assist system	J Intraoperative S Biventricular Z No qualifier
N Pericardium	0 Open 3 Percutaneous 4 Percutaneous endoscopic	0 Monitoring device, pressure sensor 2 Monitoring device J Cardiac lead, pacemaker K Cardiac lead, defibrillator M Cardiac lead Y Other device	Z No qualifier
P Pulmonary Trunk Q Pulmonary Artery, Right R Pulmonary Artery, Left S Pulmonary Vein, Right T Pulmonary Vein, Left V Superior Vena Cava W Thoracic Aorta, Descending	0 Open 3 Percutaneous 4 Percutaneous endoscopic	0 Monitoring device, pressure sensor 2 Monitoring device 3 Infusion device D Intraluminal device Y Other device	Z No qualifier
X Thoracic Aorta, Ascending/Arch	0 Open 3 Percutaneous 4 Percutaneous endoscopic	0 Monitoring device, pressure sensor 2 Monitoring device 3 Infusion device D Intraluminal device	Z No qualifier

NC*LC* – Some procedures are considered non-covered or limited coverage by Medicare. See current Medicare Code Editor for details.

1ST - 0 Medical and Surgical
2ND - 2 Heart and Great Vessels
3RD - J INSPECTION

EXAMINATION GROUP: Inspection, Map
Root Operations involving examination only.

INSPECTION: Visually and/or manually exploring a body part.

Explanation: Direct or instrumental visualization ...
Examples: Thoracoscopic visualization heart – CMS Ex: Exploratory laparotomy

Body Part – 4TH	Approach – 5TH	Device – 6TH	Qualifier – 7TH
A Heart Y Great Vessel	0 Open 3 Percutaneous 4 Percutaneous endoscopic	Z No device	Z No qualifier

© 2018 Channel Publishing, Ltd.

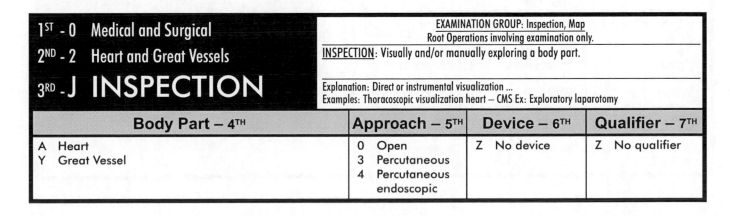

1ST - 0 Medical and Surgical
2ND - 2 Heart and Great Vessels
3RD - K MAP

EXAMINATION GROUP: Inspection, Map
Root Operations involving examination only.

MAP: Locating the route of passage of electrical impulses and/or locating functional areas in a body part.

Explanation: Applicable only to the cardiac conduction mechanism and the central nervous system
Examples: Cardiac mapping – CMS Ex: Cardiac mapping

Body Part – 4TH	Approach – 5TH	Device – 6TH	Qualifier – 7TH
8 Conduction Mechanism	0 Open 3 Percutaneous 4 Percutaneous endoscopic	Z No device	Z No qualifier

1ST - 0 Medical and Surgical
2ND - 2 Heart and Great Vessels
3RD - L OCCLUSION

TUBULAR GROUP: Bypass, Dilation, Occlusion, Restriction
Root Operations that alter the diameter/route of a tubular body part.

OCCLUSION: Completely closing an orifice or the lumen of a tubular body part.

Explanation: The orifice can be a natural orifice or an artificially created orifice
Examples: Suture closure left atrial appendage – CMS Ex: Fallopian tube ligation

Body Part – 4TH	Approach – 5TH	Device – 6TH	Qualifier – 7TH
7 Atrium, Left	0 Open 3 Percutaneous 4 Percutaneous endoscopic	C Extraluminal device D Intraluminal device Z No device	K Left Atrial Appendage
H Pulmonary Valve P Pulmonary Trunk Q Pulmonary Artery, Right S Pulmonary Vein, Right T Pulmonary Vein, Left V Superior Vena Cava	0 Open 3 Percutaneous 4 Percutaneous endoscopic	C Extraluminal device D Intraluminal device Z No device	Z No qualifier
R Pulmonary Artery, Left	0 Open 3 Percutaneous 4 Percutaneous endoscopic	C Extraluminal device D Intraluminal device Z No device	T Ductus Arteriosus Z No qualifier
W Thoracic Aorta, Descending	3 Percutaneous	D Intraluminal device	J Temporary

HEART & GREAT V. 0 2 K

1ST - 0 Medical and Surgical
2ND - 2 Heart and Great Vessels
3RD - N RELEASE

DIVISION GROUP: Division, Release
Root Operations involving cutting or separation only.

RELEASE: Freeing a body part from an abnormal physical constraint by cutting or by the use of force.

Explanation: Some of the restraining tissue may be taken out but none of the body part is taken out
Examples: Mitral valvulotomy fused leaflets – CMS Ex: Carpal tunnel release

Body Part – 4TH	Approach – 5TH	Device – 6TH	Qualifier – 7TH
0 Coronary Artery, One Artery 1 Coronary Artery, Two Arteries 2 Coronary Artery, Three Arteries 3 Coronary Artery, Four or More Arteries 4 Coronary Vein 5 Atrial Septum 6 Atrium, Right 7 Atrium, Left 8 Conduction Mechanism 9 Chordae Tendineae D Papillary Muscle F Aortic Valve G Mitral Valve H Pulmonary Valve J Tricuspid Valve K Ventricle, Right L Ventricle, Left M Ventricular Septum N Pericardium P Pulmonary Trunk Q Pulmonary Artery, Right R Pulmonary Artery, Left S Pulmonary Vein, Right T Pulmonary Vein, Left V Superior Vena Cava W Thoracic Aorta, Descending X Thoracic Aorta, Ascending/Arch	0 Open 3 Percutaneous 4 Percutaneous endoscopic	Z No device	Z No qualifier

© 2018 Channel Publishing, Ltd.

1ST - 0 Medical and Surgical
2ND - 2 Heart and Great Vessels
3RD - P REMOVAL

DEVICE GROUP: (Change), Insertion, Removal, Replacement, Revision, Supplement
Root Operations that always involve a device.

REMOVAL: Taking out or off a device from a body part.

Explanation: Removal device without reinsertion ...
Examples: Removal Swan Ganz catheter – CMS Ex: Cardiac pacemaker removal

Body Part – 4TH	Approach – 5TH	Device – 6TH	Qualifier – 7TH
A Heart	0 Open 3 Percutaneous 4 Percutaneous endoscopic	2 Monitoring device 3 Infusion device 7 Autologous tissue substitute 8 Zooplastic tissue C Extraluminal device D Intraluminal device J Synthetic substitute K Nonautologous tissue substitute M Cardiac lead N Intracardiac pacemaker Q Implantable heart assist system Y Other device	Z No qualifier
A Heart	0 Open 3 Percutaneous 4 Percutaneous endoscopic	R Short-term external heart assist system	S Biventricular Z No qualifier
A Heart	X External	2 Monitoring device 3 Infusion device D Intraluminal device M Cardiac lead	Z No qualifier
Y Great Vessel	0 Open 3 Percutaneous 4 Percutaneous endoscopic	2 Monitoring device 3 Infusion device 7 Autologous tissue substitute 8 Zooplastic tissue C Extraluminal device D Intraluminal device J Synthetic substitute K Nonautologous tissue substitute Y Other device	Z No qualifier
Y Great Vessel	X External	2 Monitoring device 3 Infusion device D Intraluminal device	Z No qualifier

© 2018 Channel Publishing, Ltd.

1ST - 0 Medical and Surgical
2ND - 2 Heart and Great Vessels
3RD - Q REPAIR

OTHER REPAIRS GROUP: (Control), Repair
Root Operations that define other repairs.

REPAIR: Restoring, to the extent possible, a body part to its normal anatomic structure and function.

Explanation: Used only when the method to accomplish the repair is not one of the other root operations
Examples: Suture pericardial injury – CMS Ex: Suture of laceration

Body Part – 4TH	Approach – 5TH	Device – 6TH	Qualifier – 7TH
0 Coronary Artery, One Artery 1 Coronary Artery, Two Arteries 2 Coronary Artery, Three Arteries 3 Coronary Artery, Four or More Arteries 4 Coronary Vein 5 Atrial Septum 6 Atrium, Right 7 Atrium, Left 8 Conduction Mechanism 9 Chordae Tendineae A Heart B Heart, Right C Heart, Left D Papillary Muscle H Pulmonary Valve K Ventricle, Right L Ventricle, Left M Ventricular Septum N Pericardium P Pulmonary Trunk Q Pulmonary Artery, Right R Pulmonary Artery, Left S Pulmonary Vein, Right T Pulmonary Vein, Left V Superior Vena Cava W Thoracic Aorta, Descending X Thoracic Aorta, Ascending/Arch	0 Open 3 Percutaneous 4 Percutaneous endoscopic	Z No device	Z No qualifier
F Aortic Valve	0 Open 3 Percutaneous 4 Percutaneous endoscopic	Z No device	J Truncal valve Z No qualifier
G Mitral Valve	0 Open 3 Percutaneous 4 Percutaneous endoscopic	Z No device	E Atrioventricular valve, left Z No qualifier
J Tricuspid Valve	0 Open 3 Percutaneous 4 Percutaneous endoscopic	Z No device	G Atrioventricular valve, right Z No qualifier

1ST - 0 Medical and Surgical
2ND - 2 Heart and Great Vessels
3RD - R REPLACEMENT

DEVICE GROUP: (Change), Insertion, Removal, Replacement, Revision, Supplement
Root Operations that always involve a device.

REPLACEMENT: Putting in or on biological or synthetic material that physically takes the place and/or function of all or a portion of a body part.

Explanation: Includes taking out or eradicating, or rendering non-functional, the body part ...
Examples: Mitral valve replacement – CMS Ex: Total hip replacement

Body Part – 4TH	Approach – 5TH	Device – 6TH	Qualifier – 7TH
5 Atrial Septum 6 Atrium, Right 7 Atrium, Left 9 Chordae Tendineae D Papillary Muscle K Ventricle, Right NC*LC* L Ventricle, Left NC*LC* M Ventricular Septum N Pericardium P Pulmonary Trunk Q Pulmonary Artery, Right R Pulmonary Artery, Left S Pulmonary Vein, Right T Pulmonary Vein, Left V Superior Vena Cava W Thoracic Aorta, Descending X Thoracic Aorta, Ascending/Arch	0 Open 4 Percutaneous endoscopic	7 Autologous tissue substitute 8 Zooplastic tissue J Synthetic substitute K Nonautologous tissue substitute	Z No qualifier
F Aortic Valve G Mitral Valve H Pulmonary Valve J Tricuspid Valve	0 Open 4 Percutaneous endoscopic	7 Autologous tissue substitute 8 Zooplastic tissue J Synthetic substitute K Nonautologous tissue substitute	Z No qualifier
F Aortic Valve G Mitral Valve H Pulmonary Valve J Tricuspid Valve	3 Percutaneous	7 Autologous tissue substitute 8 Zooplastic tissue J Synthetic substitute K Nonautologous tissue substitute	H Transapical Z No qualifier

NC*LC* – Some procedures are considered non-covered or limited coverage by Medicare. See current Medicare Code Editor for details.

© 2018 Channel Publishing, Ltd.

1ST - 0 Medical and Surgical
2ND - 2 Heart and Great Vessels
3RD - S REPOSITION

MOVE GROUP: (Reattachment), Reposition, (Transfer), Transplantation
Root Operations that put in/put back or move some/all of a body part.

REPOSITION: Moving to its normal location, or other suitable location, all or a portion of a body part.

Explanation: The body part may or may not be cut out or off to be moved to the new location ...
Examples: Relocation pulmonary vein – CMS Ex: Fracture reduction

Body Part – 4TH	Approach – 5TH	Device – 6TH	Qualifier – 7TH
0 Coronary Artery, One Artery 1 Coronary Artery, Two Arteries P Pulmonary Trunk Q Pulmonary Artery, Right R Pulmonary Artery, Left S Pulmonary Vein, Right T Pulmonary Vein, Left V Superior Vena Cava W Thoracic Aorta, Descending X Thoracic Aorta, Ascending/Arch	0 Open	Z No device	Z No qualifier

1ST - 0 Medical and Surgical
2ND - 2 Heart and Great Vessels
3RD - T RESECTION

EXCISION GROUP: Excision, Resection, Destruction, (Extraction), (Detachment)
Root Operations that take out some or all of a body part.

RESECTION: Cutting out or off, without replacement, all of a body part.

Explanation: None
Examples: Atrial septectomy – CMS Ex: Total lobectomy of lung

Body Part – 4TH	Approach – 5TH	Device – 6TH	Qualifier – 7TH
5 Atrial Septum 8 Conduction Mechanism 9 Chordae Tendineae D Papillary Muscle H Pulmonary Valve M Ventricular Septum N Pericardium	0 Open 3 Percutaneous 4 Percutaneous endoscopic	Z No device	Z No qualifier

1ST - 0 Medical and Surgical
2ND - 2 Heart and Great Vessels
3RD - U SUPPLEMENT

DEVICE GROUP: (Change), Insertion, Removal, Replacement, Revision, Supplement
Root Operations that always involve a device.

SUPPLEMENT: Putting in or on biological or synthetic material that physically reinforces and/or augments the function of a portion of a body part.

Explanation: Biological material is non-living, or is living and from the same individual ...
Examples: Valve graft annuloplasty – CMS Ex: Herniorrhaphy using mesh

Body Part – 4TH	Approach – 5TH	Device – 6TH	Qualifier – 7TH
5 Atrial Septum 6 Atrium, Right 7 Atrium, Left 9 Chordae Tendineae A Heart D Papillary Muscle H Pulmonary Valve K Ventricle, Right L Ventricle, Left M Ventricular Septum N Pericardium P Pulmonary Trunk Q Pulmonary Artery, Right R Pulmonary Artery, Left S Pulmonary Vein, Right T Pulmonary Vein, Left V Superior Vena Cava W Thoracic Aorta, Descending X Thoracic Aorta, Ascending/Arch	0 Open 3 Percutaneous 4 Percutaneous endoscopic	7 Autologous tissue substitute 8 Zooplastic tissue J Synthetic substitute K Nonautologous tissue substitute	Z No qualifier
F Aortic Valve	0 Open 3 Percutaneous 4 Percutaneous endoscopic	7 Autologous tissue substitute 8 Zooplastic tissue J Synthetic substitute K Nonautologous tissue substitute	J Truncal valve Z No qualifier
G Mitral Valve	0 Open 3 Percutaneous 4 Percutaneous endoscopic	7 Autologous tissue substitute 8 Zooplastic tissue J Synthetic substitute K Nonautologous tissue substitute	E Atrioventricular valve, left Z No qualifier
J Tricuspid Valve	0 Open 3 Percutaneous 4 Percutaneous endoscopic	7 Autologous tissue substitute 8 Zooplastic tissue J Synthetic substitute K Nonautologous tissue substitute	G Atrioventricular valve, right Z No qualifier

HEART & GREAT V. 0 2 U

© 2018 Channel Publishing, Ltd.

1ST - 0 Medical and Surgical
2ND - 2 Heart and Great Vessels
3RD - V RESTRICTION

TUBULAR GROUP: Bypass, Dilation, Occlusion, Restriction
Root Operations that alter the diameter/route of a tubular body part.

RESTRICTION: Partially closing an orifice or the lumen of a tubular body part.

Explanation: The orifice can be a natural orifice or an artificially created orifice.
Examples: Banding left pulmonary artery – CMS Ex: Cervical cerclage

Body Part – 4TH	Approach – 5TH	Device – 6TH	Qualifier – 7TH
A Heart	0 Open 3 Percutaneous 4 Percutaneous endoscopic	C Extraluminal device Z No device	Z No qualifier
G Mitral Valve	0 Open 3 Percutaneous 4 Percutaneous endoscopic	Z No device	Z No qualifier
P Pulmonary Trunk Q Pulmonary Artery, Right S Pulmonary Vein, Right T Pulmonary Vein, Left V Superior Vena Cava	0 Open 3 Percutaneous 4 Percutaneous endoscopic	C Extraluminal device D Intraluminal device Z No device	Z No qualifier
R Pulmonary Artery, Left	0 Open 3 Percutaneous 4 Percutaneous endoscopic	C Extraluminal device D Intraluminal device Z No device	T Ductus Arteriosus Z No qualifier
W Thoracic Aorta, Descending X Thoracic Aorta, Ascending/Arch	0 Open 3 Percutaneous 4 Percutaneous endoscopic	C Extraluminal device D Intraluminal device E Intraluminal device, branched or fenestrated, one or two arteries F Intraluminal device, branched or fenestrated, three or more arteries Z No device	Z No qualifier

© 2018 Channel Publishing, Ltd.

1ST - 0 Medical and Surgical
2ND - 2 Heart and Great Vessels
3RD - W REVISION

DEVICE GROUP: (Change), Insertion, Removal, Replacement, Revision, Supplement
Root Operations that always involve a device.

REVISION: Correcting, to the extent possible, a portion of a malfunctioning device or the position of a displaced device.

Explanation: Correcting by taking out or putting in components of a device such as a screw or pin ...
Examples: Reposition cardiac lead – CMS Ex: Recementing of hip prosthesis

Body Part – 4TH	Approach – 5TH	Device – 6TH	Qualifier – 7TH
5 Atrial Septum M Ventricular Septum	0 Open 4 Percutaneous endoscopic	J Synthetic substitute	Z No qualifier
A Heart	0 Open 3 Percutaneous 4 Percutaneous endoscopic	2 Monitoring device 3 Infusion device 7 Autologous tissue substitute 8 Zooplastic tissue C Extraluminal device D Intraluminal device J Synthetic substitute LC* K Nonautologous tissue substitute M Cardiac lead N Intracardiac pacemaker Q Implantable heart assist system NC*LC* Y Other device	Z No qualifier
A Heart	0 Open 3 Percutaneous 4 Percutaneous endoscopic	R Short-term external heart assist system	S Biventricular Z No qualifier
A Heart	X External	2 Monitoring device 3 Infusion device 7 Autologous tissue substitute 8 Zooplastic tissue C Extraluminal device D Intraluminal device J Synthetic substitute K Nonautologous tissue substitute M Cardiac lead N Intracardiac pacemaker Q Implantable heart assist system	Z No qualifier
A Heart	X External	R Short-term external heart assist system	S Biventricular Z No qualifier
F Aortic Valve G Mitral Valve H Pulmonary Valve J Tricuspid Valve	0 Open 3 Percutaneous 4 Percutaneous endoscopic	7 Autologous tissue substitute 8 Zooplastic tissue J Synthetic substitute K Nonautologous tissue substitute	Z No qualifier
Y Great Vessel	0 Open 3 Percutaneous 4 Percutaneous endoscopic	2 Monitoring device 3 Infusion device 7 Autologous tissue substitute 8 Zooplastic tissue C Extraluminal device D Intraluminal device J Synthetic substitute K Nonautologous tissue substitute Y Other device	Z No qualifier
Y Great Vessel	X External	2 Monitoring device 3 Infusion device 7 Autologous tissue substitute 8 Zooplastic tissue C Extraluminal device D Intraluminal device J Synthetic substitute K Nonautologous tissue substitute	Z No qualifier

NC*LC* – Some procedures are considered non-covered or limited coverage by Medicare. See current Medicare Code Editor for details.

© 2018 Channel Publishing, Ltd.

1ST - 0 Medical and Surgical
2ND - 2 Heart and Great Vessels
3RD - Y TRANSPLANTATION

MOVE GROUP: (Reattachment), Reposition, (Transfer), Transplantation
Root Operations that put in/put back or move some/all of a body part.

TRANSPLANTATION: Putting in or on all or a portion of a living body part taken from another individual or animal to physically take the place and/or function of all or a portion of a similar body part.

Explanation: The native body part may or may not be taken out ...
Examples: Heart transplant – CMS Ex: Kidney transplant

Body Part – 4TH	Approach – 5TH	Device – 6TH	Qualifier – 7TH
A Heart LC*	0 Open	Z No device	0 Allogeneic 1 Syngeneic 2 Zooplastic

LC* – Some procedures are considered limited coverage by Medicare. See current Medicare Code Editor for details.

© 2018 Channel Publishing, Ltd.

Educational Annotations | 3 – Upper Arteries

Body System Specific Educational Annotations for the Upper Arteries include:

- Anatomy and Physiology Review
- Anatomical Illustrations
- Definitions of Common Procedures
- AHA Coding Clinic® Reference Notations
- Body Part Key Listings
- Device Key Listings
- Device Aggregation Table Listings
- Coding Notes

Anatomy and Physiology Review of Upper Arteries

BODY PART VALUES – 3 - UPPER ARTERIES

Artery – Blood vessels that carry oxygenated (arterial) blood away from the heart and to the organs and tissues of the body. Arteries have a higher blood pressure than other parts of the circulatory system in order to adequately perfuse all the tissues with oxygenated red blood cells.
Axillary Artery – The axillary artery branches from the subclavian artery and serves the lateral thorax and upper limb.
Brachial Artery – The brachial artery branches from the axillary artery and serves the upper limb.
Common Carotid Artery – The left common carotid artery branches from the aortic arch and serves the head and brain. The right common carotid artery branches from the innominate artery (also known as the brachiocephalic artery) and serves the head and brain.
External Carotid Artery – The external carotid artery branches from the common carotid artery and serves the head.
Face Artery – Any of the smaller arterial branches that serves the face.
Hand Artery – Any of the smaller arterial branches that serves the hand.
Innominate Artery – The innominate artery (also known as the brachiocephalic artery) branches from the aortic arch and branches to the right common carotid artery, the internal mammary artery, and the subclavian artery.
Internal Carotid Artery – The internal carotid artery branches from the common carotid artery and serves primarily the brain.
Internal Mammary Artery – The internal mammary artery branches from the innominate artery and serves the anterior chest wall and breasts.
Intracranial Artery – Any of the smaller arterial branches that lies within the skull.
Radial Artery – The radial artery branches from the brachial artery and serves the forearm, wrist, and hand.
Subclavian Artery – The left subclavian artery branches from the aortic arch and serves the thorax, head, and left upper limb. The right subclavian artery branches from the innominate artery (also known as the brachiocephalic artery) and serves the thorax, head, and right upper limb.
Temporal Artery – The temporal artery branches from the external carotid artery and serves the head.
Thyroid Artery – The thyroid artery branches from the thyrocervical trunk of the subclavian artery and serves the thyroid gland.
Ulnar Artery – The ulnar artery branches from the brachial artery and serves the forearm and wrist.
Upper Artery – The arteries located above the diaphragm (see Coding Guideline B2.1b).
Vertebral Artery – The vertebral artery branches from the subclavian artery and serves the brain.

UPPER ARTERIES 0 3

Anatomical Illustrations of Upper Arteries

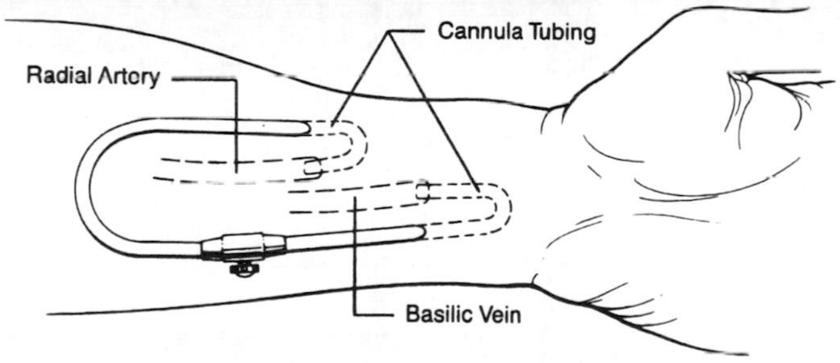

VESSEL-TO-VESSEL CANNULA

Continued on next page

© 2018 Channel Publishing, Ltd.

Educational Annotations | 3 – Upper Arteries

Anatomical Illustrations of Upper Arteries

Continued from previous page

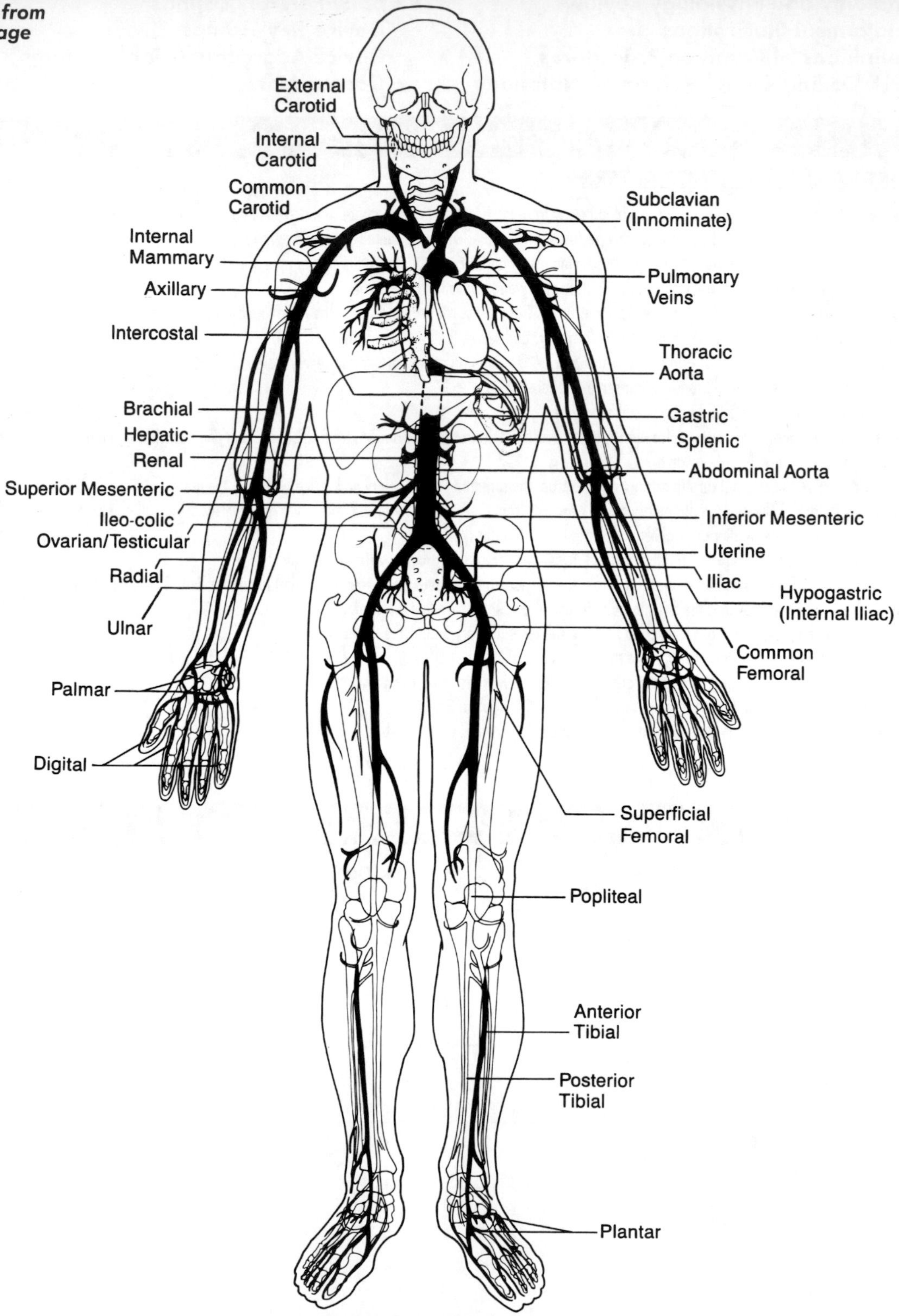

ARTERIES OF HUMAN BODY

© 2018 Channel Publishing, Ltd.

Educational Annotations | 3 – Upper Arteries

Definitions of Common Procedures of Upper Arteries

Balloon angioplasty – The surgical restoration of a narrowed arterial lumen using a balloon-dilating catheter.
Carotid artery to vertebral artery bypass – The restoration of vertebral artery blood flow by using a tubular graft (tissue or synthetic) from a carotid artery to bypass the diseased section of a vertebral artery.
Carotid endarterectomy – The surgical removal of lumen-reducing plaque from a carotid artery to increase the blood flow to the head and reduce the risk of stroke.
Creation of arteriovenous (AV) fistula – The surgical re-routing of an artery in the forearm directly into a vein in the forearm to create an easy and reliable access for repeated hemodialysis.

AHA Coding Clinic® Reference Notations of Upper Arteries

ROOT OPERATION SPECIFIC - 3 - UPPER ARTERIES

BYPASS - 1
- Anastomosis between an artery and a vein for hemodialysis access ....AHA 13:1Q:p27
- Anastomosis between common carotid artery and subclavian artery ....AHA 17:2Q:p22
- Arteriovenous anastomosis of brachial artery ....AHA 13:4Q:p125
- Carotid-carotid bypass ....AHA 17:4Q:p65
- Creation of AV graft using HeRO device via jugular vein..........AHA 16:3Q:p37
- Left to right common carotid artery bypass ....AHA 17:1Q:p31

DESTRUCTION - 5
DILATION - 7
DRAINAGE - 9
EXCISION - B
- Infratemporal fossa malignancy with excision of carotid artery ....AHA 16:2Q:p12

EXTIRPATION - C
- Carotid endarterectomy ....AHA 17:4Q:p65
- Carotid endarterectomy with patch angioplasty ....AHA 16:2Q:p11

INSERTION - H
- Arterial line placement..........AHA 16:2Q:p32

INSPECTION - J
- Discontinued carotid artery procedure ....AHA 15:1Q:p29

OCCLUSION - L
- Clipping occlusion of cerebral artery aneurysm..........AHA 16:2Q:p30
- Endovascular Onyx-18 liquid embolization ....AHA 14:4Q:p37

RELEASE - N
REMOVAL - P
REPAIR - Q
- Epistaxis control using sutures ....AHA 14:4Q:p20

REPLACEMENT - R
REPOSITION - S
- Creation of superficial temporal artery cuff..........AHA 15:3Q:p27

SUPPLEMENT - U
- Carotid endarterectomy with patch angioplasty ....AHA 16:2Q:p11

RESTRICTION - V
- Stent assisted coil embolization of carotid artery..........AHA 16:1Q:p19

REVISION - W
- New AV graft sewn to existing AV graft..........AHA 16:3Q:p39
- Stent to trap herniated/migrated coil in basilar artery..........AHA 15:1Q:p32

© 2018 Channel Publishing, Ltd.

Educational Annotations | 3 – Upper Arteries

Body Part Key Listings of Upper Arteries

See also Body Part Key in Appendix C

Angular artery ....use Face Artery
Anterior cerebral artery ....use Intracranial Artery
Anterior choroidal artery ....use Intracranial Artery
Anterior circumflex humeral artery ....use Axillary Artery, Left/Right
Anterior communicating artery ....use Intracranial Artery
Anterior intercostal artery ....use Internal Mammary Artery, Left/Right
Anterior spinal artery ....use Vertebral Artery, Left/Right
Anterior ulnar recurrent artery ....use Ulnar Artery, Left/Right
Aortic intercostal artery ....use Upper Artery
Ascending palatine artery ....use Face Artery
Ascending pharyngeal artery ....use External Carotid Artery, Left/Right
Basilar artery ....use Intracranial Artery
Brachiocephalic artery ....use Innominate Artery
Brachiocephalic trunk ....use Innominate Artery
Bronchial artery ....use Upper Artery
Caroticotympanic artery ....use Internal Carotid Artery, Left/Right
Carotid sinus ....use Internal Carotid Artery, Left/Right
Circle of Willis ....use Intracranial Artery
Common interosseous artery ....use Ulnar Artery, Left/Right
Costocervical trunk ....use Subclavian Artery, Left/Right
Cricothyroid artery ....use Thyroid Artery, Left/Right
Deep palmar arch ....use Hand Artery, Left/Right
Dorsal scapular artery ....use Subclavian Artery, Left/Right
Esophageal artery ....use Upper Artery
External maxillary artery ....use Face Artery
Facial artery ....use Face Artery
Hyoid artery ....use Thyroid Artery, Left/Right
Inferior labial artery ....use Face Artery
Inferior ulnar collateral artery ....use Brachial Artery, Left/Right
Internal carotid artery, intracranial portion ....use Intracranial Artery
Internal maxillary artery ....use External Carotid Artery, Left/Right
Internal thoracic artery ....use Internal Mammary Artery, Left/Right
....use Subclavian Artery, Left/Right
Lateral thoracic artery ....use Axillary Artery, Left/Right
Lingual artery ....use External Carotid Artery, Left/Right
Maxillary artery ....use External Carotid Artery, Left/Right
Middle cerebral artery ....use Intracranial Artery
Middle temporal artery ....use Temporal Artery, Left/Right
Musculophrenic artery ....use Internal Mammary Artery, Left/Right
Occipital artery ....use External Carotid Artery, Left/Right
Ophthalmic artery ....use Intracranial Artery
Pericardiophrenic artery ....use Internal Mammary Artery, Left/Right
Posterior auricular artery ....use External Carotid Artery, Left/Right
Posterior cerebral artery ....use Intracranial Artery
Posterior circumflex humeral artery ....use Axillary Artery, Left/Right
Posterior communicating artery ....use Intracranial Artery
Posterior inferior cerebellar artery (PICA) ....use Intracranial Artery
Posterior spinal artery ....use Vertebral Artery, Left/Right
Posterior ulnar recurrent artery ....use Ulnar Artery, Left/Right
Princeps pollicis artery ....use Hand Artery, Left/Right
Profunda brachii ....use Brachial Artery, Left/Right
Radial recurrent artery ....use Radial Artery, Left/Right
Radialis indicis ....use Hand Artery, Left/Right
Sternocleidomastoid artery ....use Thyroid Artery, Left/Right
Subcostal artery ....use Upper Artery
Submental artery ....use Face Artery
Subscapular artery ....use Axillary Artery, Left/Right
Superficial palmar arch ....use Hand Artery, Left/Right
Superficial temporal artery ....use Temporal Artery, Left/Right
Superior epigastric artery ....use Internal Mammary Artery, Left/Right
Superior labial artery ....use Face Artery
Superior laryngeal artery ....use Thyroid Artery, Left/Right
Superior thoracic artery ....use Axillary Artery, Left/Right
Superior thyroid artery ....use External Carotid Artery, Left/Right
....use Thyroid Artery, Left/Right
Superior ulnar collateral artery ....use Brachial Artery, Left/Right
Thoracoacromial artery ....use Axillary Artery, Left/Right
Thyrocervical trunk ....use Thyroid Artery, Left/Right
Transverse facial artery ....use Temporal Artery, Left/Right

Device Key Listings of Upper Arteries

See also Device Key in Appendix D

Absolute Pro Vascular (OTW) Self-Expanding Stent System ....use Intraluminal Device
Acculink (RX) Carotid Stent System ....use Intraluminal Device
AneuRx® AAA Advantage® ....use Intraluminal Device
Autograft ....use Autologous Tissue Substitute
Autologous artery graft ....use Autologous Arterial Tissue in Upper Arteries
Autologous vein graft ....use Autologous Venous Tissue in Upper Arteries
Baroreflex Activation Therapy® (BAT®) ....use Stimulator Lead in Upper Arteries
Bioactive embolization coil(s) ....use Intraluminal Device, Bioactive in Upper Arteries
Carotid (artery) sinus (baroreceptor) lead ....use Stimulator Lead in Upper Arteries
Carotid WALLSTENT® Monorail® Endoprosthesis ....use Intraluminal Device
Embolization coil(s) ....use Intraluminal Device
FLAIR® Endovascular Stent Graft ....use Intraluminal Device
GORE TAG® Thoracic Endoprosthesis ....use Intraluminal Device
Micrus CERECYTE microcoil ....use Intraluminal Device, Bioactive in Upper Arteries
Paclitaxel-eluting peripheral stent ....use Intraluminal Device, Drug-eluting in Upper Arteries, Lower Arteries
Pipeline™ Embolization device (PED) ....use Intraluminal Device
Protégé® RX Carotid Stent System ....use Intraluminal Device
Rheos® System lead ....use Stimulator Lead in Upper Arteries

Continued on next page

© 2018 Channel Publishing, Ltd.

Educational Annotations | 3 – Upper Arteries

Device Key Listings of Upper Arteries

Continued from previous page

Stent, intraluminal (cardiovascular) (gastrointestinal) (hepatobiliary) (urinary) ....use Intraluminal Device
Talent® Converter ....use Intraluminal Device
Talent® Occluder ....use Intraluminal Device
Talent® Stent Graft (abdominal) (thoracic) ....use Intraluminal Device
Therapeutic occlusion coil(s) ....use Intraluminal Device
Tissue bank graft ....use Nonautologous Tissue Substitute
WALLSTENT® Endoprosthesis ....use Intraluminal Device
Xact Carotid Stent System ....use Intraluminal Device
Zilver® PTX® (paclitaxel) Drug-Eluting Peripheral Stent ....use Intraluminal Device, Drug-eluting in Upper Arteries, Lower Arteries

Device Aggregation Table Listings of Upper Arteries

See also Device Aggregation Table in Appendix E

Specific Device	For Operation	In Body System	General Device
Autologous Arterial Tissue	All applicable	Upper Arteries	Autologous Tissue Substitute
Autologous Venous Tissue	All applicable	Upper Arteries	Autologous Tissue Substitute
Intraluminal Device, Bioactive	All applicable	Upper Arteries	Intraluminal Device
Intraluminal Device, Drug-eluting	All applicable	Upper Arteries	Intraluminal Device
Intraluminal Device, Drug-eluting, Four or More	All applicable	Heart and Great Vessels	Intraluminal Device
Intraluminal Device, Drug-eluting, Three	All applicable	Heart and Great Vessels	Intraluminal Device
Intraluminal Device, Drug-eluting, Two	All applicable	Heart and Great Vessels	Intraluminal Device
Intraluminal Device, Four or More	All applicable	Heart and Great Vessels	Intraluminal Device
Intraluminal Device, Three	All applicable	Heart and Great Vessels	Intraluminal Device
Intraluminal Device, Two	All applicable	Heart and Great Vessels	Intraluminal Device

Coding Notes of Upper Arteries

Body System Relevant Coding Guidelines

General Guidelines

B2.1b

Where the general body part values "upper" and "lower" are provided as an option in the Upper Arteries, Lower Arteries, Upper Veins, Lower Veins, Muscles and Tendons body systems, "upper" or "lower "specifies body parts located above or below the diaphragm respectively.

Example: Vein body parts above the diaphragm are found in the Upper Veins body system; vein body parts below the diaphragm are found in the Lower Veins body system.

Body part, General guidelines

B4.1c

If a procedure is performed on a continuous section of a tubular body part, code the body part value corresponding to the furthest anatomical site from the point of entry.

Example: A procedure performed on a continuous section of artery from the femoral artery to the external iliac artery with the point of entry at the femoral artery is coded to the external iliac body part.

Branches of body parts

B4.2

Where a specific branch of a body part does not have its own body part value in PCS, the body part is typically coded to the closest proximal branch that has a specific body part value. In the cardiovascular body systems, if a general body part is available in the correct root operation table, and coding to a proximal branch would require assigning a code in a different body system, the procedure is coded using the general body part value.

Examples: A procedure performed on the mandibular branch of the trigeminal nerve is coded to the trigeminal nerve body part value.

Occlusion of the bronchial artery is coded to the body part value Upper Artery in the body system Upper Arteries, and not to the body part value Thoracic Aorta, Descending in the body system Heart and Great Vessels.

© 2018 Channel Publishing, Ltd.

1ST - 0 Medical and Surgical
2ND - 3 Upper Arteries
3RD - 1 BYPASS

TUBULAR GROUP: Bypass, Dilation, Occlusion, Restriction
Root Operations that alter the diameter/route of a tubular body part.

BYPASS: Altering the route of passage of the contents of a tubular body part.

Explanation: Rerouting contents to a downstream part ... with or without the use of a device ...
Examples: Arteriovenous hemodialysis fistula – CMS Ex: Coronary artery bypass

Body Part – 4TH	Approach – 5TH	Device – 6TH	Qualifier – 7TH
2 Innominate Artery	0 Open	9 Autologous venous tissue A Autologous arterial tissue J Synthetic substitute K Nonautologous tissue substitute Z No device	0 Upper Arm Artery, Right 1 Upper Arm Artery, Left 2 Upper Arm Artery, Bilateral 3 Lower Arm Artery, Right 4 Lower Arm Artery, Left 5 Lower Arm Artery, Bilateral 6 Upper Leg Artery, Right 7 Upper Leg Artery, Left 8 Upper Leg Artery, Bilateral 9 Lower Leg Artery, Right B Lower Leg Artery, Left C Lower Leg Artery, Bilateral D Upper Arm Vein F Lower Arm Vein J Extracranial Artery, Right K Extracranial Artery, Left
3 Subclavian Artery, Right 4 Subclavian Artery, Left	0 Open	9 Autologous venous tissue A Autologous arterial tissue J Synthetic substitute K Nonautologous tissue substitute Z No device	0 Upper Arm Artery, Right 1 Upper Arm Artery, Left 2 Upper Arm Artery, Bilateral 3 Lower Arm Artery, Right 4 Lower Arm Artery, Left 5 Lower Arm Artery, Bilateral 6 Upper Leg Artery, Right 7 Upper Leg Artery, Left 8 Upper Leg Artery, Bilateral 9 Lower Leg Artery, Right B Lower Leg Artery, Left C Lower Leg Artery, Bilateral D Upper Arm Vein F Lower Arm Vein J Extracranial Artery, Right K Extracranial Artery, Left M Pulmonary Artery, Right N Pulmonary Artery, Left
5 Axillary Artery, Right 6 Axillary Artery, Left	0 Open	9 Autologous venous tissue A Autologous arterial tissue J Synthetic substitute K Nonautologous tissue substitute Z No device	0 Upper Arm Artery, Right 1 Upper Arm Artery, Left 2 Upper Arm Artery, Bilateral 3 Lower Arm Artery, Right 4 Lower Arm Artery, Left 5 Lower Arm Artery, Bilateral 6 Upper Leg Artery, Right 7 Upper Leg Artery, Left 8 Upper Leg Artery, Bilateral 9 Lower Leg Artery, Right B Lower Leg Artery, Left C Lower Leg Artery, Bilateral D Upper Arm Vein F Lower Arm Vein J Extracranial Artery, Right K Extracranial Artery, Left T Abdominal Artery V Superior Vena Cava

continued ⇨

© 2018 Channel Publishing, Ltd.

0 3 1 BYPASS – continued

Body Part – 4TH	Approach – 5TH	Device – 6TH	Qualifier – 7TH
7 Brachial Artery, Right	0 Open	9 Autologous venous tissue A Autologous arterial tissue J Synthetic substitute K Nonautologous tissue substitute Z No device	0 Upper Arm Artery, Right 3 Lower Arm Artery, Right D Upper Arm Vein F Lower Arm Vein V Superior Vena Cava
8 Brachial Artery, Left	0 Open	9 Autologous venous tissue A Autologous arterial tissue J Synthetic substitute K Nonautologous tissue substitute Z No device	1 Upper Arm Artery, Left 4 Lower Arm Artery, Left D Upper Arm Vein F Lower Arm Vein V Superior Vena Cava
9 Ulnar Artery, Right B Radial Artery, Right	0 Open	9 Autologous venous tissue A Autologous arterial tissue J Synthetic substitute K Nonautologous tissue substitute Z No device	3 Lower Arm Artery, Right F Lower Arm Vein
A Ulnar Artery, Left C Radial Artery, Left	0 Open	9 Autologous venous tissue A Autologous arterial tissue J Synthetic substitute K Nonautologous tissue substitute Z No device	4 Lower Arm Artery, Left F Lower Arm Vein
G Intracranial Artery S Temporal Artery, Right T Temporal Artery, Left	0 Open	9 Autologous venous tissue A Autologous arterial tissue J Synthetic substitute K Nonautologous tissue substitute Z No device	G Intracranial Artery
H Common Carotid Artery, Right J Common Carotid Artery, Left	0 Open	9 Autologous venous tissue A Autologous arterial tissue J Synthetic substitute K Nonautologous tissue substitute Z No device	G Intracranial Artery J Extracranial Artery, Right K Extracranial Artery, Left Y Upper Artery
K Internal Carotid Artery, Right L Internal Carotid Artery, Left M External Carotid Artery, Right N External Carotid Artery, Left	0 Open	9 Autologous venous tissue A Autologous arterial tissue J Synthetic substitute K Nonautologous tissue substitute Z No device	J Extracranial Artery, Right K Extracranial Artery, Left

1ST - 0 Medical and Surgical
2ND - 3 Upper Arteries
3RD - 5 DESTRUCTION

EXCISION GROUP: Excision, (Resection), Destruction, (Extraction), (Detachment)
Root Operations that take out some or all of a body part.

DESTRUCTION: Physical eradication of all or a portion of a body part by the direct use of energy, force, or a destructive agent.

Explanation: None of the body part is physically taken out
Examples: Fulguration arterial lesion – CMS Ex: Fulguration of rectal polyp

Body Part – 4TH			Approach – 5TH	Device – 6TH	Qualifier – 7TH
0 Internal Mammary Artery, Right 1 Internal Mammary Artery, Left 2 Innominate Artery 3 Subclavian Artery, Right 4 Subclavian Artery, Left 5 Axillary Artery, Right 6 Axillary Artery, Left 7 Brachial Artery, Right 8 Brachial Artery, Left 9 Ulnar Artery, Right A Ulnar Artery, Left	B Radial Artery, Right C Radial Artery, Left D Hand Artery, Right F Hand Artery, Left G Intracranial Artery H Common Carotid Artery, Right J Common Carotid Artery, Left K Internal Carotid Artery, Right L Internal Carotid Artery, Left	M External Carotid Artery, Right N External Carotid Artery, Left P Vertebral Artery, Right Q Vertebral Artery, Left R Face Artery S Temporal Artery, Right T Temporal Artery, Left U Thyroid Artery, Right V Thyroid Artery, Left Y Upper Artery	0 Open 3 Percutaneous 4 Percutaneous endoscopic	Z No device	Z No qualifier

© 2018 Channel Publishing, Ltd.

1ST - 0 Medical and Surgical
2ND - 3 Upper Arteries
3RD - 7 **DILATION**

TUBULAR GROUP: Bypass, Dilation, Occlusion, Restriction
Root Operations that alter the diameter/route of a tubular body part.

DILATION: Expanding an orifice or the lumen of a tubular body part.

Explanation: Accomplished by stretching or cutting ... tubular body part or orifice ...
Examples: PTA common carotid artery – CMS Ex: Percutaneous transluminal angioplasty

Body Part – 4TH		Approach - 5TH	Device - 6TH	Qualifier - 7TH
0 Internal Mammary Artery, Right 1 Internal Mammary Artery, Left 2 Innominate Artery 3 Subclavian Artery, Right 4 Subclavian Artery, Left 5 Axillary Artery, Right	6 Axillary Artery, Left 7 Brachial Artery, Right 8 Brachial Artery, Left 9 Ulnar Artery, Right A Ulnar Artery, Left B Radial Artery, Right C Radial Artery, Left	0 Open 3 Percutaneous 4 Percutaneous endoscopic	4 Drug-eluting intraluminal device 5 Drug-eluting intraluminal device, two 6 Drug-eluting intraluminal device, three 7 Drug-eluting intraluminal device, four or more E Intraluminal device, two F Intraluminal device, three G Intraluminal device, four or more	6 Bifurcation Z No qualifier
0 Internal Mammary Artery, Right 1 Internal Mammary Artery, Left 2 Innominate Artery 3 Subclavian Artery, Right 4 Subclavian Artery, Left 5 Axillary Artery, Right	6 Axillary Artery, Left 7 Brachial Artery, Right 8 Brachial Artery, Left 9 Ulnar Artery, Right A Ulnar Artery, Left B Radial Artery, Right C Radial Artery, Left	0 Open 3 Percutaneous 4 Percutaneous endoscopic	D Intraluminal device Z No device	1 Drug-Coated Balloon 6 Bifurcation Z No qualifier
D Hand Artery, Right F Hand Artery, Left G Intracranial Artery NC* H Common Carotid Artery, Right J Common Carotid Artery, Left K Internal Carotid Artery, Right L Internal Carotid Artery, Left M External Carotid Artery, Right N External Carotid Artery, Left	P Vertebral Artery, Right Q Vertebral Artery, Left R Face Artery S Temporal Artery, Right T Temporal Artery, Left U Thyroid Artery, Right V Thyroid Artery, Left Y Upper Artery	0 Open 3 Percutaneous 4 Percutaneous endoscopic	4 Drug-eluting intraluminal device 5 Drug-eluting intraluminal device, two 6 Drug-eluting intraluminal device, three 7 Drug-eluting intraluminal device, four or more D Intraluminal device E Intraluminal device, two F Intraluminal device, three G Intraluminal device, four or more Z No device	6 Bifurcation Z No qualifier

NC* – Some procedures are considered non-covered by Medicare. See current Medicare Code Editor for details.

© 2018 Channel Publishing, Ltd.

1ST - 0 Medical and Surgical
2ND - 3 Upper Arteries
3RD - 9 DRAINAGE

DRAINAGE GROUP: Drainage, Extirpation, (Fragmentation)
Root Operations that take out solids/fluids/gases from a body part.

DRAINAGE: Taking or letting out fluids and/or gases from a body part.

Explanation: Qualifier "X Diagnostic" indicates drainage procedures that are biopsies
Examples: Aspiration arterial abscess – CMS Ex: Thoracentesis

Body Part – 4TH	Approach – 5TH	Device – 6TH	Qualifier – 7TH
0 Internal Mammary Artery, Right 1 Internal Mammary Artery, Left 2 Innominate Artery 3 Subclavian Artery, Right 4 Subclavian Artery, Left 5 Axillary Artery, Right 6 Axillary Artery, Left 7 Brachial Artery, Right 8 Brachial Artery, Left 9 Ulnar Artery, Right A Ulnar Artery, Left B Radial Artery, Right C Radial Artery, Left D Hand Artery, Right F Hand Artery, Left G Intracranial Artery H Common Carotid Artery, Right J Common Carotid Artery, Left K Internal Carotid Artery, Right L Internal Carotid Artery, Left M External Carotid Artery, Right N External Carotid Artery, Left P Vertebral Artery, Right Q Vertebral Artery, Left R Face Artery S Temporal Artery, Right T Temporal Artery, Left U Thyroid Artery, Right V Thyroid Artery, Left Y Upper Artery	0 Open 3 Percutaneous 4 Percutaneous endoscopic	0 Drainage device	Z No qualifier
0 Internal Mammary Artery, Right 1 Internal Mammary Artery, Left 2 Innominate Artery 3 Subclavian Artery, Right 4 Subclavian Artery, Left 5 Axillary Artery, Right 6 Axillary Artery, Left 7 Brachial Artery, Right 8 Brachial Artery, Left 9 Ulnar Artery, Right A Ulnar Artery, Left B Radial Artery, Right C Radial Artery, Left D Hand Artery, Right F Hand Artery, Left G Intracranial Artery H Common Carotid Artery, Right J Common Carotid Artery, Left K Internal Carotid Artery, Right L Internal Carotid Artery, Left M External Carotid Artery, Right N External Carotid Artery, Left P Vertebral Artery, Right Q Vertebral Artery, Left R Face Artery S Temporal Artery, Right T Temporal Artery, Left U Thyroid Artery, Right V Thyroid Artery, Left Y Upper Artery	0 Open 3 Percutaneous 4 Percutaneous endoscopic	Z No device	X Diagnostic Z No qualifier

UPPER ARTERIES 0 3 B

1ST - 0 Medical and Surgical
2ND - 3 Upper Arteries
3RD - B EXCISION

EXCISION GROUP: Excision, (Resection), Destruction, (Extraction), (Detachment)
Root Operations that take out some or all of a body part.

EXCISION: Cutting out or off, without replacement, a portion of a body part.

Explanation: Qualifier "X Diagnostic" indicates excision procedures that are biopsies
Examples: Temporal artery biopsy – CMS Ex: Liver biopsy

Body Part – 4TH	Approach – 5TH	Device – 6TH	Qualifier – 7TH
0 Internal Mammary Artery, Right 1 Internal Mammary Artery, Left 2 Innominate Artery 3 Subclavian Artery, Right 4 Subclavian Artery, Left 5 Axillary Artery, Right 6 Axillary Artery, Left 7 Brachial Artery, Right 8 Brachial Artery, Left 9 Ulnar Artery, Right A Ulnar Artery, Left B Radial Artery, Right C Radial Artery, Left D Hand Artery, Right F Hand Artery, Left G Intracranial Artery H Common Carotid Artery, Right J Common Carotid Artery, Left K Internal Carotid Artery, Right L Internal Carotid Artery, Left M External Carotid Artery, Right N External Carotid Artery, Left P Vertebral Artery, Right Q Vertebral Artery, Left R Face Artery S Temporal Artery, Right T Temporal Artery, Left U Thyroid Artery, Right V Thyroid Artery, Left Y Upper Artery	0 Open 3 Percutaneous 4 Percutaneous endoscopic	Z No device	X Diagnostic Z No qualifier

© 2018 Channel Publishing, Ltd.

1ST - 0 Medical and Surgical
2ND - 3 Upper Arteries
3RD - C EXTIRPATION

DRAINAGE GROUP: Drainage, Extirpation, (Fragmentation)
Root Operations that take out solids/fluids/gases from a body part.

EXTIRPATION: Taking or cutting out solid matter from a body part.

Explanation: Abnormal byproduct or foreign body ...
Examples: Carotid artery endarterectomy – CMS Ex: Thrombectomy

Body Part – 4TH	Approach – 5TH	Device – 6TH	Qualifier – 7TH
0 Internal Mammary Artery, Right 1 Internal Mammary Artery, Left 2 Innominate Artery 3 Subclavian Artery, Right 4 Subclavian Artery, Left 5 Axillary Artery, Right 6 Axillary Artery, Left 7 Brachial Artery, Right 8 Brachial Artery, Left 9 Ulnar Artery, Right A Ulnar Artery, Left B Radial Artery, Right C Radial Artery, Left D Hand Artery, Right F Hand Artery, Left R Face Artery S Temporal Artery, Right T Temporal Artery, Left U Thyroid Artery, Right V Thyroid Artery, Left Y Upper Artery	0 Open 3 Percutaneous 4 Percutaneous endoscopic	Z No device	6 Bifurcation Z No qualifier
G Intracranial Artery H Common Carotid Artery, Right J Common Carotid Artery, Left K Internal Carotid Artery, Right L Internal Carotid Artery, Left M External Carotid Artery, Right N External Carotid Artery, Left P Vertebral Artery, Right Q Vertebral Artery, Left	0 Open 4 Percutaneous endoscopic	Z No device	6 Bifurcation Z No qualifier
G Intracranial Artery H Common Carotid Artery, Right J Common Carotid Artery, Left K Internal Carotid Artery, Right L Internal Carotid Artery, Left M External Carotid Artery, Right N External Carotid Artery, Left P Vertebral Artery, Right Q Vertebral Artery, Left	3 Percutaneous	Z No device	6 Bifurcation 7 Stent retriever Z No qualifier

1ST - 0 Medical and Surgical
2ND - 3 Upper Arteries
3RD - H INSERTION

DEVICE GROUP: (Change), Insertion, Removal, Replacement, Revision, Supplement
Root Operations that always involve a device.

INSERTION: Putting in a nonbiological appliance that monitors, assists, performs, or prevents a physiological function but does not physically take the place of a body part.

Explanation: None
Examples: Carotid artery stimulator lead – CMS Ex: Insertion of central venous catheter

Body Part – 4TH	Approach – 5TH	Device – 6TH	Qualifier – 7TH
0 Internal Mammary Artery, Right 1 Internal Mammary Artery, Left 2 Innominate Artery 3 Subclavian Artery, Right 4 Subclavian Artery, Left 5 Axillary Artery, Right 6 Axillary Artery, Left 7 Brachial Artery, Right 8 Brachial Artery, Left 9 Ulnar Artery, Right A Ulnar Artery, Left B Radial Artery, Right C Radial Artery, Left D Hand Artery, Right F Hand Artery, Left G Intracranial Artery H Common Carotid Artery, Right J Common Carotid Artery, Left M External Carotid Artery, Right N External Carotid Artery, Left P Vertebral Artery, Right Q Vertebral Artery, Left R Face Artery S Temporal Artery, Right T Temporal Artery, Left U Thyroid Artery, Right V Thyroid Artery, Left	0 Open 3 Percutaneous 4 Percutaneous endoscopic	3 Infusion device D Intraluminal device	Z No qualifier
K Internal Carotid Artery, Right L Internal Carotid Artery, Left	0 Open 3 Percutaneous 4 Percutaneous endoscopic	3 Infusion device D Intraluminal device M Stimulator lead	Z No qualifier
Y Upper Artery	0 Open 3 Percutaneous 4 Percutaneous endoscopic	2 Monitoring device 3 Infusion device D Intraluminal device Y Other device	Z No qualifier

© 2018 Channel Publishing, Ltd.

1ST - 0 Medical and Surgical
2ND - 3 Upper Arteries
3RD - J INSPECTION

EXAMINATION GROUP: Inspection, (Map)
Root Operations involving examination only.

INSPECTION: Visually and/or manually exploring a body part.

Explanation: Direct or instrumental visualization ...
Examples: Exploration arterial catheter removal site – CMS Ex: Exploratory laparotomy

Body Part – 4TH	Approach – 5TH	Device – 6TH	Qualifier – 7TH
Y Upper Artery	0 Open 3 Percutaneous 4 Percutaneous endoscopic X External	Z No device	Z No qualifier

1ST - 0 Medical and Surgical
2ND - 3 Upper Arteries
3RD - L OCCLUSION

TUBULAR GROUP: Bypass, Dilation, Occlusion, Restriction
Root Operations that alter the diameter/route of a tubular body part.

OCCLUSION: Completely closing an orifice or the lumen of a tubular body part.

Explanation: The orifice can be a natural orifice or an artificially created orifice
Examples: Embolization carotid fistula – CMS Ex: Fallopian tube ligation

Body Part – 4TH	Approach – 5TH	Device – 6TH	Qualifier – 7TH
0 Internal Mammary Artery, Right 1 Internal Mammary Artery, Left 2 Innominate Artery 3 Subclavian Artery, Right 4 Subclavian Artery, Left 5 Axillary Artery, Right 6 Axillary Artery, Left 7 Brachial Artery, Right 8 Brachial Artery, Left 9 Ulnar Artery, Right A Ulnar Artery, Left B Radial Artery, Right C Radial Artery, Left D Hand Artery, Right F Hand Artery, Left R Face Artery S Temporal Artery, Right T Temporal Artery, Left U Thyroid Artery, Right V Thyroid Artery, Left Y Upper Artery	0 Open 3 Percutaneous 4 Percutaneous endoscopic	C Extraluminal device D Intraluminal device Z No device	Z No qualifier
G Intracranial Artery H Common Carotid Artery, Right J Common Carotid Artery, Left K Internal Carotid Artery, Right L Internal Carotid Artery, Left M External Carotid Artery, Right N External Carotid Artery, Left P Vertebral Artery, Right Q Vertebral Artery, Left	0 Open 3 Percutaneous 4 Percutaneous endoscopic	B Bioactive intraluminal device C Extraluminal device D Intraluminal device Z No device	Z No qualifier

1ST - 0 Medical and Surgical
2ND - 3 Upper Arteries
3RD - N RELEASE

DIVISION GROUP: (Division), Release
Root Operations involving cutting or separation only.

RELEASE: Freeing a body part from an abnormal physical constraint by cutting or by the use of force.

Explanation: Some of the restraining tissue may be taken out but none of the body part is taken out
Examples: Arterial adhesiolysis – CMS Ex: Carpal tunnel release

Body Part – 4TH	Approach – 5TH	Device – 6TH	Qualifier – 7TH
0 Internal Mammary Artery, Right 1 Internal Mammary Artery, Left 2 Innominate Artery 3 Subclavian Artery, Right 4 Subclavian Artery, Left 5 Axillary Artery, Right 6 Axillary Artery, Left 7 Brachial Artery, Right 8 Brachial Artery, Left 9 Ulnar Artery, Right A Ulnar Artery, Left B Radial Artery, Right C Radial Artery, Left D Hand Artery, Right F Hand Artery, Left G Intracranial Artery H Common Carotid Artery, Right J Common Carotid Artery, Left K Internal Carotid Artery, Right L Internal Carotid Artery, Left M External Carotid Artery, Right N External Carotid Artery, Left P Vertebral Artery, Right Q Vertebral Artery, Left R Face Artery S Temporal Artery, Right T Temporal Artery, Left U Thyroid Artery, Right V Thyroid Artery, Left Y Upper Artery	0 Open 3 Percutaneous 4 Percutaneous endoscopic	Z No device	Z No qualifier

© 2018 Channel Publishing, Ltd.

1ST - 0 Medical and Surgical
2ND - 3 Upper Arteries
3RD - P REMOVAL

DEVICE GROUP: (Change), Insertion, Removal, Replacement, Revision, Supplement
Root Operations that always involve a device.

REMOVAL: Taking out or off a device from a body part.

Explanation: Removal device without reinsertion ...
Examples: Removal vascular clip – CMS Ex: Cardiac pacemaker removal

Body Part – 4TH	Approach – 5TH	Device – 6TH	Qualifier – 7TH
Y Upper Artery	0 Open 3 Percutaneous 4 Percutaneous endoscopic	0 Drainage device 2 Monitoring device 3 Infusion device 7 Autologous tissue substitute C Extraluminal device D Intraluminal device J Synthetic substitute K Nonautologous tissue substitute M Stimulator lead Y Other device	Z No qualifier
Y Upper Artery	X External	0 Drainage device 2 Monitoring device 3 Infusion device D Intraluminal device M Stimulator lead	Z No qualifier

1ST - 0 Medical and Surgical
2ND - 3 Upper Arteries
3RD - Q REPAIR

OTHER REPAIRS GROUP: (Control), Repair
Root Operations that define other repairs.

REPAIR: Restoring, to the extent possible, a body part to its normal anatomic structure and function.

Explanation: Used only when the method to accomplish the repair is not one of the other root operations
Examples: Suture arterial laceration – CMS Ex: Suture of laceration

Body Part – 4TH			Approach – 5TH	Device – 6TH	Qualifier – 7TH
0 Internal Mammary Artery, Right 1 Internal Mammary Artery, Left 2 Innominate Artery 3 Subclavian Artery, Right 4 Subclavian Artery, Left 5 Axillary Artery, Right 6 Axillary Artery, Left 7 Brachial Artery, Right 8 Brachial Artery, Left 9 Ulnar Artery, Right A Ulnar Artery, Left	B Radial Artery, Right C Radial Artery, Left D Hand Artery, Right F Hand Artery, Left G Intracranial Artery H Common Carotid Artery, Right J Common Carotid Artery, Left K Internal Carotid Artery, Right L Internal Carotid Artery, Left	M External Carotid Artery, Right N External Carotid Artery, Left P Vertebral Artery, Right Q Vertebral Artery, Left R Face Artery S Temporal Artery, Right T Temporal Artery, Left U Thyroid Artery, Right V Thyroid Artery, Left Y Upper Artery	0 Open 3 Percutaneous 4 Percutaneous endoscopic	Z No device	Z No qualifier

© 2018 Channel Publishing, Ltd.

1ST - 0 Medical and Surgical
2ND - 3 Upper Arteries
3RD - R REPLACEMENT

DEVICE GROUP: (Change), Insertion, Removal, Replacement, Revision, Supplement
Root Operations that always involve a device.

REPLACEMENT: Putting in or on biological or synthetic material that physically takes the place and/or function of all or a portion of a body part.

Explanation: Includes taking out or eradicating, or rendering non-functional, the body part ...
Examples: Reconstruction artery using graft – CMS Ex: Total hip replacement

Body Part – 4TH			Approach – 5TH	Device – 6TH	Qualifier – 7TH
0 Internal Mammary Artery, Right 1 Internal Mammary Artery, Left 2 Innominate Artery 3 Subclavian Artery, Right 4 Subclavian Artery, Left 5 Axillary Artery, Right 6 Axillary Artery, Left 7 Brachial Artery, Right 8 Brachial Artery, Left 9 Ulnar Artery, Right A Ulnar Artery, Left	B Radial Artery, Right C Radial Artery, Left D Hand Artery, Right F Hand Artery, Left G Intracranial Artery H Common Carotid Artery, Right J Common Carotid Artery, Left K Internal Carotid Artery, Right L Internal Carotid Artery, Left	M External Carotid Artery, Right N External Carotid Artery, Left P Vertebral Artery, Right Q Vertebral Artery, Left R Face Artery S Temporal Artery, Right T Temporal Artery, Left U Thyroid Artery, Right V Thyroid Artery, Left Y Upper Artery	0 Open 4 Percutaneous endoscopic	7 Autologous tissue substitute J Synthetic substitute K Nonautologous tissue substitute	Z No qualifier

1ST - 0 Medical and Surgical
2ND - 3 Upper Arteries
3RD - S REPOSITION

MOVE GROUP: (Reattachment), Reposition, (Transfer), (Transplantation)
Root Operations that put in/put back or move some/all of a body part.

REPOSITION: Moving to its normal location, or other suitable location, all or a portion of a body part.

Explanation: The body part may or may not be cut out or off to be moved to the new location ...
Examples: Relocation ulnar artery – CMS Ex: Fracture reduction

Body Part – 4TH			Approach – 5TH	Device – 6TH	Qualifier – 7TH
0 Internal Mammary Artery, Right 1 Internal Mammary Artery, Left 2 Innominate Artery 3 Subclavian Artery, Right 4 Subclavian Artery, Left 5 Axillary Artery, Right 6 Axillary Artery, Left 7 Brachial Artery, Right 8 Brachial Artery, Left 9 Ulnar Artery, Right A Ulnar Artery, Left	B Radial Artery, Right C Radial Artery, Left D Hand Artery, Right F Hand Artery, Left G Intracranial Artery H Common Carotid Artery, Right J Common Carotid Artery, Left K Internal Carotid Artery, Right L Internal Carotid Artery, Left	M External Carotid Artery, Right N External Carotid Artery, Left P Vertebral Artery, Right Q Vertebral Artery, Left R Face Artery S Temporal Artery, Right T Temporal Artery, Left U Thyroid Artery, Right V Thyroid Artery, Left Y Upper Artery	0 Open 3 Percutaneous 4 Percutaneous endoscopic	Z No device	Z No qualifier

© 2018 Channel Publishing, Ltd.

1ST - 0 Medical and Surgical
2ND - 3 Upper Arteries
3RD - U SUPPLEMENT

DEVICE GROUP: (Change), Insertion, Removal, Replacement, Revision, Supplement
Root Operations that always involve a device.

SUPPLEMENT: Putting in or on biological or synthetic material that physically reinforces and/or augments the function of a portion of a body part.

Explanation: Biological material is non-living, or is living and from the same individual ...
Examples: Bovine patch angioplasty – CMS Ex: Herniorrhaphy using mesh

Body Part – 4TH	Approach – 5TH	Device – 6TH	Qualifier – 7TH
0 Internal Mammary Artery, Right 1 Internal Mammary Artery, Left 2 Innominate Artery 3 Subclavian Artery, Right 4 Subclavian Artery, Left 5 Axillary Artery, Right 6 Axillary Artery, Left 7 Brachial Artery, Right 8 Brachial Artery, Left 9 Ulnar Artery, Right A Ulnar Artery, Left B Radial Artery, Right C Radial Artery, Left D Hand Artery, Right F Hand Artery, Left G Intracranial Artery H Common Carotid Artery, Right J Common Carotid Artery, Left K Internal Carotid Artery, Right L Internal Carotid Artery, Left M External Carotid Artery, Right N External Carotid Artery, Left P Vertebral Artery, Right Q Vertebral Artery, Left R Face Artery S Temporal Artery, Right T Temporal Artery, Left U Thyroid Artery, Right V Thyroid Artery, Left Y Upper Artery	0 Open 3 Percutaneous 4 Percutaneous endoscopic	7 Autologous tissue substitute J Synthetic substitute K Nonautologous tissue substitute	Z No qualifier

1ST - 0 Medical and Surgical
2ND - 3 Upper Arteries
3RD - V RESTRICTION

TUBULAR GROUP: Bypass, Dilation, Occlusion, Restriction
Root Operations that alter the diameter/route of a tubular body part.

RESTRICTION: Partially closing an orifice or the lumen of a tubular body part.

Explanation: The orifice can be a natural orifice or an artificially created orifice.
Examples: Clipping cerebral aneurysm – CMS Ex: Cervical cerclage

Body Part – 4TH	Approach – 5TH	Device – 6TH	Qualifier – 7TH
0 Internal Mammary Artery, Right 1 Internal Mammary Artery, Left 2 Innominate Artery 3 Subclavian Artery, Right 4 Subclavian Artery, Left 5 Axillary Artery, Right 6 Axillary Artery, Left 7 Brachial Artery, Right 8 Brachial Artery, Left 9 Ulnar Artery, Right A Ulnar Artery, Left B Radial Artery, Right C Radial Artery, Left D Hand Artery, Right F Hand Artery, Left R Face Artery S Temporal Artery, Right T Temporal Artery, Left U Thyroid Artery, Right V Thyroid Artery, Left Y Upper Artery	0 Open 3 Percutaneous 4 Percutaneous endoscopic	C Extraluminal device D Intraluminal device Z No device	Z No qualifier
G Intracranial Artery H Common Carotid Artery, Right J Common Carotid Artery, Left K Internal Carotid Artery, Right L Internal Carotid Artery, Left M External Carotid Artery, Right N External Carotid Artery, Left P Vertebral Artery, Right Q Vertebral Artery, Left	0 Open 3 Percutaneous 4 Percutaneous endoscopic	B Bioactive intraluminal device C Extraluminal device D Intraluminal device Z No device	Z No qualifier

© 2018 Channel Publishing, Ltd.

1ST - 0 Medical and Surgical
2ND - 3 Upper Arteries
3RD - W REVISION

DEVICE GROUP: (Change), Insertion, Removal, Replacement, Revision, Supplement
Root Operations that always involve a device.

REVISION: Correcting, to the extent possible, a portion of a malfunctioning device or the position of a displaced device.

Explanation: Correcting by taking out or putting in components of a device such as a screw or pin ...
Examples: Repair ruptured arterial graft – CMS Ex: Recementing of hip prosthesis

Body Part – 4TH	Approach – 5TH	Device – 6TH	Qualifier – 7TH
Y Upper Artery	0 Open 3 Percutaneous 4 Percutaneous endoscopic	0 Drainage device 2 Monitoring device 3 Infusion device 7 Autologous tissue substitute C Extraluminal device D Intraluminal device J Synthetic substitute K Nonautologous tissue substitute M Stimulator lead Y Other device	Z No qualifier
Y Upper Artery	X External	0 Drainage device 2 Monitoring device 3 Infusion device 7 Autologous tissue substitute C Extraluminal device D Intraluminal device J Synthetic substitute K Nonautologous tissue substitute M Stimulator lead	Z No qualifier

© 2018 Channel Publishing, Ltd.

NOTES

© 2018 Channel Publishing, Ltd.

Educational Annotations | 4 – Lower Arteries

Body System Specific Educational Annotations for the Lower Arteries include:

- Anatomy and Physiology Review
- Anatomical Illustrations
- Definitions of Common Procedures
- AHA Coding Clinic® Reference Notations
- Body Part Key Listings
- Device Key Listings
- Device Aggregation Table Listings
- Coding Notes

Anatomy and Physiology Review of Lower Arteries

BODY PART VALUES – 4 - LOWER ARTERIES

Abdominal Aorta – The abdominal aorta is continuous from the thoracic aorta artery and ends by branching into the right and left common iliac arteries. Many abdominal arteries branch off from the abdominal aorta.
Anterior Tibial Artery – The anterior tibial artery branches from the popliteal artery and serves the anterior portion of the lower leg and dorsal portion of the foot.
Artery – Blood vessels that carry oxygenated (arterial) blood away from the heart and to the organs and tissues of the body. Arteries have a higher blood pressure than other parts of the circulatory system in order to adequately perfuse all the tissues with oxygenated red blood cells.
Celiac Artery – The celiac artery (also known as the celiac trunk) branches from the abdominal aorta and then almost immediately (1-2cm) branches into the common hepatic artery, the splenic artery, and left gastric artery.
Colic Artery – The colic artery branches from the superior mesenteric artery and serves the colon, ileum, appendix.
Common Iliac Artery – The common iliac artery branches from the aortic bifurcation of the abdominal aorta and branch almost immediately (4 cm in length) into the internal and external iliac arteries.
External Iliac Artery – The external iliac artery branches from the common iliac artery and serves the legs.
Femoral Artery – The femoral artery branches from the external iliac artery and serves the legs.
Foot Artery – Any of the smaller arterial branches that serve the foot.
Gastric Artery – The gastric artery branches from the celiac artery and serves the stomach and esophagus.
Hepatic Artery – The hepatic artery branches from the celiac artery and serves the gallbladder, liver, duodenum, pylorus, and pancreas.
Inferior Mesenteric Artery – The inferior mesenteric artery branches from the abdominal aorta and serves the descending colon, part of the transverse colon, sigmoid colon, and the upper part of the rectum.
Internal Iliac Artery – The internal iliac artery branches from the common iliac artery and serves the pelvic viscera, buttocks, and reproductive organs.
Lower Artery – The arteries located below the diaphragm (see Coding Guideline B2.1b).
Peroneal Artery – The peroneal artery (also known as the fibular artery) branches from the posterior tibial artery and serves the lateral portion of the leg.
Popliteal Artery – The popliteal artery branches from the femoral artery and serves the knee and lower leg.
Posterior Tibial Artery – The posterior tibial artery branches from the popliteal artery and serves the posterior portion of the lower leg and the plantar portion of the foot.
Renal Artery – The renal artery branches from the abdominal aorta and serves the kidney.
Splenic Artery – The splenic artery branches from the celiac artery and serves the spleen.
Superior Mesenteric Artery – The superior mesenteric artery branches from the abdominal aorta and serves the duodenum, ascending colon, part of the transverse colon, and pancreas.
Uterine Artery – The uterine artery branches from the internal iliac artery and serves the uterus.

Anatomical Illustrations of Lower Arteries

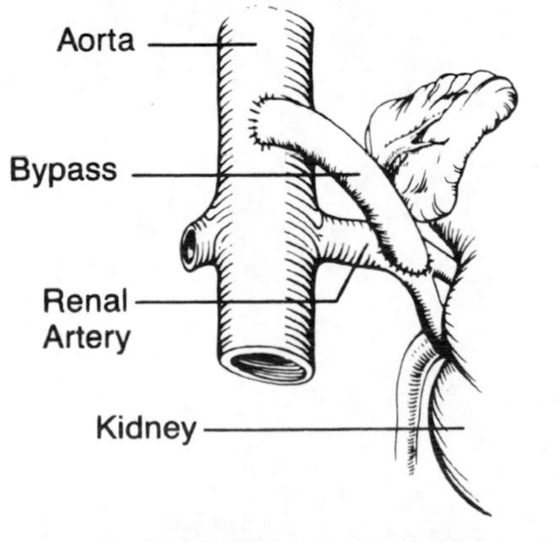

AORTA-RENAL BYPASS

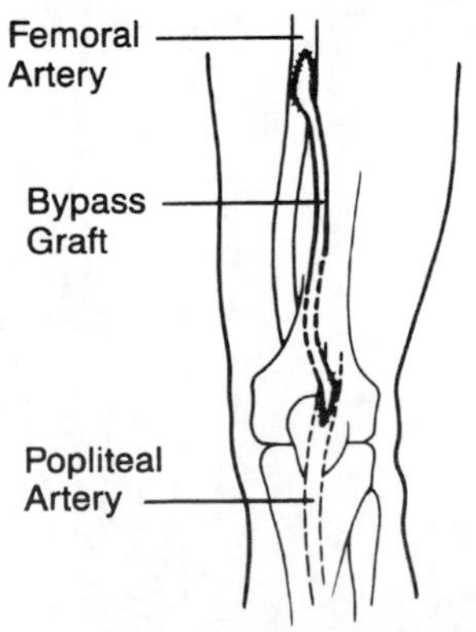

FEMORAL-POPLITEAL BYPASS

Continued on next page

© 2018 Channel Publishing, Ltd.

Educational Annotations | 4 – Lower Arteries

Anatomical Illustrations of Lower Arteries

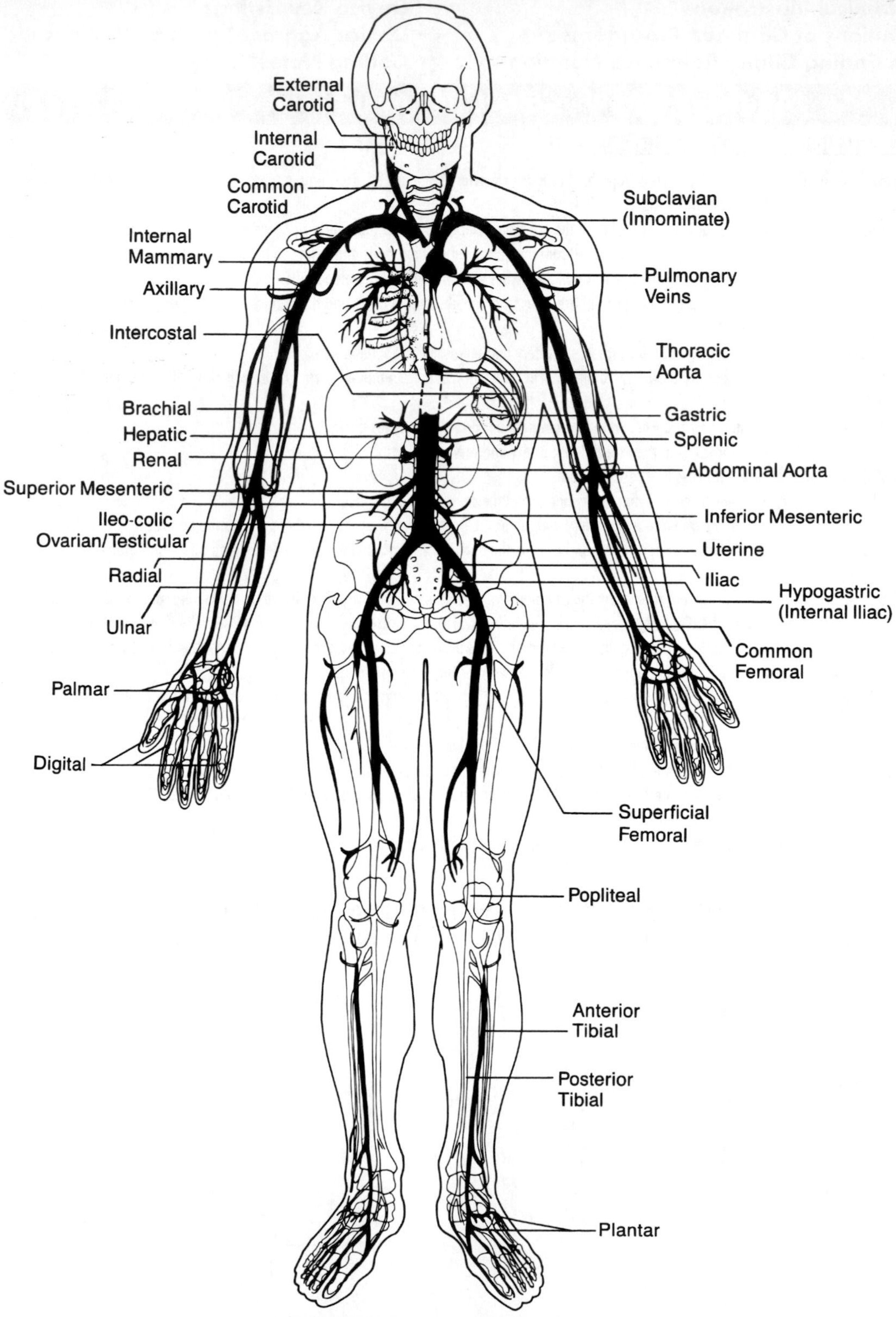

ARTERIES OF HUMAN BODY

Continued on next page

© 2018 Channel Publishing, Ltd.

Educational Annotations | 4 – Lower Arteries

Anatomical Illustrations of Lower Arteries

Continued from previous page

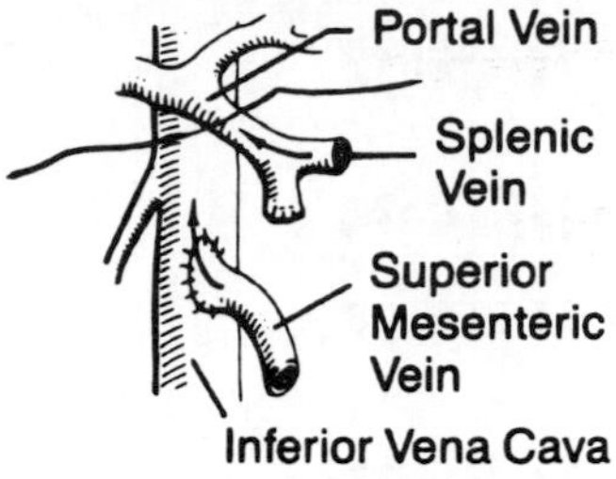

MESOCAVAL SHUNT

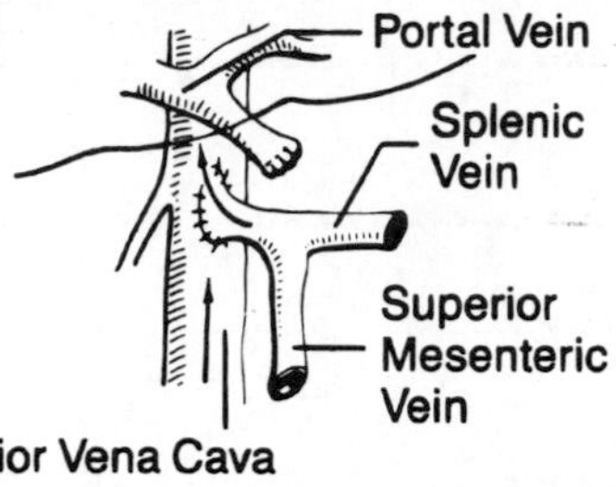

PORTACAVAL ANASTOMOSIS

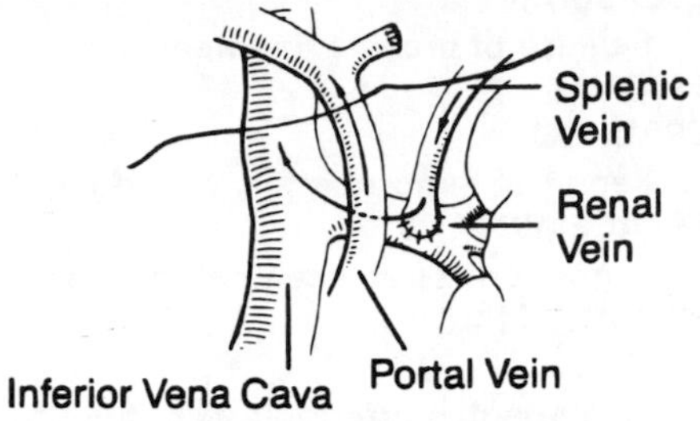

SPLENORENAL SHUNT

Definitions of Common Procedures of Lower Arteries

Aorto-bifemoral bypass – The restoration of blood flow to the legs by replacing the aortic-femoral bifurcation with a replacement graft that is usually synthetic, or the addition of a bypass graft sewn to the distal aorta and to the femoral arteries distal to the blockage site(s).
Abdominal aortic aneurysmectomy – The resection of an enlarged abdominal aortic wall protrusion and replacement with a graft that is usually synthetic. An endovascular version inserts a synthetic graft intravascularly to reinforce the weakened section without resecting any of the native aorta.
Femoral-popliteal bypass – The restoration of blood flow to the popliteal artery by using a bypass graft from the femoral artery.
Percutaneous mechanical thrombectomy – A minimally invasive approach to remove an acute thrombus in a lower extremity artery or graft by an endovascular approach using attachments to break up and remove the clot.

AHA Coding Clinic® Reference Notations of Lower Arteries

ROOT OPERATION SPECIFIC - 4 - LOWER ARTERIES

BYPASS - 1
- Bilateral renal artery bypass ....AHA 17:4Q:p47
- Bypass from gastroduodenal and splenic arteries to renal arteries ....AHA 15:3Q:p28
- Debranching bypass procedures ....AHA 17:3Q:p16
- Femoral artery bypass using in-situ saphenous vein direct bypass ....AHA 16:3Q:p31
- Femoral artery bypass using vein and synthetic grafts ....AHA 17:3Q:p5
- Peroneal artery to dorsalis pedis artery bypass ....AHA 17:1Q:p32
- Tibial artery bypass using saphenous vein graft and vein cuff ....AHA 16:2Q:p18

DESTRUCTION - 5

DILATION - 7
- Dilation of femoral artery using drug-coated balloon ....AHA 15:4Q:p15
- Drug-coated balloon angioplasty in femoral and popliteal arteries ....AHA 15:4Q:p4-7
- Femoral artery bifurcation ....AHA 16:4Q:p89

DRAINAGE - 9

EXCISION - B

EXTIRPATION - C
- Iliofemoral endarterectomy with bovine patch repair ....AHA 16:1Q:p31
- Thrombectomy of femoral popliteal bypass graft ....AHA 15:1Q:p36

INSERTION - H
- Placement of umbilical artery (UAC) catheter ....AHA 17:1Q:p30

INSPECTION - J

OCCLUSION - L
- Coil embolization of gastroduodenal artery, and chemoembolization of hepatic artery ....AHA 14:3Q:p26
- Endovascular embolization using microcoils of colic artery ....AHA 14:1Q:p24
- Gelfoam embolization of uterine artery ....AHA 15:2Q:p27
- Ligation of deep epigastric vessels before TRAM flap reconstruction ....AHA 18:2Q:p18
- Microbead embolization to the inferior mesenteric artery ....AHA 14:1Q:p24

Continued on next page

© 2018 Channel Publishing, Ltd.

Educational Annotations | 4 – Lower Arteries

AHA Coding Clinic® Reference Notations of Lower Arteries

ROOT OPERATION SPECIFIC - 4 - LOWER ARTERIES

Continued from previous page

RELEASE - N

- Release of arcuate ligament syndrome .... AHA 15:2Q:p28

REMOVAL - P

REPAIR - Q

- Repair of femoral artery pseudoaneurysm .... AHA 14:1Q:p21

REPLACEMENT - R

- Bypass graft (replacement) of celiac artery .... AHA 15:2Q:p28

REPOSITION - S

SUPPLEMENT - U

- Bovine patch arterioplasty of femoral artery .... AHA 14:4Q:p37
- Iliofemoral endarterectomy with bovine patch repair .... AHA 16:1Q:p31
- Placement of stent graft in saphenous vein graft .... AHA 14:1Q:p22
- Tibial artery bypass using saphenous vein graft and vein cuff .... AHA 16:2Q:p18

RESTRICTION - V

- Endovascular Abdominal Aortic Aneurysm Repair (EVAR) .... AHA 16:3Q:p39
- Stent graft repair of abdominal aortic aneurysm .... AHA 14:1Q:p9

REVISION - W

- Reanastomosed femoral popliteal bypass graft .... AHA 15:1Q:p36
- Reattachment of abdominal aortic stent graft .... AHA 14:1Q:p9
- Repair of ruptured femoral-popliteal bypass graft .... AHA 14:1Q:p22

Body Part Key Listings of Lower Arteries

See also Body Part Key in Appendix C

Anterior lateral malleolar artery	use Anterior Tibial Artery, Left/Right
Anterior medial malleolar artery	use Anterior Tibial Artery, Left/Right
Anterior tibial recurrent artery	use Anterior Tibial Artery, Left/Right
Arcuate artery	use Foot Artery, Left/Right
Celiac trunk	use Celiac Artery
Circumflex iliac artery	use Femoral Artery, Left/Right
Common hepatic artery	use Hepatic Artery
Deep circumflex iliac artery	use External Iliac Artery, Left/Right
Deep femoral artery	use Femoral Artery, Left/Right
Deferential artery	use Internal Iliac Artery, Left/Right
Descending genicular artery	use Femoral Artery, Left/Right
Dorsal metatarsal artery	use Foot Artery, Left/Right
Dorsalis pedis artery	use Anterior Tibial Artery, Left/Right
External pudendal artery	use Femoral Artery, Left/Right
Fibular artery	use Peroneal Artery, Left/Right
Gastroduodenal artery	use Hepatic Artery
Hepatic artery proper	use Hepatic Artery
Hypogastric artery	use Internal Iliac Artery, Left/Right
Ileal artery	use Superior Mesenteric Artery
Ileocolic artery	use Superior Mesenteric Artery
Iliolumbar artery	use Internal Iliac Artery, Left/Right
Inferior epigastric artery	use External Iliac Artery, Left/Right
Inferior genicular artery	use Popliteal Artery, Left/Right
Inferior gluteal artery	use Internal Iliac Artery, Left/Right
Inferior pancreaticoduodenal artery	use Superior Mesenteric Artery
Inferior phrenic artery	use Abdominal Aorta
Inferior suprarenal artery	use Renal Artery, Left/Right
Inferior vesical artery	use Internal Iliac Artery, Left/Right
Internal pudendal artery	use Internal Iliac Artery, Left/Right
Internal thoracic artery	use Internal Mammary Artery, Left/Right
	use Subclavian Artery, Left/Right
Jejunal artery	use Superior Mesenteric Artery
Lateral plantar artery	use Foot Artery, Left/Right
Lateral sacral artery	use Internal Iliac Artery, Left/Right
Lateral tarsal artery	use Foot Artery, Left/Right
Left gastric artery	use Gastric Artery
Left gastric artery	use Gastric Artery
Left gastroepiploic artery	use Splenic Artery
Lumbar artery	use Abdominal Aorta
Medial plantar artery	use Foot Artery, Left/Right
Median sacral artery	use Abdominal Aorta
Middle genicular artery	use Popliteal Artery, Left/Right
Middle rectal artery	use Internal Iliac Artery, Left/Right
Middle suprarenal artery	use Abdominal Aorta
Obturator artery	use Internal Iliac Artery, Left/Right
Ovarian artery	use Abdominal Aorta
Pancreatic artery	use Splenic Artery
Posterior tibial recurrent artery	use Anterior Tibial Artery, Left/Right
Renal segmental artery	use Renal Artery, Left/Right
Right gastric artery	use Gastric Artery
Short gastric artery	use Splenic Artery
Sigmoid artery	use Inferior Mesenteric Artery
Superficial epigastric artery	use Femoral Artery, Left/Right
Superior genicular artery	use Popliteal Artery, Left/Right
Superior gluteal artery	use Internal Iliac Artery, Left/Right
Superior rectal artery	use Inferior Mesenteric Artery
Sural artery	use Popliteal Artery, Left/Right
Testicular artery	use Abdominal Aorta
Umbilical artery	use Internal Iliac Artery, Left/Right
	use Lower Artery
Uterine artery	use Internal Iliac Artery, Left/Right
Vaginal artery	use Internal Iliac Artery, Left/Right

© 2018 Channel Publishing, Ltd.

Educational Annotations | 4 – Lower Arteries

Device Key Listings of Lower Arteries

See also Device Key in Appendix D

Absolute Pro Vascular (OTW) Self-Expanding Stent System ....use Intraluminal Device
AFX® Endovascular AAA System ....use Intraluminal Device
AneuRx® AAA Advantage® ....use Intraluminal Device
Assurant (Cobalt) stent ....use Intraluminal Device
Autograft ....use Autologous Tissue Substitute
Autologous artery graft ....use Autologous Arterial Tissue in Lower Arteries
Autologous vein graft....use Autologous Venous Tissue in Lower Arteries
Brachytherapy seeds ....use Radioactive Element
CoAxia NeuroFlo catheter ....use Intraluminal Device
Complete (SE) stent ....use Intraluminal Device
Cook Zenith AAA Endovascular Graft....use Intraluminal Device; Intraluminal Device, Branched or Fenestrated, One or Two Arteries for Restriction in Lower Arteries; Intraluminal Device, Branched or Fenestrated, Three or More Arteries for Restriction in Lower Arteries
E-Luminexx™ (Biliary) (Vascular) Stent....use Intraluminal Device
Embolization coil(s)....use Intraluminal Device
Endologix AFX® Endovascular AAA System....use Intraluminal Device
Endurant® II AAA stent graft system....use Intraluminal Device
Endurant® Endovascular Stent Graft....use Intraluminal Device
EXCLUDER® AAA Endoprothesis ....use Intraluminal Device, Intraluminal Device, Branched or Fenestrated, One or Two Arteries for Restriction in Lower Arteries; Intraluminal Device, Branched or Fenestrated, Three or More Arteries for Restriction in Lower Arteries
EXCLUDER® IBE Endoprothesis ....use Intraluminal Device; Intraluminal Device, Branched or Fenestrated, One or Two Arteries for Restriction in Lower Arteries
Express® (LD) Premounted Stent System ....use Intraluminal Device
Express® Biliary SD Monorail® Premounted Stent System ....use Intraluminal Device
Express® SD Renal Monorail® Premounted Stent System ....use Intraluminal Device
Formula™ Balloon-Expandable Renal Stent System ....use Intraluminal Device
GORE EXCLUDER® AAA Endoprothesis ....use Intraluminal Device; Intraluminal Device, Branched or Fenestrated, One or Two Arteries for Restriction in Lower Arteries; Intraluminal Device, Branched or Fenestrated, Three or More Arteries for Restriction in Lower Arteries
GORE EXCLUDER® IBE Endoprothesis....use Intraluminal Device, Branched or Fenestrated, One or Two Arteries for Restriction in Lower Arteries
Herculink (RX) Elite Renal Stent System ....use Intraluminal Device
LifeStent® (Flexstar) (XL) Vascular Stent System ....use Intraluminal Device
Medtronic Endurant® II AAA stent graft system....use Intraluminal Device
Omnilink Elite Vascular Balloon Expandable Stent System....use Intraluminal Device
Paclitaxel-eluting peripheral stent ....use Intraluminal Device, Drug-eluting in Upper Arteries, Lower Arteries
Stent, intraluminal (cardiovascular) (gastrointestinal) (hepatobiliary) (urinary) ....use Intraluminal Device
Talent® Converter ....use Intraluminal Device
Talent® Occluder ....use Intraluminal Device
Talent® Stent Graft (abdominal) (thoracic)....use Intraluminal Device
Tissue bank graft ....use Nonautologous Tissue Substitute
Zenith AAA Endovascular Graft ....use Intraluminal Device; Intraluminal Device, Branched or Fenestrated, One or Two Arteries for Restriction in Lower Arteries; Intraluminal Device, Branched or Fenestrated, Three or More Arteries for Restriction in Lower Arteries
Zenith Flex® AAA Endovascular Graft ....use Intraluminal Device
Zenith® Renu™ AAA Ancillary Graft....use Intraluminal Device
Zilver® PTX® (paclitaxel) Drug-Eluting Peripheral Stent ....use Intraluminal Device, Drug-eluting in Upper Arteries, Lower Arteries

© 2018 Channel Publishing, Ltd.

Educational Annotations | 4 – Lower Arteries

Device Aggregation Table Listings of Lower Arteries

See also Device Aggregation Table in Appendix E

Specific Device	For Operation	In Body System	General Device
Autologous Arterial Tissue	All applicable	Lower Arteries	Autologous Tissue Substitute
Autologous Venous Tissue	All applicable	Lower Arteries	Autologous Tissue Substitute
Intraluminal Device, Branched or Fenestrated, One or Two Arteries	All applicable	Heart and Great Vessels	Intraluminal Device
Intraluminal Device, Branched or Fenestrated, Three or More Arteries	All applicable	Heart and Great Vessels	Intraluminal Device
Intraluminal Device, Drug-eluting	All applicable	Lower Arteries	Intraluminal Device
Intraluminal Device, Drug-eluting, Four or More	All applicable	Heart and Great Vessels	Intraluminal Device
Intraluminal Device, Drug-eluting, Three	All applicable	Heart and Great Vessels	Intraluminal Device
Intraluminal Device, Drug-eluting, Two	All applicable	Heart and Great Vessels	Intraluminal Device
Intraluminal Device, Four or More	All applicable	Heart and Great Vessels	Intraluminal Device
Intraluminal Device, Three	All applicable	Heart and Great Vessels	Intraluminal Device
Intraluminal Device, Two	All applicable	Heart and Great Vessels	Intraluminal Device

Coding Notes of Lower Arteries

Body System Relevant Coding Guidelines

General Guidelines

B2.1b

Where the general body part values "upper" and "lower" are provided as an option in the Upper Arteries, Lower Arteries, Upper Veins, Lower Veins, Muscles and Tendons body systems, "upper" or "lower "specifies body parts located above or below the diaphragm respectively.

Example: Vein body parts above the diaphragm are found in the Upper Veins body system; vein body parts below the diaphragm are found in the Lower Veins body system.

Body part, General guidelines

B4.1c

If a procedure is performed on a continuous section of a tubular body part, code the body part value corresponding to the furthest anatomical site from the point of entry.

Example: A procedure performed on a continuous section of artery from the femoral artery to the external iliac artery with the point of entry at the femoral artery is coded to the external iliac body part.

Branches of body parts

B4.2

Where a specific branch of a body part does not have its own body part value in PCS, the body part is typically coded to the closest proximal branch that has a specific body part value. In the cardiovascular body systems, if a general body part is available in the correct root operation table, and coding to a proximal branch would require assigning a code in a different body system, the procedure is coded using the general body part value.

Examples: A procedure performed on the mandibular branch of the trigeminal nerve is coded to the trigeminal nerve body part value.

Occlusion of the bronchial artery is coded to the body part value Upper Artery in the body system Upper Arteries, and not to the body part value Thoracic Aorta, Descending in the body system Heart and Great Vessels.

© 2018 Channel Publishing, Ltd.

1ST - 0 Medical and Surgical

2ND - 4 Lower Arteries

3RD - 1 BYPASS

TUBULAR GROUP: Bypass, Dilation, Occlusion, Restriction
Root Operations that alter the diameter/route of a tubular body part.

BYPASS: Altering the route of passage of the contents of a tubular body part.

Explanation: Rerouting contents to a downstream part ... with or without the use of a device ...
Examples: Aorto-bifemoral bypass – CMS Ex: Coronary artery bypass

Body Part – 4TH	Approach – 5TH	Device – 6TH	Qualifier – 7TH
0 Abdominal Aorta C Common Iliac Artery, Right D Common Iliac Artery, Left	0 Open 4 Percutaneous endoscopic	9 Autologous venous tissue A Autologous arterial tissue J Synthetic substitute K Nonautologous tissue substitute Z No device	0 Abdominal Aorta 1 Celiac Artery 2 Mesenteric Artery 3 Renal Artery, Right 4 Renal Artery, Left 5 Renal Artery, Bilateral 6 Common Iliac Artery, Right 7 Common Iliac Artery, Left 8 Common Iliac Arteries, Bilateral 9 Internal Iliac Artery, Right B Internal Iliac Artery, Left C Internal Iliac Arteries, Bilateral D External Iliac Artery, Right F External Iliac Artery, Left G External Iliac Arteries, Bilateral H Femoral Artery, Right J Femoral Artery, Left K Femoral Arteries, Bilateral Q Lower Extremity Artery R Lower Artery
3 Hepatic Artery 4 Splenic Artery	0 Open 4 Percutaneous endoscopic	9 Autologous venous tissue A Autologous arterial tissue J Synthetic substitute K Nonautologous tissue substitute Z No device	3 Renal Artery, Right 4 Renal Artery, Left 5 Renal Artery, Bilateral
E Internal Iliac Artery, Right F Internal Iliac Artery, Left H External Iliac Artery, Right J External Iliac Artery, Left	0 Open 4 Percutaneous endoscopic	9 Autologous venous tissue A Autologous arterial tissue J Synthetic substitute K Nonautologous tissue substitute Z No device	9 Internal Iliac Artery, Right B Internal Iliac Artery, Left C Internal Iliac Arteries, Bilateral D External Iliac Artery, Right F External Iliac Artery, Left G External Iliac Arteries, Bilateral H Femoral Artery, Right J Femoral Artery, Left K Femoral Arteries, Bilateral P Foot Artery Q Lower Extremity Artery
K Femoral Artery, Right L Femoral Artery, Left	0 Open 4 Percutaneous endoscopic	9 Autologous venous tissue A Autologous arterial tissue J Synthetic substitute K Nonautologous tissue substitute Z No device	H Femoral Artery, Right J Femoral Artery, Left K Femoral Arteries, Bilateral L Popliteal Artery M Peroneal Artery N Posterior Tibial Artery P Foot Artery Q Lower Extremity Artery S Lower Extremity Vein
K Femoral Artery, Right L Femoral Artery, Left	3 Percutaneous	J Synthetic substitute	Q Lower Extremity Artery S Lower Extremity Vein

continued ⇨

© 2018 Channel Publishing, Ltd.

0 4 1 BYPASS – *continued*

Body Part – 4TH	Approach – 5TH	Device – 6TH	Qualifier – 7TH
M Popliteal Artery, Right N Popliteal Artery, Left	0 Open 4 Percutaneous endoscopic	9 Autologous venous tissue A Autologous arterial tissue J Synthetic substitute K Nonautologous tissue substitute Z No device	L Popliteal Artery M Peroneal Artery P Foot Artery Q Lower Extremity Artery S Lower Extremity Vein
M Popliteal Artery, Right N Popliteal Artery, Left	3 Percutaneous	J Synthetic substitute	Q Lower Extremity Artery S Lower Extremity Vein
P Anterior Tibial Artery, Right Q Anterior Tibial Artery, Left R Posterior Tibial Artery, Right S Posterior Tibial Artery, Left	0 Open 3 Percutaneous 4 Percutaneous endoscopic	J Synthetic substitute	Q Lower Extremity Artery S Lower Extremity Vein
T Peroneal Artery, Right U Peroneal Artery, Left V Foot Artery, Right W Foot Artery, Left	0 Open 4 Percutaneous endoscopic	9 Autologous venous tissue A Autologous arterial tissue J Synthetic substitute K Nonautologous tissue substitute Z No device	P Foot Artery Q Lower Extremity Artery S Lower Extremity Vein
T Peroneal Artery, Right U Peroneal Artery, Left V Foot Artery, Right W Foot Artery, Left	3 Percutaneous	J Synthetic substitute	Q Lower Extremity Artery S Lower Extremity Vein

1ST - 0 Medical and Surgical
2ND - 4 Lower Arteries
3RD - 5 DESTRUCTION

EXCISION GROUP: Excision, (Resection), Destruction, (Extraction), (Detachment)
Root Operations that take out some or all of a body part.

DESTRUCTION: Physical eradication of all or a portion of a body part by the direct use of energy, force, or a destructive agent.

Explanation: None of the body part is physically taken out
Examples: Fulguration arterial lesion – CMS Ex: Fulguration of rectal polyp

Body Part – 4TH			Approach – 5TH	Device – 6TH	Qualifier – 7TH
0 Abdominal Aorta 1 Celiac Artery 2 Gastric Artery 3 Hepatic Artery 4 Splenic Artery 5 Superior Mesenteric Artery 6 Colic Artery, Right 7 Colic Artery, Left 8 Colic Artery, Middle 9 Renal Artery, Right A Renal Artery, Left B Inferior Mesenteric Artery	C Common Iliac Artery, Right D Common Iliac Artery, Left E Internal Iliac Artery, Right F Internal Iliac Artery, Left H External Iliac Artery, Right J External Iliac Artery, Left K Femoral Artery, Right L Femoral Artery, Left M Popliteal Artery, Right N Popliteal Artery, Left	P Anterior Tibial Artery, Right Q Anterior Tibial Artery, Left R Posterior Tibial Artery, Right S Posterior Tibial Artery, Left T Peroneal Artery, Right U Peroneal Artery, Left V Foot Artery, Right W Foot Artery, Left Y Lower Artery	0 Open 3 Percutaneous 4 Percutaneous endoscopic	Z No device	Z No qualifier

© 2018 Channel Publishing, Ltd.

1ST - 0 Medical and Surgical 2ND - 4 Lower Arteries 3RD - 7 DILATION	TUBULAR GROUP: Bypass, Dilation, Occlusion, Restriction Root Operations that alter the diameter/route of a tubular body part. DILATION: Expanding an orifice or the lumen of a tubular body part. Explanation: Accomplished by stretching or cutting ... tubular body part or orifice ... Examples: PTA femoral artery – CMS Ex: Percutaneous transluminal angioplasty		

Body Part – 4TH	Approach – 5TH	Device – 6TH	Qualifier – 7TH
0 Abdominal Aorta 1 Celiac Artery 2 Gastric Artery 3 Hepatic Artery 4 Splenic Artery 5 Superior Mesenteric Artery 6 Colic Artery, Right 7 Colic Artery, Left 8 Colic Artery, Middle 9 Renal Artery, Right A Renal Artery, Left B Inferior Mesenteric Artery C Common Iliac Artery, Right D Common Iliac Artery, Left E Internal Iliac Artery, Right F Internal Iliac Artery, Left H External Iliac Artery, Right J External Iliac Artery, Left K Femoral Artery, Right L Femoral Artery, Left M Popliteal Artery, Right N Popliteal Artery, Left P Anterior Tibial Artery, Right Q Anterior Tibial Artery, Left R Posterior Tibial Artery, Right S Posterior Tibial Artery, Left T Peroneal Artery, Right U Peroneal Artery, Left V Foot Artery, Right W Foot Artery, Left Y Lower Artery	0 Open 3 Percutaneous 4 Percutaneous endoscopic	4 Drug-eluting intraluminal device D Intraluminal device Z No device	1 Drug-coated balloon 6 Bifurcation Z No qualifier
0 Abdominal Aorta 1 Celiac Artery 2 Gastric Artery 3 Hepatic Artery 4 Splenic Artery 5 Superior Mesenteric Artery 6 Colic Artery, Right 7 Colic Artery, Left 8 Colic Artery, Middle 9 Renal Artery, Right A Renal Artery, Left B Inferior Mesenteric Artery C Common Iliac Artery, Right D Common Iliac Artery, Left E Internal Iliac Artery, Right F Internal Iliac Artery, Left H External Iliac Artery, Right J External Iliac Artery, Left K Femoral Artery, Right L Femoral Artery, Left M Popliteal Artery, Right N Popliteal Artery, Left P Anterior Tibial Artery, Right Q Anterior Tibial Artery, Left R Posterior Tibial Artery, Right S Posterior Tibial Artery, Left T Peroneal Artery, Right U Peroneal Artery, Left V Foot Artery, Right W Foot Artery, Left Y Lower Artery	0 Open 3 Percutaneous 4 Percutaneous endoscopic	5 Drug-eluting intraluminal device, two 6 Drug-eluting intraluminal device,three 7 Drug-eluting intraluminal device, four or more E Intraluminal device, two F Intraluminal device, three G Intraluminal device, four or more	6 Bifurcation Z No qualifier

LOWER ARTERIES 047

© 2018 Channel Publishing, Ltd.

1ST - 0 Medical and Surgical
2ND - 4 Lower Arteries
3RD - 9 DRAINAGE

DRAINAGE GROUP: Drainage, Extirpation, (Fragmentation)
Root Operations that take out solids/fluids/gases from a body part.

DRAINAGE: Taking or letting out fluids and/or gases from a body part.

Explanation: Qualifier "X Diagnostic" indicates drainage procedures that are biopsies
Examples: Aspiration arterial abscess – CMS Ex: Thoracentesis

Body Part – 4TH	Approach – 5TH	Device – 6TH	Qualifier – 7TH
0 Abdominal Aorta 1 Celiac Artery 2 Gastric Artery 3 Hepatic Artery 4 Splenic Artery 5 Superior Mesenteric Artery 6 Colic Artery, Right 7 Colic Artery, Left 8 Colic Artery, Middle 9 Renal Artery, Right A Renal Artery, Left B Inferior Mesenteric Artery C Common Iliac Artery, Right D Common Iliac Artery, Left E Internal Iliac Artery, Right F Internal Iliac Artery, Left H External Iliac Artery, Right J External Iliac Artery, Left K Femoral Artery, Right L Femoral Artery, Left M Popliteal Artery, Right N Popliteal Artery, Left P Anterior Tibial Artery, Right Q Anterior Tibial Artery, Left R Posterior Tibial Artery, Right S Posterior Tibial Artery, Left T Peroneal Artery, Right U Peroneal Artery, Left V Foot Artery, Right W Foot Artery, Left Y Lower Artery	0 Open 3 Percutaneous 4 Percutaneous endoscopic	0 Drainage device	Z No qualifier
0 Abdominal Aorta 1 Celiac Artery 2 Gastric Artery 3 Hepatic Artery 4 Splenic Artery 5 Superior Mesenteric Artery 6 Colic Artery, Right 7 Colic Artery, Left 8 Colic Artery, Middle 9 Renal Artery, Right A Renal Artery, Left B Inferior Mesenteric Artery C Common Iliac Artery, Right D Common Iliac Artery, Left E Internal Iliac Artery, Right F Internal Iliac Artery, Left H External Iliac Artery, Right J External Iliac Artery, Left K Femoral Artery, Right L Femoral Artery, Left M Popliteal Artery, Right N Popliteal Artery, Left P Anterior Tibial Artery, Right Q Anterior Tibial Artery, Left R Posterior Tibial Artery, Right S Posterior Tibial Artery, Left T Peroneal Artery, Right U Peroneal Artery, Left V Foot Artery, Right W Foot Artery, Left Y Lower Artery	0 Open 3 Percutaneous 4 Percutaneous endoscopic	Z No device	X Diagnostic Z No qualifier

1ST - 0 Medical and Surgical
2ND - 4 Lower Arteries
3RD - B EXCISION

EXCISION GROUP: Excision, (Resection), Destruction, (Extraction), (Detachment)
Root Operations that take out some or all of a body part.

EXCISION: Cutting out or off, without replacement, a portion of a body part.

Explanation: Qualifier "X Diagnostic" indicates excision procedures that are biopsies
Examples: Femoral artery biopsy – CMS Ex: Liver biopsy

Body Part – 4TH	Approach – 5TH	Device – 6TH	Qualifier – 7TH
0 Abdominal Aorta 1 Celiac Artery 2 Gastric Artery 3 Hepatic Artery 4 Splenic Artery 5 Superior Mesenteric Artery 6 Colic Artery, Right 7 Colic Artery, Left 8 Colic Artery, Middle 9 Renal Artery, Right A Renal Artery, Left B Inferior Mesenteric Artery C Common Iliac Artery, Right D Common Iliac Artery, Left E Internal Iliac Artery, Right F Internal Iliac Artery, Left H External Iliac Artery, Right J External Iliac Artery, Left K Femoral Artery, Right L Femoral Artery, Left M Popliteal Artery, Right N Popliteal Artery, Left P Anterior Tibial Artery, Right Q Anterior Tibial Artery, Left R Posterior Tibial Artery, Right S Posterior Tibial Artery, Left T Peroneal Artery, Right U Peroneal Artery, Left V Foot Artery, Right W Foot Artery, Left Y Lower Artery	0 Open 3 Percutaneous 4 Percutaneous endoscopic	Z No device	X Diagnostic Z No qualifier

© 2018 Channel Publishing, Ltd.

1ST - 0 Medical and Surgical
2ND - 4 Lower Arteries
3RD - C EXTIRPATION

DRAINAGE GROUP: Drainage, Extirpation, (Fragmentation)
Root Operations that take out solids/fluids/gases from a body part.

EXTIRPATION: Taking or cutting out solid matter from a body part.

Explanation: Abnormal byproduct or foreign body ...
Examples: Iliac artery thrombectomy – CMS Ex: Thrombectomy

Body Part – 4TH	Approach – 5TH	Device – 6TH	Qualifier – 7TH
0 Abdominal Aorta 1 Celiac Artery 2 Gastric Artery 3 Hepatic Artery 4 Splenic Artery 5 Superior Mesenteric Artery 6 Colic Artery, Right 7 Colic Artery, Left 8 Colic Artery, Middle 9 Renal Artery, Right A Renal Artery, Left B Inferior Mesenteric Artery C Common Iliac Artery, Right D Common Iliac Artery, Left E Internal Iliac Artery, Right F Internal Iliac Artery, Left H External Iliac Artery, Right J External Iliac Artery, Left K Femoral Artery, Right L Femoral Artery, Left M Popliteal Artery, Right N Popliteal Artery, Left P Anterior Tibial Artery, Right Q Anterior Tibial Artery, Left R Posterior Tibial Artery, Right S Posterior Tibial Artery, Left T Peroneal Artery, Right U Peroneal Artery, Left V Foot Artery, Right W Foot Artery, Left Y Lower Artery	0 Open 3 Percutaneous 4 Percutaneous endoscopic	Z No device	6 Bifurcation Z No qualifier

1ST - 0 Medical and Surgical
2ND - 4 Lower Arteries
3RD - H INSERTION

DEVICE GROUP: (Change), Insertion, Removal, Replacement, Revision, Supplement
Root Operations that always involve a device.

INSERTION: Putting in a nonbiological appliance that monitors, assists, performs, or prevents a physiological function but does not physically take the place of a body part.

Explanation: None
Examples: Arterial infusion catheter – CMS Ex: Insertion of central venous catheter

Body Part – 4TH	Approach – 5TH	Device – 6TH	Qualifier – 7TH
0 Abdominal Aorta	0 Open 3 Percutaneous 4 Percutaneous endoscopic	2 Monitoring device 3 Infusion device D Intraluminal device	Z No qualifier
1 Celiac Artery 2 Gastric Artery 3 Hepatic Artery 4 Splenic Artery 5 Superior Mesenteric Artery 6 Colic Artery, Right 7 Colic Artery, Left 8 Colic Artery, Middle 9 Renal Artery, Right A Renal Artery, Left B Inferior Mesenteric Artery C Common Iliac Artery, Right D Common Iliac Artery, Left E Internal Iliac Artery, Right F Internal Iliac Artery, Left H External Iliac Artery, Right J External Iliac Artery, Left K Femoral Artery, Right L Femoral Artery, Left M Popliteal Artery, Right N Popliteal Artery, Left P Anterior Tibial Artery, Right Q Anterior Tibial Artery, Left R Posterior Tibial Artery, Right S Posterior Tibial Artery, Left T Peroneal Artery, Right U Peroneal Artery, Left V Foot Artery, Right W Foot Artery, Left	0 Open 3 Percutaneous 4 Percutaneous endoscopic	3 Infusion device D Intraluminal device	Z No qualifier
Y Lower Artery	0 Open 3 Percutaneous 4 Percutaneous endoscopic	2 Monitoring device 3 Infusion device D Intraluminal device Y Other device	Z No qualifier

© 2018 Channel Publishing, Ltd.

1ST - 0 Medical and Surgical
2ND - 4 Lower Arteries
3RD - J INSPECTION

EXAMINATION GROUP: Inspection, (Map)
Root Operations involving examination only.

INSPECTION: Visually and/or manually exploring a body part.

Explanation: Direct or instrumental visualization ...
Examples: Exploration arterial catheter removal site – CMS Ex: Exploratory laparotomy

Body Part – 4TH	Approach – 5TH	Device – 6TH	Qualifier – 7TH
Y Lower Artery	0 Open 3 Percutaneous 4 Percutaneous endoscopic X External	Z No device	Z No qualifier

1ST - 0 Medical and Surgical
2ND - 4 Lower Arteries
3RD - L OCCLUSION

TUBULAR GROUP: Bypass, Dilation, Occlusion, Restriction
Root Operations that alter the diameter/route of a tubular body part.

OCCLUSION: Completely closing an orifice or the lumen of a tubular body part.

Explanation: The orifice can be a natural orifice or an artificially created orifice
Examples: Renal artery embolization – CMS Ex: Fallopian tube ligation

Body Part – 4TH	Approach – 5TH	Device – 6TH	Qualifier – 7TH
0 Abdominal Aorta	0 Open 4 Percutaneous endoscopic	C Extraluminal device D Intraluminal device Z No device	Z No qualifier
0 Abdominal Aorta	3 Percutaneous	C Extraluminal device Z No device	Z No qualifier
0 Abdominal Aorta	3 Percutaneous	D Intraluminal device	J Temporary Z No qualifier
1 Celiac Artery 2 Gastric Artery 3 Hepatic Artery 4 Splenic Artery 5 Superior Mesenteric Artery 6 Colic Artery, Right 7 Colic Artery, Left 8 Colic Artery, Middle 9 Renal Artery, Right A Renal Artery, Left B Inferior Mesenteric Artery C Common Iliac Artery, Right D Common Iliac Artery, Left H External Iliac Artery, Right J External Iliac Artery, Left K Femoral Artery, Right L Femoral Artery, Left M Popliteal Artery, Right N Popliteal Artery, Left P Anterior Tibial Artery, Right Q Anterior Tibial Artery, Left R Posterior Tibial Artery, Right S Posterior Tibial Artery, Left T Peroneal Artery, Right U Peroneal Artery, Left V Foot Artery, Right W Foot Artery, Left Y Lower Artery	0 Open 3 Percutaneous 4 Percutaneous endoscopic	C Extraluminal device D Intraluminal device Z No device	Z No qualifier
E Internal Iliac Artery, Right	0 Open 3 Percutaneous 4 Percutaneous endoscopic	C Extraluminal device D Intraluminal device Z No device	T Uterine artery, right ♀ Z No qualifier
F Internal Iliac Artery, Left	0 Open 3 Percutaneous 4 Percutaneous endoscopic	C Extraluminal device D Intraluminal device Z No device	U Uterine artery, left ♀ Z No qualifier

© 2018 Channel Publishing, Ltd.

1ST - 0 Medical and Surgical
2ND - 4 Lower Arteries
3RD - N RELEASE

DIVISION GROUP: (Division), Release
Root Operations involving cutting or separation only.

RELEASE: Freeing a body part from an abnormal physical constraint by cutting or by the use of force.

Explanation: Some of the restraining tissue may be taken out but none of the body part is taken out
Examples: Arterial adhesiolysis – CMS Ex: Carpal tunnel release

Body Part – 4TH			Approach – 5TH	Device – 6TH	Qualifier – 7TH
0 Abdominal Aorta 1 Celiac Artery 2 Gastric Artery 3 Hepatic Artery 4 Splenic Artery 5 Superior Mesenteric Artery 6 Colic Artery, Right 7 Colic Artery, Left 8 Colic Artery, Middle 9 Renal Artery, Right A Renal Artery, Left B Inferior Mesenteric Artery	C Common Iliac Artery, Right D Common Iliac Artery, Left E Internal Iliac Artery, Right F Internal Iliac Artery, Left H External Iliac Artery, Right J External Iliac Artery, Left K Femoral Artery, Right L Femoral Artery, Left M Popliteal Artery, Right N Popliteal Artery, Left	P Anterior Tibial Artery, Right Q Anterior Tibial Artery, Left R Posterior Tibial Artery, Right S Posterior Tibial Artery, Left T Peroneal Artery, Right U Peroneal Artery, Left V Foot Artery, Right W Foot Artery, Left Y Lower Artery	0 Open 3 Percutaneous 4 Percutaneous endoscopic	Z No device	Z No qualifier

1ST - 0 Medical and Surgical
2ND - 4 Lower Arteries
3RD - P REMOVAL

DEVICE GROUP: (Change), Insertion, Removal, Replacement, Revision, Supplement
Root Operations that always involve a device.

REMOVAL: Taking out or off a device from a body part.

Explanation: Removal device without reinsertion ...
Examples: Removal arterial catheter – CMS Ex: Cardiac pacemaker removal

Body Part – 4TH	Approach – 5TH	Device – 6TH	Qualifier – 7TH
Y Lower Artery	0 Open 3 Percutaneous 4 Percutaneous endoscopic	0 Drainage device 2 Monitoring device 3 Infusion device 7 Autologous tissue substitute C Extraluminal device D Intraluminal device J Synthetic substitute K Nonautologous tissue substitute Y Other device	Z No qualifier
Y Lower Artery	X External	0 Drainage device 1 Radioactive element 2 Monitoring device 3 Infusion device D Intraluminal device	Z No qualifier

© 2018 Channel Publishing, Ltd.

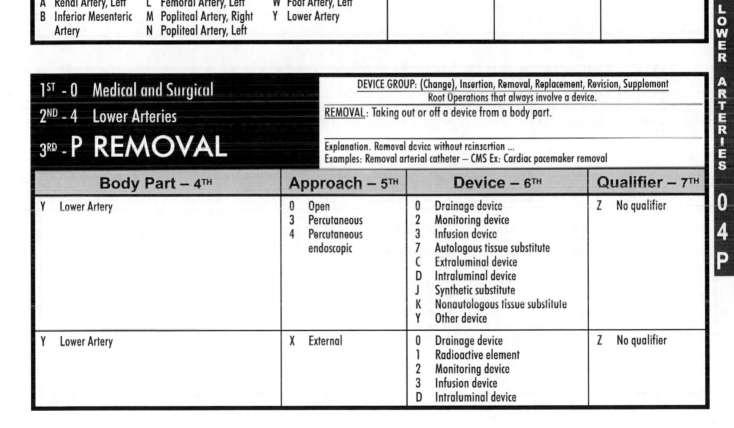

1ST - 0 Medical and Surgical
2ND - 4 Lower Arteries
3RD - Q REPAIR

OTHER REPAIRS GROUP: (Control), Repair
Root Operations that define other repairs.

REPAIR: Restoring, to the extent possible, a body part to its normal anatomic structure and function.

Explanation: Used only when the method to accomplish the repair is not one of the other root operations
Examples: Suture arterial injury – CMS Ex: Suture of laceration

Body Part – 4TH	Approach – 5TH	Device – 6TH	Qualifier – 7TH
0 Abdominal Aorta 1 Celiac Artery 2 Gastric Artery 3 Hepatic Artery 4 Splenic Artery 5 Superior Mesenteric Artery 6 Colic Artery, Right 7 Colic Artery, Left 8 Colic Artery, Middle 9 Renal Artery, Right A Renal Artery, Left B Inferior Mesenteric Artery C Common Iliac Artery, Right D Common Iliac Artery, Left E Internal Iliac Artery, Right F Internal Iliac Artery, Left H External Iliac Artery, Right J External Iliac Artery, Left K Femoral Artery, Right L Femoral Artery, Left M Popliteal Artery, Right N Popliteal Artery, Left P Anterior Tibial Artery, Right Q Anterior Tibial Artery, Left R Posterior Tibial Artery, Right S Posterior Tibial Artery, Left T Peroneal Artery, Right U Peroneal Artery, Left V Foot Artery, Right W Foot Artery, Left Y Lower Artery	0 Open 3 Percutaneous 4 Percutaneous endoscopic	Z No device	Z No qualifier

1ST - 0 Medical and Surgical
2ND - 4 Lower Arteries
3RD - R REPLACEMENT

DEVICE GROUP: (Change), Insertion, Removal, Replacement, Revision, Supplement
Root Operations that always involve a device.

REPLACEMENT: Putting in or on biological or synthetic material that physically takes the place and/or function of all or a portion of a body part.

Explanation: Includes taking out or eradicating, or rendering non-functional, the body part ...
Examples: Reconstruction artery using graft – CMS Ex: Total hip replacement

Body Part – 4TH	Approach – 5TH	Device – 6TH	Qualifier – 7TH
0 Abdominal Aorta 1 Celiac Artery 2 Gastric Artery 3 Hepatic Artery 4 Splenic Artery 5 Superior Mesenteric Artery 6 Colic Artery, Right 7 Colic Artery, Left 8 Colic Artery, Middle 9 Renal Artery, Right A Renal Artery, Left B Inferior Mesenteric Artery C Common Iliac Artery, Right D Common Iliac Artery, Left E Internal Iliac Artery, Right F Internal Iliac Artery, Left H External Iliac Artery, Right J External Iliac Artery, Left K Femoral Artery, Right L Femoral Artery, Left M Popliteal Artery, Right N Popliteal Artery, Left P Anterior Tibial Artery, Right Q Anterior Tibial Artery, Left R Posterior Tibial Artery, Right S Posterior Tibial Artery, Left T Peroneal Artery, Right U Peroneal Artery, Left V Foot Artery, Right W Foot Artery, Left Y Lower Artery	0 Open 4 Percutaneous endoscopic	7 Autologous tissue substitute J Synthetic substitute K Nonautologous tissue substitute	Z No qualifier

© 2018 Channel Publishing, Ltd.

1ST - 0 Medical and Surgical
2ND - 4 Lower Arteries
3RD - S REPOSITION

MOVE GROUP: (Reattachment), Reposition, (Transfer), (Transplantation)
Root Operations that put in/put back or move some/all of a body part.

REPOSITION: Moving to its normal location, or other suitable location, all or a portion of a body part.

Explanation: The body part may or may not be cut out or off to be moved to the new location ...
Examples: Relocation peroneal artery – CMS Ex: Fracture reduction

Body Part – 4TH			Approach – 5TH	Device – 6TH	Qualifier – 7TH
0 Abdominal Aorta 1 Celiac Artery 2 Gastric Artery 3 Hepatic Artery 4 Splenic Artery 5 Superior Mesenteric Artery 6 Colic Artery, Right 7 Colic Artery, Left 8 Colic Artery, Middle 9 Renal Artery, Right A Renal Artery, Left B Inferior Mesenteric Artery	C Common Iliac Artery, Right D Common Iliac Artery, Left E Internal Iliac Artery, Right F Internal Iliac Artery, Left H External Iliac Artery, Right J External Iliac Artery, Left K Femoral Artery, Right L Femoral Artery, Left M Popliteal Artery, Right N Popliteal Artery, Left	P Anterior Tibial Artery, Right Q Anterior Tibial Artery, Left R Posterior Tibial Artery, Right S Posterior Tibial Artery, Left T Peroneal Artery, Right U Peroneal Artery, Left V Foot Artery, Right W Foot Artery, Left Y Lower Artery	0 Open 3 Percutaneous 4 Percutaneous endoscopic	Z No device	Z No qualifier

1ST - 0 Medical and Surgical
2ND - 4 Lower Arteries
3RD - U SUPPLEMENT

DEVICE GROUP: (Change), Insertion, Removal, Replacement, Revision, Supplement
Root Operations that always involve a device.

SUPPLEMENT: Putting in or on biological or synthetic material that physically reinforces and/or augments the function of a portion of a body part.

Explanation: Biological material is non-living, or is living and from the same individual ...
Examples: Bovine graft angioplasty – CMS Ex: Herniorrhaphy using mesh

Body Part – 4TH			Approach – 5TH	Device – 6TH	Qualifier – 7TH
0 Abdominal Aorta 1 Celiac Artery 2 Gastric Artery 3 Hepatic Artery 4 Splenic Artery 5 Superior Mesenteric Artery 6 Colic Artery, Right 7 Colic Artery, Left 8 Colic Artery, Middle 9 Renal Artery, Right A Renal Artery, Left B Inferior Mesenteric Artery	C Common Iliac Artery, Right D Common Iliac Artery, Left E Internal Iliac Artery, Right F Internal Iliac Artery, Left H External Iliac Artery, Right J External Iliac Artery, Left K Femoral Artery, Right L Femoral Artery, Left M Popliteal Artery, Right N Popliteal Artery, Left	P Anterior Tibial Artery, Right Q Anterior Tibial Artery, Left R Posterior Tibial Artery, Right S Posterior Tibial Artery, Left T Peroneal Artery, Right U Peroneal Artery, Left V Foot Artery, Right W Foot Artery, Left Y Lower Artery	0 Open 3 Percutaneous 4 Percutaneous endoscopic	7 Autologous tissue substitute J Synthetic substitute K Nonautologous tissue substitute	Z No qualifier

© 2018 Channel Publishing, Ltd.

1ST - 0 Medical and Surgical
2ND - 4 Lower Arteries
3RD - V RESTRICTION

TUBULAR GROUP: Bypass, Dilation, Occlusion, Restriction
Root Operations that alter the diameter/route of a tubular body part.

RESTRICTION: Partially closing an orifice or the lumen of a tubular body part.

Explanation: The orifice can be a natural orifice or an artificially created orifice.
Examples: Stent graft repair aneurysm – CMS Ex: Cervical cerclage

Body Part – 4TH	Approach – 5TH	Device – 6TH	Qualifier – 7TH
0 Abdominal Aorta	0 Open 3 Percutaneous 4 Percutaneous endoscopic	C Extraluminal device E Intraluminal device, branched or fenestrated, one or two arteries F Intraluminal device, branched or fenestrated, three or more arteries Z No device	6 Bifurcation Z No qualifier
0 Abdominal Aorta	0 Open 3 Percutaneous 4 Percutaneous endoscopic	D Intraluminal device	6 Bifurcation J Temporary Z No qualifier
1 Celiac Artery 2 Gastric Artery 3 Hepatic Artery 4 Splenic Artery 5 Superior Mesenteric Artery 6 Colic Artery, Right 7 Colic Artery, Left 8 Colic Artery, Middle 9 Renal Artery, Right A Renal Artery, Left B Inferior Mesenteric Artery E Internal Iliac Artery, Right F Internal Iliac Artery, Left H External Iliac Artery, Right J External Iliac Artery, Left K Femoral Artery, Right L Femoral Artery, Left M Popliteal Artery, Right N Popliteal Artery, Left P Anterior Tibial Artery, Right Q Anterior Tibial Artery, Left R Posterior Tibial Artery, Right S Posterior Tibial Artery, Left T Peroneal Artery, Right U Peroneal Artery, Left V Foot Artery, Right W Foot Artery, Left Y Lower Artery	0 Open 3 Percutaneous 4 Percutaneous endoscopic	C Extraluminal device D Intraluminal device Z No device	Z No qualifier
C Common Iliac Artery, Right D Common Iliac Artery, Left	0 Open 3 Percutaneous 4 Percutaneous endoscopic	C Extraluminal device D Intraluminal device E Intraluminal device, branched or fenestrated, one or two arteries Z No device	Z No qualifier

LOWER ARTERIES 0 4 V

1ST - 0 Medical and Surgical
2ND - 4 Lower Arteries
3RD - W REVISION

DEVICE GROUP: (Change), Insertion, Removal, Replacement, Revision, Supplement
Root Operations that always involve a device.

REVISION: Correcting, to the extent possible, a portion of a malfunctioning device or the position of a displaced device.

Explanation: Correcting by taking out or putting in components of a device such as a screw or pin ...
Examples: Repair ruptured graft – CMS Ex: Recementing of hip prosthesis

Body Part – 4TH	Approach – 5TH	Device – 6TH	Qualifier – 7TH
Y Lower Artery	0 Open 3 Percutaneous 4 Percutaneous endoscopic	0 Drainage device 2 Monitoring device 3 Infusion device 7 Autologous tissue substitute C Extraluminal device D Intraluminal device J Synthetic substitute K Nonautologous tissue substitute Y Other device	Z No qualifier
Y Lower Artery	X External	0 Drainage device 2 Monitoring device 3 Infusion device 7 Autologous tissue substitute C Extraluminal device D Intraluminal device J Synthetic substitute K Nonautologous tissue substitute	Z No qualifier

© 2018 Channel Publishing, Ltd.

Educational Annotations | 5 – Upper Veins

Body System Specific Educational Annotations for the Upper Veins include:

- Anatomical Illustrations
- Anatomy and Physiology Review
- Definitions of Common Procedures
- AHA Coding Clinic® Reference Notations
- Body Part Key Listings
- Device Key Listings
- Device Aggregation Table Listings
- Coding Notes

Anatomical Illustrations of Upper Veins

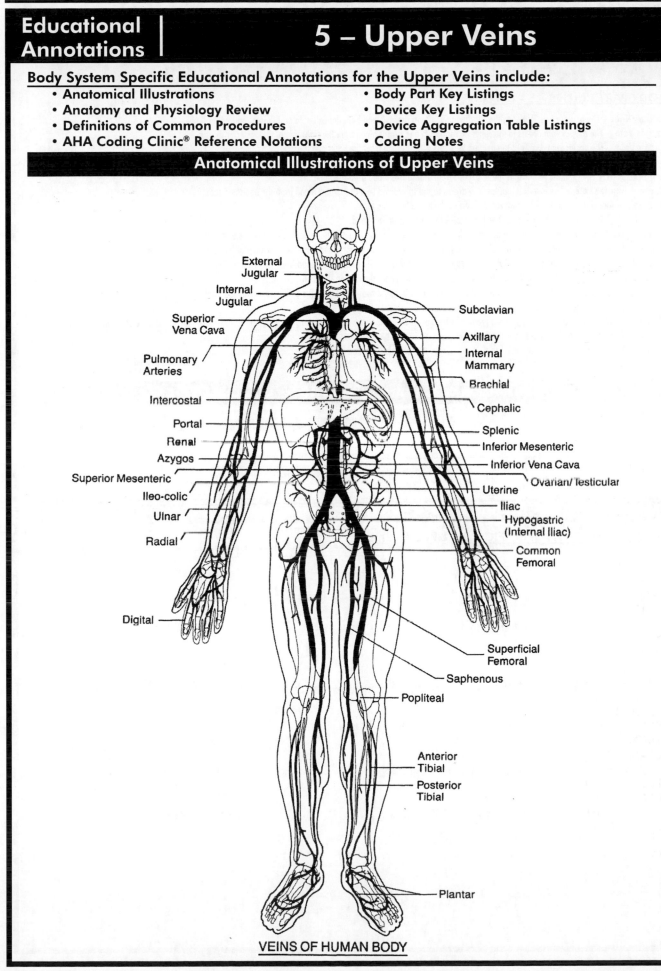

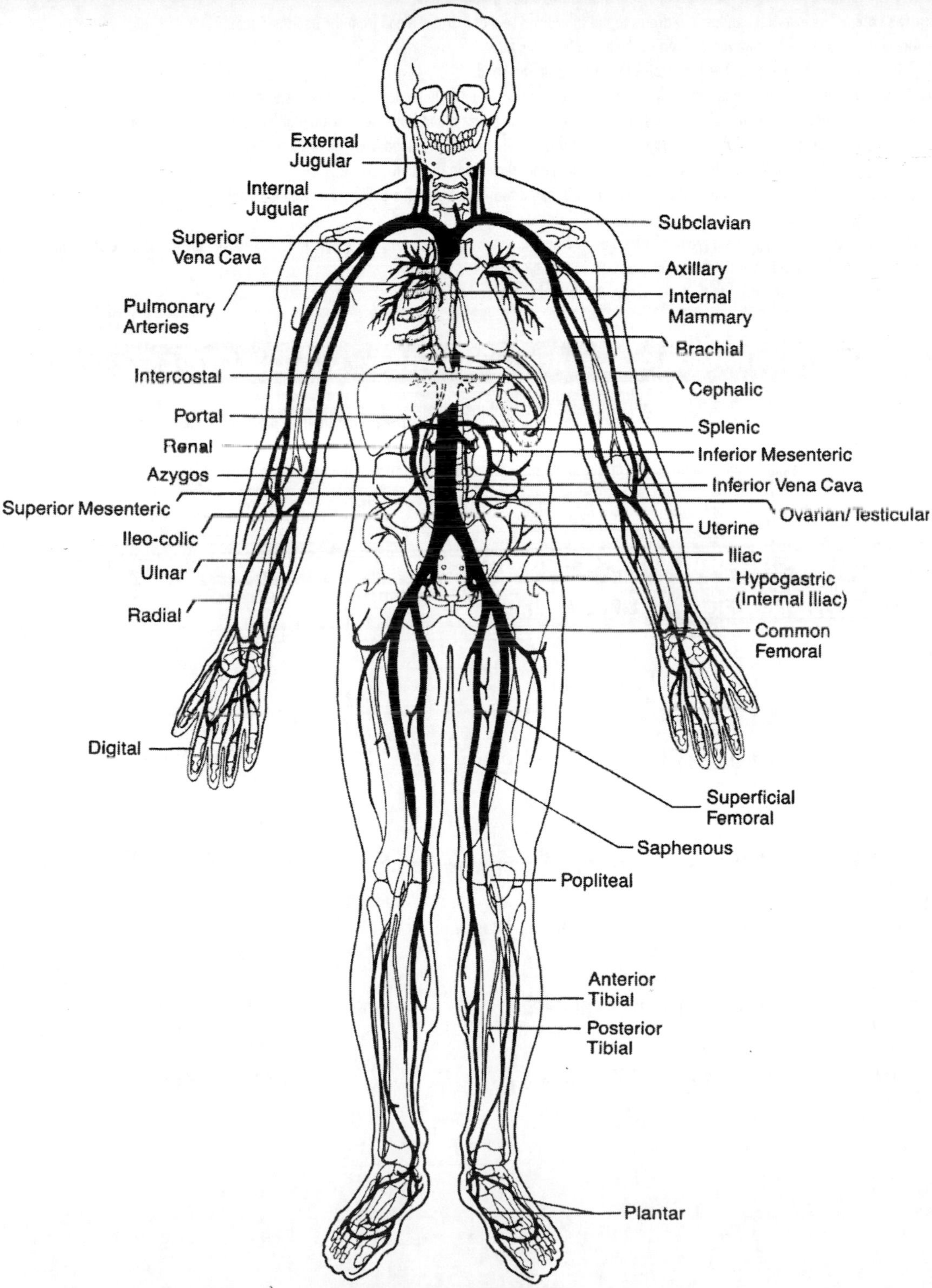

VEINS OF HUMAN BODY

© 2018 Channel Publishing, Ltd.

Educational Annotations | 5 – Upper Veins

Anatomy and Physiology Review of Upper Veins

BODY PART VALUES – 5 - UPPER VEINS

Axillary Vein – The axillary vein drains to the subclavian vein and drains blood from the axilla, lateral thorax, and upper limb.
Azygos Vein – The azygos vein drains to the superior vena cava and drains blood from the right side of the posterior thorax.
Basilic Vein – The basilic vein drains to the axillary vein and drains blood from the hand and forearm.
Brachial Vein – The brachial vein drains to the axillary vein and drains blood from the upper limb.
Cephalic Vein – The cephalic vein drains to the axillary vein and drains blood from the hand.
External Jugular Vein – The external jugular vein drains to the subclavian vein and drains blood from the head and face.
Face Vein – Any of the smaller vein branches that drains the blood from the face.
Hand Vein – Any of the smaller vein branches that drains the blood from the hand.
Hemiazygos Vein – The hemiazygos vein drains to the azygos vein and drains blood from the left side of the posterior thorax.
Innominate Vein – The innominate vein drains to the superior vena cava and drains blood from the internal jugular vein and subclavian vein.
Internal Jugular Vein – The internal jugular vein drains to the subclavian vein and drains blood from the brain and face.
Intracranial Vein – Any of the smaller vein branches that drains the blood from within the skull.
Subclavian Vein – The subclavian vein drains to the innominate vein and drains blood from the axillary vein and external jugular vein.
Upper Vein – The veins located above the diaphragm (see Coding Guideline B2.1b).
Vein – Blood vessels that carry de-oxygenated (venous) blood away from the organs and tissues of the body and to the heart. Most veins have one-way valves to prevent backflow of venous blood and to assist the lower-pressure venous blood back to the heart.
Vertebral Vein – The vertebral vein drains to the innominate vein and drains blood from the neck.

Definitions of Common Procedures of Upper Veins

Excision of damaged vein – The surgical removal of a damaged vein segment.
Mobilization/superficialization of vein – The surgical elevation of a vein to a location just under the skin from a deeper tissue location for easier and safer cannulation access.
Superior vena cava filter – The placement of a wire filter device in the superior vena cava to prevent pulmonary emboli (PE) from upper-extremity deep vein thrombosis.

AHA Coding Clinic® Reference Notations of Upper Veins

ROOT OPERATION SPECIFIC - 5 - UPPER VEINS

BYPASS - 1
DESTRUCTION - 5
DILATION - 7
DRAINAGE - 9
EXCISION - B
Infratemporal fossa malignancy with excision of jugular vein ....AHA 16:2Q:p12
EXTIRPATION - C
EXTRACTION - D
INSERTION - H
Insertion of phrenic neurostimulator...AHA 16:4Q:p97
INSPECTION - J
OCCLUSION - L
RELEASE - N
REMOVAL - P
REPAIR - Q
Bypass innominate vein to right atrial appendage......................................AHA 17:3Q:p15
REPLACEMENT - R
REPOSITION - S
Superficialization of cephalic vein..AHA 13:4Q:p125
SUPPLEMENT - U
RESTRICTION - V
REVISION - W

UPPER VEINS 0 5

© 2018 Channel Publishing, Ltd.

Educational Annotations | 5 – Upper Veins

Body Part Key Listings of Upper Veins

See also Body Part Key in Appendix C

Accessory cephalic vein....use Cephalic Vein, Left/Right
Angular vein....use Face Vein, Left/Right
Anterior cerebral vein....use Intracranial Vein
Anterior facial vein....use Face Vein, Left/Right
Basal (internal) cerebral vein....use Intracranial Vein
Brachiocephalic vein....use Innominate Vein, Left/Right
Common facial vein....use Face Vein, Left/Right
Deep cervical vein....use Vertebral Vein, Left/Right
Deep facial vein....use Face Vein, Left/Right
Dorsal metacarpal vein....use Hand Vein, Left/Right
Dural venous sinus....use Intracranial Vein
Frontal vein....use Face Vein, Left/Right
Great cerebral vein....use Intracranial Vein
Inferior cerebellar vein....use Intracranial Vein
Inferior cerebral vein....use Intracranial Vein
Inferior thyroid vein....use Innominate Vein, Left/Right
Internal (basal) cerebral vein....use Intracranial Vein
Left ascending lumbar vein....use Hemiazygos Vein
Left subcostal vein....use Hemiazygos Vein
Median antebrachial vein....use Basilic Vein, Left/Right
Median cubital vein....use Basilic Vein, Left/Right
Middle cerebral vein....use Intracranial Vein
Ophthalmic vein....use Intracranial Vein
Palmar (volar) digital vein....use Hand Vein, Left/Right
Palmar (volar) metacarpal vein....use Hand Vein, Left/Right
Posterior auricular vein....use External Jugular Vein, Left/Right
Posterior facial (retromandibular) vein....use Face Vein, Left/Right
Radial vein....use Brachial Vein, Left/Right
Right ascending lumbar vein....use Azygos Vein
Right subcostal vein....use Azygos Vein
Suboccipital venous plexus....use Vertebral Vein, Left/Right
Superficial palmar venous arch....use Hand Vein, Left/Right
Superior cerebellar vein....use Intracranial Vein
Superior cerebral vein....use Intracranial Vein
Supraorbital vein....use Face Vein, Left/Right
Ulnar vein....use Brachial Vein, Left/Right
Volar (palmar) digital vein....use Hand Vein, Left/Right
Volar (palmar) metacarpal vein....use Hand Vein, Left/Right

Device Key Listings of Upper Veins

See also Device Key in Appendix D

Autograft....use Autologous Tissue Substitute
Autologous artery graft....use Autologous Arterial Tissue in Upper Veins
Autologous vein graft....use Autologous Venous Tissue in Upper Veins
Non-tunneled central venous catheter....use Infusion Device
Peripherally inserted central catheter (PICC)....use Infusion Device
Tissue bank graft....use Nonautologous Tissue Substitute

Device Aggregation Table Listings of Upper Veins

See also Device Aggregation Table in Appendix E

Specific Device	For Operation	In Body System	General Device
Autologous Arterial Tissue	All applicable	Upper Veins	Autologous Tissue Substitute
Autologous Venous Tissue	All applicable	Upper Veins	Autologous Tissue Substitute

UPPER VEINS 05

© 2018 Channel Publishing, Ltd.

Educational Annotations | 5 – Upper Veins

Coding Notes of Upper Veins

Body System Relevant Coding Guidelines

General Guidelines

B2.1b

Where the general body part values "upper" and "lower" are provided as an option in the Upper Arteries, Lower Arteries, Upper Veins, Lower Veins, Muscles and Tendons body systems, "upper" or "lower "specifies body parts located above or below the diaphragm respectively.

Example: Vein body parts above the diaphragm are found in the Upper Veins body system; vein body parts below the diaphragm are found in the Lower Veins body system.

Body part, General guidelines

B4.1c

If a procedure is performed on a continuous section of a tubular body part, code the body part value corresponding to the furthest anatomical site from the point of entry.

Example: A procedure performed on a continuous section of artery from the femoral artery to the external iliac artery with the point of entry at the femoral artery is coded to the external iliac body part.

Branches of body parts

B4.2

Where a specific branch of a body part does not have its own body part value in PCS, the body part is typically coded to the closest proximal branch that has a specific body part value. In the cardiovascular body systems, if a general body part is available in the correct root operation table, and coding to a proximal branch would require assigning a code in a different body system, the procedure is coded using the general body part value.

Examples: A procedure performed on the mandibular branch of the trigeminal nerve is coded to the trigeminal nerve body part value.

Occlusion of the bronchial artery is coded to the body part value Upper Artery in the body system Upper Arteries, and not to the body part value Thoracic Aorta, Descending in the body system Heart and Great Vessels.

© 2018 Channel Publishing, Ltd.

1ST - 0 Medical and Surgical
2ND - 5 Upper Veins
3RD - 1 BYPASS

TUBULAR GROUP: Bypass, Dilation, Occlusion, Restriction
Root Operations that alter the diameter/route of a tubular body part.

BYPASS: Altering the route of passage of the contents of a tubular body part.

Explanation: Rerouting contents to a downstream part ... with or without the use of a device ...
Examples: Bypass damaged subclavian vein – CMS Ex: Coronary artery bypass

Body Part – 4TH	Approach – 5TH	Device – 6TH	Qualifier – 7TH
0 Azygos Vein 1 Hemiazygos Vein 3 Innominate Vein, Right 4 Innominate Vein, Left 5 Subclavian Vein, Right 6 Subclavian Vein, Left 7 Axillary Vein, Right 8 Axillary Vein, Left 9 Brachial Vein, Right A Brachial Vein, Left B Basilic Vein, Right C Basilic Vein, Left D Cephalic Vein, Right F Cephalic Vein, Left G Hand Vein, Right H Hand Vein, Left L Intracranial Vein M Internal Jugular Vein, Right N Internal Jugular Vein, Left P External Jugular Vein, Right Q External Jugular Vein, Left R Vertebral Vein, Right S Vertebral Vein, Left T Face Vein, Right V Face Vein, Left	0 Open 4 Percutaneous endoscopic	7 Autologous tissue substitute 9 Autologous venous tissue A Autologous arterial tissue J Synthetic substitute K Nonautologous tissue substitute Z No device	Y Upper Vein

1ST - 0 Medical and Surgical
2ND - 5 Upper Veins
3RD - 5 DESTRUCTION

EXCISION GROUP: Excision, (Resection), Destruction, Extraction, (Detachment)
Root Operations that take out some or all of a body part.

DESTRUCTION: Physical eradication of all or a portion of a body part by the direct use of energy, force, or a destructive agent.

Explanation: None of the body part is physically taken out
Examples: Fulguration venous lesion – CMS Ex: Fulguration of rectal polyp

Body Part – 4TH	Approach – 5TH	Device – 6TH	Qualifier – 7TH
0 Azygos Vein 1 Hemiazygos Vein 3 Innominate Vein, Right 4 Innominate Vein, Left 5 Subclavian Vein, Right 6 Subclavian Vein, Left 7 Axillary Vein, Right 8 Axillary Vein, Left 9 Brachial Vein, Right A Brachial Vein, Left B Basilic Vein, Right C Basilic Vein, Left D Cephalic Vein, Right F Cephalic Vein, Left G Hand Vein, Right H Hand Vein, Left L Intracranial Vein M Internal Jugular Vein, Right N Internal Jugular Vein, Left P External Jugular Vein, Right Q External Jugular Vein, Left R Vertebral Vein, Right S Vertebral Vein, Left T Face Vein, Right V Face Vein, Left Y Upper Vein	0 Open 3 Percutaneous 4 Percutaneous endoscopic	Z No device	Z No qualifier

1ST - 0 Medical and Surgical
2ND - 5 Upper Veins
3RD - 7 DILATION

TUBULAR GROUP: Bypass, Dilation, Occlusion, Restriction
Root Operations that alter the diameter/route of a tubular body part.

DILATION: Expanding an orifice or the lumen of a tubular body part.

Explanation: Accomplished by stretching or cutting ... tubular body part or orifice ...
Examples: Balloon dilation axillary vein – CMS Ex: Percutaneous transluminal angioplasty

Body Part – 4TH	Approach – 5TH	Device – 6TH	Qualifier – 7TH
0 Azygos Vein 1 Hemiazygos Vein G Hand Vein, Right H Hand Vein, Left L Intracranial Vein NC* M Internal Jugular Vein, Right N Internal Jugular Vein, Left P External Jugular Vein, Right Q External Jugular Vein, Left R Vertebral Vein, Right S Vertebral Vein, Left T Face Vein, Right V Face Vein, Left Y Upper Vein	0 Open 3 Percutaneous 4 Percutaneous endoscopic	D Intraluminal device Z No device	Z No qualifier
3 Innominate Vein, Right 4 Innominate Vein, Left 5 Subclavian Vein, Right 6 Subclavian Vein, Left 7 Axillary Vein, Right 8 Axillary Vein, Left 9 Brachial Vein, Right A Brachial Vein, Left B Basilic Vein, Right C Basilic Vein, Left D Cephalic Vein, Right F Cephalic Vein, Left	0 Open 3 Percutaneous 4 Percutaneous endoscopic	D Intraluminal device Z No device	1 Drug-coated balloon Z No qualifier

NC* – Some procedures are considered non-covered by Medicare. See current Medicare Code Editor for details.

© 2018 Channel Publishing, Ltd.

1ST - 0 Medical and Surgical
2ND - 5 Upper Veins
3RD - 9 DRAINAGE

DRAINAGE GROUP: Drainage, Extirpation, (Fragmentation)
Root Operations that take out solids/fluids/gases from a body part.

DRAINAGE: Taking or letting out fluids and/or gases from a body part.

Explanation: Qualifier "X Diagnostic" indicates drainage procedures that are biopsies
Examples: Phlebotomy basilic vein – CMS Ex: Thoracentesis

Body Part – 4TH	Approach – 5TH	Device – 6TH	Qualifier – 7TH
0 Azygos Vein 1 Hemiazygos Vein 3 Innominate Vein, Right 4 Innominate Vein, Left 5 Subclavian Vein, Right 6 Subclavian Vein, Left 7 Axillary Vein, Right 8 Axillary Vein, Left 9 Brachial Vein, Right A Brachial Vein, Left B Basilic Vein, Right C Basilic Vein, Left D Cephalic Vein, Right F Cephalic Vein, Left G Hand Vein, Right H Hand Vein, Left L Intracranial Vein M Internal Jugular Vein, Right N Internal Jugular Vein, Left P External Jugular Vein, Right Q External Jugular Vein, Left R Vertebral Vein, Right S Vertebral Vein, Left T Face Vein, Right V Face Vein, Left Y Upper Vein	0 Open 3 Percutaneous 4 Percutaneous endoscopic	0 Drainage device	Z No qualifier
0 Azygos Vein 1 Hemiazygos Vein 3 Innominate Vein, Right 4 Innominate Vein, Left 5 Subclavian Vein, Right 6 Subclavian Vein, Left 7 Axillary Vein, Right 8 Axillary Vein, Left 9 Brachial Vein, Right A Brachial Vein, Left B Basilic Vein, Right C Basilic Vein, Left D Cephalic Vein, Right F Cephalic Vein, Left G Hand Vein, Right H Hand Vein, Left L Intracranial Vein M Internal Jugular Vein, Right N Internal Jugular Vein, Left P External Jugular Vein, Right Q External Jugular Vein, Left R Vertebral Vein, Right S Vertebral Vein, Left T Face Vein, Right V Face Vein, Left Y Upper Vein	0 Open 3 Percutaneous 4 Percutaneous endoscopic	Z No device	X Diagnostic Z No qualifier

1ST - 0 Medical and Surgical
2ND - 5 Upper Veins
3RD - B EXCISION

EXCISION GROUP: Excision, (Resection), Destruction, Extraction, (Detachment)
Root Operations that take out some or all of a body part.

EXCISION: Cutting out or off, without replacement, a portion of a body part.

Explanation: Qualifier "X Diagnostic" indicates excision procedures that are biopsies
Examples: Harvest brachial vein – CMS Ex: Liver biopsy

Body Part – 4TH	Approach – 5TH	Device – 6TH	Qualifier – 7TH
0 Azygos Vein 1 Hemiazygos Vein 3 Innominate Vein, Right 4 Innominate Vein, Left 5 Subclavian Vein, Right 6 Subclavian Vein, Left 7 Axillary Vein, Right 8 Axillary Vein, Left 9 Brachial Vein, Right A Brachial Vein, Left B Basilic Vein, Right C Basilic Vein, Left D Cephalic Vein, Right F Cephalic Vein, Left G Hand Vein, Right H Hand Vein, Left L Intracranial Vein M Internal Jugular Vein, Right N Internal Jugular Vein, Left P External Jugular Vein, Right Q External Jugular Vein, Left R Vertebral Vein, Right S Vertebral Vein, Left T Face Vein, Right V Face Vein, Left Y Upper Vein	0 Open 3 Percutaneous 4 Percutaneous endoscopic	Z No device	X Diagnostic Z No qualifier

© 2018 Channel Publishing, Ltd.

1ST - 0 Medical and Surgical
2ND - 5 Upper Veins
3RD - C EXTIRPATION

DRAINAGE GROUP: Drainage, Extirpation, (Fragmentation)
Root Operations that take out solids/fluids/gases from a body part.

EXTIRPATION: Taking or cutting out solid matter from a body part.

Explanation: Abnormal byproduct or foreign body ...
Examples: Mechanical thrombectomy – CMS Ex: Thrombectomy

Body Part – 4TH	Approach – 5TH	Device – 6TH	Qualifier – 7TH
0 Azygos Vein 1 Hemiazygos Vein 3 Innominate Vein, Right 4 Innominate Vein, Left 5 Subclavian Vein, Right 6 Subclavian Vein, Left 7 Axillary Vein, Right 8 Axillary Vein, Left 9 Brachial Vein, Right A Brachial Vein, Left B Basilic Vein, Right C Basilic Vein, Left D Cephalic Vein, Right F Cephalic Vein, Left G Hand Vein, Right H Hand Vein, Left L Intracranial Vein M Internal Jugular Vein, Right N Internal Jugular Vein, Left P External Jugular Vein, Right Q External Jugular Vein, Left R Vertebral Vein, Right S Vertebral Vein, Left T Face Vein, Right V Face Vein, Left Y Upper Vein	0 Open 3 Percutaneous 4 Percutaneous endoscopic	Z No device	Z No qualifier

1ST - 0 Medical and Surgical
2ND - 5 Upper Veins
3RD - D EXTRACTION

EXCISION GROUP: Excision, (Resection), Destruction, Extraction, (Detachment)
Root Operations that take out some or all of a body part.

EXTRACTION: Pulling or stripping out or off all or a portion of a body part by the use of force.

Explanation: None for this Body System
Examples: Vein ligation and stripping – CMS Ex: Dilation and curettage

Body Part – 4TH	Approach – 5TH	Device – 6TH	Qualifier – 7TH
9 Brachial Vein, Right A Brachial Vein, Left B Basilic Vein, Right C Basilic Vein, Left D Cephalic Vein, Right F Cephalic Vein, Left G Hand Vein, Right H Hand Vein, Left Y Upper Vein	0 Open 3 Percutaneous	Z No device	Z No qualifier

UPPER VEINS 0 5 H

1ST - 0 Medical and Surgical
2ND - 5 Upper Veins
3RD - H INSERTION

DEVICE GROUP: (Change), Insertion, Removal, Replacement, Revision, Supplement
Root Operations that always involve a device.

INSERTION: Putting in a nonbiological appliance that monitors, assists, performs, or prevents a physiological function but does not physically take the place of a body part.

Explanation: None
Examples: Insertion central venous line – CMS Ex: Insertion of central venous catheter

Body Part – 4TH	Approach – 5TH	Device – 6TH	Qualifier – 7TH
0 Azygos Vein	0 Open 3 Percutaneous 4 Percutaneous endoscopic	2 Monitoring device 3 Infusion device D Intraluminal device M Neurostimulator lead	Z No qualifier
1 Hemiazygos Vein 5 Subclavian Vein, Right 6 Subclavian Vein, Left 7 Axillary Vein, Right 8 Axillary Vein, Left 9 Brachial Vein, Right A Brachial Vein, Left B Basilic Vein, Right C Basilic Vein, Left D Cephalic Vein, Right F Cephalic Vein, Left G Hand Vein, Right H Hand Vein, Left L Intracranial Vein M Internal Jugular Vein, Right N Internal Jugular Vein, Left P External Jugular Vein, Right Q External Jugular Vein, Left R Vertebral Vein, Right S Vertebral Vein, Left T Face Vein, Right V Face Vein, Left	0 Open 3 Percutaneous 4 Percutaneous endoscopic	3 Infusion device D Intraluminal device	Z No qualifier
3 Innominate Vein, Right 4 Innominate Vein, Left	0 Open 3 Percutaneous 4 Percutaneous endoscopic	3 Infusion device D Intraluminal device M Neurostimulator lead	Z No qualifier
Y Upper Vein	0 Open 3 Percutaneous 4 Percutaneous endoscopic	2 Monitoring device 3 Infusion device D Intraluminal device Y Other device	Z No qualifier

© 2018 Channel Publishing, Ltd.

1ST - 0 Medical and Surgical
2ND - 5 Upper Veins
3RD - J INSPECTION

EXAMINATION GROUP: Inspection, (Map)
Root Operations involving examination only.
INSPECTION: Visually and/or manually exploring a body part.

Explanation: Direct or instrumental visualization ...
Examples: Open intracranial vein examination – CMS Ex: Exploratory laparotomy

Body Part – 4TH	Approach – 5TH	Device – 6TH	Qualifier – 7TH
Y Upper Vein	0 Open 3 Percutaneous 4 Percutaneous endoscopic X External	Z No device	Z No qualifier

1ST - 0 Medical and Surgical
2ND - 5 Upper Veins
3RD - L OCCLUSION

TUBULAR GROUP: Bypass, Dilation, Occlusion, Restriction
Root Operations that alter the diameter/route of a tubular body part.
OCCLUSION: Completely closing an orifice or the lumen of a tubular body part.

Explanation: The orifice can be a natural orifice or an artificially created orifice
Examples: Ligation jugular vein – CMS Ex: Fallopian tube ligation

Body Part – 4TH			Approach – 5TH	Device – 6TH	Qualifier – 7TH
0 Azygos Vein 1 Hemiazygos Vein 3 Innominate Vein, Right 4 Innominate Vein, Left 5 Subclavian Vein, Right 6 Subclavian Vein, Left 7 Axillary Vein, Right 8 Axillary Vein, Left 9 Brachial Vein, Right A Brachial Vein, Left	B Basilic Vein, Right C Basilic Vein, Left D Cephalic Vein, Right F Cephalic Vein, Left G Hand Vein, Right H Hand Vein, Left L Intracranial Vein M Internal Jugular Vein, Right N Internal Jugular Vein, Left	P External Jugular Vein, Right Q External Jugular Vein, Left R Vertebral Vein, Right S Vertebral Vein, Left T Face Vein, Right V Face Vein, Left Y Upper Vein	0 Open 3 Percutaneous 4 Percutaneous endoscopic	C Extraluminal device D Intraluminal device Z No device	Z No qualifier

1ST - 0 Medical and Surgical
2ND - 5 Upper Veins
3RD - N RELEASE

DIVISION GROUP: (Division), Release
Root Operations involving cutting or separation only.
RELEASE: Freeing a body part from an abnormal physical constraint by cutting or by the use of force.

Explanation: Some of the restraining tissue may be taken out but none of the body part is taken out
Examples: Adhesiolysis brachial vein – CMS Ex: Carpal tunnel release

Body Part – 4TH			Approach – 5TH	Device – 6TH	Qualifier – 7TH
0 Azygos Vein 1 Hemiazygos Vein 3 Innominate Vein, Right 4 Innominate Vein, Left 5 Subclavian Vein, Right 6 Subclavian Vein, Left 7 Axillary Vein, Right 8 Axillary Vein, Left 9 Brachial Vein, Right A Brachial Vein, Left	B Basilic Vein, Right C Basilic Vein, Left D Cephalic Vein, Right F Cephalic Vein, Left G Hand Vein, Right H Hand Vein, Left L Intracranial Vein M Internal Jugular Vein, Right N Internal Jugular Vein, Left	P External Jugular Vein, Right Q External Jugular Vein, Left R Vertebral Vein, Right S Vertebral Vein, Left T Face Vein, Right V Face Vein, Left Y Upper Vein	0 Open 3 Percutaneous 4 Percutaneous endoscopic	Z No device	Z No qualifier

© 2018 Channel Publishing, Ltd.

1ST - 0 Medical and Surgical
2ND - 5 Upper Veins
3RD - P REMOVAL

DEVICE GROUP: (Change), Insertion, Removal, Replacement, Revision, Supplement
Root Operations that always involve a device.

REMOVAL: Taking out or off a device from a body part.

Explanation: Removal device without reinsertion ...
Examples: Removal central venous line – CMS Ex: Cardiac pacemaker removal

Body Part – 4TH	Approach – 5TH	Device – 6TH	Qualifier – 7TH
0 Azygos Vein	0 Open 3 Percutaneous 4 Percutaneous endoscopic X External	2 Monitoring device M Neurostimulator lead	Z No qualifier
3 Innominate Vein, Right 4 Innominate Vein, Left	0 Open 3 Percutaneous 4 Percutaneous endoscopic X External	M Neurostimulator lead	Z No qualifier
Y Upper Vein	0 Open 3 Percutaneous 4 Percutaneous endoscopic	0 Drainage device 2 Monitoring device 3 Infusion device 7 Autologous tissue substitute C Extraluminal device D Intraluminal device J Synthetic substitute K Nonautologous tissue substitute Y Other device	Z No qualifier
Y Upper Vein	X External	0 Drainage device 2 Monitoring device 3 Infusion device D Intraluminal device	Z No qualifier

1ST - 0 Medical and Surgical
2ND - 5 Upper Veins
3RD - Q REPAIR

OTHER REPAIRS GROUP: (Control), Repair
Root Operations that define other repairs.

REPAIR: Restoring, to the extent possible, a body part to its normal anatomic structure and function.

Explanation: Used only when the method to accomplish the repair is not one of the other root operations
Examples: Suture lacerated cephalic vein – CMS Ex: Suture of laceration

Body Part – 4TH			Approach – 5TH	Device – 6TH	Qualifier – 7TH
0 Azygos Vein 1 Hemiazygos Vein 3 Innominate Vein, Right 4 Innominate Vein, Left 5 Subclavian Vein, Right 6 Subclavian Vein, Left 7 Axillary Vein, Right 8 Axillary Vein, Left 9 Brachial Vein, Right A Brachial Vein, Left	B Basilic Vein, Right C Basilic Vein, Left D Cephalic Vein, Right F Cephalic Vein, Left G Hand Vein, Right H Hand Vein, Left L Intracranial Vein M Internal Jugular Vein, Right N Internal Jugular Vein, Left	P External Jugular Vein, Right Q External Jugular Vein, Left R Vertebral Vein, Right S Vertebral Vein, Left T Face Vein, Right V Face Vein, Left Y Upper Vein	0 Open 3 Percutaneous 4 Percutaneous endoscopic	Z No device	Z No qualifier

UPPER VEINS 05Q

© 2018 Channel Publishing, Ltd.

1ST - 0 Medical and Surgical
2ND - 5 Upper Veins
3RD - R REPLACEMENT

DEVICE GROUP: (Change), Insertion, Removal, Replacement, Revision, Supplement
Root Operations that always involve a device.

REPLACEMENT: Putting in or on biological or synthetic material that physically takes the place and/or function of all or a portion of a body part.

Explanation: Includes taking out or eradicating, or rendering non-functional, the body part ...
Examples: Spiral jugular vein replacement graft – CMS Ex: Total hip replacement

Body Part – 4TH			Approach – 5TH	Device – 6TH	Qualifier – 7TH
0 Azygos Vein 1 Hemiazygos Vein 3 Innominate Vein, Right 4 Innominate Vein, Left 5 Subclavian Vein, Right 6 Subclavian Vein, Left 7 Axillary Vein, Right 8 Axillary Vein, Left 9 Brachial Vein, Right A Brachial Vein, Left	B Basilic Vein, Right C Basilic Vein, Left D Cephalic Vein, Right F Cephalic Vein, Left G Hand Vein, Right H Hand Vein, Left L Intracranial Vein M Internal Jugular Vein, Right N Internal Jugular Vein, Left	P External Jugular Vein, Right Q External Jugular Vein, Left R Vertebral Vein, Right S Vertebral Vein, Left T Face Vein, Right V Face Vein, Left Y Upper Vein	0 Open 4 Percutaneous endoscopic	7 Autologous tissue substitute J Synthetic substitute K Nonautologous tissue substitute	Z No qualifier

1ST - 0 Medical and Surgical
2ND - 5 Upper Veins
3RD - S REPOSITION

MOVE GROUP: (Reattachment), Reposition, (Transfer), (Transplantation)
Root Operations that put in/put back or move some/all of a body part.

REPOSITION: Moving to its normal location, or other suitable location, all or a portion of a body part.

Explanation: The body part may or may not be cut out or off to be moved to the new location ...
Examples: Superficialization cephalic vein – CMS Ex: Fracture reduction

Body Part – 4TH			Approach – 5TH	Device – 6TH	Qualifier – 7TH
0 Azygos Vein 1 Hemiazygos Vein 3 Innominate Vein, Right 4 Innominate Vein, Left 5 Subclavian Vein, Right 6 Subclavian Vein, Left 7 Axillary Vein, Right 8 Axillary Vein, Left 9 Brachial Vein, Right A Brachial Vein, Left	B Basilic Vein, Right C Basilic Vein, Left D Cephalic Vein, Right F Cephalic Vein, Left G Hand Vein, Right H Hand Vein, Left L Intracranial Vein M Internal Jugular Vein, Right N Internal Jugular Vein, Left	P External Jugular Vein, Right Q External Jugular Vein, Left R Vertebral Vein, Right S Vertebral Vein, Left T Face Vein, Right V Face Vein, Left Y Upper Vein	0 Open 3 Percutaneous 4 Percutaneous endoscopic	Z No device	Z No qualifier

1ST - 0 Medical and Surgical
2ND - 5 Upper Veins
3RD - U SUPPLEMENT

DEVICE GROUP: (Change), Insertion, Removal, Replacement, Revision, Supplement
Root Operations that always involve a device.

SUPPLEMENT: Putting in or on biological or synthetic material that physically reinforces and/or augments the function of a portion of a body part.

Explanation: Biological material is non-living, or is living and from the same individual ...
Examples: Patch graft venoplasty – CMS Ex: Herniorrhaphy using mesh

Body Part – 4TH			Approach – 5TH	Device – 6TH	Qualifier – 7TH
0 Azygos Vein 1 Hemiazygos Vein 3 Innominate Vein, Right 4 Innominate Vein, Left 5 Subclavian Vein, Right 6 Subclavian Vein, Left 7 Axillary Vein, Right 8 Axillary Vein, Left 9 Brachial Vein, Right A Brachial Vein, Left	B Basilic Vein, Right C Basilic Vein, Left D Cephalic Vein, Right F Cephalic Vein, Left G Hand Vein, Right H Hand Vein, Left L Intracranial Vein M Internal Jugular Vein, Right N Internal Jugular Vein, Left	P External Jugular Vein, Right Q External Jugular Vein, Left R Vertebral Vein, Right S Vertebral Vein, Left T Face Vein, Right V Face Vein, Left Y Upper Vein	0 Open 3 Percutaneous 4 Percutaneous endoscopic	7 Autologous tissue substitute J Synthetic substitute K Nonautologous tissue substitute	Z No qualifier

© 2018 Channel Publishing, Ltd.

1ST - 0 Medical and Surgical
2ND - 5 Upper Veins
3RD - V RESTRICTION

TUBULAR GROUP: Bypass, Dilation, Occlusion, Restriction
Root Operations that alter the diameter/route of a tubular body part.

RESTRICTION: Partially closing an orifice or the lumen of a tubular body part.

Explanation: The orifice can be a natural orifice or an artificially created orifice.
Examples: Restrictive venous stent – CMS Ex: Cervical cerclage

Body Part – 4TH			Approach – 5TH	Device – 6TH	Qualifier – 7TH
0 Azygos Vein 1 Hemiazygos Vein 3 Innominate Vein, Right 4 Innominate Vein, Left 5 Subclavian Vein, Right 6 Subclavian Vein, Left 7 Axillary Vein, Right 8 Axillary Vein, Left 9 Brachial Vein, Right A Brachial Vein, Left	B Basilic Vein, Right C Basilic Vein, Left D Cephalic Vein, Right F Cephalic Vein, Left G Hand Vein, Right H Hand Vein, Left L Intracranial Vein M Internal Jugular Vein, Right N Internal Jugular Vein, Left	P External Jugular Vein, Right Q External Jugular Vein, Left R Vertebral Vein, Right S Vertebral Vein, Left T Face Vein, Right V Face Vein, Left Y Upper Vein	0 Open 3 Percutaneous 4 Percutaneous endoscopic	C Extraluminal device D Intraluminal device Z No device	Z No qualifier

1ST - 0 Medical and Surgical
2ND - 5 Upper Veins
3RD - W REVISION

DEVICE GROUP: (Change), Insertion, Removal, Replacement, Revision, Supplement
Root Operations that always involve a device.

REVISION: Correcting, to the extent possible, a portion of a malfunctioning device or the position of a displaced device.

Explanation: Correcting by taking out or putting in components of a device such as a screw or pin ...
Examples: Reposition central line – CMS Ex: Recementing of hip prosthesis

Body Part – 4TH	Approach – 5TH	Device – 6TH	Qualifier – 7TH
0 Azygos Vein	0 Open 3 Percutaneous 4 Percutaneous endoscopic X External	2 Monitoring device M Neurostimulator lead	Z No qualifier
3 Innominate Vein, Right 4 Innominate Vein, Left	0 Open 3 Percutaneous 4 Percutaneous endoscopic X External	M Neurostimulator lead	Z No qualifier
Y Upper Vein	0 Open 3 Percutaneous 4 Percutaneous endoscopic	0 Drainage device 2 Monitoring device 3 Infusion device 7 Autologous tissue substitute C Extraluminal device D Intraluminal device J Synthetic substitute K Nonautologous tissue substitute Y Other device	Z No qualifier
Y Upper Vein	X External	0 Drainage device 2 Monitoring device 3 Infusion device 7 Autologous tissue substitute C Extraluminal device D Intraluminal device J Synthetic substitute K Nonautologous tissue substitute	Z No qualifier

© 2018 Channel Publishing, Ltd.

NOTES

© 2018 Channel Publishing, Ltd.

Educational Annotations | 6 – Lower Veins

Body System Specific Educational Annotations for the Lower Veins include:

- Anatomical Illustrations
- Anatomy and Physiology Review
- Definitions of Common Procedures
- AHA Coding Clinic® Reference Notations
- Body Part Key Listings
- Device Key Listings
- Device Aggregation Table Listings
- Coding Notes

Anatomical Illustrations of Lower Veins

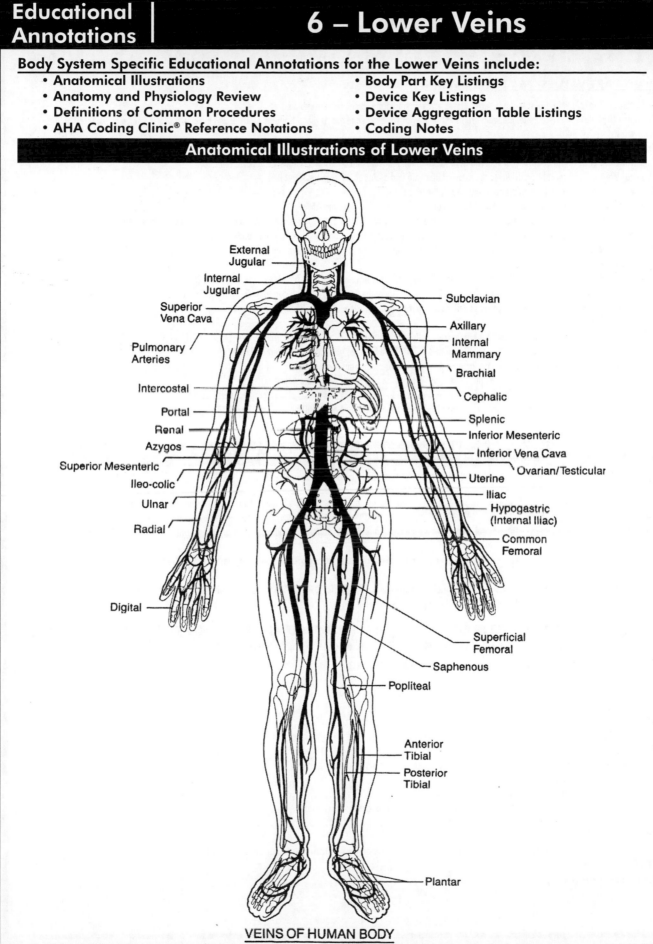

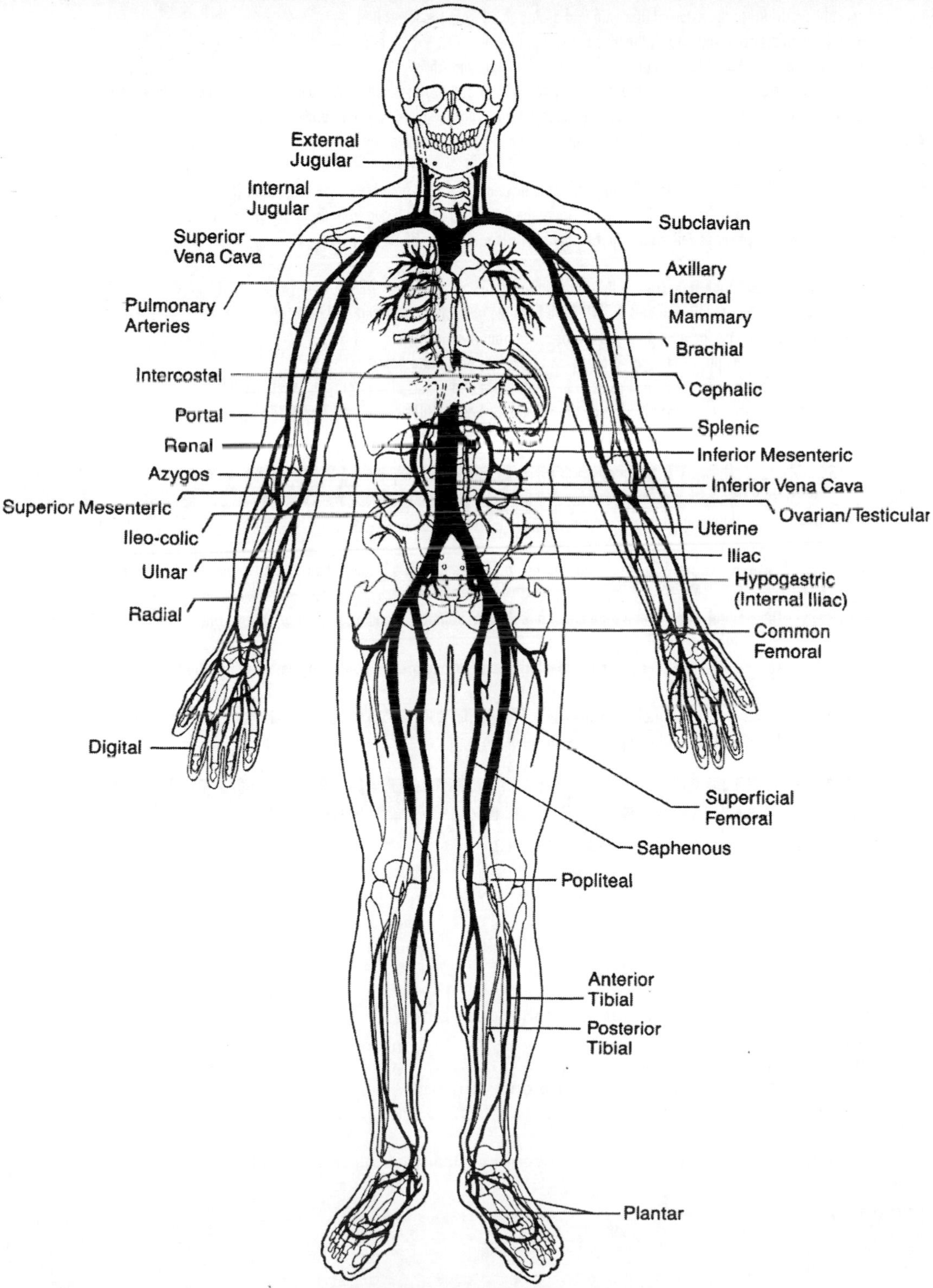

VEINS OF HUMAN BODY

© 2018 Channel Publishing, Ltd.

Educational Annotations | 6 – Lower Veins

Anatomy and Physiology Review of Lower Veins

BODY PART VALUES – 6 - LOWER VEINS

Colic Vein – The colic vein drains to the superior mesenteric vein and drains blood from the colon.
Common Iliac Vein – The common iliac vein drains to the inferior vena cava and drains blood from the external and hypogastric (also known as the internal iliac vein) veins.
Esophageal Vein – The esophageal vein drains to the azygos vein and drains blood from the esophagus.
External Iliac Vein – The external iliac vein drains to the common iliac vein and drains blood from the femoral veins.
Femoral Vein – The femoral vein drains to the external iliac vein and drains blood from the lower limb.
Foot Vein – Any of the smaller vein branches that drains the blood from the foot.
Gastric Vein – The gastric vein drains to the portal vein and drains blood from the stomach.
Greater Saphenous Vein – The greater saphenous vein drains to the femoral vein and drains blood from the lower limb including the plantar portion of the foot.
Hepatic Vein – The hepatic vein drains to the inferior vena cava and drains blood from the liver, pancreas, and small intestine.
Hypogastric Vein – The hypogastric vein (also known as the internal iliac vein) drains to the common iliac vein and drains blood from the pelvic viscera and reproductive organs.
Inferior Mesenteric Vein – The inferior mesenteric vein drains to the splenic vein and drains blood from the large intestine.
Inferior Vena Cava – The inferior vena cava drains to the right atrium of the heart and drains blood from the common iliac veins.
Lesser Saphenous Vein – The lesser saphenous vein drains to the popliteal vein and drains blood from the dorsal portion of the foot.
Lower Vein – The veins located below the diaphragm (see Coding Guideline B2.1b).
Portal Vein – The portal vein drains to the hepatic vein and drains blood from the gastrointestinal tract and liver.
Renal Vein – The renal vein drains to the inferior vena cava and drains blood from the kidney.
Splenic Vein – The splenic vein drains to the portal vein and drains blood from the spleen and pancreas.
Superior Mesenteric Vein – The superior mesenteric vein drains to the portal vein and drains blood from the small intestine.
Vein – Blood vessels that carry de-oxygenated (venous) blood away from the organs and tissues of the body and to the heart. Most veins have one-way valves to prevent backflow of venous blood and to assist the lower-pressure venous blood back to the heart.

Definitions of Common Procedures of Lower Veins

Endovenous laser vein ablation – The placement of a laser-tipped catheter into the targeted vein, using the laser energy to destroy the vein by causing it to collapse and seal shut without removing it.
External light laser treatment of varicose veins – The use of an external laser to send strong bursts of light to small, superficial varicose veins and spider veins that make the veins slowly fade away.
Harvesting of saphenous vein – The surgical removal of a segment of a saphenous vein to be used as a vessel graft (e.g., coronary artery bypass, femoral-popliteal bypass).
Inferior vena cava filter – The placement of a wire filter device in the inferior vena cava to prevent pulmonary emboli (PE) from lower-extremity deep vein thrombosis.
Ligation and stripping of varicose veins – The surgical removal of enlarged, painful lower leg veins that is performed by making small incisions at the distal and proximal locations and using an attached endovenous wire to pull the vein out of the leg.

AHA Coding Clinic® Reference Notations of Lower Veins

ROOT OPERATION SPECIFIC - 6 - LOWER VEINS

BYPASS - 1
Fontan completion procedure....................AHA 17:4Q:p36
DESTRUCTION - 5
DILATION - 7
DIVISION - 8
EXCISION - B
Coronary artery bypass graft, using greater saphenous vein....................AHA 14:3Q:p20
....................AHA 14:1Q:p10
Harvesting of sphenous vein graft....................AHA 17:3Q:p5
Tibial artery bypass using saphenous vein graft and vein cuff....................AHA 16:2Q:p18
Unspecified saphenous vein harvested....................AHA 14:3Q:p8
EXTIRPATION - C
Pharmacomechanical thrombolysis of femoral venous thrombus....................AHA 13:4Q:p115
EXTRACTION - D

Continued on next page

© 2018 Channel Publishing, Ltd.

Educational Annotations | 6 – Lower Veins

AHA Coding Clinic® Reference Notations of Lower Veins

ROOT OPERATION SPECIFIC - 6 - LOWER VEINS

Continued from previous page

INSERTION - H

- Insertion of a Mahurkar catheter into inferior vena cava (IVC) .... AHA 13:3Q:p18
- Insertion of central line catheter via the femoral vein .... AHA 17:1Q:p31
- Insertion of umbilical vein catheter in newborn .... AHA 17:1Q:p31

INSPECTION - J

OCCLUSION - L

- Endoscopic ligation of esophageal varices using bands .... AHA 13:4Q:p112
- Ligation of deep epigastric vessels before TRAM flap reconstruction .... AHA 18:2Q:p18
- Transorifice endoscopic ligation of esophageal varices .... AHA 17:4Q:p57

RELEASE - N

REMOVAL - P

REPAIR - Q

REPLACEMENT - R

REPOSITION - S

SUPPLEMENT - U

RESTRICTION - T

REVISION - W

- Removal of clots from transjugular intrahepatic portosystemic shunt (TIPS) AHA 14:3Q:p25
- Stent exchange with a different diameter stent .... AHA 18:1Q:p10

Body Part Key Listings of Lower Veins

See also Body Part Key in Appendix C

Common digital vein ....use Foot Vein, Left/Right
Deep femoral (profunda femoris) vein use Femoral Vein, Left/Right
Dorsal metatarsal vein ....use Foot Vein, Left/Right
Dorsal venous arch ....use Foot Vein, Left/Right
External pudendal vein ....use Saphenous Vein, Left/Right
Gluteal vein ....use Hypogastric Vein, Left/Right
Great(er) saphenous vein ....use Saphenous Vein, Left/Right
Hepatic portal vein ....use Portal Vein
Ileocolic vein ....use Colic Vein
Internal iliac vein.................................use Hypogastric Vein, Left/Right
Internal pudendal vein ....use Hypogastric Vein, Left/Right
Lateral sacral vein ....use Hypogastric Vein, Left/Right
Left colic vein ....use Colic Vein
Left gastroepiploic vein ....use Splenic Vein
Left inferior phrenic vein ....use Renal Vein, Left
Left ovarian vein ....use Renal Vein, Left
Left second lumbar vein.........................use Renal Vein, Left
Left suprarenal vein..............................use Renal Vein, Left
Left testicular vein ....use Renal Vein, Left
Lesser saphenous vein ....use Saphenous Vein, Left/Right
Middle colic vein ....use Colic Vein
Middle hemorrhoidal vein ....use Hypogastric Vein, Left/Right
Obturator vein ....use Hypogastric Vein, Left/Right
Pancreatic vein.....................................use Splenic Vein
Plantar digital vein ....use Foot Vein, Left/Right
Plantar metatarsal vein ....use Foot Vein, Left/Right
Plantar venous arch..............................use Foot Vein, Left/Right
Popliteal vein..use Femoral Vein, Left/Right
Postcava ....use Inferior Vena Cava
Profunda femoris (deep femoral) vein use Femoral Vein, Left/Right
Right colic vein.....................................use Colic Vein
Right gastroepiploic vein ....use Superior Mesenteric Vein
Right inferior phrenic vein.....................use Inferior Vena Cava
Right ovarian vein ....use Inferior Vena Cava
Right second lumbar vein ....use Inferior Vena Cava
Right suprarenal vein ....use Inferior Vena Cava
Right testicular vein..............................use Inferior Vena Cava
Sigmoid vein ....use Inferior Mesenteric Vein
Small saphenous vein ....use Saphenous Vein, Left/Right
Superficial circumflex iliac vein ....use Saphenous Vein, Left/Right
Superficial epigastric vein ....use Saphenous Vein, Left/Right
Superior rectal vein ....use Inferior Mesenteric Vein
Uterine vein ....use Hypogastric Vein, Left/Right
Vaginal vein..use Hypogastric Vein, Left/Right
Vesical vein ....use Hypogastric Vein, Left/Right

Device Key Listings of Lower Veins

See also Device Key in Appendix D

Autograft ....use Autologous Tissue Substitute
Autologous artery graft ....use Autologous Arterial Tissue in Lower Veins
Autologous vein graft...use Autologous Venous Tissue in Lower Veins
Non-tunneled central venous catheter.....................use Infusion Device
Tissue bank graft ....use Nonautologous Tissue Substitute

© 2018 Channel Publishing, Ltd.

Educational Annotations | 6 – Lower Veins

Device Aggregation Table Listings of Lower Veins

See also Device Aggregation Table in Appendix E

Specific Device	For Operation	In Body System	General Device
Autologous Arterial Tissue	All applicable	Lower Veins	Autologous Tissue Substitute
Autologous Venous Tissue	All applicable	Lower Veins	Autologous Tissue Substitute

Coding Notes of Lower Veins

Body System Relevant Coding Guidelines

General Guidelines

B2.1b

Where the general body part values "upper" and "lower" are provided as an option in the Upper Arteries, Lower Arteries, Upper Veins, Lower Veins, Muscles and Tendons body systems, "upper" or "lower "specifies body parts located above or below the diaphragm respectively.

Example: Vein body parts above the diaphragm are found in the Upper Veins body system; vein body parts below the diaphragm are found in the Lower Veins body system.

Body part, General guidelines

B4.1c

If a procedure is performed on a continuous section of a tubular body part, code the body part value corresponding to the furthest anatomical site from the point of entry.

Example: A procedure performed on a continuous section of artery from the femoral artery to the external iliac artery with the point of entry at the femoral artery is coded to the external iliac body part.

Branches of body parts

B4.2

Where a specific branch of a body part does not have its own body part value in PCS, the body part is typically coded to the closest proximal branch that has a specific body part value. In the cardiovascular body systems, if a general body part is available in the correct root operation table, and coding to a proximal branch would require assigning a code in a different body system, the procedure is coded using the general body part value.

Examples: A procedure performed on the mandibular branch of the trigeminal nerve is coded to the trigeminal nerve body part value.

Occlusion of the bronchial artery is coded to the body part value Upper Artery in the body system Upper Arteries, and not to the body part value Thoracic Aorta, Descending in the body system Heart and Great Vessels.

© 2018 Channel Publishing, Ltd.

1ST - 0 Medical and Surgical
2ND - 6 Lower Veins
3RD - 1 BYPASS

TUBULAR GROUP: Bypass, Dilation, Occlusion, Restriction
Root Operations that alter the diameter/route of a tubular body part.

BYPASS: Altering the route of passage of the contents of a tubular body part.

Explanation: Rerouting contents to a downstream part ... with or without the use of a device ...
Examples: Bypass damaged splenic vein – CMS Ex: Coronary artery bypass

Body Part – 4TH	Approach – 5TH	Device – 6TH	Qualifier – 7TH
0 Inferior Vena Cava	0 Open 4 Percutaneous endoscopic	7 Autologous tissue substitute 9 Autologous venous tissue A Autologous arterial tissue J Synthetic substitute K Nonautologous tissue substitute Z No device	5 Superior Mesenteric Vein 6 Inferior Mesenteric Vein P Pulmonary Trunk Q Pulmonary Artery, Right R Pulmonary Artery, Left Y Lower Vein
1 Splenic Vein	0 Open 4 Percutaneous endoscopic	7 Autologous tissue substitute 9 Autologous venous tissue A Autologous arterial tissue J Synthetic substitute K Nonautologous tissue substitute Z No device	9 Renal Vein, Right B Renal Vein, Left Y Lower Vein
2 Gastric Vein 3 Esophageal Vein 4 Hepatic Vein 5 Superior Mesenteric Vein 6 Inferior Mesenteric Vein 7 Colic Vein 9 Renal Vein, Right B Renal Vein, Left C Common Iliac Vein, Right D Common Iliac Vein, Left F External Iliac Vein, Right G External Iliac Vein, Left H Hypogastric Vein, Right J Hypogastric Vein, Left M Femoral Vein, Right N Femoral Vein, Left P Saphenous Vein, Right Q Saphenous Vein, Left T Foot Vein, Right V Foot Vein, Left	0 Open 4 Percutaneous endoscopic	7 Autologous tissue substitute 9 Autologous venous tissue A Autologous arterial tissue J Synthetic substitute K Nonautologous tissue substitute Z No device	Y Lower Vein
8 Portal Vein	0 Open	7 Autologous tissue substitute 9 Autologous venous tissue A Autologous arterial tissue J Synthetic substitute K Nonautologous tissue substitute Z No device	9 Renal Vein, Right B Renal Vein, Left Y Lower Vein
8 Portal Vein	3 Percutaneous	J Synthetic substitute	4 Hepatic Vein Y Lower Vein
8 Portal Vein	4 Percutaneous endoscopic	7 Autologous tissue substitute 9 Autologous venous tissue A Autologous arterial tissue K Nonautologous tissue substitute Z No device	9 Renal Vein, Right B Renal Vein, Left Y Lower Vein
8 Portal Vein	4 Percutaneous endoscopic	J Synthetic substitute	4 Hepatic Vein 9 Renal Vein, Right B Renal Vein, Left Y Lower Vein

© 2018 Channel Publishing, Ltd.

1ST - 0 Medical and Surgical
2ND - 6 Lower Veins
3RD - 5 DESTRUCTION

EXCISION GROUP: Excision, (Resection), Destruction, Extraction, (Detachment)
Root Operations that take out some or all of a body part.

DESTRUCTION: Physical eradication of all or a portion of a body part by the direct use of energy, force, or a destructive agent.

Explanation: None of the body part is physically taken out
Examples: Fulguration venous lesion – CMS Ex: Fulguration of rectal polyp

Body Part – 4TH	Approach – 5TH	Device – 6TH	Qualifier – 7TH
0 Inferior Vena Cava 1 Splenic Vein 2 Gastric Vein 3 Esophageal Vein 4 Hepatic Vein 5 Superior Mesenteric Vein 6 Inferior Mesenteric Vein 7 Colic Vein 8 Portal Vein 9 Renal Vein, Right B Renal Vein, Left C Common Iliac Vein, Right D Common Iliac Vein, Left F External Iliac Vein, Right G External Iliac Vein, Left H Hypogastric Vein, Right J Hypogastric Vein, Left M Femoral Vein, Right N Femoral Vein, Left P Saphenous Vein, Right Q Saphenous Vein, Left T Foot Vein, Right V Foot Vein, Left	0 Open 3 Percutaneous 4 Percutaneous endoscopic	Z No device	Z No qualifier
Y Lower Vein	0 Open 3 Percutaneous 4 Percutaneous endoscopic	Z No device	C Hemorrhoidal Plexus Z No qualifier

1ST - 0 Medical and Surgical
2ND - 6 Lower Veins
3RD - 7 DILATION

TUBULAR GROUP: Bypass, Dilation, Occlusion, Restriction
Root Operations that alter the diameter/route of a tubular body part.

DILATION: Expanding an orifice or the lumen of a tubular body part.

Explanation: Accomplished by stretching or cutting ... tubular body part or orifice ...
Examples: Balloon dilation hepatic vein – CMS Ex: Percutaneous transluminal angioplasty

Body Part – 4TH	Approach – 5TH	Device – 6TH	Qualifier – 7TH
0 Inferior Vena Cava 1 Splenic Vein 2 Gastric Vein 3 Esophageal Vein 4 Hepatic Vein 5 Superior Mesenteric Vein 6 Inferior Mesenteric Vein 7 Colic Vein 8 Portal Vein 9 Renal Vein, Right B Renal Vein, Left C Common Iliac Vein, Right D Common Iliac Vein, Left F External Iliac Vein, Right G External Iliac Vein, Left H Hypogastric Vein, Right J Hypogastric Vein, Left M Femoral Vein, Right N Femoral Vein, Left P Saphenous Vein, Right Q Saphenous Vein, Left T Foot Vein, Right V Foot Vein, Left Y Lower Vein	0 Open 3 Percutaneous 4 Percutaneous endoscopic	D Intraluminal device Z No device	Z No qualifier

© 2018 Channel Publishing, Ltd.

1ST - 0 Medical and Surgical
2ND - 6 Lower Veins
3RD - 9 DRAINAGE

DRAINAGE GROUP: Drainage, Extirpation, (Fragmentation)
Root Operations that take out solids/fluids/gases from a body part.

DRAINAGE: Taking or letting out fluids and/or gases from a body part.

Explanation: Qualifier "X Diagnostic" indicates drainage procedures that are biopsies
Examples: Phlebotomy iliac vein – CMS Ex: Thoracentesis

Body Part – 4TH	Approach – 5TH	Device – 6TH	Qualifier – 7TH
0 Inferior Vena Cava 1 Splenic Vein 2 Gastric Vein 3 Esophageal Vein 4 Hepatic Vein 5 Superior Mesenteric Vein 6 Inferior Mesenteric Vein 7 Colic Vein 8 Portal Vein 9 Renal Vein, Right B Renal Vein, Left C Common Iliac Vein, Right D Common Iliac Vein, Left F External Iliac Vein, Right G External Iliac Vein, Left H Hypogastric Vein, Right J Hypogastric Vein, Left M Femoral Vein, Right N Femoral Vein, Left P Saphenous Vein, Right Q Saphenous Vein, Left T Foot Vein, Right V Foot Vein, Left Y Lower Vein	0 Open 3 Percutaneous 4 Percutaneous endoscopic	0 Drainage device	Z No qualifier
0 Inferior Vena Cava 1 Splenic Vein 2 Gastric Vein 3 Esophageal Vein 4 Hepatic Vein 5 Superior Mesenteric Vein 6 Inferior Mesenteric Vein 7 Colic Vein 8 Portal Vein 9 Renal Vein, Right B Renal Vein, Left C Common Iliac Vein, Right D Common Iliac Vein, Left F External Iliac Vein, Right G External Iliac Vein, Left H Hypogastric Vein, Right J Hypogastric Vein, Left M Femoral Vein, Right N Femoral Vein, Left P Saphenous Vein, Right Q Saphenous Vein, Left T Foot Vein, Right V Foot Vein, Left Y Lower Vein	0 Open 3 Percutaneous 4 Percutaneous endoscopic	Z No device	X Diagnostic Z No qualifier

1ST - 0 Medical and Surgical
2ND - 6 Lower Veins
3RD - B EXCISION

EXCISION GROUP. Excision, (Resection), Destruction, Extraction, (Detachment)
Root Operations that take out some or all of a body part.

EXCISION: Cutting out or off, without replacement, a portion of a body part.

Explanation: Qualifier "X Diagnostic" indicates excision procedures that are biopsies
Examples: Harvest saphenous vein – CMS Ex: Liver biopsy

Body Part – 4TH	Approach – 5TH	Device – 6TH	Qualifier – 7TH
0 Inferior Vena Cava 1 Splenic Vein 2 Gastric Vein 3 Esophageal Vein 4 Hepatic Vein 5 Superior Mesenteric Vein 6 Inferior Mesenteric Vein 7 Colic Vein 8 Portal Vein 9 Renal Vein, Right B Renal Vein, Left C Common Iliac Vein, Right D Common Iliac Vein, Left F External Iliac Vein, Right G External Iliac Vein, Left H Hypogastric Vein, Right J Hypogastric Vein, Left M Femoral Vein, Right N Femoral Vein, Left P Saphenous Vein, Right Q Saphenous Vein, Left T Foot Vein, Right V Foot Vein, Left	0 Open 3 Percutaneous 4 Percutaneous endoscopic	Z No device	X Diagnostic Z No qualifier
Y Lower Vein	0 Open 3 Percutaneous 4 Percutaneous endoscopic	Z No device	C Hemorrhoidal Plexus X Diagnostic Z No qualifier

© 2018 Channel Publishing, Ltd.

1ST - 0 Medical and Surgical
2ND - 6 Lower Veins
3RD - C **EXTIRPATION**

DRAINAGE GROUP: Drainage, Extirpation, (Fragmentation)
Root Operations that take out solids/fluids/gases from a body part.
EXTIRPATION: Taking or cutting out solid matter from a body part.

Explanation: Abnormal byproduct or foreign body ...
Examples: Mechanical thrombectomy – CMS Ex: Thrombectomy

Body Part – 4TH	Approach – 5TH	Device – 6TH	Qualifier – 7TH
0 Inferior Vena Cava 1 Splenic Vein 2 Gastric Vein 3 Esophageal Vein 4 Hepatic Vein 5 Superior Mesenteric Vein 6 Inferior Mesenteric Vein 7 Colic Vein 8 Portal Vein 9 Renal Vein, Right B Renal Vein, Left C Common Iliac Vein, Right D Common Iliac Vein, Left F External Iliac Vein, Right G External Iliac Vein, Left H Hypogastric Vein, Right J Hypogastric Vein, Left M Femoral Vein, Right N Femoral Vein, Left P Saphenous Vein, Right Q Saphenous Vein, Left T Foot Vein, Right V Foot Vein, Left Y Lower Vein	0 Open 3 Percutaneous 4 Percutaneous endoscopic	Z No device	Z No qualifier

1ST - 0 Medical and Surgical
2ND - 6 Lower Veins
3RD - D **EXTRACTION**

EXCISION GROUP: Excision, (Resection), Destruction, Extraction, (Detachment)
Root Operations that take out some or all of a body part.
EXTRACTION: Pulling or stripping out or off all or a portion of a body part by the use of force.

Explanation: None for this Body System
Examples: Vein ligation and stripping – CMS Ex: Dilation and curettage

Body Part – 4TH	Approach – 5TH	Device – 6TH	Qualifier – 7TH
M Femoral Vein, Right N Femoral Vein, Left P Saphenous Vein, Right Q Saphenous Vein, Left T Foot Vein, Right V Foot Vein, Left Y Lower Vein	0 Open 3 Percutaneous 4 Percutaneous endoscopic	Z No device	Z No qualifier

1ST - 0 Medical and Surgical
2ND - 6 Lower Veins
3RD - H **INSERTION**

DEVICE GROUP: (Change), Insertion, Removal, Replacement, Revision, Supplement
Root Operations that always involve a device.
INSERTION: Putting in a nonbiological appliance that monitors, assists, performs, or prevents a physiological function but does not physically take the place of a body part.
Explanation: None
Examples: Insertion inferior vena cava (IVC) filter – CMS Ex: Insertion of central venous catheter

Body Part – 4TH	Approach – 5TH	Device – 6TH	Qualifier – 7TH
0 Inferior Vena Cava	0 Open 3 Percutaneous	3 Infusion device	T Via Umbilical Vein Z No qualifier
0 Inferior Vena Cava	0 Open 3 Percutaneous	D Intraluminal device	Z No qualifier
0 Inferior Vena Cava	4 Percutaneous endoscopic	3 Infusion device D Intraluminal device	Z No qualifier
1 Splenic Vein 2 Gastric Vein 3 Esophageal Vein 4 Hepatic Vein 5 Superior Mesenteric Vein 6 Inferior Mesenteric Vein 7 Colic Vein 8 Portal Vein 9 Renal Vein, Right B Renal Vein, Left C Common Iliac Vein, Right D Common Iliac Vein, Left F External Iliac Vein, Right G External Iliac Vein, Left H Hypogastric Vein, Right J Hypogastric Vein, Left M Femoral Vein, Right N Femoral Vein, Left P Saphenous Vein, Right Q Saphenous Vein, Left T Foot Vein, Right V Foot Vein, Left	0 Open 3 Percutaneous 4 Percutaneous endoscopic	3 Infusion device D Intraluminal device	Z No qualifier
Y Lower Vein	0 Open 3 Percutaneous 4 Percutaneous endoscopic	2 Monitoring device 3 Infusion device D Intraluminal device Y Other device	Z No qualifier

© 2018 Channel Publishing, Ltd.

1ST - 0 Medical and Surgical
2ND - 6 Lower Veins
3RD - J INSPECTION

EXAMINATION GROUP: Inspection, (Map)
Root Operations involving examination only.

INSPECTION: Visually and/or manually exploring a body part.

Explanation: Direct or instrumental visualization ...
Examples: Open iliac vein examination – CMS Ex: Exploratory laparotomy

Body Part – 4TH	Approach – 5TH	Device – 6TH	Qualifier – 7TH
Y Lower Vein	0 Open 3 Percutaneous 4 Percutaneous endoscopic X External	Z No device	Z No qualifier

1ST - 0 Medical and Surgical
2ND - 6 Lower Veins
3RD - L OCCLUSION

TUBULAR GROUP: Bypass, Dilation, Occlusion, Restriction
Root Operations that alter the diameter/route of a tubular body part.

OCCLUSION: Completely closing an orifice or the lumen of a tubular body part.

Explanation: The orifice can be a natural orifice or an artificially created orifice
Examples: Ligation esophageal varices – CMS Ex: Fallopian tube ligation

Body Part – 4TH	Approach – 5TH	Device – 6TH	Qualifier – 7TH
0 Inferior Vena Cava 1 Splenic Vein 2 Gastric Vein 4 Hepatic Vein 5 Superior Mesenteric Vein 6 Inferior Mesenteric Vein 7 Colic Vein 8 Portal Vein 9 Renal Vein, Right B Renal Vein, Left C Common Iliac Vein, Right D Common Iliac Vein, Left F External Iliac Vein, Right G External Iliac Vein, Left H Hypogastric Vein, Right J Hypogastric Vein, Left M Femoral Vein, Right N Femoral Vein, Left P Saphenous Vein, Right Q Saphenous Vein, Left T Foot Vein, Right V Foot Vein, Left	0 Open 3 Percutaneous 4 Percutaneous endoscopic	C Extraluminal device D Intraluminal device Z No device	Z No qualifier
3 Esophageal Vein	0 Open 3 Percutaneous 4 Percutaneous endoscopic 7 Via natural or artificial opening 8 Via natural or artificial opening endoscopic	C Extraluminal device D Intraluminal device Z No device	Z No qualifier
Y Lower Vein	0 Open 3 Percutaneous 4 Percutaneous endoscopic	C Extraluminal device D Intraluminal device Z No device	C Hemorrhoidal Plexus Z No qualifier

LOWER VEINS 0 6 N

1ST - 0 Medical and Surgical
2ND - 6 Lower Veins
3RD - N RELEASE

DIVISION GROUP: (Division), Release
Root Operations involving cutting or separation only.

RELEASE: Freeing a body part from an abnormal physical constraint by cutting or by the use of force.

Explanation: Some of the restraining tissue may be taken out but none of the body part is taken out
Examples: Adhesiolysis hepatic vein – CMS Ex: Carpal tunnel release

Body Part – 4TH	Approach – 5TH	Device – 6TH	Qualifier – 7TH
0 Inferior Vena Cava 1 Splenic Vein 2 Gastric Vein 3 Esophageal Vein 4 Hepatic Vein 5 Superior Mesenteric Vein 6 Inferior Mesenteric Vein 7 Colic Vein 8 Portal Vein 9 Renal Vein, Right B Renal Vein, Left C Common Iliac Vein, Right D Common Iliac Vein, Left F External Iliac Vein, Right G External Iliac Vein, Left H Hypogastric Vein, Right J Hypogastric Vein, Left M Femoral Vein, Right N Femoral Vein, Left P Saphenous Vein, Right Q Saphenous Vein, Left T Foot Vein, Right V Foot Vein, Left Y Lower Vein	0 Open 3 Percutaneous 4 Percutaneous endoscopic	Z No device	Z No qualifier

© 2018 Channel Publishing, Ltd.

1ST - 0 Medical and Surgical
2ND - 6 Lower Veins
3RD - P REMOVAL

DEVICE GROUP: (Change), Insertion, Removal, Replacement, Revision, Supplement
Root Operations that always involve a device.

REMOVAL: Taking out or off a device from a body part.

Explanation: Removal device without reinsertion ...
Examples: Removal inferior vena cava (IVC) filter – CMS Ex: Cardiac pacemaker removal

Body Part – 4TH	Approach – 5TH	Device – 6TH	Qualifier – 7TH
Y Lower Vein	0 Open 3 Percutaneous 4 Percutaneous endoscopic	0 Drainage device 2 Monitoring device 3 Infusion device 7 Autologous tissue substitute C Extraluminal device D Intraluminal device J Synthetic substitute K Nonautologous tissue substitute Y Other device	Z No qualifier
Y Lower Vein	X External	0 Drainage device 2 Monitoring device 3 Infusion device D Intraluminal device	Z No qualifier

1ST - 0 Medical and Surgical
2ND - 6 Lower Veins
3RD - Q REPAIR

OTHER REPAIRS GROUP: (Control), Repair
Root Operations that define other repairs.

REPAIR: Restoring, to the extent possible, a body part to its normal anatomic structure and function.

Explanation: Used only when the method to accomplish the repair is not one of the other root operations
Examples: Suture varicose vein – CMS Ex: Suture of laceration

Body Part – 4TH	Approach – 5TH	Device – 6TH	Qualifier – 7TH
0 Inferior Vena Cava 1 Splenic Vein 2 Gastric Vein 3 Esophageal Vein 4 Hepatic Vein 5 Superior Mesenteric Vein 6 Inferior Mesenteric Vein 7 Colic Vein 8 Portal Vein 9 Renal Vein, Right B Renal Vein, Left C Common Iliac Vein, Right D Common Iliac Vein, Left F External Iliac Vein, Right G External Iliac Vein, Left H Hypogastric Vein, Right J Hypogastric Vein, Left M Femoral Vein, Right N Femoral Vein, Left P Saphenous Vein, Right Q Saphenous Vein, Left T Foot Vein, Right V Foot Vein, Left Y Lower Vein	0 Open 3 Percutaneous 4 Percutaneous endoscopic	Z No device	Z No qualifier

1ST - 0 Medical and Surgical
2ND - 6 Lower Veins
3RD - R REPLACEMENT

DEVICE GROUP: (Change), Insertion, Removal, Replacement, Revision, Supplement
Root Operations that always involve a device.

REPLACEMENT: Putting in or on biological or synthetic material that physically takes the place and/or function of all or a portion of a body part.

Explanation: Includes taking out or eradicating, or rendering non-functional, the body part ...
Examples: Portal vein reconstruction graft – CMS Ex: Total hip replacement

Body Part – 4TH	Approach – 5TH	Device – 6TH	Qualifier – 7TH
0 Inferior Vena Cava 1 Splenic Vein 2 Gastric Vein 3 Esophageal Vein 4 Hepatic Vein 5 Superior Mesenteric Vein 6 Inferior Mesenteric Vein 7 Colic Vein 8 Portal Vein 9 Renal Vein, Right B Renal Vein, Left C Common Iliac Vein, Right D Common Iliac Vein, Left F External Iliac Vein, Right G External Iliac Vein, Left H Hypogastric Vein, Right J Hypogastric Vein, Left M Femoral Vein, Right N Femoral Vein, Left P Saphenous Vein, Right Q Saphenous Vein, Left T Foot Vein, Right V Foot Vein, Left Y Lower Vein	0 Open 4 Percutaneous endoscopic	7 Autologous tissue substitute J Synthetic substitute K Nonautologous tissue substitute	Z No qualifier

LOWER VEINS 06P

© 2018 Channel Publishing, Ltd.

1ST - 0 Medical and Surgical
2ND - 6 Lower Veins
3RD - S REPOSITION

MOVE GROUP: (Reattachment), Reposition, (Transfer), (Transplantation)
Root Operations that put in/put back or move some/all of a body part.

REPOSITION: Moving to its normal location, or other suitable location, all or a portion of a body part.

Explanation: The body part may or may not be cut out or off to be moved to the new location ...
Examples: Relocation hypogastric vein – CMS Ex: Fracture reduction

Body Part – 4TH	Approach – 5TH	Device – 6TH	Qualifier – 7TH
0 Inferior Vena Cava 1 Splenic Vein 2 Gastric Vein 3 Esophageal Vein 4 Hepatic Vein 5 Superior Mesenteric Vein 6 Inferior Mesenteric Vein 7 Colic Vein 8 Portal Vein 9 Renal Vein, Right B Renal Vein, Left C Common Iliac Vein, Right D Common Iliac Vein, Left F External Iliac Vein, Right G External Iliac Vein, Left H Hypogastric Vein, Right J Hypogastric Vein, Left M Femoral Vein, Right N Femoral Vein, Left P Saphenous Vein, Right Q Saphenous Vein, Left T Foot Vein, Right V Foot Vein, Left Y Lower Vein	0 Open 3 Percutaneous 4 Percutaneous endoscopic	Z No device	Z No qualifier

1ST - 0 Medical and Surgical
2ND - 6 Lower Veins
3RD - U SUPPLEMENT

DEVICE GROUP: (Change), Insertion, Removal, Replacement, Revision, Supplement
Root Operations that always involve a device.

SUPPLEMENT: Putting in or on biological or synthetic material that physically reinforces and/or augments the function of a portion of a body part.

Explanation: Biological material is non-living, or is living and from the same individual ...
Examples: Patch graft venoplasty – CMS Ex: Herniorrhaphy using mesh

Body Part – 4TH	Approach – 5TH	Device – 6TH	Qualifier – 7TH
0 Inferior Vena Cava 1 Splenic Vein 2 Gastric Vein 3 Esophageal Vein 4 Hepatic Vein 5 Superior Mesenteric Vein 6 Inferior Mesenteric Vein 7 Colic Vein 8 Portal Vein 9 Renal Vein, Right B Renal Vein, Left C Common Iliac Vein, Right D Common Iliac Vein, Left F External Iliac Vein, Right G External Iliac Vein, Left H Hypogastric Vein, Right J Hypogastric Vein, Left M Femoral Vein, Right N Femoral Vein, Left P Saphenous Vein, Right Q Saphenous Vein, Left T Foot Vein, Right V Foot Vein, Left Y Lower Vein	0 Open 3 Percutaneous 4 Percutaneous endoscopic	7 Autologous tissue substitute J Synthetic substitute K Nonautologous tissue substitute	Z No qualifier

1ST - 0 Medical and Surgical
2ND - 6 Lower Veins
3RD - V RESTRICTION

TUBULAR GROUP: Bypass, Dilation, Occlusion, Restriction
Root Operations that alter the diameter/route of a tubular body part.

RESTRICTION: Partially closing an orifice or the lumen of a tubular body part.

Explanation: The orifice can be a natural orifice or an artificially created orifice.
Examples: Restrictive venous stent – CMS Ex: Cervical cerclage

Body Part – 4TH	Approach – 5TH	Device – 6TH	Qualifier – 7TH
0 Inferior Vena Cava 1 Splenic Vein 2 Gastric Vein 3 Esophageal Vein 4 Hepatic Vein 5 Superior Mesenteric Vein 6 Inferior Mesenteric Vein 7 Colic Vein 8 Portal Vein 9 Renal Vein, Right B Renal Vein, Left C Common Iliac Vein, Right D Common Iliac Vein, Left F External Iliac Vein, Right G External Iliac Vein, Left H Hypogastric Vein, Right J Hypogastric Vein, Left M Femoral Vein, Right N Femoral Vein, Left P Saphenous Vein, Right Q Saphenous Vein, Left T Foot Vein, Right V Foot Vein, Left Y Lower Vein	0 Open 3 Percutaneous 4 Percutaneous endoscopic	C Extraluminal device D Intraluminal device Z No device	Z No qualifier

© 2018 Channel Publishing, Ltd.

1ST - 0 Medical and Surgical
2ND - 6 Lower Veins
3RD - W REVISION

DEVICE GROUP: (Change), Insertion, Removal, Replacement, Revision, Supplement
Root Operations that always involve a device.

REVISION: Correcting, to the extent possible, a portion of a malfunctioning device or the position of a displaced device.

Explanation: Correcting by taking out or putting in components of a device such as a screw or pin ...
Examples: Reposition inferior vena cava (IVC) filter – CMS Ex: Recementing of hip prosthesis

Body Part – 4TH	Approach – 5TH	Device – 6TH	Qualifier – 7TH
Y Lower Vein	0 Open 3 Percutaneous 4 Percutaneous endoscopic	0 Drainage device 2 Monitoring device 3 Infusion device 7 Autologous tissue substitute C Extraluminal device D Intraluminal device J Synthetic substitute K Nonautologous tissue substitute Y Other device	Z No qualifier
Y Lower Vein	X External	0 Drainage device 2 Monitoring device 3 Infusion device 7 Autologous tissue substitute C Extraluminal device D Intraluminal device J Synthetic substitute K Nonautologous tissue substitute	Z No qualifier

© 2018 Channel Publishing, Ltd.

Educational Annotations | 7 – Lymphatic and Hemic Systems

Body System Specific Educational Annotations for the Lymphatic and Hemic Systems include:

- Anatomy and Physiology Review
- Anatomical Illustrations
- Definitions of Common Procedures
- AHA Coding Clinic® Reference Notations
- Body Part Key Listings
- Device Key Listings
- Device Aggregation Table Listings
- Coding Notes

Anatomy and Physiology Review of Lymphatic and Hemic Systems

BODY PART VALUES – 7 - LYMPHATIC AND HEMIC SYSTEMS

Bone Marrow – ANATOMY – The soft tissue on the inside of bones that is comprised of red and yellow bone marrow tissue. PHYSIOLOGY – Red bone marrow produces red blood cells, platelets, and most white blood cells. Yellow bone marrow has a minor role in cell production and consists primarily of fat cells.

Cisterna Chyli – ANATOMY – The cisterna chyli is a sac-like structure formed by the junction of the lumbar, intestinal, and descending intercostal lymphatic trunks that empties into the thoracic duct. PHYSIOLOGY – The cisterna chyli collects the lymph from the lower body and chyle from the intestines.

Lymphatic – ANATOMY – The general term for structures and tissues of the lymphatic system. The lymphatic system is part of the circulatory system and its major components include: Thymus, spleen, bone marrow, cisterna chyli, thoracic duct, lymph vessels, lymph nodes, and lymph node chains. PHYSIOLOGY – The lymphatic system serves multiple functions including: Immune system defense, draining the interstitial fluid, removing waste products and cellular debris, and maintaining the balance of body fluids.

Spleen – ANATOMY – The spleen is a gland-like organ, located in the upper abdomen behind the stomach and at the tail of the pancreas, and is about 5 inches (13 cm) in length. The spleen contains both white pulp and red pulp. PHYSIOLOGY – The spleen functions as both a large lymph node (white pulp) that filters the blood and produces lymphocytes and monocytes, and as a red blood cell reservoir (red pulp) and disintegrator of worn-out red blood cells. It also plays a role in producing antibodies. Although important, the spleen is not essential to life.

Thoracic Duct – ANATOMY – The largest of the lymphatic vessels extending from the middle lumbar region to the base of the neck. PHYSIOLOGY – The thoracic duct collects most of the body's the lymphatic fluid from the chest down and drains it into the left subclavian vein.

Thymus – ANATOMY – The thymus is the small, flat bi-lobed organ lying behind the sternum, and is composed of lymphoid material. PHYSIOLOGY – The thymus functions substantially during childhood by producing lymphocytes and aids in the development of the individual's immunity.

Anatomical Illustrations of Lymphatic and Hemic Systems

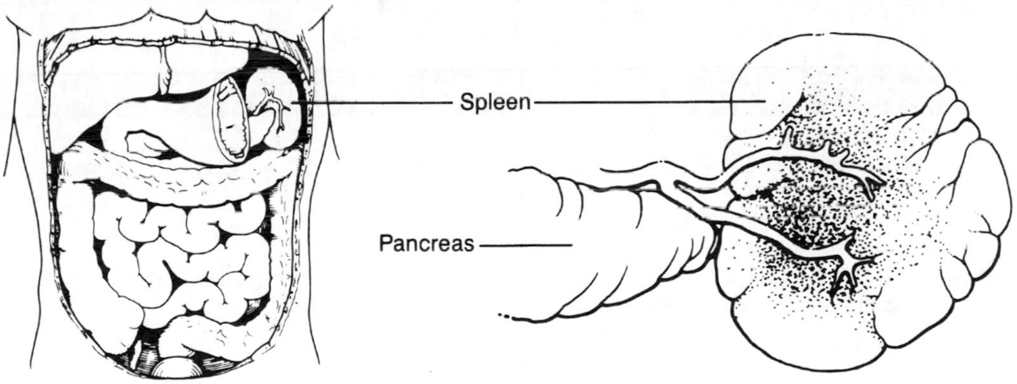

SPLEEN

Continued on next page

© 2018 Channel Publishing, Ltd.

LYMPHATIC & HEMIC 07

Educational Annotations | 7 – Lymphatic and Hemic Systems

Anatomical Illustrations of Lymphatic and Hemic Systems

Continued from previous page

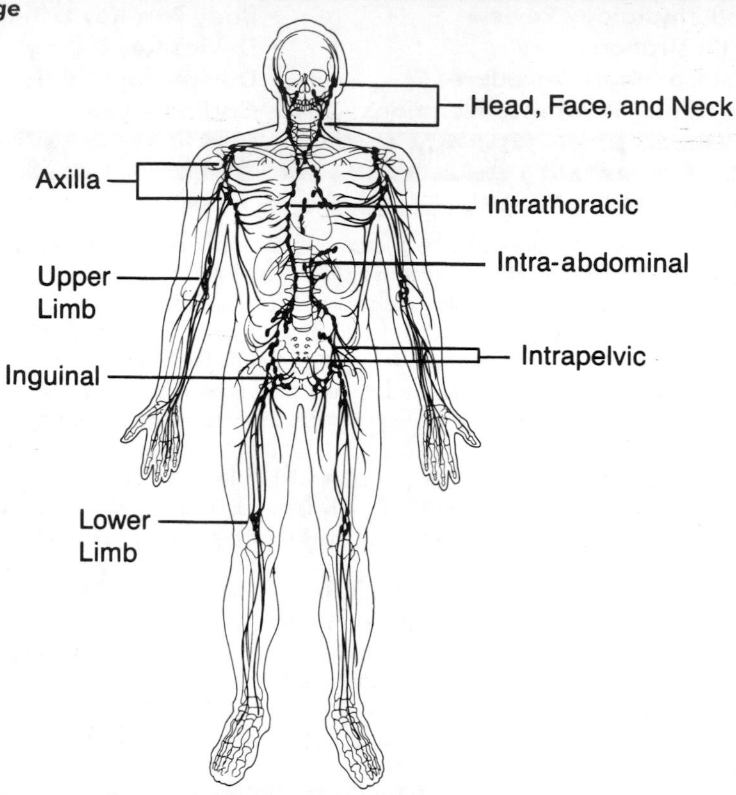

LYMPH NODES

Definitions of Common Procedures of Lymphatic and Hemic Systems

Bone marrow biopsy – The removal of living bone marrow tissue for microscopic examination using a special needle that extracts a core (cylindrical sample) of tissue.
Lymphadenectomy – The surgical removal of a lymph node or several lymph nodes in the same group.
Radical lymph node dissection – The surgical removal of an entire lymph node chain.
Splenectomy – The surgical removal of the spleen.
Thymectomy – The surgical removal of the thymus.
Transbronchial needle aspiration (TBNA) biopsy of lymph node – The lymph node biopsy that is performed using a bronchoscopic-guided technique that inserts the biopsy needle through the bronchial or tracheal wall and into the lymph node.

© 2018 Channel Publishing, Ltd.

Educational Annotations | 7 – Lymphatic and Hemic Systems

AHA Coding Clinic® Reference Notations of Lymphatic and Hemic Systems

ROOT OPERATION SPECIFIC - 7 - LYMPHATIC AND HEMIC SYSTEMS

CHANGE - 2
DESTRUCTION - 5
DRAINAGE - 9
EXCISION - B
- Removal of some paratracheal lymph nodes .... AHA 14:3Q:p10
- Transbronchial endoscopic needle aspiration biopsy of right lung lymph nodes .... AHA 14:1Q:p20
- Transbronchial endoscopic lymph node aspiration biopsy (*see also* AHA 13:4Q:p111) .... AHA 14:1Q:p26

EXTIRPATION - C
EXTRACTION - D
- Bone marrow biopsy .... AHA 13:4Q:p111

INSERTION - H
INSPECTION - J
OCCLUSION - L
RELEASE - N
REMOVAL - P
REPAIR - Q
- Lymphovenous bypass procedure .... AHA 17:1Q:p34

REPOSITION - S
RESECTION - T
- Infratemporal fossa malignancy with lymph node level resection .... AHA 16:2Q:p12
- Radical resection of level I lymph nodes, bilateral .... AHA 14:3Q:p9
- Resection of lymph node levels .... AHA 16:1Q:p30
- Resection of lymph node levels - Official Clarification .... AHA 18:1Q:p22
- Resection of thymus .... AHA 14:3Q:p16

SUPPLEMENT - U
RESTRICTION - V
REVISION - W
TRANSPLANTATION - Y

© 2018 Channel Publishing, Ltd.

Educational Annotations | 7 – Lymphatic and Hemic Systems

Body Part Key Listings of Lymphatic and Hemic Systems

See also Body Part Key in Appendix C

Accessory spleen ... use Spleen
Anterior (pectoral) lymph node ... use Lymphatic, Axillary, Left/Right
Apical (subclavicular) lymph node ... use Lymphatic, Axillary, Left/Right
Brachial (lateral) lymph node ... use Lymphatic, Axillary, Left/Right
Buccinator lymph node ... use Lymphatic, Head
Celiac lymph node ... use Lymphatic, Aortic
Central axillary lymph node ... use Lymphatic, Axillary, Left/Right
Cervical lymph node ... use Lymphatic, Neck, Left/Right
Common iliac (subaortic) lymph node ... use Lymphatic, Pelvis
Cubital lymph node ... use Lymphatic, Upper Extremity, Left/Right
Deltopectoral (infraclavicular) lymph node ... use Lymphatic, Upper Extremity, Left/Right
Epitrochlear lymph node ... use Lymphatic, Upper Extremity, Left/Right
Femoral lymph node ... use Lymphatic, Lower Extremity, Left/Right
Gastric lymph node ... use Lymphatic, Aortic
Gluteal lymph node ... use Lymphatic, Pelvis
Hepatic lymph node ... use Lymphatic, Aortic
Iliac lymph node ... use Lymphatic, Pelvis
Inferior epigastric lymph node ... use Lymphatic, Pelvis
Inferior mesenteric lymph node ... use Lymphatic, Mesenteric
Infraauricular lymph node ... use Lymphatic, Head
Infraclavicular (deltopectoral) lymph node ... use Lymphatic, Upper Extremity, Left/Right
Infraparotid lymph node ... use Lymphatic, Head
Intercostal lymph node ... use Lymphatic, Thorax
Intestinal lymphatic trunk ... use Cisterna Chyli
Jugular lymph node ... use Lymphatic, Neck, Left/Right
Lateral (brachial) lymph node ... use Lymphatic, Axillary, Left/Right
Left jugular trunk ... use Thoracic Duct
Left subclavian trunk ... use Thoracic Duct
Lumbar lymph node ... use Lymphatic, Aortic
Lumbar lymphatic trunk ... use Cisterna Chyli
Mastoid (postauricular) lymph node ... use Lymphatic, Neck, Left/Right
Mediastinal lymph node ... use Lymphatic, Thorax
Obturator lymph node ... use Lymphatic, Pelvis
Occipital lymph node ... use Lymphatic, Neck, Left/Right
Pancreaticosplenic lymph node ... use Lymphatic, Aortic
Paraaortic lymph node ... use Lymphatic, Aortic
Pararectal lymph node ... use Lymphatic, Mesenteric
Parasternal lymph node ... use Lymphatic, Thorax
Paratracheal lymph node ... use Lymphatic, Thorax
Parotid lymph node ... use Lymphatic, Head
Pectoral (anterior) lymph node ... use Lymphatic, Axillary, Left/Right
Popliteal lymph node ... use Lymphatic, Lower Extremity, Left/Right
Postauricular (mastoid) lymph node ... use Lymphatic, Neck, Left/Right
Posterior (subscapular) lymph node ... use Lymphatic, Axillary, Left/Right
Preauricular lymph node ... use Lymphatic, Head
Retroperitoneal lymph node ... use Lymphatic, Aortic
Retropharyngeal lymph node ... use Lymphatic, Neck, Left/Right
Right jugular trunk ... use Lymphatic, Right Neck
Right lymphatic duct ... use Lymphatic, Right Neck
Right subclavian trunk ... use Lymphatic, Right Neck
Sacral lymph node ... use Lymphatic, Pelvis
Subaortic (common iliac) lymph node use Lymphatic, Pelvis
Subclavicular (apical) lymph node ... use Lymphatic, Axillary, Left/Right
Submandibular lymph node ... use Lymphatic, Head
Submaxillary lymph node ... use Lymphatic, Head
Submental lymph node ... use Lymphatic, Head
Subparotid lymph node ... use Lymphatic, Head
Subscapular (posterior) lymph node ... use Lymphatic, Axillary, Left/Right
Superior mesenteric lymph node ... use Lymphatic, Mesenteric
Supraclavicular (Virchow's) lymph node ... use Lymphatic, Neck, Left/Right
Suprahyoid lymph node ... use Lymphatic, Head
Suprainguinal lymph node ... use Lymphatic, Pelvis
Supratrochlear lymph node ... use Lymphatic, Upper Extremity, Left/Right
Thymus gland ... use Thymus
Tracheobronchial lymph node ... use Lymphatic, Thorax
Virchow's (supraclavicular) lymph node ... use Lymphatic, Neck, Left/Right

Device Key Listings of Lymphatic and Hemic Systems

See also Device Key in Appendix D

Autograft ... use Autologous Tissue Substitute
Tissue bank graft ... use Nonautologous Tissue Substitute

Device Aggregation Table Listings of Lymphatic and Hemic Systems

See also Device Aggregation Table in Appendix E

Specific Device	For Operation	In Body System	General Device
None Listed in Device Aggregation Table for this Body System			

Coding Notes of Lymphatic and Hemic Systems

LYMPHATIC & HEMIC 0 7

© 2018 Channel Publishing, Ltd.

1ST - 0 Medical and Surgical
2ND - 7 Lymphatic and Hemic Systems
3RD - 2 CHANGE

DEVICE GROUP: Change, Insertion, Removal, (Replacement), Revision, Supplement
Root Operations that always involve a device.

CHANGE: Taking out or off a device from a body part and putting back an identical or similar device in or on the same body part without cutting or puncturing the skin or a mucous membrane.

Explanation: All CHANGE procedures are coded using the approach External
Examples: Exchange drain tube – CMS Ex: Urinary catheter change

Body Part – 4TH		Approach – 5TH	Device – 6TH	Qualifier – 7TH
K Thoracic Duct L Cisterna Chyli M Thymus	N Lymphatic P Spleen T Bone Marrow	X External	0 Drainage device Y Other device	Z No qualifier

1ST - 0 Medical and Surgical
2ND - 7 Lymphatic and Hemic Systems
3RD - 5 DESTRUCTION

EXCISION GROUP: Excision, Resection, Destruction, Extraction, (Detachment)
Root Operations that take out some or all of a body part.

DESTRUCTION: Physical eradication of all or a portion of a body part by the direct use of energy, force, or a destructive agent.

Explanation: None of the body part is physically taken out
Examples: Radiofrequency node ablation – CMS Ex: Fulguration of rectal polyp

Body Part – 4TH			Approach – 5TH	Device – 6TH	Qualifier – 7TH
0 Lymphatic, Head 1 Lymphatic, Right Neck 2 Lymphatic, Left Neck 3 Lymphatic, Right Upper Extremity 4 Lymphatic, Left Upper Extremity 5 Lymphatic, Right Axillary 6 Lymphatic, Left Axillary	7 Lymphatic, Thorax 8 Lymphatic, Internal Mammary, Right 9 Lymphatic, Internal Mammary, Left B Lymphatic, Mesenteric C Lymphatic, Pelvis D Lymphatic, Aortic	F Lymphatic, Right Lower Extremity G Lymphatic, Left Lower Extremity H Lymphatic, Right Inguinal J Lymphatic, Left Inguinal K Thoracic Duct L Cisterna Chyli M Thymus P Spleen	0 Open 3 Percutaneous 4 Percutaneous endoscopic	Z No device	Z No qualifier

© 2018 Channel Publishing, Ltd.

1ST - 0 Medical and Surgical
2ND - 7 Lymphatic and Hemic Systems
3RD - 9 DRAINAGE

DRAINAGE GROUP: Drainage, Extirpation, (Fragmentation)
Root Operations that take out solids/fluids/gases from a body part.

DRAINAGE: Taking or letting out fluids and/or gases from a body part.

Explanation: Qualifier "X Diagnostic" indicates drainage procedures that are biopsies
Examples: Drainage Cisterna Chyli – CMS Ex: Thoracentesis

Body Part – 4TH	Approach – 5TH	Device – 6TH	Qualifier – 7TH
0 Lymphatic, Head 1 Lymphatic, Right Neck 2 Lymphatic, Left Neck 3 Lymphatic, Right Upper Extremity 4 Lymphatic, Left Upper Extremity 5 Lymphatic, Right Axillary 6 Lymphatic, Left Axillary 7 Lymphatic, Thorax 8 Lymphatic, Internal Mammary, Right 9 Lymphatic, Internal Mammary, Left B Lymphatic, Mesenteric C Lymphatic, Pelvis D Lymphatic, Aortic F Lymphatic, Right Lower Extremity G Lymphatic, Left Lower Extremity H Lymphatic, Right Inguinal J Lymphatic, Left Inguinal K Thoracic Duct L Cisterna Chyli	0 Open 3 Percutaneous 4 Percutaneous endoscopic 8 Via natural or artificial opening endoscopic	0 Drainage device	Z No qualifier
0 Lymphatic, Head 1 Lymphatic, Right Neck 2 Lymphatic, Left Neck 3 Lymphatic, Right Upper Extremity 4 Lymphatic, Left Upper Extremity 5 Lymphatic, Right Axillary 6 Lymphatic, Left Axillary 7 Lymphatic, Thorax 8 Lymphatic, Internal Mammary, Right 9 Lymphatic, Internal Mammary, Left B Lymphatic, Mesenteric C Lymphatic, Pelvis D Lymphatic, Aortic F Lymphatic, Right Lower Extremity G Lymphatic, Left Lower Extremity H Lymphatic, Right Inguinal J Lymphatic, Left Inguinal K Thoracic Duct L Cisterna Chyli	0 Open 3 Percutaneous 4 Percutaneous endoscopic 8 Via natural or artificial opening endoscopic	Z No device	X Diagnostic Z No qualifier
M Thymus P Spleen T Bone Marrow	0 Open 3 Percutaneous 4 Percutaneous endoscopic	0 Drainage device	Z No qualifier
M Thymus P Spleen T Bone Marrow	0 Open 3 Percutaneous 4 Percutaneous endoscopic	Z No device	X Diagnostic Z No qualifier

LYMPHATIC & HEMIC 079

1ST - 0 Medical and Surgical
2ND - 7 Lymphatic and Hemic Systems
3RD - B EXCISION

EXCISION GROUP: Excision, Resection, Destruction, Extraction, (Detachment)
Root Operations that take out some or all of a body part.

EXCISION: Cutting out or off, without replacement, a portion of a body part.

Explanation: Qualifier "X Diagnostic" indicates excision procedures that are biopsies
Examples: Removal single lymph node – CMS Ex: Liver biopsy

Body Part – 4TH	Approach – 5TH	Device – 6TH	Qualifier – 7TH
0 Lymphatic, Head 1 Lymphatic, Right Neck 2 Lymphatic, Left Neck 3 Lymphatic, Right Upper Extremity 4 Lymphatic, Left Upper Extremity 5 Lymphatic, Right Axillary 6 Lymphatic, Left Axillary 7 Lymphatic, Thorax 8 Lymphatic, Internal Mammary, Right 9 Lymphatic, Internal Mammary, Left B Lymphatic, Mesenteric C Lymphatic, Pelvis D Lymphatic, Aortic F Lymphatic, Right Lower Extremity G Lymphatic, Left Lower Extremity H Lymphatic, Right Inguinal J Lymphatic, Left Inguinal K Thoracic Duct L Cisterna Chyli M Thymus P Spleen	0 Open 3 Percutaneous 4 Percutaneous endoscopic	Z No device	X Diagnostic Z No qualifier

© 2018 Channel Publishing, Ltd.

1ST - 0 Medical and Surgical
2ND - 7 Lymphatic and Hemic Systems
3RD - C EXTIRPATION

DRAINAGE GROUP: Drainage, Extirpation, (Fragmentation)
Root Operations that take out solids/fluids/gases from a body part.

EXTIRPATION: Taking or cutting out solid matter from a body part.

Explanation: Abnormal byproduct or foreign body ...
Examples: Removal foreign body spleen – CMS Ex: Thrombectomy

Body Part – 4TH			Approach – 5TH	Device – 6TH	Qualifier – 7TH
0 Lymphatic, Head 1 Lymphatic, Right Neck 2 Lymphatic, Left Neck 3 Lymphatic, Right Upper Extremity 4 Lymphatic, Left Upper Extremity 5 Lymphatic, Right Axillary 6 Lymphatic, Left Axillary	7 Lymphatic, Thorax 8 Lymphatic, Internal Mammary, Right 9 Lymphatic, Internal Mammary, Left B Lymphatic, Mesenteric C Lymphatic, Pelvis D Lymphatic, Aortic	F Lymphatic, Right Lower Extremity G Lymphatic, Left Lower Extremity H Lymphatic, Right Inguinal J Lymphatic, Left Inguinal K Thoracic Duct L Cisterna Chyli M Thymus P Spleen	0 Open 3 Percutaneous 4 Percutaneous endoscopic	Z No device	Z No qualifier

1ST - 0 Medical and Surgical
2ND - 7 Lymphatic and Hemic Systems
3RD - D EXTRACTION

EXCISION GROUP: Excision, Resection, Destruction, Extraction, (Detachment)
Root Operations that take out some or all of a body part.

EXTRACTION: Pulling or stripping out or off all or a portion of a body part by the use of force.

Explanation: Qualifier "X Diagnostic" indicates extraction procedures that are biopsies
Examples: Bone marrow biopsy – CMS Ex: Dilation and curettage

Body Part – 4TH			Approach – 5TH	Device – 6TH	Qualifier – 7TH
0 Lymphatic, Head 1 Lymphatic, Right Neck 2 Lymphatic, Left Neck 3 Lymphatic, Right Upper Extremity 4 Lymphatic, Left Upper Extremity 5 Lymphatic, Right Axillary 6 Lymphatic, Left Axillary	7 Lymphatic, Thorax 8 Lymphatic, Internal Mammary, Right 9 Lymphatic, Internal Mammary, Left B Lymphatic, Mesenteric C Lymphatic, Pelvis D Lymphatic, Aortic	F Lymphatic, Right Lower Extremity G Lymphatic, Left Lower Extremity H Lymphatic, Right Inguinal J Lymphatic, Left Inguinal K Thoracic Duct L Cisterna Chyli	3 Percutaneous 4 Percutaneous endoscopic 8 Via natural or artificial opening endoscopic	Z No device	X Diagnostic
M Thymus P Spleen			3 Percutaneous 4 Percutaneous endoscopic	Z No device	X Diagnostic
Q Bone Marrow, Sternum R Bone Marrow, Iliac S Bone Marrow, Vertebral			0 Open 3 Percutaneous	Z No device	X Diagnostic Z No qualifier

1ST - 0 Medical and Surgical
2ND - 7 Lymphatic and Hemic Systems
3RD - H INSERTION

DEVICE GROUP: Change, Insertion, Removal, (Replacement), Revision, Supplement
Root Operations that always involve a device.

INSERTION: Putting in a nonbiological appliance that monitors, assists, performs, or prevents a physiological function but does not physically take the place of a body part.

Explanation: None
Examples: Insertion infusion device – CMS Ex: Insertion of central venous catheter

Body Part – 4TH		Approach – 5TH	Device – 6TH	Qualifier – 7TH
K Thoracic Duct L Cisterna Chyli M Thymus	N Lymphatic P Spleen	0 Open 3 Percutaneous 4 Percutaneous endoscopic	3 Infusion device Y Other device	Z No qualifier

LYMPHATIC & HEMIC 0 7 H

© 2018 Channel Publishing, Ltd.

1ST - 0 Medical and Surgical
2ND - 7 Lymphatic and Hemic Systems
3RD - J INSPECTION

EXAMINATION GROUP: Inspection, (Map)
Root Operations involving examination only.

INSPECTION: Visually and/or manually exploring a body part.

Explanation: Direct or instrumental visualization ...
Examples: Examination spleen – CMS Ex: Exploratory laparotomy

Body Part – 4TH	Approach – 5TH	Device – 6TH	Qualifier – 7TH
K Thoracic Duct L Cisterna Chyli M Thymus T Bone Marrow	0 Open 3 Percutaneous 4 Percutaneous endoscopic	Z No device	Z No qualifier
N Lymphatic	0 Open 3 Percutaneous 4 Percutaneous endoscopic 8 Via natural or artificial opening endoscopic X External	Z No device	Z No qualifier
P Spleen	0 Open 3 Percutaneous 4 Percutaneous endoscopic X External	Z No device	Z No qualifier

1ST - 0 Medical and Surgical
2ND - 7 Lymphatic and Hemic Systems
3RD - L OCCLUSION

TUBULAR GROUP: (Bypass), (Dilation), Occlusion, Restriction
Root Operations that alter the diameter/route of a tubular body part.

OCCLUSION: Completely closing an orifice or the lumen of a tubular body part.

Explanation: The orifice can be a natural orifice or an artificially created orifice
Examples: Occlusion para-aortic lymph – CMS Ex: Fallopian tube ligation

Body Part – 4TH	Approach – 5TH	Device – 6TH	Qualifier – 7TH
0 Lymphatic, Head 1 Lymphatic, Right Neck 2 Lymphatic, Left Neck 3 Lymphatic, Right Upper Extremity 4 Lymphatic, Left Upper Extremity 5 Lymphatic, Right Axillary 6 Lymphatic, Left Axillary 7 Lymphatic, Thorax 8 Lymphatic, Internal Mammary, Right 9 Lymphatic, Internal Mammary, Left B Lymphatic, Mesenteric C Lymphatic, Pelvis D Lymphatic, Aortic F Lymphatic, Right Lower Extremity G Lymphatic, Left Lower Extremity H Lymphatic, Right Inguinal J Lymphatic, Left Inguinal K Thoracic Duct L Cisterna Chyli	0 Open 3 Percutaneous 4 Percutaneous endoscopic	C Extraluminal device D Intraluminal device Z No device	Z No qualifier

1ST - 0 Medical and Surgical
2ND - 7 Lymphatic and Hemic Systems
3RD - N RELEASE

DIVISION GROUP: (Division), Release
Root Operations involving cutting or separation only.

RELEASE: Freeing a body part from an abnormal physical constraint by cutting or by the use of force.

Explanation: Some of the restraining tissue may be taken out but none of the body part is taken out
Examples: Lysis adhesions spleen – CMS Ex: Carpal tunnel release

Body Part – 4TH	Approach – 5TH	Device – 6TH	Qualifier – 7TH
0 Lymphatic, Head 1 Lymphatic, Right Neck 2 Lymphatic, Left Neck 3 Lymphatic, Right Upper Extremity 4 Lymphatic, Left Upper Extremity 5 Lymphatic, Right Axillary 6 Lymphatic, Left Axillary 7 Lymphatic, Thorax 8 Lymphatic, Internal Mammary, Right 9 Lymphatic, Internal Mammary, Left B Lymphatic, Mesenteric C Lymphatic, Pelvis D Lymphatic, Aortic F Lymphatic, Right Lower Extremity G Lymphatic, Left Lower Extremity H Lymphatic, Right Inguinal J Lymphatic, Left Inguinal K Thoracic Duct L Cisterna Chyli M Thymus P Spleen	0 Open 3 Percutaneous 4 Percutaneous endoscopic	Z No device	Z No qualifier

© 2018 Channel Publishing, Ltd.

1ST - 0 Medical and Surgical
2ND - 7 Lymphatic and Hemic Systems
3RD - P REMOVAL

DEVICE GROUP: Change, Insertion, Removal, (Replacement), Revision, Supplement
Root Operations that always involve a device.

REMOVAL: Taking out or off a device from a body part.

Explanation: Removal device without reinsertion ...
Examples: Removal drain tube – CMS Ex: Cardiac pacemaker removal

Body Part – 4TH	Approach – 5TH	Device – 6TH	Qualifier – 7TH
K Thoracic Duct L Cisterna Chyli N Lymphatic	0 Open 3 Percutaneous 4 Percutaneous endoscopic	0 Drainage device 3 Infusion device 7 Autologous tissue substitute C Extraluminal device D Intraluminal device J Synthetic substitute K Nonautologous tissue substitute Y Other device	Z No qualifier
K Thoracic Duct L Cisterna Chyli N Lymphatic	X External	0 Drainage device 3 Infusion device D Intraluminal device	Z No qualifier
M Thymus P Spleen	0 Open 3 Percutaneous 4 Percutaneous endoscopic	0 Drainage device 3 Infusion device Y Other device	Z No qualifier
M Thymus P Spleen	X External	0 Drainage device 3 Infusion device	Z No qualifier
T Bone Marrow	0 Open 3 Percutaneous 4 Percutaneous endoscopic X External	0 Drainage device	Z No qualifier

1ST - 0 Medical and Surgical
2ND - 7 Lymphatic and Hemic Systems
3RD - Q REPAIR

OTHER REPAIRS GROUP: (Control), Repair
Root Operations that define other repairs.

REPAIR: Restoring, to the extent possible, a body part to its normal anatomic structure and function.

Explanation: Used only when the method to accomplish the repair is not one of the other root operations
Examples: Splenorrhaphy – CMS Ex: Suture of laceration

Body Part – 4TH	Approach – 5TH	Device – 6TH	Qualifier – 7TH
0 Lymphatic, Head 1 Lymphatic, Right Neck 2 Lymphatic, Left Neck 3 Lymphatic, Right Upper Extremity 4 Lymphatic, Left Upper Extremity 5 Lymphatic, Right Axillary 6 Lymphatic, Left Axillary 7 Lymphatic, Thorax 8 Lymphatic, Internal Mammary, Right 9 Lymphatic, Internal Mammary, Left B Lymphatic, Mesenteric C Lymphatic, Pelvis D Lymphatic, Aortic F Lymphatic, Right Lower Extremity G Lymphatic, Left Lower Extremity H Lymphatic, Right Inguinal J Lymphatic, Left Inguinal K Thoracic Duct L Cisterna Chyli	0 Open 3 Percutaneous 4 Percutaneous endoscopic 8 Via natural or artificial opening endoscopic	Z No device	Z No qualifier
M Thymus P Spleen	0 Open 3 Percutaneous 4 Percutaneous endoscopic	Z No device	Z No qualifier

LYMPHATIC & HEMIC 07Q

© 2018 Channel Publishing, Ltd.

1ST - 0 Medical and Surgical
2ND - 7 Lymphatic and Hemic Systems
3RD - S REPOSITION

MOVE GROUP: (Reattachment), Reposition, (Transfer), Transplantation
Root Operations that put in/put back or move some/all of a body part.

REPOSITION: Moving to its normal location, or other suitable location, all or a portion of a body part.

Explanation: The body part may or may not be cut out or off to be moved to the new location ...
Examples: Relocation spleen – CMS Ex: Fracture reduction

Body Part – 4TH	Approach – 5TH	Device – 6TH	Qualifier – 7TH
M Thymus P Spleen	0 Open	Z No device	Z No qualifier

1ST - 0 Medical and Surgical
2ND - 7 Lymphatic and Hemic Systems
3RD - T RESECTION

EXCISION GROUP: Excision, Resection, Destruction, Extraction, (Detachment)
Root Operations that take out some or all of a body part.

RESECTION: Cutting out or off, without replacement, all of a body part.

Explanation: None
Examples: Excision axillary lymph node chain – CMS Ex: Total lobectomy of lung

Body Part – 4TH			Approach – 5TH	Device – 6TH	Qualifier – 7TH
0 Lymphatic, Head 1 Lymphatic, Right Neck 2 Lymphatic, Left Neck 3 Lymphatic, Right Upper Extremity 4 Lymphatic, Left Upper Extremity 5 Lymphatic, Right Axillary 6 Lymphatic, Left Axillary	7 Lymphatic, Thorax 8 Lymphatic, Internal Mammary, Right 9 Lymphatic, Internal Mammary, Left B Lymphatic, Mesenteric C Lymphatic, Pelvis D Lymphatic, Aortic	F Lymphatic, Right Lower Extremity G Lymphatic, Left Lower Extremity H Lymphatic, Right Inguinal J Lymphatic, Left Inguinal K Thoracic Duct L Cisterna Chyli M Thymus P Spleen	0 Open 4 Percutaneous endoscopic	Z No device	Z No qualifier

1ST - 0 Medical and Surgical
2ND - 7 Lymphatic and Hemic Systems
3RD - U SUPPLEMENT

DEVICE GROUP: Change, Insertion, Removal, (Replacement), Revision, Supplement
Root Operations that always involve a device.

SUPPLEMENT: Putting in or on biological or synthetic material that physically reinforces and/or augments the function of a portion of a body part.

Explanation: Biological material is non-living, or is living and from the same individual ...
Examples: Overlay splenic graft – CMS Ex: Herniorrhaphy using mesh

Body Part – 4TH			Approach – 5TH	Device – 6TH	Qualifier – 7TH
0 Lymphatic, Head 1 Lymphatic, Right Neck 2 Lymphatic, Left Neck 3 Lymphatic, Right Upper Extremity 4 Lymphatic, Left Upper Extremity 5 Lymphatic, Right Axillary 6 Lymphatic, Left Axillary	7 Lymphatic, Thorax 8 Lymphatic, Internal Mammary, Right 9 Lymphatic, Internal Mammary, Left B Lymphatic, Mesenteric C Lymphatic, Pelvis D Lymphatic, Aortic	F Lymphatic, Right Lower Extremity G Lymphatic, Left Lower Extremity H Lymphatic, Right Inguinal J Lymphatic, Left Inguinal K Thoracic Duct L Cisterna Chyli	0 Open 4 Percutaneous endoscopic	7 Autologous tissue substitute J Synthetic substitute K Nonautologous tissue substitute	Z No qualifier

© 2018 Channel Publishing, Ltd.

1ST - 0 Medical and Surgical
2ND - 7 Lymphatic and Hemic Systems
3RD - V RESTRICTION

TUBULAR GROUP: (Bypass), (Dilation), Occlusion, Restriction
Root Operations that alter the diameter/route of a tubular body part.

RESTRICTION: Partially closing an orifice or the lumen of a tubular body part.

Explanation: The orifice can be a natural orifice or an artificially created orifice.
Examples: Thoracic duct restrictive stent – CMS Ex: Cervical cerclage

Body Part – 4TH			Approach – 5TH	Device – 6TH	Qualifier – 7TH
0 Lymphatic, Head 1 Lymphatic, Right Neck 2 Lymphatic, Left Neck 3 Lymphatic, Right Upper Extremity 4 Lymphatic, Left Upper Extremity 5 Lymphatic, Right Axillary 6 Lymphatic, Left Axillary	7 Lymphatic, Thorax 8 Lymphatic, Internal Mammary, Right 9 Lymphatic, Internal Mammary, Left B Lymphatic, Mesenteric C Lymphatic, Pelvis D Lymphatic, Aortic	F Lymphatic, Right Lower Extremity G Lymphatic, Left Lower Extremity H Lymphatic, Right Inguinal J Lymphatic, Left Inguinal K Thoracic Duct L Cisterna Chyli	0 Open 3 Percutaneous 4 Percutaneous endoscopic	C Extraluminal device D Intraluminal device Z No device	Z No qualifier

1ST - 0 Medical and Surgical
2ND - 7 Lymphatic and Hemic Systems
3RD - W REVISION

DEVICE GROUP: Change, Insertion, Removal, (Replacement), Revision, Supplement
Root Operations that always involve a device.

REVISION: Correcting, to the extent possible, a portion of a malfunctioning device or the position of a displaced device.

Explanation: Correcting by taking out or putting in components of a device such as a screw or pin ...
Examples: Reposition drainage tube – CMS Ex: Recementing of hip prosthesis

Body Part – 4TH	Approach – 5TH	Device – 6TH	Qualifier – 7TH
K Thoracic Duct L Cisterna Chyli N Lymphatic	0 Open 3 Percutaneous 4 Percutaneous endoscopic	0 Drainage device 3 Infusion device 7 Autologous tissue substitute C Extraluminal device D Intraluminal device J Synthetic substitute K Nonautologous tissue substitute Y Other device	Z No qualifier
K Thoracic Duct L Cisterna Chyli N Lymphatic	X External	0 Drainage device 3 Infusion device 7 Autologous tissue substitute C Extraluminal device D Intraluminal device J Synthetic substitute K Nonautologous tissue substitute	Z No qualifier
M Thymus P Spleen	0 Open 3 Percutaneous 4 Percutaneous endoscopic	0 Drainage device 3 Infusion device Y Other device	Z No qualifier
M Thymus P Spleen	X External	0 Drainage device 3 Infusion device	Z No qualifier
T Bone Marrow	0 Open 3 Percutaneous 4 Percutaneous endoscopic X External	0 Drainage device	Z No qualifier

© 2018 Channel Publishing, Ltd.

1ST - 0 Medical and Surgical
2ND - 7 Lymphatic and Hemic Systems
3RD - Y TRANSPLANTATION

MOVE GROUP: (Reattachment), Reposition, (Transfer), Transplantation
Root Operations that put in/put back or move some/all of a body part.

TRANSPLANTATION: Putting in or on all or a portion of a living body part taken from another individual or animal to physically take the place and/or function of all or a portion of a similar body part.

Explanation: The native body part may or may not be taken out ...
Examples: Spleen transplant – CMS Ex: Kidney transplant

Body Part – 4TH	Approach – 5TH	Device – 6TH	Qualifier – 7TH
M Thymus P Spleen	0 Open	Z No device	0 Allogeneic 1 Syngeneic 2 Zooplastic

© 2018 Channel Publishing, Ltd.

Educational Annotations | 8 – Eye

Body System Specific Educational Annotations for the Eye include:

- Anatomy and Physiology Review
- Anatomical Illustrations
- Definitions of Common Procedures
- AHA Coding Clinic® Reference Notations
- Body Part Key Listings
- Device Key Listings
- Device Aggregation Table Listings
- Coding Notes

Anatomy and Physiology Review of Eye

BODY PART VALUES – 8 - EYE

Anterior Chamber – The anterior chamber contains the watery fluid between the iris and cornea.
Choroid – ANATOMY – The choroid is the vascular layer lying between the retina and the sclera that contains the dark brown pigment. PHYSIOLOGY – The choroid functions as a vascular blood supply to most eye structures and absorbs excess light through its dark pigment.
Ciliary Body – The ciliary body consists of smooth muscle with suspensory ligaments which holds the lens in place and adjusts the focus of the lens.
Conjunctiva – ANATOMY – The conjunctiva is the delicate mucous membrane that lines the eyelids and covers the exposed surface of the sclera. PHYSIOLOGY – The conjunctiva is the protective mucous-producing membrane covering the eyelids and exposed portion of the sclera. In addition to providing lubrication, it helps prevent the entry of microorganisms.
Cornea – ANATOMY – The transparent tissue layer that covers the front part of the eye including the iris, pupil, and anterior chamber. PHYSIOLOGY – The cornea refracts and focuses most of the light entering the eye.
Extraocular Muscle – ANATOMY – The extraocular muscles attach the eyeball to the orbit by 6 different muscles. PHYSIOLOGY – The extraocular muscles function to rotate the eyeballs to look at desired objects. Four muscles move the eyeball up, down, right, and left. The other two muscles control the adjustments involved in counteracting head movement while maintaining the target.
Eye – ANATOMY – The eyes are hollow spherical structures about 1 inch (2.5 cm) in diameter, located in and protected by the orbital socket in the skull. PHYSIOLOGY – The eyes are the primary organ of sight, and are directly connected to the brain through the retina and optic nerve.
Eyelid – ANATOMY – The thin folds of skin that cover the eye when muscles draw the eyelids together. PHYSIOLOGY – The eyelids protect the eye from injury and foreign objects and aid in tear flow and distribution.
Iris – ANATOMY – The iris is a muscular diaphragm that controls the dilation of the pupil. PHYSIOLOGY – The iris contracts or dilates, allowing for varying amounts of light to enter the eye and retina.
Lacrimal Duct – ANATOMY – The lacrimal duct is located at the inner lower corner of each eye and connects the lacrimal sac with the nasal cavity. PHYSIOLOGY – The lacrimal duct drains the tears from the eyes into the nasal cavities.
Lacrimal Gland – ANATOMY – The lacrimal glands are almond-shaped glands located in the upper outer corner of each orbit. PHYSIOLOGY – The lacrimal glands produce the tears that function to keep protective fluid on the conjunctiva and cornea.
Lens – ANATOMY – The crystalline lens is a transparent elastic, biconvex structure whose shape is controlled by the action of ciliary muscles. PHYSIOLOGY – The lens and cornea refract light waves to focus them on the retina.
Retina – ANATOMY – The retina is the inner layer of the eye and is continuous with the optic nerve. It contains the visual receptor cells including the rods and cones. PHYSIOLOGY – The rods are responsible for colorless vision, like in dim light, and the cones are responsible for color vision through their light-sensitive pigment sets.
Retinal Vessels – The small arteries and veins that circulate the blood to the retina. The retinal arteries are branches of the ophthalmic artery.
Sclera – ANATOMY – The protective, outer layer of the eye (white of the eye). PHYSIOLOGY – The sclera maintains the shape of the globe and serves as the attachment insertions for the extraocular muscles. Its anterior portion, the cornea, is transparent so that it can refract light entering the eye.
Vitreous – ANATOMY – The clear, gelatinous substance filling the globe of the eye between the lens and retina. PHYSIOLOGY – The thick, gel-like substance maintains the shape of the eye globe.

Anatomical Illustrations of Eye

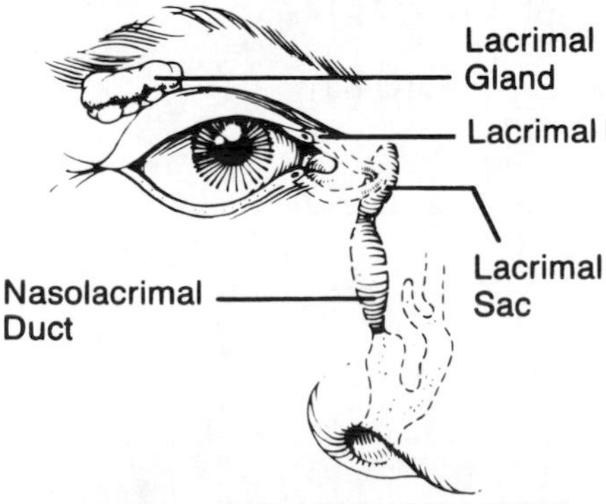

EYE AND LACRIMAL SYSTEM

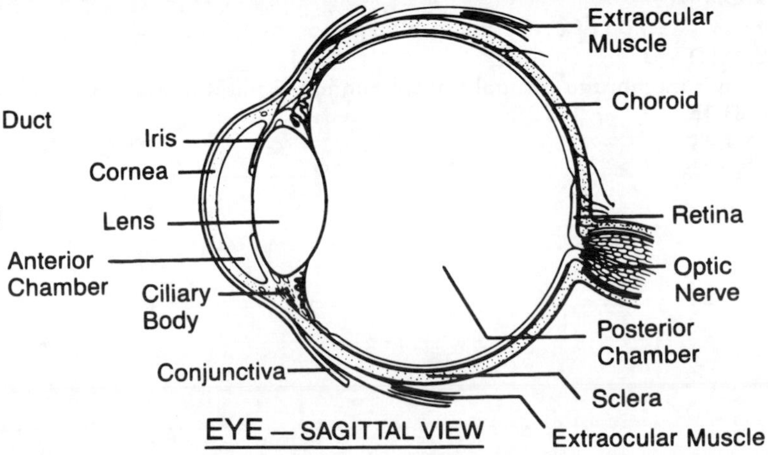

EYE — SAGITTAL VIEW

EYE
08

© 2018 Channel Publishing, Ltd.

Educational Annotations | 8 – Eye

Definitions of Common Procedures – Body System Specific

Blepharoplasty – The plastic surgical correction of eyelid defects and deformities. It may also be done for cosmetic reasons.
Cataract extraction – The surgical removal of a cloudy lens (normally clear) that is most often immediately replaced with an artificial lens substitute.
Conjunctivoplasty – The surgical procedure to correct a conjunctival defect or conjunctivochalasis.
Corneal transplant – The replacement of the cornea with a donor cornea graft. Also referred to as a keratoplasty.
Dacryocystorhinostomy – The surgical creation of a communicating passage between the lacrimal sac and the nasal cavity to restore the flow of tears.
Enucleation of eyeball – The surgical removal of the entire eyeball (globe) that leaves the eyelids and eye socket structures intact.
Evisceration of eyeball – The surgical removal of the iris, cornea, lens, retina, and vitreous while leaving the sclera, optic nerve, and extraocular eye muscles intact so that an artificial eye prosthesis (integrated orbital implant) moves naturally with the other eye.
Exenteration of eyeball – The surgical removal of all of the contents of the eye socket including the extraocular muscles and often including the eyelids.
Scleral buckling – The surgical placement of synthetic material around the eyeball to create an inward indentation of the sclera from the exterior creating a ridge (or buckle) that corrects the effects of retinal detachment.
Strabismus surgery – The surgical correction of strabismus by repositioning, shortening, or lengthening of one or more of the extraocular eye muscles.

AHA Coding Clinic® Reference Notations of Eye

ROOT OPERATION SPECIFIC - 8 - EYE

ALTERATION - 0
BYPASS - 1
CHANGE - 2
DESTRUCTION - 5
DILATION - 7
DRAINAGE - 9
Laser trabeculoplasty .... AHA 16:2Q:p21
EXCISION - B
Core vitrectomy with gas replacement .... AHA 14:4Q:p35
Posterior pars plana vitrectomy .... AHA 14:4Q:p36
EXTIRPATION - C
EXTRACTION - D
FRAGMENTATION - F
INSERTION - H
INSPECTION - J
Unsuccessful removal of foreign body of eye .... AHA 15:1Q:p35
OCCLUSION - L
REATTACHMENT - M
RELEASE - N
Lysis of iris adhesions .... AHA 15:2Q:p24
REMOVAL - P
REPAIR - Q
REPLACEMENT - R
Penetrating keratoplasty with anterior segment reconstruction .... AHA 15:2Q:p24
Penetrating keratoplasty with viscoelastic filling .... AHA 15:2Q:p25
REPOSITION - S
RESECTION - T
Radical resection of eyelid and orbital tumor .... AHA 15:2Q:p12
SUPPLEMENT - U
Amniotic membrane corneal transplantation .... AHA 14:3Q:p31
RESTRICTION - V
REVISION - W
TRANSFER - X

© 2018 Channel Publishing, Ltd.

Educational Annotations | 8 – Eye

Body Part Key Listings of Eye

See also Body Part Key in Appendix C

Aqueous humour	use Anterior Chamber, Left/Right
Ciliary body	use Eye, Left/Right
Fovea	use Retina, Left/Right
Inferior oblique muscle	use Extraocular Muscle, Left/Right
Inferior rectus muscle	use Extraocular Muscle, Left/Right
Inferior tarsal plate	use Lower Eyelid, Left/Right
Lacrimal canaliculus	use Lacrimal Duct, Left/Right
Lacrimal punctum	use Lacrimal Duct, Left/Right
Lacrimal sac	use Lacrimal Duct, Left/Right
Lateral canthus	use Upper Eyelid, Left/Right
Lateral rectus muscle	use Extraocular Muscle, Left/Right
Levator palpebrae superioris muscle	use Upper Eyelid, Left/Right
Macula	use Retina, Left/Right
Medial canthus	use Lower Eyelid, Left/Right
Medial rectus muscle	use Extraocular Muscle, Left/Right
Nasolacrimal duct	use Lacrimal Duct, Left/Right
Optic disc	use Retina, Left/Right
Orbicularis oculi muscle	use Upper Eyelid, Left/Right
Plica semilunaris	use Conjunctiva, Left/Right
Posterior chamber	use Eye, Left/Right
Superior oblique muscle	use Extraocular Muscle, Left/Right
Superior rectus muscle	use Extraocular Muscle, Left/Right
Superior tarsal plate	use Upper Eyelid, Left/Right
Vitreous body	use Vitreous, Left/Right
Zonule of Zinn	use Lens, Left/Right

Device Key Listings of Eye

See also Device Key in Appendix D

Autograft	use Autologous Tissue Substitute
Brachytherapy seeds	use Radioactive Element
Ex-PRESS™ mini glaucoma shunt	use Synthetic Substitute
Implantable Miniature Telescope™ (IMT)	use Synthetic Substitute, Intraocular Telescope for Replacement in Eye
Tissue bank graft	use Nonautologous Tissue Substitute

Device Aggregation Table Listings of Eye

See also Device Aggregation Table in Appendix E

Specific Device	For Operation	In Body System	General Device
Epiretinal Visual Prosthesis	All applicable	Eye	Synthetic Substitute
Synthetic Substitute, Intraocular Telescope	Replacement	Eye	Synthetic Substitute

Coding Notes of Eye

EYE

0 8

© 2018 Channel Publishing, Ltd.

1ST - 0 Medical and Surgical
2ND - 8 Eye
3RD - 0 ALTERATION

OTHER OBJECTIVES GROUP: Alteration, (Creation), (Fusion)
Root Operations that define other objectives.

ALTERATION: Modifying the anatomic structure of a body part without affecting the function of the body part.

Explanation: Principal purpose is to improve appearance
Examples: Cosmetic blepharoplasty – CMS Ex: Face lift

Body Part – 4TH	Approach – 5TH	Device – 6TH	Qualifier – 7TH
N Upper Eyelid, Right P Upper Eyelid, Left Q Lower Eyelid, Right R Lower Eyelid, Left	0 Open 3 Percutaneous X External	7 Autologous tissue substitute J Synthetic substitute K Nonautologous tissue substitute Z No device	Z No qualifier

1ST - 0 Medical and Surgical
2ND - 8 Eye
3RD - 1 BYPASS

TUBULAR GROUP: Bypass, Dilation, Occlusion, Restriction
Root Operations that alter the diameter/route of a tubular body part.

BYPASS: Altering the route of passage of the contents of a tubular body part.

Explanation: Rerouting contents to a downstream part ... with or without the use of a device ...
Examples: Dacryocystorhinostomy – CMS Ex: Coronary artery bypass

Body Part – 4TH	Approach – 5TH	Device – 6TH	Qualifier – 7TH
2 Anterior Chamber, Right 3 Anterior Chamber, Left	3 Percutaneous	J Synthetic substitute K Nonautologous tissue substitute Z No device	4 Sclera
X Lacrimal Duct, Right Y Lacrimal Duct, Left	0 Open 3 Percutaneous	J Synthetic substitute K Nonautologous tissue substitute Z No device	3 Nasal Cavity

1ST - 0 Medical and Surgical
2ND - 8 Eye
3RD - 2 CHANGE

DEVICE GROUP: Change, Insertion, Removal, Replacement, Revision, Supplement
Root Operations that always involve a device.

CHANGE: Taking out or off a device from a body part and putting back an identical or similar device in or on the same body part without cutting or puncturing the skin or a mucous membrane.

Explanation: All CHANGE procedures are coded using the approach External
Examples: Exchange drainage tube – CMS Ex: Urinary catheter change

Body Part – 4TH	Approach – 5TH	Device – 6TH	Qualifier – 7TH
0 Eye, Right 1 Eye, Left	X External	0 Drainage device Y Other device	Z No qualifier

© 2018 Channel Publishing, Ltd.

1ST - 0 Medical and Surgical
2ND - 8 Eye
3RD - 5 DESTRUCTION

EXCISION GROUP: Excision, Resection, Destruction, Extraction, (Detachment)
Root Operations that take out some or all of a body part.

DESTRUCTION: Physical eradication of all or a portion of a body part by the direct use of energy, force, or a destructive agent.

Explanation: None of the body part is physically taken out
Examples: Cryoablation eyelid lesion – CMS Ex: Fulguration of rectal polyp

Body Part – 4TH	Approach – 5TH	Device – 6TH	Qualifier – 7TH
0 Eye, Right 1 Eye, Left 6 Sclera, Right 7 Sclera, Left 8 Cornea, Right 9 Cornea, Left S Conjunctiva, Right T Conjunctiva, Left	X External	Z No device	Z No qualifier
2 Anterior Chamber, Right 3 Anterior Chamber, Left 4 Vitreous, Right 5 Vitreous, Left C Iris, Right D Iris, Left E Retina, Right F Retina, Left G Retinal Vessel, Right H Retinal Vessel, Left J Lens, Right K Lens, Left	3 Percutaneous	Z No device	Z No qualifier
A Choroid, Right B Choroid, Left L Extraocular Muscle, Right M Extraocular Muscle, Left V Lacrimal Gland, Right W Lacrimal Gland, Left	0 Open 3 Percutaneous	Z No device	Z No qualifier
N Upper Eyelid, Right P Upper Eyelid, Left Q Lower Eyelid, Right R Lower Eyelid, Left	0 Open 3 Percutaneous X External	Z No device	Z No qualifier
X Lacrimal Duct, Right Y Lacrimal Duct, Left	0 Open 3 Percutaneous 7 Via natural or artificial opening 8 Via natural or artificial opening endoscopic	Z No device	Z No qualifier

1ST - 0 Medical and Surgical
2ND - 8 Eye
3RD - 7 DILATION

TUBULAR GROUP: Bypass, Dilation, Occlusion, Restriction
Root Operations that alter the diameter/route of a tubular body part.

DILATION: Expanding an orifice or the lumen of a tubular body part.

Explanation: Accomplished by stretching or cutting ... tubular body part or orifice ...
Examples: Dilation lacrimal duct – CMS Ex: Percutaneous transluminal angioplasty

Body Part – 4TH	Approach – 5TH	Device – 6TH	Qualifier – 7TH
X Lacrimal Duct, Right Y Lacrimal Duct, Left	0 Open 3 Percutaneous 7 Via natural or artificial opening 8 Via natural or artificial opening endoscopic	D Intraluminal device Z No device	Z No qualifier

EYE 0

© 2018 Channel Publishing, Ltd.

1ST - 0 Medical and Surgical
2ND - 8 Eye
3RD - 9 DRAINAGE

DRAINAGE GROUP: Drainage, Extirpation, Fragmentation
Root Operations that take out solids/fluids/gases from a body part.
DRAINAGE: Taking or letting out fluids and/or gases from a body part.

Explanation: Qualifier "X Diagnostic" indicates drainage procedures that are biopsies
Examples: Drainage lacrimal duct – CMS Ex: Thoracentesis

Body Part – 4TH	Approach – 5TH	Device – 6TH	Qualifier – 7TH
0 Eye, Right 1 Eye, Left 6 Sclera, Right 7 Sclera, Left 8 Cornea, Right 9 Cornea, Left S Conjunctiva, Right T Conjunctiva, Left	X External	0 Drainage device	Z No qualifier
0 Eye, Right 1 Eye, Left 6 Sclera, Right 7 Sclera, Left 8 Cornea, Right 9 Cornea, Left S Conjunctiva, Right T Conjunctiva, Left	X External	Z No device	X Diagnostic Z No qualifier
2 Anterior Chamber, Right 3 Anterior Chamber, Left 4 Vitreous, Right 5 Vitreous, Left C Iris, Right D Iris, Left E Retina, Right F Retina, Left G Retinal Vessel, Right H Retinal Vessel, Left J Lens, Right K Lens, Left	3 Percutaneous	0 Drainage device	Z No qualifier
2 Anterior Chamber, Right 3 Anterior Chamber, Left 4 Vitreous, Right 5 Vitreous, Left C Iris, Right D Iris, Left E Retina, Right F Retina, Left G Retinal Vessel, Right H Retinal Vessel, Left J Lens, Right K Lens, Left	3 Percutaneous	Z No device	X Diagnostic Z No qualifier
A Choroid, Right B Choroid, Left L Extraocular Muscle, Right M Extraocular Muscle, Left V Lacrimal Gland, Right W Lacrimal Gland, Left	0 Open 3 Percutaneous	0 Drainage device	Z No qualifier
A Choroid, Right B Choroid, Left L Extraocular Muscle, Right M Extraocular Muscle, Left V Lacrimal Gland, Right W Lacrimal Gland, Left	0 Open 3 Percutaneous	Z No device	X Diagnostic Z No qualifier
N Upper Eyelid, Right P Upper Eyelid, Left Q Lower Eyelid, Right R Lower Eyelid, Left	0 Open 3 Percutaneous X External	0 Drainage device	Z No qualifier
N Upper Eyelid, Right P Upper Eyelid, Left Q Lower Eyelid, Right R Lower Eyelid, Left	0 Open 3 Percutaneous X External	Z No device	X Diagnostic Z No qualifier
X Lacrimal Duct, Right Y Lacrimal Duct, Left	0 Open 3 Percutaneous 7 Via natural or artificial opening 8 Via natural or artificial opening endoscopic	0 Drainage device	Z No qualifier
X Lacrimal Duct, Right Y Lacrimal Duct, Left	0 Open 3 Percutaneous 7 Via natural or artificial opening 8 Via natural or artificial opening endoscopic	Z No device	X Diagnostic Z No qualifier

EYE

0
8
9

© 2018 Channel Publishing, Ltd.

1ST - 0 Medical and Surgical
2ND - 8 Eye
3RD - B EXCISION

EXCISION GROUP: Excision, Resection, Destruction, Extraction, (Detachment)
Root Operations that take out some or all of a body part.

EXCISION: Cutting out or off, without replacement, a portion of a body part.

Explanation: Qualifier "X Diagnostic" indicates excision procedures that are biopsies
Examples: Sclerectomy – CMS Ex: Liver biopsy

Body Part – 4TH	Approach – 5TH	Device – 6TH	Qualifier – 7TH
0 Eye, Right 1 Eye, Left N Upper Eyelid, Right P Upper Eyelid, Left Q Lower Eyelid, Right R Lower Eyelid, Left	0 Open 3 Percutaneous X External	Z No device	X Diagnostic Z No qualifier
4 Vitreous, Right 5 Vitreous, Left C Iris, Right D Iris, Left E Retina, Right F Retina, Left J Lens, Right K Lens, Left	3 Percutaneous	Z No device	X Diagnostic Z No qualifier
6 Sclera, Right 7 Sclera, Left 8 Cornea, Right 9 Cornea, Left S Conjunctiva, Right T Conjunctiva, Left	X External	Z No device	X Diagnostic Z No qualifier
A Choroid, Right B Choroid, Left L Extraocular Muscle, Right M Extraocular Muscle, Left V Lacrimal Gland, Right W Lacrimal Gland, Left	0 Open 3 Percutaneous	Z No device	X Diagnostic Z No qualifier
X Lacrimal Duct, Right Y Lacrimal Duct, Left	0 Open 3 Percutaneous 7 Via natural or artificial opening 8 Via natural or artificial opening endoscopic	Z No device	X Diagnostic Z No qualifier

1ST - 0 Medical and Surgical
2ND - 8 Eye
3RD - C EXTIRPATION

DRAINAGE GROUP: Drainage, Extirpation, Fragmentation
Root Operations that take out solids/fluids/gases from a body part.

EXTIRPATION: Taking or cutting out solid matter from a body part.

Explanation: Abnormal byproduct or foreign body ...
Examples: Magnetic extraction metal splinter – CMS Ex: Thrombectomy

Body Part – 4TH	Approach – 5TH	Device – 6TH	Qualifier – 7TH
0 Eye, Right 1 Eye, Left 6 Sclera, Right 7 Sclera, Left 8 Cornea, Right 9 Cornea, Left S Conjunctiva, Right T Conjunctiva, Left	X External	Z No device	Z No qualifier
2 Anterior Chamber, Right 3 Anterior Chamber, Left 4 Vitreous, Right 5 Vitreous, Left C Iris, Right D Iris, Left E Retina, Right F Retina, Left G Retinal Vessel, Right H Retinal Vessel, Left J Lens, Right K Lens, Left	3 Percutaneous X External	Z No device	Z No qualifier
A Choroid, Right B Choroid, Left L Extraocular Muscle, Right M Extraocular Muscle, Left N Upper Eyelid, Right P Upper Eyelid, Left Q Lower Eyelid, Right R Lower Eyelid, Left V Lacrimal Gland, Right W Lacrimal Gland, Left	0 Open 3 Percutaneous X External	Z No device	Z No qualifier
X Lacrimal Duct, Right Y Lacrimal Duct, Left	0 Open 3 Percutaneous 7 Via natural or artificial opening 8 Via natural or artificial opening endoscopic	Z No device	Z No qualifier

© 2018 Channel Publishing, Ltd.

1ST - 0 Medical and Surgical
2ND - 8 Eye
3RD - D EXTRACTION

EXCISION GROUP: Excision, Resection, Destruction, Extraction, (Detachment)
Root Operations that take out some or all of a body part.

EXTRACTION: Pulling or stripping out or off all or a portion of a body part by the use of force.

Explanation: Qualifier "X Diagnostic" indicates extraction procedures that are biopsies
Examples: Lens extraction without replacement – CMS Ex: Dilation and curettage

Body Part – 4TH	Approach – 5TH	Device – 6TH	Qualifier – 7TH
8 Cornea, Right 9 Cornea, Left	X External	Z No device	X Diagnostic Z No qualifier
J Lens, Right K Lens, Left	3 Percutaneous	Z No device	Z No qualifier

1ST - 0 Medical and Surgical
2ND - 8 Eye
3RD - F FRAGMENTATION

DRAINAGE GROUP: Drainage, Extirpation, Fragmentation
Root Operations that take out solids/fluids/gases from a body part.

FRAGMENTATION: Breaking solid matter in a body part into pieces.

Explanation: Pieces are not taken out during the procedure ...
Examples: Lithotripsy vitreous – CMS Ex: Extracorporeal shockwave lithotripsy

Body Part – 4TH	Approach – 5TH	Device – 6TH	Qualifier – 7TH
4 Vitreous, Right 5 Vitreous, Left	3 Percutaneous X External NC*	Z No device	Z No qualifier

NC* – Non-covered by Medicare. See current Medicare Code Editor for details.

1ST - 0 Medical and Surgical
2ND - 8 Eye
3RD - H INSERTION

DEVICE GROUP: Change, Insertion, Removal, Replacement, Revision, Supplement
Root Operations that always involve a device.

INSERTION: Putting in a nonbiological appliance that monitors, assists, performs, or prevents a physiological function but does not physically take the place of a body part.

Explanation: None
Examples: Implantation EpiRet – CMS Ex: Insertion of central venous catheter

Body Part – 4TH	Approach – 5TH	Device – 6TH	Qualifier – 7TH
0 Eye, Right 1 Eye, Left	0 Open	5 Epiretinal visual prosthesis Y Other device	Z No qualifier
0 Eye, Right 1 Eye, Left	3 Percutaneous	1 Radioactive element 3 Infusion device Y Other device	Z No qualifier
0 Eye, Right 1 Eye, Left	7 Via natural or artificial opening 8 Via natural or artificial opening endoscopic	Y Other device	Z No qualifier
0 Eye, Right 1 Eye, Left	X External	1 Radioactive element 3 Infusion device	Z No qualifier

© 2018 Channel Publishing, Ltd.

1ST - 0 Medical and Surgical
2ND - 8 Eye
3RD - J INSPECTION

EXAMINATION GROUP: Inspection, (Map)
Root Operations involving examination only.

INSPECTION: Visually and/or manually exploring a body part.

Explanation: Direct or instrumental visualization ...
Examples: Eye examination – CMS Ex: Exploratory laparotomy

Body Part – 4TH	Approach – 5TH	Device – 6TH	Qualifier – 7TH
0 Eye, Right 1 Eye, Left J Lens, Right K Lens, Left	X External	Z No device	Z No qualifier
L Extraocular Muscle, Right M Extraocular Muscle, Left	0 Open X External	Z No device	Z No qualifier

1ST - 0 Medical and Surgical
2ND - 8 Eye
3RD - L OCCLUSION

TUBULAR GROUP: Bypass, Dilation, Occlusion, Restriction
Root Operations that alter the diameter/route of a tubular body part.

OCCLUSION: Completely closing an orifice or the lumen of a tubular body part.

Explanation: The orifice can be a natural orifice or an artificially created orifice
Examples: Punctal occlusion – CMS Ex: Fallopian tube ligation

Body Part – 4TH	Approach – 5TH	Device – 6TH	Qualifier – 7TH
X Lacrimal Duct, Right Y Lacrimal Duct, Left	0 Open 3 Percutaneous	C Extraluminal device D Intraluminal device Z No device	Z No qualifier
X Lacrimal Duct, Right Y Lacrimal Duct, Left	7 Via natural or artificial opening 8 Via natural or artificial opening endoscopic	D Intraluminal device Z No device	Z No qualifier

1ST - 0 Medical and Surgical
2ND - 8 Eye
3RD - M REATTACHMENT

MOVE GROUP: Reattachment, Reposition, Transfer, (Transplantation)
Root Operations that put in/put back or move some/all of a body part.

REATTACHMENT: Putting back in or on all or a portion of a separated body part to its normal location or other suitable location.

Explanation: Vascular circulation and nervous pathways may or may not be reestablished
Examples: Reattachment avulsed eyelid – CMS Ex: Reattachment of hand

Body Part – 4TH	Approach – 5TH	Device – 6TH	Qualifier – 7TH
N Upper Eyelid, Right P Upper Eyelid, Left Q Lower Eyelid, Right R Lower Eyelid, Left	X External	Z No device	Z No qualifier

© 2018 Channel Publishing, Ltd.

1ST - 0 Medical and Surgical
2ND - 8 Eye
3RD - N RELEASE

DIVISION GROUP: (Division), Release
Root Operations involving cutting or separation only.

RELEASE: Freeing a body part from an abnormal physical constraint by cutting or by the use of force.

Explanation: Some of the restraining tissue may be taken out but none of the body part is taken out
Examples: Adhesiolysis lateral rectus – CMS Ex: Carpal tunnel release

Body Part – 4TH		Approach – 5TH	Device – 6TH	Qualifier – 7TH
0 Eye, Right 1 Eye, Left 6 Sclera, Right 7 Sclera, Left	8 Cornea, Right 9 Cornea, Left S Conjunctiva, Right T Conjunctiva, Left	X External	Z No device	Z No qualifier
2 Anterior Chamber, Right 3 Anterior Chamber, Left 4 Vitreous, Right 5 Vitreous, Left C Iris, Right D Iris, Left	E Retina, Right F Retina, Left G Retinal Vessel, Right H Retinal Vessel, Left J Lens, Right K Lens, Left	3 Percutaneous	Z No device	Z No qualifier
A Choroid, Right B Choroid, Left L Extraocular Muscle, Right	M Extraocular Muscle, Left V Lacrimal Gland, Right W Lacrimal Gland, Left	0 Open 3 Percutaneous	Z No device	Z No qualifier
N Upper Eyelid, Right P Upper Eyelid, Left Q Lower Eyelid, Right R Lower Eyelid, Left		0 Open 3 Percutaneous X External	Z No device	Z No qualifier
X Lacrimal Duct, Right Y Lacrimal Duct, Left		0 Open 3 Percutaneous 7 Via natural or artificial opening 8 Via natural or artificial opening endoscopic	Z No device	Z No qualifier

© 2018 Channel Publishing, Ltd.

1ST - 0 Medical and Surgical
2ND - 8 Eye
3RD - P REMOVAL

DEVICE GROUP: Change, Insertion, Removal, Replacement, Revision, Supplement
Root Operations that always involve a device.

REMOVAL: Taking out or off a device from a body part.

Explanation: Removal device without reinsertion ...
Examples: Removal eye drain tube – CMS Ex: Cardiac pacemaker removal

Body Part – 4TH	Approach – 5TH	Device – 6TH	Qualifier – 7TH
0 Eye, Right 1 Eye, Left	0 Open 3 Percutaneous 7 Via natural or artificial opening 8 Via natural or artificial opening endoscopic	0 Drainage device 1 Radioactive element 3 Infusion device 7 Autologous tissue substitute C Extraluminal device D Intraluminal device J Synthetic substitute K Nonautologous tissue substitute Y Other device	Z No qualifier
0 Eye, Right 1 Eye, Left	X External	0 Drainage device 1 Radioactive element 3 Infusion device 7 Autologous tissue substitute C Extraluminal device D Intraluminal device J Synthetic substitute K Nonautologous tissue substitute	Z No qualifier
J Lens, Right K Lens, Left	3 Percutaneous	J Synthetic substitute Y Other device	Z No qualifier
L Extraocular Muscle, Right M Extraocular Muscle, Left	0 Open 3 Percutaneous	0 Drainage device 7 Autologous tissue substitute J Synthetic substitute K Nonautologous tissue substitute Y Other device	Z No qualifier

1ST - 0 Medical and Surgical
2ND - 8 Eye
3RD - Q REPAIR

OTHER REPAIRS GROUP: (Control), Repair
Root Operations that define other repairs.

REPAIR: Restoring, to the extent possible, a body part to its normal anatomic structure and function.

Explanation: Used only when the method to accomplish the repair is not one of the other root operations
Examples: Iris mattress suture – CMS Ex: Suture of laceration

Body Part – 4TH	Approach – 5TH	Device – 6TH	Qualifier – 7TH
0 Eye, Right 1 Eye, Left 6 Sclera, Right 7 Sclera, Left 8 Cornea, Right NC* 9 Cornea, Left NC* S Conjunctiva, Right T Conjunctiva, Left	X External	Z No device	Z No qualifier
2 Anterior Chamber, Right 3 Anterior Chamber, Left 4 Vitreous, Right 5 Vitreous, Left C Iris, Right D Iris, Left E Retina, Right F Retina, Left G Retinal Vessel, Right H Retinal Vessel, Left J Lens, Right K Lens, Left	3 Percutaneous	Z No device	Z No qualifier
A Choroid, Right B Choroid, Left L Extraocular Muscle, Right M Extraocular Muscle, Left V Lacrimal Gland, Right W Lacrimal Gland, Left	0 Open 3 Percutaneous	Z No device	Z No qualifier
N Upper Eyelid, Right P Upper Eyelid, Left Q Lower Eyelid, Right R Lower Eyelid, Left	0 Open 3 Percutaneous X External	Z No device	Z No qualifier
X Lacrimal Duct, Right Y Lacrimal Duct, Left	0 Open 3 Percutaneous 7 Via natural or artificial opening 8 Via natural or artificial opening endoscopic	Z No device	Z No qualifier

NC* – Non-covered by Medicare. See current Medicare Code Editor for details.

© 2018 Channel Publishing, Ltd.

1ST - 0 Medical and Surgical
2ND - 8 Eye
3RD - R REPLACEMENT

DEVICE GROUP: Change, Insertion, Removal, Replacement, Revision, Supplement
Root Operations that always involve a device.

REPLACEMENT: Putting in or on biological or synthetic material that physically takes the place and/or function of all or a portion of a body part.

Explanation: Includes taking out or eradicating, or rendering non-functional, the body part ...
Examples: Lens extraction with prosthetic implant – CMS Ex: Total hip replacement

Body Part – 4TH	Approach – 5TH	Device – 6TH	Qualifier – 7TH
0 Eye, Right 1 Eye, Left A Choroid, Right B Choroid, Left	0 Open 3 Percutaneous	7 Autologous tissue substitute J Synthetic substitute K Nonautologous tissue substitute	Z No qualifier
4 Vitreous, Right 5 Vitreous, Left C Iris, Right D Iris, Left G Retinal Vessel, Right H Retinal Vessel, Left	3 Percutaneous	7 Autologous tissue substitute J Synthetic substitute K Nonautologous tissue substitute	Z No qualifier
6 Sclera, Right 7 Sclera, Left S Conjunctiva, Right T Conjunctiva, Left	X External	7 Autologous tissue substitute J Synthetic substitute K Nonautologous tissue substitute	Z No qualifier
8 Cornea, Right 9 Cornea, Left	3 Percutaneous X External	7 Autologous tissue substitute J Synthetic substitute K Nonautologous tissue substitute	Z No qualifier
J Lens, Right K Lens, Left	3 Percutaneous	0 Synthetic substitute, intraocular telescope 7 Autologous tissue substitute J Synthetic substitute K Nonautologous tissue substitute	Z No qualifier
N Upper Eyelid, Right P Upper Eyelid, Left Q Lower Eyelid, Right R Lower Eyelid, Left	0 Open 3 Percutaneous X External	7 Autologous tissue substitute J Synthetic substitute K Nonautologous tissue substitute	Z No qualifier
X Lacrimal Duct, Right Y Lacrimal Duct, Left	0 Open 3 Percutaneous 7 Via natural or artificial opening 8 Via natural or artificial opening endoscopic	7 Autologous tissue substitute J Synthetic substitute K Nonautologous tissue substitute	Z No qualifier

1ST - 0 Medical and Surgical
2ND - 8 Eye
3RD - S REPOSITION

MOVE GROUP: Reattachment, Reposition, Transfer, (Transplantation)
Root Operations that put in/put back or move some/all of a body part.

REPOSITION: Moving to its normal location, or other suitable location, all or a portion of a body part.

Explanation: The body part may or may not be cut out or off to be moved to the new location ...
Examples: Relocation eye muscle – CMS Ex: Fracture reduction

Body Part – 4TH	Approach – 5TH	Device – 6TH	Qualifier – 7TH
C Iris, Right D Iris, Left G Retinal Vessel, Right H Retinal Vessel, Left J Lens, Right K Lens, Left	3 Percutaneous	Z No device	Z No qualifier
L Extraocular Muscle, Right M Extraocular Muscle, Left V Lacrimal Gland, Right W Lacrimal Gland, Left	0 Open 3 Percutaneous	Z No device	Z No qualifier
N Upper Eyelid, Right P Upper Eyelid, Left Q Lower Eyelid, Right R Lower Eyelid, Left	0 Open 3 Percutaneous X External	Z No device	Z No qualifier
X Lacrimal Duct, Right Y Lacrimal Duct, Left	0 Open 3 Percutaneous 7 Via natural or artificial opening 8 Via natural or artificial opening endoscopic	Z No device	Z No qualifier

© 2018 Channel Publishing, Ltd.

1ST - 0 Medical and Surgical
2ND - 8 Eye
3RD - T RESECTION

EXCISION GROUP: Excision, Resection, Destruction, Extraction, (Detachment)
Root Operations that take out some or all of a body part.

RESECTION: Cutting out or off, without replacement, all of a body part.

Explanation: None
Examples: Enucleation eyeball – CMS Ex: Total lobectomy of lung

Body Part – 4TH	Approach – 5TH	Device – 6TH	Qualifier – 7TH
0 Eye, Right 1 Eye, Left 8 Cornea, Right 9 Cornea, Left	X External	Z No device	Z No qualifier
4 Vitreous, Right 5 Vitreous, Left C Iris, Right D Iris, Left J Lens, Right K Lens, Left	3 Percutaneous	Z No device	Z No qualifier
L Extraocular Muscle, Right M Extraocular Muscle, Left V Lacrimal Gland, Right W Lacrimal Gland, Left	0 Open 3 Percutaneous	Z No device	Z No qualifier
N Upper Eyelid, Right P Upper Eyelid, Left Q Lower Eyelid, Right R Lower Eyelid, Left	0 Open X External	Z No device	Z No qualifier
X Lacrimal Duct, Right Y Lacrimal Duct, Left	0 Open 3 Percutaneous 7 Via natural or artificial opening 8 Via natural or artificial opening endoscopic	Z No device	Z No qualifier

1ST - 0 Medical and Surgical
2ND - 8 Eye
3RD - U SUPPLEMENT

DEVICE GROUP: Change, Insertion, Removal, Replacement, Revision, Supplement
Root Operations that always involve a device.

SUPPLEMENT: Putting in or on biological or synthetic material that physically reinforces and/or augments the function of a portion of a body part.

Explanation: Biological material is non-living, or is living and from the same individual ...
Examples: Scleral buckle with implant – CMS Ex: Herniorrhaphy using mesh

Body Part – 4TH	Approach – 5TH	Device – 6TH	Qualifier – 7TH
0 Eye, Right 1 Eye, Left C Iris, Right D Iris, Left E Retina, Right F Retina, Left G Retinal Vessel, Right H Retinal Vessel, Left L Extraocular Muscle, Right M Extraocular Muscle, Left	0 Open 3 Percutaneous	7 Autologous tissue substitute J Synthetic substitute K Nonautologous tissue substitute	Z No qualifier
8 Cornea, Right NC* 9 Cornea, Left NC* N Upper Eyelid, Right P Upper Eyelid, Left Q Lower Eyelid, Right R Lower Eyelid, Left	0 Open 3 Percutaneous X External	7 Autologous tissue substitute J Synthetic substitute K Nonautologous tissue substitute	Z No qualifier
X Lacrimal Duct, Right Y Lacrimal Duct, Left	0 Open 3 Percutaneous 7 Via natural or artificial opening 8 Via natural or artificial opening endoscopic	7 Autologous tissue substitute J Synthetic substitute K Nonautologous tissue substitute	Z No qualifier

NC* – Some procedures are considered non-covered by Medicare. See current Medicare Code Editor for details.

© 2018 Channel Publishing, Ltd.

1ST - 0 Medical and Surgical
2ND - 8 Eye
3RD - V RESTRICTION

TUBULAR GROUP: Bypass, Dilation, Occlusion, Restriction
Root Operations that alter the diameter/route of a tubular body part.

RESTRICTION: Partially closing an orifice or the lumen of a tubular body part.

Explanation: The orifice can be a natural orifice or an artificially created orifice.
Examples: Lacrimal duct restrictive stent – CMS Ex: Cervical cerclage

Body Part – 4TH	Approach – 5TH	Device – 6TH	Qualifier – 7TH
X Lacrimal Duct, Right Y Lacrimal Duct, Left	0 Open 3 Percutaneous	C Extraluminal device D Intraluminal device Z No device	Z No qualifier
X Lacrimal Duct, Right Y Lacrimal Duct, Left	7 Via natural or artificial opening 8 Via natural or artificial opening endoscopic	D Intraluminal device Z No device	Z No qualifier

1ST - 0 Medical and Surgical
2ND - 8 Eye
3RD - W REVISION

DEVICE GROUP: Change, Insertion, Removal, Replacement, Revision, Supplement
Root Operations that always involve a device.

REVISION: Correcting, to the extent possible, a portion of a malfunctioning device or the position of a displaced device.

Explanation: Correcting by taking out or putting in components of a device such as a screw or pin ...
Examples: Reposition prosthetic lens – CMS Ex: Recementing of hip prosthesis

Body Part – 4TH	Approach – 5TH	Device – 6TH	Qualifier – 7TH
0 Eye, Right 1 Eye, Left	0 Open 3 Percutaneous 7 Via natural or artificial opening 8 Via natural or artificial opening endoscopic	0 Drainage device 3 Infusion device 7 Autologous tissue substitute C Extraluminal device D Intraluminal device J Synthetic substitute K Nonautologous tissue substitute Y Other device	Z No qualifier
0 Eye, Right 1 Eye, Left	X External	0 Drainage device 3 Infusion device 7 Autologous tissue substitute C Extraluminal device D Intraluminal device J Synthetic substitute K Nonautologous tissue substitute	Z No qualifier
J Lens, Right K Lens, Left	3 Percutaneous	J Synthetic substitute Y Other device	Z No qualifier
J Lens, Right K Lens, Left	X External	J Synthetic substitute	Z No qualifier
L Extraocular Muscle, Right M Extraocular Muscle, Left	0 Open 3 Percutaneous	0 Drainage device 7 Autologous tissue substitute J Synthetic substitute K Nonautologous tissue substitute Y Other device	Z No qualifier

1ST - 0 Medical and Surgical
2ND - 8 Eye
3RD - X TRANSFER

MOVE GROUP: Reattachment, Reposition, Transfer, (Transplantation)
Root Operations that put in/put back or move some/all of a body part.

TRANSFER: Moving, without taking out, all or a portion of a body part to another location to take over the function of all or a portion of a body part.

Explanation: The body part transferred remains connected to its vascular and nervous supply
Examples: Transfer medial rectus muscle – CMS Ex: Tendon transfer

Body Part – 4TH	Approach – 5TH	Device – 6TH	Qualifier – 7TH
L Extraocular Muscle, Right M Extraocular Muscle, Left	0 Open 3 Percutaneous	Z No device	Z No qualifier

© 2018 Channel Publishing, Ltd.

Educational Annotations | 9 – Ear, Nose, Sinus

Body System Specific Educational Annotations for the Ear, Nose, Sinus include:

- Anatomy and Physiology Review
- Definitions of Common Procedures
- Anatomical Illustrations
- AHA Coding Clinic® Reference Notations
- Body Part Key Listings
- Device Key Listings
- Device Aggregation Table Listings
- Coding Notes

Anatomy and Physiology Review of Ear, Nose, Sinus

BODY PART VALUES – 9 - EAR, NOSE, SINUS

Accessory Sinus – A paranasal sinus that is not identified as one of the four paired nasal sinuses (maxillary, frontal, ethmoid, and sphenoid).
Auditory Ossicle – ANATOMY – The three small bones of the middle ear (malleus, incus, and stapes). PHYSIOLOGY – These bones transfer the sound waves from the tympanic membrane to the oval window of the inner ear while modulating and amplifying the sound.
Ear – ANATOMY – The organ of hearing comprised of the external ear (auricle or pinna), middle ear (malleus, incus, and stapes bones), and inner ear (cochlea). PHYSIOLOGY – The external ear collects the sound, the middle ear transfers and amplifies the sound to the inner ear, and the inner ear converts it into neural impulses.
Ethmoid Sinus – The one of four paired, air-filled paranasal sinuses located within the ethmoid bone cavities that lies between the nose and the eyes.
Eustachian Tube – ANATOMY – The Eustachian (auditory) tube connects the middle ear with the nasopharynx. PHYSIOLOGY – The tube allows for proper equalization of atmospheric pressure between the atmosphere and the middle ear, and for mucous drainage from the middle ear.
External Auditory Canal – That cylindrical portion of the external ear that focuses the sound waves onto the tympanic membrane.
External Ear – ANATOMY – The visible outer portion of the ear (auricle or pinna) that includes the ear canal and outer tympanic membrane (ear drum). PHYSIOLOGY – The external ear collects the sound onto the tympanic membrane.
Frontal Sinus – The one of four paired, air-filled paranasal sinuses located above the eye in the frontal bone.
Inner Ear – ANATOMY – The fluid-filled (endolymph) inner ear is that portion behind the middle ear and comprised of the cochlea and the semicircular canals. PHYSIOLOGY – The sound waves travel through the endolymph of the cochlea stimulating millions of hairs that in turn send neural signals through the vestibulocochlear nerve to the brain where the brain interprets it as sound. The semicircular canals allow the individual to sense physical balance and motion.
Mastoid Sinus – The numerous, small air-filled cavities within the mastoid process of the temporal bone.
Maxillary Sinus – The largest of the one of four paired, air-filled paranasal sinuses located under the eye in the maxillary bone.
Middle Ear – ANATOMY – The middle ear is the air-filled space behind the tympanic membrane of the external ear that connects the inner ear, mastoid cells, and Eustachian tube. PHYSIOLOGY – The middle ear transfers, modulates, and amplifies the sound to the inner ear.
Nasal Septum – The bone and cartilage that divides the left and right nasal cavities and airways.
Nasal Turbinate – ANATOMY – The cartilage-like mucosal tissue grooves that divide the nasal airways into passages. PHYSIOLOGY – The turbinates assist in directing and smoothing the airflow through the nasal airways. They also sense heat and cold and help regulate the temperature and humidity of the inhaled air.
Nasopharynx – The upper portion of the pharynx from the base of skull and the nasal cavities to the top of the soft palate and the oral portion of the pharynx.
Nose – ANATOMY – The organ of sense of smell in the middle of the face and skull with the external portion extending out from the face. PHYSIOLOGY – The nose contains the organs and tissues (olfactory epithelium) that collect scent molecules and transmit impulses to the brain. The nose also warms, filters, and humidifies the air inhaled into the lungs.
Sinus – ANATOMY – The group of four paired, air-filled mucous-membrane-lined skull bone cavities (maxillary, frontal, ethmoid, and sphenoid) that are linked to the nasal airways and the mastoid and accessory sinus bone cavities. PHYSIOLOGY – The sinuses function to warm and humidify the inhaled air, filter airborne pathogens, increase the resonance of the voice, lighten the weight of the skull, and provide a role in immunological response.
Sphenoid Sinus – The one of four paired, air-filled paranasal sinuses in the sphenoid bone and located behind the eye and nose.
Tympanic Membrane – ANATOMY – The membrane at the innermost portion of the ear canal that separates the external ear from the middle ear. PHYSIOLOGY – Transmits sound waves to the middle ear bones, and serves as a barrier to organisms and microorganisms.

Definitions of Common Procedures of Ear, Nose, Sinus

Cochlear implant – The surgical implantation of a small, complex electronic hearing device (microphone, speech processor, transmitter, and electrical array) that can help to provide a sense of sound to individuals that are profoundly deaf. It is implanted behind the ear and connected to the auditory nerve.
Mastoidectomy – The surgical procedure to remove diseased mastoid air cells (chronic mastoiditis, cholesteatoma). A radical mastoidectomy also involves removing portions of the middle ear and tympanic membrane.
Rhinoplasty – The surgical repair of nasal defects or cosmetic reconstruction of the exterior shape of the nose.
Septoplasty – The surgical correction of a nasal septum defect (deviated nasal septum).
Sinusectomy – The surgical excision of paranasal sinus tissue to remove diseased or excessive tissue and/or to create a larger sinus cavity and promote more efficient drainage.
Sinusotomy (antrostomy) – The surgical incision/excision of paranasal sinus tissue to increase the drainage passage opening.
Stapedectomy/stapedotomy – The surgical correction of a dysfunctional stapes (middle ear) bone by implanting a small, movable prosthesis to allow the transfer of sound vibrations from the tympanic membrane to the middle ear and then on to the inner ear.
Turbinectomy – The surgical procedure to remove the turbinate bones of the nasal cavity that are causing nasal cavity obstruction.

© 2018 Channel Publishing, Ltd.

Educational Annotations | 9 – Ear, Nose, Sinus

Anatomical Illustrations of Ear, Nose, Sinus

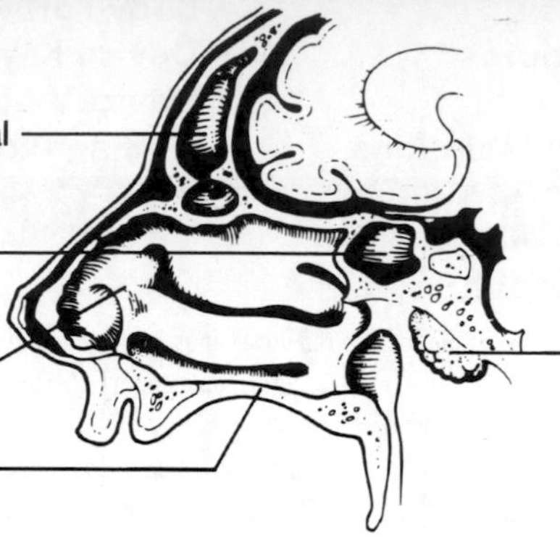

NASOPHARYNX

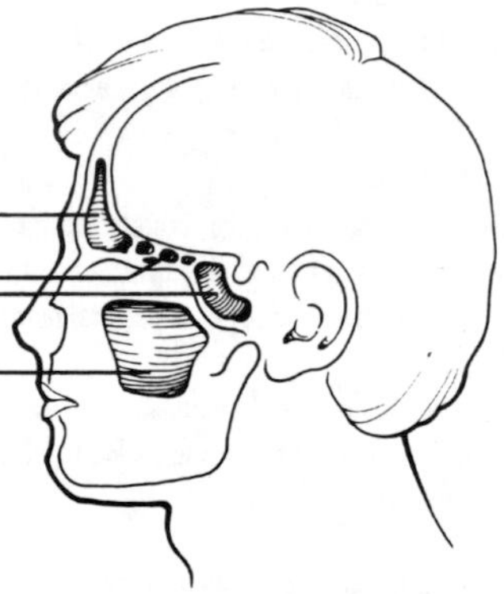

ACCESSORY SINUSES

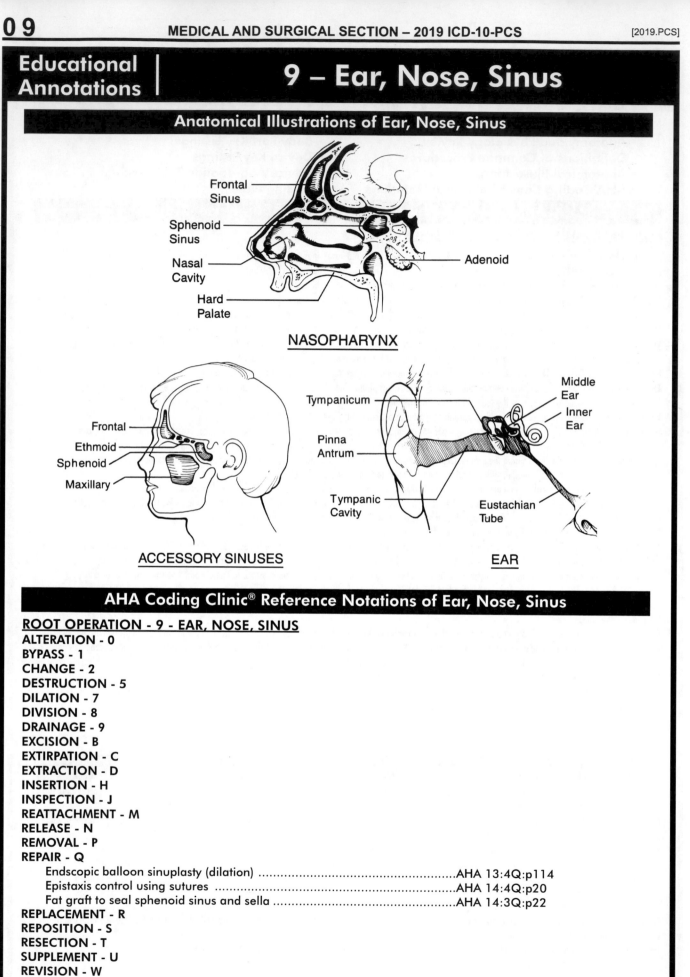

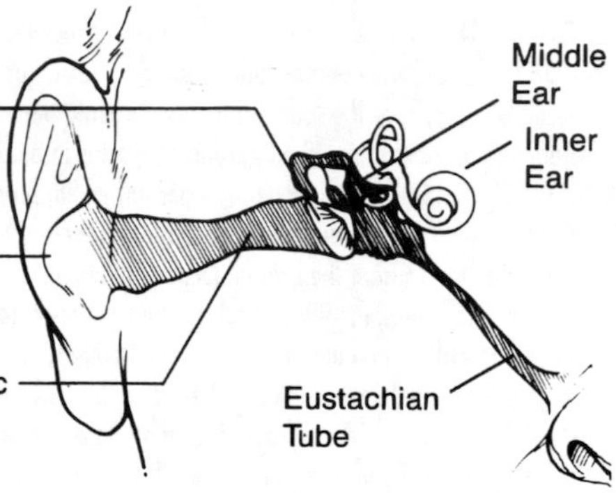

EAR

AHA Coding Clinic® Reference Notations of Ear, Nose, Sinus

ROOT OPERATION - 9 - EAR, NOSE, SINUS

ALTERATION - 0
BYPASS - 1
CHANGE - 2
DESTRUCTION - 5
DILATION - 7
DIVISION - 8
DRAINAGE - 9
EXCISION - B
EXTIRPATION - C
EXTRACTION - D
INSERTION - H
INSPECTION - J
REATTACHMENT - M
RELEASE - N
REMOVAL - P
REPAIR - Q

- Endscopic balloon sinuplasty (dilation) ....AHA 13:4Q:p114
- Epistaxis control using sutures ....AHA 14:4Q:p20
- Fat graft to seal sphenoid sinus and sella ....AHA 14:3Q:p22

REPLACEMENT - R
REPOSITION - S
RESECTION - T
SUPPLEMENT - U
REVISION - W

EAR NOSE SINUS 09

© 2018 Channel Publishing, Ltd.

Educational Annotations | 9 – Ear, Nose, Sinus

Body Part Key Listings of Ear, Nose, Sinus

See also Body Part Key in Appendix C

Antihelix	use External Ear, Bilateral/Left/Right
Antitragus	use External Ear, Bilateral/Left/Right
Antrum of Highmore	use Maxillary Sinus, Left/Right
Auditory tube	use Eustachian Tube, Left/Right
Auricle	use External Ear, Bilateral/Left/Right
Bony labyrinth	use Inner Ear, Left/Right
Bony vestibule	use Inner Ear, Left/Right
Choana	use Nasopharynx
Cochlea	use Inner Ear, Left/Right
Columella	use Nasal Mucosa and Soft Tissue
Earlobe	use External Ear, Bilateral/Left/Right
Ethmoidal air cell	use Ethmoid Sinus, Left/Right
External auditory meatus	use External Auditory Canal, Left/Right
External naris	use Nasal Mucosa and Soft Tissue
Fossa of Rosenmuller	use Nasopharynx
Greater alar cartilage	use Nasal Mucosa and Soft Tissue
Helix	use External Ear, Bilateral/Left/Right
Incus	use Auditory Ossicle, Left/Right
Inferior turbinate	use Nasal Turbinate
Internal naris	use Nasal Mucosa and Soft Tissue
Lateral nasal cartilage	use Nasal Mucosa and Soft Tissue
Lesser alar cartilage	use Nasal Mucosa and Soft Tissue
Malleus	use Auditory Ossicle, Left/Right
Mastoid air cells	use Mastoid Sinus, Left/Right
Middle turbinate	use Nasal Turbinate
Nasal cavity	use Nasal Mucosa and Soft Tissue
Nasal concha	use Nasal Turbinate
Nostril	use Nasal Mucosa and Soft Tissue
Oval window	use Middle Ear, Left/Right
Pars flaccida	use Tympanic Membrane, Left/Right
Pharyngeal recess	use Nasopharynx
Pharyngotympanic tube	use Eustachian Tube, Left/Right
Pinna	use External Ear, Bilateral/Left/Right
Quadrangular cartilage	use Nasal Septum
Rhinopharynx	use Nasopharynx
Round window	use Inner Ear, Left/Right
Semicircular canal	use Inner Ear, Left/Right
Septal cartilage	use Nasal Septum
Stapes	use Auditory Ossicle, Left/Right
Superior turbinate	use Nasal Turbinate
Tragus	use External Ear, Bilateral/Left/Right
Tympanic cavity	use Middle Ear, Left/Right
Vomer bone	use Nasal Septum

Device Key Listings of Ear, Nose, Sinus

See also Device Key in Appendix D

Autograft	use Autologous Tissue Substitute
Bone anchored hearing device	use Hearing Device, Bone Conduction for Insertion in Ear, Nose, Sinus
Cochlear implant (CI), multiple channel (electrode)	use Hearing Device, Multiple Channel Cochlear Prosthesis for Insertion in Ear, Nose, Sinus
Cochlear implant (CI), single channel (electrode)	use Hearing Device, Single Channel Cochlear Prosthesis for Insertion in Ear, Nose, Sinus
Esteem® implantable hearing system	use Hearing Device in Ear, Nose, Sinus
Nasopharyngeal airway (NPA)	use Intraluminal Device, Airway in Ear, Nose, Sinus
Tissue bank graft	use Nonautologous Tissue Substitute

Device Aggregation Table Listings of Ear, Nose, Sinus

See also Device Aggregation Table in Appendix E

Specific Device	For Operation	In Body System	General Device
Hearing Device, Bone Conduction	Insertion	Ear, Nose, Sinus	Hearing Device
Hearing Device, Multiple Channel Cochlear Prosthesis	Insertion	Ear, Nose, Sinus	Hearing Device
Hearing Device, Single Channel Cochlear Prosthesis	Insertion	Ear, Nose, Sinus	Hearing Device
Intraluminal Device, Airway	All applicable	Ear, Nose, Sinus	Intraluminal Device

Coding Notes of Ear, Nose, Sinus

Body System Relevant Coding Guidelines

Control vs. more definitive root operations

B3.7

The root operation Control is defined as, "Stopping, or attempting to stop, postprocedural or other acute bleeding." If an attempt to stop postprocedural or other acute bleeding is unsuccessful, and to stop the bleeding requires performing a more definitive root operation, such as Bypass, Detachment, Excision, Extraction, Reposition, Replacement, or Resection, then the more definitive root operation is coded instead of Control.

Example: Resection of spleen to stop bleeding is coded to Resection instead of Control.

© 2018 Channel Publishing, Ltd.

1ST - 0 Medical and Surgical
2ND - 9 Ear, Nose, Sinus
3RD - 0 ALTERATION

OTHER OBJECTIVES GROUP: Alteration, (Creation), (Fusion)
Root Operations that define other objectives.

ALTERATION: Modifying the anatomic structure of a body part without affecting the function of the body part.

Explanation: Principal purpose is to improve appearance
Examples: Cosmetic rhinoplasty – CMS Ex: Face lift

Body Part – 4TH	Approach – 5TH	Device – 6TH	Qualifier – 7TH
0 External Ear, Right 1 External Ear, Left 2 External Ear, Bilateral K Nasal Mucosa and Soft Tissue	0 Open 3 Percutaneous 4 Percutaneous endoscopic X External	7 Autologous tissue substitute J Synthetic substitute K Nonautologous tissue substitute Z No device	Z No qualifier

1ST - 0 Medical and Surgical
2ND - 9 Ear, Nose, Sinus
3RD - 1 BYPASS

TUBULAR GROUP: Bypass, Dilation, (Occlusion), (Restriction)
Root Operations that alter the diameter/route of a tubular body part.

BYPASS: Altering the route of passage of the contents of a tubular body part.

Explanation: Rerouting contents to a downstream part ... with or without the use of a device ...
Examples: Endolymphatic bypass – CMS Ex: Coronary artery bypass

Body Part – 4TH	Approach – 5TH	Device – 6TH	Qualifier – 7TH
D Inner Ear, Right E Inner Ear, Left	0 Open	7 Autologous tissue substitute J Synthetic substitute K Nonautologous tissue substitute Z No device	0 Endolymphatic

1ST - 0 Medical and Surgical
2ND - 9 Ear, Nose, Sinus
3RD - 2 CHANGE

DEVICE GROUP: Change, Insertion, Removal, Replacement, Revision, Supplement
Root Operations that always involve a device.

CHANGE: Taking out or off a device from a body part and putting back an identical or similar device in or on the same body part without cutting or puncturing the skin or a mucous membrane.

Explanation: All CHANGE procedures are coded using the approach External
Examples: Exchange drain tube – CMS Ex: Urinary catheter change

Body Part – 4TH		Approach – 5TH	Device – 6TH	Qualifier – 7TH
H Ear, Right J Ear, Left	K Nasal Mucosa and Soft Tissue Y Sinus	X External	0 Drainage device Y Other device	Z No qualifier

1ST - 0 Medical and Surgical
2ND - 9 Ear, Nose, Sinus
3RD - 3 CONTROL

OTHER REPAIRS GROUP: Control, Repair
Root Operations that define other repairs.

CONTROL: Stopping, or attempting to stop, postprocedural or other acute bleeding.

Explanation: The site of the bleeding is coded as an anatomical region and not to a specific body part
Examples: Control epistaxis (nosebleed) – CMS Ex: Control of bleeding duodenal ulcer

Body Part – 4TH	Approach – 5TH	Device – 6TH	Qualifier – 7TH
K Nasal Mucosa and Soft Tissue	7 Via natural or artificial opening 8 Via natural or artificial opening endoscopic	Z No device	Z No qualifier

© 2018 Channel Publishing, Ltd.

1ST - 0 Medical and Surgical
2ND - 9 Ear, Nose, Sinus
3RD - 5 DESTRUCTION

EXCISION GROUP: Excision, Resection, Destruction, Extraction, (Detachment)
Root Operations that take out some or all of a body part.

DESTRUCTION: Physical eradication of all or a portion of a body part by the direct use of energy, force, or a destructive agent.

Explanation: None of the body part is physically taken out
Examples: Cryoablation external ear lesion – CMS Ex: Fulguration of rectal polyp

Body Part – 4TH	Approach – 5TH	Device – 6TH	Qualifier – 7TH
0 External Ear, Right 1 External Ear, Left	0 Open 3 Percutaneous 4 Percutaneous endoscopic X External	Z No device	Z No qualifier
3 External Auditory Canal, Right 4 External Auditory Canal, Left	0 Open 3 Percutaneous 4 Percutaneous endoscopic 7 Via natural or artificial opening 8 Via natural or artificial opening endoscopic X External	Z No device	Z No qualifier
5 Middle Ear, Right 6 Middle Ear, Left 9 Auditory Ossicle, Right A Auditory Ossicle, Left D Inner Ear, Right E Inner Ear, Left	0 Open 8 Via natural or artificial opening endoscopic	Z No device	Z No qualifier
7 Tympanic Membrane, Right 8 Tympanic Membrane, Left F Eustachian Tube, Right G Eustachian Tube, Left L Nasal Turbinate N Nasopharynx	0 Open 3 Percutaneous 4 Percutaneous endoscopic 7 Via natural or artificial opening 8 Via natural or artificial opening endoscopic	Z No device	Z No qualifier
B Mastoid Sinus, Right C Mastoid Sinus, Left M Nasal Septum P Accessory Sinus Q Maxillary Sinus, Right R Maxillary Sinus, Left S Frontal Sinus, Right T Frontal Sinus, Left U Ethmoid Sinus, Right V Ethmoid Sinus, Left W Sphenoid Sinus, Right X Sphenoid Sinus, Left	0 Open 3 Percutaneous 4 Percutaneous endoscopic 8 Via natural or artificial opening endoscopic	Z No device	Z No qualifier
K Nasal Mucosa and Soft Tissue	0 Open 3 Percutaneous 4 Percutaneous endoscopic 8 Via natural or artificial opening endoscopic X External	Z No device	Z No qualifier

EAR NOSE SINUS 0 9 7

1ST - 0 Medical and Surgical
2ND - 9 Ear, Nose, Sinus
3RD - 7 DILATION

TUBULAR GROUP: Bypass, Dilation, (Occlusion), (Restriction)
Root Operations that alter the diameter/route of a tubular body part.

DILATION: Expanding an orifice or the lumen of a tubular body part.

Explanation: Accomplished by stretching or cutting ... tubular body part or orifice ...
Examples: Balloon dilation Eustachian tube – CMS Ex: Percutaneous transluminal angioplasty

Body Part – 4TH	Approach – 5TH	Device – 6TH	Qualifier – 7TH
F Eustachian Tube, Right G Eustachian Tube, Left	0 Open 7 Via natural or artificial opening 8 Via natural or artificial opening endoscopic	D Intraluminal device Z No device	Z No qualifier
F Eustachian Tube, Right G Eustachian Tube, Left	3 Percutaneous 4 Percutaneous endoscopic	Z No device	Z No qualifier

© 2018 Channel Publishing, Ltd.

1ST - 0 Medical and Surgical
2ND - 9 Ear, Nose, Sinus
3RD - 8 DIVISION

DIVISION GROUP: Division, Release
Root Operations involving cutting or separation only.

DIVISION: Cutting into a body part, without draining fluids and/or gases from the body part, in order to separate or transect a body part.

Explanation: All or a portion of the body part is separated into two or more portions
Examples: Division nasal turbinate – CMS Ex: Spinal cordotomy

Body Part – 4TH	Approach – 5TH	Device – 6TH	Qualifier – 7TH
L Nasal Turbinate	0 Open 3 Percutaneous 4 Percutaneous endoscopic 7 Via natural or artificial opening 8 Via natural or artificial opening endoscopic	Z No device	Z No qualifier

1ST - 0 Medical and Surgical
2ND - 9 Ear, Nose, Sinus
3RD - 9 DRAINAGE

DRAINAGE GROUP: Drainage, Extirpation, (Fragmentation)
Root Operations that take out solids/fluids/gases from a body part.

DRAINAGE: Taking or letting out fluids and/or gases from a body part.

Explanation: Qualifier "X Diagnostic" indicates drainage procedures that are biopsies
Examples: Sinusotomy for drainage – CMS Ex: Thoracentesis

Body Part – 4TH	Approach – 5TH	Device – 6TH	Qualifier – 7TH
0 External Ear, Right 1 External Ear, Left	0 Open 3 Percutaneous 4 Percutaneous endoscopic X External	0 Drainage device	Z No qualifier
0 External Ear, Right 1 External Ear, Left	0 Open 3 Percutaneous 4 Percutaneous endoscopic X External	Z No device	X Diagnostic Z No qualifier
3 External Auditory Canal, Right 4 External Auditory Canal, Left K Nasal Mucosa and Soft Tissue	0 Open 3 Percutaneous 4 Percutaneous endoscopic 7 Via natural or artificial opening 8 Via natural or artificial opening endoscopic X External	0 Drainage device	Z No qualifier
3 External Auditory Canal, Right 4 External Auditory Canal, Left K Nasal Mucosa and Soft Tissue	0 Open 3 Percutaneous 4 Percutaneous endoscopic 7 Via natural or artificial opening 8 Via natural or artificial opening endoscopic X External	Z No device	X Diagnostic Z No qualifier
5 Middle Ear, Right 6 Middle Ear, Left 9 Auditory Ossicle, Right A Auditory Ossicle, Left D Inner Ear, Right E Inner Ear, Left	0 Open 7 Via natural or artificial opening 8 Via natural or artificial opening endoscopic	0 Drainage device	Z No qualifier
5 Middle Ear, Right 6 Middle Ear, Left 9 Auditory Ossicle, Right A Auditory Ossicle, Left D Inner Ear, Right E Inner Ear, Left	0 Open 7 Via natural or artificial opening 8 Via natural or artificial opening endoscopic	Z No device	X Diagnostic Z No qualifier
7 Tympanic Membrane, Right 8 Tympanic Membrane, Left B Mastoid Sinus, Right C Mastoid Sinus, Left F Eustachian Tube, Right G Eustachian Tube, Left L Nasal Turbinate M Nasal Septum N Nasopharynx P Accessory Sinus Q Maxillary Sinus, Right R Maxillary Sinus, Left S Frontal Sinus, Right T Frontal Sinus, Left U Ethmoid Sinus, Right V Ethmoid Sinus, Left W Sphenoid Sinus, Right X Sphenoid Sinus, Left	0 Open 3 Percutaneous 4 Percutaneous endoscopic 7 Via natural or artificial opening 8 Via natural or artificial opening endoscopic	0 Drainage device	Z No qualifier

continued ⇨

© 2018 Channel Publishing, Ltd.

0 9 9 DRAINAGE – *continued*

Body Part – 4TH	Approach – 5TH	Device – 6TH	Qualifier – 7TH
7 Tympanic Membrane, Right 8 Tympanic Membrane, Left B Mastoid Sinus, Right C Mastoid Sinus, Left F Eustachian Tube, Right G Eustachian Tube, Left L Nasal Turbinate M Nasal Septum N Nasopharynx P Accessory Sinus Q Maxillary Sinus, Right R Maxillary Sinus, Left S Frontal Sinus, Right T Frontal Sinus, Left U Ethmoid Sinus, Right V Ethmoid Sinus, Left W Sphenoid Sinus, Right X Sphenoid Sinus, Left	0 Open 3 Percutaneous 4 Percutaneous endoscopic 7 Via natural or artificial opening 8 Via natural or artificial opening endoscopic	Z No device	X Diagnostic Z No qualifier

1ST - 0 Medical and Surgical

2ND - 9 Ear, Nose, Sinus

3RD - B EXCISION

EXCISION GROUP: Excision, Resection, Destruction, Extraction, (Detachment)
Root Operations that take out some or all of a body part.

EXCISION: Cutting out or off, without replacement, a portion of a body part.

Explanation: Qualifier "X Diagnostic" indicates excision procedures that are biopsies
Examples: Excision lesion nose – CMS Ex: Liver biopsy

Body Part – 4TH	Approach – 5TH	Device – 6TH	Qualifier – 7TH
0 External Ear, Right 1 External Ear, Left	0 Open 3 Percutaneous 4 Percutaneous endoscopic X External	Z No device	X Diagnostic Z No qualifier
3 External Auditory Canal, Right 4 External Auditory Canal, Left	0 Open 3 Percutaneous 4 Percutaneous endoscopic 7 Via natural or artificial opening 8 Via natural or artificial opening endoscopic X External	Z No device	X Diagnostic Z No qualifier
5 Middle Ear, Right 6 Middle Ear, Left 9 Auditory Ossicle, Right A Auditory Ossicle, Left D Inner Ear, Right E Inner Ear, Left	0 Open 8 Via natural or artificial opening endoscopic	Z No device	X Diagnostic Z No qualifier
7 Tympanic Membrane, Right 8 Tympanic Membrane, Left F Eustachian Tube, Right G Eustachian Tube, Left L Nasal Turbinate N Nasopharynx	0 Open 3 Percutaneous 4 Percutaneous endoscopic 7 Via natural or artificial opening 8 Via natural or artificial opening endoscopic	Z No device	X Diagnostic Z No qualifier
B Mastoid Sinus, Right C Mastoid Sinus, Left M Nasal Septum P Accessory Sinus Q Maxillary Sinus, Right R Maxillary Sinus, Left S Frontal Sinus, Right T Frontal Sinus, Left U Ethmoid Sinus, Right V Ethmoid Sinus, Left W Sphenoid Sinus, Right X Sphenoid Sinus, Left	0 Open 3 Percutaneous 4 Percutaneous endoscopic 8 Via natural or artificial opening endoscopic	Z No device	X Diagnostic Z No qualifier
K Nasal Mucosa and Soft Tissue	0 Open 3 Percutaneous 4 Percutaneous endoscopic 8 Via natural or artificial opening endoscopic X External	Z No device	X Diagnostic Z No qualifier

EAR NOSE SINUS 0 9 B

© 2018 Channel Publishing, Ltd.

1ST - 0 Medical and Surgical
2ND - 9 Ear, Nose, Sinus
3RD - C EXTIRPATION

DRAINAGE GROUP: Drainage, Extirpation, (Fragmentation)
Root Operations that take out solids/fluids/gases from a body part.

EXTIRPATION: Taking or cutting out solid matter from a body part.

Explanation: Abnormal byproduct or foreign body ...
Examples: Removal foreign body nose – CMS Ex: Thrombectomy

Body Part – 4TH	Approach – 5TH	Device – 6TH	Qualifier – 7TH
0 External Ear, Right 1 External Ear, Left	0 Open 3 Percutaneous 4 Percutaneous endoscopic X External	Z No device	Z No qualifier
3 External Auditory Canal, Right 4 External Auditory Canal, Left	0 Open 3 Percutaneous 4 Percutaneous endoscopic 7 Via natural or artificial opening 8 Via natural or artificial opening endoscopic X External	Z No device	Z No qualifier
5 Middle Ear, Right 6 Middle Ear, Left 9 Auditory Ossicle, Right A Auditory Ossicle, Left D Inner Ear, Right E Inner Ear, Left	0 Open 8 Via natural or artificial opening endoscopic	Z No device	Z No qualifier
7 Tympanic Membrane, Right 8 Tympanic Membrane, Left F Eustachian Tube, Right G Eustachian Tube, Left L Nasal Turbinate N Nasopharynx	0 Open 3 Percutaneous 4 Percutaneous endoscopic 7 Via natural or artificial opening 8 Via natural or artificial opening endoscopic	Z No device	Z No qualifier
B Mastoid Sinus, Right C Mastoid Sinus, Left M Nasal Septum P Accessory Sinus Q Maxillary Sinus, Right R Maxillary Sinus, Left S Frontal Sinus, Right T Frontal Sinus, Left U Ethmoid Sinus, Right V Ethmoid Sinus, Left W Sphenoid Sinus, Right X Sphenoid Sinus, Left	0 Open 3 Percutaneous 4 Percutaneous endoscopic 8 Via natural or artificial opening endoscopic	Z No device	Z No qualifier
K Nasal Mucosa and Soft Tissue	0 Open 3 Percutaneous 4 Percutaneous endoscopic 8 Via natural or artificial opening endoscopic X External	Z No device	Z No qualifier

1ST - 0 Medical and Surgical
2ND - 9 Ear, Nose, Sinus
3RD - D EXTRACTION

EXCISION GROUP: Excision, Resection, Destruction, Extraction, (Detachment)
Root Operations that take out some or all of a body part.

EXTRACTION: Pulling or stripping out or off all or a portion of a body part by the use of force.

Explanation: None for this Body System
Examples: Removal lining membrane sinus – CMS Ex: Dilation and curettage

Body Part – 4TH	Approach – 5TH	Device – 6TH	Qualifier – 7TH
7 Tympanic Membrane, Right 8 Tympanic Membrane, Left L Nasal Turbinate	0 Open 3 Percutaneous 4 Percutaneous endoscopic 7 Via natural or artificial opening 8 Via natural or artificial opening endoscopic	Z No device	Z No qualifier
9 Auditory Ossicle, Right A Auditory Ossicle, Left	0 Open	Z No device	Z No qualifier
B Mastoid Sinus, Right C Mastoid Sinus, Left M Nasal Septum P Accessory Sinus Q Maxillary Sinus, Right R Maxillary Sinus, Left S Frontal Sinus, Right T Frontal Sinus, Left U Ethmoid Sinus, Right V Ethmoid Sinus, Left W Sphenoid Sinus, Right X Sphenoid Sinus, Left	0 Open 3 Percutaneous 4 Percutaneous endoscopic	Z No device	Z No qualifier

© 2018 Channel Publishing, Ltd.

1ST - 0 Medical and Surgical
2ND - 9 Ear, Nose, Sinus
3RD - H INSERTION

DEVICE GROUP: Change, Insertion, Removal, Replacement, Revision, Supplement
Root Operations that always involve a device.

INSERTION: Putting in a nonbiological appliance that monitors, assists, performs, or prevents a physiological function but does not physically take the place of a body part.

Explanation: None
Examples: Cochlear implant – CMS Ex: Insertion of central venous catheter

Body Part – 4TH	Approach – 5TH	Device – 6TH	Qualifier – 7TH
D Inner Ear, Right E Inner Ear, Left	0 Open 3 Percutaneous 4 Percutaneous endoscopic	4 Hearing device, bone conduction 5 Hearing device, single channel cochlear prosthesis 6 Hearing device, multiple channel cochlear prosthesis S Hearing device	Z No qualifier
H Ear, Right J Ear, Left K Nasal Mucosa and Soft Tissue Y Sinus	0 Open 3 Percutaneous 4 Percutaneous endoscopic 7 Via natural or artificial opening 8 Via natural or artificial opening endoscopic	Y Other device	Z No qualifier
N Nasopharynx	7 Via natural or artificial opening 8 Via natural or artificial opening endoscopic	B Intraluminal device, airway	Z No qualifier

1ST - 0 Medical and Surgical
2ND - 9 Ear, Nose, Sinus
3RD - J INSPECTION

EXAMINATION GROUP: Inspection, (Map)
Root Operations involving examination only.

INSPECTION: Visually and/or manually exploring a body part.

Explanation: Direct or instrumental visualization ...
Examples: Sinus endoscopy – CMS Ex: Exploratory laparotomy

Body Part – 4TH	Approach – 5TH	Device – 6TH	Qualifier – 7TH
7 Tympanic Membrane, Right 8 Tympanic Membrane, Left H Ear, Right J Ear, Left	0 Open 3 Percutaneous 4 Percutaneous endoscopic 7 Via natural or artificial opening 8 Via natural or artificial opening endoscopic X External	Z No device	Z No qualifier
D Inner Ear, Right E Inner Ear, Left K Nasal Mucosa and Soft Tissue Y Sinus	0 Open 3 Percutaneous 4 Percutaneous endoscopic 8 Via natural or artificial opening endoscopic X External	Z No device	Z No qualifier

1ST - 0 Medical and Surgical
2ND - 9 Ear, Nose, Sinus
3RD - M REATTACHMENT

MOVE GROUP: Reattachment, Reposition, (Transfer), (Transplantation)
Root Operations that put in/put back or move some/all of a body part.

REATTACHMENT: Putting back in or on all or a portion of a separated body part to its normal location or other suitable location.

Explanation: Vascular circulation and nervous pathways may or may not be reestablished
Examples: Reattachment severed ear – CMS Ex: Reattachment of hand

Body Part – 4TH	Approach – 5TH	Device – 6TH	Qualifier – 7TH
0 External Ear, Right 1 External Ear, Left K Nasal Mucosa and Soft Tissue	X External	Z No device	Z No qualifier

© 2018 Channel Publishing, Ltd.

1ST - 0 Medical and Surgical
2ND - 9 Ear, Nose, Sinus
3RD - N RELEASE

DIVISION GROUP: Division, Release
Root Operations involving cutting or separation only.

RELEASE: Freeing a body part from an abnormal physical constraint by cutting or by the use of force.

Explanation: Some of the restraining tissue may be taken out but none of the body part is taken out
Examples: Adhesiolysis middle ear – CMS Ex: Carpal tunnel release

Body Part – 4TH	Approach – 5TH	Device – 6TH	Qualifier – 7TH
0 External Ear, Right 1 External Ear, Left	0 Open 3 Percutaneous 4 Percutaneous endoscopic X External	Z No device	Z No qualifier
3 External Auditory Canal, Right 4 External Auditory Canal, Left	0 Open 3 Percutaneous 4 Percutaneous endoscopic 7 Via natural or artificial opening 8 Via natural or artificial opening endoscopic X External	Z No device	Z No qualifier
5 Middle Ear, Right 6 Middle Ear, Left 9 Auditory Ossicle, Right A Auditory Ossicle, Left D Inner Ear, Right E Inner Ear, Left	0 Open 8 Via natural or artificial opening endoscopic	Z No device	Z No qualifier
7 Tympanic Membrane, Right 8 Tympanic Membrane, Left F Eustachian Tube, Right G Eustachian Tube, Left L Nasal Turbinate N Nasopharynx	0 Open 3 Percutaneous 4 Percutaneous endoscopic 7 Via natural or artificial opening 8 Via natural or artificial opening endoscopic	Z No device	Z No qualifier
B Mastoid Sinus, Right C Mastoid Sinus, Left M Nasal Septum P Accessory Sinus Q Maxillary Sinus, Right R Maxillary Sinus, Left S Frontal Sinus, Right T Frontal Sinus, Left U Ethmoid Sinus, Right V Ethmoid Sinus, Left W Sphenoid Sinus, Right X Sphenoid Sinus, Left	0 Open 3 Percutaneous 4 Percutaneous endoscopic 8 Via natural or artificial opening endoscopic	Z No device	Z No qualifier
K Nasal Mucosa and Soft Tissue	0 Open 3 Percutaneous 4 Percutaneous endoscopic 8 Via natural or artificial opening endoscopic X External	Z No device	Z No qualifier

© 2018 Channel Publishing, Ltd.

1ST - 0 Medical and Surgical
2ND - 9 Ear, Nose, Sinus
3RD - P REMOVAL

DEVICE GROUP: Change, Insertion, Removal, Replacement, Revision, Supplement
Root Operations that always involve a device.

REMOVAL: Taking out or off a device from a body part.

Explanation: Removal device without reinsertion ...
Examples: Removal drain tube – CMS Ex: Cardiac pacemaker removal

Body Part – 4TH	Approach – 5TH	Device – 6TH	Qualifier – 7TH
7 Tympanic Membrane, Right 8 Tympanic Membrane, Left	0 Open 7 Via natural or artificial opening 8 Via natural or artificial opening endoscopic X External	0 Drainage device	Z No qualifier
D Inner Ear, Right E Inner Ear, Left	0 Open 7 Via natural or artificial opening 8 Via natural or artificial opening endoscopic	S Hearing device	Z No qualifier
H Ear, Right J Ear, Left K Nasal Mucosa and Soft Tissue	0 Open 3 Percutaneous 4 Percutaneous endoscopic 7 Via natural or artificial opening 8 Via natural or artificial opening endoscopic	0 Drainage device 7 Autologous tissue substitute D Intraluminal device J Synthetic substitute K Nonautologous tissue substitute Y Other device	Z No qualifier
H Ear, Right J Ear, Left K Nasal Mucosa and Soft Tissue	X External	0 Drainage device 7 Autologous tissue substitute D Intraluminal device J Synthetic substitute K Nonautologous tissue substitute	Z No qualifier
Y Sinus	0 Open 3 Percutaneous 4 Percutaneous endoscopic	0 Drainage device Y Other device	Z No qualifier
Y Sinus	7 Via natural or artificial opening 8 Via natural or artificial opening endoscopic	Y Other device	Z No qualifier
Y Sinus	X External	0 Drainage device	Z No qualifier

© 2018 Channel Publishing, Ltd.

1ST - 0 Medical and Surgical
2ND - 9 Ear, Nose, Sinus
3RD - Q REPAIR

OTHER REPAIRS GROUP: Control, Repair
Root Operations that define other repairs.

REPAIR: Restoring, to the extent possible, a body part to its normal anatomic structure and function.

Explanation: Used only when the method to accomplish the repair is not one of the other root operations
Examples: Suture lacerated external ear – CMS Ex: Suture of laceration

Body Part – 4TH	Approach – 5TH	Device – 6TH	Qualifier – 7TH
0 External Ear, Right 1 External Ear, Left 2 External Ear, Bilateral	0 Open 3 Percutaneous 4 Percutaneous endoscopic X External	Z No device	Z No qualifier
3 External Auditory Canal, Right 4 External Auditory Canal, Left F Eustachian Tube, Right G Eustachian Tube, Left	0 Open 3 Percutaneous 4 Percutaneous endoscopic 7 Via natural or artificial opening 8 Via natural or artificial opening endoscopic X External	Z No device	Z No qualifier
5 Middle Ear, Right 6 Middle Ear, Left 9 Auditory Ossicle, Right A Auditory Ossicle, Left D Inner Ear, Right E Inner Ear, Left	0 Open 8 Via natural or artificial opening endoscopic	Z No device	Z No qualifier
7 Tympanic Membrane, Right 8 Tympanic Membrane, Left L Nasal Turbinate N Nasopharynx	0 Open 3 Percutaneous 4 Percutaneous endoscopic 7 Via natural or artificial opening 8 Via natural or artificial opening endoscopic	Z No device	Z No qualifier
B Mastoid Sinus, Right C Mastoid Sinus, Left M Nasal Septum P Accessory Sinus Q Maxillary Sinus, Right R Maxillary Sinus, Left S Frontal Sinus, Right T Frontal Sinus, Left U Ethmoid Sinus, Right V Ethmoid Sinus, Left W Sphenoid Sinus, Right X Sphenoid Sinus, Left	0 Open 3 Percutaneous 4 Percutaneous endoscopic 8 Via natural or artificial opening endoscopic	Z No device	Z No qualifier
K Nasal Mucosa and Soft Tissue	0 Open 3 Percutaneous 4 Percutaneous endoscopic 8 Via natural or artificial opening endoscopic X External	Z No device	Z No qualifier

© 2018 Channel Publishing, Ltd.

1ST - 0 Medical and Surgical
2ND - 9 Ear, Nose, Sinus
3RD - R REPLACEMENT

DEVICE GROUP: Change, Insertion, Removal, Replacement, Revision, Supplement
Root Operations that always involve a device.

REPLACEMENT: Putting in or on biological or synthetic material that physically takes the place and/or function of all or a portion of a body part.

Explanation: Includes taking out or eradicating, or rendering non-functional, the body part ...
Examples: External ear reconstruction – CMS Ex: Total hip replacement

Body Part – 4TH	Approach – 5TH	Device – 6TH	Qualifier – 7TH
0 External Ear, Right 1 External Ear, Left 2 External Ear, Bilateral K Nasal Mucosa and Soft Tissue	0 Open X External	7 Autologous tissue substitute J Synthetic substitute K Nonautologous tissue substitute	Z No qualifier
5 Middle Ear, Right 6 Middle Ear, Left 9 Auditory Ossicle, Right A Auditory Ossicle, Left D Inner Ear, Right E Inner Ear, Left	0 Open	7 Autologous tissue substitute J Synthetic substitute K Nonautologous tissue substitute	Z No qualifier
7 Tympanic Membrane, Right 8 Tympanic Membrane, Left N Nasopharynx	0 Open 7 Via natural or artificial opening 8 Via natural or artificial opening endoscopic	7 Autologous tissue substitute J Synthetic substitute K Nonautologous tissue substitute	Z No qualifier
L Nasal Turbinate	0 Open 3 Percutaneous 4 Percutaneous endoscopic 7 Via natural or artificial opening 8 Via natural or artificial opening endoscopic	7 Autologous tissue substitute J Synthetic substitute K Nonautologous tissue substitute	Z No qualifier
M Nasal Septum	0 Open 3 Percutaneous 4 Percutaneous endoscopic	7 Autologous tissue substitute J Synthetic substitute K Nonautologous tissue substitute	Z No qualifier

1ST - 0 Medical and Surgical
2ND - 9 Ear, Nose, Sinus
3RD - S REPOSITION

MOVE GROUP: Reattachment, Reposition, (Transfer), (Transplantation)
Root Operations that put in/put back or move some/all of a body part.

REPOSITION: Moving to its normal location, or other suitable location, all or a portion of a body part.

Explanation: The body part may or may not be cut out or off to be moved to the new location ...
Examples: Deviated septum septoplasty – CMS Ex: Fracture reduction

Body Part – 4TH	Approach – 5TH	Device – 6TH	Qualifier – 7TH
0 External Ear, Right 1 External Ear, Left 2 External Ear, Bilateral K Nasal Mucosa and Soft Tissue	0 Open 4 Percutaneous endoscopic X External	Z No device	Z No qualifier
7 Tympanic Membrane, Right 8 Tympanic Membrane, Left F Eustachian Tube, Right G Eustachian Tube, Left L Nasal Turbinate	0 Open 4 Percutaneous endoscopic 7 Via natural or artificial opening 8 Via natural or artificial opening endoscopic	Z No device	Z No qualifier
9 Auditory Ossicle, Right A Auditory Ossicle, Left M Nasal Septum	0 Open 4 Percutaneous endoscopic	Z No device	Z No qualifier

© 2018 Channel Publishing, Ltd.

1ST - 0 Medical and Surgical
2ND - 9 Ear, Nose, Sinus
3RD - T RESECTION

EXCISION GROUP: Excision, Resection, Destruction, Extraction, (Detachment)
Root Operations that take out some or all of a body part.

RESECTION: Cutting out or off, without replacement, all of a body part.

Explanation: None
Examples: Total maxillary sinusectomy – CMS Ex: Total lobectomy of lung

Body Part – 4TH	Approach – 5TH	Device – 6TH	Qualifier – 7TH
0 External Ear, Right 1 External Ear, Left	0 Open 4 Percutaneous endoscopic X External	Z No device	Z No qualifier
5 Middle Ear, Right 6 Middle Ear, Left 9 Auditory Ossicle, Right A Auditory Ossicle, Left D Inner Ear, Right E Inner Ear, Left	0 Open 8 Via natural or artificial opening endoscopic	Z No device	Z No qualifier
7 Tympanic Membrane, Right 8 Tympanic Membrane, Left F Eustachian Tube, Right G Eustachian Tube, Left L Nasal Turbinate N Nasopharynx	0 Open 4 Percutaneous endoscopic 7 Via natural or artificial opening 8 Via natural or artificial opening endoscopic	Z No device	Z No qualifier
B Mastoid Sinus, Right C Mastoid Sinus, Left M Nasal Septum P Accessory Sinus Q Maxillary Sinus, Right R Maxillary Sinus, Left S Frontal Sinus, Right T Frontal Sinus, Left U Ethmoid Sinus, Right V Ethmoid Sinus, Left W Sphenoid Sinus, Right X Sphenoid Sinus, Left	0 Open 4 Percutaneous endoscopic 8 Via natural or artificial opening endoscopic	Z No device	Z No qualifier
K Nasal Mucosa and Soft Tissue	0 Open 4 Percutaneous endoscopic 8 Via natural or artificial opening endoscopic X External	Z No device	Z No qualifier

© 2018 Channel Publishing, Ltd.

1ST - 0 Medical and Surgical
2ND - 9 Ear, Nose, Sinus
3RD - U SUPPLEMENT

DEVICE GROUP: Change, Insertion, Removal, Replacement, Revision, Supplement
Root Operations that always involve a device.

SUPPLEMENT: Putting in or on biological or synthetic material that physically reinforces and/or augments the function of a portion of a body part.

Explanation: Biological material is non-living, or is living and from the same individual ...
Examples: Overlay graft myringoplasty – CMS Ex: Herniorrhaphy using mesh

Body Part – 4TH	Approach – 5TH	Device – 6TH	Qualifier – 7TH
0 External Ear, Right 1 External Ear, Left 2 External Ear, Bilateral	0 Open X External	7 Autologous tissue substitute J Synthetic substitute K Nonautologous tissue substitute	Z No qualifier
5 Middle Ear, Right 6 Middle Ear, Left 9 Auditory Ossicle, Right A Auditory Ossicle, Left D Inner Ear, Right E Inner Ear, Left	0 Open 8 Via natural or artificial opening endoscopic	7 Autologous tissue substitute J Synthetic substitute K Nonautologous tissue substitute	Z No qualifier
7 Tympanic Membrane, Right 8 Tympanic Membrane, Left N Nasopharynx	0 Open 7 Via natural or artificial opening 8 Via natural or artificial opening endoscopic	7 Autologous tissue substitute J Synthetic substitute K Nonautologous tissue substitute	Z No qualifier
K Nasal Mucosa and Soft Tissue	0 Open 8 Via natural or artificial opening endoscopic X External	7 Autologous tissue substitute J Synthetic substitute K Nonautologous tissue substitute	Z No qualifier
L Nasal Turbinate	0 Open 3 Percutaneous 4 Percutaneous endoscopic 7 Via natural or artificial opening 8 Via natural or artificial opening endoscopic	7 Autologous tissue substitute J Synthetic substitute K Nonautologous tissue substitute	Z No qualifier
M Nasal Septum	0 Open 3 Percutaneous 4 Percutaneous endoscopic 8 Via natural or artificial opening endoscopic	7 Autologous tissue substitute J Synthetic substitute K Nonautologous tissue substitute	Z No qualifier

© 2018 Channel Publishing, Ltd.

1ST - 0 Medical and Surgical
2ND - 9 Ear, Nose, Sinus
3RD - W REVISION

DEVICE GROUP: Change, Insertion, Removal, Replacement, Revision, Supplement
Root Operations that always involve a device.

REVISION: Correcting, to the extent possible, a portion of a malfunctioning device or the position of a displaced device.

Explanation: Correcting by taking out or putting in components of a device such as a screw or pin ...
Examples: Reposition cochlear implant – CMS Ex: Recementing of hip prosthesis

Body Part – 4TH	Approach – 5TH	Device – 6TH	Qualifier – 7TH
7 Tympanic Membrane, Right 8 Tympanic Membrane, Left 9 Auditory Ossicle, Right A Auditory Ossicle, Left	0 Open 7 Via natural or artificial opening 8 Via natural or artificial opening endoscopic	7 Autologous tissue substitute J Synthetic substitute K Nonautologous tissue substitute	Z No qualifier
D Inner Ear, Right E Inner Ear, Left	0 Open 7 Via natural or artificial opening 8 Via natural or artificial opening endoscopic	S Hearing device	Z No qualifier
H Ear, Right J Ear, Left K Nasal Mucosa and Soft Tissue	0 Open 3 Percutaneous 4 Percutaneous endoscopic 7 Via natural or artificial opening 8 Via natural or artificial opening endoscopic	0 Drainage device 7 Autologous tissue substitute D Intraluminal device J Synthetic substitute K Nonautologous tissue substitute Y Other device	Z No qualifier
H Ear, Right J Ear, Left K Nasal Mucosa and Soft Tissue	X External	0 Drainage device 7 Autologous tissue substitute D Intraluminal device J Synthetic substitute K Nonautologous tissue substitute	Z No qualifier
Y Sinus	0 Open 3 Percutaneous 4 Percutaneous endoscopic	0 Drainage device Y Other device	Z No qualifier
Y Sinus	7 Via natural or artificial opening 8 Via natural or artificial opening endoscopic	Y Other device	Z No qualifier
Y Sinus	X External	0 Drainage device	Z No qualifier

© 2018 Channel Publishing, Ltd.

Educational Annotations | B – Respiratory System

Body System Specific Educational Annotations for the Respiratory System include:

- Anatomy and Physiology Review
- Definitions of Common Procedures
- Anatomical Illustrations
- AHA Coding Clinic® Reference Notations
- Body Part Key Listings
- Device Key Listings
- Device Aggregation Table Listings
- Coding Notes

Anatomy and Physiology Review of Respiratory System

BODY PART VALUES - B - RESPIRATORY SYSTEM

Carina – ANATOMY – The carina is a ridge of cartilaginous tissue within the trachea at the tracheal bifurcation at the lower end of the trachea. PHYSIOLOGY – The sensitive mucous membrane of the carina is responsible for triggering a cough reflex.

Diaphragm – ANATOMY – The diaphragm is dome-shaped sheet of skeletal muscle between the thoracic and abdominal cavities. PHYSIOLOGY – The diaphragm is the primary muscle in respiration and when it contracts, air is drawn into the lungs.

Lingula Bronchus – The secondary bronchi serving a lung lingula.

Lower Lobe Bronchus – The secondary bronchi serving a lower lung lobe (left or right).

Lower Lobe Lung – The lower lung lobes are soft, spongy, cone-shaped organs of respiration (left or right).

Lung – ANATOMY – The lungs are soft, spongy, cone-shaped organs located in the thoracic cavity. The right and left lungs are separated medially by the heart and the mediastinum, and they are enclosed by the diaphragm and the thoracic cage. The right lung is divided into 3 lobes called the upper (superior), middle, and lower (inferior). The left lung is divided into 2 lobes, the upper and lower. The lobes are subdivided into lobules which are composed of bronchioles, alveolar sacs, alveoli, nerves, and associated blood and lymphatic vessels. The alveoli are thin-walled, microscopic air sacs that open only on the side communicating with the inhaled air. PHYSIOLOGY – The lungs are organs that perform pulmonary ventilation. The alveoli are the microscopic structures responsible for the exchange of oxygen into the blood and carbon dioxide out of the body. Inspiration (inhalation) and expiration (exhalation) are complex central nervous system functions. Two groups of nerve cell bodies in the medulla of the brain compose the inspiratory center and the expiratory center. These two centers act reciprocally; that is, when one is stimulated and discharging, the other is inhibited. Both centers discharge nerve impulses to the intercostal muscles. When the inspiration center discharges nerve impulses, the diaphragm moves down and the external intercostal muscles contract, causing inflation. Inflation of the lungs causes stimulation of stretch receptors, which send impulses to the medulla, which in turn stimulates the expiratory center. Two other respiratory centers are contained in the pons which modify and control the medullary centers' activities, and are called the apneustic center and the pneumotaxic center. In addition to the above centers, there is also a chemical reaction which helps to control pulmonary ventilation. The carbon dioxide level in the blood is directly measured by the medulla, and respiration is adjusted accordingly. A decrease in the oxygen level, sensed by nerve endings in the common carotid artery and the aortic arch, will also stimulate a respiratory adjustment, but it does not play a noticeable difference in pulmonary ventilation.

Lung Lingula – The downward projection of the upper lobe of the left lung.

Main Bronchus – ANATOMY – The bronchial tree consists of branched airways leading from the trachea to the microscopic air sacs. The two main branches, the right and left bronchi, subdivide into secondary or lobar bronchi, which in turn branch into finer tubes down to the bronchioles. PHYSIOLOGY – The trachea and bronchi allow for the rapid transport of air to and from the lung tissue.

Middle Lobe Bronchus – The secondary bronchi serving a middle lung lobe (right).

Middle Lobe Lung – The middle lung lobe is the soft, spongy, cone-shaped organ of respiration (right).

Pleura – ANATOMY – The pleura are closed, double-layered serous membranous sacs surrounding the lungs. The parietal pleura is the layer which lines the thoracic walls opposite to the visceral pleura. The visceral pleura is the layer which adheres to the lungs and together with the parietal, forms the pleural cavity. PHYSIOLOGY – The pleura functions to prevent friction of the lungs against the thoracic wall during respiration. There is a small amount of serous fluid in the pleural cavity which lubricates the facing membranes.

Trachea – ANATOMY – The trachea is a cylindrical tube about 1 inch (2.5 cm) in diameter. It extends downward from the larynx in front of the esophagus and into the thoracic cavity, where it splits into the right and left main bronchi. PHYSIOLOGY – The trachea and bronchi allow for the rapid transport of air to and from the lung tissue.

Tracheobronchial Tree – The trachea, main bronchi, secondary (lobar) bronchi, and bronchioles.

Upper Lobe Bronchus – The secondary bronchi serving a lower lung lobe (left or right).

Upper Lobe Lung – The upper lung lobes are soft, spongy, cone-shaped organs of respiration (left or right).

Definitions of Common Procedures of Respiratory System

Bronchoscopy – The use of a flexible bronchoscope to visualize and perform procedures on the bronchi and lungs.

Endobronchial valve insertion – The bronchoscopic placement of one-way bronchial airflow valves that prevent air from entering the designated lobe segments while allowing trapped air and secretions to flow out. The valves are used primarily to treat emphysema by not allowing that segment to inflate and thus allowing other healthier segments to inflate and exhale more easily and efficiently.

Endotracheal intubation – The placement of a flexible, plastic breathing tube into the trachea through the oral cavity and occasionally through the nose.

Lobectomy of lung – The surgical removal of an entire lobe of a lung.

Lung transplant – The surgical replacement of a diseased lung by implantation of a donor lung.

Pleurodesis – The medical procedure to eliminate the pleural cavity space by instilling a substance (chemical, talc, etc.) through a chest tube that adheres the visceral and parietal pleura together.

Tracheostomy – The creation of a surgical opening in the front of neck and into the trachea with the placement of a tube through the opening and into the trachea to maintain the patency of the new airway for breathing and secretion removal.

© 2018 Channel Publishing, Ltd.

Educational Annotations | B – Respiratory System

Anatomical Illustrations of Respiratory System

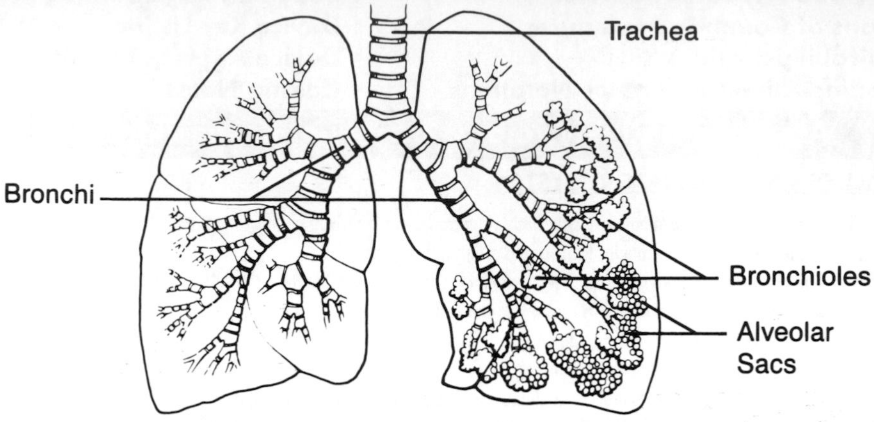

LUNGS — ANTERIOR (CUT-AWAY) VIEW

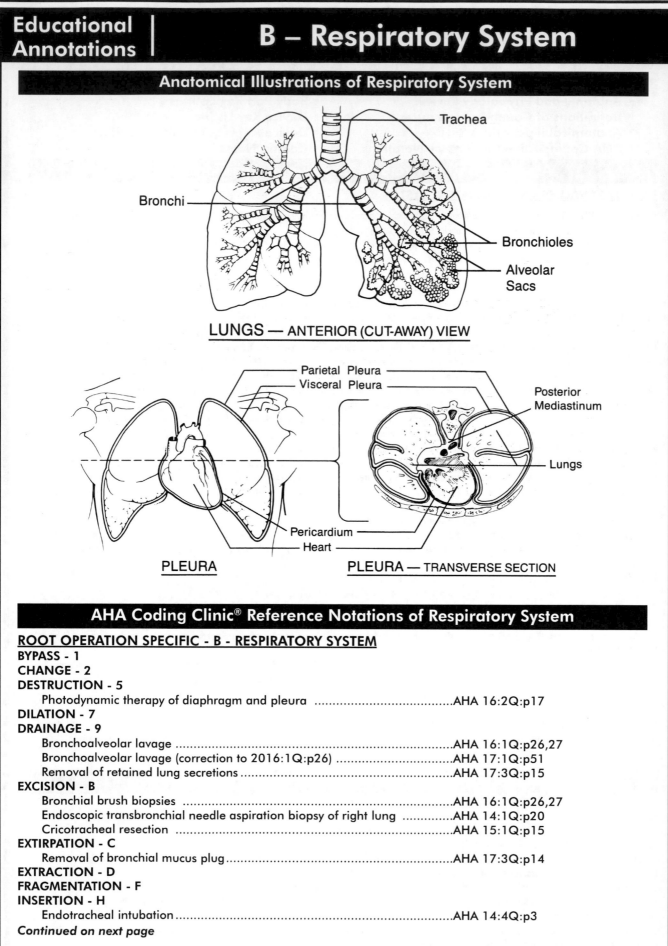

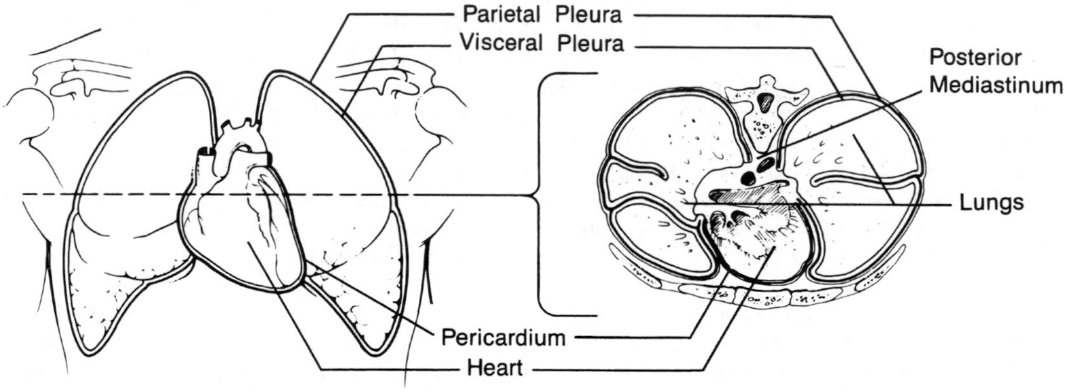

PLEURA

PLEURA — TRANSVERSE SECTION

AHA Coding Clinic® Reference Notations of Respiratory System

ROOT OPERATION SPECIFIC - B - RESPIRATORY SYSTEM

BYPASS - 1

CHANGE - 2

DESTRUCTION - 5

Photodynamic therapy of diaphragm and pleura ....AHA 16:2Q:p17

DILATION - 7

DRAINAGE - 9

Bronchoalveolar lavage ....AHA 16:1Q:p26,27
Bronchoalveolar lavage (correction to 2016:1Q:p26) ....AHA 17:1Q:p51
Removal of retained lung secretions ....AHA 17:3Q:p15

EXCISION - B

Bronchial brush biopsies ....AHA 16:1Q:p26,27
Endoscopic transbronchial needle aspiration biopsy of right lung ....AHA 14:1Q:p20
Cricotracheal resection ....AHA 15:1Q:p15

EXTIRPATION - C

Removal of bronchial mucus plug ....AHA 17:3Q:p14

EXTRACTION - D

FRAGMENTATION - F

INSERTION - H

Endotracheal intubation ....AHA 14:4Q:p3

Continued on next page

© 2018 Channel Publishing, Ltd.

Educational Annotations | B – Respiratory System

AHA Coding Clinic® Reference Notations of Respiratory System

Continued from previous page

INSPECTION - J

Bronchoscopic placement of fiducial marker ....AHA 14:1Q:p20
Endoscopic viewing of talc placement in pleural cavity ....AHA 15:2Q:p31

OCCLUSION - L

REATTACHMENT - M

RELEASE - N

Release of tracheal vascular ring ....AHA 15:3Q:p15

REMOVAL - P

REPAIR - Q

Diaphragm hiatal hernia repair ....AHA 16:2Q:p22
Repair of midline diaphragm (paraesophageal) hernia ....AHA 14:3Q:p28

REPOSITION - S

RESECTION - T

SUPPLEMENT - U

Omental flap repair of bronchopleural fistula ....AHA 15:1Q:p28

RESTRICTION - V

REVISION - W

TRANSPLANTATION - Y

Body Part Key Listings of Respiratory System

See also Body Part Key in Appendix C

Bronchus intermedius ....use Main Bronchus, Right
Cricoid cartilage..........................use Trachea
Intermediate bronchus ....use Main Bronchus, Right

Device Key Listings of Respiratory System

See also Device Key in Appendix D

Autograft ....use Autologous Tissue Substitute
Brachytherapy seeds ....use Radioactive Element
Endotracheal tube (cuffed) (double-lumen) ....use Intraluminal Device, Endotracheal Airway in Respiratory System
Phrenic nerve stimulator lead ....use Diaphragmatic Pacemaker Lead in Respiratory System
Spiration IBV™ Valve System ....use Intraluminal Device, Endobronchial Valve in Respiratory System
Tissue bank graft..........................use Nonautologous Tissue Substitute
Tracheostomy tube ....use Tracheostomy Device in Respiratory System

Device Aggregation Table Listings of Respiratory System

See also Device Aggregation Table in Appendix E

Specific Device	For Operation	In Body System	General Device
Intraluminal Device, Endobronchial Valve	All applicable	Respiratory System	Intraluminal Device
Intraluminal Device, Endotracheal Airway	All applicable	Respiratory System	Intraluminal Device

RESPIRATORY 0 B

© 2018 Channel Publishing, Ltd.

Educational Annotations | B – Respiratory System

Coding Notes of Respiratory System

Body System Relevant Coding Guidelines

Body part, General guidelines

B4.1c

If a procedure is performed on a continuous section of a tubular body part, code the body part value corresponding to the furthest anatomical site from the point of entry.

Example: A procedure performed on a continuous section of artery from the femoral artery to the external iliac artery with the point of entry at the femoral artery is coded to the external iliac body part.

Branches of body parts

B4.2

Where a specific branch of a body part does not have its own body part value in PCS, the body part is typically coded to the closest proximal branch that has a specific body part value. In the cardiovascular body systems, if a general body part is available in the correct root operation table, and coding to a proximal branch would require assigning a code in a different body system, the procedure is coded using the general body part value.

Examples: A procedure performed on the mandibular branch of the trigeminal nerve is coded to the trigeminal nerve body part value.

Occlusion of the bronchial artery is coded to the body part value Upper Artery in the body system Upper Arteries, and not to the body part value Thoracic Aorta, Descending in the body system Heart and Great Vessels.

© 2018 Channel Publishing, Ltd.

1ST - 0 Medical and Surgical
2ND - B Respiratory System
3RD - 1 BYPASS

TUBULAR GROUP: Bypass, Dilation, Occlusion, Restriction
Root Operations that alter the diameter/route of a tubular body part.
BYPASS: Altering the route of passage of the contents of a tubular body part.

Explanation: Rerouting contents to a downstream part ... with or without the use of a device ...
Examples: Tracheostomy tube placement – CMS Ex: Coronary artery bypass

Body Part – 4TH	Approach – 5TH	Device – 6TH	Qualifier – 7TH
1 Trachea	0 Open	D Intraluminal device	6 Esophagus
1 Trachea	0 Open	F Tracheostomy device Z No device	4 Cutaneous
1 Trachea	3 Percutaneous 4 Percutaneous endoscopic	F Tracheostomy device Z No device	4 Cutaneous

1ST - 0 Medical and Surgical
2ND - B Respiratory System
3RD - 2 CHANGE

DEVICE GROUP: Change, Insertion, Removal, Replacement, Revision, Supplement
Root Operations that always involve a device.
CHANGE: Taking out or off a device from a body part and putting back an identical or similar device in or on the same body part without cutting or puncturing the skin or a mucous membrane.
Explanation: All CHANGE procedures are coded using the approach External
Examples: Exchange trachea tube – CMS Ex. Urinary catheter change

Body Part – 4TH	Approach – 5TH	Device – 6TH	Qualifier – 7TH
0 Tracheobronchial Tree K Lung, Right L Lung, Left Q Pleura T Diaphragm	X External	0 Drainage device Y Other device	Z No qualifier
1 Trachea	X External	0 Drainage device E Intraluminial device, endotracheal airway F Tracheostomy device Y Other device	Z No qualifier

1ST - 0 Medical and Surgical
2ND - B Respiratory System
3RD - 5 DESTRUCTION

EXCISION GROUP: Excision, Resection, Destruction, Extraction, (Detachment)
Root Operations that take out some or all of a body part.
DESTRUCTION: Physical eradication of all or a portion of a body part by the direct use of energy, force, or a destructive agent.
Explanation: None of the body part is physically taken out
Examples: Pleurodesis using talc – CMS Ex: Fulguration of rectal polyp

Body Part – 4TH	Approach – 5TH	Device – 6TH	Qualifier – 7TH
1 Trachea 2 Carina 3 Main Bronchus, Right 4 Upper Lobe Bronchus, Right 5 Middle Lobe Bronchus, Right 6 Lower Lobe Bronchus, Right 7 Main Bronchus, Left 8 Upper Lobe Bronchus, Left 9 Lingula Bronchus B Lower Lobe Bronchus, Left C Upper Lung Lobe, Right D Middle Lung Lobe, Right F Lower Lung Lobe, Right G Upper Lung Lobe, Left H Lung Lingula J Lower Lung Lobe, Left K Lung, Right L Lung, Left M Lungs, Bilateral	0 Open 3 Percutaneous 4 Percutaneous endoscopic 7 Via natural or artificial opening 8 Via natural or artificial opening endoscopic	Z No device	Z No qualifier
N Pleura, Right P Pleura, Left T Diaphragm	0 Open 3 Percutaneous 4 Percutaneous endoscopic	Z No device	Z No qualifier

RESPIRATORY 0B5

© 2018 Channel Publishing, Ltd.

1ST - 0 Medical and Surgical
2ND - B Respiratory System
3RD - 7 DILATION

TUBULAR GROUP: Bypass, Dilation, Occlusion, Restriction
Root Operations that alter the diameter/route of a tubular body part.

DILATION: Expanding an orifice or the lumen of a tubular body part.

Explanation: Accomplished by stretching or cutting ... tubular body part or orifice ...
Examples: Dilation tracheal stenosis – CMS Ex: Percutaneous transluminal angioplasty

Body Part – 4TH	Approach – 5TH	Device – 6TH	Qualifier – 7TH
1 Trachea 2 Carina 3 Main Bronchus, Right 4 Upper Lobe Bronchus, Right 5 Middle Lobe Bronchus, Right 6 Lower Lobe Bronchus, Right 7 Main Bronchus, Left 8 Upper Lobe Bronchus, Left 9 Lingula Bronchus B Lower Lobe Bronchus, Left	0 Open 3 Percutaneous 4 Percutaneous endoscopic 7 Via natural or artificial opening 8 Via natural or artificial opening endoscopic	D Intraluminal device Z No device	Z No qualifier

1ST - 0 Medical and Surgical
2ND - B Respiratory System
3RD - 9 DRAINAGE

DRAINAGE GROUP: Drainage, Extirpation, Fragmentation
Root Operations that take out solids/fluids/gases from a body part.

DRAINAGE: Taking or letting out fluids and/or gases from a body part.

Explanation: Qualifier "X Diagnostic" indicates drainage procedures that are biopsies
Examples: Needle aspiration lung abscess – CMS Ex: Thoracentesis

Body Part – 4TH	Approach – 5TH	Device – 6TH	Qualifier – 7TH
1 Trachea 2 Carina 3 Main Bronchus, Right 4 Upper Lobe Bronchus, Right 5 Middle Lobe Bronchus, Right 6 Lower Lobe Bronchus, Right 7 Main Bronchus, Left 8 Upper Lobe Bronchus, Left 9 Lingula Bronchus B Lower Lobe Bronchus, Left C Upper Lung Lobe, Right D Middle Lung Lobe, Right F Lower Lung Lobe, Right G Upper Lung Lobe, Left H Lung Lingula J Lower Lung Lobe, Left K Lung, Right L Lung, Left M Lungs, Bilateral	0 Open 3 Percutaneous 4 Percutaneous endoscopic 7 Via natural or artificial opening 8 Via natural or artificial opening endoscopic	0 Drainage device	Z No qualifier
1 Trachea 2 Carina 3 Main Bronchus, Right 4 Upper Lobe Bronchus, Right 5 Middle Lobe Bronchus, Right 6 Lower Lobe Bronchus, Right 7 Main Bronchus, Left 8 Upper Lobe Bronchus, Left 9 Lingula Bronchus B Lower Lobe Bronchus, Left C Upper Lung Lobe, Right D Middle Lung Lobe, Right F Lower Lung Lobe, Right G Upper Lung Lobe, Left H Lung Lingula J Lower Lung Lobe, Left K Lung, Right L Lung, Left M Lungs, Bilateral	0 Open 3 Percutaneous 4 Percutaneous endoscopic 7 Via natural or artificial opening 8 Via natural or artificial opening endoscopic	Z No device	X Diagnostic Z No qualifier
N Pleura, Right P Pleura, Left	0 Open 3 Percutaneous 4 Percutaneous endoscopic 8 Via natural or artificial opening endoscopic	0 Drainage device	Z No qualifier
N Pleura, Right P Pleura, Left	0 Open 3 Percutaneous 4 Percutaneous endoscopic 8 Via natural or artificial opening endoscopic	Z No device	X Diagnostic Z No qualifier
T Diaphragm	0 Open 3 Percutaneous 4 Percutaneous endoscopic	0 Drainage device	Z No qualifier
T Diaphragm	0 Open 3 Percutaneous 4 Percutaneous endoscopic	Z No device	X Diagnostic Z No qualifier

© 2018 Channel Publishing, Ltd.

1ST - 0 Medical and Surgical
2ND - B Respiratory System
3RD - B EXCISION

EXCISION GROUP: Excision, Resection, Destruction, Extraction, (Detachment)
Root Operations that take out some or all of a body part.

EXCISION: Cutting out or off, without replacement, a portion of a body part.

Explanation: Qualifier "X Diagnostic" indicates excision procedures that are biopsies
Examples: Endoscopic biopsy lung – CMS Ex: Liver biopsy

Body Part – 4TH	Approach – 5TH	Device – 6TH	Qualifier – 7TH
1 Trachea 2 Carina 3 Main Bronchus, Right 4 Upper Lobe Bronchus, Right 5 Middle Lobe Bronchus, Right 6 Lower Lobe Bronchus, Right 7 Main Bronchus, Left 8 Upper Lobe Bronchus, Left 9 Lingula Bronchus B Lower Lobe Bronchus, Left C Upper Lung Lobe, Right D Middle Lung Lobe, Right F Lower Lung Lobe, Right G Upper Lung Lobe, Left H Lung Lingula J Lower Lung Lobe, Left K Lung, Right L Lung, Left M Lungs, Bilateral	0 Open 3 Percutaneous 4 Percutaneous endoscopic 7 Via natural or artificial opening 8 Via natural or artificial opening endoscopic	Z No device	X Diagnostic Z No qualifier
N Pleura, Right P Pleura, Left	0 Open 3 Percutaneous 4 Percutaneous endoscopic 8 Via natural or artificial opening endoscopic	Z No device	X Diagnostic Z No qualifier
T Diaphragm	0 Open 3 Percutaneous 4 Percutaneous endoscopic	Z No device	X Diagnostic Z No qualifier

1ST - 0 Medical and Surgical
2ND - B Respiratory System
3RD - C EXTIRPATION

DRAINAGE GROUP: Drainage, Extirpation, Fragmentation
Root Operations that take out solids/fluids/gases from a body part.

EXTIRPATION: Taking or cutting out solid matter from a body part.

Explanation: Abnormal byproduct or foreign body ...
Examples: Removal bronchial foreign body – CMS Ex: Thrombectomy

Body Part – 4TH	Approach – 5TH	Device – 6TH	Qualifier – 7TH
1 Trachea 2 Carina 3 Main Bronchus, Right 4 Upper Lobe Bronchus, Right 5 Middle Lobe Bronchus, Right 6 Lower Lobe Bronchus, Right 7 Main Bronchus, Left 8 Upper Lobe Bronchus, Left 9 Lingula Bronchus B Lower Lobe Bronchus, Left C Upper Lung Lobe, Right D Middle Lung Lobe, Right F Lower Lung Lobe, Right G Upper Lung Lobe, Left H Lung Lingula J Lower Lung Lobe, Left K Lung, Right L Lung, Left M Lungs, Bilateral	0 Open 3 Percutaneous 4 Percutaneous endoscopic 7 Via natural or artificial opening 8 Via natural or artificial opening endoscopic	Z No device	Z No qualifier
N Pleura, Right P Pleura, Left T Diaphragm	0 Open 3 Percutaneous 4 Percutaneous endoscopic	Z No device	Z No qualifier

© 2018 Channel Publishing, Ltd.

1ST - 0 Medical and Surgical
2ND - B Respiratory System
3RD - D EXTRACTION

EXCISION GROUP: Excision, Resection, Destruction, Extraction, (Detachment)
Root Operations that take out some or all of a body part.

EXTRACTION: Pulling or stripping out or off all or a portion of a body part by the use of force.

Explanation: Qualifier "X Diagnostic" indicates extraction procedures that are biopsies
Examples: Pleural extraction – CMS Ex: Dilation and curettage

Body Part – 4TH		Approach – 5TH	Device – 6TH	Qualifier–7TH
1 Trachea 2 Carina 3 Main Bronchus, Right 4 Upper Lobe Bronchus, Right 5 Middle Lobe Bronchus, Right 6 Lower Lobe Bronchus, Right 7 Main Bronchus, Left 8 Upper Lobe Bronchus, Left 9 Lingula Bronchus B Lower Lobe Bronchus, Left	C Upper Lung Lobe, Right D Middle Lung Lobe, Right F Lower Lung Lobe, Right G Upper Lung Lobe, Left H Lung Lingula J Lower Lung Lobe, Left K Lung, Right L Lung, Left M Lungs, Bilateral	4 Percutaneous endoscopic 8 Via natural or artificial opening endoscopic	Z No device	X Diagnostic
N Pleura, Right P Pleura, Left		0 Open 3 Percutaneous 4 Percutaneous endoscopic	Z No device	X Diagnostic Z No qualifier

1ST - 0 Medical and Surgical
2ND - B Respiratory System
3RD - F FRAGMENTATION

DRAINAGE GROUP: Drainage, Extirpation, Fragmentation
Root Operations that take out solids/fluids/gases from a body part.

FRAGMENTATION: Breaking solid matter in a body part into pieces.

Explanation: Pieces are not taken out during the procedure ...
Examples: Lithotripsy broncholithiasis – CMS Ex: Extracorporeal shockwave lithotripsy

Body Part – 4TH		Approach – 5TH	Device – 6TH	Qualifier–7TH
1 Trachea 2 Carina 3 Main Bronchus, Right 4 Upper Lobe Bronchus, Right 5 Middle Lobe Bronchus, Right	6 Lower Lobe Bronchus, Right 7 Main Bronchus, Left 8 Upper Lobe Bronchus, Left 9 Lingula Bronchus B Lower Lobe Bronchus, Left	0 Open 3 Percutaneous 4 Percutaneous endoscopic 7 Via natural or artificial opening 8 Via natural or artificial opening endoscopic X External NC*	Z No device	Z No qualifier

NC* – Non-covered by Medicare. See current Medicare Code Editor for details.

1ST - 0 Medical and Surgical
2ND - B Respiratory System
3RD - H INSERTION

DEVICE GROUP: Change, Insertion, Removal, Replacement, Revision, Supplement
Root Operations that always involve a device.

INSERTION: Putting in a nonbiological appliance that monitors, assists, performs, or prevents a physiological function but does not physically take the place of a body part.

Explanation: None
Examples: Endotracheal intubation – CMS Ex: Insertion of central venous catheter

Body Part – 4TH	Approach – 5TH	Device – 6TH	Qualifier 7TH
0 Tracheobronchial Tree	0 Open 3 Percutaneous 4 Percutaneous endoscopic 7 Via natural or artificial opening 8 Via natural or artificial opening endoscopic	1 Radioactive element 2 Monitoring device 3 Infusion device D Intraluminal device Y Other device	Z No qualifier
1 Trachea	0 Open	2 Monitoring device D Intraluminal device Y Other device	Z No qualifier

continued ⇨

© 2018 Channel Publishing, Ltd.

0 B H INSERTION – *continued*

Body Part – 4TH	Approach – 5TH	Device – 6TH	Qualifier 7TH
1 Trachea	3 Percutaneous	D Intraluminal device E Intraluminal device, endotracheal airway Y Other device	Z No qualifier
1 Trachea	4 Percutaneous endoscopic	D Intraluminal device Y Other device	Z No qualifier
1 Trachea	7 Via natural or artificial opening 8 Via natural or artificial opening endoscopic	2 Monitoring device D Intraluminal device E Intraluminal device, endotracheal airway Y Other device	Z No qualifier
3 Main Bronchus, Right 4 Upper Lobe Bronchus, Right 5 Middle Lobe Bronchus, Right 6 Lower Lobe Bronchus, Right 7 Main Bronchus, Left 8 Upper Lobe Bronchus, Left 9 Lingula Bronchus B Lower Lobe Bronchus, Left	0 Open 3 Percutaneous 4 Percutaneous endoscopic 7 Via natural or artificial opening 8 Via natural or artificial opening endoscopic	G Intraluminal device, endobronchial valve	Z No qualifier
K Lung, Right L Lung, Left	0 Open 3 Percutaneous 4 Percutaneous endoscopic 7 Via natural or artificial opening 8 Via natural or artificial opening endoscopic	1 Radioactive element 2 Monitoring device 3 Infusion device Y Other device	Z No qualifier
Q Pleura	0 Open 3 Percutaneous 4 Percutaneous endoscopic 7 Via natural or artificial opening 8 Via natural or artificial opening endoscopic	Y Other device	Z No qualifier
T Diaphragm	0 Open 3 Percutaneous 4 Percutaneous endoscopic	2 Monitoring device M Diaphragmatic pacemaker lead Y Other device	Z No qualifier
T Diaphragm	7 Via natural or artificial opening 8 Via natural or artificial opening endoscopic	Y Other device	Z No qualifier

1ST - 0 Medical and Surgical
2ND - B Respiratory System
3RD - J INSPECTION

EXAMINATION GROUP: Inspection, (Map)
Root Operations involving examination only.

INSPECTION: Visually and/or manually exploring a body part.

Explanation: Direct or instrumental visualization ...
Examples: Diagnostic bronchoscopy – CMS Ex: Exploratory laparotomy

Body Part – 4TH	Approach – 5TH	Device – 6TH	Qualifier –7TH
0 Tracheobronchial Tree 1 Trachea K Lung, Right L Lung, Left Q Pleura T Diaphragm	0 Open 3 Percutaneous 4 Percutaneous endoscopic 7 Via natural or artificial opening 8 Via natural or artificial opening endoscopic X External	Z No device	Z No qualifier

RESPIRATORY 0 B J

© 2018 Channel Publishing, Ltd.

1ST - 0 Medical and Surgical
2ND - B Respiratory System
3RD - L OCCLUSION

TUBULAR GROUP: Bypass, Dilation, Occlusion, Restriction
Root Operations that alter the diameter/route of a tubular body part.

OCCLUSION: Completely closing an orifice or the lumen of a tubular body part.

Explanation: The orifice can be a natural orifice or an artificially created orifice
Examples: Suture closure bronchus – CMS Ex: Fallopian tube ligation

Body Part – 4TH	Approach – 5TH	Device – 6TH	Qualifier – 7TH
1 Trachea 2 Carina 3 Main Bronchus, Right 4 Upper Lobe Bronchus, Right 5 Middle Lobe Bronchus, Right 6 Lower Lobe Bronchus, Right 7 Main Bronchus, Left 8 Upper Lobe Bronchus, Left 9 Lingula Bronchus B Lower Lobe Bronchus, Left	0 Open 3 Percutaneous 4 Percutaneous endoscopic	C Extraluminal device D Intraluminal device Z No device	Z No qualifier
1 Trachea 2 Carina 3 Main Bronchus, Right 4 Upper Lobe Bronchus, Right 5 Middle Lobe Bronchus, Right 6 Lower Lobe Bronchus, Right 7 Main Bronchus, Left 8 Upper Lobe Bronchus, Left 9 Lingula Bronchus B Lower Lobe Bronchus, Left	7 Via natural or artificial opening 8 Via natural or artificial opening endoscopic	D Intraluminal device Z No device	Z No qualifier

RESPIRATORY 0BL

1ST - 0 Medical and Surgical
2ND - B Respiratory System
3RD - M REATTACHMENT

MOVE GROUP: Reattachment, Reposition, (Transfer), Transplantation
Root Operations that put in/put back or move some/all of a body part.

REATTACHMENT: Putting back in or on all or a portion of a separated body part to its normal location or other suitable location.

Explanation: Vascular circulation and nervous pathways may or may not be reestablished
Examples: Reattachment ruptured diaphragm – CMS Ex: Reattachment of hand

Body Part – 4TH	Approach – 5TH	Device – 6TH	Qualifier – 7TH
1 Trachea 2 Carina 3 Main Bronchus, Right 4 Upper Lobe Bronchus, Right 5 Middle Lobe Bronchus, Right 6 Lower Lobe Bronchus, Right 7 Main Bronchus, Left 8 Upper Lobe Bronchus, Left 9 Lingula Bronchus B Lower Lobe Bronchus, Left C Upper Lung Lobe, Right D Middle Lung Lobe, Right F Lower Lung Lobe, Right G Upper Lung Lobe, Left H Lung Lingula J Lower Lung Lobe, Left K Lung, Right L Lung, Left T Diaphragm	0 Open	Z No device	Z No qualifier

1ST - 0 Medical and Surgical
2ND - B Respiratory System
3RD - N RELEASE

DIVISION GROUP: (Division), Release
Root Operations involving cutting or separation only.

RELEASE: Freeing a body part from an abnormal physical constraint by cutting or by the use of force.

Explanation: Some of the restraining tissue may be taken out but none of the body part is taken out
Examples: Lysis adhesions lung – CMS Ex: Carpal tunnel release

Body Part – 4TH	Approach – 5TH	Device – 6TH	Qualifier – 7TH
1 Trachea 2 Carina 3 Main Bronchus, Right 4 Upper Lobe Bronchus, Right 5 Middle Lobe Bronchus, Right 6 Lower Lobe Bronchus, Right 7 Main Bronchus, Left 8 Upper Lobe Bronchus, Left 9 Lingula Bronchus B Lower Lobe Bronchus, Left C Upper Lung Lobe, Right D Middle Lung Lobe, Right F Lower Lung Lobe, Right G Upper Lung Lobe, Left H Lung Lingula J Lower Lung Lobe, Left K Lung, Right L Lung, Left M Lungs, Bilateral	0 Open 3 Percutaneous 4 Percutaneous endoscopic 7 Via natural or artificial opening 8 Via natural or artificial opening endoscopic	Z No device	Z No qualifier
N Pleura, Right P Pleura, Left T Diaphragm	0 Open 3 Percutaneous 4 Percutaneous endoscopic	Z No device	Z No qualifier

© 2018 Channel Publishing, Ltd.

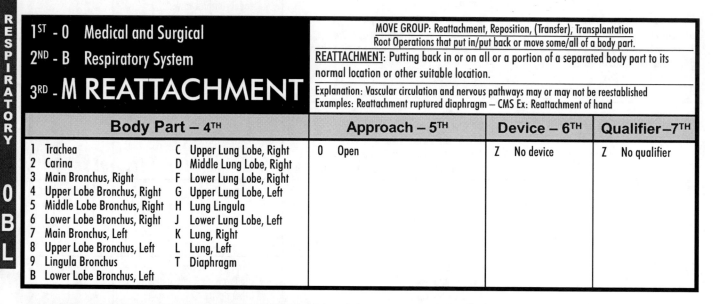

1ST - 0 Medical and Surgical
2ND - B Respiratory System
3RD - P REMOVAL

DEVICE GROUP: Change, Insertion, Removal, Replacement, Revision, Supplement
Root Operations that always involve a device.

REMOVAL: Taking out or off a device from a body part.

Explanation: Removal device without reinsertion ...
Examples: Removal tracheostomy tube – CMS Ex: Cardiac pacemaker removal

Body Part – 4TH	Approach – 5TH	Device – 6TH	Qualifier 7TH
0 Tracheobronchial Tree	0 Open 3 Percutaneous 4 Percutaneous endoscopic 7 Via natural or artificial opening 8 Via natural or artificial opening endoscopic	0 Drainage device 1 Radioactive element 2 Monitoring device 3 Infusion device 7 Autologous tissue substitute C Extraluminal device D Intraluminal device J Synthetic substitute K Nonautologous tissue substitute Y Other device	Z No qualifier
0 Tracheobronchial Tree	X External	0 Drainage device 1 Radioactive element 2 Monitoring device 3 Infusion device D Intraluminal device	Z No qualifier
1 Trachea	0 Open 3 Percutaneous 4 Percutaneous endoscopic 7 Via natural or artificial opening 8 Via natural or artificial opening endoscopic	0 Drainage device 2 Monitoring device 7 Autologous tissue substitute C Extraluminal device D Intraluminal device F Tracheostomy device J Synthetic substitute K Nonautologous tissue substitute	Z No qualifier
1 Trachea	X External	0 Drainage device 2 Monitoring device D Intraluminal device F Tracheostomy device	Z No qualifier
K Lung, Right L Lung, Left	0 Open 3 Percutaneous 4 Percutaneous endoscopic 7 Via natural or artificial opening 8 Via natural or artificial opening endoscopic	0 Drainage device 1 Radioactive element 2 Monitoring device 3 Infusion device Y Other device	Z No qualifier
K Lung, Right L Lung, Left	X External	0 Drainage device 1 Radioactive element 2 Monitoring device 3 Infusion device	Z No qualifier
Q Pleura	0 Open 3 Percutaneous 4 Percutaneous endoscopic 7 Via natural or artificial opening 8 Via natural or artificial opening endoscopic	0 Drainage device 1 Radioactive element 2 Monitoring device Y Other device	Z No qualifier
Q Pleura	X External	0 Drainage device 1 Radioactive element 2 Monitoring device	Z No qualifier
T Diaphragm	0 Open 3 Percutaneous 4 Percutaneous endoscopic 7 Via natural or artificial opening 8 Via natural or artificial opening endoscopic	0 Drainage device 2 Monitoring device 7 Autologous tissue substitute J Synthetic substitute K Nonautologous tissue substitute M Diaphragmatic pacemaker lead Y Other device	Z No qualifier
T Diaphragm	X External	0 Drainage device 2 Monitoring device M Diaphragmatic pacemaker lead	Z No qualifier

© 2018 Channel Publishing, Ltd.

1ST - 0 Medical and Surgical
2ND - B Respiratory System
3RD - Q REPAIR

OTHER REPAIRS GROUP: (Control), Repair
Root Operations that define other repairs.

REPAIR: Restoring, to the extent possible, a body part to its normal anatomic structure and function.

Explanation: Used only when the method to accomplish the repair is not one of the other root operations
Examples: Repair diaphragmatic hernia – CMS Ex: Suture of laceration

Body Part – 4TH	Approach – 5TH	Device – 6TH	Qualifier – 7TH
1 Trachea 2 Carina 3 Main Bronchus, Right 4 Upper Lobe Bronchus, Right 5 Middle Lobe Bronchus, Right 6 Lower Lobe Bronchus, Right 7 Main Bronchus, Left 8 Upper Lobe Bronchus, Left 9 Lingula Bronchus B Lower Lobe Bronchus, Left C Upper Lung Lobe, Right D Middle Lung Lobe, Right F Lower Lung Lobe, Right G Upper Lung Lobe, Left H Lung Lingula J Lower Lung Lobe, Left K Lung, Right L Lung, Left M Lungs, Bilateral	0 Open 3 Percutaneous 4 Percutaneous endoscopic 7 Via natural or artificial opening 8 Via natural or artificial opening endoscopic	Z No device	Z No qualifier
N Pleura, Right P Pleura, Left T Diaphragm	0 Open 3 Percutaneous 4 Percutaneous endoscopic	Z No device	Z No qualifier

1ST - 0 Medical and Surgical
2ND - B Respiratory System
3RD - R REPLACEMENT

DEVICE GROUP: Change, Insertion, Removal, Replacement, Revision, Supplement
Root Operations that always involve a device.

REPLACEMENT: Putting in or on biological or synthetic material that physically takes the place and/or function of all or a portion of a body part.

Explanation: Includes taking out or eradicating, or rendering non-functional, the body part ...
Examples: Artificial tracheal implant – CMS Ex: Total hip replacement

Body Part – 4TH	Approach – 5TH	Device – 6TH	Qualifier – 7TH
1 Trachea 2 Carina 3 Main Bronchus, Right 4 Upper Lobe Bronchus, Right 5 Middle Lobe Bronchus, Right 6 Lower Lobe Bronchus, Right 7 Main Bronchus, Left 8 Upper Lobe Bronchus, Left 9 Lingula Bronchus B Lower Lobe Bronchus, Left T Diaphragm	0 Open 4 Percutaneous endoscopic	7 Autologous tissue substitute J Synthetic substitute K Nonautologous tissue substitute	Z No qualifier

1ST - 0 Medical and Surgical
2ND - B Respiratory System
3RD - S REPOSITION

MOVE GROUP: Reattachment, Reposition, (Transfer), Transplantation
Root Operations that put in/put back or move some/all of a body part.

REPOSITION: Moving to its normal location, or other suitable location, all or a portion of a body part.

Explanation: The body part may or may not be cut out or off to be moved to the new location ...
Examples: Tracheal relocation – CMS Ex: Fracture reduction

Body Part – 4TH	Approach – 5TH	Device – 6TH	Qualifier – 7TH
1 Trachea 2 Carina 3 Main Bronchus, Right 4 Upper Lobe Bronchus, Right 5 Middle Lobe Bronchus, Right 6 Lower Lobe Bronchus, Right 7 Main Bronchus, Left 8 Upper Lobe Bronchus, Left 9 Lingula Bronchus B Lower Lobe Bronchus, Left C Upper Lung Lobe, Right D Middle Lung Lobe, Right F Lower Lung Lobe, Right G Upper Lung Lobe, Left H Lung Lingula J Lower Lung Lobe, Left K Lung, Right L Lung, Left T Diaphragm	0 Open	Z No device	Z No qualifier

© 2018 Channel Publishing, Ltd.

1ST - 0 Medical and Surgical
2ND - B Respiratory System
3RD - T RESECTION

EXCISION GROUP: Excision, Resection, Destruction, Extraction, (Detachment)
Root Operations that take out some or all of a body part.

RESECTION: Cutting out or off, without replacement, all of a body part.

Explanation: None
Examples: Lobectomy – CMS Ex: Total lobectomy of lung

Body Part – 4TH	Approach – 5TH	Device – 6TH	Qualifier – 7TH
1 Trachea 2 Carina 3 Main Bronchus, Right 4 Upper Lobe Bronchus, Right 5 Middle Lobe Bronchus, Right 6 Lower Lobe Bronchus, Right 7 Main Bronchus, Left 8 Upper Lobe Bronchus, Left 9 Lingula Bronchus B Lower Lobe Bronchus, Left C Upper Lung Lobe, Right D Middle Lung Lobe, Right F Lower Lung Lobe, Right G Upper Lung Lobe, Left H Lung Lingula J Lower Lung Lobe, Left K Lung, Right L Lung, Left M Lungs, Bilateral T Diaphragm	0 Open 4 Percutaneous endoscopic	Z No device	Z No qualifier

1ST - 0 Medical and Surgical
2ND - B Respiratory System
3RD - U SUPPLEMENT

DEVICE GROUP: Change, Insertion, Removal, Replacement, Revision, Supplement
Root Operations that always involve a device.

SUPPLEMENT: Putting in or on biological or synthetic material that physically reinforces and/or augments the function of a portion of a body part.

Explanation: Biological material is non living, or is living and from the same individual ...
Examples: Graft repair diaphragm defect – CMS Ex: Herniorrhaphy using mesh

Body Part – 4TH	Approach – 5TH	Device – 6TH	Qualifier – 7TH
1 Trachea 2 Carina 3 Main Bronchus, Right 4 Upper Lobe Bronchus, Right 5 Middle Lobe Bronchus, Right 6 Lower Lobe Bronchus, Right 7 Main Bronchus, Left 8 Upper Lobe Bronchus, Left 9 Lingula Bronchus B Lower Lobe Bronchus, Left	0 Open 4 Percutaneous endoscopic 8 Via natural or artificial opening endoscopic	7 Autologous tissue substitute J Synthetic substitute K Nonautologous tissue substitute	Z No qualifier
T Diaphragm	0 Open 4 Percutaneous endoscopic	7 Autologous tissue substitute J Synthetic substitute K Nonautologous tissue substitute	Z No qualifier

1ST - 0 Medical and Surgical
2ND - B Respiratory System
3RD - V RESTRICTION

TUBULAR GROUP: Bypass, Dilation, Occlusion, Restriction
Root Operations that alter the diameter/route of a tubular body part.

RESTRICTION: Partially closing an orifice or the lumen of a tubular body part.

Explanation: The orifice can be a natural orifice or an artificially created orifice.
Examples: Bronchial restrictive stent – CMS Ex: Cervical cerclage

Body Part – 4TH	Approach – 5TH	Device – 6TH	Qualifier – 7TH
1 Trachea 2 Carina 3 Main Bronchus, Right 4 Upper Lobe Bronchus, Right 5 Middle Lobe Bronchus, Right 6 Lower Lobe Bronchus, Right 7 Main Bronchus, Left 8 Upper Lobe Bronchus, Left 9 Lingula Bronchus B Lower Lobe Bronchus, Left	0 Open 3 Percutaneous 4 Percutaneous endoscopic	C Extraluminal device D Intraluminal device Z No device	Z No qualifier
1 Trachea 2 Carina 3 Main Bronchus, Right 4 Upper Lobe Bronchus, Right 5 Middle Lobe Bronchus, Right 6 Lower Lobe Bronchus, Right 7 Main Bronchus, Left 8 Upper Lobe Bronchus, Left 9 Lingula Bronchus B Lower Lobe Bronchus, Left	7 Via natural or artificial opening 8 Via natural or artificial opening endoscopic	D Intraluminal device Z No device	Z No qualifier

© 2018 Channel Publishing, Ltd.

1ST - 0 Medical and Surgical
2ND - B Respiratory System
3RD - W REVISION

DEVICE GROUP: Change, Insertion, Removal, Replacement, Revision, Supplement
Root Operations that always involve a device.

REVISION: Correcting, to the extent possible, a portion of a malfunctioning device or the position of a displaced device.

Explanation: Correcting by taking out or putting in components of a device such as a screw or pin ...
Examples: Reposition diaphragmatic pacemaker lead – CMS Ex: Recementing of hip prosthesis

Body Part – 4TH	Approach – 5TH	Device – 6TH	Qualifier – 7TH
0 Tracheobronchial Tree	0 Open 3 Percutaneous 4 Percutaneous endoscopic 7 Via natural or artificial opening 8 Via natural or artificial opening endoscopic	0 Drainage device 2 Monitoring device 3 Infusion device 7 Autologous tissue substitute C Extraluminal device D Intraluminal device J Synthetic substitute K Nonautologous tissue substitute Y Other device	Z No qualifier
0 Tracheobronchial Tree	X External	0 Drainage device 2 Monitoring device 3 Infusion device 7 Autologous tissue substitute C Extraluminal device D Intraluminal device J Synthetic substitute K Nonautologous tissue substitute	Z No qualifier
1 Trachea	0 Open 3 Percutaneous 4 Percutaneous endoscopic 7 Via natural or artificial opening 8 Via natural or artificial opening endoscopic X External	0 Drainage device 2 Monitoring device 7 Autologous tissue substitute C Extraluminal device D Intraluminal device F Tracheostomy device J Synthetic substitute K Nonautologous tissue substitute	Z No qualifier
K Lung, Right L Lung, Left	0 Open 3 Percutaneous 4 Percutaneous endoscopic 7 Via natural or artificial opening 8 Via natural or artificial opening endoscopic	0 Drainage device 2 Monitoring device 3 Infusion device Y Other device	Z No qualifier
K Lung, Right L Lung, Left	X External	0 Drainage device 2 Monitoring device 3 Infusion device	Z No qualifier
Q Pleura	0 Open 3 Percutaneous 4 Percutaneous endoscopic 7 Via natural or artificial opening 8 Via natural or artificial opening endoscopic	0 Drainage device 2 Monitoring device Y Other device	Z No qualifier
Q Pleura	X External	0 Drainage device 2 Monitoring device	Z No qualifier
T Diaphragm	0 Open 3 Percutaneous 4 Percutaneous endoscopic 7 Via natural or artificial opening 8 Via natural or artificial opening endoscopic	0 Drainage device 2 Monitoring device 7 Autologous tissue substitute J Synthetic substitute K Nonautologous tissue substitute M Diaphragmatic pacemaker lead Y Other device	Z No qualifier
T Diaphragm	X External	0 Drainage device 2 Monitoring device 7 Autologous tissue substitute J Synthetic substitute K Nonautologous tissue substitute M Diaphragmatic pacemaker lead	Z No qualifier

© 2018 Channel Publishing, Ltd.

1ST - 0 Medical and Surgical 2ND - B Respiratory System 3RD - Y TRANSPLANTATION	MOVE GROUP: Reattachment, Reposition, (Transfer), Transplantation Root Operations that put in/put back or move some/all of a body part. TRANSPLANTATION: Putting in or on all or a portion of a living body part taken from another individual or animal to physically take the place and/or function of all or a portion of a similar body part. Explanation: The native body part may or may not be taken out ... Examples: Lung transplant – CMS Ex: Kidney transplant

Body Part – 4TH	Approach – 5TH	Device – 6TH	Qualifier – 7TH
C Upper Lung Lobe, Right LC* D Middle Lung Lobe, Right LC* F Lower Lung Lobe, Right LC* G Upper Lung Lobe, Left LC* H Lung Lingula LC* J Lower Lung Lobe, Left LC* K Lung, Right LC* L Lung, Left LC* M Lungs, Bilateral LC*	0 Open	Z No device	0 Allogeneic 1 Syngeneic 2 Zooplastic

LC* – Some procedures are considered limited coverage by Medicare. See current Medicare Code Editor for details.

© 2018 Channel Publishing, Ltd.

NOTES

© 2018 Channel Publishing, Ltd.

Educational Annotations | C – Mouth and Throat

Body System Specific Educational Annotations for the Mouth and Throat include:

- Anatomy and Physiology Review
- Anatomical Illustrations
- Definitions of Common Procedures
- AHA Coding Clinic® Reference Notations
- Body Part Key Listings
- Device Key Listings
- Device Aggregation Table Listings
- Coding Notes

Anatomy and Physiology Review of Mouth and Throat

BODY PART VALUES – C - MOUTH AND THROAT

Adenoids – ANATOMY – The adenoids (nasopharyngeal tonsils) are masses of lymphatic tissue located behind the nasal cavity and on roof of the nasopharynx. PHYSIOLOGY – The adenoids help in the prevention of bacteria entering the body.

Buccal Mucosa – The mucous membrane lining of the mouth and inside of cheeks.

Epiglottis – ANATOMY – The epiglottis is a mucous-membrane-covered flap of elastic cartilage tissue that is attached to the entrance of the larynx. PHYSIOLOGY – The epiglottis prevents food from going into the trachea and channels it into the esophagus.

Gingiva – ANATOMY – The gingiva (gums) are fibrous and mucous membrane tissue that surround the roots of erupted teeth and the crowns of unerupted teeth, and cover the alveolar process of the maxilla and mandible. PHYSIOLOGY – The gingiva (gums) function to help protect and support the roots of the teeth.

Hard Palate – The hard palate is the superior wall of the oral cavity formed by the palatine processes of the maxilla that separates the oral cavity from the nasal cavity.

Larynx – ANATOMY – The larynx is the musculocartilaginous structure, lined with mucous membrane located between the root of the tongue and the trachea. The glottis is the slit like opening of the larynx formed by the true vocal cords. The supraglottis is that portion of the larynx situated above the glottis. There are nine laryngeal cartilages, three paired and three single. PHYSIOLOGY – The larynx functions to guard the entrance of the trachea from food and liquids, to control the expulsion of air, and to produce sound. The glottis produces sound, controls pitch, and when closed prevents food from entering the trachea. The supraglottis is an area of the larynx which helps to prevent food and liquid from entering the trachea. The laryngeal cartilages frame and support the larynx and its muscles.

Lip – ANATOMY – The soft tissue opening of the mouth comprised of skin, connective tissue, and muscle. PHYSIOLOGY – The lips contain sensitive nerve endings that provide sensory information about food. The lips secure the closure of the mouth during chewing and swallowing. They also are involved in sound production and facial expression.

Minor Salivary Gland – Any of the large number of small salivary glands in the oral mucosa of the mouth.

Parotid Duct – The tube (Stenson's ducts) beginning in the parotid gland and emptying into the oral cavity.

Parotid Gland – The two parotid glands lie above the mouth, and below and in front of the ears, with ducts (Stenson's ducts) that run down through the cheeks and empty into the roof of the mouth opposite of the second molar.

Pharynx – ANATOMY – The portion of the throat comprised of the oropharynx and the laryngopharynx. PHYSIOLOGY – The pharynx serves as a passageway for food and air.

Salivary Gland – ANATOMY – There are three pairs of major salivary glands; the parotids, the submandibular, and the sublingual glands. Both sympathetic and parasympathetic nerves stimulate the major salivary glands. PHYSIOLOGY – The major salivary glands function to secrete saliva which moistens food particles, help to bind them together, and begin digestion of carbohydrates. Saliva also dissolves various food chemicals so they can be tasted. There are two types of secretory cells. Serous cells produce a watery fluid which contain a digestive enzyme called amylase. Mucous cells produce a thick stringy liquid that bind food together and act as a lubricant during swallowing. Sympathetic nerves stimulate the glands to secrete a small quantity of saliva to keep the mouth moist. Parasympathetic nerves stimulate the glands reflexly when the person sees, smells, or even thinks about pleasant food.

Soft Palate – ANATOMY – The soft palate is the muscular extension of the hard palate in the superior-posterior oral cavity. PHYSIOLOGY – The soft palate contracts to allow swallowing and prevents food from entering the nasal cavity.

Subligual Gland – The two sublingual glands lie beneath the tongue, with ducts opening near the frenulum of the tongue.

Submaxillary Gland – The two submaxillary (submandibular) glands lie in the floor of the mouth on the inside surface of the mandible, with ducts (Wharton's ducts) opening beneath the tongue, and with other ducts opening near the frenulum of the tongue.

Teeth – ANATOMY – The teeth consist of the bony substance dentine, which surround the soft inner pulp that contain blood vessels and nerves and are embedded in rows in the upper (maxilla) and lower (mandible) jaw bones. PHYSIOLOGY – The teeth function primarily to chew food into smaller parts in preparation for swallowing and digestion.

Tongue – ANATOMY – The tongue is the movable, muscular organ on the floor of the mouth. The lingual tonsils are a mass of lymphoid tissue at the root, and the frenulum is the mucous membrane fold which attaches the undersurface of the tongue to the floor of the mouth. PHYSIOLOGY – The tongue functions primarily as the organ of sense of taste, as well as aiding in the chewing and swallowing of food, and the articulation of sound. The lingual tonsils aid in the elimination of bacteria entering the oral cavity. The frenulum somewhat restricts the movement of the tongue.

Tonsils – ANATOMY – The tonsils (palatine tonsils) are masses of lymphatic tissue located on either side of the tongue in the posterior oral cavity. The tonsillar fossa is the depression in which the tonsils are located. The tonsillar pillars are the mucous membrane folds attached to the soft palate. PHYSIOLOGY – The tonsils function to help fight off bacteria by releasing bacteria-consuming phagocytes.

Uvula – The uvula is the cone-shaped projection of the soft palate.

Vocal Cord – ANATOMY – The vocal cords are folds of mucous membranes located within the larynx. PHYSIOLOGY – The vocal cords are primarily responsible for voice production. Sound is produced by the vibration of the folds as air is exhaled from the lungs.

© 2018 Channel Publishing, Ltd.

Educational Annotations | C – Mouth and Throat

Anatomical Illustrations of Mouth and Throat

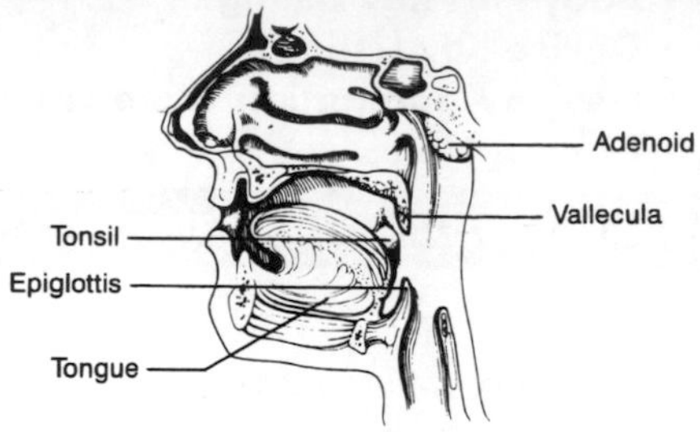

OROPHARYNX

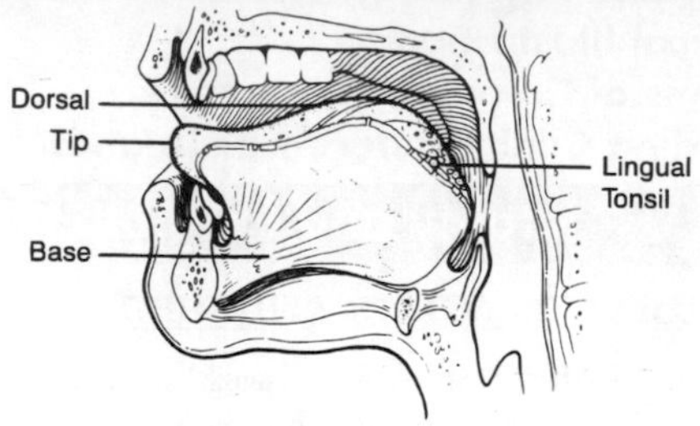

TONGUE — SAGITTAL VIEW

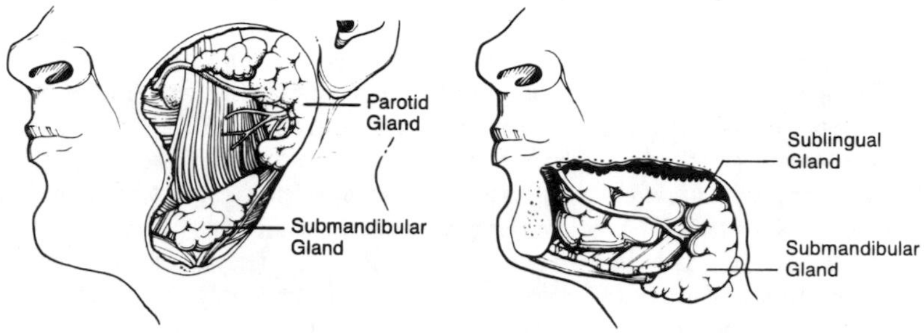

MAJOR SALIVARY GLANDS

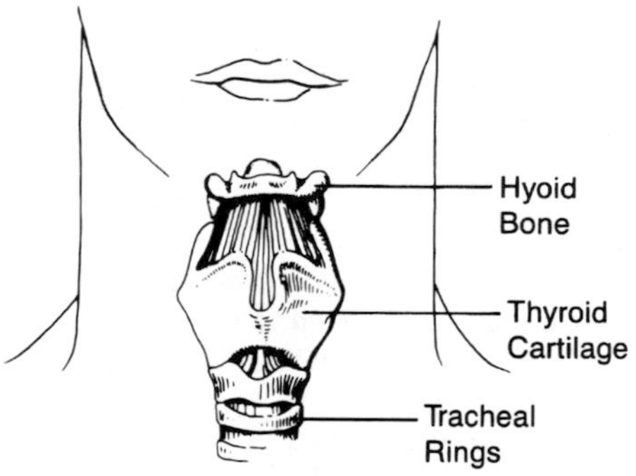

LARYNX

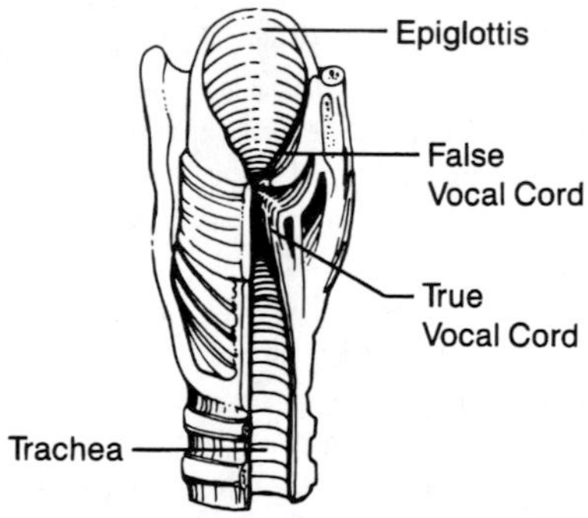

LARYNX — ANTERIOR (CUT-AWAY) VIEW

Definitions of Common Procedures of Mouth and Throat

Ablation of vocal cord lesion – The destruction of a vocal cord lesion using a tissue destroying technique (laser, radiofrequency heat, etc.).
Cleft palate repair – The reconstructing surgical repair of a cleft palate (defect in the roof of the mouth) by excising and moving tissue from the palate and other oral tissues and closing in layers while realigning the palatal muscles.
Glossectomy – The excision of all or a portion of the tongue.
Laser-assisted uvuloplasty – The use of repeated laser treatments to destroy and modify the uvula tissue in order to reduce or eliminate snoring.
Sialoadenectomy – The excision of a salivary gland.
Sialolithotomy – The incision of a salivary gland to remove a stone from the gland or its duct.
Tonsillectomy – The excision of the tonsils performed by a direct approach (external).
Total laryngectomy – The surgical removal of all of the larynx and usually with the insertion of an artificial voice box prosthesis.
Uvulopalatopharyngoplasty – The reconstructing surgical repair of the back of the oral cavity by removing the tonsils, and reshaping the uvula, pharynx, and soft palate to correct obstructive sleep apnea.

© 2018 Channel Publishing, Ltd.

Educational Annotations | C – Mouth and Throat

AHA Coding Clinic® Reference Notations of Mouth and Throat

ROOT OPERATION SPECIFIC - C - MOUTH AND THROAT

ALTERATION - 0
CHANGE - 2
DESTRUCTION - 5
DILATION - 7
DRAINAGE - 9
EXCISION - B
- Biopsy of base of tongue ....AHA 16:2Q:p19
- Lingual tonsillectomy ....AHA 16:3Q:p28
- Superficial parotidectomy....AHA 14:3Q:p21

EXTIRPATION - C
- Submandibular gland stone removal with sialoendoscope ....AHA 16:2Q:p20

EXTRACTION - D
FRAGMENTATION - F
INSERTION - H
INSPECTION - J
OCCLUSION - L
REATTACHMENT - M
RELEASE - N
REMOVAL - P
REPAIR - Q
- Nasal adhesion repair of cleft lip and palate ....AHA 17:1Q:p20

REPLACEMENT - R
- Intraoral graft using Oasis® acellular matrix ....AHA 14:2Q:p5,6
- Wide local excision of soft palate with placement of a maxillary surgical obturator ....AHA 14:3Q:p25

REPOSITION - S
- Epiglottopexy ....AHA 16:3Q:p28

RESECTION - T
- Extraction of impacted teeth ....AHA 14:3Q:p23
- Infratemporal fossa malignancy with parotidectomy ....AHA 16:2Q:p12

SUPPLEMENT - U
RESTRICTION - V
REVISION - W
TRANSFER - X

MOUTH & THROAT 0C

© 2018 Channel Publishing, Ltd.

Educational Annotations | C – Mouth and Throat

Body Part Key Listings of Mouth and Throat

See also Body Part Key in Appendix C

Anterior lingual gland ....use Minor Salivary Gland
Aryepiglottic fold ....use Larynx
Arytenoid cartilage ....use Larynx
Base of tongue ....use Pharynx
Buccal gland ....use Buccal Mucosa
Corniculate cartilage ....use Larynx
Cuneiform cartilage ....use Larynx
False vocal cord ....use Larynx
Frenulum labii inferioris ....use Lower Lip
Frenulum labii superioris ....use Upper Lip
Frenulum linguae ....use Tongue
Glossoepiglottic fold ....use Epiglottis
Glottis ....use Larynx
Hypopharynx ....use Pharynx
Labial gland ....use Upper Lip, Lower Lip
Laryngopharynx ....use Pharynx
Lingual tonsil ....use Pharynx
Molar gland ....use Buccal Mucosa
Oropharynx ....use Pharynx
Palatine gland ....use Buccal Mucosa
Palatine tonsil ....use Tonsils
Palatine uvula ....use Uvula
Pharyngeal tonsil ....use Adenoids
Piriform recess (sinus) ....use Pharynx
Rima glottidis ....use Larynx
Stensen's duct ....use Parotid Duct, Left/Right
Submandibular gland ....use Submaxillary Gland, Left/Right
Thyroid cartilage ....use Larynx
Tongue, base of ....use Pharynx
Ventricular fold ....use Larynx
Vermilion border ....use Upper Lip, Lower Lip
Vocal fold ....use Vocal Cord, Left/Right

Device Key Listings of Mouth and Throat

See also Device Key in Appendix D

Autograft ....use Autologous Tissue Substitute
Brachytherapy seeds ....use Radioactive Element
Guedel airway ....use Intraluminal Device, Airway in Mouth and Throat
Oropharyngeal airway (OPA) ....use Intraluminal Device, Airway in Mouth and Throat
Tissue bank graft ....use Nonautologous Tissue Substitute

Device Aggregation Table Listings of Mouth and Throat

See also Device Aggregation Table in Appendix E

Specific Device	For Operation	In Body System	General Device
Intraluminal Device, Airway	All applicable	Mouth and Throat	Intraluminal Device

Coding Notes of Mouth and Throat

MOUTH & THROAT 0C

© 2018 Channel Publishing, Ltd.

1ST - 0 Medical and Surgical
2ND - C Mouth and Throat
3RD - 0 ALTERATION

OTHER OBJECTIVES GROUP: Alteration, (Creation), (Fusion)
Root Operations that define other objectives.

ALTERATION: Modifying the anatomic structure of a body part without affecting the function of the body part.

Explanation: Principal purpose is to improve appearance
Examples: Cosmetic lip augmentation – CMS Ex: Face lift

Body Part – 4TH	Approach – 5TH	Device – 6TH	Qualifier – 7TH
0 Upper Lip 1 Lower Lip	X External	7 Autologous tissue substitute J Synthetic substitute K Nonautologous tissue substitute Z No device	Z No qualifier

1ST - 0 Medical and Surgical
2ND - C Mouth and Throat
3RD - 2 CHANGE

DEVICE GROUP: Change, Insertion, Removal, Replacement, Revision, Supplement
Root Operations that always involve a device.

CHANGE: Taking out or off a device from a body part and putting back an identical or similar device in or on the same body part without cutting or puncturing the skin or a mucous membrane.

Explanation: All CHANGE procedures are coded using the approach External
Examples: Exchange drain tube – CMS Ex: Urinary catheter change

Body Part – 4TH	Approach – 5TH	Device – 6TH	Qualifier – 7TH
A Salivary Gland S Larynx Y Mouth and Throat	X External	0 Drainage device Y Other device	Z No qualifier

1ST - 0 Medical and Surgical
2ND - C Mouth and Throat
3RD - 5 DESTRUCTION

EXCISION GROUP: Excision, Resection, Destruction, Extraction, (Detachment)
Root Operations that take out some or all of a body part.

DESTRUCTION: Physical eradication of all or a portion of a body part by the direct use of energy, force, or a destructive agent.

Explanation: None of the body part is physically taken out
Examples: Ablation voccal cord lesion – CMS Ex: Fulguration of rectal polyp

Body Part – 4TH		Approach – 5TH	Device – 6TH	Qualifier – 7TH
0 Upper Lip 1 Lower Lip 2 Hard Palate 3 Soft Palate 4 Buccal Mucosa	5 Upper Gingiva 6 Lower Gingiva 7 Tongue N Uvula P Tonsils Q Adenoids	0 Open 3 Percutaneous X External	Z No device	Z No qualifier
8 Parotid Gland, Right 9 Parotid Gland, Left B Parotid Duct, Right C Parotid Duct, Left	D Sublingual Gland, Right F Sublingual Gland, Left G Submaxillary Gland, Right H Submaxillary Gland, Left J Minor Salivary Gland	0 Open 3 Percutaneous	Z No device	Z No qualifier
M Pharynx R Epiglottis S Larynx T Vocal Cord, Right V Vocal Cord, Left		0 Open 3 Percutaneous 4 Percutaneous endoscopic 7 Via natural or artificial opening 8 Via natural or artificial opening endoscopic	Z No device	Z No qualifier
W Upper Tooth X Lower Tooth		0 Open X External	Z No device	0 Single 1 Multiple 2 All

© 2018 Channel Publishing, Ltd.

1ST - 0 Medical and Surgical
2ND - C Mouth and Throat
3RD - 7 **DILATION**

TUBULAR GROUP: (Bypass), Dilation, Occlusion, Restriction
Root Operations that alter the diameter/route of a tubular body part.

DILATION: Expanding an orifice or the lumen of a tubular body part.

Explanation: Accomplished by stretching or cutting ... tubular body part or orifice ...
Examples: Dilation laryngeal stenosis – CMS Ex: Percutaneous transluminal angioplasty

Body Part – 4TH	Approach – 5TH	Device – 6TH	Qualifier – 7TH
B Parotid Duct, Right C Parotid Duct, Left	0 Open 3 Percutaneous 7 Via natural or artificial opening	D Intraluminal device Z No device	Z No qualifier
M Pharynx	7 Via natural or artificial opening 8 Via natural or artificial opening endoscopic	D Intraluminal device Z No device	Z No qualifier
S Larynx	0 Open 3 Percutaneous 4 Percutaneous endoscopic 7 Via natural or artificial opening 8 Via natural or artificial opening endoscopic	D Intraluminal device Z No device	Z No qualifier

1ST - 0 Medical and Surgical
2ND - C Mouth and Throat
3RD - 9 **DRAINAGE**

DRAINAGE GROUP: Drainage, Extirpation, Fragmentation
Root Operations that take out solids/fluids/gases from a body part.

DRAINAGE: Taking or letting out fluids and/or gases from a body part.

Explanation: Qualifier "X Diagnostic" indicates drainage procedures that are biopsies
Examples: I&D parotid gland abscess – CMS Ex: Thoracentesis

Body Part – 4TH	Approach – 5TH	Device – 6TH	Qualifier – 7TH
0 Upper Lip 1 Lower Lip 2 Hard Palate 3 Soft Palate 4 Buccal Mucosa 5 Upper Gingiva 6 Lower Gingiva 7 Tongue N Uvula P Tonsils Q Adenoids	0 Open 3 Percutaneous X External	0 Drainage device	Z No qualifier
0 Upper Lip 1 Lower Lip 2 Hard Palate 3 Soft Palate 4 Buccal Mucosa 5 Upper Gingiva 6 Lower Gingiva 7 Tongue N Uvula P Tonsils Q Adenoids	0 Open 3 Percutaneous X External	Z No device	X Diagnostic Z No qualifier
8 Parotid Gland, Right 9 Parotid Gland, Left B Parotid Duct, Right C Parotid Duct, Left D Sublingual Gland, Right F Sublingual Gland, Left G Submaxillary Gland, Right H Submaxillary Gland, Left J Minor Salivary Gland	0 Open 3 Percutaneous	0 Drainage device	Z No qualifier
8 Parotid Gland, Right 9 Parotid Gland, Left B Parotid Duct, Right C Parotid Duct, Left D Sublingual Gland, Right F Sublingual Gland, Left G Submaxillary Gland, Right H Submaxillary Gland, Left J Minor Salivary Gland	0 Open 3 Percutaneous	Z No device	X Diagnostic Z No qualifier
M Pharynx R Epiglottis S Larynx T Vocal Cord, Right V Vocal Cord, Left	0 Open 3 Percutaneous 4 Percutaneous endoscopic 7 Via natural or artificial opening 8 Via natural or artificial opening endoscopic	0 Drainage device	Z No qualifier
M Pharynx R Epiglottis S Larynx T Vocal Cord, Right V Vocal Cord, Left	0 Open 3 Percutaneous 4 Percutaneous endoscopic 7 Via natural or artificial opening 8 Via natural or artificial opening endoscopic	Z No device	X Diagnostic Z No qualifier
W Upper Tooth X Lower Tooth	0 Open X External	0 Drainage device Z No device	0 Single 1 Multiple 2 All

© 2018 Channel Publishing, Ltd.

1ST - 0 Medical and Surgical
2ND - C Mouth and Throat
3RD - B EXCISION

EXCISION GROUP: Excision, Resection, Destruction, Extraction, (Detachment)
Root Operations that take out some or all of a body part.

EXCISION: Cutting out or off, without replacement, a portion of a body part.

Explanation: Qualifier "X Diagnostic" indicates excision procedures that are biopsies
Examples: Excision lesion lip – CMS Ex: Liver biopsy

Body Part – 4TH		Approach – 5TH	Device – 6TH	Qualifier – 7TH
0 Upper Lip 1 Lower Lip 2 Hard Palate 3 Soft Palate 4 Buccal Mucosa	5 Upper Gingiva 6 Lower Gingiva 7 Tongue N Uvula P Tonsils Q Adenoids	0 Open 3 Percutaneous X External	Z No device	X Diagnostic Z No qualifier
8 Parotid Gland, Right 9 Parotid Gland, Left B Parotid Duct, Right C Parotid Duct, Left	D Sublingual Gland, Right F Sublingual Gland, Left G Submaxillary Gland, Right H Submaxillary Gland, Left J Minor Salivary Gland	0 Open 3 Percutaneous	Z No device	X Diagnostic Z No qualifier
M Pharynx R Epiglottis S Larynx T Vocal Cord, Right V Vocal Cord, Left		0 Open 3 Percutaneous 4 Percutaneous endoscopic 7 Via natural or artificial opening 8 Via natural or artificial opening endoscopic	Z No device	X Diagnostic Z No qualifier
W Upper Tooth X Lower Tooth		0 Open X External	Z No device	0 Single 1 Multiple 2 All

1ST - 0 Medical and Surgical
2ND - C Mouth and Throat
3RD - C EXTIRPATION

DRAINAGE GROUP: Drainage, Extirpation, Fragmentation
Root Operations that take out solids/fluids/gases from a body part.

EXTIRPATION: Taking or cutting out solid matter from a body part.

Explanation: Abnormal byproduct or foreign body ...
Examples: Sialolithotomy – CMS Ex: Thrombectomy

Body Part – 4TH		Approach – 5TH	Device – 6TH	Qualifier – 7TH
0 Upper Lip 1 Lower Lip 2 Hard Palate 3 Soft Palate 4 Buccal Mucosa	5 Upper Gingiva 6 Lower Gingiva 7 Tongue N Uvula P Tonsils Q Adenoids	0 Open 3 Percutaneous X External	Z No device	Z No qualifier
8 Parotid Gland, Right 9 Parotid Gland, Left B Parotid Duct, Right C Parotid Duct, Left	D Sublingual Gland, Right F Sublingual Gland, Left G Submaxillary Gland, Right H Submaxillary Gland, Left J Minor Salivary Gland	0 Open 3 Percutaneous	Z No device	Z No qualifier
M Pharynx R Epiglottis S Larynx T Vocal Cord, Right V Vocal Cord, Left		0 Open 3 Percutaneous 4 Percutaneous endoscopic 7 Via natural or artificial opening 8 Via natural or artificial opening endoscopic	Z No device	Z No qualifier
W Upper Tooth X Lower Tooth		0 Open X External	Z No device	0 Single 1 Multiple 2 All

© 2018 Channel Publishing, Ltd.

1ST - 0 Medical and Surgical
2ND - C Mouth and Throat
3RD - D EXTRACTION

EXCISION GROUP: Excision, Resection, Destruction, Extraction, (Detachment)
Root Operations that take out some or all of a body part.

EXTRACTION: Pulling or stripping out or off all or a portion of a body part by the use of force.

Explanation: None for this Body System
Examples: Tooth extraction – CMS Ex: Dilation and curettage

Body Part – 4TH	Approach – 5TH	Device – 6TH	Qualifier – 7TH
T Vocal Cord, Right V Vocal Cord, Left	0 Open 3 Percutaneous 4 Percutaneous endoscopic 7 Via natural or artificial opening 8 Via natural or artificial opening endoscopic	Z No device	Z No qualifier
W Upper Tooth X Lower Tooth	X External	Z No device	0 Single 1 Multiple 2 All

1ST - 0 Medical and Surgical
2ND - C Mouth and Throat
3RD - F FRAGMENTATION

DRAINAGE GROUP: Drainage, Extirpation, Fragmentation
Root Operations that take out solids/fluids/gases from a body part.

FRAGMENTATION: Breaking solid matter in a body part into pieces.

Explanation: Pieces are not taken out during the procedure ...
Examples: Lithotripsy parotid stone – CMS Ex: Extracorporeal shockwave lithotripsy

Body Part – 4TH	Approach – 5TH	Device – 6TH	Qualifier – 7TH
B Parotid Duct, Right C Parotid Duct, Left	0 Open 3 Percutaneous 7 Via natural or artificial opening X External NC*	Z No device	Z No qualifier

NC* – Non-covered by Medicare. See current Medicare Code Editor for details.

1ST - 0 Medical and Surgical
2ND - C Mouth and Throat
3RD - H INSERTION

DEVICE GROUP: Change, Insertion, Removal, Replacement, Revision, Supplement
Root Operations that always involve a device.

INSERTION: Putting in a nonbiological appliance that monitors, assists, performs, or prevents a physiological function but does not physically take the place of a body part.

Explanation: None
Examples: Insertion oral airway – CMS Ex: Insertion of central venous catheter

Body Part – 4TH	Approach – 5TH	Device – 6TH	Qualifier – 7TH
7 Tongue	0 Open 3 Percutaneous X External	1 Radioactive element	Z No qualifier
A Salivary Gland S Larynx	0 Open 3 Percutaneous 7 Via natural or artificial opening 8 Via natural or artificial opening endoscopic	Y Other device	Z No qualifier
Y Mouth and Throat	0 Open 3 Percutaneous	Y Other device	Z No qualifier
Y Mouth and Throat	7 Via natural or artificial opening 8 Via natural or artificial opening endoscopic	B Intraluminal device, airway Y Other device	Z No qualifier

© 2018 Channel Publishing, Ltd.

1ST - 0 Medical and Surgical
2ND - C Mouth and Throat
3RD - J INSPECTION

EXAMINATION GROUP: Inspection, (Map)
Root Operations involving examination only.

INSPECTION: Visually and/or manually exploring a body part.

Explanation: Direct or instrumental visualization ...
Examples: Diagnostic laryngoscopy – CMS Ex: Exploratory laparotomy

Body Part – 4TH	Approach – 5TH	Device – 6TH	Qualifier – 7TH
A Salivary Gland	0 Open 3 Percutaneous X External	Z No device	Z No qualifier
S Larynx Y Mouth and Throat	0 Open 3 Percutaneous 4 Percutaneous endoscopic 7 Via natural or artificial opening 8 Via natural or artificial opening endoscopic X External	Z No device	Z No qualifier

1ST - 0 Medical and Surgical
2ND - C Mouth and Throat
3RD - L OCCLUSION

TUBULAR GROUP: (Bypass), Dilation, Occlusion, Restriction
Root Operations that alter the diameter/route of a tubular body part.

OCCLUSION: Completely closing an orifice or the lumen of a tubular body part.

Explanation: The orifice can be a natural orifice or an artificially created orifice
Examples: Ligation Stensen's duct – CMS Ex: Fallopian tube ligation

Body Part – 4TH	Approach – 5TH	Device – 6TH	Qualifier – 7TH
B Parotid Duct, Right C Parotid Duct, Left	0 Open 3 Percutaneous 4 Percutaneous endoscopic	C Extraluminal device D Intraluminal device Z No device	Z No qualifier
B Parotid Duct, Right C Parotid Duct, Left	7 Via natural or artificial opening 8 Via natural or artificial opening endoscopic	D Intraluminal device Z No device	Z No qualifier

1ST - 0 Medical and Surgical
2ND - C Mouth and Throat
3RD - M REATTACHMENT

MOVE GROUP: Reattachment, Reposition, Transfer, (Transplantation)
Root Operations that put in/put back or move some/all of a body part.

REATTACHMENT: Putting back in or on all or a portion of a separated body part to its normal location or other suitable location.

Explanation: Vascular circulation and nervous pathways may or may not be reestablished
Examples: Replantation tooth – CMS Ex: Reattachment of hand

Body Part – 4TH	Approach – 5TH	Device – 6TH	Qualifier – 7TH
0 Upper Lip 1 Lower Lip 3 Soft Palate 7 Tongue N Uvula	0 Open	Z No device	Z No qualifier
W Upper Tooth X Lower Tooth	0 Open X External	Z No device	0 Single 1 Multiple 2 All

MOUTH & THROAT 0CM

© 2018 Channel Publishing, Ltd.

1ST - 0 Medical and Surgical
2ND - C Mouth and Throat
3RD - N RELEASE

DIVISION GROUP: (Division), Release
Root Operations involving cutting or separation only.

RELEASE: Freeing a body part from an abnormal physical constraint by cutting or by the use of force.

Explanation: Some of the restraining tissue may be taken out but none of the body part is taken out
Examples: Lysis vocal cord adhesions – CMS Ex: Carpal tunnel release

Body Part – 4TH		Approach – 5TH	Device – 6TH	Qualifier – 7TH
0 Upper Lip 1 Lower Lip 2 Hard Palate 3 Soft Palate 4 Buccal Mucosa	5 Upper Gingiva 6 Lower Gingiva 7 Tongue N Uvula P Tonsils Q Adenoids	0 Open 3 Percutaneous X External	Z No device	Z No qualifier
8 Parotid Gland, Right 9 Parotid Gland, Left B Parotid Duct, Right C Parotid Duct, Left	D Sublingual Gland, Right F Sublingual Gland, Left G Submaxillary Gland, Right H Submaxillary Gland, Left J Minor Salivary Gland	0 Open 3 Percutaneous	Z No device	Z No qualifier
M Pharynx R Epiglottis S Larynx T Vocal Cord, Right V Vocal Cord, Left		0 Open 3 Percutaneous 4 Percutaneous endoscopic 7 Via natural or artificial opening 8 Via natural or artificial opening endoscopic	Z No device	Z No qualifier
W Upper Tooth X Lower Tooth		0 Open X External	Z No device	0 Single 1 Multiple 2 All

© 2018 Channel Publishing, Ltd.

1ST - 0 Medical and Surgical
2ND - C Mouth and Throat
3RD - P REMOVAL

DEVICE GROUP: Change, Insertion, Removal, Replacement, Revision, Supplement
Root Operations that always involve a device.

REMOVAL: Taking out or off a device from a body part.

Explanation: Removal device without reinsertion ...
Examples: Removal drain tube – CMS Ex: Cardiac pacemaker removal

Body Part – 4TH	Approach – 5TH	Device – 6TH	Qualifier – 7TH
A Salivary Gland	0 Open 3 Percutaneous	0 Drainage device C Extraluminal device Y Other device	Z No qualifier
A Salivary Gland	7 Via natural or artificial opening 8 Via natural or artificial opening endoscopic	Y Other device	Z No qualifier
S Larynx	0 Open 3 Percutaneous 7 Via natural or artificial opening 8 Via natural or artificial opening endoscopic	0 Drainage device 7 Autologous tissue substitute D Intraluminal device J Synthetic substitute K Nonautologous tissue substitute Y Other device	Z No qualifier
S Larynx	X External	0 Drainage device 7 Autologous tissue substitute D Intraluminal device J Synthetic substitute K Nonautologous tissue substitute	Z No qualifier
Y Mouth and Throat	0 Open 3 Percutaneous 7 Via natural or artificial opening 8 Via natural or artificial opening endoscopic	0 Drainage device 1 Radioactive element 7 Autologous tissue substitute D Intraluminal device J Synthetic substitute K Nonautologous tissue substitute Y Other device	Z No qualifier
Y Mouth and Throat	X External	0 Drainage device 1 Radioactive element 7 Autologous tissue substitute D Intraluminal device J Synthetic substitute K Nonautologous tissue substitute	Z No qualifier

© 2018 Channel Publishing, Ltd.

1ST - 0 Medical and Surgical
2ND - C Mouth and Throat
3RD - Q REPAIR

OTHER REPAIRS GROUP: (Control), Repair
Root Operations that define other repairs.

REPAIR: Restoring, to the extent possible, a body part to its normal anatomic structure and function.

Explanation: Used only when the method to accomplish the repair is not one of the other root operations
Examples: Cleft palate repair – CMS Ex: Suture of laceration

Body Part – 4TH	Approach – 5TH	Device – 6TH	Qualifier – 7TH
0 Upper Lip 1 Lower Lip 2 Hard Palate 3 Soft Palate 4 Buccal Mucosa 5 Upper Gingiva 6 Lower Gingiva 7 Tongue N Uvula P Tonsils Q Adenoids	0 Open 3 Percutaneous X External	Z No device	Z No qualifier
8 Parotid Gland, Right 9 Parotid Gland, Left B Parotid Duct, Right C Parotid Duct, Left D Sublingual Gland, Right F Sublingual Gland, Left G Submaxillary Gland, Right H Submaxillary Gland, Left J Minor Salivary Gland	0 Open 3 Percutaneous	Z No device	Z No qualifier
M Pharynx R Epiglottis S Larynx T Vocal Cord, Right V Vocal Cord, Left	0 Open 3 Percutaneous 4 Percutaneous endoscopic 7 Via natural or artificial opening 8 Via natural or artificial opening endoscopic	Z No device	Z No qualifier
W Upper Tooth X Lower Tooth	0 Open X External	Z No device	0 Single 1 Multiple 2 All

1ST - 0 Medical and Surgical
2ND - C Mouth and Throat
3RD - R REPLACEMENT

DEVICE GROUP: Change, Insertion, Removal, Replacement, Revision, Supplement
Root Operations that always involve a device.

REPLACEMENT: Putting in or on biological or synthetic material that physically takes the place and/or function of all or a portion of a body part.

Explanation: Includes taking out or eradicating, or rendering non-functional, the body part ...
Examples: Parotid duct replacement – CMS Ex: Total hip replacement

Body Part – 4TH	Approach – 5TH	Device – 6TH	Qualifier – 7TH
0 Upper Lip 1 Lower Lip 2 Hard Palate 3 Soft Palate 4 Buccal Mucosa 5 Upper Gingiva 6 Lower Gingiva 7 Tongue N Uvula	0 Open 3 Percutaneous X External	7 Autologous tissue substitute J Synthetic substitute K Nonautologous tissue substitute	Z No qualifier
B Parotid Duct, Right C Parotid Duct, Left	0 Open 3 Percutaneous	7 Autologous tissue substitute J Synthetic substitute K Nonautologous tissue substitute	Z No qualifier
M Pharynx R Epiglottis S Larynx T Vocal Cord, Right V Vocal Cord, Left	0 Open 7 Via natural or artificial opening 8 Via natural or artificial opening endoscopic	7 Autologous tissue substitute J Synthetic substitute K Nonautologous tissue substitute	Z No qualifier
W Upper Tooth X Lower Tooth	0 Open X External	7 Autologous tissue substitute J Synthetic substitute K Nonautologous tissue substitute	0 Single 1 Multiple 2 All

© 2018 Channel Publishing, Ltd.

1ST - 0 Medical and Surgical
2ND - C Mouth and Throat
3RD - S REPOSITION

MOVE GROUP: Reattachment, Reposition, Transfer, (Transplantation)
Root Operations that put in/put back or move some/all of a body part.

REPOSITION: Moving to its normal location, or other suitable location, all or a portion of a body part.

Explanation: The body part may or may not be cut out or off to be moved to the new location ...
Examples: Reposition tongue – CMS Ex: Fracture reduction

Body Part – 4TH	Approach – 5TH	Device – 6TH	Qualifier – 7TH
0 Upper Lip 1 Lower Lip 2 Hard Palate 3 Soft Palate 7 Tongue N Uvula	0 Open X External	Z No device	Z No qualifier
B Parotid Duct, Right C Parotid Duct, Left	0 Open 3 Percutaneous	Z No device	Z No qualifier
R Epiglottis T Vocal Cord, Right V Vocal Cord, Left	0 Open 7 Via natural or artificial opening 8 Via natural or artificial opening endoscopic	Z No device	Z No qualifier
W Upper Tooth X Lower Tooth	0 Open X External	5 External fixation device Z No device	0 Single 1 Multiple 2 All

1ST - 0 Medical and Surgical
2ND - C Mouth and Throat
3RD - T RESECTION

EXCISION GROUP: Excision, Resection, Destruction, Extraction, (Detachment)
Root Operations that take out some or all of a body part.

RESECTION: Cutting out or off, without replacement, all of a body part.

Explanation: None
Examples: Tonsillectomy – CMS Ex: Total lobectomy of lung

Body Part – 4TH	Approach – 5TH	Device – 6TH	Qualifier – 7TH
0 Upper Lip 1 Lower Lip 2 Hard Palate 3 Soft Palate 7 Tongue N Uvula P Tonsils Q Adenoids	0 Open X External	Z No device	Z No qualifier
8 Parotid Gland, Right 9 Parotid Gland, Left B Parotid Duct, Right C Parotid Duct, Left D Sublingual Gland, Right F Sublingual Gland, Left G Submaxillary Gland, Right H Submaxillary Gland, Left J Minor Salivary Gland	0 Open	Z No device	Z No qualifier
M Pharynx R Epiglottis S Larynx T Vocal Cord, Right V Vocal Cord, Left	0 Open 4 Percutaneous endoscopic 7 Via natural or artificial opening 8 Via natural or artificial opening endoscopic	Z No device	Z No qualifier
W Upper Tooth X Lower Tooth	0 Open	Z No device	0 Single 1 Multiple 2 All

© 2018 Channel Publishing, Ltd.

1ST - 0 Medical and Surgical
2ND - C Mouth and Throat
3RD - U SUPPLEMENT

DEVICE GROUP: Change, Insertion, Removal, Replacement, Revision, Supplement
Root Operations that always involve a device.

SUPPLEMENT: Putting in or on biological or synthetic material that physically reinforces and/or augments the function of a portion of a body part.

Explanation: Biological material is non-living, or is living and from the same individual ...
Examples: Palatoplasty with graft – CMS Ex: Herniorrhaphy using mesh

Body Part – 4TH	Approach – 5TH	Device – 6TH	Qualifier – 7TH
0 Upper Lip 1 Lower Lip 2 Hard Palate 3 Soft Palate 4 Buccal Mucosa 5 Upper Gingiva 6 Lower Gingiva 7 Tongue N Uvula	0 Open 3 Percutaneous X External	7 Autologous tissue substitute J Synthetic substitute K Nonautologous tissue substitute	Z No qualifier
M Pharynx R Epiglottis S Larynx T Vocal Cord, Right V Vocal Cord, Left	0 Open 7 Via natural or artificial opening 8 Via natural or artificial opening endoscopic	7 Autologous tissue substitute J Synthetic substitute K Nonautologous tissue substitute	Z No qualifier

1ST - 0 Medical and Surgical
2ND - C Mouth and Throat
3RD - V RESTRICTION

TUBULAR GROUP: (Bypass), Dilation, Occlusion, Restriction
Root Operations that alter the diameter/route of a tubular body part.

RESTRICTION: Partially closing an orifice or the lumen of a tubular body part.

Explanation: The orifice can be a natural orifice or an artificially created orifice.
Examples: Parotid duct restrictive stent – CMS Ex: Cervical cerclage

Body Part – 4TH	Approach – 5TH	Device – 6TH	Qualifier – 7TH
B Parotid Duct, Right C Parotid Duct, Left	0 Open 3 Percutaneous	C Extraluminal device D Intraluminal device Z No device	Z No qualifier
B Parotid Duct, Right C Parotid Duct, Left	7 Via natural or artificial opening 8 Via natural or artificial opening endoscopic	D Intraluminal device Z No device	Z No qualifier

© 2018 Channel Publishing, Ltd.

1ST - 0 Medical and Surgical
2ND - C Mouth and Throat
3RD - W REVISION

DEVICE GROUP: Change, Insertion, Removal, Replacement, Revision, Supplement
Root Operations that always involve a device.

REVISION: Correcting, to the extent possible, a portion of a malfunctioning device or the position of a displaced device.

Explanation: Correcting by taking out or putting in components of a device such as a screw or pin ...
Examples: Trimming palatoplasty graft – CMS Ex: Recementing of hip prosthesis

Body Part – 4TH	Approach – 5TH	Device – 6TH	Qualifier – 7TH
A Salivary Gland	0 Open 3 Percutaneous	0 Drainage device C Extraluminal device Y Other device	Z No qualifier
A Salivary Gland	7 Via natural or artificial opening 8 Via natural or artificial opening endoscopic	Y Other device	Z No qualifier
A Salivary Gland	X External	0 Drainage device C Extraluminal device	Z No qualifier
S Larynx	0 Open 3 Percutaneous 7 Via natural or artificial opening 8 Via natural or artificial opening endoscopic	0 Drainage device 7 Autologous tissue substitute D Intraluminal device J Synthetic substitute K Nonautologous tissue substitute Y Other device	Z No qualifier
S Larynx	X External	0 Drainage device 7 Autologous tissue substitute D Intraluminal device J Synthetic substitute K Nonautologous tissue substitute	Z No qualifier
Y Mouth and Throat	0 Open 3 Percutaneous 7 Via natural or artificial opening 8 Via natural or artificial opening endoscopic	0 Drainage device 1 Radioactive element 7 Autologous tissue substitute D Intraluminal device J Synthetic substitute K Nonautologous tissue substitute Y Other device	Z No qualifier
Y Mouth and Throat	X External	0 Drainage device 1 Radioactive element 7 Autologous tissue substitute D Intraluminal device J Synthetic substitute K Nonautologous tissue substitute	Z No qualifier

1ST - 0 Medical and Surgical
2ND - C Mouth and Throat
3RD - X TRANSFER

MOVE GROUP: Reattachment, Reposition, Transfer, (Transplantation)
Root Operations that put in/put back or move some/all of a body part.

TRANSFER: Moving, without taking out, all or a portion of a body part to another location to take over the function of all or a portion of a body part.

Explanation: The body part transferred remains connected to its vascular and nervous supply
Examples: Gingival pedicle graft – CMS Ex: Tendon transfer

Body Part – 4TH		Approach – 5TH	Device – 6TH	Qualifier – 7TH
0 Upper Lip 1 Lower Lip 3 Soft Palate 4 Buccal Mucosa	5 Upper Gingiva 6 Lower Gingiva 7 Tongue	0 Open X External	Z No device	Z No qualifier

© 2018 Channel Publishing, Ltd.

MOUTH & THROAT 0CX

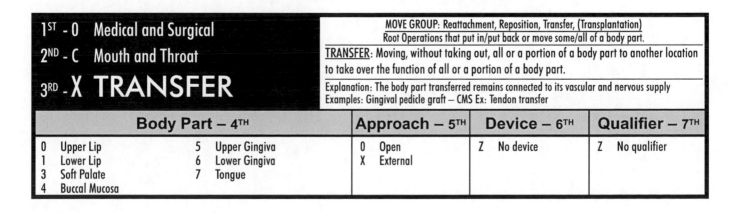

NOTES

© 2018 Channel Publishing, Ltd.

Educational Annotations | D – Gastrointestinal System

Body System Specific Educational Annotations for the Gastrointestinal System include:

- Anatomy and Physiology Review
- Definitions of Common Procedures
- Anatomical Illustrations
- AHA Coding Clinic® Reference Notations
- Body Part Key Listings
- Device Key Listings
- Device Aggregation Table Listings
- Coding Notes

Anatomy and Physiology Review of Gastrointestinal System

BODY PART VALUES – D - GASTROINTESTINAL SYSTEM

Anal Sphincter – ANATOMY – The anal sphincter is a group of muscles (internal and external) that surrounds the anus. PHYSIOLOGY – Maintains continence by controlling the release of stool from the rectum.

Anus – ANATOMY – The anus is the internal canal from the rectum which ends the alimentary tract at the anal opening. PHYSIOLOGY – The rectum and anus function to eliminate feces from the alimentary tract. A reflex signal is sent when the rectum fills and urgency to defecate is perceived. The external voluntary muscle is voluntarily relaxed to defecate.

Appendix – The appendix is a closed appendage of the colon and projects downward from the cecum.

Ascending Colon – The ascending colon arises from the cecum (the pouch-like structure) and continues upwards where it turns (hepatic flexure) and connects to the transverse colon.

Cecum – ANATOMY – The cecum is an enlarged pouch of the ascending intestine at the junction with the ileum. PHYSIOLOGY – Receives the contents from the small intestine.

Descending Colon – The descending colon extends downward to the rectum, and is called the sigmoid (flexure) colon where it makes an S-shaped curve over the pelvic brim.

Duodenum – The duodenum is the first portion about 10 inches (25 cm) long connected at its proximal end to the stomach.

Esophagogastric Junction – ANATOMY – The lower end of the esophagus at the transition to the stomach identified by the abrupt change from esophageal epithelium to the gastric folds.

Esophagus – ANATOMY – The esophagus, located between the pharynx and stomach, is a collapsible musculomembranous alimentary tract tube about 10 inches (25 cm) long. The esophagus is lined with mucous glands. PHYSIOLOGY – The esophagus is the passageway for food from the mouth to the stomach. The mucous glands moisten and lubricate the inner lining to facilitate the passage of food. Situated just above the stomach opening lie the contracted circular muscles which prevent regurgitation.

Esophagus, Lower – The distal lower one-third of the esophagus (also known as the abdominal esophagus).

Esophagus, Middle – The middle one-third of the esophagus (also known as the thoracic esophagus).

Esophagus, Upper – The proximal upper one-third of the esophagus (also known as the cervical esophagus).

Greater Omentum – The double layer of the peritoneum that extends from the greater curvature of the stomach to the transverse colon.

Ileocecal Valve – ANATOMY – The ileocecal valve is the sphincter muscle valve that separates the small intestine and the large intestine. PHYSIOLOGY – The ileocecal valve prevents contents from the large intestine from backflowing into the small intestine.

Ileum – The ileum is the distal portion of the small intestine which connects with the large intestine.

Jejunum – The jejunum is the middle portion of the small intestine, comprising approximately two-fifths of the intestine.

Large Intestine – ANATOMY – The large intestine (colon) is the tubular organ of the alimentary tract between the small intestine and the rectum, and is about 5 feet (1.5 m) long. The colon has four main segments: Ascending, transverse, descending, and sigmoid. The rectosigmoid junction is that portion of the alimentary tract between the distal end of the sigmoid colon and the proximal end of the rectum. PHYSIOLOGY – The large intestine (colon) functions to absorb water and electrolytes, and to move by peristalsis nonabsorbed substances to the rectum for defecation. Many bacteria normally inhabit the colon and serve to further break down substances for colonic absorption.

Large Intestine, Left – In general, the descending colon and part of the transverse colon.

Large Intestine, Right – In general, the ascending colon and part of the transverse colon.

Lesser Omentum – The double layer of the peritoneum that extends from the liver to lesser curvature of the stomach.

Lower Intestinal Tract – The gastrointestinal tract from the jejunum down to and including the rectum and anus (see Coding Guideline B4.8).

Mesentery – The mesentery is a fold of membranous tissue that arises from the posterior wall of the peritoneal cavity and attaches the intestine to the abdominal wall and holds it in place.

Omentum – The double layer of the peritoneum that encompasses most of the organs in the abdominal cavity.

Peritoneum – ANATOMY – The peritoneum is the serous membrane (visceral and parietal) which contains most of the abdominal contents, and where doubled upon itself forms supporting structures called ligaments. PHYSIOLOGY – The peritoneum encapsules and protects the abdominal visceral organs allowing them to move slightly without damaging function.

Rectum – ANATOMY – The rectum is the musculomembranous portion of the alimentary tract between the colon and anus, approximately 5 inches (13 cm) long. The rectosigmoid junction is that portion of the alimentary tract between the distal end of the sigmoid colon and the proximal end of the rectum. PHYSIOLOGY – The rectum and anus function to eliminate feces from the alimentary tract. A reflex signal is sent when the rectum fills and urgency to defecate is perceived. The external voluntary muscle is voluntarily relaxed to defecate.

Sigmoid Colon – The descending colon extends downward to the rectum, and is called the sigmoid (flexure) colon where it makes an S-shaped curve over the pelvic brim.

Continued on next page

© 2018 Channel Publishing, Ltd.

Educational Annotations | D – Gastrointestinal System

Anatomy and Physiology Review of Gastrointestinal System

BODY PART VALUES – D - GASTROINTESTINAL SYSTEM

Continued from previous page

Small Intestine – ANATOMY – The small intestine is the tubular organ of the alimentary tract between the stomach and large intestine and is about 16 to 20 feet (5 to 6 m) long, and has 3 parts: Duodenum, jejunum, and ileum. Both the jejunum and ileum are suspended from the posterior abdominal wall by the mesentery. PHYSIOLOGY – The small intestine functions to absorb the nutrients produced through digestion. The food is passed through the small intestine by the contraction (peristalsis) of its circular smooth muscle layer. The duodenum releases several enzymes and mixes the pancreatic and bile juices with food from the stomach. The jejunum and ileum continue mixing and absorbing until the remaining substances pass into the large intestine.

Stomach – ANATOMY – The stomach, located in the upper abdomen, is a pouch-like organ of the alimentary tract connecting with the esophagus in the proximal (upper) portion and the duodenum in the distal (lower) portion and is about 10 to 12 inches (25 to 30 cm) long. The cardia lies at the opening of the esophagus at the fundus of the stomach. The fundus is the upper ballooned area of the stomach. The body is the main part of the stomach and is located between the fundus and the pyloric antrum and the duodenum. When empty, the mucous membrane on the interior surface forms longitudinal folds (rugae). There are three mucosal glands which secrete digestive juices and mucous. These are the gastric glands, which are located throughout the body of the stomach; the cardiac glands, which are found near the esophageal opening; and the pyloric glands, which are located in the pyloric (distal) region. The vagus nerve stimulates the gastric glands. There are three layers of smooth muscle and a serosal covering of the visceral peritoneum. The stomach has a rich arterial blood supply through the celiac artery. The venous blood is drained into the hepatic portal system. PHYSIOLOGY – The stomach functions to receive food from the esophagus, mixes it with the gastric juice, initiates the digestion of proteins with pepsin, carries on a limited amount of absorption, and moves food into the small intestine by peristaltic muscle action. The gastric glands produce mucous, digestive enzymes (pepsin), hydrochloric acid, and an intrinsic factor, forming the gastric juice. The mucous is thought to help prevent the pepsin and hydrochloric acid from digesting the stomach surface. The stomach may absorb small quantities of water, glucose, certain salts, and alcohol. The parasympathetic vagus nerve stimulates the gastric glands to secrete large amounts of gastric juice, which in turn releases gastrin, a hormone that causes the gastric glands to increase their secretory activity.

Stomach, Pylorus – The pylorus is the lower section of the stomach that connects to the duodenum and allows emptying of the contents into the small intestine.

Transverse Colon – The transverse colon extends horizontally and turns (splenic flexure) downward connecting to the descending colon.

Upper Intestinal Tract – The gastrointestinal tract from the esophagus down to and including the duodenum (see Coding Guideline B4.8).

Definitions of Common Procedures of Gastrointestinal System

Anal sphincterotomy – The incision of the anal sphincter muscle to prevent spasms and intentionally weaken the muscle during healing.

Colostomy – The creation of an artificial opening of the colon through the abdominal wall.

Gastrojejunostomy – The surgical creation of an anastomosis between the stomach and the jejunum (the second portion of the small intestine) to bypass and relieve gastric outlet obstruction.

Nissen's fundoplication – The surgical wrapping of the fundus of the stomach around the lower portion of the esophagus to prevent reflux of the stomach contents back into the esophagus.

Percutaneous endoscopic gastrostomy (PEG) – The placement of a tube through an abdominal wall incision from inside the stomach by using an endoscope and a pull-through technique.

Pyloromyotomy – The incision in the muscular layers of the pylorus to treat hypertrophic pyloric stenosis.

Right hemicolectomy – The surgical removal of the cecum, ascending colon, and hepatic flexure portion of the tranverse colon, and usually end-to-end anastomosis between the small intestine and the transverse colon.

Vertical sleeve gastrectomy – The surgical excision of a large portion of the stomach along a vertical line of the stomach to reduce the stomach volume and limit the amount of food that can be consumed at one time.

Anatomical Illustrations of Gastrointestinal System

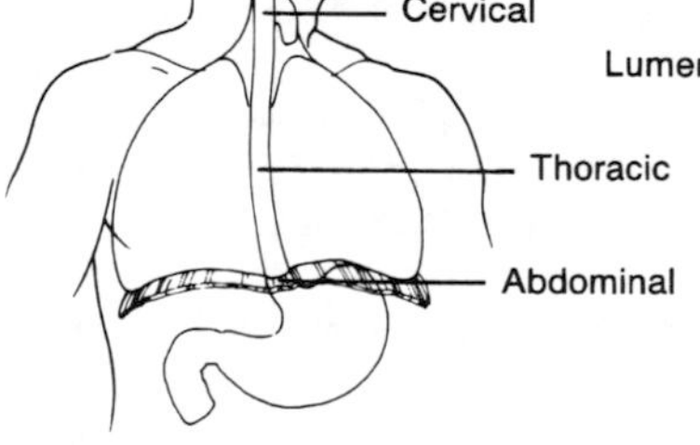

ESOPHAGUS — ANTERIOR VIEW

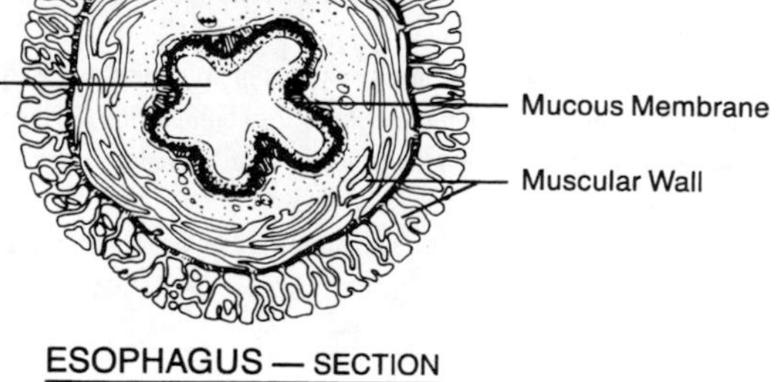

ESOPHAGUS — SECTION

Continued on next page

GASTROINTESTINAL 0 D

© 2018 Channel Publishing, Ltd.

Educational Annotations | D – Gastrointestinal System

Anatomical Illustrations of Gastrointestinal System

Continued from previous page

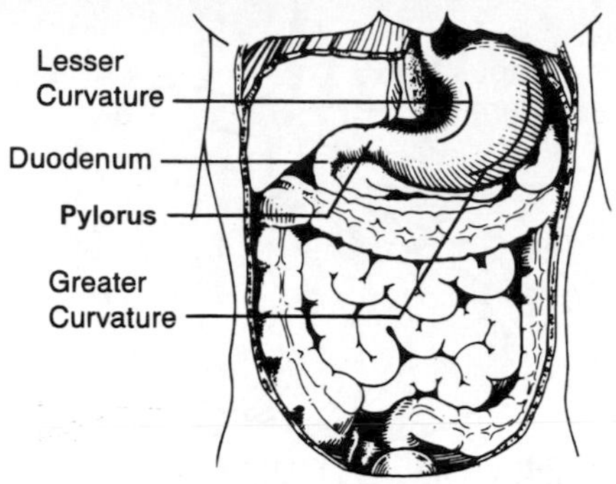

STOMACH

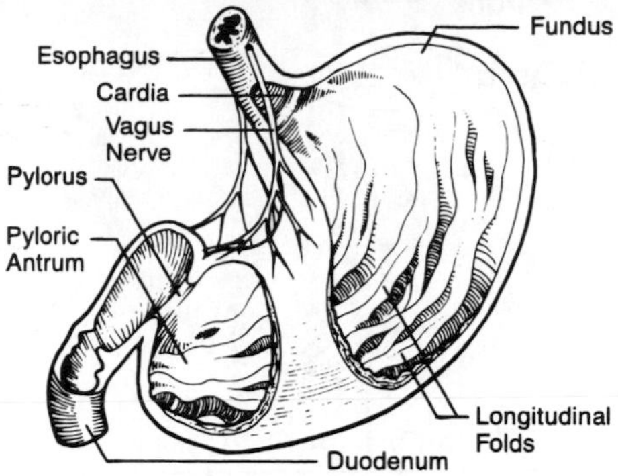

STOMACH — ANTERIOR (CUT-AWAY) VIEW

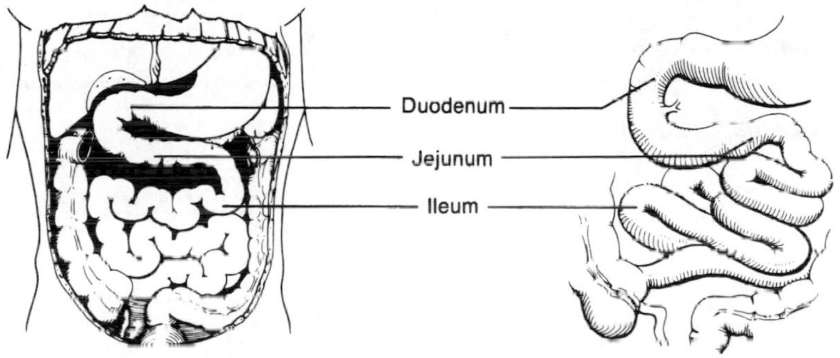

SMALL INTESTINE

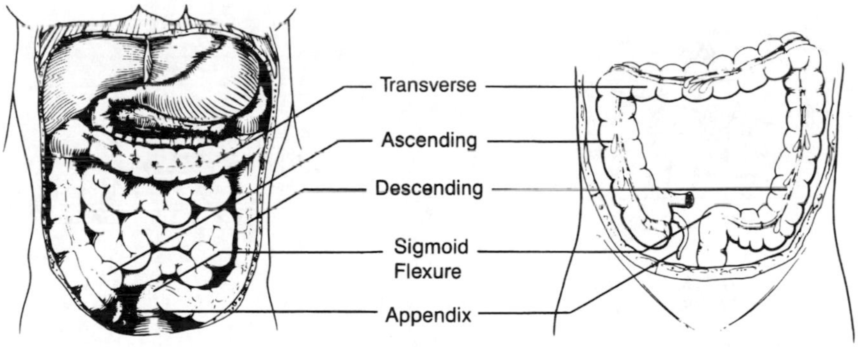

LARGE INTESTINE (COLON)

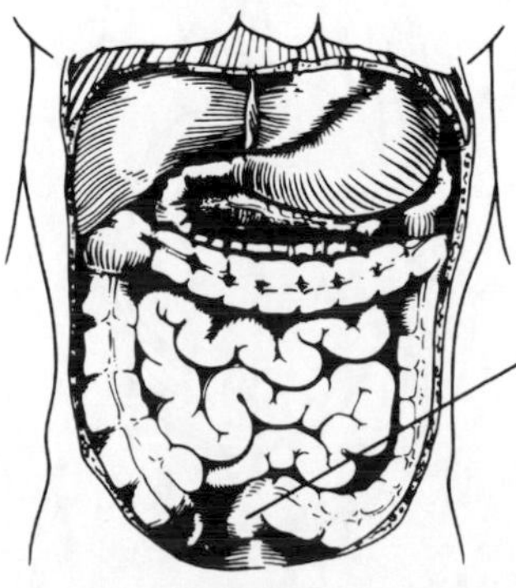

RECTUM

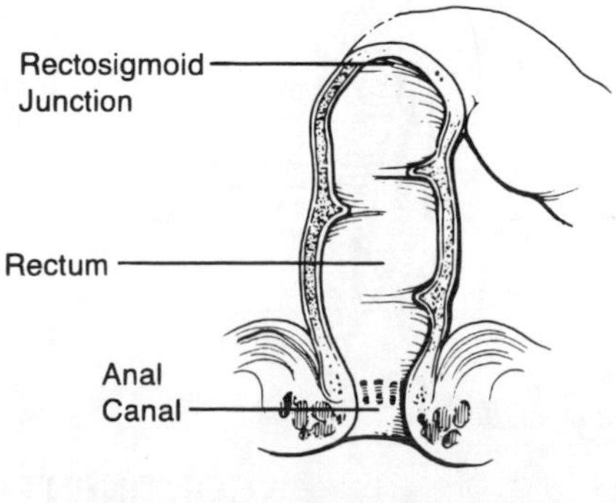

RECTUM — ANTERIOR (CUT-AWAY) VIEW

Continued on next page

© 2018 Channel Publishing, Ltd.

GASTROINTESTINAL 0 D

Educational Annotations | D – Gastrointestinal System

Anatomical Illustrations of Gastrointestinal System

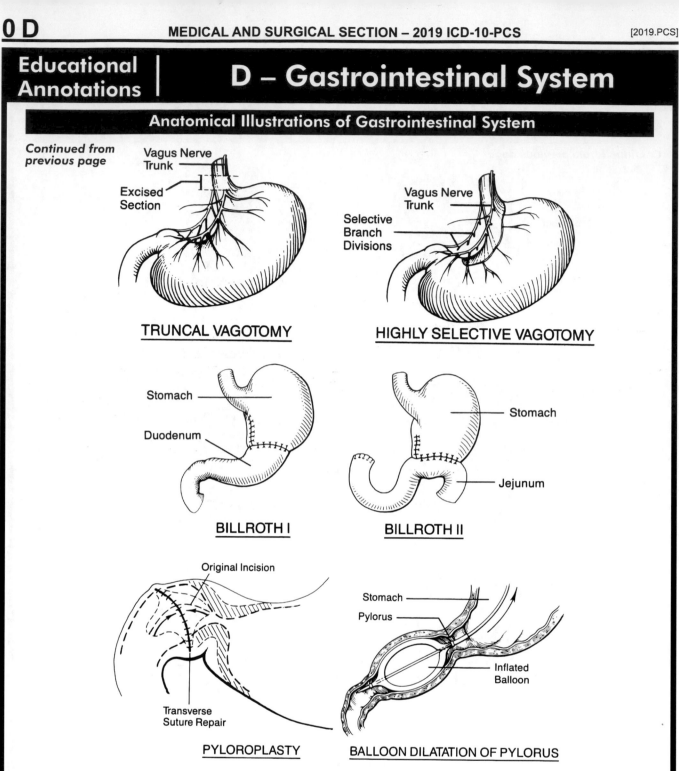

Continued from previous page

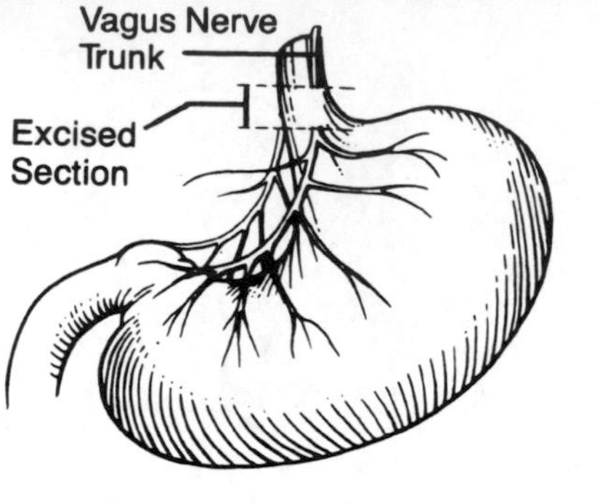

TRUNCAL VAGOTOMY

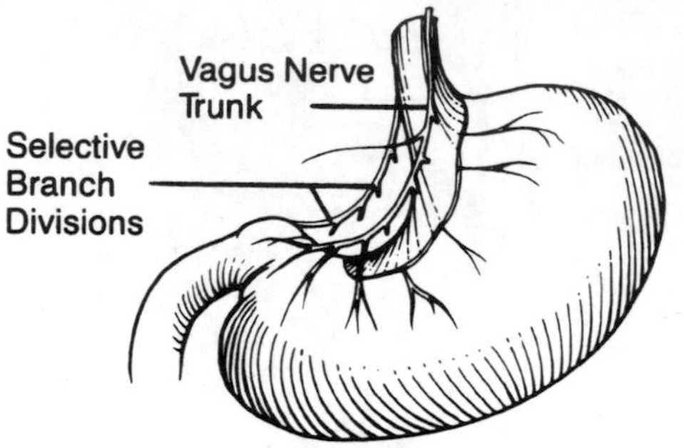

HIGHLY SELECTIVE VAGOTOMY

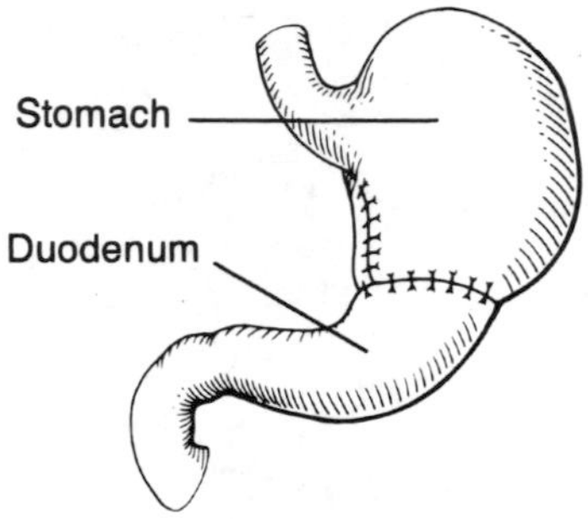

BILLROTH I

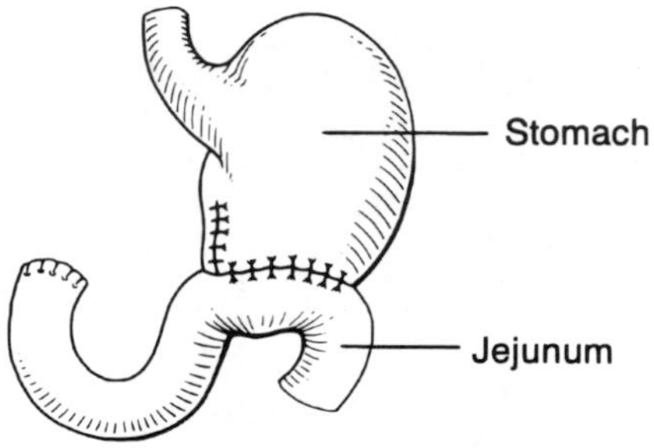

BILLROTH II

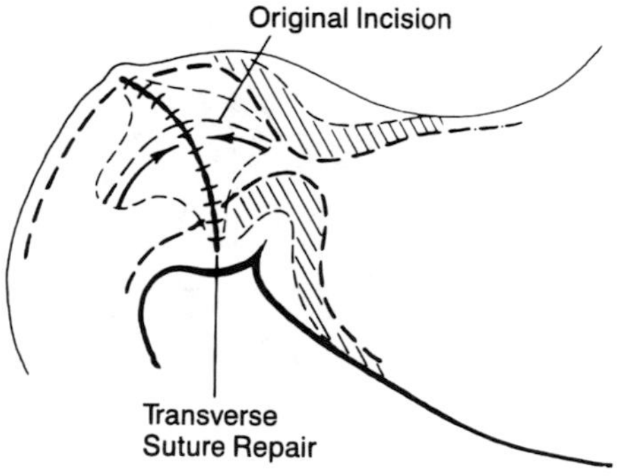

PYLOROPLASTY

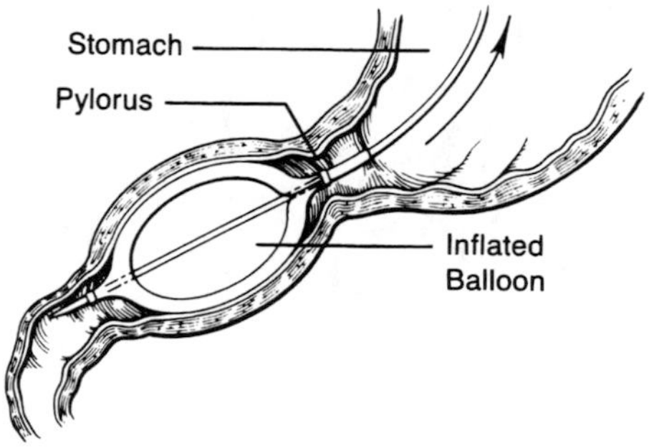

BALLOON DILATATION OF PYLORUS

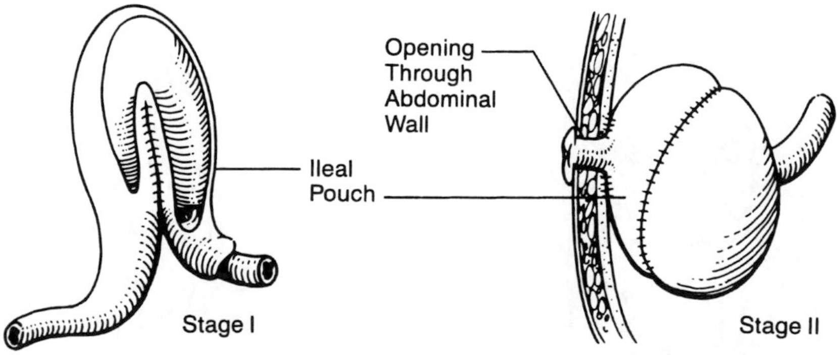

CONTINENT ILEOSTOMY

Continued on next page

© 2018 Channel Publishing, Ltd.

GASTROINTESTINAL 0 D

Educational Annotations | D – Gastrointestinal System

Anatomical Illustrations of Gastrointestinal System

Continued from previous page

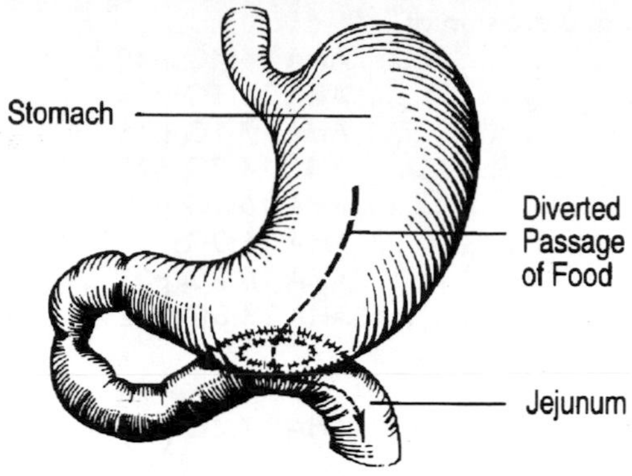

GASTROJEJUNOSTOMY

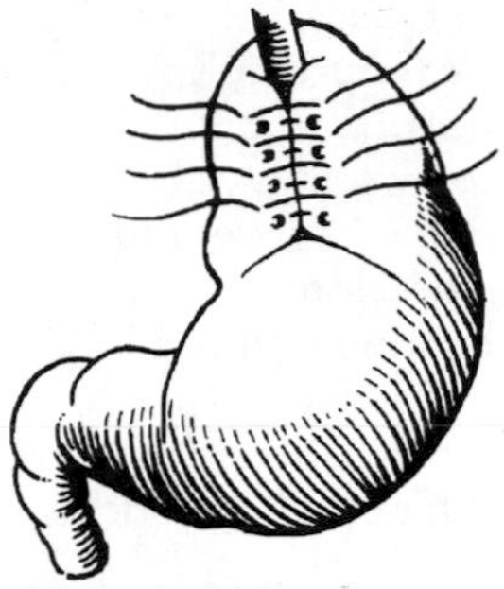

NISSEN'S FUNDOPLICATION

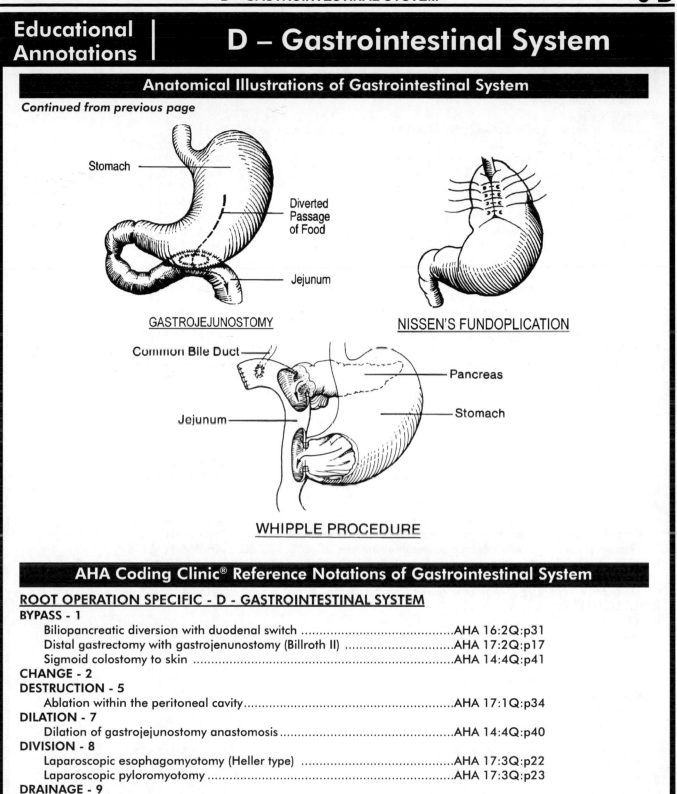

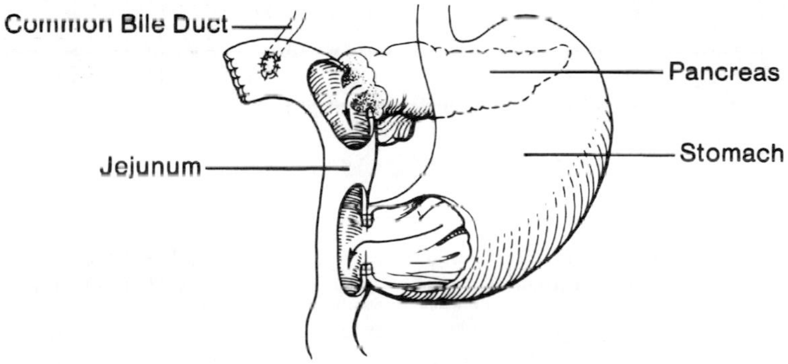

WHIPPLE PROCEDURE

AHA Coding Clinic® Reference Notations of Gastrointestinal System

ROOT OPERATION SPECIFIC - D - GASTROINTESTINAL SYSTEM

BYPASS - 1

Biliopancreatic diversion with duodenal switch ....AHA 16:2Q:p31
Distal gastrectomy with gastrojenunostomy (Billroth II) ....AHA 17:2Q:p17
Sigmoid colostomy to skin ....AHA 14:4Q:p41

CHANGE - 2

DESTRUCTION - 5

Ablation within the peritoneal cavity...AHA 17:1Q:p34

DILATION - 7

Dilation of gastrojejunostomy anastomosis...AHA 14:4Q:p40

DIVISION - 8

Laparoscopic esophagomyotomy (Heller type) ....AHA 17:3Q:p22
Laparoscopic pyloromyotomy ....AHA 17:3Q:p23

DRAINAGE - 9

Nasogastric (NG) tube used for both drainage and feeding ....AHA 15:2Q:p2

Continued on next page

© 2018 Channel Publishing, Ltd.

Educational Annotations | D – Gastrointestinal System

AHA Coding Clinic® Reference Notations of Gastrointestinal System

Continued from previous page

EXCISION - B

Abdominoperineal resection (APR) of rectum and anus, and excision of sigmoid colon ....AHA 14:4Q:p40
Esophageal brush biopsy ....AHA 16:1Q:p24
Excision of hepatic flexure polyp ....AHA 17:1Q:p16
Ileostomy takedown ....AHA 14:3Q:p28
Perineal proctectomy ....AHA 16:1Q:p22
Stoma creation and takedown procedures ....AHA 16:3Q:p3-7
Vertical sleeve gastrectomy ....AHA 16:2Q:p31
Whipple pyloric sparing pancreaticoduodenectomy ....AHA 14:3Q:p32

EXTIRPATION - C

EXTRACTION - D

Endoscopic brush biopsy of stomach ....AHA 17:4Q:p42

FRAGMENTATION - F

INSERTION - H

Percutaneous endoscopic gastrostomy (PEG) placement ....AHA 13:4Q:p117

INSPECTION - J

Capsule endoscopy ....AHA 16:2Q:p20
EGD with epinephrine injection ....AHA 15:3Q:p24
Sigmoidoscopy to check anastomosis following low anterior resection ....AHA 17:2Q:p15

OCCLUSION - L

REATTACHMENT - M

RELEASE - N

Lysis of adhesions, integral or code separately ....AHA 14:1Q:p3
Release of esophageal vascular ring ....AHA 15:3Q:p15,16
Take down of adhesions of omentum and peritoneum ....AHA 17:1Q:p35

REMOVAL - P

REPAIR - Q

Clips to control bleeding duodenal ulcer ....AHA 14:4Q:p20
Repair internal hernia at Peterson mesentery space ....AHA 18:1Q:p11
Repair of third and fourth degree perineal lacerations ....AHA 16:1Q:p6-8
Repair of third and fourth degree perineal lacerations - Official Clarification AHA 18:2Q:p25
Stoma creation and takedown procedures ....AHA 16:3Q:p3-7
Takedown of ileostomy without excision ....AHA 16:3Q:p3-7

REPLACEMENT - R

REPOSITION - S

Hartmann end colostomy reversal ....AHA 16:3Q:p5
Posterior sagittal anorectoplasty ....AHA 17:3Q:p17
Reduction of intussusception via air enema ....AHA 17:3Q:p9
Repair of small and large bowel malrotation ....AHA 17:4Q:p49

RESECTION - T

Abdominoperineal resection (APR) of rectum and anus, and excision of sigmoid colon ....AHA 14:4Q:p40
Colectomy, right ....AHA 14:3Q:p6
Colectomy with side-to-side anastomosis ....AHA 14:4Q:p42
Ileocecectomy ....AHA 14:3Q:p6

SUPPLEMENT - U

RESTRICTION - V

Nissen fundoplication ....AHA 14:3Q:p28
........AHA 16:2Q:p22
Toupet fundoplication ....AHA 17:3Q:p22

REVISION - W

Removal of fluid from gastric band stenosis ....AHA 18:1Q:p20

TRANSFER - X

Cervical esophagogastrostomy ....AHA 17:2Q:p18
Collis gastroplasty ....AHA 16:2Q:p22

TRANSPLANTATION - Y

© 2018 Channel Publishing, Ltd.

Educational Annotations | D – Gastrointestinal System

Body Part Key Listings of Gastrointestinal System

See also Body Part Key in Appendix C

Abdominal esophagus .... use Esophagus, Lower
Anal orifice .... use Anus
Anorectal junction .... use Rectum
Cardia .... use Esophagogastric Junction
Cardioesophageal junction .... use Esophagogastric Junction
Cervical esophagus .... use Esophagus, Upper
Duodenojejunal flexure .... use Jejunum
Epiploic foramen .... use Peritoneum
External anal sphincter .... use Anal Sphincter
Gastrocolic ligament .... use Omentum
Gastrocolic omentum .... use Omentum
Gastroesophageal (GE) junction .... use Esophagogastric Junction
Gastrohepatic omentum .... use Omentum
Gastrophrenic ligament .... use Omentum
Gastrosplenic ligament .... use Omentum
Greater omentum .... use Omentum
Hepatic flexure .... use Transverse Colon
Hepatogastric ligament .... use Omentum
Internal anal sphincter .... use Anal Sphincter
Lesser omentum .... use Omentum
Mesoappendix .... use Mesentery
Mesocolon .... use Mesentery
Pyloric antrum .... use Stomach, Pylorus
Pyloric canal .... use Stomach, Pylorus
Pyloric sphincter .... use Stomach, Pylorus
Rectosigmoid junction .... use Sigmoid Colon
Sigmoid flexure .... use Sigmoid Colon
Splenic flexure .... use Transverse Colon
Thoracic esophagus .... use Esophagus, Middle
Vermiform appendix .... use Appendix

Device Key Listings of Gastrointestinal System

See also Device Key in Appendix D

Artificial anal sphincter (AAS) .... use Artificial Sphincter in Gastrointestinal System
Artificial bowel sphincter (neosphincter) .... use Artificial Sphincter in Gastrointestinal System
Autograft .... use Autologous Tissue Substitute
Brachytherapy seeds .... use Radioactive Element
Colonic Z-Stent® .... use Intraluminal Device
Cook Biodesign® Fistula Plug(s) .... use Nonautologous Tissue Substitute
Esophageal obturator airway (EOA) .... use Intraluminal Device, Airway in Gastrointestinal System
Gastric electrical stimulation (GES) lead .... use Stimulator Lead in Gastrointestinal System
Gastric pacemaker lead .... use Stimulator Lead in Gastrointestinal System
LAP-BAND® adjustable gastric banding system .... use Extraluminal Device
Percutaneous endoscopic gastrojejunostomy (PEG/J) tube .... use Feeding Device in Gastrointestinal System
Percutaneous endoscopic gastrostomy (PEG) tube .... use Feeding Device in Gastrointestinal System
REALIZE® Adjustable Gastric Band .... use Extraluminal Device
Tissue bank graft .... use Nonautologous Tissue Substitute
Ultraflex™ Precision Colonic Stent System .... use Intraluminal Device

Device Aggregation Table Listings of Gastrointestinal System

See also Device Aggregation Table in Appendix E

Specific Device	For Operation	In Body System	General Device
Intraluminal Device, Airway	All applicable	Gastrointestinal System	Intraluminal Device

Coding Notes of Gastrointestinal System

Body System Relevant Coding Guidelines

Upper and lower intestinal tract

B4.8

In the Gastrointestinal body system, the general body part values Upper Intestinal Tract and Lower Intestinal Tract are provided as an option for the root operations Change, Inspection, Removal and Revision. Upper Intestinal Tract includes the portion of the gastrointestinal tract from the esophagus down to and including the duodenum, and Lower Intestinal Tract includes the portion of the gastrointestinal tract from the jejunum down to and including the rectum and anus.

Example: In the root operation Change table, change of a device in the jejunum is coded using the body part Lower Intestinal Tract.

© 2018 Channel Publishing, Ltd.

1ST - 0 Medical and Surgical
2ND - D Gastrointestinal System
3RD - 1 BYPASS

TUBULAR GROUP: Bypass, Dilation, Occlusion, Restriction
Root Operations that alter the diameter/route of a tubular body part.
BYPASS: Altering the route of passage of the contents of a tubular body part.

Explanation: Rerouting contents to a downstream part ... with or without the use of a device ...
Examples: Colostomy formation – CMS Ex: Coronary artery bypass

Body Part – 4TH	Approach – 5TH	Device – 6TH	Qualifier–7TH
1 Esophagus, Upper 2 Esophagus, Middle 3 Esophagus, Lower 5 Esophagus	0 Open 4 Percutaneous endoscopic 8 Via natural or artificial opening endoscopic	7 Autologous tissue substitute J Synthetic substitute K Nonautologous tissue substitute Z No device	4 Cutaneous 6 Stomach 9 Duodenum A Jejunum B Ileum
1 Esophagus, Upper 2 Esophagus, Middle 3 Esophagus, Lower 5 Esophagus	3 Percutaneous	J Synthetic substitute	4 Cutaneous
6 Stomach 9 Duodenum	0 Open 4 Percutaneous endoscopic 8 Via natural or artificial opening endoscopic	7 Autologous tissue substitute J Synthetic substitute K Nonautologous tissue substitute Z No device	4 Cutaneous 9 Duodenum A Jejunum B Ileum L Transverse Colon
6 Stomach 9 Duodenum	3 Percutaneous	J Synthetic substitute	4 Cutaneous
A Jejunum	0 Open 4 Percutaneous endoscopic 8 Via natural or artificial opening endoscopic	7 Autologous tissue substitute J Synthetic substitute K Nonautologous tissue substitute Z No device	4 Cutaneous A Jejunum B Ileum H Cecum K Ascending Colon L Transverse Colon M Descending Colon N Sigmoid Colon P Rectum Q Anus
A Jejunum	3 Percutaneous	J Synthetic substitute	4 Cutaneous
B Ileum	0 Open 4 Percutaneous endoscopic 8 Via natural or artificial opening endoscopic	7 Autologous tissue substitute J Synthetic substitute K Nonautologous tissue substitute Z No device	4 Cutaneous B Ileum H Cecum K Ascending Colon L Transverse Colon M Descending Colon N Sigmoid Colon P Rectum Q Anus
B Ileum	3 Percutaneous	J Synthetic substitute	4 Cutaneous
H Cecum	0 Open 4 Percutaneous endoscopic 8 Via natural or artificial opening endoscopic	7 Autologous tissue substitute J Synthetic substitute K Nonautologous tissue substitute Z No device	4 Cutaneous H Cecum K Ascending Colon L Transverse Colon M Descending Colon N Sigmoid Colon P Rectum
H Cecum	3 Percutaneous	J Synthetic substitute	4 Cutaneous

continued ⇨

© 2018 Channel Publishing, Ltd.

0 D 1 BYPASS – continued

Body Part – 4TH	Approach – 5TH	Device – 6TH	Qualifier – 7TH
K Ascending Colon	0 Open 4 Percutaneous endoscopic 8 Via natural or artificial opening endoscopic	7 Autologous tissue substitute J Synthetic substitute K Nonautologous tissue substitute Z No device	4 Cutaneous K Ascending Colon L Transverse Colon M Descending Colon N Sigmoid Colon P Rectum
K Ascending Colon	3 Percutaneous	J Synthetic substitute	4 Cutaneous
L Transverse Colon	0 Open 4 Percutaneous endoscopic 8 Via natural or artificial opening endoscopic	7 Autologous tissue substitute J Synthetic substitute K Nonautologous tissue substitute Z No device	4 Cutaneous L Transverse Colon M Descending Colon N Sigmoid Colon P Rectum
L Transverse Colon	3 Percutaneous	J Synthetic substitute	4 Cutaneous
M Descending Colon	0 Open 4 Percutaneous endoscopic 8 Via natural or artificial opening endoscopic	7 Autologous tissue substitute J Synthetic substitute K Nonautologous tissue substitute Z No device	4 Cutaneous M Descending Colon N Sigmoid Colon P Rectum
M Descending Colon	3 Percutaneous	J Synthetic substitute	4 Cutaneous
N Sigmoid Colon	0 Open 4 Percutaneous endoscopic 8 Via natural or artificial opening endoscopic	7 Autologous tissue substitute J Synthetic substitute K Nonautologous tissue substitute Z No device	4 Cutaneous N Sigmoid Colon P Rectum
N Sigmoid Colon	3 Percutaneous	J Synthetic substitute	4 Cutaneous

1ST - 0 Medical and Surgical
2ND - D Gastrointestinal System
3RD - 2 CHANGE

DEVICE GROUP: Change, Insertion, Removal, Replacement, Revision, Supplement
Root Operations that always involve a device.

CHANGE: Taking out or off a device from a body part and putting back an identical or similar device in or on the same body part without cutting or puncturing the skin or a mucous membrane.

Explanation: All CHANGE procedures are coded using the approach External
Examples: Exchange feeding tube – CMS Ex: Urinary catheter change

Body Part – 4TH	Approach – 5TH	Device – 6TH	Qualifier – 7TH
0 Upper Intestinal Tract D Lower Intestinal Tract	X External	0 Drainage device U Feeding device Y Other device	Z No qualifier
U Omentum V Mesentery W Peritoneum	X External	0 Drainage device Y Other device	Z No qualifier

© 2018 Channel Publishing, Ltd.

1ST - 0 Medical and Surgical
2ND - D Gastrointestinal System
3RD - 5 DESTRUCTION

EXCISION GROUP: Excision, Resection, Destruction, Extraction, (Detachment)
Root Operations that take out some or all of a body part.

DESTRUCTION: Physical eradication of all or a portion of a body part by the direct use of energy, force, or a destructive agent.

Explanation: None of the body part is physically taken out
Examples: Ablation esophageal polyp – CMS Ex: Fulguration of rectal polyp

Body Part – 4TH	Approach – 5TH	Device – 6TH	Qualifier – 7TH
1 Esophagus, Upper 2 Esophagus, Middle 3 Esophagus, Lower 4 Esophagogastric Junction 5 Esophagus 6 Stomach 7 Stomach, Pylorus 8 Small Intestine 9 Duodenum A Jejunum B Ileum C Ileocecal Valve E Large Intestine F Large Intestine, Right G Large Intestine, Left H Cecum J Appendix K Ascending Colon L Transverse Colon M Descending Colon N Sigmoid Colon P Rectum	0 Open 3 Percutaneous 4 Percutaneous endoscopic 7 Via natural or artificial opening 8 Via natural or artificial opening endoscopic	Z No device	Z No qualifier
Q Anus	0 Open 3 Percutaneous 4 Percutaneous endoscopic 7 Via natural or artificial opening 8 Via natural or artificial opening endoscopic X External	Z No device	Z No qualifier
R Anal Sphincter U Omentum V Mesentery W Peritoneum	0 Open 3 Percutaneous 4 Percutaneous endoscopic	Z No device	Z No qualifier

GASTROINTESTINAL 0 D 5

1ST - 0 Medical and Surgical
2ND - D Gastrointestinal System
3RD - 7 DILATION

TUBULAR GROUP: Bypass, Dilation, Occlusion, Restriction
Root Operations that alter the diameter/route of a tubular body part.

DILATION: Expanding an orifice or the lumen of a tubular body part.

Explanation: Accomplished by stretching or cutting ... tubular body part or orifice ...
Examples: Dilation rectal stricture – CMS Ex: Percutaneous transluminal angioplasty

Body Part – 4TH	Approach – 5TH	Device – 6TH	Qualifier – 7TH
1 Esophagus, Upper 2 Esophagus, Middle 3 Esophagus, Lower 4 Esophagogastric Junction 5 Esophagus 6 Stomach 7 Stomach, Pylorus 8 Small Intestine 9 Duodenum A Jejunum B Ileum C Ileocecal Valve E Large Intestine F Large Intestine, Right G Large Intestine, Left H Cecum K Ascending Colon L Transverse Colon M Descending Colon N Sigmoid Colon P Rectum Q Anus	0 Open 3 Percutaneous 4 Percutaneous endoscopic 7 Via natural or artificial opening 8 Via natural or artificial opening endoscopic	D Intraluminal device Z No device	Z No qualifier

1ST - 0 Medical and Surgical
2ND - D Gastrointestinal System
3RD - 8 DIVISION

DIVISION GROUP: Division, Release
Root Operations involving cutting or separation only.

DIVISION: Cutting into a body part, without draining fluids and/or gases from the body part, in order to separate or transect a body part.

Explanation: All or a portion of the body part is separated into two or more portions
Examples: Pyloromyotomy – CMS Ex: Spinal cordotomy

Body Part – 4TH	Approach – 5TH	Device – 6TH	Qualifier – 7TH
4 Esophagogastric Junction 7 Stomach, Pylorus	0 Open 3 Percutaneous 4 Percutaneous endoscopic 7 Via natural or artificial opening 8 Via natural or artificial opening endoscopic	Z No device	Z No qualifier
R Anal Sphincter	0 Open 3 Percutaneous	Z No device	Z No qualifier

© 2018 Channel Publishing, Ltd.

1ST - 0 Medical and Surgical
2ND - D Gastrointestinal System
3RD - 9 DRAINAGE

DRAINAGE GROUP: Drainage, Extirpation, Fragmentation
Root Operations that take out solids/fluids/gases from a body part.

DRAINAGE: Taking or letting out fluids and/or gases from a body part.

Explanation: Qualifier "X Diagnostic" indicates drainage procedures that are biopsies
Examples: Incision and drainage perianal abscess – CMS Ex: Thoracentesis

Body Part – 4TH	Approach – 5TH	Device – 6TH	Qualifier–7TH
1 Esophagus, Upper 2 Esophagus, Middle 3 Esophagus, Lower 4 Esophagogastric Junction 5 Esophagus 6 Stomach 7 Stomach, Pylorus 8 Small Intestine 9 Duodenum A Jejunum B Ileum C Ileocecal Valve E Large Intestine F Large Intestine, Right G Large Intestine, Left H Cecum J Appendix K Ascending Colon L Transverse Colon M Descending Colon N Sigmoid Colon P Rectum	0 Open 3 Percutaneous 4 Percutaneous endoscopic 7 Via natural or artificial opening 8 Via natural or artificial opening endoscopic	0 Drainage device	Z No qualifier
1 Esophagus, Upper 2 Esophagus, Middle 3 Esophagus, Lower 4 Esophagogastric Junction 5 Esophagus 6 Stomach 7 Stomach, Pylorus 8 Small Intestine 9 Duodenum A Jejunum B Ileum C Ileocecal Valve E Large Intestine F Large Intestine, Right G Large Intestine, Left H Cecum J Appendix K Ascending Colon L Transverse Colon M Descending Colon N Sigmoid Colon P Rectum	0 Open 3 Percutaneous 4 Percutaneous endoscopic 7 Via natural or artificial opening 8 Via natural or artificial opening endoscopic	Z No device	X Diagnostic Z No qualifier
Q Anus	0 Open 3 Percutaneous 4 Percutaneous endoscopic 7 Via natural or artificial opening 8 Via natural or artificial opening endoscopic X External	0 Drainage device	Z No qualifier
Q Anus	0 Open 3 Percutaneous 4 Percutaneous endoscopic 7 Via natural or artificial opening 8 Via natural or artificial opening endoscopic X External	Z No device	X Diagnostic Z No qualifier
R Anal Sphincter U Omentum V Mesentery W Peritoneum	0 Open 3 Percutaneous 4 Percutaneous endoscopic	0 Drainage device	Z No qualifier
R Anal Sphincter U Omentum V Mesentery W Peritoneum	0 Open 3 Percutaneous 4 Percutaneous endoscopic	Z No device	X Diagnostic Z No qualifier

© 2018 Channel Publishing, Ltd.

1ST - 0 Medical and Surgical
2ND - D Gastrointestinal System
3RD - B EXCISION

EXCISION GROUP: Excision, Resection, Destruction, Extraction, (Detachment)
Root Operations that take out some or all of a body part.

EXCISION: Cutting out or off, without replacement, a portion of a body part.

Explanation: Qualifier "X Diagnostic" indicates excision procedures that are biopsies
Examples: Vertical sleeve gastrectomy – CMS Ex: Liver biopsy

Body Part – 4TH	Approach – 5TH	Device – 6TH	Qualifier – 7TH
1 Esophagus, Upper 2 Esophagus, Middle 3 Esophagus, Lower 4 Esophagogastric Junction 5 Esophagus 7 Stomach, Pylorus 8 Small Intestine 9 Duodenum A Jejunum B Ileum C Ileocecal Valve E Large Intestine F Large Intestine, Right H Cecum J Appendix K Ascending Colon P Rectum	0 Open 3 Percutaneous 4 Percutaneous endoscopic 7 Via natural or artificial opening 8 Via natural or artificial opening endoscopic	Z No device	X Diagnostic Z No qualifier
6 Stomach	0 Open 3 Percutaneous 4 Percutaneous endoscopic 7 Via natural or artificial opening 8 Via natural or artificial opening endoscopic	Z No device	3 Vertical X Diagnostic Z No qualifier
G Large Intestine, Left L Transverse Colon M Descending Colon N Sigmoid Colon	0 Open 3 Percutaneous 4 Percutaneous endoscopic 7 Via natural or artificial opening 8 Via natural or artificial opening endoscopic	Z No device	X Diagnostic Z No qualifier
G Large Intestine, Left L Transverse Colon M Descending Colon N Sigmoid Colon	F Via natural or artificial opening with percutaneous endoscopic assistance	Z No device	Z No qualifier
Q Anus	0 Open 3 Percutaneous 4 Percutaneous endoscopic 7 Via natural or artificial opening 8 Via natural or artificial opening endoscopic X External	Z No device	X Diagnostic Z No qualifier
R Anal Sphincter U Omentum V Mesentery W Peritoneum	0 Open 3 Percutaneous 4 Percutaneous endoscopic	Z No device	X Diagnostic Z No qualifier

© 2018 Channel Publishing, Ltd.

1ST - 0 Medical and Surgical
2ND - D Gastrointestinal System
3RD - C EXTIRPATION

DRAINAGE GROUP: Drainage, Extirpation, Fragmentation
Root Operations that take out solids/fluids/gases from a body part.

EXTIRPATION: Taking or cutting out solid matter from a body part.

Explanation: Abnormal byproduct or foreign body ...
Examples: Removal gastric bezoar – CMS Ex: Thrombectomy

Body Part – 4TH	Approach – 5TH	Device – 6TH	Qualifier–7TH
1 Esophagus, Upper 2 Esophagus, Middle 3 Esophagus, Lower 4 Esophagogastric Junction 5 Esophagus 6 Stomach 7 Stomach, Pylorus 8 Small Intestine 9 Duodenum A Jejunum B Ileum C Ileocecal Valve E Large Intestine F Large Intestine, Right G Large Intestine, Left H Cecum J Appendix K Ascending Colon L Transverse Colon M Descending Colon N Sigmoid Colon P Rectum	0 Open 3 Percutaneous 4 Percutaneous endoscopic 7 Via natural or artificial opening 8 Via natural or artificial opening endoscopic	Z No device	Z No qualifier
Q Anus	0 Open 3 Percutaneous 4 Percutaneous endoscopic 7 Via natural or artificial opening 8 Via natural or artificial opening endoscopic X External	Z No device	Z No qualifier
R Anal Sphincter U Omentum V Mesentery W Peritoneum	0 Open 3 Percutaneous 4 Percutaneous endoscopic	Z No device	Z No qualifier

1ST - 0 Medical and Surgical
2ND - D Gastrointestinal System
3RD - D EXTRACTION

EXCISION GROUP: Excision, Resection, Destruction, Extraction, (Detachment)
Root Operations that take out some or all of a body part.

EXTRACTION: Pulling or stripping out or off all or a portion of a body part by the use of force.

Explanation: Qualifier "X Diagnostic" indicates extraction procedures that are biopsies
Examples: Non-excisional debridement – CMS Ex: Dilation and curettage

Body Part – 4TH	Approach – 5TH	Device – 6TH	Qualifier–7TH
1 Esophagus, Upper 2 Esophagus, Middle 3 Esophagus, Lower 4 Esophagogastric Junction 5 Esophagus 6 Stomach 7 Stomach, Pylorus 8 Small Intestine 9 Duodenum A Jejunum B Ileum C Ileocecal Valve E Large Intestine F Large Intestine, Right G Large Intestine, Left H Cecum J Appendix K Ascending Colon L Transverse Colon M Descending Colon N Sigmoid Colon P Rectum	3 Percutaneous 4 Percutaneous endoscopic 8 Via natural or artificial opening endoscopic	Z No device	X Diagnostic
Q Anus	3 Percutaneous 4 Percutaneous endoscopic 8 Via natural or artificial opening endoscopic X External	Z No device	X Diagnostic

© 2018 Channel Publishing, Ltd.

1ST - 0 Medical and Surgical
2ND - D Gastrointestinal System
3RD - F FRAGMENTATION

DRAINAGE GROUP: Drainage, Extirpation, Fragmentation
Root Operations that take out solids/fluids/gases from a body part.

FRAGMENTATION: Breaking solid matter in a body part into pieces.

Explanation: Pieces are not taken out during the procedure ...
Examples: Breaking apart gastric bezoar – CMS Ex: Extracorporeal shockwave lithotripsy

Body Part – 4TH			Approach – 5TH	Device – 6TH	Qualifier–7TH
5 Esophagus 6 Stomach 8 Small Intestine 9 Duodenum A Jejunum B Ileum	E Large Intestine F Large Intestine, Right G Large Intestine, Left H Cecum J Appendix K Ascending Colon	L Transverse Colon M Descending Colon N Sigmoid Colon P Rectum Q Anus	0 Open 3 Percutaneous 4 Percutaneous endoscopic 7 Via natural or artificial opening 8 Via natural or artificial opening endoscopic X External NC*	Z No device	Z No qualifier

NC* – Non-covered by Medicare. See current Medicare Code Editor for details.

1ST - 0 Medical and Surgical
2ND - D Gastrointestinal System
3RD - H INSERTION

DEVICE GROUP: Change, Insertion, Removal, Replacement, Revision, Supplement
Root Operations that always involve a device.

INSERTION: Putting in a nonbiological appliance that monitors, assists, performs, or prevents a physiological function but does not physically take the place of a body part.

Explanation: None
Examples: Placement artificial sphincter – CMS Ex: Insertion of central venous catheter

Body Part – 4TH	Approach – 5TH	Device – 6TH	Qualifier–7TH
0 Upper Intestinal Tract D Lower Intestinal Tract	0 Open 3 Percutaneous 4 Percutaneous endoscopic 7 Via natural or artificial opening 8 Via natural or artificial opening endoscopic	Y Other device	Z No qualifier
5 Esophagus	0 Open 3 Percutaneous 4 Percutaneous endoscopic	1 Radioactive element 2 Monitoring device 3 Infusion device D Intraluminal device U Feeding device Y Other device	Z No qualifier
5 Esophagus	7 Via natural or artificial opening 8 Via natural or artificial opening endoscopic	1 Radioactive element 2 Monitoring device 3 Infusion device B Intraluminal device, airway D Intraluminal device U Feeding device Y Other device	Z No qualifier
6 Stomach	0 Open 3 Percutaneous 4 Percutaneous endoscopic	2 Monitoring device 3 Infusion device D Intraluminal device M Stimulator lead U Feeding device Y Other device	Z No qualifier
6 Stomach	7 Via natural or artificial opening 8 Via natural or artificial opening endoscopic	2 Monitoring device 3 Infusion device D Intraluminal device U Feeding device Y Other device	Z No qualifier
8 Small Intestine 9 Duodenum A Jejunum B Ileum	0 Open 3 Percutaneous 4 Percutaneous endoscopic 7 Via natural or artificial opening 8 Via natural or artificial opening endoscopic	2 Monitoring device 3 Infusion device D Intraluminal device U Feeding device	Z No qualifier

continued ⇨

© 2018 Channel Publishing, Ltd.

0 D H INSERTION – *continued*

Body Part – 4TH	Approach – 5TH	Device – 6TH	Qualifier – 7TH
E Large Intestine	0 Open 3 Percutaneous 4 Percutaneous endoscopic 7 Via natural or artificial opening 8 Via natural or artificial opening endoscopic	D Intraluminal device	Z No qualifier
P Rectum	0 Open 3 Percutaneous 4 Percutaneous endoscopic 7 Via natural or artificial opening 8 Via natural or artificial opening endoscopic	1 Radioactive element D Intraluminal device	Z No qualifier
Q Anus	0 Open 3 Percutaneous 4 Percutaneous endoscopic	D Intraluminal device L Artificial sphincter	Z No qualifier
Q Anus	7 Via natural or artificial opening 8 Via natural or artificial opening endoscopic	D Intraluminal device	Z No qualifier
R Anal Sphincter	0 Open 3 Percutaneous 4 Percutaneous endoscopic	M Stimulator lead	Z No qualifier

1ST - 0 Medical and Surgical

2ND - D Gastrointestinal System

3RD - J INSPECTION

EXAMINATION GROUP: Inspection, (Map)
Root Operations involving examination only.

INSPECTION: Visually and/or manually exploring a body part.

Explanation: Direct or instrumental visualization ...
Examples: Esophagogastroduodenoscopy – CMS Ex: Exploratory laparotomy

Body Part – 4TH	Approach – 5TH	Device – 6TH	Qualifier – 7TH
0 Upper Intestinal Tract 6 Stomach D Lower Intestinal Tract	0 Open 3 Percutaneous 4 Percutaneous endoscopic 7 Via natural or artificial opening 8 Via natural or artificial opening endoscopic X External	Z No device	Z No qualifier
U Omentum V Mesentery W Peritoneum	0 Open 3 Percutaneous 4 Percutaneous endoscopic X External	Z No device	Z No qualifier

© 2018 Channel Publishing, Ltd.

1ST - 0 Medical and Surgical
2ND - D Gastrointestinal System
3RD - L OCCLUSION

TUBULAR GROUP: Bypass, Dilation, Occlusion, Restriction
Root Operations that alter the diameter/route of a tubular body part.

OCCLUSION: Completely closing an orifice or the lumen of a tubular body part.

Explanation: The orifice can be a natural orifice or an artificially created orifice
Examples: Closure rectal stump – CMS Ex: Fallopian tube ligation

Body Part – 4TH	Approach – 5TH	Device – 6TH	Qualifier – 7TH
1 Esophagus, Upper 2 Esophagus, Middle 3 Esophagus, Lower 4 Esophagogastric Junction 5 Esophagus 6 Stomach 7 Stomach, Pylorus 8 Small Intestine 9 Duodenum A Jejunum B Ileum C Ileocecal Valve E Large Intestine F Large Intestine, Right G Large Intestine, Left H Cecum K Ascending Colon L Transverse Colon M Descending Colon N Sigmoid Colon P Rectum	0 Open 3 Percutaneous 4 Percutaneous endoscopic	C Extraluminal device D Intraluminal device Z No device	Z No qualifier
1 Esophagus, Upper 2 Esophagus, Middle 3 Esophagus, Lower 4 Esophagogastric Junction 5 Esophagus 6 Stomach 7 Stomach, Pylorus 8 Small Intestine 9 Duodenum A Jejunum B Ileum C Ileocecal Valve E Large Intestine F Large Intestine, Right G Large Intestine, Left H Cecum K Ascending Colon L Transverse Colon M Descending Colon N Sigmoid Colon P Rectum	7 Via natural or artificial opening 8 Via natural or artificial opening endoscopic	D Intraluminal device Z No device	Z No qualifier
Q Anus	0 Open 3 Percutaneous 4 Percutaneous endoscopic X External	C Extraluminal device D Intraluminal device Z No device	Z No qualifier
Q Anus	7 Via natural or artificial opening 8 Via natural or artificial opening endoscopic	D Intraluminal device Z No device	Z No qualifier

1ST - 0 Medical and Surgical
2ND - D Gastrointestinal System
3RD - M REATTACHMENT

MOVE GROUP: Reattachment, Reposition, Transfer, Transplantation
Root Operations that put in/put back or move some/all of a body part.

REATTACHMENT: Putting back in or on all or a portion of a separated body part to its normal location or other suitable location.

Explanation: Vascular circulation and nervous pathways may or may not be reestablished
Examples: Reattachment avulsed esophagus – CMS Ex: Reattachment of hand

Body Part – 4TH	Approach – 5TH	Device – 6TH	Qualifier – 7TH
5 Esophagus 6 Stomach 8 Small Intestine 9 Duodenum A Jejunum B Ileum E Large Intestine F Large Intestine, Right G Large Intestine, Left H Cecum K Ascending Colon L Transverse Colon M Descending Colon N Sigmoid Colon P Rectum	0 Open 4 Percutaneous endoscopic	Z No device	Z No qualifier

© 2018 Channel Publishing, Ltd.

1ST - 0 Medical and Surgical
2ND - D Gastrointestinal System
3RD - N RELEASE

DIVISION GROUP: Division, Release
Root Operations involving cutting or separation only.

RELEASE: Freeing a body part from an abnormal physical constraint by cutting or by the use of force.

Explanation: Some of the restraining tissue may be taken out but none of the body part is taken out
Examples: Adhesiolysis colon – CMS Ex: Carpal tunnel release

Body Part – 4TH	Approach – 5TH	Device – 6TH	Qualifier–7TH
1 Esophagus, Upper 2 Esophagus, Middle 3 Esophagus, Lower 4 Esophagogastric Junction 5 Esophagus 6 Stomach 7 Stomach, Pylorus 8 Small Intestine 9 Duodenum A Jejunum B Ileum C Ileocecal Valve E Large Intestine F Large Intestine, Right G Large Intestine, Left H Cecum J Appendix K Ascending Colon L Transverse Colon M Descending Colon N Sigmoid Colon P Rectum	0 Open 3 Percutaneous 4 Percutaneous endoscopic 7 Via natural or artificial opening 8 Via natural or artificial opening endoscopic	Z No device	Z No qualifier
Q Anus	0 Open 3 Percutaneous 4 Percutaneous endoscopic 7 Via natural or artificial opening 8 Via natural or artificial opening endoscopic X External	Z No device	Z No qualifier
R Anal Sphincter U Omentum V Mesentery W Peritoneum	0 Open 3 Percutaneous 4 Percutaneous endoscopic	Z No device	Z No qualifier

1ST - 0 Medical and Surgical
2ND - D Gastrointestinal System
3RD - P REMOVAL

DEVICE GROUP: Change, Insertion, Removal, Replacement, Revision, Supplement
Root Operations that always involve a device.

REMOVAL: Taking out or off a device from a body part.

Explanation: Removal device without reinsertion ...
Examples: Removal artificial sphincter – CMS Ex: Cardiac pacemaker removal

Body Part – 4TH	Approach – 5TH	Device – 6TH	Qualifier –7TH
0 Upper Intestinal Tract D Lower Intestinal Tract	0 Open 3 Percutaneous 4 Percutaneous endoscopic 7 Via natural or artificial opening 8 Via natural or artificial opening endoscopic	0 Drainage device 2 Monitoring device 3 Infusion device 7 Autologous tissue substitute C Extraluminal device D Intraluminal device J Synthetic substitute K Nonautologous tissue substitute U Feeding device Y Other device	Z No qualifier
0 Upper Intestinal Tract D Lower Intestinal Tract	X External	0 Drainage device 2 Monitoring device 3 Infusion device D Intraluminal device U Feeding device	Z No qualifier
5 Esophagus	0 Open 3 Percutaneous 4 Percutaneous endoscopic	1 Radioactive element 2 Monitoring device 3 Infusion device U Feeding device Y Other device	Z No qualifier
5 Esophagus	7 Via natural or artificial opening 8 Via natural or artificial opening endoscopic	1 Radioactive element D Intraluminal device Y Other device	Z No qualifier

continued ⇨

© 2018 Channel Publishing, Ltd.

0 D P REMOVAL – *continued*

Body Part – 4TH	Approach – 5TH	Device – 6TH	Qualifier–7TH
5 Esophagus	X External	1 Radioactive element 2 Monitoring device 3 Infusion device D Intraluminal device U Feeding device	Z No qualifier
6 Stomach	0 Open 3 Percutaneous 4 Percutaneous endoscopic	0 Drainage device 2 Monitoring device 3 Infusion device 7 Autologous tissue substitute C Extraluminal device D Intraluminal device J Synthetic substitute K Nonautologous tissue substitute M Stimulator lead U Feeding device Y Other device	Z No qualifier
6 Stomach	7 Via natural or artificial opening 8 Via natural or artificial opening endoscopic	0 Drainage device 2 Monitoring device 3 Infusion device 7 Autologous tissue substitute C Extraluminal device D Intraluminal device J Synthetic substitute K Nonautologous tissue substitute U Feeding device Y Other device	Z No qualifier
6 Stomach	X External	0 Drainage device 2 Monitoring device 3 Infusion device D Intraluminal device U Feeding device	Z No qualifier
P Rectum	0 Open 3 Percutaneous 4 Percutaneous endoscopic 7 Via natural or artificial opening 8 Via natural or artificial opening endoscopic X External	1 Radioactive element	Z No qualifier
Q Anus	0 Open 3 Percutaneous 4 Percutaneous endoscopic 7 Via natural or artificial opening 8 Via natural or artificial opening endoscopic	L Artificial sphincter	Z No qualifier
R Anal Sphincter	0 Open 3 Percutaneous 4 Percutaneous endoscopic	M Stimulator lead	Z No qualifier
U Omentum V Mesentery W Peritoneum	0 Open 3 Percutaneous 4 Percutaneous endoscopic	0 Drainage device 1 Radioactive element 7 Autologous tissue substitute J Synthetic substitute K Nonautologous tissue substitute	Z No qualifier

© 2018 Channel Publishing, Ltd.

1ST - 0 Medical and Surgical
2ND - D Gastrointestinal System
3RD - Q REPAIR

OTHER REPAIRS GROUP: (Control), Repair
Root Operations that define other repairs.

REPAIR: Restoring, to the extent possible, a body part to its normal anatomic structure and function.

Explanation: Used only when the method to accomplish the repair is not one of the other root operations
Examples: Suture duodenal laceration – CMS Ex: Suture of laceration

Body Part – 4TH	Approach – 5TH	Device – 6TH	Qualifier–7TH
1 Esophagus, Upper 2 Esophagus, Middle 3 Esophagus, Lower 4 Esophagogastric Junction 5 Esophagus 6 Stomach 7 Stomach, Pylorus 8 Small Intestine 9 Duodenum A Jejunum B Ileum C Ileocecal Valve E Large Intestine F Large Intestine, Right G Large Intestine, Left H Cecum J Appendix K Ascending Colon L Transverse Colon M Descending Colon N Sigmoid Colon P Rectum	0 Open 3 Percutaneous 4 Percutaneous endoscopic 7 Via natural or artificial opening 8 Via natural or artificial opening endoscopic	Z No device	Z No qualifier
Q Anus	0 Open 3 Percutaneous 4 Percutaneous endoscopic 7 Via natural or artificial opening 8 Via natural or artificial opening endoscopic X External	Z No device	Z No qualifier
R Anal Sphincter U Omentum V Mesentery W Peritoneum	0 Open 3 Percutaneous 4 Percutaneous endoscopic	Z No device	Z No qualifier

1ST - 0 Medical and Surgical
2ND - D Gastrointestinal System
3RD - R REPLACEMENT

DEVICE GROUP: Change, Insertion, Removal, Replacement, Revision, Supplement
Root Operations that always involve a device.

REPLACEMENT: Putting in or on biological or synthetic material that physically takes the place and/or function of all or a portion of a body part.

Explanation: Includes taking out or eradicating, or rendering non-functional, the body part ...
Examples: Esophageal segment replacement – CMS Ex: Total hip replacement

Body Part – 4TH	Approach – 5TH	Device – 6TH	Qualifier–7TH
5 Esophagus	0 Open 4 Percutaneous endoscopic 7 Via natural or artificial opening 8 Via natural or artificial opening endoscopic	7 Autologous tissue substitute J Synthetic substitute K Nonautologous tissue substitute	Z No qualifier
R Anal Sphincter U Omentum V Mesentery W Peritoneum	0 Open 4 Percutaneous endoscopic	7 Autologous tissue substitute J Synthetic substitute K Nonautologous tissue substitute	Z No qualifier

1ST - 0 Medical and Surgical
2ND - D Gastrointestinal System
3RD - S REPOSITION

MOVE GROUP: Reattachment, Reposition, Transfer, Transplantation
Root Operations that put in/put back or move some/all of a body part.

REPOSITION: Moving to its normal location, or other suitable location, all or a portion of a body part.

Explanation: The body part may or may not be cut out or off to be moved to the new location ...
Examples: Gastropexy for malrotation – CMS Ex: Fracture reduction

Body Part – 4TH	Approach – 5TH	Device – 6TH	Qualifier – 7TH
5 Esophagus 6 Stomach 9 Duodenum A Jejunum B Ileum H Cecum K Ascending Colon L Transverse Colon M Descending Colon N Sigmoid Colon P Rectum Q Anus	0 Open 4 Percutaneous endoscopic 7 Via natural or artificial opening 8 Via natural or artificial opening endoscopic X External	Z No device	Z No qualifier
8 Small Intestine E Large Intestine	0 Open 4 Percutaneous endoscopic 7 Via natural or artificial opening 8 Via natural or artificial opening endoscopic	Z No device	Z No qualifier

© 2018 Channel Publishing, Ltd.

1ST - 0 Medical and Surgical
2ND - D Gastrointestinal System
3RD - T RESECTION

EXCISION GROUP: Excision, Resection, Destruction, Extraction, (Detachment)
Root Operations that take out some or all of a body part.

RESECTION: Cutting out or off, without replacement, all of a body part.

Explanation: None
Examples: Sigmoid colectomy – CMS Ex: Total lobectomy of lung

Body Part – 4TH	Approach – 5TH	Device – 6TH	Qualifier – 7TH
1 Esophagus, Upper 2 Esophagus, Middle 3 Esophagus, Lower 4 Esophagogastric Junction 5 Esophagus 6 Stomach 7 Stomach, Pylorus 8 Small Intestine 9 Duodenum A Jejunum B Ileum C Ileocecal Valve E Large Intestine F Large Intestine, Right H Cecum J Appendix K Ascending Colon P Rectum Q Anus	0 Open 4 Percutaneous endoscopic 7 Via natural or artificial opening 8 Via natural or artificial opening endoscopic	Z No device	Z No qualifier
G Large Intestine, Left L Transverse Colon M Descending Colon N Sigmoid Colon	0 Open 4 Percutaneous endoscopic 7 Via natural or artificial opening 8 Via natural or artificial opening endoscopic F Via natural or artificial opening with percutaneous endoscopic assistance	Z No device	Z No qualifier
R Anal Sphincter U Omentum	0 Open 4 Percutaneous endoscopic	Z No device	Z No qualifier

1ST - 0 Medical and Surgical
2ND - D Gastrointestinal System
3RD - U SUPPLEMENT

DEVICE GROUP: Change, Insertion, Removal, Replacement, Revision, Supplement
Root Operations that always involve a device.

SUPPLEMENT: Putting in or on biological or synthetic material that physically reinforces and/or augments the function of a portion of a body part.

Explanation: Biological material is non-living, or is living and from the same individual ...
Examples: Repair rectum with graft – CMS Ex: Herniorrhaphy using mesh

Body Part – 4TH	Approach – 5TH	Device – 6TH	Qualifier – 7TH
1 Esophagus, Upper 2 Esophagus, Middle 3 Esophagus, Lower 4 Esophagogastric Junction 5 Esophagus 6 Stomach 7 Stomach, Pylorus 8 Small Intestine 9 Duodenum A Jejunum B Ileum C Ileocecal Valve E Large Intestine F Large Intestine, Right G Large Intestine, Left H Cecum K Ascending Colon L Transverse Colon M Descending Colon N Sigmoid Colon P Rectum	0 Open 4 Percutaneous endoscopic 7 Via natural or artificial opening 8 Via natural or artificial opening endoscopic	7 Autologous tissue substitute J Synthetic substitute K Nonautologous tissue substitute	Z No qualifier
Q Anus	0 Open 4 Percutaneous endoscopic 7 Via natural or artificial opening 8 Via natural or artificial opening endoscopic X External	7 Autologous tissue substitute J Synthetic substitute K Nonautologous tissue substitute	Z No qualifier
R Anal Sphincter U Omentum V Mesentery W Peritoneum	0 Open 4 Percutaneous endoscopic	7 Autologous tissue substitute J Synthetic substitute K Nonautologous tissue substitute	Z No qualifier

GASTROINTESTINAL 0DT

© 2018 Channel Publishing, Ltd.

1ST - 0 Medical and Surgical
2ND - D Gastrointestinal System
3RD - V RESTRICTION

TUBULAR GROUP: Bypass, Dilation, Occlusion, Restriction
Root Operations that alter the diameter/route of a tubular body part.
RESTRICTION: Partially closing an orifice or the lumen of a tubular body part.

Explanation: The orifice can be a natural orifice or an artificially created orifice.
Examples: Nissen fundoplication – CMS Ex: Cervical cerclage

Body Part – 4TH	Approach – 5TH	Device – 6TH	Qualifier -7TH
1 Esophagus, Upper 2 Esophagus, Middle 3 Esophagus, Lower 4 Esophagogastric Junction 5 Esophagus 6 Stomach 7 Stomach, Pylorus 8 Small Intestine 9 Duodenum A Jejunum B Ileum C Ileocecal Valve E Large Intestine F Large Intestine, Right G Large Intestine, Left H Cecum K Ascending Colon L Transverse Colon M Descending Colon N Sigmoid Colon P Rectum	0 Open 3 Percutaneous 4 Percutaneous endoscopic	C Extraluminal device D Intraluminal device Z No device	Z No qualifier
1 Esophagus, Upper 2 Esophagus, Middle 3 Esophagus, Lower 4 Esophagogastric Junction 5 Esophagus 6 Stomach NC* 7 Stomach, Pylorus 8 Small Intestine 9 Duodenum A Jejunum B Ileum C Ileocecal Valve E Large Intestine F Large Intestine, Right G Large Intestine, Left H Cecum K Ascending Colon L Transverse Colon M Descending Colon N Sigmoid Colon P Rectum	7 Via natural or artificial opening 8 Via natural or artificial opening endoscopic	D Intraluminal device Z No device	Z No qualifier
Q Anus	0 Open 3 Percutaneous 4 Percutaneous endoscopic X External	C Extraluminal device D Intraluminal device Z No device	Z No qualifier
Q Anus	7 Via natural or artificial opening 8 Via natural or artificial opening endoscopic	D Intraluminal device Z No device	Z No qualifier

NC* – Some procedures are considered non-covered by Medicare. See current Medicare Code Editor for details.

1ST - 0 Medical and Surgical
2ND - D Gastrointestinal System
3RD - W REVISION

DEVICE GROUP: Change, Insertion, Removal, Replacement, Revision, Supplement
Root Operations that always involve a device.
REVISION: Correcting, to the extent possible, a portion of a malfunctioning device or the position of a displaced device.

Explanation: Correcting by taking out or putting in components of a device such as a screw or pin ...
Examples: Reposition artificial anal sphincter – CMS Ex: Recementing of hip prosthesis

Body Part – 4TH	Approach – 5TH	Device – 6TH	Qualifier –7TH
0 Upper Intestinal Tract D Lower Intestinal Tract	0 Open 3 Percutaneous 4 Percutaneous endoscopic 7 Via natural or artificial opening 8 Via natural or artificial opening endoscopic	0 Drainage device 2 Monitoring device 3 Infusion device 7 Autologous tissue substitute C Extraluminal device D Intraluminal device J Synthetic substitute K Nonautologous tissue substitute U Feeding device Y Other device	Z No qualifier
0 Upper Intestinal Tract D Lower Intestinal Tract	X External	0 Drainage device 2 Monitoring device 3 Infusion device 7 Autologous tissue substitute C Extraluminal device D Intraluminal device J Synthetic substitute K Nonautologous tissue substitute U Feeding device	Z No qualifier

continued ⇨

© 2018 Channel Publishing, Ltd.

0 D W REVISION – *continued*

Body Part – 4TH	Approach – 5TH	Device – 6TH	Qualifier–7TH
5 Esophagus	0 Open 3 Percutaneous 4 Percutaneous endoscopic	Y Other device	Z No qualifier
5 Esophagus	7 Via natural or artificial opening 8 Via natural or artificial opening endoscopic	D Intraluminal device Y Other device	Z No qualifier
5 Esophagus	X External	D Intraluminal device	Z No qualifier
6 Stomach	0 Open 3 Percutaneous 4 Percutaneous endoscopic	0 Drainage device 2 Monitoring device 3 Infusion device 7 Autologous tissue substitute C Extraluminal device D Intraluminal device J Synthetic substitute K Nonautologous tissue substitute M Stimulator lead U Feeding device Y Other device	Z No qualifier
6 Stomach	7 Via natural or artificial opening 8 Via natural or artificial opening endoscopic	0 Drainage device 2 Monitoring device 3 Infusion device 7 Autologous tissue substitute C Extraluminal device D Intraluminal device J Synthetic substitute K Nonautologous tissue substitute U Feeding device Y Other device	Z No qualifier
6 Stomach	X External	0 Drainage device 2 Monitoring device 3 Infusion device 7 Autologous tissue substitute C Extraluminal device D Intraluminal device J Synthetic substitute K Nonautologous tissue substitute U Feeding device	Z No qualifier
8 Small Intestine E Large Intestine	0 Open 4 Percutaneous endoscopic 7 Via natural or artificial opening 8 Via natural or artificial opening endoscopic	7 Autologous tissue substitute J Synthetic substitute K Nonautologous tissue substitute	Z No qualifier
Q Anus	0 Open 3 Percutaneous 4 Percutaneous endoscopic 7 Via natural or artificial opening 8 Via natural or artificial opening endoscopic	L Artificial sphincter	Z No qualifier
R Anal Sphincter	0 Open 3 Percutaneous 4 Percutaneous endoscopic	M Stimulator lead	Z No qualifier
U Omentum V Mesentery W Peritoneum	0 Open 3 Percutaneous 4 Percutaneous endoscopic	0 Drainage device 7 Autologous tissue substitute J Synthetic substitute K Nonautologous tissue substitute	Z No qualifier

© 2018 Channel Publishing, Ltd.

1ST - 0 Medical and Surgical
2ND - D Gastrointestinal System
3RD - X TRANSFER

MOVE GROUP: Reattachment, Reposition, Transfer, Transplantation
Root Operations that put in/put back or move some/all of a body part.

TRANSFER: Moving, without taking out, all or a portion of a body part to another location to take over the function of all or a portion of a body part.

Explanation: The body part transferred remains connected to its vascular and nervous supply
Examples: Colon-interposition esophagus – CMS Ex: Tendon transfer

Body Part – 4TH	Approach – 5TH	Device – 6TH	Qualifier – 7TH
6 Stomach 8 Small Intestine E Large Intestine	0 Open 4 Percutaneous endoscopic	Z No device	5 Esophagus

1ST - 0 Medical and Surgical
2ND - D Gastrointestinal System
3RD - Y TRANSPLANTATION

MOVE GROUP: Reattachment, Reposition, Transfer, Transplantation
Root Operations that put in/put back or move some/all of a body part.

TRANSPLANTATION: Putting in or on all or a portion of a living body part taken from another individual or animal to physically take the place and/or function of all or a portion of a similar body part.

Explanation: The native body part may or may not be taken out ...
Examples: Esophagus transplant – CMS Ex: Kidney transplant

Body Part – 4TH	Approach – 5TH	Device – 6TH	Qualifier – 7TH
5 Esophagus 6 Stomach 8 Small Intestine LC* E Large Intestine LC*	0 Open	Z No device	0 Allogeneic 1 Syngeneic 2 Zooplastic

LC* – Some procedures are considered limited coverage by Medicare. See current Medicare Code Editor for details.

© 2018 Channel Publishing, Ltd.

NOTES

© 2018 Channel Publishing, Ltd.

Educational Annotations | F – Hepatobiliary System and Pancreas

Body System Specific Educational Annotations for the Hepatobiliary System and Pancreas include:

- Anatomy and Physiology Review
- Definitions of Common Procedures
- Anatomical Illustrations
- AHA Coding Clinic® Reference Notations
- Body Part Key Listings
- Device Key Listings
- Device Aggregation Table Listings
- Coding Notes

Anatomy and Physiology Review of Hepatobiliary System and Pancreas

BODY PART VALUES - F - HEPATOBILIARY SYSTEM AND PANCREAS

Ampulla of Vater – The common bile duct merges with the pancreatic duct in the dilated area known as the ampulla of Vater.

Common Bile Duct – ANATOMY – The common bile duct is formed by the merger of the cystic duct from the gallbladder and the common hepatic duct. PHYSIOLOGY – The cystic duct, hepatic duct, and common bile duct convey the bile into the duodenum.

Cystic Duct – ANATOMY – The cystic duct is the tubular drain of the gallbladder which merges with the hepatic duct to form the common bile duct. PHYSIOLOGY – The cystic duct, hepatic duct, and common bile duct convey the bile into the duodenum.

Gallbladder – ANATOMY – The gallbladder is the musculomembranous, pear-shaped bile reservoir located on the undersurface of the liver. PHYSIOLOGY – The gallbladder functions to store and concentrate the bile and release the bile on demand to the small intestine for the digestion of fats.

Hepatic Duct – ANATOMY – The common hepatic duct is formed by the merger of the right and left hepatic ducts that drain the smaller intrahepatic ducts. PHYSIOLOGY – The cystic duct, hepatic duct, and common bile duct convey the bile into the duodenum.

Hepatobiliary Duct – The ducts of the hepatobiliary system including the cystic duct, hepatic ducts, and common bile duct.

Liver – ANATOMY – The liver is the largest organ in the body, weighing about 3 pounds (1 kg) in the adult. Located in the upper right quadrant of the abdominal cavity, its superior surface lies under the dome of the diaphragm. There are 4 lobes of the liver; the left, right (the right lobe has two smaller lobes, the caudate and quadrate). The common bile duct is formed by the joining of the hepatic duct, which carries bile from the liver, and the cystic duct, which carries bile from the gallbladder. The common duct then carries the bile into the duodenum through an opening on the duodenal papilla. The hepatic artery furnishes arterial blood for the nourishment of the liver cells. The portal vein carries blood containing products of digestion from the intestinal tract into the liver. Internally, the liver lobules are the functional units of liver substance. Bile is secreted by the liver cells into tiny canals, or canaliculi, and then emptied into a bile duct. PHYSIOLOGY – One of the regulatory functions of the liver is controlling the blood sugar level. The liver is able to both absorb excess sugar and dispense it into the blood. The liver also stores and secretes other essential nutrients. It chemically processes these materials and detoxifies many substances that could be harmful if allowed to accumulate in the body. Its bile salts are necessary for the absorption of vitamin K from the gastrointestinal tract, which in turn are needed for the production of prothrombin. Another important liver function is producing bile. A brownish-yellow fluid, it is secreted continuously by the liver in amounts averaging about 20 fluid ounces (600 ml) per day. Bile contains the bile salts which are very important in the digestion of fat.

Liver, Left Lobe – One of the two common lobes of the liver.

Liver, Right Lobe – One of the two common lobes of the liver.

Pancreas – ANATOMY – The pancreas is a slender organ about 6 to 9 inches (15 to 23 cm) long lying horizontally and located in the abdomen behind and under the stomach. The pancreas is divided into 3 areas: The head, lying in the curve formed by the duodenum; the body, the main portion lying between the head and tail; and the tail, the most lateral portion blunting up against the spleen. The cells that produce pancreatic juice are called pancreatic acinar cells, and they make up the bulk of the pancreas. These cells are clustered around tiny tubes which drain into the pancreatic duct (duct of Wirsung). This duct connects with the duodenum at the same place where the bile ducts join the duodenum. The second type of pancreatic cells are arranged in groups closely associated with blood vessels and are called islets of Langerhans. The pancreas arterial blood is supplied via the common hepatic artery, the gastroduodenal artery, the pancreatico-duodenal arches, the splenic artery, and also from the superior mesenteric artery. PHYSIOLOGY – The pancreas functions as both an exocrine gland, producing pancreatic juice, and as an endocrine gland, producing the hormones insulin and glucagen. The pancreatic juice contains enzymes capable of digesting carbohydrates, fats, proteins, and nucleic acids, and is produced by the pancreatic acinar cells. This juice is drained into the duodenum. The pancreatic hormones which are produced by the islets of Langerhans cells regulate blood glucose level.

Pancreatic Duct – The pancreatic duct connects with the duodenum at the dilated area known as the ampulla of Vater.

Pancreatic Duct, Accessory – The presence of an additional pancreatic duct that connects directly with the duodenum.

Definitions of Common Procedures of Hepatobiliary System and Pancreas

Choledochojejunostomy – The surgical anastomosis of the common bile duct to the jejunum to relieve biliary obstruction symptoms.

Endoscopic retrograde cholangiopancreatography (ERCP) – The combination of endoscopic and fluoroscopy to visualize, obtain radiographs, and treat conditions in the biliary and/or pancreatic duct systems.

Laparoscopic gallbladder-preserving cholelithotomy – The incision and removal of gallstones that is performed laparoscopically and without removing the gallbladder.

Lobectomy of liver – The surgical excision of an anatomic lobe of the liver with its vascular connections.

Wedge resection of liver – The surgical excision of less than a whole anatomic liver segment or parts of two anatomic segments.

Whipple procedure (pancreatoduodenectomy) – The surgical excision of the head of the pancreas that usually includes a duodenectomy, cholecystectomy, and a portion of the stomach including the pylorus, with anastomosis of the common bile duct, pancreas, and stomach to the jejunum. A pyloric-sparing version keeps the stomach and pylorus intact.

© 2018 Channel Publishing, Ltd.

Educational Annotations | F – Hepatobiliary System and Pancreas

Anatomical Illustrations of Hepatobiliary System and Pancreas

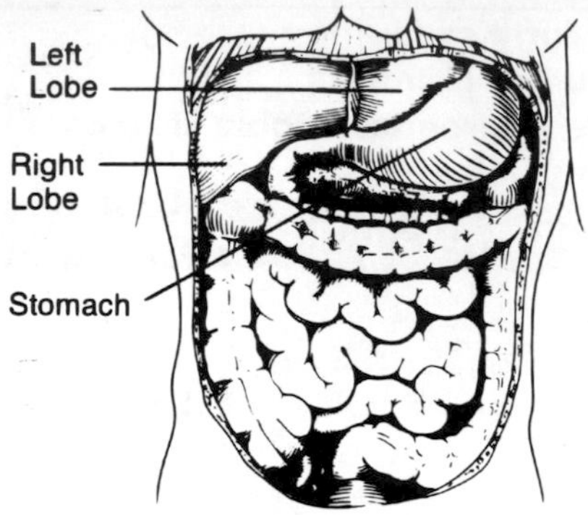

LIVER — ANTERIOR VIEW

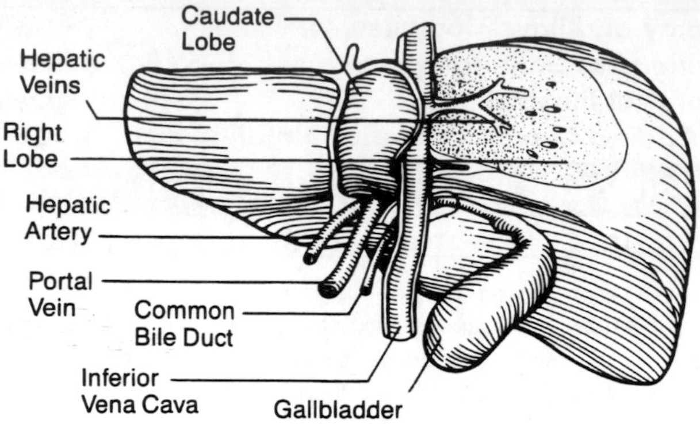

LIVER — POSTERIOR VIEW

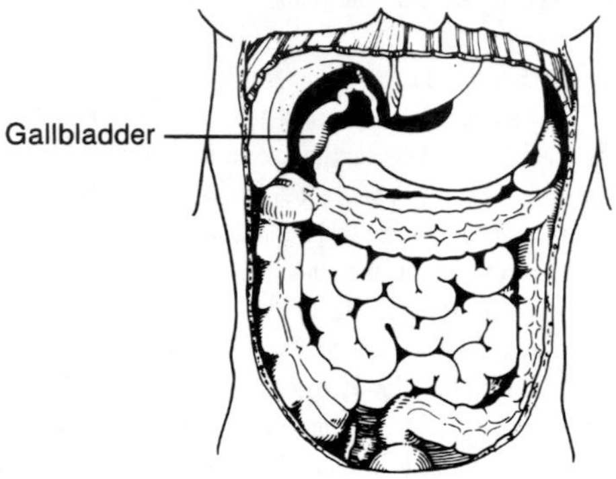

GALLBLADDER

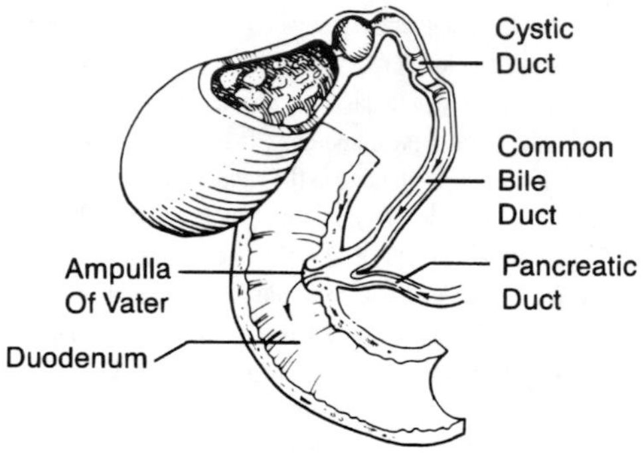

GALLBLADDER — ANTERIOR (CUT-AWAY) VIEW

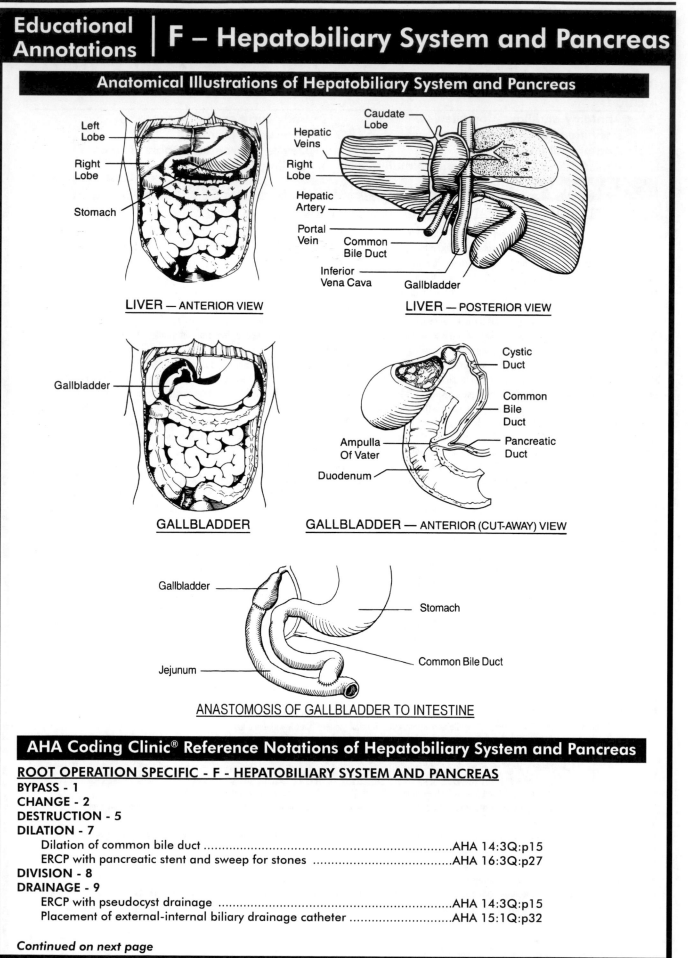

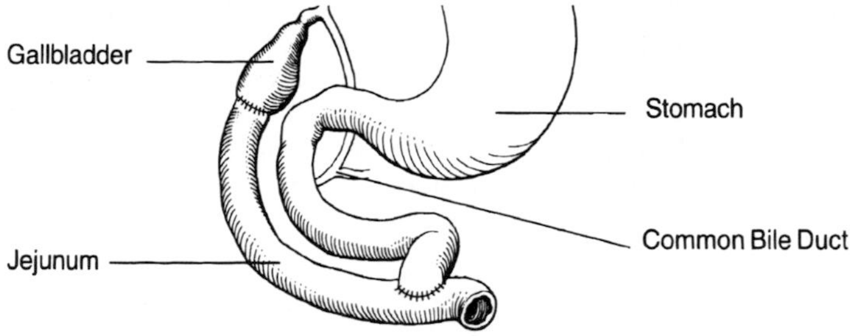

ANASTOMOSIS OF GALLBLADDER TO INTESTINE

AHA Coding Clinic® Reference Notations of Hepatobiliary System and Pancreas

ROOT OPERATION SPECIFIC - F - HEPATOBILIARY SYSTEM AND PANCREAS

BYPASS - 1
CHANGE - 2
DESTRUCTION - 5
DILATION - 7
Dilation of common bile duct ....AHA 14:3Q:p15
ERCP with pancreatic stent and sweep for stones ....AHA 16:3Q:p27
DIVISION - 8
DRAINAGE - 9
ERCP with pseudocyst drainage ....AHA 14:3Q:p15
Placement of external-internal biliary drainage catheter ....AHA 15:1Q:p32

Continued on next page

HEPATOBILIARY 0F

© 2018 Channel Publishing, Ltd.

Educational Annotations | F – Hepatobiliary System and Pancreas

AHA Coding Clinic® Reference Notations of Hepatobiliary System and Pancreas

ROOT OPERATION SPECIFIC - F - HEPATOBILIARY SYSTEM AND PANCREAS

Continued from previous page

EXCISION - B
- Brush biopsy of pancreatic and common bile ducts ....AHA 16:1Q:p25
- Needle biopsy of common hepatic duct ....AHA 16:1Q:p23
- Whipple pyloric sparing pancreaticoduodenectomy....AHA 14:3Q:p32

EXTIRPATION - C
FRAGMENTATION - F
INSERTION - H
INSPECTION - J
OCCLUSION - L
REATTACHMENT - M
RELEASE - N
REMOVAL - P
REPAIR - Q
- Redo of bile duct anastomosis ....AHA 16:3Q:p27

REPLACEMENT - R
REPOSITION - S
RESECTION - T
- Resection of liver to capture "domino liver transplant" ....AHA 12:4Q:p99

SUPPLEMENT - U
RESTRICTION - V
REVISION - W
TRANSPLANTATION - Y
- "Domino liver transplant"....AHA 12:4Q:p99
- Orthotopic liver allotransplant ....AHA 14:3Q:p13

Body Part Key Listings of Hepatobiliary System and Pancreas

See also Body Part Key in Appendix C

Duct of Santorini ....use Pancreatic Duct, Accessory
Duct of Wirsung ....use Pancreatic Duct
Duodenal ampulla....use Ampulla of Vater
Hepatopancreatic ampulla ....use Ampulla of Vater
Quadrate lobe ....use Liver

Device Key Listings of Hepatobiliary System and Pancreas

See also Device Key in Appendix D

Autograft ....use Autologous Tissue Substitute
Brachytherapy seeds ....use Radioactive Element
Stent, intraluminal (cardiovascular) (gastrointestinal) (hepatobiliary) (urinary) ....use Intraluminal Device
Tissue bank graft ....use Nonautologous Tissue Substitute

Device Aggregation Table Listings of Hepatobiliary System and Pancreas

See also Device Aggregation Table in Appendix E

Specific Device	For Operation	In Body System	General Device
None Listed in Device Aggregation Table for this Body System			

Coding Notes of Hepatobiliary System and Pancreas

© 2018 Channel Publishing, Ltd.

HEPATOBILIARY 0F

1ST - 0 Medical and Surgical
2ND - F Hepatobiliary System and Pancreas
3RD - 1 BYPASS

TUBULAR GROUP: Bypass, Dilation, Occlusion, Restriction
Root Operations that alter the diameter/route of a tubular body part.
BYPASS: Altering the route of passage of the contents of a tubular body part.
Explanation: Rerouting contents to a downstream part ... with or without the use of a device ...
Examples: Choledochojejunostomy – CMS Ex: Coronary artery bypass

Body Part – 4TH	Approach – 5TH	Device – 6TH	Qualifier – 7TH
4 Gallbladder 5 Hepatic Duct, Right 6 Hepatic Duct, Left 7 Hepatic Duct, Common 8 Cystic Duct 9 Common Bile Duct	0 Open 4 Percutaneous endoscopic	D Intraluminal device Z No device	3 Duodenum 4 Stomach 5 Hepatic Duct, Right 6 Hepatic Duct, Left 7 Hepatic Duct, Caudate 8 Cystic Duct 9 Common Bile Duct B Small Intestine
D Pancreatic Duct F Pancreatic Duct, Accessory G Pancreas	0 Open 4 Percutaneous endoscopic	D Intraluminal device Z No device	3 Duodenum B Small Intestine C Large Intestine

1ST - 0 Medical and Surgical
2ND - F Hepatobiliary System and Pancreas
3RD - 2 CHANGE

DEVICE GROUP: Change, Insertion, Removal, Replacement, Revision, Supplement
Root Operations that always involve a device.
CHANGE: Taking out or off a device from a body part and putting back an identical or similar device in or on the same body part without cutting or puncturing the skin or a mucous membrane.
Explanation: All CHANGE procedures are coded using the approach External
Examples: Exchange drainage tube – CMS Ex: Urinary catheter change

Body Part – 4TH	Approach – 5TH	Device – 6TH	Qualifier – 7TH
0 Liver 4 Gallbladder B Hepatobiliary Duct D Pancreatic Duct G Pancreas	X External	0 Drainage device Y Other device	Z No qualifier

1ST - 0 Medical and Surgical
2ND - F Hepatobiliary System and Pancreas
3RD - 5 DESTRUCTION

EXCISION GROUP: Excision, Resection, Destruction, Extraction, (Detachment)
Root Operations that take out some or all of a body part.
DESTRUCTION: Physical eradication of all or a portion of a body part by the direct use of energy, force, or a destructive agent.
Explanation: None of the body part is physically taken out
Examples: Radiofrequency ablation liver lesion – CMS Ex: Fulguration of rectal polyp

Body Part – 4TH	Approach – 5TH	Device – 6TH	Qualifier – 7TH
0 Liver 1 Liver, Right Lobe 2 Liver, Left Lobe	0 Open 3 Percutaneous 4 Percutaneous endoscopic	Z No device	F Irreversible electroporation Z No qualifier
4 Gallbladder	0 Open 3 Percutaneous 4 Percutaneous endoscopic 8 Via natural or artificial opening endoscopic	Z No device	Z No qualifier
5 Hepatic Duct, Right 6 Hepatic Duct, Left 7 Hepatic Duct, Common 8 Cystic Duct 9 Common Bile Duct C Ampulla of Vater D Pancreatic Duct F Pancreatic Duct, Accessory	0 Open 3 Percutaneous 4 Percutaneous endoscopic 7 Via natural or artificial opening 8 Via natural or artificial opening endoscopic	Z No device	Z No qualifier
G Pancreas	0 Open 3 Percutaneous 4 Percutaneous endoscopic	Z No device	F Irreversible electroporation Z No qualifier
G Pancreas	8 Via natural or artificial opening endoscopic	Z No device	Z No qualifier

© 2018 Channel Publishing, Ltd.

1ST - 0 Medical and Surgical
2ND - F Hepatobiliary System and Pancreas
3RD - 7 DILATION

TUBULAR GROUP: Bypass, Dilation, Occlusion, Restriction
Root Operations that alter the diameter/route of a tubular body part.

DILATION: Expanding an orifice or the lumen of a tubular body part.

Explanation: Accomplished by stretching or cutting ... tubular body part or orifice ...
Examples: ERCP dilation pancreatic duct – CMS Ex: Percutaneous transluminal angioplasty

Body Part – 4TH	Approach – 5TH	Device – 6TH	Qualifier -7TH
5 Hepatic Duct, Right 6 Hepatic Duct, Left 7 Hepatic Duct, Common 8 Cystic Duct 9 Common Bile Duct C Ampulla of Vater D Pancreatic Duct F Pancreatic Duct, Accessory	0 Open 3 Percutaneous 4 Percutaneous endoscopic 7 Via natural or artificial opening 8 Via natural or artificial opening endoscopic	D Intraluminal device Z No device	Z No qualifier

1ST - 0 Medical and Surgical
2ND - F Hepatobiliary System and Pancreas
3RD - 8 DIVISION

DIVISION GROUP: Division, Release
Root Operations involving cutting or separation only.

DIVISION: Cutting into a body part, without draining fluids and/or gases from the body part, in order to separate or transect a body part.

Explanation: All or a portion of the body part is separated into two or more portions
Examples: Pancreatotomy – CMS Ex: Spinal cordotomy

Body Part – 4TH	Approach – 5TH	Device – 6TH	Qualifier – 7TH
G Pancreas	0 Open 3 Percutaneous 4 Percutaneous endoscopic	Z No device	Z No qualifier

1ST - 0 Medical and Surgical
2ND - F Hepatobiliary System and Pancreas
3RD - 9 DRAINAGE

DRAINAGE GROUP: Drainage, Extirpation, Fragmentation
Root Operations that take out solids/fluids/gases from a body part.

DRAINAGE: Taking or letting out fluids and/or gases from a body part.

Explanation: Qualifier "X Diagnostic" indicates drainage procedures that are biopsies
Examples: ERCP pseudocyst drainage – CMS Ex: Thoracentesis

Body Part – 4TH	Approach – 5TH	Device – 6TH	Qualifier -7TH
0 Liver 1 Liver, Right Lobe 2 Liver, Left Lobe	0 Open 3 Percutaneous 4 Percutaneous endoscopic	0 Drainage device	Z No qualifier
0 Liver 1 Liver, Right Lobe 2 Liver, Left Lobe	0 Open 3 Percutaneous 4 Percutaneous endoscopic	Z No device	X Diagnostic Z No qualifier
4 Gallbladder G Pancreas	0 Open 3 Percutaneous 4 Percutaneous endoscopic 8 Via natural or artificial opening endoscopic	0 Drainage device	Z No qualifier
4 Gallbladder G Pancreas	0 Open 3 Percutaneous 4 Percutaneous endoscopic 8 Via natural or artificial opening endoscopic	Z No device	X Diagnostic Z No qualifier
5 Hepatic Duct, Right 6 Hepatic Duct, Left 7 Hepatic Duct, Common 8 Cystic Duct 9 Common Bile Duct C Ampulla of Vater D Pancreatic Duct F Pancreatic Duct, Accessory	0 Open 3 Percutaneous 4 Percutaneous endoscopic 7 Via natural or artificial opening 8 Via natural or artificial opening endoscopic	0 Drainage device	Z No qualifier
5 Hepatic Duct, Right 6 Hepatic Duct, Left 7 Hepatic Duct, Common 8 Cystic Duct 9 Common Bile Duct C Ampulla of Vater D Pancreatic Duct F Pancreatic Duct, Accessory	0 Open 3 Percutaneous 4 Percutaneous endoscopic 7 Via natural or artificial opening 8 Via natural or artificial opening endoscopic	Z No device	X Diagnostic Z No qualifier

© 2018 Channel Publishing, Ltd.

1ST - 0 Medical and Surgical
2ND - F Hepatobiliary System and Pancreas
3RD - B EXCISION

EXCISION GROUP: Excision, Resection, Destruction, Extraction, (Detachment)
Root Operations that take out some or all of a body part.

EXCISION: Cutting out or off, without replacement, a portion of a body part.

Explanation: Qualifier "X Diagnostic" indicates excision procedures that are biopsies
Examples: Wedge resection liver – CMS Ex: Liver biopsy

Body Part – 4TH	Approach – 5TH	Device – 6TH	Qualifier - 7TH
0 Liver 1 Liver, Right Lobe 2 Liver, Left Lobe	0 Open 3 Percutaneous 4 Percutaneous endoscopic	Z No device	X Diagnostic Z No qualifier
4 Gallbladder G Pancreas	0 Open 3 Percutaneous 4 Percutaneous endoscopic 8 Via natural or artificial opening endoscopic	Z No device	X Diagnostic Z No qualifier
5 Hepatic Duct, Right 6 Hepatic Duct, Left 7 Hepatic Duct, Common 8 Cystic Duct 9 Common Bile Duct C Ampulla of Vater D Pancreatic Duct F Pancreatic Duct, Accessory	0 Open 3 Percutaneous 4 Percutaneous endoscopic 7 Via natural or artificial opening 8 Via natural or artificial opening endoscopic	Z No device	X Diagnostic Z No qualifier

1ST - 0 Medical and Surgical
2ND - F Hepatobiliary System and Pancreas
3RD - C EXTIRPATION

DRAINAGE GROUP: Drainage, Extirpation, Fragmentation
Root Operations that take out solids/fluids/gases from a body part.

EXTIRPATION: Taking or cutting out solid matter from a body part.

Explanation: Abnormal byproduct or foreign body ...
Examples: Cholelithotomy – CMS Ex: Thrombectomy

Body Part – 4TH	Approach – 5TH	Device – 6TH	Qualifier - 7TH
0 Liver 1 Liver, Right Lobe 2 Liver, Left Lobe	0 Open 3 Percutaneous 4 Percutaneous endoscopic	Z No device	Z No qualifier
4 Gallbladder G Pancreas	0 Open 3 Percutaneous 4 Percutaneous endoscopic 8 Via natural or artificial opening endoscopic	Z No device	Z No qualifier
5 Hepatic Duct, Right 6 Hepatic Duct, Left 7 Hepatic Duct, Common 8 Cystic Duct 9 Common Bile Duct C Ampulla of Vater D Pancreatic Duct F Pancreatic Duct, Accessory	0 Open 3 Percutaneous 4 Percutaneous endoscopic 7 Via natural or artificial opening 8 Via natural or artificial opening endoscopic	Z No device	Z No qualifier

1ST - 0 Medical and Surgical
2ND - F Hepatobiliary System and Pancreas
3RD - D EXTRACTION

EXCISION GROUP: Excision, Resection, Destruction, Extraction, (Detachment)
Root Operations that take out some or all of a body part.

EXTRACTION: Pulling or stripping out or off all or a portion of a body part by the use of force.

Explanation: Qualifier "X Diagnostic" indicates extraction procedures that are biopsies
Examples: Extraction accessory pancreatic duct – CMS Ex: Dilation and curettage

Body Part – 4TH	Approach – 5TH	Device – 6TH	Qualifier - 7TH
0 Liver 1 Liver, Right Lobe 2 Liver, Left Lobe	3 Percutaneous 4 Percutaneous endoscopic	Z No device	X Diagnostic
4 Gallbladder 5 Hepatic Duct, Right 6 Hepatic Duct, Left 7 Hepatic Duct, Common 8 Cystic Duct 9 Common Bile Duct C Ampulla of Vater D Pancreatic Duct F Pancreatic Duct, Accessory G Pancreas	3 Percutaneous 4 Percutaneous endoscopic 8 Via natural or artificial opening endoscopic	Z No device	X Diagnostic

© 2018 Channel Publishing, Ltd.

1ST - 0 Medical and Surgical
2ND - F Hepatobiliary System and Pancreas
3RD - F FRAGMENTATION

DRAINAGE GROUP: Drainage, Extirpation, Fragmentation
Root Operations that take out solids/fluids/gases from a body part.

FRAGMENTATION: Breaking solid matter in a body part into pieces.

Explanation: Pieces are not taken out during the procedure ...
Examples: Lithotripsy gallstones – CMS Ex: Extracorporeal shockwave lithotripsy

Body Part – 4TH		Approach – 5TH	Device – 6TH	Qualifier -7TH
4 Gallbladder 5 Hepatic Duct, Right 6 Hepatic Duct, Left 7 Hepatic Duct, Common 8 Cystic Duct	9 Common Bile Duct C Ampulla of Vater D Pancreatic Duct F Pancreatic Duct, Accessory	0 Open 3 Percutaneous 4 Percutaneous endoscopic 7 Via natural or artificial opening 8 Via natural or artificial opening endoscopic X External NC*	Z No device	Z No qualifier

NC* – Non-covered by Medicare. See current Medicare Code Editor for details.

1ST - 0 Medical and Surgical
2ND - F Hepatobiliary System and Pancreas
3RD - H INSERTION

DEVICE GROUP: Change, Insertion, Removal, Replacement, Revision, Supplement
Root Operations that always involve a device.

INSERTION: Putting in a nonbiological appliance that monitors, assists, performs, or prevents a physiological function but does not physically take the place of a body part.

Explanation: None
Examples: Insertion infusion pump pancreas – CMS Ex: Insertion of central venous catheter

Body Part – 4TH	Approach – 5TH	Device – 6TH	Qualifier – 7TH
0 Liver 4 Gallbladder G Pancreas	0 Open 3 Percutaneous 4 Percutaneous endoscopic	2 Monitoring device 3 Infusion device Y Other device	Z No qualifier
1 Liver, Right Lobe 2 Liver, Left Lobe	0 Open 3 Percutaneous 4 Percutaneous endoscopic	2 Monitoring device 3 Infusion device	Z No qualifier
B Hepatobiliary Duct D Pancreatic Duct	0 Open 3 Percutaneous 4 Percutaneous endoscopic 7 Via natural or artificial opening 8 Via natural or artificial opening endoscopic	1 Radioactive element 2 Monitoring device 3 Infusion device D Intraluminal device Y Other device	Z No qualifier

1ST - 0 Medical and Surgical
2ND - F Hepatobiliary System and Pancreas
3RD - J INSPECTION

EXAMINATION GROUP: Inspection, (Map)
Root Operations involving examination only.

INSPECTION: Visually and/or manually exploring a body part.

Explanation: Direct or instrumental visualization ...
Examples: Exploration common bile duct – CMS Ex: Exploratory laparotomy

Body Part – 4TH	Approach – 5TH	Device – 6TH	Qualifier – 7TH
0 Liver	0 Open 3 Percutaneous 4 Percutaneous endoscopic X External	Z No device	Z No qualifier
4 Gallbladder G Pancreas	0 Open 3 Percutaneous 4 Percutaneous endoscopic 8 Via natural or artificial opening endoscopic X External	Z No device	Z No qualifier
B Hepatobiliary Duct D Pancreatic Duct	0 Open 3 Percutaneous 4 Percutaneous endoscopic 7 Via natural or artificial opening 8 Via natural or artificial opening endoscopic	Z No device	Z No qualifier

© 2018 Channel Publishing, Ltd.

1ST - 0 Medical and Surgical
2ND - F Hepatobiliary System and Pancreas
3RD - L OCCLUSION

TUBULAR GROUP: Bypass, Dilation, Occlusion, Restriction
Root Operations that alter the diameter/route of a tubular body part.

OCCLUSION: Completely closing an orifice or the lumen of a tubular body part.

Explanation: The orifice can be a natural orifice or an artificially created orifice
Examples: Clipping accessory pancreatic duct – CMS Ex: Fallopian tube ligation

Body Part – 4TH	Approach – 5TH	Device – 6TH	Qualifier - 7TH
5 Hepatic Duct, Right 6 Hepatic Duct, Left 7 Hepatic Duct, Common 8 Cystic Duct 9 Common Bile Duct C Ampulla of Vater D Pancreatic Duct F Pancreatic Duct, Accessory	0 Open 3 Percutaneous 4 Percutaneous endoscopic	C Extraluminal device D Intraluminal device Z No device	Z No qualifier
5 Hepatic Duct, Right 6 Hepatic Duct, Left 7 Hepatic Duct, Common 8 Cystic Duct 9 Common Bile Duct C Ampulla of Vater D Pancreatic Duct F Pancreatic Duct, Accessory	7 Via natural or artificial opening 8 Via natural or artificial opening endoscopic	D Intraluminal device Z No device	Z No qualifier

1ST - 0 Medical and Surgical
2ND - F Hepatobiliary System and Pancreas
3RD - M REATTACHMENT

MOVE GROUP: Reattachment, Reposition, (Transfer), Transplantation
Root Operations that put in/put back or move some/all of a body part.

REATTACHMENT: Putting back in or on all or a portion of a separated body part to its normal location or other suitable location.

Explanation: Vascular circulation and nervous pathways may or may not be reestablished
Examples: Reattachment avulsed pancreas – CMS Ex: Reattachment of hand

Body Part – 4TH	Approach – 5TH	Device – 6TH	Qualifier – 7TH
0 Liver 1 Liver, Right Lobe 2 Liver, Left Lobe 4 Gallbladder 5 Hepatic Duct, Right 6 Hepatic Duct, Left 7 Hepatic Duct, Common 8 Cystic Duct 9 Common Bile Duct C Ampulla of Vater D Pancreatic Duct F Pancreatic Duct, Accessory G Pancreas	0 Open 4 Percutaneous endoscopic	Z No device	Z No qualifier

1ST - 0 Medical and Surgical
2ND - F Hepatobiliary System and Pancreas
3RD - N RELEASE

DIVISION GROUP: Division, Release
Root Operations involving cutting or separation only.

RELEASE: Freeing a body part from an abnormal physical constraint by cutting or by the use of force.

Explanation: Some of the restraining tissue may be taken out but none of the body part is taken out
Examples: Lysis adhesions gallbladder – CMS Ex: Carpal tunnel release

Body Part – 4TH	Approach – 5TH	Device – 6TH	Qualifier – 7TH
0 Liver 1 Liver, Right Lobe 2 Liver, Left Lobe	0 Open 3 Percutaneous 4 Percutaneous endoscopic	Z No device	Z No qualifier
4 Gallbladder G Pancreas	0 Open 3 Percutaneous 4 Percutaneous endoscopic 8 Via natural or artificial opening endoscopic	Z No device	Z No qualifier
5 Hepatic Duct, Right 6 Hepatic Duct, Left 7 Hepatic Duct, Common 8 Cystic Duct 9 Common Bile Duct C Ampulla of Vater D Pancreatic Duct F Pancreatic Duct, Accessory	0 Open 3 Percutaneous 4 Percutaneous endoscopic 7 Via natural or artificial opening 8 Via natural or artificial opening endoscopic	Z No device	Z No qualifier

© 2018 Channel Publishing, Ltd.

1ST - 0 Medical and Surgical
2ND - F Hepatobiliary System and Pancreas
3RD - P REMOVAL

DEVICE GROUP: Change, Insertion, Removal, Replacement, Revision, Supplement
Root Operations that always involve a device.

REMOVAL: Taking out or off a device from a body part.

Explanation: Removal device without reinsertion ...
Examples: Removal drain tube – CMS Ex: Cardiac pacemaker removal

Body Part – 4TH	Approach – 5TH	Device – 6TH	Qualifier – 7TH
0 Liver	0 Open 3 Percutaneous 4 Percutaneous endoscopic	0 Drainage device 2 Monitoring device 3 Infusion device Y Other device	Z No qualifier
0 Liver	X External	0 Drainage device 2 Monitoring device 3 Infusion device	Z No qualifier
4 Gallbladder G Pancreas	0 Open 3 Percutaneous 4 Percutaneous endoscopic	0 Drainage device 2 Monitoring device 3 Infusion device D Intraluminal device Y Other device	Z No qualifier
4 Gallbladder G Pancreas	X External	0 Drainage device 2 Monitoring device 3 Infusion device D Intraluminal device	Z No qualifier
B Hepatobiliary Duct D Pancreatic Duct	0 Open 3 Percutaneous 4 Percutaneous endoscopic 7 Via natural or artificial opening 8 Via natural or artificial opening endoscopic	0 Drainage device 1 Radioactive element 2 Monitoring device 3 Infusion device 7 Autologous tissue substitute C Extraluminal device D Intraluminal device J Synthetic substitute K Nonautologous tissue substitute Y Other device	Z No qualifier
B Hepatobiliary Duct D Pancreatic Duct	X External	0 Drainage device 1 Radioactive element 2 Monitoring device 3 Infusion device D Intraluminal device	Z No qualifier

1ST - 0 Medical and Surgical
2ND - F Hepatobiliary System and Pancreas
3RD - Q REPAIR

OTHER REPAIRS GROUP: (Control), Repair
Root Operations that define other repairs.

REPAIR: Restoring, to the extent possible, a body part to its normal anatomic structure and function.

Explanation: Used only when the method to accomplish the repair is not one of the other root operations
Examples: Repair liver laceration – CMS Ex: Suture of laceration

Body Part – 4TH	Approach – 5TH	Device – 6TH	Qualifier -7TH
0 Liver 1 Liver, Right Lobe 2 Liver, Left Lobe	0 Open 3 Percutaneous 4 Percutaneous endoscopic	Z No device	Z No qualifier
4 Gallbladder G Pancreas	0 Open 3 Percutaneous 4 Percutaneous endoscopic 8 Via natural or artificial opening endoscopic	Z No device	Z No qualifier
5 Hepatic Duct, Right 6 Hepatic Duct, Left 7 Hepatic Duct, Common 8 Cystic Duct 9 Common Bile Duct C Ampulla of Vater D Pancreatic Duct F Pancreatic Duct, Accessory	0 Open 3 Percutaneous 4 Percutaneous endoscopic 7 Via natural or artificial opening 8 Via natural or artificial opening endoscopic	Z No device	Z No qualifier

HEPATOBILIARY 0FQ

© 2018 Channel Publishing, Ltd.

1ST - 0 Medical and Surgical
2ND - F Hepatobiliary System and Pancreas
3RD - R REPLACEMENT

DEVICE GROUP: Change, Insertion, Removal, Replacement, Revision, Supplement
Root Operations that always involve a device.

REPLACEMENT: Putting in or on biological or synthetic material that physically takes the place and/or function of all or a portion of a body part.

Explanation: Includes taking out or eradicating, or rendering non-functional, the body part ...
Examples: Hepatic duct replacement – CMS Ex: Total hip replacement

Body Part – 4TH		Approach – 5TH	Device – 6TH	Qualifier -7TH
5 Hepatic Duct, Right 6 Hepatic Duct, Left 7 Hepatic Duct, Common 8 Cystic Duct	9 Common Bile Duct C Ampulla of Vater D Pancreatic Duct F Pancreatic Duct, Accessory	0 Open 4 Percutaneous endoscopic 8 Via natural or artificial opening endoscopic	7 Autologous tissue substitute J Synthetic substitute K Nonautologous tissue substitute	Z No qualifier

1ST - 0 Medical and Surgical
2ND - F Hepatobiliary System and Pancreas
3RD - S REPOSITION

MOVE GROUP: Reattachment, Reposition, (Transfer), Transplantation
Root Operations that put in/put back or move some/all of a body part.

REPOSITION: Moving to its normal location, or other suitable location, all or a portion of a body part.

Explanation: The body part may or may not be cut out or off to be moved to the new location ...
Examples: Relocation cystic duct – CMS Ex: Fracture reduction

Body Part – 4TH		Approach – 5TH	Device – 6TH	Qualifier – 7TH
0 Liver 4 Gallbladder 5 Hepatic Duct, Right 6 Hepatic Duct, Left 7 Hepatic Duct, Common 8 Cystic Duct	9 Common Bile Duct C Ampulla of Vater D Pancreatic Duct F Pancreatic Duct, Accessory G Pancreas	0 Open 4 Percutaneous endoscopic	Z No device	Z No qualifier

1ST - 0 Medical and Surgical
2ND - F Hepatobiliary System and Pancreas
3RD - T RESECTION

EXCISION GROUP: Excision, Resection, Destruction, Extraction, (Detachment)
Root Operations that take out some or all of a body part.

RESECTION: Cutting out or off, without replacement, all of a body part.

Explanation: None
Examples: Liver lobectomy – CMS Ex: Total lobectomy of lung

Body Part – 4TH		Approach – 5TH	Device – 6TH	Qualifier -7TH
0 Liver 1 Liver, Right Lobe 2 Liver, Left Lobe 4 Gallbladder G Pancreas		0 Open 4 Percutaneous endoscopic	Z No device	Z No qualifier
5 Hepatic Duct, Right 6 Hepatic Duct, Left 7 Hepatic Duct, Common 8 Cystic Duct	9 Common Bile Duct C Ampulla of Vater D Pancreatic Duct F Pancreatic Duct, Accessory	0 Open 4 Percutaneous endoscopic 7 Via natural or artificial opening 8 Via natural or artificial opening endoscopic	Z No device	Z No qualifier

© 2018 Channel Publishing, Ltd.

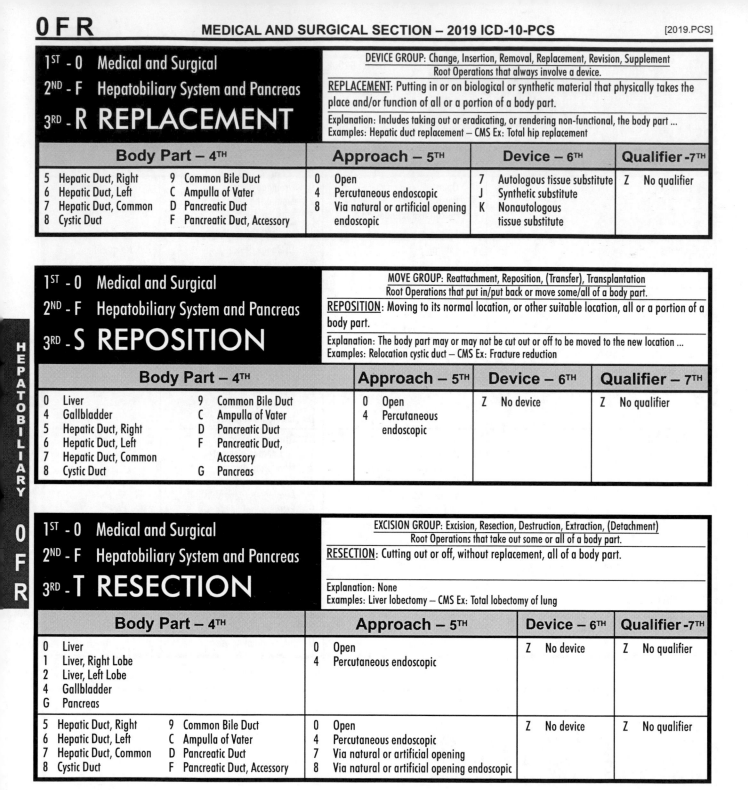

1ST - 0 Medical and Surgical
2ND - F Hepatobiliary System and Pancreas
3RD - U SUPPLEMENT

DEVICE GROUP: Change, Insertion, Removal, Replacement, Revision, Supplement
Root Operations that always involve a device.

SUPPLEMENT: Putting in or on biological or synthetic material that physically reinforces and/or augments the function of a portion of a body part.

Explanation: Biological material is non-living, or is living and from the same individual ...
Examples: Tissue graft ductal repair – CMS Ex: Herniorrhaphy using mesh

Body Part – 4TH	Approach – 5TH	Device – 6TH	Qualifier -7TH
5 Hepatic Duct, Right 6 Hepatic Duct, Left 7 Hepatic Duct, Common 8 Cystic Duct 9 Common Bile Duct C Ampulla of Vater D Pancreatic Duct F Pancreatic Duct, Accessory	0 Open 3 Percutaneous 4 Percutaneous endoscopic 8 Via natural or artificial opening endoscopic	7 Autologous tissue substitute J Synthetic substitute K Nonautologous tissue substitute	Z No qualifier

1ST - 0 Medical and Surgical
2ND - F Hepatobiliary System and Pancreas
3RD - V RESTRICTION

TUBULAR GROUP: Bypass, Dilation, Occlusion, Restriction
Root Operations that alter the diameter/route of a tubular body part.

RESTRICTION: Partially closing an orifice or the lumen of a tubular body part.

Explanation: The orifice can be a natural orifice or an artificially created orifice.
Examples: Restrictive ductal stent – CMS Ex: Cervical cerclage

Body Part – 4TH	Approach – 5TH	Device – 6TH	Qualifier -7TH
5 Hepatic Duct, Right 6 Hepatic Duct, Left 7 Hepatic Duct, Common 8 Cystic Duct 9 Common Bile Duct C Ampulla of Vater D Pancreatic Duct F Pancreatic Duct, Accessory	0 Open 3 Percutaneous 4 Percutaneous endoscopic	C Extraluminal device D Intraluminal device Z No device	Z No qualifier
5 Hepatic Duct, Right 6 Hepatic Duct, Left 7 Hepatic Duct, Common 8 Cystic Duct 9 Common Bile Duct C Ampulla of Vater D Pancreatic Duct F Pancreatic Duct, Accessory	7 Via natural or artificial opening 8 Via natural or artificial opening endoscopic	D Intraluminal device Z No device	Z No qualifier

© 2018 Channel Publishing, Ltd.

1ST - 0 Medical and Surgical
2ND - F Hepatobiliary System and Pancreas
3RD - W REVISION

DEVICE GROUP: Change, Insertion, Removal, Replacement, Revision, Supplement
Root Operations that always involve a device.

REVISION: Correcting, to the extent possible, a portion of a malfunctioning device or the position of a displaced device.

Explanation: Correcting by taking out or putting in components of a device such as a screw or pin ...
Examples: Reposition drainage tube – CMS Ex: Recementing of hip prosthesis

Body Part – 4TH	Approach – 5TH	Device – 6TH	Qualifier – 7TH
0 Liver	0 Open 3 Percutaneous 4 Percutaneous endoscopic	0 Drainage device 2 Monitoring device 3 Infusion device Y Other device	Z No qualifier
0 Liver	X External	0 Drainage device 2 Monitoring device 3 Infusion device	Z No qualifier
4 Gallbladder G Pancreas	0 Open 3 Percutaneous 4 Percutaneous endoscopic	0 Drainage device 2 Monitoring device 3 Infusion device D Intraluminal device Y Other device	Z No qualifier
4 Gallbladder G Pancreas	X External	0 Drainage device 2 Monitoring device 3 Infusion device D Intraluminal device	Z No qualifier
B Hepatobiliary Duct D Pancreatic Duct	0 Open 3 Percutaneous 4 Percutaneous endoscopic 7 Via natural or artificial opening 8 Via natural or artificial opening endoscopic	0 Drainage device 2 Monitoring device 3 Infusion device 7 Autologous tissue substitute C Extraluminal device D Intraluminal device J Synthetic substitute K Nonautologous tissue substitute Y Other device	Z No qualifier
B Hepatobiliary Duct D Pancreatic Duct	X External	0 Drainage device 2 Monitoring device 3 Infusion device 7 Autologous tissue substitute C Extraluminal device D Intraluminal device J Synthetic substitute K Nonautologous tissue substitute	Z No qualifier

1ST - 0 Medical and Surgical
2ND - F Hepatobiliary System and Pancreas
3RD - Y TRANSPLANTATION

MOVE GROUP: Reattachment, Reposition, (Transfer), Transplantation
Root Operations that put in/put back or move some/all of a body part.

TRANSPLANTATION: Putting in or on all or a portion of a living body part taken from another individual or animal to physically take the place and/or function of all or a portion of a similar body part.

Explanation: The native body part may or may not be taken out ...
Examples: Liver transplant – CMS Ex: Kidney transplant

Body Part – 4TH	Approach – 5TH	Device – 6TH	Qualifier – 7TH
0 Liver G Pancreas NC*LC*	0 Open	Z No device	0 Allogeneic 1 Syngeneic 2 Zooplastic NC*LC*

NC*LC* – Some procedures are considered non-covered or limited coverage by Medicare. See current Medicare Code Editor for details.

© 2018 Channel Publishing, Ltd.

Educational Annotations | G – Endocrine System

Body System Specific Educational Annotations for the Endocrine System include:

- Anatomy and Physiology Review
- Definitions of Common Procedures
- Anatomical Illustrations
- AHA Coding Clinic® Reference Notations
- Body Part Key Listings
- Device Key Listings
- Device Aggregation Table Listings
- Coding Notes

Anatomy and Physiology Review of Endocrine System

BODY PART VALUES – G - ENDOCRINE SYSTEM

Adrenal Gland – ANATOMY – The adrenal gland is the highly vascular, pyramid-shaped endocrine gland that sits upon the top of each kidney. PHYSIOLOGY – The adrenal gland produces several important hormones, among them: Adrenalin, noradrenalin, aldosterone, cortisol, and some sex hormones.
Aortic Body – ANATOMY – The aortic body is the small neurovascular structure located at the aortic arch. PHYSIOLOGY – The aortic body monitors and regulates the reflex respiration and blood pressure.
Carotid Body – ANATOMY – The carotid bodies are small neurovascular structures at the carotid bifurcation. PHYSIOLOGY – The carotid bodies function as a blood oxygen, carbon dioxide, and Ph sensor.
Coccygeal Glomus – The coccygeal glomus is a very small (2.5mm), oval mass exocrine gland tissue located beneath the coccyx tip.
Endocrine Gland – A gland that secretes hormones.
Glomus Jugulare – A mass of neuroendocrine cells in the jugular foramen area of the temporal bone near the middle and inner ear.
Para-aortic Body – ANATOMY – The para-aortic body is the small mass of chromaffin tissue located alongside the abdominal aorta. PHYSIOLOGY – The para-aortic body produces catecholamines.
Paraganglion Extremity – Groups of extra-adrenal neuroendocrine cells usually found in the peripheral nervous system that produce adrenaline.
Parathyroid Gland – ANATOMY – The parathyroid glands are 4 small glands, 2 on the posterior surface of the thyroid lobes. PHYSIOLOGY – The parathyroid gland secretes one hormone, the parathyroid hormone which causes an increase in the blood calcium level and a decrease in the blood phosphate level.
Pineal Gland – ANATOMY – The pineal gland is the small endocrine gland located below the posterior base of the corpus callosum, and attached to the upper portion of the thalamus. PHYSIOLOGY – The pineal gland produces the hormone melatonin.
Pituitary Gland – ANATOMY – The pituitary gland is the small endocrine gland with two lobes located in the sella turcica of the sphenoid bone at the base of the cerebrum, and is about 0.4 inches (1 cm) in diameter. PHYSIOLOGY – The pituitary gland functions as the central endocrine gland by producing hormones which stimulate many of the other endocrine glands, and has two lobes. The anterior lobe (adenohypophysis) produces the growth hormone (prolactin), thyroid-stimulating hormone, follicle-stimulating and luteinizing hormones, and adrenocorticotropic hormone. The posterior lobe (neurohypophysis) secretes the antidiuretic hormone and oxytocin.
Thyroid Gland – ANATOMY – The thyroid gland is the bi-lobed endocrine gland of the front of the neck and is connected by a narrow isthmus. PHYSIOLOGY – The thyroid gland produces the hormones thyroxine and triiodothyronine that help to regulate the metabolic rate of the body.
Thyroid Gland Isthmus – The narrow, middle portion connecting the two thyroid lobes.

Definitions of Common Procedures of Endocrine System

Adrenalectomy – The surgical removal of one or both of the adrenal glands.
Hypophysectomy – The surgical removal of the pituitary gland (hypophysis).
Thyroid lobectomy – The surgical removal of one of the two lobes of the thyroid.
Total thyroidectomy – The surgical removal of both lobes and the isthmus of the thyroid.

© 2018 Channel Publishing, Ltd.

Educational Annotations | G – Endocrine System

Anatomical Illustrations of Endocrine System

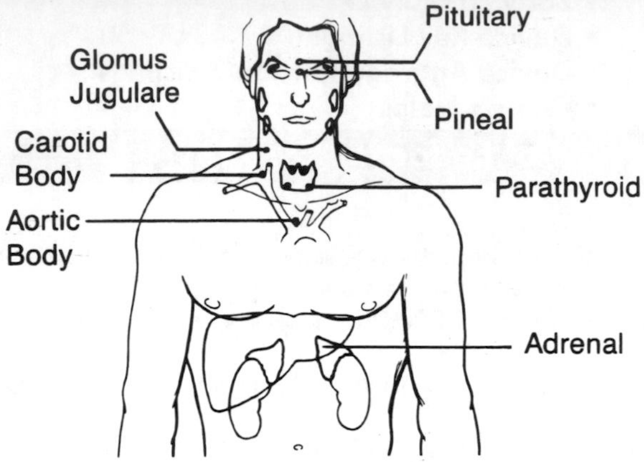

ENDOCRINE GLANDS

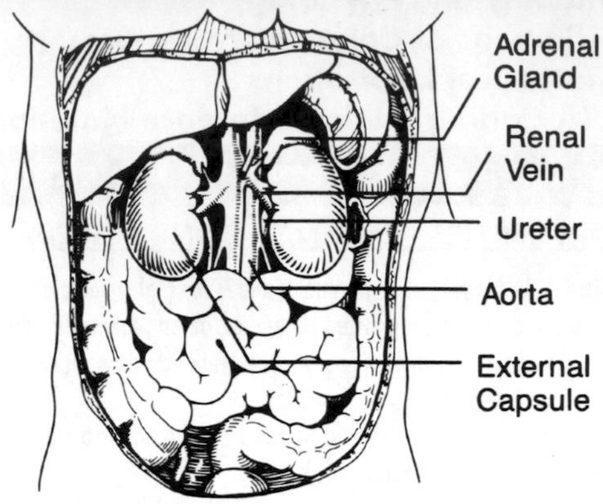

KIDNEY — ANTERIOR VIEW

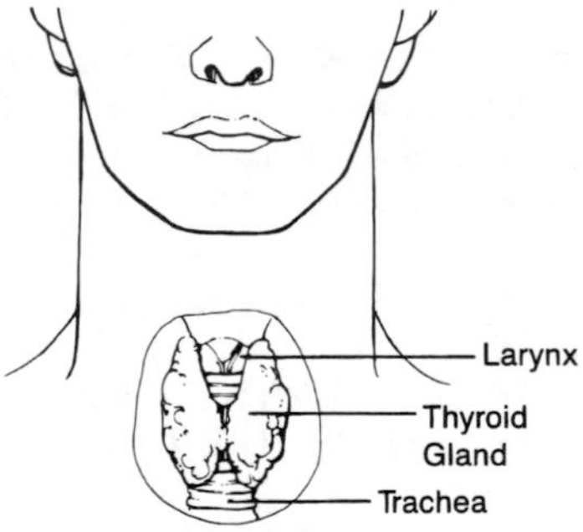

THYROID GLAND

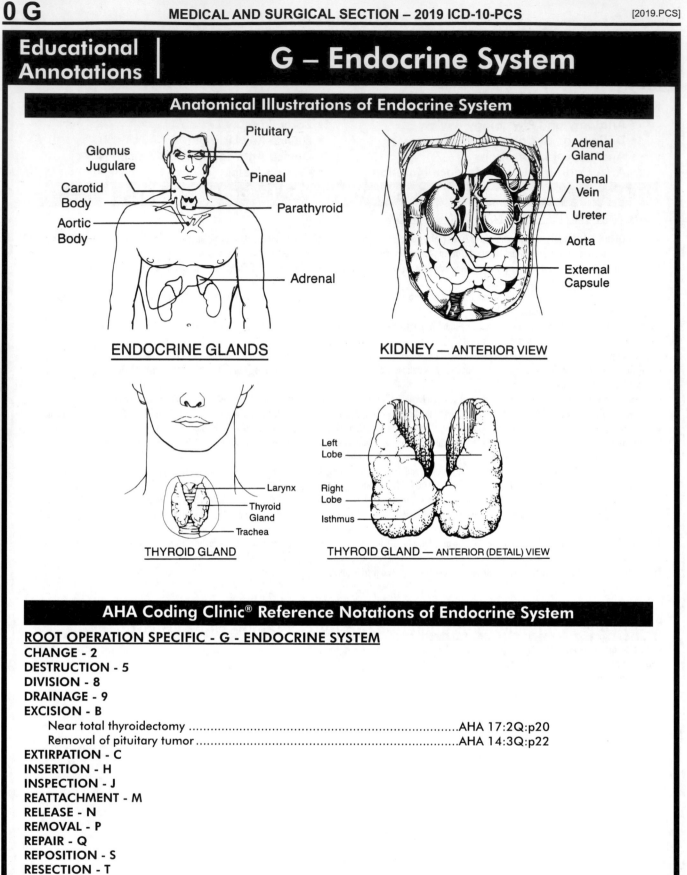

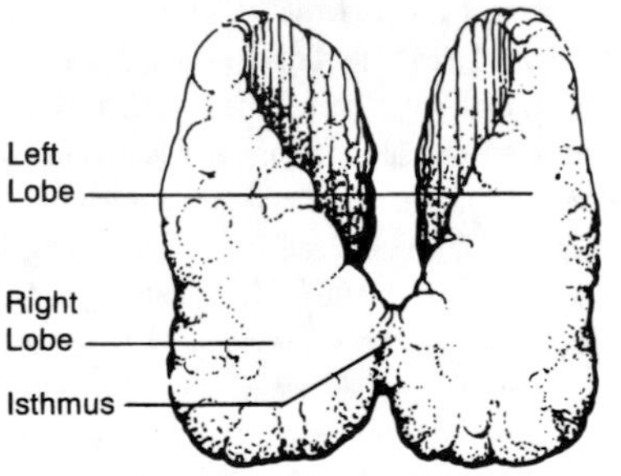

THYROID GLAND — ANTERIOR (DETAIL) VIEW

AHA Coding Clinic® Reference Notations of Endocrine System

ROOT OPERATION SPECIFIC - G - ENDOCRINE SYSTEM

CHANGE - 2
DESTRUCTION - 5
DIVISION - 8
DRAINAGE - 9
EXCISION - B
- Near total thyroidectomy .... AHA 17:2Q:p20
- Removal of pituitary tumor .... AHA 14:3Q:p22

EXTIRPATION - C
INSERTION - H
INSPECTION - J
REATTACHMENT - M
RELEASE - N
REMOVAL - P
REPAIR - Q
REPOSITION - S
RESECTION - T
REVISION - W

© 2018 Channel Publishing, Ltd.

Educational Annotations | G – Endocrine System

Body Part Key Listings of Endocrine System

See also Body Part Key in Appendix C

Adenohypophysis....use Pituitary Gland
Carotid glomus ....use Carotid Body, Bilateral/Left/Right
Coccygeal body ....use Coccygeal Glomus
Hypophysis....use Pituitary Gland
Jugular body ....use Glomus Jugulare
Neurohypophysis....use Pituitary Gland
Suprarenal gland ....use Adrenal Gland, Bilateral/Left/Right

Device Key Listings of Endocrine System

See also Device Key in Appendix D

Autograft ....use Autologous Tissue Substitute
Tissue bank graft ....use Nonautologous Tissue Substitute

Device Aggregation Table Listings of Endocrine System

See also Device Aggregation Table in Appendix E

Specific Device	For Operation	In Body System	General Device
None Listed in Device Aggregation Table for this Body System			

Coding Notes of Endocrine System

© 2018 Channel Publishing, Ltd.

1ST - 0 Medical and Surgical
2ND - G Endocrine System
3RD - 2 CHANGE

DEVICE GROUP: Change, Insertion, Removal, (Replacement), Revision, (Supplement)
Root Operations that always involve a device.

CHANGE: Taking out or off a device from a body part and putting back an identical or similar device in or on the same body part without cutting or puncturing the skin or a mucous membrane.

Explanation: All CHANGE procedures are coded using the approach External
Examples: Exchange drain tube – CMS Ex: Urinary catheter change

Body Part – 4TH	Approach – 5TH	Device – 6TH	Qualifier – 7TH
0 Pituitary Gland 1 Pineal Body 5 Adrenal Gland K Thyroid Gland R Parathyroid Gland S Endocrine Gland	X External	0 Drainage device Y Other device	Z No qualifier

1ST - 0 Medical and Surgical
2ND - G Endocrine System
3RD - 5 DESTRUCTION

EXCISION GROUP: Excision, Resection, Destruction, (Extraction), (Detachment)
Root Operations that take out some or all of a body part.

DESTRUCTION: Physical eradication of all or a portion of a body part by the direct use of energy, force, or a destructive agent.

Explanation: None of the body part is physically taken out
Examples: Radiofrequency ablation – CMS Ex: Fulguration of rectal polyp

Body Part – 4TH	Approach – 5TH	Device – 6TH	Qualifier – 7TH
0 Pituitary Gland 1 Pineal Body 2 Adrenal Gland, Left 3 Adrenal Gland, Right 4 Adrenal Glands, Bilateral 6 Carotid Body, Left 7 Carotid Body, Right 8 Carotid Bodies, Bilateral 9 Para-aortic Body B Coccygeal Glomus C Glomus Jugulare D Aortic Body F Paraganglion Extremity G Thyroid Gland Lobe, Left H Thyroid Gland Lobe, Right K Thyroid Gland L Superior Parathyroid Gland, Right M Superior Parathyroid Gland, Left N Inferior Parathyroid Gland, Right P Inferior Parathyroid Gland, Left Q Parathyroid Glands, Multiple R Parathyroid Gland	0 Open 3 Percutaneous 4 Percutaneous endoscopic	Z No device	Z No qualifier

1ST - 0 Medical and Surgical
2ND - G Endocrine System
3RD - 8 DIVISION

DIVISION GROUP: Division, Release
Root Operations involving cutting or separation only.

DIVISION: Cutting into a body part, without draining fluids and/or gases from the body part, in order to separate or transect a body part.

Explanation: All or a portion of the body part is separated into two or more portions
Examples: Transection thyroid isthmus – CMS Ex: Spinal cordotomy

Body Part – 4TH	Approach – 5TH	Device – 6TH	Qualifier – 7TH
0 Pituitary Gland J Thyroid Gland Isthmus	0 Open 3 Percutaneous 4 Percutaneous endoscopic	Z No device	Z No qualifier

© 2018 Channel Publishing, Ltd.

1ST - 0 Medical and Surgical
2ND - G Endocrine System
3RD - 9 DRAINAGE

DRAINAGE GROUP: Drainage, Extirpation, (Fragmentation)
Root Operations that take out solids/fluids/gases from a body part.
DRAINAGE: Taking or letting out fluids and/or gases from a body part.

Explanation: Qualifier "X Diagnostic" indicates drainage procedures that are biopsies
Examples: Needle aspiration adrenal abscess – CMS Ex: Thoracentesis

Body Part – 4TH			Approach – 5TH	Device – 6TH	Qualifier – 7TH
0 Pituitary Gland 1 Pineal Body 2 Adrenal Gland, Left 3 Adrenal Gland, Right 4 Adrenal Glands, Bilateral 6 Carotid Body, Left 7 Carotid Body, Right 8 Carotid Bodies, Bilateral 9 Para-aortic Body	B Coccygeal Glomus C Glomus Jugulare D Aortic Body F Paraganglion Extremity G Thyroid Gland Lobe, Left H Thyroid Gland Lobe, Right K Thyroid Gland L Superior Parathyroid Gland, Right	M Superior Parathyroid Gland, Left N Inferior Parathyroid Gland, Right P Inferior Parathyroid Gland, Left Q Parathyroid Glands, Multiple R Parathyroid Gland	0 Open 3 Percutaneous 4 Percutaneous endoscopic	0 Drainage device	Z No qualifier
0 Pituitary Gland 1 Pineal Body 2 Adrenal Gland, Left 3 Adrenal Gland, Right 4 Adrenal Glands, Bilateral 6 Carotid Body, Left 7 Carotid Body, Right 8 Carotid Bodies, Bilateral 9 Para-aortic Body	B Coccygeal Glomus C Glomus Jugulare D Aortic Body F Paraganglion Extremity G Thyroid Gland Lobe, Left H Thyroid Gland Lobe, Right K Thyroid Gland L Superior Parathyroid Gland, Right	M Superior Parathyroid Gland, Left N Inferior Parathyroid Gland, Right P Inferior Parathyroid Gland, Left Q Parathyroid Glands, Multiple R Parathyroid Gland	0 Open 3 Percutaneous 4 Percutaneous endoscopic	Z No device	X Diagnostic Z No qualifier

1ST - 0 Medical and Surgical
2ND - G Endocrine System
3RD - B EXCISION

EXCISION GROUP: Excision, Resection, Destruction, (Extraction), (Detachment)
Root Operations that take out some or all of a body part.
EXCISION: Cutting out or off, without replacement, a portion of a body part.

Explanation: Qualifier "X Diagnostic" indicates excision procedures that are biopsies
Examples: Needle biopsy parathyroid gland – CMS Ex: Liver biopsy

Body Part – 4TH			Approach – 5TH	Device – 6TH	Qualifier – 7TH
0 Pituitary Gland 1 Pineal Body 2 Adrenal Gland, Left 3 Adrenal Gland, Right 4 Adrenal Glands, Bilateral 6 Carotid Body, Left 7 Carotid Body, Right 8 Carotid Bodies, Bilateral 9 Para-aortic Body	B Coccygeal Glomus C Glomus Jugulare D Aortic Body F Paraganglion Extremity G Thyroid Gland Lobe, Left H Thyroid Gland Lobe, Right J Thyroid Gland Isthmus L Superior Parathyroid Gland, Right	M Superior Parathyroid Gland, Left N Inferior Parathyroid Gland, Right P Inferior Parathyroid Gland, Left Q Parathyroid Glands, Multiple R Parathyroid Gland	0 Open 3 Percutaneous 4 Percutaneous endoscopic	Z No device	X Diagnostic Z No qualifier

1ST - 0 Medical and Surgical
2ND - G Endocrine System
3RD - C EXTIRPATION

DRAINAGE GROUP: Drainage, Extirpation, (Fragmentation)
Root Operations that take out solids/fluids/gases from a body part.
EXTIRPATION: Taking or cutting out solid matter from a body part.

Explanation: Abnormal byproduct or foreign body ...
Examples: Removal foreign body – CMS Ex: Thrombectomy

Body Part – 4TH			Approach – 5TH	Device – 6TH	Qualifier – 7TH
0 Pituitary Gland 1 Pineal Body 2 Adrenal Gland, Left 3 Adrenal Gland, Right 4 Adrenal Glands, Bilateral 6 Carotid Body, Left 7 Carotid Body, Right 8 Carotid Bodies, Bilateral 9 Para-aortic Body	B Coccygeal Glomus C Glomus Jugulare D Aortic Body F Paraganglion Extremity G Thyroid Gland Lobe, Left H Thyroid Gland Lobe, Right K Thyroid Gland L Superior Parathyroid Gland, Right	M Superior Parathyroid Gland, Left N Inferior Parathyroid Gland, Right P Inferior Parathyroid Gland, Left Q Parathyroid Glands, Multiple R Parathyroid Gland	0 Open 3 Percutaneous 4 Percutaneous endoscopic	Z No device	Z No qualifier

© 2018 Channel Publishing, Ltd.

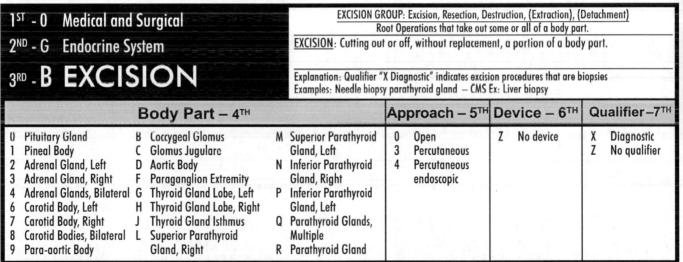

1ST - 0 Medical and Surgical
2ND - G Endocrine System
3RD - H INSERTION

DEVICE GROUP: Change, Insertion, Removal, (Replacement), Revision, (Supplement)
Root Operations that always involve a device.

INSERTION: Putting in a nonbiological appliance that monitors, assists, performs, or prevents a physiological function but does not physically take the place of a body part.

Explanation: None
Examples: Insertion infusion device – CMS Ex: Insertion of central venous catheter

Body Part – 4TH	Approach – 5TH	Device – 6TH	Qualifier – 7TH
S Endocrine Gland	0 Open 3 Percutaneous 4 Percutaneous endoscopic	2 Monitoring device 3 Infusion device Y Other device	Z No qualifier

1ST - 0 Medical and Surgical
2ND - G Endocrine System
3RD - J INSPECTION

EXAMINATION GROUP: Inspection, (Map)
Root Operations involving examination only.

INSPECTION: Visually and/or manually exploring a body part.

Explanation: Direct or instrumental visualization ...
Examples: Laparoscopic examination adrenal gland – CMS Ex: Exploratory laparotomy

Body Part – 4TH		Approach – 5TH	Device – 6TH	Qualifier – 7TH
0 Pituitary Gland 1 Pineal Body 5 Adrenal Gland	K Thyroid Gland R Parathyroid Gland S Endocrine Gland	0 Open 3 Percutaneous 4 Percutaneous endoscopic	Z No device	Z No qualifier

ENDOCRINE 0 G H

1ST - 0 Medical and Surgical
2ND - G Endocrine System
3RD - M REATTACHMENT

MOVE GROUP: Reattachment, Reposition, (Transfer), (Transplantation)
Root Operations that put in/put back or move some/all of a body part.

REATTACHMENT: Putting back in or on all or a portion of a separated body part to its normal location or other suitable location.

Explanation: Vascular circulation and nervous pathways may or may not be reestablished
Examples: Reattachment thyroid lobe – CMS Ex: Reattachment of hand

Body Part – 4TH		Approach – 5TH	Device – 6TH	Qualifier – 7TH
2 Adrenal Gland, Left 3 Adrenal Gland, Right G Thyroid Gland Lobe, Left H Thyroid Gland Lobe, Right L Superior Parathyroid Gland, Right	M Superior Parathyroid Gland, Left N Inferior Parathyroid Gland, Right P Inferior Parathyroid Gland, Left Q Parathyroid Glands, Multiple R Parathyroid Gland	0 Open 4 Percutaneous endoscopic	Z No device	Z No qualifier

1ST - 0 Medical and Surgical
2ND - G Endocrine System
3RD - N RELEASE

DIVISION GROUP: Division, Release
Root Operations involving cutting or separation only.

RELEASE: Freeing a body part from an abnormal physical constraint by cutting or by the use of force.

Explanation: Some of the restraining tissue may be taken out but none of the body part is taken out
Examples: Adhesiolysis adrenal gland – CMS Ex: Carpal tunnel release

Body Part – 4TH			Approach – 5TH	Device – 6TH	Qualifier – 7TH
0 Pituitary Gland 1 Pineal Body 2 Adrenal Gland, Left 3 Adrenal Gland, Right 4 Adrenal Glands, Bilateral 6 Carotid Body, Left 7 Carotid Body, Right 8 Carotid Bodies, Bilateral 9 Para-aortic Body	B Coccygeal Glomus C Glomus Jugulare D Aortic Body F Paraganglion Extremity G Thyroid Gland Lobe, Left H Thyroid Gland Lobe, Right K Thyroid Gland L Superior Parathyroid Gland, Right	M Superior Parathyroid Gland, Left N Inferior Parathyroid Gland, Right P Inferior Parathyroid Gland, Left Q Parathyroid Glands, Multiple R Parathyroid Gland	0 Open 3 Percutaneous 4 Percutaneous endoscopic	Z No device	Z No qualifier

© 2018 Channel Publishing, Ltd.

1ST - 0 Medical and Surgical
2ND - G Endocrine System
3RD - P REMOVAL

DEVICE GROUP: Change, Insertion, Removal, (Replacement), Revision, (Supplement)
Root Operations that always involve a device.

REMOVAL: Taking out or off a device from a body part.

Explanation: Removal device without reinsertion ...
Examples: Removal drain tube – CMS Ex: Cardiac pacemaker removal

Body Part – 4TH	Approach – 5TH	Device – 6TH	Qualifier – 7TH
0 Pituitary Gland 1 Pineal Body 5 Adrenal Gland K Thyroid Gland R Parathyroid Gland	0 Open 3 Percutaneous 4 Percutaneous endoscopic X External	0 Drainage device	Z No qualifier
S Endocrine Gland	0 Open 3 Percutaneous 4 Percutaneous endoscopic	0 Drainage device 2 Monitoring device 3 Infusion device Y Other device	Z No qualifier
S Endocrine Gland	X External	0 Drainage device 2 Monitoring device 3 Infusion device	Z No qualifier

1ST - 0 Medical and Surgical
2ND - G Endocrine System
3RD - Q REPAIR

OTHER REPAIRS GROUP: (Control), Repair
Root Operations that define other repairs.

REPAIR: Restoring, to the extent possible, a body part to its normal anatomic structure and function.

Explanation: Used only when the method to accomplish the repair is not one of the other root operations
Examples: Suture thyroid laceration – CMS Ex: Suture of laceration

Body Part – 4TH			Approach – 5TH	Device – 6TH	Qualifier –7TH
0 Pituitary Gland 1 Pineal Body 2 Adrenal Gland, Left 3 Adrenal Gland, Right 4 Adrenal Glands, Bilateral 6 Carotid Body, Left 7 Carotid Body, Right 8 Carotid Bodies, Bilateral 9 Para-aortic Body B Coccygeal Glomus	C Glomus Jugulare D Aortic Body F Paraganglion Extremity G Thyroid Gland Lobe, Left H Thyroid Gland Lobe, Right J Thyroid Gland Isthmus K Thyroid Gland L Superior Parathyroid Gland, Right	M Superior Parathyroid Gland, Left N Inferior Parathyroid Gland, Right P Inferior Parathyroid Gland, Left Q Parathyroid Glands, Multiple R Parathyroid Gland	0 Open 3 Percutaneous 4 Percutaneous endoscopic	Z No device	Z No qualifier

1ST - 0 Medical and Surgical
2ND - E Endocrine System
3RD - S REPOSITION

MOVE GROUP: Reattachment, Reposition, (Transfer), (Transplantation)
Root Operations that put in/put back or move some/all of a body part.

REPOSITION: Moving to its normal location, or other suitable location, all or a portion of a body part.

Explanation: The body part may or may not be cut out or off to be moved to the new location ...
Examples: Relocation parathyroid glands – CMS Ex: Fracture reduction

Body Part – 4TH		Approach – 5TH	Device – 6TH	Qualifier – 7TH
2 Adrenal Gland, Left 3 Adrenal Gland, Right G Thyroid Gland Lobe, Left H Thyroid Gland Lobe, Right L Superior Parathyroid Gland, Right	M Superior Parathyroid Gland, Left N Inferior Parathyroid Gland, Right P Inferior Parathyroid Gland, Left Q Parathyroid Glands Multiple R Parathyroid Gland	0 Open 4 Percutaneous endoscopic	Z No device	Z No qualifier

ENDOCRINE 0 G S

© 2018 Channel Publishing, Ltd.

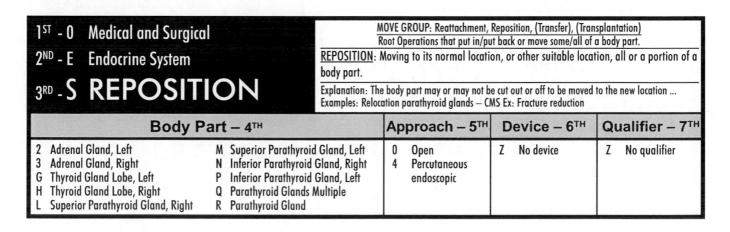

1ST - 0 Medical and Surgical
2ND - G Endocrine System
3RD - T RESECTION

EXCISION GROUP: Excision, Resection, Destruction, (Extraction), (Detachment)
Root Operations that take out some or all of a body part.

RESECTION: Cutting out or off, without replacement, all of a body part.

Explanation: None
Examples: Thyroid lobectomy – CMS Ex: Total lobectomy of lung

Body Part – 4TH			Approach – 5TH	Device – 6TH	Qualifier – 7TH
0 Pituitary Gland 1 Pineal Body 2 Adrenal Gland, Left 3 Adrenal Gland, Right 4 Adrenal Glands, Bilateral 6 Carotid Body, Left 7 Carotid Body, Right 8 Carotid Bodies, Bilateral 9 Para-aortic Body B Coccygeal Glomus	C Glomus Jugulare D Aortic Body F Paraganglion Extremity G Thyroid Gland Lobe, Left H Thyroid Gland Lobe, Right J Thyroid Gland Isthmus K Thyroid Gland L Superior Parathyroid Gland, Right	M Superior Parathyroid Gland, Left N Inferior Parathyroid Gland, Right P Inferior Parathyroid Gland, Left Q Parathyroid Glands, Multiple R Parathyroid Gland	0 Open 4 Percutaneous endoscopic	Z No device	Z No qualifier

1ST - 0 Medical and Surgical
2ND - G Endocrine System
3RD - W REVISION

DEVICE GROUP: Change, Insertion, Removal, (Replacement), Revision, (Supplement)
Root Operations that always involve a device.

REVISION: Correcting, to the extent possible, a portion of a malfunctioning device or the position of a displaced device.

Explanation: Correcting by taking out or putting in components of a device such as a screw or pin ...
Examples: Reposition drainage tube – CMS Ex: Recementing of hip prosthesis

Body Part – 4TH	Approach – 5TH	Device – 6TH	Qualifier – 7TH
0 Pituitary Gland 1 Pineal Body 5 Adrenal Gland K Thyroid Gland R Parathyroid Gland	0 Open 3 Percutaneous 4 Percutaneous endoscopic X External	0 Drainage device	Z No qualifier
S Endocrine Gland	0 Open 3 Percutaneous 4 Percutaneous endoscopic	0 Drainage device 2 Monitoring device 3 Infusion device Y Other device	Z No qualifier
S Endocrine Gland	X External	0 Drainage device 2 Monitoring device 3 Infusion device	Z No qualifier

© 2018 Channel Publishing, Ltd.

Educational Annotations | H – Skin and Breast

Body System Specific Educational Annotations for the Skin and Breast include:

- Anatomy and Physiology Review
- Anatomical Illustrations
- Definitions of Common Procedures
- AHA Coding Clinic® Reference Notations
- Body Part Key Listings
- Device Key Listings
- Device Aggregation Table Listings
- Coding Notes

Anatomy and Physiology Review of Skin and Breast

BODY PART VALUES – H - SKIN AND BREAST

Breast, Female – ANATOMY – The female breast is the modified cutaneous glandular cone-shaped prominence overlying the pectoral muscles on the anterior chest, and contains the milk-producing mammary glands. PHYSIOLOGY – The female breast functions to secrete nourishing milk for the newborn. During pregnancy, hormones increase the size of the mammary glands, and following delivery, the pituitary gland secretes prolactin, which stimulates the mammary glands to produce milk. The mammary ducts convey the milk to the nipple.

Breast, Male – ANATOMY – The male breast is the modified cutaneous glandular structure overlying the pectoral muscles of the anterior chest. PHYSIOLOGY – The male breast fails to develop due to the lack of ovarian hormones.

Finger Nail – ANATOMY – The tough keratin covering of the top and end of the fingers. PHYSIOLOGY – The nail functions to protect the end of the finger.

Hair – ANATOMY – Hair is a threadlike structure that grows from follicles found in the dermis and is made of protein. PHYSIOLOGY – Hair serves multiple functions depending on location, including: Sensory transmission, heat retention, skin protection, and protection from particles and organisms.

Nipple – ANATOMY – The nipple is the pigmented projection of the breast and contains the ends of the mammary ducts. The areola is the circular pigmented area around the nipple.

Skin – ANATOMY – The skin is the outer covering of the body, consisting of the epidermis and dermis, that rests upon the subcutaneous tissue. The epidermis is the outermost layer of the skin which develops keratin, a tough, fibrous waterproof protein, and lacks blood vessels. The dermis is the tough, elastic vascular connective tissue layer of the skin which contains the sebaceous and sweat glands. PHYSIOLOGY – The skin functions to protect the body from invading microorganisms, limits the loss of water from deep tissues, assists homeostasis, aids in the regulation of body temperature, acts as the sense organ for the cutaneous senses, and is a source of vitamin D when it is exposed to light.

Supernumerary Breast – The presence of an additional breast (accessory breast) that may or may not have an associated areola and nipple.

Toe Nail – ANATOMY – The tough keratin covering of the top and end of the toes. PHYSIOLOGY – The nail functions to protect the end of the toe.

Anatomical Illustrations of Skin and Breast

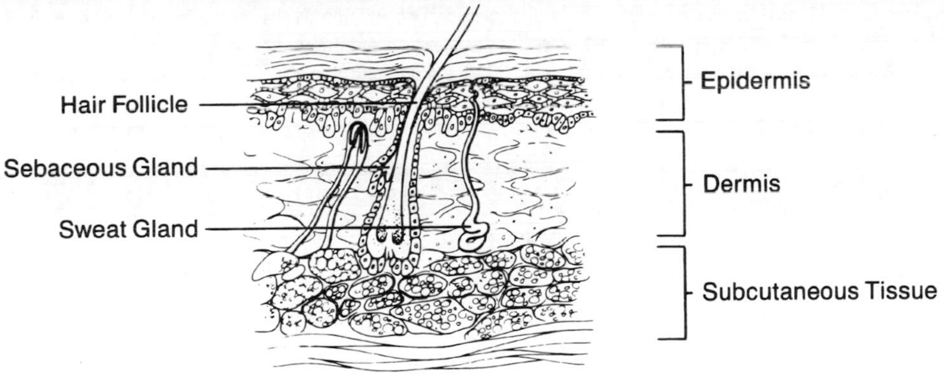

SKIN

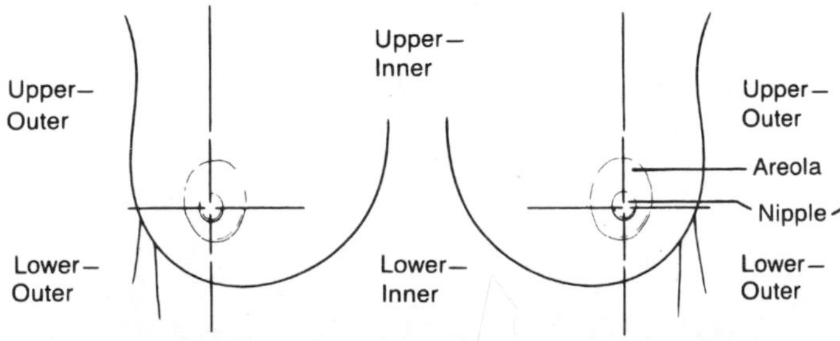

FEMALE BREASTS — ANTER R VIEW (QUADRANTS)

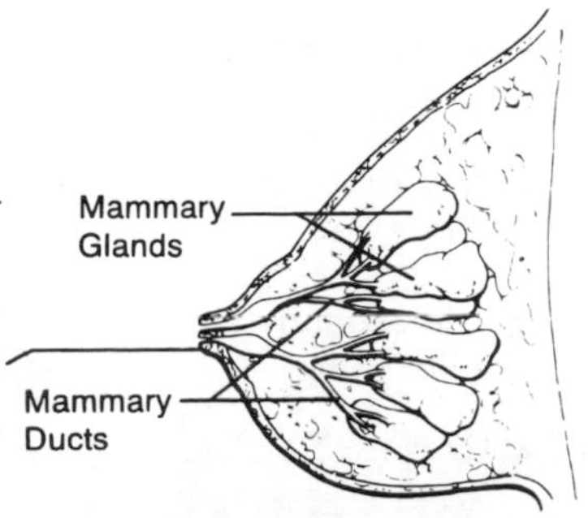

FEMALE BREAST — SAGITTAL VIEW

Continued on next page

© 2018 Channel Publishing, Ltd.

Educational Annotations | H – Skin and Breast

Anatomical Illustrations of Skin and Breast

Continued from previous page

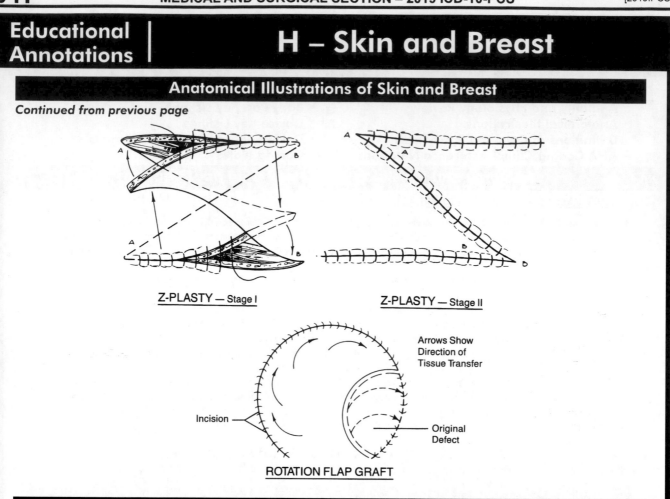

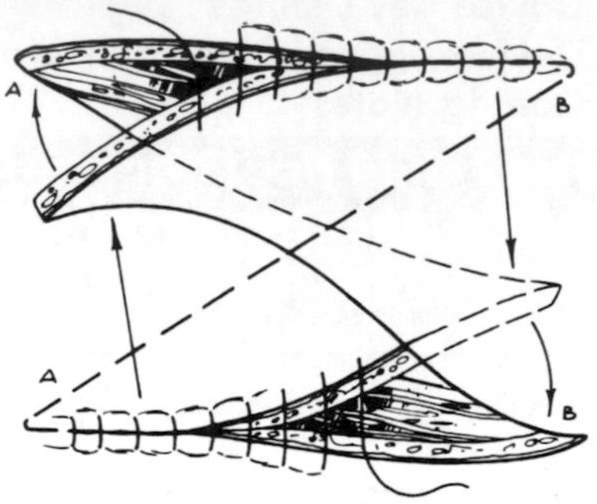

Z-PLASTY – Stage I

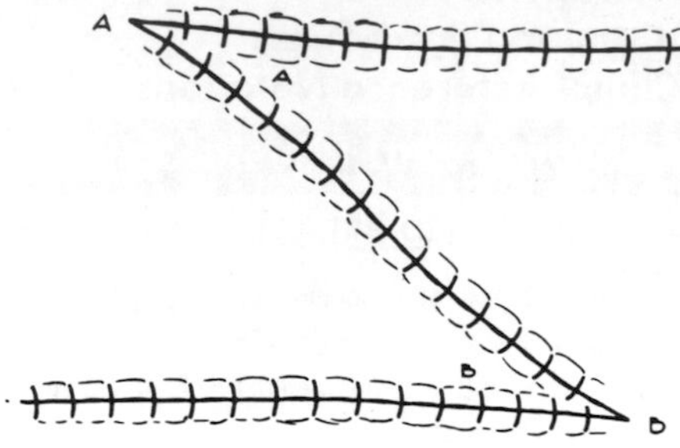

Z-PLASTY – Stage II

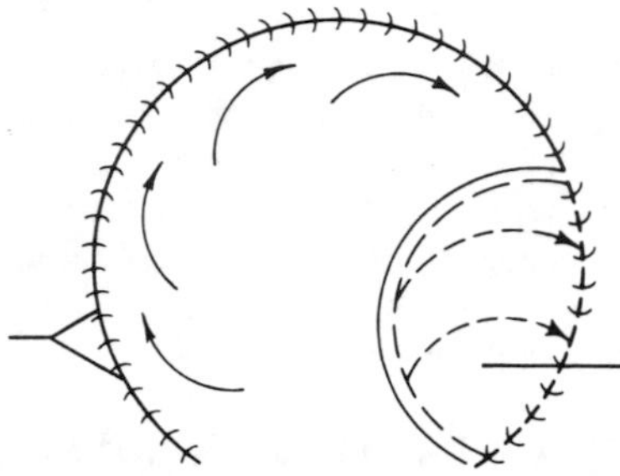

ROTATION FLAP GRAFT

Definitions of Common Procedures of Skin and Breast

Full-thickness skin graft – The surgical removal and placement of a layer of skin that includes the epidermis and entire thickness of the dermis.
Mastectomy with placement of breast tissue expander – The surgical removal of a breast with the placement of an inflatable breast implant to stretch the skin and muscle that is slowly inflated over time (2 to 3 months) to make room for a permanent breast implant.
Mastectomy with TRAM (transverse rectus abdominis myocutaneous) flap breast replacement – The surgical removal of a breast with the replacement of the breast using the rectus abdominis muscle that is raised (including the overlying fat and skin) and transferred to the mastectomy site.
Split-thickness skin graft – The surgical removal and placement of a layer of skin that includes the epidermis and part of the dermis.

AHA Coding Clinic® Reference Notations of Skin and Breast

ROOT OPERATION SPECIFIC - H - SKIN AND BREAST
ALTERATION - 0
CHANGE - 2
DESTRUCTION - 5
DIVISION - 8
DRAINAGE - 9
EXCISION - B
- Excisional debridement ....AHA 15:3Q:p3-8
- Excisional debridement of skin necrosis, right breast ....AHA 18:1Q:p14

EXTIRPATION - C
EXTRACTION - D
- Gastrostomy tube insertion following tube falling out ....AHA 16:3Q:p26
- Non-excisional debridement ....AHA 15:3Q:p3-8

INSERTION - H
- Bilateral breast tissue expanders ....AHA 14:2Q:p12
- Breast tissue expander using acellular dermal matrix ....AHA 13:4Q:p107

INSPECTION - J
REATTACHMENT - M
RELEASE - N

Continued on next page

SKIN & BREAST 0H

© 2018 Channel Publishing, Ltd.

Educational Annotations | H – Skin and Breast

AHA Coding Clinic® Reference Notations of Skin and Breast

ROOT OPERATION SPECIFIC - H - SKIN AND BREAST

Continued from previous page

REMOVAL - P
- Removal of bilateral nonviable TRAM flap ....AHA 16:2Q:p27

REPAIR - Q
- Delayed closure of wound using skin clips ....AHA 14:4Q:p31
- Repair of first degree perineal laceration ....AHA 16:1Q:p6-8

REPLACEMENT - R
- Application of TheraSkin® ....AHA 14:3Q:p14
- Biologically derived skin substitutes ....AHA 14:2Q:p5
- Placement of an EpiFix® graft to skin ....AHA 17:1Q:p35

REPOSITION - S

RESECTION - T
- Skin-sparing mastectomy ....AHA 14:4Q:p34

SUPPLEMENT - U

REVISION - W

TRANSFER - X

Body Part Key Listings of Skin and Breast

See also Body Part Key in Appendix C

Areola ....use Nipple, Left/Right
Dermis ....use Skin
Epidermis ....use Skin
Mammary duct ....use Breast, Bilateral/Left/Right
Mammary gland ....use Breast, Bilateral/Left/Right
Nail bed, Nail plate ....use Finger Nail, Toe Nail
Sebaceous gland ....use Skin
Sweat gland ....use Skin

Device Key Listings of Skin and Breast

See also Device Key in Appendix D

Acellular Hydrated Dermis ....use Nonautologous Tissue Substitute
Autograft ....use Autologous Tissue Substitute
Blood glucose monitoring system ....use Monitoring Device
Brachytherapy seeds ....use Radioactive Element
Continuous Glucose Monitoring (CGM) device ....use Monitoring Device
Cultured epidermal cell autograft ....use Autologous Tissue Substitute
Epicel® cultured epidermal autograft ....use Autologous Tissue Substitute
Implantable glucose monitoring device ....use Monitoring Device
Tissue bank graft ....use Nonautologous Tissue Substitute
Tissue expander (inflatable) (injectable) ....use Tissue Expander in Skin and Breast

Device Aggregation Table Listings of Skin and Breast

See also Device Aggregation Table in Appendix E

Specific Device	For Operation	In Body System	General Device
None Listed in Device Aggregation Table for this Body System			

SKIN & BREAST 0 H

© 2018 Channel Publishing, Ltd.

Educational Annotations | H – Skin and Breast

Coding Notes of Skin and Breast

Body System Relevant Coding Guidelines

Transfer procedures using multiple tissue layers

B3.17

The root operation Transfer contains qualifiers that can be used to specify when a transfer flap is composed of more than one tissue layer, such as a musculocutaneous flap. For procedures involving transfer of multiple tissue layers including skin, subcutaneous tissue, fascia or muscle, the procedure is coded to the body part value that describes the deepest tissue layer in the flap, and the qualifier can be used to describe the other tissue layer(s) in the transfer flap.

Example: A musculocutaneous flap transfer is coded to the appropriate body part value in the body system Muscles, and the qualifier is used to describe the additional tissue layer(s) in the transfer flap.

Skin, subcutaneous tissue and fascia overlying a joint

B4.6

If a procedure is performed on the skin, subcutaneous tissue or fascia overlying a joint, the procedure is coded to the following body part:

- Shoulder is coded to Upper Arm
- Elbow is coded to Lower Arm
- Wrist is coded to Lower Arm
- Hip is coded to Upper Leg
- Knee is coded to Lower Leg
- Ankle is coded to Foot

© 2018 Channel Publishing, Ltd.

1ST - 0 Medical and Surgical
2ND - H Skin and Breast
3RD - 0 ALTERATION

OTHER OBJECTIVES GROUP: Alteration, (Creation), (Fusion)
Root Operations that define other objectives.

ALTERATION: Modifying the anatomic structure of a body part without affecting the function of the body part.

Explanation: Principal purpose is to improve appearance
Examples: Breast augmentation with implants – CMS Ex: Face lift

Body Part – 4TH	Approach – 5TH	Device – 6TH	Qualifier – 7TH
T Breast, Right U Breast, Left V Breast, Bilateral	0 Open 3 Percutaneous X External	7 Autologous tissue substitute J Synthetic substitute K Nonautologous tissue substitute Z No device	Z No qualifier

1ST - 0 Medical and Surgical
2ND - H Skin and Breast
3RD - 2 CHANGE

DEVICE GROUP: Change, Insertion, Removal, Replacement, Revision, Supplement
Root Operations that always involve a device.

CHANGE: Taking out or off a device from a body part and putting back an identical or similar device in or on the same body part without cutting or puncturing the skin or a mucous membrane.

Explanation: All CHANGE procedures are coded using the approach External
Examples: Exchange drain tube – CMS Ex: Urinary catheter change

Body Part – 4TH	Approach – 5TH	Device – 6TH	Qualifier – 7TH
P Skin T Breast, Right U Breast, Left	X External	0 Drainage device Y Other device	Z No qualifier

1ST - 0 Medical and Surgical
2ND - H Skin and Breast
3RD - 5 DESTRUCTION

EXCISION GROUP: Excision, Resection, Destruction, Extraction, (Detachment)
Root Operations that take out some or all of a body part.

DESTRUCTION: Physical eradication of all or a portion of a body part by the direct use of energy, force, or a destructive agent.

Explanation: None of the body part is physically taken out
Examples: Cryoablation skin lesion – CMS Ex: Fulguration of rectal polyp

Body Part – 4TH			Approach – 5TH	Device – 6TH	Qualifier-7TH
0 Skin, Scalp 1 Skin, Face 2 Skin, Right Ear 3 Skin, Left Ear 4 Skin, Neck 5 Skin, Chest 6 Skin, Back 7 Skin, Abdomen	8 Skin, Buttock 9 Skin, Perineum A Skin, Inguinal B Skin, Right Upper Arm C Skin, Left Upper Arm D Skin, Right Lower Arm E Skin, Left Lower Arm F Skin, Right Hand	G Skin, Left Hand H Skin, Right Upper Leg J Skin, Left Upper Leg K Skin, Right Lower Leg L Skin, Left Lower Leg M Skin, Right Foot N Skin, Left Foot	X External	Z No device	D Multiple Z No qualifier
Q Finger Nail R Toe Nail			X External	Z No device	Z No qualifier
T Breast, Right U Breast, Left V Breast, Bilateral W Nipple, Right X Nipple, Left			0 Open 3 Percutaneous 7 Via natural or artificial opening 8 Via natural or artificial opening endoscopic X External	Z No device	Z No qualifier

© 2018 Channel Publishing, Ltd.

1ST - 0 Medical and Surgical
2ND - H Skin and Breast
3RD - 8 DIVISION

DIVISION GROUP: Division, Release
Root Operations involving cutting or separation only.

DIVISION: Cutting into a body part, without draining fluids and/or gases from the body part, in order to separate or transect a body part.

Explanation: All or a portion of the body part is separated into two or more portions
Examples: Division skin back – CMS Ex: Spinal cordotomy

Body Part – 4TH	Approach – 5TH	Device – 6TH	Qualifier-7TH
0 Skin, Scalp 1 Skin, Face 2 Skin, Right Ear 3 Skin, Left Ear 4 Skin, Neck 5 Skin, Chest 6 Skin, Back 7 Skin, Abdomen 8 Skin, Buttock 9 Skin, Perineum A Skin, Inguinal B Skin, Right Upper Arm C Skin, Left Upper Arm D Skin, Right Lower Arm E Skin, Left Lower Arm F Skin, Right Hand G Skin, Left Hand H Skin, Right Upper Leg J Skin, Left Upper Leg K Skin, Right Lower Leg L Skin, Left Lower Leg M Skin, Right Foot N Skin, Left Foot	X External	Z No device	Z No qualifier

1ST - 0 Medical and Surgical
2ND - H Skin and Breast
3RD - 9 DRAINAGE

DRAINAGE GROUP: Drainage, Extirpation, (Fragmentation)
Root Operations that take out solids/fluids/gases from a body part.

DRAINAGE: Taking or letting out fluids and/or gases from a body part.

Explanation: Qualifier "X Diagnostic" indicates drainage procedures that are biopsies
Examples: Incision and drainage boil – CMS Ex: Thoracentesis

Body Part – 4TH	Approach – 5TH	Device – 6TH	Qualifier-7TH
0 Skin, Scalp 1 Skin, Face 2 Skin, Right Ear 3 Skin, Left Ear 4 Skin, Neck 5 Skin, Chest 6 Skin, Back 7 Skin, Abdomen 8 Skin, Buttock 9 Skin, Perineum A Skin, Inguinal B Skin, Right Upper Arm C Skin, Left Upper Arm D Skin, Right Lower Arm E Skin, Left Lower Arm F Skin, Right Hand G Skin, Left Hand H Skin, Right Upper Leg J Skin, Left Upper Leg K Skin, Right Lower Leg L Skin, Left Lower Leg M Skin, Right Foot N Skin, Left Foot Q Finger Nail R Toe Nail	X External	0 Drainage device	Z No qualifier
0 Skin, Scalp 1 Skin, Face 2 Skin, Right Ear 3 Skin, Left Ear 4 Skin, Neck 5 Skin, Chest 6 Skin, Back 7 Skin, Abdomen 8 Skin, Buttock 9 Skin, Perineum A Skin, Inguinal B Skin, Right Upper Arm C Skin, Left Upper Arm D Skin, Right Lower Arm E Skin, Left Lower Arm F Skin, Right Hand G Skin, Left Hand H Skin, Right Upper Leg J Skin, Left Upper Leg K Skin, Right Lower Leg L Skin, Left Lower Leg M Skin, Right Foot N Skin, Left Foot Q Finger Nail R Toe Nail	X External	Z No device	X Diagnostic Z No qualifier
T Breast, Right U Breast, Left V Breast, Bilateral W Nipple, Right X Nipple, Left	0 Open 3 Percutaneous 7 Via natural or artificial opening 8 Via natural or artificial opening endoscopic X External	0 Drainage device	Z No qualifier
T Breast, Right U Breast, Left V Breast, Bilateral W Nipple, Right X Nipple, Left	0 Open 3 Percutaneous 7 Via natural or artificial opening 8 Via natural or artificial opening endoscopic X External	Z No device	X Diagnostic Z No qualifier

© 2018 Channel Publishing, Ltd.

1ST - 0 Medical and Surgical 2ND - H Skin and Breast 3RD - B EXCISION	EXCISION GROUP: Excision, Resection, Destruction, Extraction, (Detachment) Root Operations that take out some or all of a body part. EXCISION: Cutting out or off, without replacement, a portion of a body part. Explanation: Qualifier "X Diagnostic" indicates excision procedures that are biopsies Examples: Partial mastectomy – CMS Ex: Liver biopsy		
Body Part – 4TH	**Approach – 5TH**	**Device – 6TH**	**Qualifier-7TH**
0 Skin, Scalp 1 Skin, Face 2 Skin, Right Ear 3 Skin, Left Ear 4 Skin, Neck 5 Skin, Chest 6 Skin, Back 7 Skin, Abdomen 8 Skin, Buttock 9 Skin, Perineum A Skin, Inguinal B Skin, Right Upper Arm C Skin, Left Upper Arm D Skin, Right Lower Arm E Skin, Left Lower Arm F Skin, Right Hand G Skin, Left Hand H Skin, Right Upper Leg J Skin, Left Upper Leg K Skin, Right Lower Leg L Skin, Left Lower Leg M Skin, Right Foot N Skin, Left Foot Q Finger Nail R Toe Nail	X External	Z No device	X Diagnostic Z No qualifier
T Breast, Right U Breast, Left V Breast, Bilateral W Nipple, Right X Nipple, Left Y Supernumerary Breast	0 Open 3 Percutaneous 7 Via natural or artificial opening 8 Via natural or artificial opening endoscopic X External	Z No device	X Diagnostic Z No qualifier

1ST - 0 Medical and Surgical 2ND - H Skin and Breast 3RD - C EXTIRPATION	DRAINAGE GROUP: Drainage, Extirpation, (Fragmentation) Root Operations that take out solids/fluids/gases from a body part. EXTIRPATION: Taking or cutting out solid matter from a body part. Explanation: Abnormal byproduct or foreign body ... Examples: Removal splinter scalp – CMS Ex: Thrombectomy		
Body Part – 4TH	**Approach – 5TH**	**Device – 6TH**	**Qualifier-7TH**
0 Skin, Scalp 1 Skin, Face 2 Skin, Right Ear 3 Skin, Left Ear 4 Skin, Neck 5 Skin, Chest 6 Skin, Back 7 Skin, Abdomen 8 Skin, Buttock 9 Skin, Perineum A Skin, Inguinal B Skin, Right Upper Arm C Skin, Left Upper Arm D Skin, Right Lower Arm E Skin, Left Lower Arm F Skin, Right Hand G Skin, Left Hand H Skin, Right Upper Leg J Skin, Left Upper Leg K Skin, Right Lower Leg L Skin, Left Lower Leg M Skin, Right Foot N Skin, Left Foot Q Finger Nail R Toe Nail	X External	Z No device	Z No qualifier
T Breast, Right U Breast, Left V Breast, Bilateral W Nipple, Right X Nipple, Left	0 Open 3 Percutaneous 7 Via natural or artificial opening 8 Via natural or artificial opening endoscopic X External	Z No device	Z No qualifier

© 2018 Channel Publishing, Ltd.

1ST - 0 Medical and Surgical
2ND - H Skin and Breast
3RD - D EXTRACTION

EXCISION GROUP: Excision, Resection, Destruction, Extraction, (Detachment)
Root Operations that take out some or all of a body part.

EXTRACTION: Pulling or stripping out or off all or a portion of a body part by the use of force.

Explanation: None for this Body System
Examples: Non-excisional debridement skin – CMS Ex: Dilation and curettage

Body Part – 4TH	Approach – 5TH	Device – 6TH	Qualifier-7TH
0 Skin, Scalp 1 Skin, Face 2 Skin, Right Ear 3 Skin, Left Ear 4 Skin, Neck 5 Skin, Chest 6 Skin, Back 7 Skin, Abdomen 8 Skin, Buttock 9 Skin, Perineum A Skin, Inguinal B Skin, Right Upper Arm C Skin, Left Upper Arm D Skin, Right Lower Arm E Skin, Left Lower Arm F Skin, Right Hand G Skin, Left Hand H Skin, Right Upper Leg J Skin, Left Upper Leg K Skin, Right Lower Leg L Skin, Left Lower Leg M Skin, Right Foot N Skin, Left Foot Q Finger Nail R Toe Nail S Hair	X External	Z No device	Z No qualifier

1ST - 0 Medical and Surgical
2ND - H Skin and Breast
3RD - H INSERTION

DEVICE GROUP: Change, Insertion, Removal, Replacement, Revision, Supplement
Root Operations that always involve a device.

INSERTION: Putting in a nonbiological appliance that monitors, assists, performs, or prevents a physiological function but does not physically take the place of a body part.

Explanation: None
Examples: Insertion breast tissue expander – CMS Ex: Insertion of central venous catheter

Body Part – 4TH	Approach – 5TH	Device – 6TH	Qualifier – 7TH
P Skin	X External	Y Other device	Z No qualifier
T Breast, Right U Breast, Left	0 Open 3 Percutaneous 7 Via natural or artificial opening 8 Via natural or artificial opening endoscopic	1 Radioactive element N Tissue expander Y Other device	Z No qualifier
T Breast, Right U Breast, Left	X External	1 Radioactive element	Z No qualifier
V Breast, Bilateral W Nipple, Right X Nipple, Left	0 Open 3 Percutaneous 7 Via natural or artificial opening 8 Via natural or artificial opening endoscopic	1 Radioactive element N Tissue expander	Z No qualifier
V Breast, Bilateral W Nipple, Right X Nipple, Left	X External	1 Radioactive element	Z No qualifier

1ST - 0 Medical and Surgical
2ND - H Skin and Breast
3RD - J INSPECTION

EXAMINATION GROUP: Inspection, (Map)
Root Operations involving examination only.

INSPECTION: Visually and/or manually exploring a body part.

Explanation: Direct or instrumental visualization ...
Examples: Breast exam – CMS Ex: Exploratory laparotomy

Body Part – 4TH	Approach – 5TH	Device – 6TH	Qualifier – 7TH
P Skin Q Finger Nail R Toe Nail	X External	Z No device	Z No qualifier
T Breast, Right U Breast, Left	0 Open 3 Percutaneous 7 Via natural or artificial opening 8 Via natural or artificial opening endoscopic X External	Z No device	Z No qualifier

© 2018 Channel Publishing, Ltd.

1ST - 0 Medical and Surgical
2ND - H Skin and Breast
3RD - M REATTACHMENT

MOVE GROUP: Reattachment, Reposition, Transfer, (Transplantation)
Root Operations that put in/put back or move some/all of a body part.

REATTACHMENT: Putting back in or on all or a portion of a separated body part to its normal location or other suitable location.

Explanation: Vascular circulation and nervous pathways may or may not be reestablished
Examples: Reattachment avulsed scalp – CMS Ex: Reattachment of hand

Body Part – 4TH	Approach – 5TH	Device – 6TH	Qualifier-7TH
0 Skin, Scalp 1 Skin, Face 2 Skin, Right Ear 3 Skin, Left Ear 4 Skin, Neck 5 Skin, Chest 6 Skin, Back 7 Skin, Abdomen 8 Skin, Buttock 9 Skin, Perineum A Skin, Inguinal B Skin, Right Upper Arm C Skin, Left Upper Arm D Skin, Right Lower Arm E Skin, Left Lower Arm F Skin, Right Hand G Skin, Left Hand H Skin, Right Upper Leg J Skin, Left Upper Leg K Skin, Right Lower Leg L Skin, Left Lower Leg M Skin, Right Foot N Skin, Left Foot T Breast, Right U Breast, Left V Breast, Bilateral W Nipple, Right X Nipple, Left	X External	Z No device	Z No qualifier

1ST - 0 Medical and Surgical
2ND - H Skin and Breast
3RD - N RELEASE

DIVISION GROUP: Division, Release
Root Operations involving cutting or separation only.

RELEASE: Freeing a body part from an abnormal physical constraint by cutting or by the use of force.

Explanation: Some of the restraining tissue may be taken out but none of the body part is taken out
Examples: Incision scar contracture – CMS Ex: Carpal tunnel release

Body Part – 4TH	Approach – 5TH	Device – 6TH	Qualifier-7TH
0 Skin, Scalp 1 Skin, Face 2 Skin, Right Ear 3 Skin, Left Ear 4 Skin, Neck 5 Skin, Chest 6 Skin, Back 7 Skin, Abdomen 8 Skin, Buttock 9 Skin, Perineum A Skin, Inguinal B Skin, Right Upper Arm C Skin, Left Upper Arm D Skin, Right Lower Arm E Skin, Left Lower Arm F Skin, Right Hand G Skin, Left Hand H Skin, Right Upper Leg J Skin, Left Upper Leg K Skin, Right Lower Leg L Skin, Left Lower Leg M Skin, Right Foot N Skin, Left Foot Q Finger Nail R Toe Nail	X External	Z No device	Z No qualifier
T Breast, Right U Breast, Left V Breast, Bilateral W Nipple, Right X Nipple, Left	0 Open 3 Percutaneous 7 Via natural or artificial opening 8 Via natural or artificial opening endoscopic X External	Z No device	Z No qualifier

SKIN & BREAST 0HN

© 2018 Channel Publishing, Ltd.

1ST - 0 Medical and Surgical
2ND - H Skin and Breast
3RD - P REMOVAL

DEVICE GROUP: Change, Insertion, Removal, Replacement, Revision, Supplement
Root Operations that always involve a device.

REMOVAL: Taking out or off a device from a body part.

Explanation: Removal device without reinsertion ...
Examples: Removal tissue expander – CMS Ex: Cardiac pacemaker removal

Body Part – 4TH	Approach – 5TH	Device – 6TH	Qualifier – 7TH
P Skin	X External	0 Drainage device 7 Autologous tissue substitute J Synthetic substitute K Nonautologous tissue substitute Y Other device	Z No qualifier
Q Finger Nail R Toe Nail	X External	0 Drainage device 7 Autologous tissue substitute J Synthetic substitute K Nonautologous tissue substitute	Z No qualifier
S Hair	X External	7 Autologous tissue substitute J Synthetic substitute K Nonautologous tissue substitute	Z No qualifier
T Breast, Right U Breast, Left	0 Open 3 Percutaneous 7 Via natural or artificial opening 8 Via natural or artificial opening endoscopic	0 Drainage device 1 Radioactive element 7 Autologous tissue substitute J Synthetic substitute K Nonautologous tissue substitute N Tissue expander Y Other device	Z No qualifier
T Breast, Right U Breast, Left	X External	0 Drainage device 1 Radioactive element 7 Autologous tissue substitute J Synthetic substitute K Nonautologous tissue substitute	Z No qualifier

SKIN & BREAST 0HP

1ST - 0 Medical and Surgical
2ND - H Skin and Breast
3RD - Q REPAIR

OTHER REPAIRS GROUP: (Control), Repair
Root Operations that define other repairs.

REPAIR: Restoring, to the extent possible, a body part to its normal anatomic structure and function.

Explanation: Used only when the method to accomplish the repair is not one of the other root operations
Examples: Repair first degree perineum laceration – CMS Ex: Suture of laceration

Body Part – 4TH	Approach – 5TH	Device – 6TH	Qualifier-7TH
0 Skin, Scalp 1 Skin, Face 2 Skin, Right Ear 3 Skin, Left Ear 4 Skin, Neck 5 Skin, Chest 6 Skin, Back 7 Skin, Abdomen 8 Skin, Buttock 9 Skin, Perineum A Skin, Inguinal B Skin, Right Upper Arm C Skin, Left Upper Arm D Skin, Right Lower Arm E Skin, Left Lower Arm F Skin, Right Hand G Skin, Left Hand H Skin, Right Upper Leg J Skin, Left Upper Leg K Skin, Right Lower Leg L Skin, Left Lower Leg M Skin, Right Foot N Skin, Left Foot Q Finger Nail R Toe Nail	X External	Z No device	Z No qualifier
T Breast, Right U Breast, Left V Breast, Bilateral W Nipple, Right X Nipple, Left Y Supernumerary Breast	0 Open 3 Percutaneous 7 Via natural or artificial opening 8 Via natural or artificial opening endoscopic X External	Z No device	Z No qualifier

© 2018 Channel Publishing, Ltd.

1ST - 0 Medical and Surgical
2ND - H Skin and Breast
3RD - R REPLACEMENT

DEVICE GROUP: Change, Insertion, Removal, Replacement, Revision, Supplement
Root Operations that always involve a device.

REPLACEMENT: Putting in or on biological or synthetic material that physically takes the place and/or function of all or a portion of a body part.

Explanation: Includes taking out or eradicating, or rendering non-functional, the body part ...
Examples: Mastectomy with implant – CMS Ex: Total hip replacement

Body Part – 4TH	Approach -5TH	Device – 6TH	Qualifier-7TH
0 Skin, Scalp 1 Skin, Face 2 Skin, Right Ear 3 Skin, Left Ear 4 Skin, Neck 5 Skin, Chest 6 Skin, Back 7 Skin, Abdomen 8 Skin, Buttock 9 Skin, Perineum A Skin, Inguinal B Skin, Right Upper Arm C Skin, Left Upper Arm D Skin, Right Lower Arm E Skin, Left Lower Arm F Skin, Right Hand G Skin, Left Hand H Skin, Right Upper Leg J Skin, Left Upper Leg K Skin, Right Lower Leg L Skin, Left Lower Leg M Skin, Right Foot N Skin, Left Foot	X External	7 Autologous tissue substitute K Nonautologous tissue substitute	3 Full thickness 4 Partial thickness
0 Skin, Scalp 1 Skin, Face 2 Skin, Right Ear 3 Skin, Left Ear 4 Skin, Neck 5 Skin, Chest 6 Skin, Back 7 Skin, Abdomen 8 Skin, Buttock 9 Skin, Perineum A Skin, Inguinal B Skin, Right Upper Arm C Skin, Left Upper Arm D Skin, Right Lower Arm E Skin, Left Lower Arm F Skin, Right Hand G Skin, Left Hand H Skin, Right Upper Leg J Skin, Left Upper Leg K Skin, Right Lower Leg L Skin, Left Lower Leg M Skin, Right Foot N Skin, Left Foot	X External	J Synthetic substitute	3 Full thickness 4 Partial thickness Z No qualifier
Q Finger Nail R Toe Nail S Hair	X External	7 Autologous tissue substitute J Synthetic substitute K Nonautologous tissue substitute	Z No qualifier
T Breast, Right U Breast, Left V Breast, Bilateral	0 Open	7 Autologous tissue substitute	5 Latissimus Dorsi Myocutaneous Flap 6 Transverse Rectus Abdominis Myocutaneous Flap 7 Deep Inferior Epigastric Artery Perforator Flap 8 Superficial Inferior Epigastric Artery Flap 9 Gluteal Artery Perforator Flap Z No qualifier
T Breast, Right U Breast, Left V Breast, Bilateral	0 Open	J Synthetic substitute K Nonautologous tissue substitute	Z No qualifier
T Breast, Right U Breast, Left V Breast, Bilateral	3 Percutaneous X External	7 Autologous tissue substitute J Synthetic substitute K Nonautologous tissue substitute	Z No qualifier
W Nipple, Right X Nipple, Left	0 Open 3 Percutaneous X External	7 Autologous tissue substitute J Synthetic substitute K Nonautologous tissue substitute	Z No qualifier

SKIN & BREAST 0 H R

© 2018 Channel Publishing, Ltd.

1ST - 0 Medical and Surgical
2ND - H Skin and Breast
3RD - S REPOSITION

MOVE GROUP: Reattachment, Reposition, Transfer, (Transplantation)
Root Operations that put in/put back or move some/all of a body part.

REPOSITION: Moving to its normal location, or other suitable location, all or a portion of a body part.

Explanation: The body part may or may not be cut out or off to be moved to the new location ...
Examples: Reposition nipple location – CMS Ex: Fracture reduction

Body Part – 4TH	Approach – 5TH	Device – 6TH	Qualifier – 7TH
S Hair W Nipple, Right X Nipple, Left	X External	Z No device	Z No qualifier
T Breast, Right U Breast, Left V Breast, Bilateral	0 Open	Z No device	Z No qualifier

1ST - 0 Medical and Surgical
2ND - H Skin and Breast
3RD - T RESECTION

EXCISION GROUP: Excision, Resection, Destruction, Extraction, (Detachment)
Root Operations that take out some or all of a body part.

RESECTION: Cutting out or off, without replacement, all of a body part.

Explanation: None
Examples: Skin-sparing total mastectomy – CMS Ex: Total lobectomy of lung

Body Part – 4TH	Approach – 5TH	Device – 6TH	Qualifier – 7TH
Q Finger Nail R Toe Nail W Nipple, Right X Nipple, Left	X External	Z No device	Z No qualifier
T Breast, Right U Breast, Left V Breast, Bilateral Y Supernumerary Breast	0 Open	Z No device	Z No qualifier

1ST - 0 Medical and Surgical
2ND - H Skin and Breast
3RD - U SUPPLEMENT

DEVICE GROUP: Change, Insertion, Removal, Replacement, Revision, Supplement
Root Operations that always involve a device.

SUPPLEMENT: Putting in or on biological or synthetic material that physically reinforces and/or augments the function of a portion of a body part.

Explanation: Biological material is non-living, or is living and from the same individual ...
Examples: Repair inverted nipple with graft – CMS Ex: Herniorrhaphy using mesh

Body Part – 4TH	Approach – 5TH	Device – 6TH	Qualifier – 7TH
T Breast, Right U Breast, Left V Breast, Bilateral W Nipple, Right X Nipple, Left	0 Open 3 Percutaneous 7 Via natural or artificial opening 8 Via natural or artificial opening endoscopic X External	7 Autologous tissue substitute J Synthetic substitute K Nonautologous tissue substitute	Z No qualifier

© 2018 Channel Publishing, Ltd.

1ST - 0 Medical and Surgical
2ND - H Skin and Breast
3RD - W REVISION

DEVICE GROUP: Change, Insertion, Removal, Replacement, Revision, Supplement
Root Operations that always involve a device.

REVISION: Correcting, to the extent possible, a portion of a malfunctioning device or the position of a displaced device.

Explanation: Correcting by taking out or putting in components of a device such as a screw or pin ...
Examples: Reposition tissue expander – CMS Ex: Recementing of hip prosthesis

Body Part – 4TH	Approach – 5TH	Device – 6TH	Qualifier – 7TH
P Skin	X External	0 Drainage device 7 Autologous tissue substitute J Synthetic substitute K Nonautologous tissue substitute Y Other device	Z No qualifier
Q Finger Nail R Toe Nail	X External	0 Drainage device 7 Autologous tissue substitute J Synthetic substitute K Nonautologous tissue substitute	Z No qualifier
S Hair	X External	7 Autologous tissue substitute J Synthetic substitute K Nonautologous tissue substitute	Z No qualifier
T Breast, Right U Breast, Left	0 Open 3 Percutaneous 7 Via natural or artificial opening 8 Via natural or artificial opening endoscopic	0 Drainage device 7 Autologous tissue substitute J Synthetic substitute K Nonautologous tissue substitute N Tissue expander Y Other device	Z No qualifier
T Breast, Right U Breast, Left	X External	0 Drainage device 7 Autologous tissue substitute J Synthetic substitute K Nonautologous tissue substitute	Z No qualifier

1ST - 0 Medical and Surgical
2ND - H Skin and Breast
3RD - X TRANSFER

MOVE GROUP: Reattachment, Reposition, Transfer, (Transplantation)
Root Operations that put in/put back or move some/all of a body part.

TRANSFER: Moving, without taking out, all or a portion of a body part to another location to take over the function of all or a portion of a body part.

Explanation: The body part transferred remains connected to its vascular and nervous supply
Examples: Scalp advancement flap – CMS Ex: Tendon transfer

Body Part – 4TH	Approach – 5TH	Device – 6TH	Qualifier-7TH
0 Skin, Scalp 1 Skin, Face 2 Skin, Right Ear 3 Skin, Left Ear 4 Skin, Neck 5 Skin, Chest 6 Skin, Back 7 Skin, Abdomen 8 Skin, Buttock 9 Skin, Perineum A Skin, Inguinal B Skin, Right Upper Arm C Skin, Left Upper Arm D Skin, Right Lower Arm E Skin, Left Lower Arm F Skin, Right Hand G Skin, Left Hand H Skin, Right Upper Leg J Skin, Left Upper Leg K Skin, Right Lower Leg L Skin, Left Lower Leg M Skin, Right Foot N Skin, Left Foot	X External	Z No device	Z No qualifier

SKIN & BREAST 0 H X

© 2018 Channel Publishing, Ltd.

NOTES

© 2018 Channel Publishing, Ltd.

Educational Annotations | J – Subcutaneous Tissue and Fascia

Body System Specific Educational Annotations for the Subcutaneous Tissue and Fascia include:

- Anatomy and Physiology Review
- Anatomical Illustrations
- Definitions of Common Procedures
- AHA Coding Clinic® Reference Notations
- Body Part Key Listings
- Device Key Listings
- Device Aggregation Table Listings
- Coding Notes

Anatomy and Physiology Review of Subcutaneous Tissue and Fascia

BODY PART VALUES – J - SUBCUTANEOUS TISSUE AND FASCIA

Fascia – ANATOMY – The sheets or bands of dense connective tissue located beneath the skin between muscles, organs, and other structures. PHYSIOLOGY – The fascia is strong but flexible and functions to separate, protect, and reduce friction of muscule movement on the organs, blood vessels, nerves, muscles, and other structures within the body.

Subcutaneous Tissue – ANATOMY – The innermost layer of the three layers of the skin (also known as the hypodermis) and comprised of fibous tissue, adipose tissue, elastic fibers, connective tissue, and hair follicle roots. PHYSIOLOGY – The subcutaneous tissue is responsible for regulating body temperature, plays a role in pigmentation, and protects the inner organs and bones.

Anatomical Illustrations of Subcutaneous Tissue and Fascia

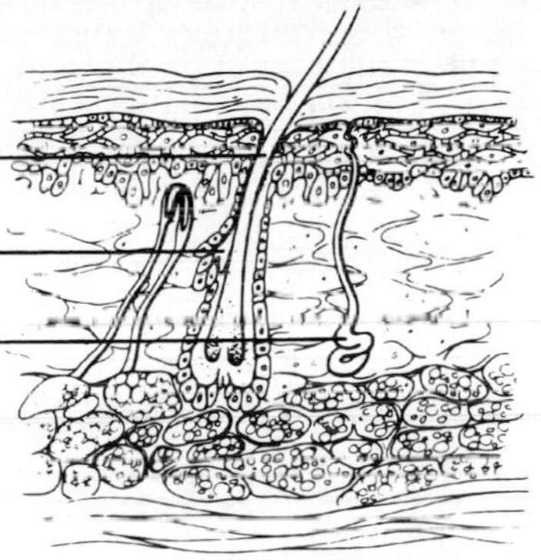

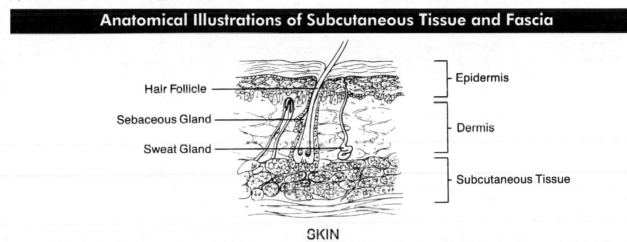

SKIN

Definitions of Common Procedures of Subcutaneous Tissue and Fascia

Free fascia graft – The implantation of fascia to fill a defect using an allograft or donor tissue.

Insertion of pacemaker generator – The surgical placement of a pacemaker generator just under the skin in the subcutaneous tissue.

Liposuction – The surgical removal of excess fat deposits using a hollow cannula that is connected to a strong suction pump.

Pedicle fascia graft – The transfer of fascia to fill a defect without dissecting the graft tissue free from its vascular and nervous supply.

AHA Coding Clinic® Reference Notations of Subcutaneous Tissue and Fascia

ROOT OPERATION SPECIFIC - J - SUBCUTANEOUS TISSUE AND FASCIA

ALTERATION - 0

CHANGE - 2

Change of tunneled hemodialysis catheter ....AHA 17:2Q:p26

DESTRUCTION - 5

DIVISION - 8

DRAINAGE - 9

Drainage of subcutaneous abscesses ....AHA 15:3Q:p23

EXCISION - B

Excision of abdominal subcutaneous fat during hernia repair ....AHA 14:4Q:p38

Excision of inclusion cyst of perineum ....AHA 13:4Q:p119

Excisional repair of perineal fistula ....AHA 15:1Q:p29

Graft excision, forearm free flap....................AHA 15:2Q:p13

Harvesting of fat graft from abdomen ....AHA 14:3Q:p22

Continued on next page

© 2018 Channel Publishing, Ltd.

SUBCUTANEOUS 0 J

Educational Annotations | J – Subcutaneous Tissue and Fascia

AHA Coding Clinic® Reference Notations of Subcutaneous Tissue and Fascia

ROOT OPERATION SPECIFIC - J - SUBCUTANEOUS TISSUE AND FASCIA

Continued from previous page

EXTIRPATION - C
- Removal of bone flap from abdominal wall .... AHA 17:3Q:p22

EXTRACTION - D
- Non-excisional debridement .... AHA 15:3Q:p3-8
- Non-excisional debridement using Pulsavac .... AHA 15:1Q:p23

INSERTION - H
- Exchange of tunneled hemodialysis catheter with chest port .... AHA 15:4Q:p31
- Insertion of infusion pump in chest pocket .... AHA 15:4Q:p14
- Insertion of subcutaneous port-a-cath .... AHA 17:4Q:p63
- Insertion of tunneled hemodialysis catheter into superior vena cava with port chest pocket .... AHA 15:4Q:p30
- Insertion of various cardiac devices and components .... AHA 12:4Q:p104
- Insertion of vascular access device into chest .... AHA 17:2Q:p24
- Insertion of venous access port .... AHA 13:4Q:p116
  - Official Clarification of 13:4Q:p116 .... AHA 15:2Q:p34
- Peritoneal port-a-cath insertion .... AHA 16:2Q:p14
- Removal with new insertion of jugular tunneled catheter in right atrium .... AHA 16:2Q:p15
- Replacement of Baclofen medication pump/spinal canal catheter .... AHA 14:3Q:p19

INSPECTION - J

RELEASE - N
- Escharotomy to release underlying tissue .... AHA 17:3Q:p11

REMOVAL - P
- Exchange of tunneled hemodialysis catheter with chest port .... AHA 15:4Q:p31
- Removal of various cardiac devices and components .... AHA 12:4Q:p104
- Removal with new insertion of jugular tunneled catheter in right atrium .... AHA 16:2Q:p15
- Replacement of Baclofen medication pump/spinal canal catheter .... AHA 14:3Q:p19

REPAIR - Q
- Anterior cystocele repair .... AHA 17:3Q:p19
- Posterior colporrhaphy/rectocele repair .... AHA 14:4Q:p44

REPLACEMENT - R
- Reconstruction of orbital defect using forearm free flap .... AHA 15:2Q:p13

SUPPLEMENT - U
- AlloDerm™ first stage forearm free flap graft .... AHA 18:2Q:p20
- Fat graft .... AHA 18:1Q:p7

REVISION - W
- Externalization of peritoneal dialysis catheter .... AHA 15:4Q:p33
- Ligation of catheter portion of ventricular peritoneal shunt .... AHA 18:1Q:p8
- Retunneling and reconnection of VP shunt in periauricular subcutaneous tissue .... AHA 15:2Q:p9
- Revision of various cardiac devices and components .... AHA 12:4Q:p104

TRANSFER - X
- Closure of scalp wound using pericranial flap .... AHA 18:1Q:p10
- Reverse sural fasciocutaneous pedicle flap .... AHA 14:3Q:p18

Body Part Key Listings of Subcutaneous Tissue and Fascia

See also Body Part Key in Appendix C

- Antebrachial fascia .... use Subcutaneous Tissue and Fascia, Lower Arm, Left/Right
- Axillary fascia .... use Subcutaneous Tissue and Fascia, Upper Arm, Left/Right
- Bicipital aponeurosis .... use Subcutaneous Tissue and Fascia, Lower Arm, Left/Right
- Crural fascia .... use Subcutaneous Tissue and Fascia, Upper Leg, Left/Right
- Deep cervical fascia .... use Subcutaneous Tissue and Fascia, Neck, Left/Right
- Deltoid fascia .... use Subcutaneous Tissue and Fascia, Upper Arm, Left/Right

Continued on next page

© 2018 Channel Publishing, Ltd.

Educational Annotations | J – Subcutaneous Tissue and Fascia

Body Part Key Listings of Subcutaneous Tissue and Fascia

Continued from previous page

External oblique aponeurosis .... use Subcutaneous Tissue and Fascia, Trunk
Fascia lata .... use Subcutaneous Tissue and Fascia, Upper Leg, Left/Right
Galea aponeurotica .... use Subcutaneous Tissue and Fascia, Scalp
Iliac fascia .... use Subcutaneous Tissue and Fascia, Upper Leg, Left/Right
Iliotibial tract (band) .... use Subcutaneous Tissue and Fascia, Upper Leg, Left/Right
Infraspinatus fascia .... use Subcutaneous Tissue and Fascia, Upper Arm, Left/Right
Masseteric fascia .... use Subcutaneous Tissue and Fascia, Face
Orbital fascia .... use Subcutaneous Tissue and Fascia, Face
Palmar fascia (aponeurosis) .... use Subcutaneous Tissue and Fascia, Hand, Left/Right
Pectoral fascia .... use Subcutaneous Tissue and Fascia, Chest
Plantar fascia (aponeurosis) .... use Subcutaneous Tissue and Fascia, Foot, Left/Right
Pretracheal fascia .... use Subcutaneous Tissue and Fascia, Neck, Left/Right
Prevertebral fascia .... use Subcutaneous Tissue and Fascia, Neck, Left/Right
Subscapular aponeurosis .... use Subcutaneous Tissue and Fascia, Upper Arm, Left/Right
Supraspinatus fascia .... use Subcutaneous Tissue and Fascia, Upper Arm, Left/Right
Transversalis fascia .... use Subcutaneous Tissue and Fascia, Trunk

Device Key Listings of Subcutaneous Tissue and Fascia

See also Device Key in Appendix D

Activa PC neurostimulator .... use Stimulator Generator, Multiple Array for Insertion in Subcutaneous Tissue and Fascia
Activa RC neurostimulator .... use Stimulator Generator, Multiple Array Rechargeable for Insertion in Subcutaneous Tissue and Fascia
Activa SC neurostimulator .... use Stimulator Generator, Single Array for Insertion in Subcutaneous Tissue and Fascia
Advisa (MRI) .... use Pacemaker, Dual Chamber for Insertion in Subcutaneous Tissue and Fascia
Autograft .... use Autologous Tissue Substitute
Baroreflex Activation Therapy® (BAT®) .... use Stimulator Generator in Subcutaneous Tissue and Fascia
Brachytherapy seeds .... use Radioactive Element
COGNIS® CRT-D .... use Cardiac Resynchronization Defibrillator Pulse Generator for Insertion in Subcutaneous Tissue and Fascia
Concerto II CRT-D .... use Cardiac Resynchronization Defibrillator Pulse Generator for Insertion in Subcutaneous Tissue and Fascia
Consulta CRT-D .... use Cardiac Resynchronization Defibrillator Pulse Generator for Insertion in Subcutaneous Tissue and Fascia
Consulta CRT-P .... use Cardiac Resynchronization Pacemaker Pulse Generator for Insertion in Subcutaneous Tissue and Fascia
CONTAK RENEWAL® 3 RF (HE) CRT-D .... use Cardiac Resynchronization Defibrillator Pulse Generator for Insertion in Subcutaneous Tissue and Fascia
Cook Biodesign® Fistula Plug(s) .... use Nonautologous Tissue Substitute
Cook Biodesign® Hernia Graft(s) .... use Nonautologous Tissue Substitute
Cook Biodesign® Layered Graft(s) .... use Nonautologous Tissue Substitute
Cook Zenapro™ Layered Graft(s) .... use Nonautologous Tissue Substitute
Diaphragmatic pacemaker generator .... use Stimulator Generator in Subcutaneous Tissue and Fascia
EnRhythm .... use Pacemaker, Dual Chamber for Insertion in Subcutaneous Tissue and Fascia
Enterra gastric neurostimulator .... use Stimulator Generator, Multiple Array for Insertion in Subcutaneous Tissue and Fascia
Evera (XT) (S) (DR/VR) .... use Defibrillator Generator for Insertion in Subcutaneous Tissue and Fascia
Implantable cardioverter-defibrillator (ICD) .... use Defibrillator Generator for Insertion in Subcutaneous Tissue and Fascia
Implantable drug infusion pump (anti-spasmodic) (chemotherapy) (pain) .... use Infusion Device, Pump in Subcutaneous Tissue and Fascia
Implantable hemodynamic monitor (IHM) .... use Monitoring Device, Hemodynamic for Insertion in Subcutaneous Tissue and Fascia
Implantable hemodynamic monitoring system (IHMS) .... use Monitoring Device, Hemodynamic for Insertion in Subcutaneous Tissue and Fascia
Implanted (venous) (access) port .... use Vascular Access Device, Totally Implantable in Subcutaneous Tissue and Fascia
Injection reservoir, port .... use Vascular Access Device, Totally Implantable in Subcutaneous Tissue andFascia
Injection reservoir, pump .... use Infusion Device, Pump in Subcutaneous Tissue and Fascia
InterStim® Therapy neurostimulator .... use Stimulator Generator, Single Array for Insertion in Subcutaneous Tissue and Fascia
Itrel (3) (4) neurostimulator .... use Stimulator Generator, Single Array for Insertion in Subcutaneous Tissue and Fascia
Kappa .... use Pacemaker, Dual Chamber for Insertion in Subcutaneous Tissue and Fascia
LIVIAN™ CRT-D .... use Cardiac Resynchronization Defibrillator Pulse Generator for Insertion in Subcutaneous Tissue and Fascia
Loop recorder, implantable .... use Monitoring Device
Mark IV Breathing Pacemaker System .... use Stimulator Generator in Subcutaneous Tissue and Fascia
Maximo II DR (VR) .... use Defibrillator Generator for Insertion in Subcutaneous Tissue and Fascia
Maximo II DR CRT-D .... use Cardiac Resynchronization Defibrillator Pulse Generator for Insertion in Subcutaneous Tissue and Fascia

Continued on next page

© 2018 Channel Publishing, Ltd.

Educational Annotations | J – Subcutaneous Tissue and Fascia

Device Key Listings of Subcutaneous Tissue and Fascia

Continued from previous page

Neurostimulator generator, multiple channel ....use Stimulator Generator, Multiple Array for Insertion in Subcutaneous Tissue and Fascia
Neurostimulator generator, multiple channel rechargeable ....use Stimulator Generator, Multiple Array Rechargeable for Insertion in Subcutaneous Tissue and Fascia
Neurostimulator generator, single channel ....use Stimulator Generator, Single Array for Insertion in Subcutaneous Tissue and Fascia
Neurostimulator generator, single channel rechargeable ....use Stimulator Generator, Single Array Rechargeable for Insertion in Subcutaneous Tissue and Fascia
Optimizer™ III implantable pulse generator ....use Contractility Modulation Device for Insertion in Subcutaneous Tissue and Fascia
Ovatio™ CRT-D ....use Cardiac Resynchronization Defibrillator Pulse Generator for Insertion in Subcutaneous Tissue and Fascia
Phrenic nerve stimulator generator ....use Stimulator Generator in Subcutaneous Tissue and Fascia
PrimeAdvanced neurostimulator (SureScan) (MRI Safe) ....use Stimulator Generator, Multiple Array for Insertion in Subcutaneous Tissue and Fascia
Protecta XT CRT-D..........use Cardiac Resynchronization Defibrillator Pulse Generator for Insertion in Subcutaneous Tissue and Fascia
Protecta XT DR (XT VR) ....use Defibrillator Generator for Insertion in Subcutaneous Tissue and Fascia
Pump reservoir..........use Infusion Device, Pump in Subcutaneous Tissue and Fascia
RestoreAdvanced neurostimulator (SureScan) (MRI Safe) ....use Stimulator Generator, Multiple Array Rechargeable for Insertion in Subcutaneous Tissue and Fascia
RestoreSensor neurostimulator (SureScan) (MRI Safe) ....use Stimulator Generator, Multiple Array Rechargeable for Insertion in Subcutaneous Tissue and Fascia
RestoreUltra neurostimulator (SureScan) (MRI Safe) use Stimulator Generator, Multiple Array Rechargeable for Insertion in Subcutaneous Tissue and Fascia
Reveal (DX) (XT)..........use Monitoring Device
Revo MRI™ SureScan® pacemaker ....use Pacemaker, Dual Chamber for Insertion in Subcutaneous Tissue and Fascia
Rheos® System device ....use Stimulator Generator in Subcutaneous Tissue and Fascia
Secura (DR) (VR) ....use Defibrillator Generator for Insertion in Subcutaneous Tissue and Fascia
Single lead pacemaker (atrium) (ventricle)..........use Pacemaker, Single Chamber for Insertion in Subcutaneous Tissue and Fascia
Single lead rate responsive pacemaker (atrium) (ventricle) ....use Pacemaker, Single Chamber Rate Responsive for Insertionin Subcutaneous Tissue and Fascia
Stratos LV ....use Cardiac Resynchronization Pacemaker Pulse Generator for Insertion in Subcutaneous Tissue and Fascia
Subcutaneous injection reservoir, port ....use Vascular Access Device, Totally Implantable in Subcutaneous Tissue and Fascia
Subcutaneous injection reservoir, pump..........use Infusion Device, Pump in Subcutaneous Tissue and Fascia
Subdermal progesterone implant ....use Contraceptive Device in Subcutaneous Tissue and Fascia
Synchra CRT-P ....use Cardiac Resynchronization Pacemaker Pulse Generator for Insertion in Subcutaneous Tissue and Fascia
SynchroMed pump ....use Infusion Device, Pump in Subcutaneous Tissue and Fascia
Tissue bank graft ....use Nonautologous Tissue Substitute
Tissue expander (inflatable) (injectable) ....use Tissue Expander in Subcutaneous Tissue and Fascia
Tunneled central venous catheter..........use Vascular Access Device, Tunneled in Subcutaneous Tissue and Fascia
Two lead pacemaker..........use Pacemaker, Dual Chamber for Insertion in Subcutaneous Tissue and Fascia
Vectra® Vascular Access Graft..........use Vascular Access Device, Tunneled in Subcutaneous Tissue and Fascia
Versa ....use Pacemaker, Dual Chamber for Insertion in Subcutaneous Tissue and Fascia
Virtuoso (II) (DR) (VR) ....use Defibrillator Generator for Insertion in Subcutaneous Tissue and Fascia
Viva (XT) (S)..........use Cardiac Resynchronization Defibrillator Pulse Generator for Insertion in Subcutaneous Tissue and Fascia

Device Aggregation Table Listings of Subcutaneous Tissue and Fascia

See also Device Aggregation Table in Appendix E

Specific Device	For Operation	In Body System	General Device
Cardiac Resynchronization Defibrillator Pulse Generator	Insertion	Subcutaneous Tissue and Fascia	Cardiac Rhythm Related Device
Cardiac Resynchronization Pacemaker Pulse Generator	Insertion	Subcutaneous Tissue and Fascia	Cardiac Rhythm Related Device
Contractility Modulation Device	Insertion	Subcutaneous Tissue and Fascia	Cardiac Rhythm Related Device
Defibrillator Generator	Insertion	Subcutaneous Tissue and Fascia	Cardiac Rhythm Related Device
Monitoring Device, Hemodynamic	Insertion	Subcutaneous Tissue and Fascia	Monitoring Device
Pacemaker, Dual Chamber	Insertion	Subcutaneous Tissue and Fascia	Cardiac Rhythm Related Device
Pacemaker, Single Chamber	Insertion	Subcutaneous Tissue and Fascia	Cardiac Rhythm Related Device
Pacemaker, Single Chamber Rate Responsive	Insertion	Subcutaneous Tissue and Fascia	Cardiac Rhythm Related Device
Stimulator Generator, Multiple Array	Insertion	Subcutaneous Tissue and Fascia	Stimulator Generator
Stimulator Generator, Multiple Array Rechargeable	Insertion	Subcutaneous Tissue and Fascia	Stimulator Generator
Stimulator Generator, Single Array	Insertion	Subcutaneous Tissue and Fascia	Stimulator Generator
Stimulator Generator, Single Array Rechargeable	Insertion	Subcutaneous Tissue and Fascia	Stimulator Generator

© 2018 Channel Publishing, Ltd.

Educational Annotations | J – Subcutaneous Tissue and Fascia

Coding Notes of Subcutaneous Tissue and Fascia

Body System Relevant Coding Guidelines

Transfer procedures using multiple tissue layers

B3.17

The root operation Transfer contains qualifiers that can be used to specify when a transfer flap is composed of more than one tissue layer, such as a musculocutaneous flap. For procedures involving transfer of multiple tissue layers including skin, subcutaneous tissue, fascia or muscle, the procedure is coded to the body part value that describes the deepest tissue layer in the flap, and the qualifier can be used to describe the other tissue layer(s) in the transfer flap.

Example: A musculocutaneous flap transfer is coded to the appropriate body part value in the body system Muscles, and the qualifier is used to describe the additional tissue layer(s) in the transfer flap.

Tendons, ligaments, bursae and fascia near a joint

B4.5

Procedures performed on tendons, ligaments, bursae and fascia supporting a joint are coded to the body part in the respective body system that is the focus of the procedure. Procedures performed on joint structures themselves are coded to the body part in the joint body systems.

Examples: Repair of the anterior cruciate ligament of the knee is coded to the knee bursa and ligament body part in the bursae and ligaments body system.

Knee arthroscopy with shaving of articular cartilage is coded to the knee joint body part in the Lower Joints body system.

Skin, subcutaneous tissue and fascia overlying a joint

B4.6

If a procedure is performed on the skin, subcutaneous tissue or fascia overlying a joint, the procedure is coded to the following body part:

- Shoulder is coded to Upper Arm
- Elbow is coded to Lower Arm
- Wrist is coded to Lower Arm
- Hip is coded to Upper Leg
- Knee is coded to Lower Leg
- Ankle is coded to Foot

© 2018 Channel Publishing, Ltd.

1ST - 0 Medical and Surgical
2ND - J Subcutaneous Tissue and Fascia
3RD - 0 ALTERATION

OTHER OBJECTIVES GROUP: Alteration, (Creation), (Fusion)
Root Operations that define other objectives.

ALTERATION: Modifying the anatomic structure of a body part without affecting the function of the body part.

Explanation: Principal purpose is to improve appearance
Examples: Liposuction thighs – CMS Ex: Face lift

Body Part – 4TH	Approach – 5TH	Device – 6TH	Qualifier – 7TH
Subcutaneous Tissue and Fascia, ... 1 ... Face 4 ... Right Neck 5 ... Left Neck 6 ... Chest 7 ... Back 8 ... Abdomen 9 ... Buttock D ... Right Upper Arm F ... Left Upper Arm G ... Right Lower Arm H ... Left Lower Arm L ... Right Upper Leg M ... Left Upper Leg N ... Right Lower Leg P ... Left Lower Leg	0 Open 3 Percutaneous	Z No device	Z No qualifier

1ST - 0 Medical and Surgical
2ND - J Subcutaneous Tissue and Fascia
3RD - 2 CHANGE

DEVICE GROUP: Change, Insertion, Removal, Replacement, Revision, Supplement
Root Operations that always involve a device.

CHANGE: Taking out or off a device from a body part and putting back an identical or similar device in or on the same body part without cutting or puncturing the skin or a mucous membrane.

Explanation: All CHANGE procedures are coded using the approach External
Examples: Exchange drain tube – CMS Ex: Urinary catheter change

Body Part – 4TH	Approach – 5TH	Device – 6TH	Qualifier – 7TH
Subcutaneous Tissue and Fascia, ... S ... Head and Neck T ... Trunk V ... Upper Extremity W ... Lower Extremity	X External	0 Drainage device Y Other device	Z No qualifier

1ST - 0 Medical and Surgical
2ND - J Subcutaneous Tissue and Fascia
3RD - 5 DESTRUCTION

EXCISION GROUP: Excision, (Resection), Destruction, Extraction, (Detachment)
Root Operations that take out some or all of a body part.

DESTRUCTION: Physical eradication of all or a portion of a body part by the direct use of energy, force, or a destructive agent.

Explanation: None of the body part is physically taken out
Examples: Radiofrquency ablation – CMS Ex: Fulguration of rectal polyp

Body Part – 4TH	Approach – 5TH	Device – 6TH	Qualifier – 7TH
Subcutaneous Tissue and Fascia, ... 0 ... Scalp 1 ... Face 4 ... Right Neck 5 ... Left Neck 6 ... Chest 7 ... Back 8 ... Abdomen 9 ... Buttock B ... Perineum C ... Pelvic Region D ... Right Upper Arm F ... Left Upper Arm G ... Right Lower Arm H ... Left Lower Arm J ... Right Hand K ... Left Hand L ... Right Upper Leg M ... Left Upper Leg N ... Right Lower Leg P ... Left Lower Leg Q ... Right Foot R ... Left Foot	0 Open 3 Percutaneous	Z No device	Z No qualifier

© 2018 Channel Publishing, Ltd.

1ST - 0 Medical and Surgical
2ND - J Subcutaneous Tissue and Fascia
3RD - 8 DIVISION

DIVISION GROUP: Division, Release
Root Operations involving cutting or separation only.

DIVISION: Cutting into a body part, without draining fluids and/or gases from the body part, in order to separate or transect a body part.

Explanation: All or a portion of the body part is separated into two or more portions
Examples: Division plantar fascia – CMS Ex: Spinal cordotomy

Body Part – 4TH	Approach – 5TH	Device – 6TH	Qualifier – 7TH
Subcutaneous Tissue and Fascia, ... 0 ... Scalp 1 ... Face 4 ... Right Neck 5 ... Left Neck 6 ... Chest 7 ... Back 8 ... Abdomen 9 ... Buttock B ... Perineum C ... Pelvic Region D ... Right Upper Arm F ... Left Upper Arm G ... Right Lower Arm H ... Left Lower Arm J ... Right Hand K ... Left Hand L ... Right Upper Leg M ... Left Upper Leg N ... Right Lower Leg P ... Left Lower Leg Q ... Right Foot R ... Left Foot S ... Head and Neck T ... Trunk V ... Upper Extremity W ... Lower Extremity	0 Open 3 Percutaneous	Z No device	Z No qualifier

1ST - 0 Medical and Surgical
2ND - J Subcutaneous Tissue and Fascia
3RD - 9 DRAINAGE

DRAINAGE GROUP: Drainage, Extirpation, (Fragmentation)
Root Operations that take out solids/fluids/gases from a body part.

DRAINAGE: Taking or letting out fluids and/or gases from a body part.

Explanation: Qualifier "X Diagnostic" indicates drainage procedures that are biopsies
Examples: Incision and drainage fascial abscess – CMS Ex: Thoracentesis

Body Part – 4TH	Approach – 5TH	Device – 6TH	Qualifier – 7TH
Subcutaneous Tissue and Fascia, ... 0 ... Scalp 1 ... Face 4 ... Right Neck 5 ... Left Neck 6 ... Chest 7 ... Back 8 ... Abdomen 9 ... Buttock B ... Perineum C ... Pelvic Region D ... Right Upper Arm F ... Left Upper Arm G ... Right Lower Arm H ... Left Lower Arm J ... Right Hand K ... Left Hand L ... Right Upper Leg M ... Left Upper Leg N ... Right Lower Leg P ... Left Lower Leg Q ... Right Foot R ... Left Foot	0 Open 3 Percutaneous	0 Drainage device	Z No qualifier
Subcutaneous Tissue and Fascia, ... 0 ... Scalp 1 ... Face 4 ... Right Neck 5 ... Left Neck 6 ... Chest 7 ... Back 8 ... Abdomen 9 ... Buttock B ... Perineum C ... Pelvic Region D ... Right Upper Arm F ... Left Upper Arm G ... Right Lower Arm H ... Left Lower Arm J ... Right Hand K ... Left Hand L ... Right Upper Leg M ... Left Upper Leg N ... Right Lower Leg P ... Left Lower Leg Q ... Right Foot R ... Left Foot	0 Open 3 Percutaneous	Z No device	X Diagnostic Z No qualifier

© 2018 Channel Publishing, Ltd.

1ST - 0 Medical and Surgical
2ND - J Subcutaneous Tissue and Fascia
3RD - B EXCISION

EXCISION GROUP: Excision, (Resection), Destruction, Extraction, (Detachment)
Root Operations that take out some or all of a body part.
EXCISION: Cutting out or off, without replacement, a portion of a body part.

Explanation: Qualifier "X Diagnostic" indicates excision procedures that are biopsies
Examples: Harvesting fat for graft – CMS Ex: Liver biopsy

Body Part – 4TH	Approach – 5TH	Device – 6TH	Qualifier – 7TH
Subcutaneous Tissue and Fascia, ... 0 ... Scalp 1 ... Face 4 ... Right Neck 5 ... Left Neck 6 ... Chest 7 ... Back 8 ... Abdomen 9 ... Buttock B ... Perineum C ... Pelvic Region D ... Right Upper Arm F ... Left Upper Arm G ... Right Lower Arm H ... Left Lower Arm J ... Right Hand K ... Left Hand L ... Right Upper Leg M ... Left Upper Leg N ... Right Lower Leg P ... Left Lower Leg Q ... Right Foot R ... Left Foot	0 Open 3 Percutaneous	Z No device	X Diagnostic Z No qualifier

1ST - 0 Medical and Surgical
2ND - J Subcutaneous Tissue and Fascia
3RD - C EXTIRPATION

DRAINAGE GROUP: Drainage, Extirpation, (Fragmentation)
Root Operations that take out solids/fluids/gases from a body part.
EXTIRPATION: Taking or cutting out solid matter from a body part.

Explanation: Abnormal byproduct or foreign body ...
Examples: Removal foreign body – CMS Ex: Thrombectomy

Body Part – 4TH	Approach – 5TH	Device – 6TH	Qualifier – 7TH
Subcutaneous Tissue and Fascia, ... 0 ... Scalp 1 ... Face 4 ... Right Neck 5 ... Left Neck 6 ... Chest 7 ... Back 8 ... Abdomen 9 ... Buttock B ... Perineum C ... Pelvic Region D ... Right Upper Arm F ... Left Upper Arm G ... Right Lower Arm H ... Left Lower Arm J ... Right Hand K ... Left Hand L ... Right Upper Leg M ... Left Upper Leg N ... Right Lower Leg P ... Left Lower Leg Q ... Right Foot R ... Left Foot	0 Open 3 Percutaneous	Z No device	Z No qualifier

1ST - 0 Medical and Surgical
2ND - J Subcutaneous Tissue and Fascia
3RD - D EXTRACTION

EXCISION GROUP: Excision, (Resection), Destruction, Extraction, (Detachment)
Root Operations that take out some or all of a body part.
EXTRACTION: Pulling or stripping out or off all or a portion of a body part by the use of force.

Explanation: None for this Body System
Examples: Non-excisional debridement – CMS Ex: Dilation and curettage

Body Part – 4TH	Approach – 5TH	Device – 6TH	Qualifier – 7TH
Subcutaneous Tissue and Fascia, ... 0 ... Scalp 1 ... Face 4 ... Right Neck 5 ... Left Neck 6 ... Chest 7 ... Back 8 ... Abdomen 9 ... Buttock B ... Perineum C ... Pelvic Region D ... Right Upper Arm F ... Left Upper Arm G ... Right Lower Arm H ... Left Lower Arm J ... Right Hand K ... Left Hand L ... Right Upper Leg M ... Left Upper Leg N ... Right Lower Leg P ... Left Lower Leg Q ... Right Foot R ... Left Foot	0 Open 3 Percutaneous	Z No device	Z No qualifier

© 2018 Channel Publishing, Ltd.

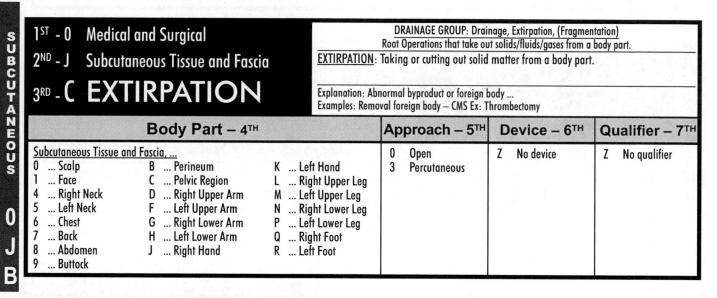

1ST - 0 Medical and Surgical
2ND - J Subcutaneous Tissue and Fascia
3RD - H INSERTION

DEVICE GROUP: Change, Insertion, Removal, Replacement, Revision, Supplement
Root Operations that always involve a device.

INSERTION: Putting in a nonbiological appliance that monitors, assists, performs, or prevents a physiological function but does not physically take the place of a body part.

Explanation: None
Examples: Placement pacemaker generator – CMS Ex: Insertion of central venous catheter

Body Part – 4TH	Approach – 5TH	Device – 6TH	Qualifier – 7TH
Subcutaneous Tissue and Fascia, ... 0 ... Scalp 1 ... Face 4 ... Right Neck 5 ... Left Neck 9 ... Buttock B ... Perineum C ... Pelvic Region J ... Right Hand K ... Left Hand Q ... Right Foot R ... Left Foot	0 Open 3 Percutaneous	N Tissue Expander	Z No qualifier
Subcutaneous Tissue and Fascia, ... 6 ... Chest 8 ... Abdomen	0 Open 3 Percutaneous	0 Monitoring device, hemodynamic 2 Monitoring device 4 Pacemaker, single chamber 5 Pacemaker, single chamber rate responsive 6 Pacemaker, dual chamber 7 Cardiac resynchronization pacemaker pulse generator 8 Defibrillator generator 9 Cardiac resynchronization defibrillator pulse generator A Contractility modulation device B Stimulator generator, single array C Stimulator generator, single array rechargeable D Stimulator generator, multiple array E Stimulator generator, multiple array rechargeable H Contraceptive device M Stimulator generator NC* N Tissue expander P Cardiac rhythm related device V Infusion device, pump W Vascular access device, totally implantable X Vascular access device, tunneled	Z No qualifier
Subcutaneous Tissue and Fascia, ... 7 ... Back	0 Open 3 Percutaneous	B Stimulator generator, single array C Stimulator generator, single array rechargeable D Stimulator generator, multiple array E Stimulator generator, multiple array rechargeable M Stimulator generator NC* N Tissue expander V Infusion device, pump	Z No qualifier
Subcutaneous Tissue and Fascia, ... D ... Right Upper Arm F ... Left Upper Arm G ... Right Lower Arm H ... Left Lower Arm L ... Right Upper Leg M ... Left Upper Leg N ... Right Lower Leg P ... Left Lower Leg	0 Open 3 Percutaneous	H Contraceptive device N Tissue expander V Infusion device, pump W Vascular access device, totally implantable X Vascular access device, tunneled	Z No qualifier
Subcutaneous Tissue and Fascia, ... S ... Head and Neck V ... Upper Extremity W ... Lower Extremity	0 Open 3 Percutaneous	1 Radioactive element 3 Infusion device Y Other device	Z No qualifier
Subcutaneous Tissue and Fascia, ... T ... Trunk	0 Open 3 Percutaneous	1 Radioactive element 3 Infusion device V Infusion device, pump Y Other device	Z No qualifier

NC* – Some procedures are considered non-covered by Medicare. See current Medicare Code Editor for details.

SUBCUTANEOUS 0 J H

© 2018 Channel Publishing, Ltd.

1ST - 0 Medical and Surgical
2ND - J Subcutaneous Tissue and Fascia
3RD - J INSPECTION

EXAMINATION GROUP: Inspection, (Map)
Root Operations involving examination only.

INSPECTION: Visually and/or manually exploring a body part.

Explanation: Direct or instrumental visualization ...
Examples: Exploration abdominal fascia – CMS Ex: Exploratory laparotomy

Body Part – 4TH		Approach – 5TH	Device – 6TH	Qualifier – 7TH
Subcutaneous Tissue and Fascia, ...		0 Open	Z No device	Z No qualifier
S ... Head and Neck	V ... Upper Extremity	3 Percutaneous		
T ... Trunk	W ... Lower Extremity	X External		

1ST - 0 Medical and Surgical
2ND - J Subcutaneous Tissue and Fascia
3RD - N RELEASE

DIVISION GROUP: Division, Release
Root Operations involving cutting or separation only.

RELEASE: Freeing a body part from an abnormal physical constraint by cutting or by the use of force.

Explanation: Some of the restraining tissue may be taken out but none of the body part is taken out
Examples: Lysis fascial adhesions – CMS Ex: Carpal tunnel release

Body Part – 4TH			Approach – 5TH	Device – 6TH	Qualifier – 7TH
Subcutaneous Tissue and Fascia, ...			0 Open	Z No device	Z No qualifier
0 ... Scalp	B ... Perineum	K ... Left Hand	3 Percutaneous		
1 ... Face	C ... Pelvic Region	L ... Right Upper Leg	X External		
4 ... Right Neck	D ... Right Upper Arm	M ... Left Upper Leg			
5 ... Left Neck	F ... Left Upper Arm	N ... Right Lower Leg			
6 ... Chest	G ... Right Lower Arm	P ... Left Lower Leg			
7 ... Back	H ... Left Lower Arm	Q ... Right Foot			
8 ... Abdomen	J ... Right Hand	R ... Left Foot			
9 ... Buttock					

SUBCUTANEOUS 0 J J

© 2018 Channel Publishing, Ltd.

1ST - 0 Medical and Surgical
2ND - J Subcutaneous Tissue and Fascia
3RD - P REMOVAL

DEVICE GROUP: Change, Insertion, Removal, Replacement, Revision, Supplement
Root Operations that always involve a device.

REMOVAL: Taking out or off a device from a body part.

Explanation: Removal device without reinsertion ...
Examples: Removal vascular access device – CMS Ex: Cardiac pacemaker removal

Body Part – 4TH	Approach – 5TH	Device – 6TH	Qualifier – 7TH
Subcutaneous Tissue and Fascia, ... S ... Head and Neck	0 Open 3 Percutaneous	0 Drainage device 1 Radioactive element 3 Infusion device 7 Autologous tissue substitute J Synthetic substitute K Nonautologous tissue substitute N Tissue expander Y Other device	Z No qualifier
Subcutaneous Tissue and Fascia, ... S ... Head and Neck	X External	0 Drainage device 1 Radioactive element 3 Infusion device	Z No qualifier
Subcutaneous Tissue and Fascia, ... T ... Trunk	0 Open 3 Percutaneous	0 Drainage device 1 Radioactive element 2 Monitoring device 3 Infusion device 7 Autologous tissue substitute H Contraceptive device J Synthetic substitute K Nonautologous tissue substitute M Stimulator generator N Tissue expander P Cardiac rhythm related device V Infusion device, pump W Vascular access device, totally implantable X Vascular access device, tunneled Y Other device	Z No qualifier
Subcutaneous Tissue and Fascia, ... T ... Trunk	X External	0 Drainage device 1 Radioactive element 2 Monitoring device 3 Infusion device H Contraceptive device V Infusion device, pump X Vascular access device, tunneled	Z No qualifier
Subcutaneous Tissue and Fascia, ... V ... Upper Extremity W ... Lower Extremity	0 Open 3 Percutaneous	0 Drainage device 1 Radioactive element 3 Infusion device 7 Autologous tissue substitute H Contraceptive device J Synthetic substitute K Nonautologous tissue substitute N Tissue expander V Infusion device, pump W Vascular access device, totally implantable X Vascular access device, tunneled Y Other device	Z No qualifier
Subcutaneous Tissue and Fascia, ... V ... Upper Extremity W ... Lower Extremity	X External	0 Drainage device 1 Radioactive element 3 Infusion device H Contraceptive device V Infusion device, pump X Vascular access device, tunneled	Z No qualifier

© 2018 Channel Publishing, Ltd.

1ST - 0 Medical and Surgical
2ND - J Subcutaneous Tissue and Fascia
3RD - Q REPAIR

OTHER REPAIRS GROUP: (Control), Repair
Root Operations that define other repairs.

REPAIR: Restoring, to the extent possible, a body part to its normal anatomic structure and function.

Explanation: Used only when the method to accomplish the repair is not one of the other root operations
Examples: Rectocele repair with sutures – CMS Ex: Suture of laceration

Body Part – 4TH			Approach – 5TH	Device – 6TH	Qualifier – 7TH
Subcutaneous Tissue and Fascia, ...			0 Open	Z No device	Z No qualifier
0 ... Scalp	B ... Perineum	K ... Left Hand	3 Percutaneous		
1 ... Face	C ... Pelvic Region	L ... Right Upper Leg			
4 ... Right Neck	D ... Right Upper Arm	M ... Left Upper Leg			
5 ... Left Neck	F ... Left Upper Arm	N ... Right Lower Leg			
6 ... Chest	G ... Right Lower Arm	P ... Left Lower Leg			
7 ... Back	H ... Left Lower Arm	Q ... Right Foot			
8 ... Abdomen	J ... Right Hand	R ... Left Foot			
9 ... Buttock					

1ST - 0 Medical and Surgical
2ND - J Subcutaneous Tissue and Fascia
3RD - R REPLACEMENT

DEVICE GROUP: Change, Insertion, Removal, Replacement, Revision, Supplement
Root Operations that always involve a device.

REPLACEMENT: Putting in or on biological or synthetic material that physically takes the place and/or function of all or a portion of a body part.

Explanation: Includes taking out or eradicating, or rendering non-functional, the body part ...
Examples: Free fascia lata graft – CMS Ex: Total hip replacement

Body Part – 4TH			Approach – 5TH	Device – 6TH	Qualifier – 7TH
Subcutaneous Tissue and Fascia, ...			0 Open	7 Autologous tissue substitute	Z No qualifier
0 ... Scalp	B ... Perineum	K ... Left Hand	3 Percutaneous	J Synthetic substitute	
1 ... Face	C ... Pelvic Region	L ... Right Upper Leg		K Nonautologous tissue substitute	
4 ... Right Neck	D ... Right Upper Arm	M ... Left Upper Leg			
5 ... Left Neck	F ... Left Upper Arm	N ... Right Lower Leg			
6 ... Chest	G ... Right Lower Arm	P ... Left Lower Leg			
7 ... Back	H ... Left Lower Arm	Q ... Right Foot			
8 ... Abdomen	J ... Right Hand	R ... Left Foot			
9 ... Buttock					

1ST - 0 Medical and Surgical
2ND - J Subcutaneous Tissue and Fascia
3RD - U SUPPLEMENT

DEVICE GROUP: Change, Insertion, Removal, Replacement, Revision, Supplement
Root Operations that always involve a device.

SUPPLEMENT: Putting in or on biological or synthetic material that physically reinforces and/or augments the function of a portion of a body part.

Explanation: Biological material is non-living, or is living and from the same individual ...
Examples: Rectocele repair with mesh – CMS Ex: Herniorrhaphy using mesh

Body Part – 4TH			Approach – 5TH	Device – 6TH	Qualifier – 7TH
Subcutaneous Tissue and Fascia, ...			0 Open	7 Autologous tissue substitute	Z No qualifier
0 ... Scalp	B ... Perineum	K ... Left Hand	3 Percutaneous	J Synthetic substitute	
1 ... Face	C ... Pelvic Region	L ... Right Upper Leg		K Nonautologous tissue substitute	
4 ... Right Neck	D ... Right Upper Arm	M ... Left Upper Leg			
5 ... Left Neck	F ... Left Upper Arm	N ... Right Lower Leg			
6 ... Chest	G ... Right Lower Arm	P ... Left Lower Leg			
7 ... Back	H ... Left Lower Arm	Q ... Right Foot			
8 ... Abdomen	J ... Right Hand	R ... Left Foot			
9 ... Buttock					

© 2018 Channel Publishing, Ltd.

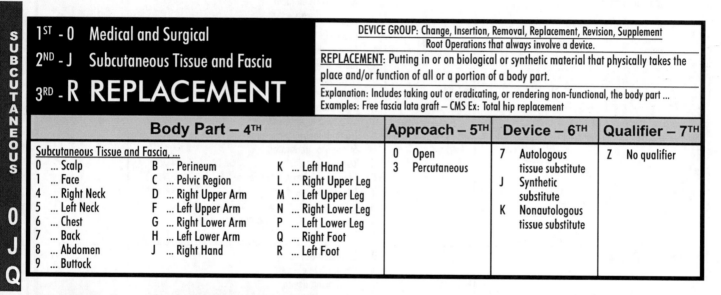

1ST - 0 Medical and Surgical
2ND - J Subcutaneous Tissue and Fascia
3RD - W REVISION

DEVICE GROUP: Change, Insertion, Removal, Replacement, Revision, Supplement
Root Operations that always involve a device.

REVISION: Correcting, to the extent possible, a portion of a malfunctioning device or the position of a displaced device.

Explanation: Correcting by taking out or putting in components of a device such as a screw or pin ...
Examples: Reposition stimulator generator – CMS Ex: Recementing of hip prosthesis

Body Part – 4TH	Approach – 5TH	Device – 6TH	Qualifier – 7TH
Subcutaneous Tissue and Fascia, ... S ... Head and Neck	0 Open 3 Percutaneous	0 Drainage device 3 Infusion device 7 Autologous tissue substitute J Synthetic substitute K Nonautologous tissue substitute N Tissue expander Y Other device	Z No qualifier
Subcutaneous Tissue and Fascia, ... S ... Head and Neck	X External	0 Drainage device 3 Infusion device 7 Autologous tissue substitute J Synthetic substitute K Nonautologous tissue substitute N Tissue expander	Z No qualifier
Subcutaneous Tissue and Fascia, ... T ... Trunk	0 Open 3 Percutaneous	0 Drainage device 2 Monitoring device 3 Infusion device 7 Autologous tissue substitute H Contraceptive device J Synthetic substitute K Nonautologous tissue substitute M Stimulator generator N Tissue expander P Cardiac rhythm related device V Infusion device, pump W Vascular access device, totally implantable X Vascular access device, tunneled Y Other device	Z No qualifier
Subcutaneous Tissue and Fascia, ... T ... Trunk	X External	0 Drainage device 2 Monitoring device 3 Infusion device 7 Autologous tissue substitute H Contraceptive device J Synthetic substitute K Nonautologous tissue substitute M Stimulator generator N Tissue expander P Cardiac rhythm related device V Infusion device, pump W Vascular access device, totally implantable X Vascular access device, tunneled	Z No qualifier
Subcutaneous Tissue and Fascia, ... V ... Upper Extremity W ... Lower Extremity	0 Open 3 Percutaneous	0 Drainage device 3 Infusion device 7 Autologous tissue substitute H Contraceptive device J Synthetic substitute K Nonautologous tissue substitute N Tissue expander V Infusion device, pump W Vascular access device, totally implantable X Vascular access device, tunneled Y Other device	Z No qualifier
Subcutaneous Tissue and Fascia, ... V ... Upper Extremity W ... Lower Extremity	X External	0 Drainage device 3 Infusion device 7 Autologous tissue substitute H Contraceptive device J Synthetic substitute K Nonautologous tissue substitute N Tissue expander V Infusion device, pump W Vascular access device, totally implantable X Vascular access device, tunneled	Z No qualifier

© 2018 Channel Publishing, Ltd.

1ST - 0 Medical and Surgical
2ND - J Subcutaneous Tissue and Fascia
3RD - X TRANSFER

MOVE GROUP: (Reattachment), (Reposition), Transfer, (Transplantation)
Root Operations that put in/put back or move some/all of a body part.

TRANSFER: Moving, without taking out, all or a portion of a body part to another location to take over the function of all or a portion of a body part.

Explanation: The body part transferred remains connected to its vascular and nervous supply
Examples: Fasciocutaneous pedicle flap graft – CMS Ex: Tendon transfer

Body Part – 4TH	Approach – 5TH	Device – 6TH	Qualifier – 7TH
Subcutaneous Tissue and Fascia, ... 0 ... Scalp 1 ... Face 4 ... Right Neck 5 ... Left Neck 6 ... Chest 7 ... Back 8 ... Abdomen 9 ... Buttock B ... Perineum C ... Pelvic Region D ... Right Upper Arm F ... Left Upper Arm G ... Right Lower Arm H ... Left Lower Arm J ... Right Hand K ... Left Hand L ... Right Upper Leg M ... Left Upper Leg N ... Right Lower Leg P ... Left Lower Leg Q ... Right Foot R ... Left Foot	0 Open 3 Percutaneous	Z No device	B Skin and Subcutaneous Tissue C Skin, Subcutaneous Tissue and Fascia Z No qualifier

© 2018 Channel Publishing, Ltd.

Educational Annotations | K – Muscles

Body System Specific Educational Annotations for the Muscles include:

- Anatomy and Physiology Review
- Anatomical Illustrations
- Definitions of Common Procedures
- AHA Coding Clinic® Reference Notations
- Body Part Key Listings
- Device Key Listings
- Device Aggregation Table Listings
- Coding Notes

Anatomy and Physiology Review of Muscles

BODY PART VALUES – K - MUSCLES

Lower Muscle – The muscles located below the diaphragm (see Coding Guideline B2.1b).
Muscle – ANATOMY – Muscles are groups of skeletal muscle tissue, blood vessels, and nerves that are attached to the skeletal bones. Cardiac and smooth muscle tissue is also found in the heart and other organs. PHYSIOLOGY – The muscles contract to allow the movement of the human body.
Upper Muscle – The muscles located above the diaphragm (see Coding Guideline B2.1b).

Anatomical Illustrations of Muscles

None for the Muscles Body System

Definitions of Common Procedures of Muscles

Muscle transfer – The surgical detachment of the distal end of a muscle and subsequent connection to another nearby site while maintaining its vascular and nervous supply.
Muscle transplant – The surgical removal of a muscle with transplantation to a different site and, through microsurgery, connected to blood vessels and a nerve.
TRAM (transverse rectus abdominis myocutaneous) flap breast reconstruction – The post-mastectomy reconstruction of the breast using the transverse rectus abdominis muscle that is raised (including the overlying fat and skin) and transferred to the mastectomy site.

MUSCLES 0K

AHA Coding Clinic® Reference Notations of Muscles

ROOT OPERATION SPECIFIC - K - MUSCLES

CHANGE - 2
DESTRUCTION - 5
DIVISION - 8
DRAINAGE - 9
EXCISION - B
Debridement of sacral decubitus ulcer including muscle ....AHA 16:3Q:p20
EXTIRPATION - C
EXTRACTION - D
Jet lavage removal of necrotic muscle tissue ....AHA 17:4Q:p42
INSERTION - H
INSPECTION - J
REATTACHMENT - M
RELEASE - N
Biceps tenotomy............................AHA 15:2Q:p22
Fasciotomy for compartment syndrome, foot, multiple sites............................AHA 17:2Q:p12,13
Repair of incisional hernia with component release and mesh............................AHA 14:4Q:p39
REMOVAL - P
REPAIR - Q
Repair of second degree perineal laceration ....AHA 14:4Q:p43
............................AHA 16:1Q:p6-8
Repair of second degree perineal laceration including muscle............................AHA 13:4Q:p120
Repair perineum muscle............................AHA 16:2Q:p34
REPOSITION - S
RESECTION - T
Infratemporal fossa malignancy with neck muscle............................AHA 16:2Q:p12
Resection of perineum muscle ....AHA 15:1Q:p38
SUPPLEMENT - U
REVISION - W

Continued on next page

© 2018 Channel Publishing, Ltd.

Educational Annotations | K – Muscles

AHA Coding Clinic® Reference Notations of Muscles

Continued from previous page

TRANSFER - X

- Cleft lip repair, Millard technique ....AHA 15:3Q:p33
- Ipsilateral pedicle transverse abdominomyocutaneous (TRAM) flap breast reconstruction ....AHA 14:2Q:p10
- Pedicle latissimus myocutaneous flap ....AHA 17:4Q:p67
- Pedicle latissimus myocutaneous flap breast reconstruction ....AHA 14:2Q:p12
- Perineal myocutaneous flap closure of abdominoperineal resection ....AHA 14:4Q:p41
- Posterior pharyngeal flap to the soft palate ....AHA 15:2Q:p26

Body Part Key Listings of Muscles

See also Body Part Key in Appendix C

Abductor hallucis muscle ....use Foot Muscle, Left/Right
Adductor brevis muscle ....use Upper Leg Muscle, Left/Right
Adductor hallucis muscle ....use Foot Muscle, Left/Right
Adductor longus muscle ....use Upper Leg Muscle, Left/Right
Adductor magnus muscle ....use Upper Leg Muscle, Left/Right
Anatomical snuffbox ....use Lower Arm and Wrist Muscle, Left/Right
Anterior vertebral muscle ....use Neck Muscle, Left/Right
Arytenoid muscle ....use Neck Muscle, Left/Right
Auricularis muscle ....use Head Muscle
Biceps brachii muscle ....use Upper Arm Muscle, Left/Right
Biceps femoris muscle ....use Upper Leg Muscle, Left/Right
Brachialis muscle ....use Upper Arm Muscle, Left/Right
Brachioradialis muscle ....use Lower Arm and Wrist Muscle, Left/Right
Buccinator muscle ....use Facial Muscle
Bulbospongiosus muscle ....use Perineum Muscle
Chondroglossus muscle ....use Tongue, Palate, Pharynx Muscle
Coccygeus muscle ....use Trunk Muscle, Left/Right
Coracobrachialis muscle ....use Upper Arm Muscle, Left/Right
Corrugator supercilii muscle ....use Facial Muscle
Cremaster muscle ....use Perineum Muscle
Cricothyroid muscle ....use Neck Muscle, Left/Right
Deep transverse perineal muscle ....use Perineum Muscle
Deltoid muscle ....use Shoulder Muscle, Left/Right
Depressor anguli oris muscle ....use Facial Muscle
Depressor labii inferioris muscle ....use Facial Muscle
Depressor septi nasi muscle ....use Facial Muscle
Depressor supercilii muscle ....use Facial Muscle
Erector spinae muscle ....use Trunk Muscle, Left/Right
Extensor carpi radialis muscle ....use Lower Arm and Wrist Muscle, Left/Right
Extensor carpi ulnaris muscle ....use Lower Arm and Wrist Muscle, Left/Right
Extensor digitorum brevis muscle ....use Foot Muscle, Left/Right
Extensor digitorum longus muscle ....use Lower Leg Muscle, Left/Right
Extensor hallucis brevis muscle ....use Foot Muscle, Left/Right
Extensor hallucis longus muscle ....use Lower Leg Muscle, Left/Right
External oblique muscle ....use Abdomen Muscle, Left/Right
Fibularis brevis muscle ....use Lower Leg Muscle, Left/Right
Fibularis longus muscle ....use Lower Leg Muscle, Left/Right
Flexor carpi radialis muscle ....use Lower Arm and Wrist Muscle, Left/Right
Flexor carpi ulnaris muscle ....use Lower Arm and Wrist Muscle, Left/Right
Flexor digitorum brevis muscle ....use Foot Muscle, Left/Right
Flexor digitorum longus muscle ....use Lower Leg Muscle, Left/Right
Flexor hallucis brevis muscle ....use Foot Muscle, Left/Right
Flexor hallucis longus muscle ....use Lower Leg Muscle, Left/Right
Flexor pollicis longus muscle ....use Lower Arm and Wrist Muscle, Left/Right
Gastrocnemius muscle ....use Lower Leg Muscle, Left/Right
Gemellus muscle ....use Hip Muscle, Left/Right
Genioglossus muscle ....use Tongue, Palate, Pharynx Muscle
Gluteus maximus muscle ....use Hip Muscle, Left/Right
Gluteus medius muscle ....use Hip Muscle, Left/Right
Gluteus minimus muscle ....use Hip Muscle, Left/Right
Gracilis muscle ....use Upper Leg Muscle, Left/Right
Hyoglossus muscle ....use Tongue, Palate, Pharynx Muscle
Hypothenar muscle ....use Hand Muscle, Left/Right
Iliacus muscle ....use Hip Muscle, Left/Right
Inferior longitudinal muscle ....use Tongue, Palate, Pharynx Muscle
Infrahyoid muscle ....use Neck Muscle, Left/Right
Infraspinatus muscle ....use Shoulder Muscle, Left/Right
Intercostal muscle ....use Thorax Muscle, Left/Right
Internal oblique muscle ....use Abdomen Muscle, Left/Right
Interspinalis muscle ....use Trunk Muscle, Left/Right
Intertransversarius muscle ....use Trunk Muscle, Left/Right
Ischiocavernosus muscle ....use Perineum Muscle
Latissimus dorsi muscle ....use Trunk Muscle, Left/Right
Levator anguli oris muscle ....use Facial Muscle
Levator ani muscle ....use Perineum Muscle
Levator labii superioris alaeque nasi muscle ....use Facial Muscle
Levator labii superioris muscle ....use Facial Muscle
Levator scapulae muscle ....use Neck Muscle, Left/Right
Levator veli palatini muscle ....use Tongue, Palate, Pharynx Muscle
Levatores costarum muscle ....use Thorax Muscle, Left/Right
Masseter muscle ....use Head Muscle
Mentalis muscle ....use Facial Muscle
Nasalis muscle ....use Facial Muscle
Obturator muscle ....use Hip Muscle, Left/Right
Occipitofrontalis muscle ....use Facial Muscle
Orbicularis oris muscle ....use Facial Muscle
Palatoglossal muscle ....use Tongue, Palate, Pharynx Muscle
Palatopharyngeal muscle ....use Tongue, Palate, Pharynx Muscle
Palmar interosseous muscle ....use Hand Muscle, Left/Right
Palmaris longus muscle ....use Lower Arm and Wrist Muscle, Left/Right
Pectineus muscle ....use Upper Leg Muscle, Left/Right
Pectoralis major muscle ....use Thorax Muscle, Left/Right
Pectoralis minor muscle ....use Thorax Muscle, Left/Right
Peroneus brevis muscle ....use Lower Leg Muscle, Left/Right
Peroneus longus muscle ....use Lower Leg Muscle, Left/Right
Pharyngeal constrictor muscle ....use Tongue, Palate, Pharynx Muscle
Piriformis muscle ....use Hip Muscle, Left/Right
Platysma muscle ....use Neck Muscle, Left/Right
Popliteus muscle ....use Lower Leg Muscle, Left/Right
Procerus muscle ....use Facial Muscle
Pronator quadratus muscle ....use Lower Arm and Wrist Muscle, Left/Right
Pronator teres muscle ....use Lower Arm and Wrist Muscle, Left/Right
Psoas muscle ....use Hip Muscle, Left/Right
Pterygoid muscle ....use Head Muscle

Continued on next page

© 2018 Channel Publishing, Ltd.

Educational Annotations | K – Muscles

Body Part Key Listings of Muscles

Continued from previous page

Pyramidalis muscle	use Abdomen Muscle, Left/Right
Quadratus femoris muscle	use Hip Muscle, Left/Right
Quadratus lumborum muscle	use Trunk Muscle, Left/Right
Quadratus plantae muscle	use Foot Muscle, Left/Right
Quadriceps (femoris)	use Upper Leg Muscle, Left/Right
Rectus abdominis muscle	use Abdomen Muscle, Left/Right
Rectus femoris muscle	use Upper Leg Muscle, Left/Right
Rhomboid major muscle	use Trunk Muscle, Left/Right
Rhomboid minor muscle	use Trunk Muscle, Left/Right
Risorius muscle	use Facial Muscle
Salpingopharyngeus muscle	use Tongue, Palate, Pharynx Muscle
Sartorius muscle	use Upper Leg Muscle, Left/Right
Scalene muscle	use Neck Muscle, Left/Right
Semimembranosus muscle	use Upper Leg Muscle, Left/Right
Semitendinosus muscle	use Upper Leg Muscle, Left/Right
Serratus anterior muscle	use Thorax Muscle, Left/Right
Serratus posterior muscle	use Trunk Muscle, Left/Right
Soleus muscle	use Lower Leg Muscle, Left/Right
Splenius capitis muscle	use Head Muscle
Splenius cervicis muscle	use Neck Muscle, Left/Right
Sternocleidomastoid muscle	use Neck Muscle, Left/Right
Styloglossus muscle	use Tongue, Palate, Pharynx Muscle
Stylopharyngeus muscle	use Tongue, Palate, Pharynx Muscle
Subclavius muscle	use Thorax Muscle, Left/Right
Subcostal muscle	use Thorax Muscle, Left/Right
Subscapularis muscle	use Shoulder Muscle, Left/Right
Superficial transverse perineal muscle	use Perineum Muscle
Superior longitudinal muscle	use Tongue, Palate, Pharynx Muscle
Suprahyoid muscle	use Neck Muscle, Left/Right
Supraspinatus muscle	use Shoulder Muscle, Left/Right
Temporalis muscle	use Head Muscle
Temporoparietalis muscle	use Head Muscle
Tensor fasciae latae muscle	use Hip Muscle, Left/Right
Tensor veli palatini muscle	use Tongue, Palate, Pharynx Muscle
Teres major muscle	use Shoulder Muscle, Left/Right
Teres minor muscle	use Shoulder Muscle, Left/Right
Thenar muscle	use Hand Muscle, Left/Right
Thyroarytenoid muscle	use Neck Muscle, Left/Right
Tibialis anterior muscle	use Lower Leg Muscle, Left/Right
Tibialis posterior muscle	use Lower Leg Muscle, Left/Right
Transverse thoracis muscle	use Thorax Muscle, Left/Right
Transversospinalis muscle	use Trunk Muscle, Left/Right
Transversus abdominis muscle	use Abdomen Muscle, Left/Right
Trapezius muscle	use Trunk Muscle, Left/Right
Triceps brachii muscle	use Upper Arm Muscle, Left/Right
Vastus intermedius muscle	use Upper Leg Muscle, Left/Right
Vastus lateralis muscle	use Upper Leg Muscle, Left/Right
Vastus medialis muscle	use Upper Leg Muscle, Left/Right
Zygomaticus muscle	use Facial Muscle

Device Key Listings of Muscles

See also Device Key in Appendix D

Autograft	use Autologous Tissue Substitute
Electrical muscle stimulation (EMS) lead	use Stimulator Lead in Muscles
Electronic muscle stimulator lead	use Stimulator Lead in Muscles
Neuromuscular electrical stimulation (NEMS) lead	use Stimulator Lead in Muscles
Tissue bank graft	use Nonautologous Tissue Substitute

Device Aggregation Table Listings of Muscles

See also Device Aggregation Table in Appendix E

Specific Device	For Operation	In Body System	General Device
None Listed in Device Aggregation Table for this Body System			

Coding Notes of Muscles

Body System Relevant Coding Guidelines

General Guidelines

B2.1b

Where the general body part values "upper" and "lower" are provided as an option in the Upper Arteries, Lower Arteries, Upper Veins, Lower Veins, Muscles and Tendons body systems, "upper" or "lower "specifies body parts located above or below the diaphragm respectively.

Example: Vein body parts above the diaphragm are found in the Upper Veins body system; vein body parts below the diaphragm are found in the Lower Veins body system.

Transfer procedures using multiple tissue layers

B3.17

The root operation Transfer contains qualifiers that can be used to specify when a transfer flap is composed of more than one tissue layer, such as a musculocutaneous flap. For procedures involving transfer of multiple tissue layers including skin, subcutaneous tissue, fascia or muscle, the procedure is coded to the body part value that describes the deepest tissue layer in the flap, and the qualifier can be used to describe the other tissue layer(s) in the transfer flap.

Example: A musculocutaneous flap transfer is coded to the appropriate body part value in the body system Muscles, and the qualifier is used to describe the additional tissue layer(s) in the transfer flap.

MUSCLES 0K

© 2018 Channel Publishing, Ltd.

1ST - 0 Medical and Surgical
2ND - K Muscles
3RD - 2 CHANGE

DEVICE GROUP: Change, Insertion, Removal, Replacement, Revision, Supplement
Root Operations that always involve a device.

CHANGE: Taking out or off a device from a body part and putting back an identical or similar device in or on the same body part without cutting or puncturing the skin or a mucous membrane.

Explanation: All CHANGE procedures are coded using the approach External
Examples: Exchange drain tube – CMS Ex: Urinary catheter change

Body Part – 4TH	Approach – 5TH	Device – 6TH	Qualifier – 7TH
X Upper Muscle Y Lower Muscle	X External	0 Drainage device Y Other device	Z No qualifier

1ST - 0 Medical and Surgical
2ND - K Muscles
3RD - 5 DESTRUCTION

EXCISION GROUP: Excision, Resection, Destruction, Extraction, (Detachment)
Root Operations that take out some or all of a body part.

DESTRUCTION: Physical eradication of all or a portion of a body part by the direct use of energy, force, or a destructive agent.

Explanation: None of the body part is physically taken out
Examples: Radiofrequency ablation – CMS Ex: Fulguration of rectal polyp

Body Part – 4TH			Approach – 5TH	Device – 6TH	Qualifier–7TH
0 Head Muscle 1 Facial Muscle 2 Neck Muscle, Right 3 Neck Muscle, Left 4 Tongue, Palate, Pharynx Muscle 5 Shoulder Muscle, Right 6 Shoulder Muscle, Left 7 Upper Arm Muscle, Right 8 Upper Arm Muscle, Left	9 Lower Arm and Wrist Muscle, Right B Lower Arm and Wrist Muscle, Left C Hand Muscle, Right D Hand Muscle, Left F Trunk Muscle, Right G Trunk Muscle, Left H Thorax Muscle, Right J Thorax Muscle, Left	K Abdomen Muscle, Right L Abdomen Muscle, Left M Perineum Muscle N Hip Muscle, Right P Hip Muscle, Left Q Upper Leg Muscle, Right R Upper Leg Muscle, Left S Lower Leg Muscle, Right T Lower Leg Muscle, Left V Foot Muscle, Right W Foot Muscle, Left	0 Open 3 Percutaneous 4 Percutaneous endoscopic	Z No device	Z No qualifier

1ST - 0 Medical and Surgical
2ND - K Muscles
3RD - 8 DIVISION

DIVISION GROUP: Division, Release
Root Operations involving cutting or separation only.

DIVISION: Cutting into a body part, without draining fluids and/or gases from the body part, in order to separate or transect a body part.

Explanation: All or a portion of the body part is separated into two or more portions
Examples: Myotomy hand muscle – CMS Ex: Spinal cordotomy

Body Part – 4TH			Approach – 5TH	Device – 6TH	Qualifier–7TH
0 Head Muscle 1 Facial Muscle 2 Neck Muscle, Right 3 Neck Muscle, Left 4 Tongue, Palate, Pharynx Muscle 5 Shoulder Muscle, Right 6 Shoulder Muscle, Left 7 Upper Arm Muscle, Right 8 Upper Arm Muscle, Left	9 Lower Arm and Wrist Muscle, Right B Lower Arm and Wrist Muscle, Left C Hand Muscle, Right D Hand Muscle, Left F Trunk Muscle, Right G Trunk Muscle, Left H Thorax Muscle, Right J Thorax Muscle, Left	K Abdomen Muscle, Right L Abdomen Muscle, Left M Perineum Muscle N Hip Muscle, Right P Hip Muscle, Left Q Upper Leg Muscle, Right R Upper Leg Muscle, Left S Lower Leg Muscle, Right T Lower Leg Muscle, Left V Foot Muscle, Right W Foot Muscle, Left	0 Open 3 Percutaneous 4 Percutaneous endoscopic	Z No device	Z No qualifier

© 2018 Channel Publishing, Ltd.

1ST - 0 Medical and Surgical
2ND - K Muscles
3RD - 9 DRAINAGE

DRAINAGE GROUP: Drainage, Extirpation, (Fragmentation)
Root Operations that take out solids/fluids/gases from a body part.

DRAINAGE: Taking or letting out fluids and/or gases from a body part.

Explanation: Qualifier "X Diagnostic" indicates drainage procedures that are biopsies
Examples: Aspiration psoas muscle abscess – CMS Ex: Thoracentesis

Body Part – 4TH	Approach – 5TH	Device – 6TH	Qualifier–7TH
0 Head Muscle 1 Facial Muscle 2 Neck Muscle, Right 3 Neck Muscle, Left 4 Tongue, Palate, Pharynx Muscle 5 Shoulder Muscle, Right 6 Shoulder Muscle, Left 7 Upper Arm Muscle, Right 8 Upper Arm Muscle, Left 9 Lower Arm and Wrist Muscle, Right B Lower Arm and Wrist Muscle, Left C Hand Muscle, Right D Hand Muscle, Left F Trunk Muscle, Right G Trunk Muscle, Left H Thorax Muscle, Right J Thorax Muscle, Left K Abdomen Muscle, Right L Abdomen Muscle, Left M Perineum Muscle N Hip Muscle, Right P Hip Muscle, Left Q Upper Leg Muscle, Right R Upper Leg Muscle, Left S Lower Leg Muscle, Right T Lower Leg Muscle, Left V Foot Muscle, Right W Foot Muscle, Left	0 Open 3 Percutaneous 4 Percutaneous endoscopic	0 Drainage device	Z No qualifier
0 Head Muscle 1 Facial Muscle 2 Neck Muscle, Right 3 Neck Muscle, Left 4 Tongue, Palate, Pharynx Muscle 5 Shoulder Muscle, Right 6 Shoulder Muscle, Left 7 Upper Arm Muscle, Right 8 Upper Arm Muscle, Left 9 Lower Arm and Wrist Muscle, Right B Lower Arm and Wrist Muscle, Left C Hand Muscle, Right D Hand Muscle, Left F Trunk Muscle, Right G Trunk Muscle, Left H Thorax Muscle, Right J Thorax Muscle, Left K Abdomen Muscle, Right L Abdomen Muscle, Left M Perineum Muscle N Hip Muscle, Right P Hip Muscle, Left Q Upper Leg Muscle, Right R Upper Leg Muscle, Left S Lower Leg Muscle, Right T Lower Leg Muscle, Left V Foot Muscle, Right W Foot Muscle, Left	0 Open 3 Percutaneous 4 Percutaneous endoscopic	Z No device	X Diagnostic Z No qualifier

1ST - 0 Medical and Surgical
2ND - K Muscles
3RD - B EXCISION

EXCISION GROUP: Excision, Resection, Destruction, Extraction, (Detachment)
Root Operations that take out some or all of a body part.

EXCISION: Cutting out or off, without replacement, a portion of a body part.

Explanation: Qualifier "X Diagnostic" indicates excision procedures that are biopsies
Examples: Muscle biopsy – CMS Ex: Liver biopsy

Body Part – 4TH	Approach – 5TH	Device – 6TH	Qualifier–7TH
0 Head Muscle 1 Facial Muscle 2 Neck Muscle, Right 3 Neck Muscle, Left 4 Tongue, Palate, Pharynx Muscle 5 Shoulder Muscle, Right 6 Shoulder Muscle, Left 7 Upper Arm Muscle, Right 8 Upper Arm Muscle, Left 9 Lower Arm and Wrist Muscle, Right B Lower Arm and Wrist Muscle, Left C Hand Muscle, Right D Hand Muscle, Left F Trunk Muscle, Right G Trunk Muscle, Left H Thorax Muscle, Right J Thorax Muscle, Left K Abdomen Muscle, Right L Abdomen Muscle, Left M Perineum Muscle N Hip Muscle, Right P Hip Muscle, Left Q Upper Leg Muscle, Right R Upper Leg Muscle, Left S Lower Leg Muscle, Right T Lower Leg Muscle, Left V Foot Muscle, Right W Foot Muscle, Left	0 Open 3 Percutaneous 4 Percutaneous endoscopic	Z No device	X Diagnostic Z No qualifier

© 2018 Channel Publishing, Ltd.

1ST - 0 Medical and Surgical
2ND - K Muscles
3RD - C EXTIRPATION

DRAINAGE GROUP: Drainage, Extirpation, (Fragmentation)
Root Operations that take out solids/fluids/gases from a body part.

EXTIRPATION: Taking or cutting out solid matter from a body part.

Explanation: Abnormal byproduct or foreign body ...
Examples: Removal foreign body – CMS Ex: Thrombectomy

Body Part – 4TH			Approach – 5TH	Device – 6TH	Qualifier–7TH
0 Head Muscle 1 Facial Muscle 2 Neck Muscle, Right 3 Neck Muscle, Left 4 Tongue, Palate, Pharynx Muscle 5 Shoulder Muscle, Right 6 Shoulder Muscle, Left 7 Upper Arm Muscle, Right 8 Upper Arm Muscle, Left	9 Lower Arm and Wrist Muscle, Right B Lower Arm and Wrist Muscle, Left C Hand Muscle, Right D Hand Muscle, Left F Trunk Muscle, Right G Trunk Muscle, Left H Thorax Muscle, Right J Thorax Muscle, Left	K Abdomen Muscle, Right L Abdomen Muscle, Left M Perineum Muscle N Hip Muscle, Right P Hip Muscle, Left Q Upper Leg Muscle, Right R Upper Leg Muscle, Left S Lower Leg Muscle, Right T Lower Leg Muscle, Left V Foot Muscle, Right W Foot Muscle, Left	0 Open 3 Percutaneous 4 Percutaneous endoscopic	Z No device	Z No qualifier

1ST - 0 Medical and Surgical
2ND - K Muscles
3RD - D EXTRACTION

EXCISION GROUP: Excision, Resection, Destruction, Extraction, (Detachment)
Root Operations that take out some or all of a body part.

EXTRACTION: Pulling or stripping out or off all or a portion of a body part by the use of force.

Explanation: None for this Body System
Examples: Non-excisional debridement – CMS Ex: Dilation and curettage

Body Part – 4TH			Approach – 5TH	Device – 6TH	Qualifier–7TH
0 Head Muscle 1 Facial Muscle 2 Neck Muscle, Right 3 Neck Muscle, Left 4 Tongue, Palate, Pharynx Muscle 5 Shoulder Muscle, Right 6 Shoulder Muscle, Left 7 Upper Arm Muscle, Right 8 Upper Arm Muscle, Left	9 Lower Arm and Wrist Muscle, Right B Lower Arm and Wrist Muscle, Left C Hand Muscle, Right D Hand Muscle, Left F Trunk Muscle, Right G Trunk Muscle, Left H Thorax Muscle, Right J Thorax Muscle, Left	K Abdomen Muscle, Right L Abdomen Muscle, Left M Perineum Muscle N Hip Muscle, Right P Hip Muscle, Left Q Upper Leg Muscle, Right R Upper Leg Muscle, Left S Lower Leg Muscle, Right T Lower Leg Muscle, Left V Foot Muscle, Right W Foot Muscle, Left	0 Open	Z No device	Z No qualifier

1ST - 0 Medical and Surgical
2ND - K Muscles
3RD - H INSERTION

DEVICE GROUP: Change, Insertion, Removal, Replacement, Revision, Supplement
Root Operations that always involve a device.

INSERTION: Putting in a nonbiological appliance that monitors, assists, performs, or prevents a physiological function but does not physically take the place of a body part.

Explanation: None
Examples: Insertion stimulator lead – CMS Ex: Insertion of central venous catheter

Body Part – 4TH	Approach – 5TH	Device – 6TH	Qualifier – 7TH
X Upper Muscle Y Lower Muscle	0 Open 3 Percutaneous 4 Percutaneous endoscopic	M Stimulator lead Y Other device	Z No qualifier

© 2018 Channel Publishing, Ltd.

1ST - 0 Medical and Surgical
2ND - K Muscles
3RD - J INSPECTION

EXAMINATION GROUP: Inspection, (Map)
Root Operations involving examination only.

INSPECTION: Visually and/or manually exploring a body part.

Explanation: Direct or instrumental visualization ...
Examples: Examination pelvic floor muscle – CMS Ex: Exploratory laparotomy

Body Part – 4TH	Approach – 5TH	Device – 6TH	Qualifier – 7TH
X Upper Muscle Y Lower Muscle	0 Open 3 Percutaneous 4 Percutaneous endoscopic X External	Z No device	Z No qualifier

1ST - 0 Medical and Surgical
2ND - K Muscles
3RD - M REATTACHMENT

MOVE GROUP: Reattachment, Reposition, Transfer, (Transplantation)
Root Operations that put in/put back or move some/all of a body part.

REATTACHMENT: Putting back in or on all or a portion of a separated body part to its normal location or other suitable location.

Explanation: Vascular circulation and nervous pathways may or may not be reestablished
Examples: Reattachment biceps muscle – CMS Ex: Reattachment of hand

Body Part – 4TH			Approach – 5TH	Device – 6TH	Qualifier–7TH
0 Head Muscle 1 Facial Muscle 2 Neck Muscle, Right 3 Neck Muscle, Left 4 Tongue, Palate, Pharynx Muscle 5 Shoulder Muscle, Right 6 Shoulder Muscle, Left 7 Upper Arm Muscle, Right 8 Upper Arm Muscle, Left	9 Lower Arm and Wrist Muscle, Right B Lower Arm and Wrist Muscle, Left C Hand Muscle, Right D Hand Muscle, Left F Trunk Muscle, Right G Trunk Muscle, Left H Thorax Muscle, Right J Thorax Muscle, Left	K Abdomen Muscle, Right L Abdomen Muscle, Left M Perineum Muscle N Hip Muscle, Right P Hip Muscle, Left Q Upper Leg Muscle, Right R Upper Leg Muscle, Left S Lower Leg Muscle, Right T Lower Leg Muscle, Left V Foot Muscle, Right W Foot Muscle, Left	0 Open 4 Percutaneous endoscopic	Z No device	Z No qualifier

1ST - 0 Medical and Surgical
2ND - K Muscles
3RD - N RELEASE

DIVISION GROUP: Division, Release
Root Operations involving cutting or separation only.

RELEASE: Freeing a body part from an abnormal physical constraint by cutting or by the use of force.

Explanation: Some of the restraining tissue may be taken out but none of the body part is taken out
Examples: Component muscle separation – CMS Ex: Carpal tunnel release

Body Part – 4TH			Approach – 5TH	Device – 6TH	Qualifier–7TH
0 Head Muscle 1 Facial Muscle 2 Neck Muscle, Right 3 Neck Muscle, Left 4 Tongue, Palate, Pharynx Muscle 5 Shoulder Muscle, Right 6 Shoulder Muscle, Left 7 Upper Arm Muscle, Right 8 Upper Arm Muscle, Left	9 Lower Arm and Wrist Muscle, Right B Lower Arm and Wrist Muscle, Left C Hand Muscle, Right D Hand Muscle, Left F Trunk Muscle, Right G Trunk Muscle, Left H Thorax Muscle, Right J Thorax Muscle, Left	K Abdomen Muscle, Right L Abdomen Muscle, Left M Perineum Muscle N Hip Muscle, Right P Hip Muscle, Left Q Upper Leg Muscle, Right R Upper Leg Muscle, Left S Lower Leg Muscle, Right T Lower Leg Muscle, Left V Foot Muscle, Right W Foot Muscle, Left	0 Open 3 Percutaneous 4 Percutaneous endoscopic X External	Z No device	Z No qualifier

© 2018 Channel Publishing, Ltd.

1ST - 0 Medical and Surgical
2ND - K Muscles
3RD - P REMOVAL

DEVICE GROUP: Change, Insertion, Removal, Replacement, Revision, Supplement
Root Operations that always involve a device.

REMOVAL: Taking out or off a device from a body part.

Explanation: Removal device without reinsertion ...
Examples: Removal stimulator lead – CMS Ex: Cardiac pacemaker removal

Body Part – 4TH	Approach – 5TH	Device – 6TH	Qualifier – 7TH
X Upper Muscle Y Lower Muscle	0 Open 3 Percutaneous 4 Percutaneous endoscopic	0 Drainage device 7 Autologous tissue substitute J Synthetic substitute K Nonautologous tissue substitute M Stimulator lead Y Other device	Z No qualifier
X Upper Muscle Y Lower Muscle	X External	0 Drainage device M Stimulator lead	Z No qualifier

1ST - 0 Medical and Surgical
2ND - K Muscles
3RD - Q REPAIR

OTHER REPAIRS GROUP: (Control), Repair
Root Operations that define other repairs.

REPAIR: Restoring, to the extent possible, a body part to its normal anatomic structure and function.

Explanation: Used only when the method to accomplish the repair is not one of the other root operations
Examples: Repair second degree laceration perineum muscle – CMS Ex: Suture of laceration

Body Part – 4TH			Approach – 5TH	Device – 6TH	Qualifier–7TH
0 Head Muscle 1 Facial Muscle 2 Neck Muscle, Right 3 Neck Muscle, Left 4 Tongue, Palate, Pharynx Muscle 5 Shoulder Muscle, Right 6 Shoulder Muscle, Left 7 Upper Arm Muscle, Right 8 Upper Arm Muscle, Left	9 Lower Arm and Wrist Muscle, Right B Lower Arm and Wrist Muscle, Left C Hand Muscle, Right D Hand Muscle, Left F Trunk Muscle, Right G Trunk Muscle, Left H Thorax Muscle, Right J Thorax Muscle, Left	K Abdomen Muscle, Right L Abdomen Muscle, Left M Perineum Muscle N Hip Muscle, Right P Hip Muscle, Left Q Upper Leg Muscle, Right R Upper Leg Muscle, Left S Lower Leg Muscle, Right T Lower Leg Muscle, Left V Foot Muscle, Right W Foot Muscle, Left	0 Open 3 Percutaneous 4 Percutaneous endoscopic	Z No device	Z No qualifier

1ST - 0 Medical and Surgical
2ND - K Muscles
3RD - R REPLACEMENT

DEVICE GROUP: Change, Insertion, Removal, Replacement, Revision, Supplement
Root Operations that always involve a device.

REPLACEMENT: Putting in or on biological or synthetic material that physically takes the place and/or function of all or a portion of a body part.

Explanation: Includes taking out or eradicating, or rendering non-functional, the body part ...
Examples: Foot muscle replacement – CMS Ex: Total hip replacement

Body Part – 4TH			Approach – 5TH	Device – 6TH	Qualifier–7TH
0 Head Muscle 1 Facial Muscle 2 Neck Muscle, Right 3 Neck Muscle, Left 4 Tongue, Palate, Pharynx Muscle 5 Shoulder Muscle, Right 6 Shoulder Muscle, Left 7 Upper Arm Muscle, Right 8 Upper Arm Muscle, Left	9 Lower Arm and Wrist Muscle, Right B Lower Arm and Wrist Muscle, Left C Hand Muscle, Right D Hand Muscle, Left F Trunk Muscle, Right G Trunk Muscle, Left H Thorax Muscle, Right J Thorax Muscle, Left	K Abdomen Muscle, Right L Abdomen Muscle, Left M Perineum Muscle N Hip Muscle, Right P Hip Muscle, Left Q Upper Leg Muscle, Right R Upper Leg Muscle, Left S Lower Leg Muscle, Right T Lower Leg Muscle, Left V Foot Muscle, Right W Foot Muscle, Left	0 Open 4 Percutaneous endoscopic	7 Autologous tissue substitute J Synthetic substitute K Nonautologous tissue substitute	Z No qualifier

© 2018 Channel Publishing, Ltd.

1ST - 0 Medical and Surgical
2ND - K Muscles
3RD - S REPOSITION

MOVE GROUP: Reattachment, Reposition, Transfer, (Transplantation)
Root Operations that put in/put back or move some/all of a body part.

REPOSITION: Moving to its normal location, or other suitable location, all or a portion of a body part.

Explanation: The body part may or may not be cut out or off to be moved to the new location ...
Examples: Relocation shoulder muscle – CMS Ex: Fracture reduction

Body Part – 4TH			Approach – 5TH	Device – 6TH	Qualifier–7TH
0 Head Muscle 1 Facial Muscle 2 Neck Muscle, Right 3 Neck Muscle, Left 4 Tongue, Palate, Pharynx Muscle 5 Shoulder Muscle, Right 6 Shoulder Muscle, Left 7 Upper Arm Muscle, Right 8 Upper Arm Muscle, Left	9 Lower Arm and Wrist Muscle, Right B Lower Arm and Wrist Muscle, Left C Hand Muscle, Right D Hand Muscle, Left F Trunk Muscle, Right G Trunk Muscle, Left H Thorax Muscle, Right J Thorax Muscle, Left	K Abdomen Muscle, Right L Abdomen Muscle, Left M Perineum Muscle N Hip Muscle, Right P Hip Muscle, Left Q Upper Leg Muscle, Right R Upper Leg Muscle, Left S Lower Leg Muscle, Right T Lower Leg Muscle, Left V Foot Muscle, Right W Foot Muscle, Left	0 Open 4 Percutaneous endoscopic	Z No device	Z No qualifier

1ST - 0 Medical and Surgical
2ND - K Muscles
3RD - T RESECTION

EXCISION GROUP: Excision, Resection, Destruction, Extraction, (Detachment)
Root Operations that take out some or all of a body part.

RESECTION: Cutting out or off, without replacement, all of a body part.

Explanation: None
Examples: Complete removal thenar muscle hand – CMS Ex: Total lobectomy of lung

Body Part – 4TH			Approach – 5TH	Device – 6TH	Qualifier–7TH
0 Head Muscle 1 Facial Muscle 2 Neck Muscle, Right 3 Neck Muscle, Left 4 Tongue, Palate, Pharynx Muscle 5 Shoulder Muscle, Right 6 Shoulder Muscle, Left 7 Upper Arm Muscle, Right 8 Upper Arm Muscle, Left	9 Lower Arm and Wrist Muscle, Right B Lower Arm and Wrist Muscle, Left C Hand Muscle, Right D Hand Muscle, Left F Trunk Muscle, Right G Trunk Muscle, Left H Thorax Muscle, Right J Thorax Muscle, Left	K Abdomen Muscle, Right L Abdomen Muscle, Left M Perineum Muscle N Hip Muscle, Right P Hip Muscle, Left Q Upper Leg Muscle, Right R Upper Leg Muscle, Left S Lower Leg Muscle, Right T Lower Leg Muscle, Left V Foot Muscle, Right W Foot Muscle, Left	0 Open 4 Percutaneous endoscopic	Z No device	Z No qualifier

1ST - 0 Medical and Surgical
2ND - K Muscles
3RD - U SUPPLEMENT

DEVICE GROUP: Change, Insertion, Removal, Replacement, Revision, Supplement
Root Operations that always involve a device.

SUPPLEMENT: Putting in or on biological or synthetic material that physically reinforces and/or augments the function of a portion of a body part.

Explanation: Biological material is non-living, or is living and from the same individual ...
Examples: Gracilis muscle graft to face – CMS Ex: Herniorrhaphy using mesh

Body Part – 4TH			Approach – 5TH	Device – 6TH	Qualifier–7TH
0 Head Muscle 1 Facial Muscle 2 Neck Muscle, Right 3 Neck Muscle, Left 4 Tongue, Palate, Pharynx Muscle 5 Shoulder Muscle, Right 6 Shoulder Muscle, Left 7 Upper Arm Muscle, Right 8 Upper Arm Muscle, Left	9 Lower Arm and Wrist Muscle, Right B Lower Arm and Wrist Muscle, Left C Hand Muscle, Right D Hand Muscle, Left F Trunk Muscle, Right G Trunk Muscle, Left H Thorax Muscle, Right J Thorax Muscle, Left	K Abdomen Muscle, Right L Abdomen Muscle, Left M Perineum Muscle N Hip Muscle, Right P Hip Muscle, Left Q Upper Leg Muscle, Right R Upper Leg Muscle, Left S Lower Leg Muscle, Right T Lower Leg Muscle, Left V Foot Muscle, Right W Foot Muscle, Left	0 Open 4 Percutaneous endoscopic	7 Autologous tissue substitute J Synthetic substitute K Nonautologous tissue substitute	Z No qualifier

© 2018 Channel Publishing, Ltd.

1ST - 0 Medical and Surgical
2ND - K Muscles
3RD - W REVISION

DEVICE GROUP: Change, Insertion, Removal, Replacement, Revision, Supplement
Root Operations that always involve a device.

REVISION: Correcting, to the extent possible, a portion of a malfunctioning device or the position of a displaced device.

Explanation: Correcting by taking out or putting in components of a device such as a screw or pin ...
Examples: Reposition stimulator lead – CMS Ex: Recementing of hip prosthesis

Body Part – 4TH	Approach – 5TH	Device – 6TH	Qualifier – 7TH
X Upper Muscle Y Lower Muscle	0 Open 3 Percutaneous 4 Percutaneous endoscopic	0 Drainage device 7 Autologous tissue substitute J Synthetic substitute K Nonautologous tissue substitute M Stimulator lead Y Other device	Z No qualifier
X Upper Muscle Y Lower Muscle	X External	0 Drainage device 7 Autologous tissue substitute J Synthetic substitute K Nonautologous tissue substitute M Stimulator lead	Z No qualifier

1ST - 0 Medical and Surgical
2ND - K Muscles
3RD - X TRANSFER

MOVE GROUP: Reattachment, Reposition, Transfer, (Transplantation)
Root Operations that put in/put back or move some/all of a body part.

TRANSFER: Moving, without taking out, all or a portion of a body part to another location to take over the function of all or a portion of a body part.

Explanation: The body part transferred remains connected to its vascular and nervous supply
Examples: TRAM flap breast reconstruction – CMS Ex: Tendon transfer

Body Part – 4TH	Approach - 5TH	Device - 6TH	Qualifier–7TH
0 Head Muscle 1 Facial Muscle 2 Neck Muscle, Right 3 Neck Muscle, Left 4 Tongue, Palate, Pharynx Muscle 5 Shoulder Muscle, Right 6 Shoulder Muscle, Left 7 Upper Arm Muscle, Right 8 Upper Arm Muscle, Left 9 Lower Arm and Wrist Muscle, Right B Lower Arm and Wrist Muscle, Left C Hand Muscle, Right D Hand Muscle, Left H Thorax Muscle, Right J Thorax Muscle, Left M Perineum Muscle N Hip Muscle, Right P Hip Muscle, Left Q Upper Leg Muscle, Right R Upper Leg Muscle, Left S Lower Leg Muscle, Right T Lower Leg Muscle, Left V Foot Muscle, Right W Foot Muscle, Left	0 Open 4 Percutaneous endoscopic	Z No device	0 Skin 1 Subcutaneous Tissue 2 Skin and Subcutaneous Tissue Z No qualifier
F Trunk Muscle, Right G Trunk Muscle, Left	0 Open 4 Percutaneous endoscopic	Z No device	0 Skin 1 Subcutaneous Tissue 2 Skin and Subcutaneous Tissue 5 Latissimus Dorsi Myocutaneous Flap 7 Deep Inferior Epigastric Artery Perforator Flap 8 Superficial Inferior Epigastric Artery Flap 9 Gluteal Artery Perforator Flap Z No qualifier
K Abdomen Muscle, Right L Abdomen Muscle, Left	0 Open 4 Percutaneous endoscopic	Z No device	0 Skin 1 Subcutaneous Tissue 2 Skin and Subcutaneous Tissue 6 Transverse Rectus Abdominis Myocutaneous Flap Z No qualifier

© 2018 Channel Publishing, Ltd.

Educational Annotations | L – Tendons

Body System Specific Educational Annotations for the Tendons include:

- Anatomy and Physiology Review
- Anatomical Illustrations
- Definitions of Common Procedures
- AHA Coding Clinic® Reference Notations
- Body Part Key Listings
- Device Key Listings
- Device Aggregation Table Listings
- Coding Notes

Anatomy and Physiology Review of Tendons

BODY PART VALUES – L - TENDONS

Lower Tendon – The tendons located below the diaphragm (see Coding Guideline B2.1b).

Tendon – ANATOMY – A tendon is a strong, yet somewhat flexible cord or band of fibrous connective tissue that most often connects muscle to bone. PHYSIOLOGY – Tendons and muscles work together to move the bones.

Upper Tendon – The tendons located above the diaphragm (see Coding Guideline B2.1b).

Anatomical Illustrations of Tendons

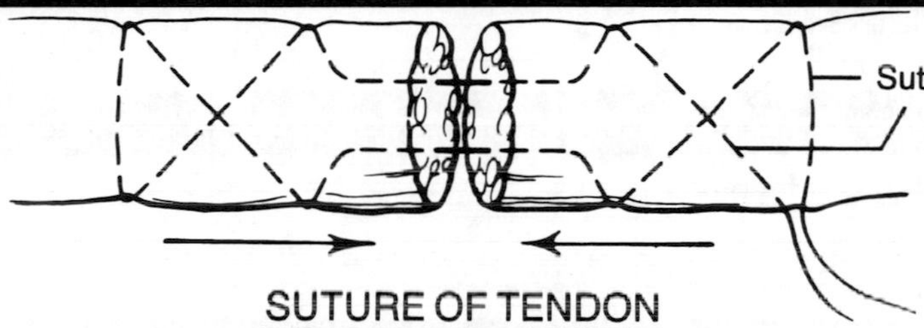

SUTURE OF TENDON

Definitions of Common Procedures of Tendons

Bridle procedure tendon transfer – The surgical transfer of the distal ends of the posterior tibial, peroneus longus, and the anterior tibialis tendons in a "bridle" configuration to correct the condition of foot drop.

Free tendon graft – The surgical placement of a section of tendon (from another part of the body or donor) to repair a damaged tendon.

AHA Coding Clinic® Reference Notations of Tendons

ROOT OPERATION SPECIFIC - L - TENDONS

CHANGE - 2
DESTRUCTION - 5
DIVISION - 8
DRAINAGE - 9
EXCISION - B
- Excision of tendon for graft ....AHA 15:3Q:p26
- Excisional debridement of nonhealing wound that included tendon........AHA 14:3Q:p18
- Excisional debridement of ulceration that included tendon ....AHA 14:3Q:p14

EXTIRPATION - C
INSPECTION - H
REATTACHMENT - M
RELEASE - N
REMOVAL - P
REPAIR - Q
- Arthroscopic rotator cuff suture repair ....AHA 13:3Q:p20

REPLACEMENT - R
REPOSITION - S
- Repair by reposition of torn biceps muscle ....AHA 15:3Q:p14

RESECTION - T
SUPPLEMENT - U
- Patellar tendon augmentation with allograft ....AHA 15:2Q:p11

REVISION - W
TRANSFER - X

TENDONS 0 L

© 2018 Channel Publishing, Ltd.

Educational Annotations | L – Tendons

Body Part Key Listings of Tendons

See also Body Part Key in Appendix C

Achilles tendon ....use Lower Leg Tendon, Left/Right
Patellar tendon ....use Knee Tendon, Left/Right

Device Key Listings of Tendons

See also Device Key in Appendix D

Autograft ....use Autologous Tissue Substitute
Tissue bank graft ....use Nonautologous Tissue Substitute

Device Aggregation Table Listings of Tendons

See also Device Aggregation Table in Appendix E

Specific Device	For Operation	In Body System	General Device
None Listed in Device Aggregation Table for this Body System			

Coding Notes of Tendons

Body System Relevant Coding Guidelines

General Guidelines

B2.1b

Where the general body part values "upper" and "lower" are provided as an option in the Upper Arteries, Lower Arteries, Upper Veins, Lower Veins, Muscles and Tendons body systems, "upper" or "lower "specifies body parts located above or below the diaphragm respectively.

Example: Vein body parts above the diaphragm are found in the Upper Veins body system; vein body parts below the diaphragm are found in the Lower Veins body system.

Tendons, ligaments, bursae and fascia near a joint

B4.5

Procedures performed on tendons, ligaments, bursae and fascia supporting a joint are coded to the body part in the respective body system that is the focus of the procedure. Procedures performed on joint structures themselves are coded to the body part in the joint body systems.

Examples: Repair of the anterior cruciate ligament of the knee is coded to the knee bursa and ligament body part in the bursae and ligaments body system.

Knee arthroscopy with shaving of articular cartilage is coded to the knee joint body part in the Lower Joints body system.

© 2018 Channel Publishing, Ltd.

1ST - 0 Medical and Surgical
2ND - L Tendons
3RD - 2 CHANGE

DEVICE GROUP: Change, Insertion, Removal, Replacement, Revision, Supplement
Root Operations that always involve a device.

CHANGE: Taking out or off a device from a body part and putting back an identical or similar device in or on the same body part without cutting or puncturing the skin or a mucous membrane.

Explanation: All CHANGE procedures are coded using the approach External
Examples: Exchange drain tube – CMS Ex: Urinary catheter change

Body Part – 4TH	Approach – 5TH	Device – 6TH	Qualifier – 7TH
X Upper Tendon Y Lower Tendon	X External	0 Drainage device Y Other device	Z No qualifier

1ST - 0 Medical and Surgical
2ND - L Tendons
3RD - 5 DESTRUCTION

EXCISION GROUP: Excision, Resection, Destruction, Extraction, (Detachment)
Root Operations that take out some or all of a body part.

DESTRUCTION: Physical eradication of all or a portion of a body part by the direct use of energy, force, or a destructive agent.

Explanation: None of the body part is physically taken out
Examples: Cryoablation tendon lesion – CMS Ex: Fulguration of rectal polyp

Body Part – 4TH			Approach – 5TH	Device – 6TH	Qualifier – 7TH
0 Head and Neck Tendon 1 Shoulder Tendon, Right 2 Shoulder Tendon, Left 3 Upper Arm Tendon, Right 4 Upper Arm Tendon, Left 5 Lower Arm and Wrist Tendon, Right 6 Lower Arm and Wrist Tendon, Left 7 Hand Tendon, Right	8 Hand Tendon, Left 9 Trunk Tendon, Right B Trunk Tendon, Left C Thorax Tendon, Right D Thorax Tendon, Left F Abdomen Tendon, Right G Abdomen Tendon, Left H Perineum Tendon J Hip Tendon, Right K Hip Tendon, Left	L Upper Leg Tendon, Right M Upper Leg Tendon, Left N Lower Leg Tendon, Right P Lower Leg Tendon, Left Q Knee Tendon, Right R Knee Tendon, Left S Ankle Tendon, Right T Ankle Tendon, Left V Foot Tendon, Right W Foot Tendon, Left	0 Open 3 Percutaneous 4 Percutaneous endoscopic	Z No device	Z No qualifier

1ST - 0 Medical and Surgical
2ND - L Tendons
3RD - 8 DIVISION

DIVISION GROUP: Division, Release
Root Operations involving cutting or separation only.

DIVISION: Cutting into a body part, without draining fluids and/or gases from the body part, in order to separate or transect a body part.

Explanation: All or a portion of the body part is separated into two or more portions
Examples: Division Achilles tendon – CMS Ex: Spinal cordotomy

Body Part – 4TH			Approach – 5TH	Device – 6TH	Qualifier – 7TH
0 Head and Neck Tendon 1 Shoulder Tendon, Right 2 Shoulder Tendon, Left 3 Upper Arm Tendon, Right 4 Upper Arm Tendon, Left 5 Lower Arm and Wrist Tendon, Right 6 Lower Arm and Wrist Tendon, Left 7 Hand Tendon, Right	8 Hand Tendon, Left 9 Trunk Tendon, Right B Trunk Tendon, Left C Thorax Tendon, Right D Thorax Tendon, Left F Abdomen Tendon, Right G Abdomen Tendon, Left H Perineum Tendon J Hip Tendon, Right K Hip Tendon, Left	L Upper Leg Tendon, Right M Upper Leg Tendon, Left N Lower Leg Tendon, Right P Lower Leg Tendon, Left Q Knee Tendon, Right R Knee Tendon, Left S Ankle Tendon, Right T Ankle Tendon, Left V Foot Tendon, Right W Foot Tendon, Left	0 Open 3 Percutaneous 4 Percutaneous endoscopic	Z No device	Z No qualifier

© 2018 Channel Publishing, Ltd.

1ST - 0 Medical and Surgical
2ND - L Tendons
3RD - 9 DRAINAGE

DRAINAGE GROUP: Drainage, Extirpation, (Fragmentation)
Root Operations that take out solids/fluids/gases from a body part.

DRAINAGE: Taking or letting out fluids and/or gases from a body part.

Explanation: Qualifier "X Diagnostic" indicates drainage procedures that are biopsies
Examples: Incision and drainage tendon sheath abscess – CMS Ex: Thoracentesis

Body Part – 4TH			Approach – 5TH	Device – 6TH	Qualifier – 7TH
0 Head and Neck Tendon 1 Shoulder Tendon, Right 2 Shoulder Tendon, Left 3 Upper Arm Tendon, Right 4 Upper Arm Tendon, Left 5 Lower Arm and Wrist Tendon, Right 6 Lower Arm and Wrist Tendon, Left 7 Hand Tendon, Right	8 Hand Tendon, Left 9 Trunk Tendon, Right B Trunk Tendon, Left C Thorax Tendon, Right D Thorax Tendon, Left F Abdomen Tendon, Right G Abdomen Tendon, Left H Perineum Tendon J Hip Tendon, Right K Hip Tendon, Left	L Upper Leg Tendon, Right M Upper Leg Tendon, Left N Lower Leg Tendon, Right P Lower Leg Tendon, Left Q Knee Tendon, Right R Knee Tendon, Left S Ankle Tendon, Right T Ankle Tendon, Left V Foot Tendon, Right W Foot Tendon, Left	0 Open 3 Percutaneous 4 Percutaneous endoscopic	0 Drainage device	Z No qualifier
0 Head and Neck Tendon 1 Shoulder Tendon, Right 2 Shoulder Tendon, Left 3 Upper Arm Tendon, Right 4 Upper Arm Tendon, Left 5 Lower Arm and Wrist Tendon, Right 6 Lower Arm and Wrist Tendon, Left 7 Hand Tendon, Right	8 Hand Tendon, Left 9 Trunk Tendon, Right B Trunk Tendon, Left C Thorax Tendon, Right D Thorax Tendon, Left F Abdomen Tendon, Right G Abdomen Tendon, Left H Perineum Tendon J Hip Tendon, Right K Hip Tendon, Left	L Upper Leg Tendon, Right M Upper Leg Tendon, Left N Lower Leg Tendon, Right P Lower Leg Tendon, Left Q Knee Tendon, Right R Knee Tendon, Left S Ankle Tendon, Right T Ankle Tendon, Left V Foot Tendon, Right W Foot Tendon, Left	0 Open 3 Percutaneous 4 Percutaneous endoscopic	Z No device	X Diagnostic Z No qualifier

1ST - 0 Medical and Surgical
2ND - L Tendons
3RD - B EXCISION

EXCISION GROUP: Excision, Resection, Destruction, Extraction, (Detachment)
Root Operations that take out some or all of a body part.

EXCISION: Cutting out or off, without replacement, a portion of a body part.

Explanation: Qualifier "X Diagnostic" indicates excision procedures that are biopsies
Examples: Ganglionectomy tendon sheath wrist – CMS Ex: Liver biopsy

Body Part – 4TH			Approach – 5TH	Device – 6TH	Qualifier – 7TH
0 Head and Neck Tendon 1 Shoulder Tendon, Right 2 Shoulder Tendon, Left 3 Upper Arm Tendon, Right 4 Upper Arm Tendon, Left 5 Lower Arm and Wrist Tendon, Right 6 Lower Arm and Wrist Tendon, Left 7 Hand Tendon, Right	8 Hand Tendon, Left 9 Trunk Tendon, Right B Trunk Tendon, Left C Thorax Tendon, Right D Thorax Tendon, Left F Abdomen Tendon, Right G Abdomen Tendon, Left H Perineum Tendon J Hip Tendon, Right K Hip Tendon, Left	L Upper Leg Tendon, Right M Upper Leg Tendon, Left N Lower Leg Tendon, Right P Lower Leg Tendon, Left Q Knee Tendon, Right R Knee Tendon, Left S Ankle Tendon, Right T Ankle Tendon, Left V Foot Tendon, Right W Foot Tendon, Left	0 Open 3 Percutaneous 4 Percutaneous endoscopic	Z No device	X Diagnostic Z No qualifier

© 2018 Channel Publishing, Ltd.

1ST - 0 Medical and Surgical
2ND - L Tendons
3RD - C EXTIRPATION

DRAINAGE GROUP: Drainage, Extirpation, (Fragmentation)
Root Operations that take out solids/fluids/gases from a body part.

EXTIRPATION: Taking or cutting out solid matter from a body part.

Explanation: Abnormal byproduct or foreign body ...
Examples: Removal calcium tendon deposit – CMS Ex: Thrombectomy

Body Part – 4TH			Approach – 5TH	Device – 6TH	Qualifier – 7TH
0 Head and Neck Tendon 1 Shoulder Tendon, Right 2 Shoulder Tendon, Left 3 Upper Arm Tendon, Right 4 Upper Arm Tendon, Left 5 Lower Arm and Wrist Tendon, Right 6 Lower Arm and Wrist Tendon, Left 7 Hand Tendon, Right	8 Hand Tendon, Left 9 Trunk Tendon, Right B Trunk Tendon, Left C Thorax Tendon, Right D Thorax Tendon, Left F Abdomen Tendon, Right G Abdomen Tendon, Left H Perineum Tendon J Hip Tendon, Right K Hip Tendon, Left	L Upper Leg Tendon, Right M Upper Leg Tendon, Left N Lower Leg Tendon, Right P Lower Leg Tendon, Left Q Knee Tendon, Right R Knee Tendon, Left S Ankle Tendon, Right T Ankle Tendon, Left V Foot Tendon, Right W Foot Tendon, Left	0 Open 3 Percutaneous 4 Percutaneous endoscopic	Z No device	Z No qualifier

1ST - 0 Medical and Surgical
2ND - L Tendons
3RD - D EXTRACTION

EXCISION GROUP: Excision, Resection, Destruction, Extraction, (Detachment)
Root Operations that take out some or all of a body part.

EXTRACTION: Pulling or stripping out or off all or a portion of a body part by the use of force.

Explanation: None for this Body System
Examples: Non-excisional debridement – CMS Ex: Dilation and curettage

Body Part – 4TH			Approach – 5TH	Device – 6TH	Qualifier – 7TH
0 Head and Neck Tendon 1 Shoulder Tendon, Right 2 Shoulder Tendon, Left 3 Upper Arm Tendon, Right 4 Upper Arm Tendon, Left 5 Lower Arm and Wrist Tendon, Right 6 Lower Arm and Wrist Tendon, Left 7 Hand Tendon, Right	8 Hand Tendon, Left 9 Trunk Tendon, Right B Trunk Tendon, Left C Thorax Tendon, Right D Thorax Tendon, Left F Abdomen Tendon, Right G Abdomen Tendon, Left H Perineum Tendon J Hip Tendon, Right K Hip Tendon, Left	L Upper Leg Tendon, Right M Upper Leg Tendon, Left N Lower Leg Tendon, Right P Lower Leg Tendon, Left Q Knee Tendon, Right R Knee Tendon, Left S Ankle Tendon, Right T Ankle Tendon, Left V Foot Tendon, Right W Foot Tendon, Left	0 Open	Z No device	Z No qualifier

1ST - 0 Medical and Surgical
2ND - L Tendons
3RD - H INSERTION

DEVICE GROUP: Change, Insertion, Removal, Replacement, Revision, Supplement
Root Operations that always involve a device.

INSERTION: Putting in a nonbiological appliance that monitors, assists, performs, or prevents a physiological function but does not physically take the place of a body part.

Explanation: None
Examples: Insertion tendon device – CMS Ex: Insertion of central venous catheter

Body Part – 4TH	Approach – 5TH	Device – 6TH	Qualifier – 7TH
X Upper Tendon Y Lower Tendon	0 Open 3 Percutaneous 4 Percutaneous endoscopic	Y Other device	Z No qualifier

© 2018 Channel Publishing, Ltd.

1ST - 0 Medical and Surgical
2ND - L Tendons
3RD - J INSPECTION

EXAMINATION GROUP: Inspection, (Map)
Root Operations involving examination only.

INSPECTION: Visually and/or manually exploring a body part.

Explanation: Direct or instrumental visualization ...
Examples: Exploration tendon attachments – CMS Ex: Exploratory laparotomy

Body Part – 4TH	Approach – 5TH	Device – 6TH	Qualifier – 7TH
X Upper Tendon Y Lower Tendon	0 Open 3 Percutaneous 4 Percutaneous endoscopic X External	Z No device	Z No qualifier

1ST - 0 Medical and Surgical
2ND - L Tendons
3RD - M REATTACHMENT

MOVE GROUP: Reattachment, Reposition, Transfer, (Transplantation)
Root Operations that put in/put back or move some/all of a body part.

REATTACHMENT: Putting back in or on all or a portion of a separated body part to its normal location or other suitable location.

Explanation: Vascular circulation and nervous pathways may or may not be reestablished
Examples: Re-anchor torn tendon – CMS Ex: Reattachment of hand

Body Part – 4TH			Approach – 5TH	Device – 6TH	Qualifier – 7TH
0 Head and Neck Tendon 1 Shoulder Tendon, Right 2 Shoulder Tendon, Left 3 Upper Arm Tendon, Right 4 Upper Arm Tendon, Left 5 Lower Arm and Wrist Tendon, Right 6 Lower Arm and Wrist Tendon, Left 7 Hand Tendon, Right	8 Hand Tendon, Left 9 Trunk Tendon, Right B Trunk Tendon, Left C Thorax Tendon, Right D Thorax Tendon, Left F Abdomen Tendon, Right G Abdomen Tendon, Left H Perineum Tendon J Hip Tendon, Right K Hip Tendon, Left	L Upper Leg Tendon, Right M Upper Leg Tendon, Left N Lower Leg Tendon, Right P Lower Leg Tendon, Left Q Knee Tendon, Right R Knee Tendon, Left S Ankle Tendon, Right T Ankle Tendon, Left V Foot Tendon, Right W Foot Tendon, Left	0 Open 4 Percutaneous endoscopic	Z No device	Z No qualifier

1ST - 0 Medical and Surgical
2ND - L Tendons
3RD - N RELEASE

DIVISION GROUP: Division, Release
Root Operations involving cutting or separation only.

RELEASE: Freeing a body part from an abnormal physical constraint by cutting or by the use of force.

Explanation: Some of the restraining tissue may be taken out but none of the body part is taken out
Examples: Extensor tenolysis – CMS Ex: Carpal tunnel release

Body Part – 4TH			Approach – 5TH	Device – 6TH	Qualifier – 7TH
0 Head and Neck Tendon 1 Shoulder Tendon, Right 2 Shoulder Tendon, Left 3 Upper Arm Tendon, Right 4 Upper Arm Tendon, Left 5 Lower Arm and Wrist Tendon, Right 6 Lower Arm and Wrist Tendon, Left 7 Hand Tendon, Right	8 Hand Tendon, Left 9 Trunk Tendon, Right B Trunk Tendon, Left C Thorax Tendon, Right D Thorax Tendon, Left F Abdomen Tendon, Right G Abdomen Tendon, Left H Perineum Tendon J Hip Tendon, Right K Hip Tendon, Left	L Upper Leg Tendon, Right M Upper Leg Tendon, Left N Lower Leg Tendon, Right P Lower Leg Tendon, Left Q Knee Tendon, Right R Knee Tendon, Left S Ankle Tendon, Right T Ankle Tendon, Left V Foot Tendon, Right W Foot Tendon, Left	0 Open 3 Percutaneous 4 Percutaneous endoscopic X External	Z No device	Z No qualifier

© 2018 Channel Publishing, Ltd.

1ST - 0 Medical and Surgical
2ND - L Tendons
3RD - P REMOVAL

DEVICE GROUP: Change, Insertion, Removal, Replacement, Revision, Supplement
Root Operations that always involve a device.

REMOVAL: Taking out or off a device from a body part.

Explanation: Removal device without reinsertion ...
Examples: Removal drain tube – CMS Ex: Cardiac pacemaker removal

Body Part – 4TH	Approach – 5TH	Device – 6TH	Qualifier – 7TH
X Upper Tendon Y Lower Tendon	0 Open 3 Percutaneous 4 Percutaneous endoscopic	0 Drainage device 7 Autologous tissue substitute J Synthetic substitute K Nonautologous tissue substitute Y Other device	Z No qualifier
X Upper Tendon Y Lower Tendon	X External	0 Drainage device	Z No qualifier

1ST - 0 Medical and Surgical
2ND - L Tendons
3RD - Q REPAIR

OTHER REPAIRS GROUP: (Control), Repair
Root Operations that define other repairs.

REPAIR: Restoring, to the extent possible, a body part to its normal anatomic structure and function.

Explanation: Used only when the method to accomplish the repair is not one of the other root operations
Examples: Tenorrhpahy – CMS Ex: Suture of laceration

Body Part – 4TH			Approach – 5TH	Device – 6TH	Qualifier – 7TH
0 Head and Neck Tendon 1 Shoulder Tendon, Right 2 Shoulder Tendon, Left 3 Upper Arm Tendon, Right 4 Upper Arm Tendon, Left 5 Lower Arm and Wrist Tendon, Right 6 Lower Arm and Wrist Tendon, Left 7 Hand Tendon, Right	8 Hand Tendon, Left 9 Trunk Tendon, Right B Trunk Tendon, Left C Thorax Tendon, Right D Thorax Tendon, Left F Abdomen Tendon, Right G Abdomen Tendon, Left H Perineum Tendon J Hip Tendon, Right K Hip Tendon, Left	L Upper Leg Tendon, Right M Upper Leg Tendon, Left N Lower Leg Tendon, Right P Lower Leg Tendon, Left Q Knee Tendon, Right R Knee Tendon, Left S Ankle Tendon, Right T Ankle Tendon, Left V Foot Tendon, Right W Foot Tendon, Left	0 Open 3 Percutaneous 4 Percutaneous endoscopic	Z No device	Z No qualifier

1ST - 0 Medical and Surgical
2ND - L Tendons
3RD - R REPLACEMENT

DEVICE GROUP: Change, Insertion, Removal, Replacement, Revision, Supplement
Root Operations that always involve a device.

REPLACEMENT: Putting in or on biological or synthetic material that physically takes the place and/or function of all or a portion of a body part.

Explanation: Includes taking out or eradicating, or rendering non-functional, the body part ...
Examples: Tendon replacement with cadaver graft – CMS Ex: Total hip replacement

Body Part – 4TH			Approach – 5TH	Device – 6TH	Qualifier – 7TH
0 Head and Neck Tendon 1 Shoulder Tendon, Right 2 Shoulder Tendon, Left 3 Upper Arm Tendon, Right 4 Upper Arm Tendon, Left 5 Lower Arm and Wrist Tendon, Right 6 Lower Arm and Wrist Tendon, Left 7 Hand Tendon, Right	8 Hand Tendon, Left 9 Trunk Tendon, Right B Trunk Tendon, Left C Thorax Tendon, Right D Thorax Tendon, Left F Abdomen Tendon, Right G Abdomen Tendon, Left H Perineum Tendon J Hip Tendon, Right K Hip Tendon, Left	L Upper Leg Tendon, Right M Upper Leg Tendon, Left N Lower Leg Tendon, Right P Lower Leg Tendon, Left Q Knee Tendon, Right R Knee Tendon, Left S Ankle Tendon, Right T Ankle Tendon, Left V Foot Tendon, Right W Foot Tendon, Left	0 Open 4 Percutaneous endoscopic	7 Autologous tissue substitute J Synthetic substitute K Nonautologous tissue substitute	Z No qualifier

© 2018 Channel Publishing, Ltd.

1ST - 0 Medical and Surgical
2ND - L Tendons
3RD - S REPOSITION

MOVE GROUP: Reattachment, Reposition, Transfer, (Transplantation)
Root Operations that put in/put back or move some/all of a body part.

REPOSITION: Moving to its normal location, or other suitable location, all or a portion of a body part.

Explanation: The body part may or may not be cut out or off to be moved to the new location ...
Examples: Relocation extensor tendon hand – CMS Ex: Fracture reduction

Body Part – 4TH			Approach – 5TH	Device – 6TH	Qualifier – 7TH
0 Head and Neck Tendon 1 Shoulder Tendon, Right 2 Shoulder Tendon, Left 3 Upper Arm Tendon, Right 4 Upper Arm Tendon, Left 5 Lower Arm and Wrist Tendon, Right 6 Lower Arm and Wrist Tendon, Left 7 Hand Tendon, Right	8 Hand Tendon, Left 9 Trunk Tendon, Right B Trunk Tendon, Left C Thorax Tendon, Right D Thorax Tendon, Left F Abdomen Tendon, Right G Abdomen Tendon, Left H Perineum Tendon J Hip Tendon, Right K Hip Tendon, Left	L Upper Leg Tendon, Right M Upper Leg Tendon, Left N Lower Leg Tendon, Right P Lower Leg Tendon, Left Q Knee Tendon, Right R Knee Tendon, Left S Ankle Tendon, Right T Ankle Tendon, Left V Foot Tendon, Right W Foot Tendon, Left	0 Open 4 Percutaneous endoscopic	Z No device	Z No qualifier

1ST - 0 Medical and Surgical
2ND - L Tendons
3RD - T RESECTION

EXCISION GROUP: Excision, Resection, Destruction, Extraction, (Detachment)
Root Operations that take out some or all of a body part.

RESECTION: Cutting out or off, without replacement, all of a body part.

Explanation: None
Examples: Complete removal flexor tendon hand – CMS Ex: Total lobectomy of lung

Body Part – 4TH			Approach – 5TH	Device – 6TH	Qualifier – 7TH
0 Head and Neck Tendon 1 Shoulder Tendon, Right 2 Shoulder Tendon, Left 3 Upper Arm Tendon, Right 4 Upper Arm Tendon, Left 5 Lower Arm and Wrist Tendon, Right 6 Lower Arm and Wrist Tendon, Left 7 Hand Tendon, Right	8 Hand Tendon, Left 9 Trunk Tendon, Right B Trunk Tendon, Left C Thorax Tendon, Right D Thorax Tendon, Left F Abdomen Tendon, Right G Abdomen Tendon, Left H Perineum Tendon J Hip Tendon, Right K Hip Tendon, Left	L Upper Leg Tendon, Right M Upper Leg Tendon, Left N Lower Leg Tendon, Right P Lower Leg Tendon, Left Q Knee Tendon, Right R Knee Tendon, Left S Ankle Tendon, Right T Ankle Tendon, Left V Foot Tendon, Right W Foot Tendon, Left	0 Open 4 Percutaneous endoscopic	Z No device	Z No qualifier

1ST - 0 Medical and Surgical
2ND - L Tendons
3RD - U SUPPLEMENT

DEVICE GROUP: Change, Insertion, Removal, Replacement, Revision, Supplement
Root Operations that always involve a device.

SUPPLEMENT: Putting in or on biological or synthetic material that physically reinforces and/or augments the function of a portion of a body part.

Explanation: Biological material is non-living, or is living and from the same individual ...
Examples: Tenoplasty augmentation graft – CMS Ex: Herniorrhaphy using mesh

Body Part – 4TH			Approach – 5TH	Device – 6TH	Qualifier – 7TH
0 Head and Neck Tendon 1 Shoulder Tendon, Right 2 Shoulder Tendon, Left 3 Upper Arm Tendon, Right 4 Upper Arm Tendon, Left 5 Lower Arm and Wrist Tendon, Right 6 Lower Arm and Wrist Tendon, Left 7 Hand Tendon, Right	8 Hand Tendon, Left 9 Trunk Tendon, Right B Trunk Tendon, Left C Thorax Tendon, Right D Thorax Tendon, Left F Abdomen Tendon, Right G Abdomen Tendon, Left H Perineum Tendon J Hip Tendon, Right K Hip Tendon, Left	L Upper Leg Tendon, Right M Upper Leg Tendon, Left N Lower Leg Tendon, Right P Lower Leg Tendon, Left Q Knee Tendon, Right R Knee Tendon, Left S Ankle Tendon, Right T Ankle Tendon, Left V Foot Tendon, Right W Foot Tendon, Left	0 Open 4 Percutaneous endoscopic	7 Autologous tissue substitute J Synthetic substitute K Nonautologous tissue substitute	Z No qualifier

© 2018 Channel Publishing, Ltd.

1ST - 0 Medical and Surgical
2ND - L Tendons
3RD - W REVISION

DEVICE GROUP: Change, Insertion, Removal, Replacement, Revision, Supplement
Root Operations that always involve a device.

REVISION: Correcting, to the extent possible, a portion of a malfunctioning device or the position of a displaced device.

Explanation: Correcting by taking out or putting in components of a device such as a screw or pin ...
Examples: Reposition drainage tube – CMS Ex: Recementing of hip prosthesis

Body Part – 4TH	Approach – 5TH	Device – 6TH	Qualifier – 7TH
X Upper Tendon Y Lower Tendon	0 Open 3 Percutaneous 4 Percutaneous endoscopic	0 Drainage device 7 Autologous tissue substitute J Synthetic substitute K Nonautologous tissue substitute Y Other device	Z No qualifier
X Upper Tendon Y Lower Tendon	X External	0 Drainage device 7 Autologous tissue substitute J Synthetic substitute K Nonautologous tissue substitute	Z No qualifier

1ST - 0 Medical and Surgical
2ND - L Tendons
3RD - X TRANSFER

MOVE GROUP: Reattachment, Reposition, Transfer, (Transplantation)
Root Operations that put in/put back or move some/all of a body part.

TRANSFER: Moving, without taking out, all or a portion of a body part to another location to take over the function of all or a portion of a body part.

Explanation: The body part transferred remains connected to its vascular and nervous supply
Examples: Pedicled tendon graft – CMS Ex: Tendon transfer

Body Part – 4TH			Approach – 5TH	Device – 6TH	Qualifier – 7TH
0 Head and Neck Tendon 1 Shoulder Tendon, Right 2 Shoulder Tendon, Left 3 Upper Arm Tendon, Right 4 Upper Arm Tendon, Left 5 Lower Arm and Wrist Tendon, Right 6 Lower Arm and Wrist Tendon, Left 7 Hand Tendon, Right	8 Hand Tendon, Left 9 Trunk Tendon, Right B Trunk Tendon, Left C Thorax Tendon, Right D Thorax Tendon, Left F Abdomen Tendon, Right G Abdomen Tendon, Left H Perineum Tendon J Hip Tendon, Right K Hip Tendon, Left	L Upper Leg Tendon, Right M Upper Leg Tendon, Left N Lower Leg Tendon, Right P Lower Leg Tendon, Left Q Knee Tendon, Right R Knee Tendon, Left S Ankle Tendon, Right T Ankle Tendon, Left V Foot Tendon, Right W Foot Tendon, Left	0 Open 4 Percutaneous endoscopic	Z No device	Z No qualifier

TENDONS

0 L X

© 2018 Channel Publishing, Ltd.

NOTES

© 2018 Channel Publishing, Ltd.

Educational Annotations | M – Bursae and Ligaments

Body System Specific Educational Annotations for the Bursae and Ligaments include:

- Anatomy and Physiology Review
- Anatomical Illustrations
- Definitions of Common Procedures
- AHA Coding Clinic® Reference Notations
- Body Part Key Listings
- Device Key Listings
- Device Aggregation Table Listings
- Coding Notes

Anatomy and Physiology Review of Bursae and Ligaments

BODY PART VALUES – M - BURSAE AND LIGAMENTS

Bursa – ANATOMY – Bursa are small, synovial fluid-filled sacs that lie between bones, tendons, and muscles around joints. PHYSIOLOGY – Bursa function to allow less friction between the bones, tendons, and muscles around joints during movement.

Ligament – ANATOMY – A ligament is a strong band or sheath of connective tissue that connects bones to bones. PHYSIOLOGY – Ligaments hold bones and joints in proper alignment and allow some flexibility.

Lower Bursa and Ligament – The bursa and ligaments located below the diaphragm (see Coding Guideline B2.1b)

Upper Bursa and Ligament – The bursa and ligaments located above the diaphragm (see Coding Guideline B2.1b).

Anatomical Illustrations of Bursae and Ligaments

None for the Bursae and Ligaments Body System

Definitions of Common Procedures of Bursae and Ligaments

Prepatellar bursectomy – The surgical removal of a prepatellar (knee) bursal sac.

Reattach severed ankle ligament – The repair of a torn ankle ligament using sutures to a small hole drilled in the fibula.

Tommy John surgery – The surgical reconstruction of a torn ulnar collateral ligament by using a tendon graft sewn through small drill holes in the medial epicondyle of the humerus and sublime tubercle of the ulna in a figure 8 pattern with any remnants of the original ligament attached to the tendon.

AHA Coding Clinic® Reference Notations of Bursae and Ligaments

ROOT OPERATION SPECIFIC - M - BURSAE AND LIGAMENTS

CHANGE - 2
DESTRUCTION - 5
DIVISION - 7
DRAINAGE - 9
EXCISION - B
EXTIRPATION - C
EXTRACTION - D
INSPECTION - J
REATTACHMENT - M
    Arthroscopic type 2 SLAP repair .... AHA 13:3Q:p20
RELEASE - N
REMOVAL - P
REPAIR - Q
    Cervical interspinous ligamentoplasty .... AHA 14:3Q:p9
REPOSITION - S
RESECTION - T
SUPPLEMENT - U
REVISION - W
TRANSFER - X

BURSAE & LIGAMENTS 0 M

© 2018 Channel Publishing, Ltd.

Educational Annotations | M – Bursae and Ligaments

Body Part Key Listings of Bursae and Ligaments

See also Body Part Key in Appendix C

Acromioclavicular ligament ....use Shoulder Bursa and Ligament, Left/Right
Alar ligament of axis ....use Head and Neck Bursa and Ligament
Annular ligament ....use Elbow Bursa and Ligament, Left/Right
Anterior cruciate ligament (ACL) ....use Knee Bursa and Ligament, Left/Right
Calcaneocuboid ligament....use Foot Bursa and Ligament, Left/Right
Calcaneofibular ligament ....use Ankle Bursa and Ligament, Left/Right
Carpometacarpal ligament ....use Hand Bursa and Ligament, Left/Right
Cervical interspinous ligament ....use Head and Neck Bursa and Ligament
Cervical intertransverse ligament ....use Head and Neck Bursa and Ligament
Cervical ligamentum flavum ....use Head and Neck Bursa and Ligament
Coracoacromial ligament....use Shoulder Bursa and Ligament, Left/Right
Coracoclavicular ligament ....use Shoulder Bursa and Ligament, Left/Right
Coracohumeral ligament....use Shoulder Bursa and Ligament, Left/Right
Costoclavicular ligament ....use Shoulder Bursa and Ligament, Left/Right
Costotransverse ligament....use Sternum Bursa and Ligament
....use Rib(s) Bursa and Ligament
Costoxiphoid ligament....use Sternum Bursa and Ligament
....use Rib(s) Bursa and Ligament
Cuneonavicular ligament....use Foot Bursa and Ligament, Left/Right
Deltoid ligament ....use Ankle Bursa and Ligament, Left/Right
Glenohumeral ligament ....use Shoulder Bursa and Ligament, Left/Right
Iliofemoral ligament ....use Hip Bursa and Ligament, Left/Right
Iliolumbar ligament ....use Lower Spine Bursa and Ligament
Intercarpal ligament ....use Hand Bursa and Ligament, Left/Right
Interclavicular ligament....use Shoulder Bursa and Ligament, Left/Right
Intercuneiform ligament ....use Foot Bursa and Ligament, Left/Right
Interphalangeal ligament ....use Hand Bursa and Ligament, Left/Right
....use Foot Bursa and Ligament, Left/Right
Interspinous ligament ....use Head and Neck Bursa and Ligament
....use Lower Spine/Upper Spine Bursa and Ligament
Intertransverse ligament ....use Lower Spine/Upper Spine Bursa and Ligament
Ischiofemoral ligament ....use Hip Bursa and Ligament, Left/Right
Lateral collateral ligament (LCL) ....use Knee Bursa and Ligament, Left/Right
Lateral temporomandibular ligament..use Head and Neck Bursa and Ligament
Ligament of head of fibula ....use Knee Bursa and Ligament, Left/Right
Ligament of the lateral malleolus ....use Ankle Bursa and Ligament, Left/Right
Ligamentum flavum ....use Lower Spine/Upper Spine Bursa and Ligament
Lunotriquetral ligament ....use Hand Bursa and Ligament, Left/Right
Medial collateral ligament (MCL) ....use Knee Bursa and Ligament, Left/Right
Metacarpal ligament ....use Hand Bursa and Ligament, Left/Right
Metacarpophalangeal ligament ....use Hand Bursa and Ligament, Left/Right
Metatarsal ligament ....use Foot Bursa and Ligament, Left/Right
Metatarsophalangeal ligament ....use Foot Bursa and Ligament, Left/Right
Olecranon bursa ....use Elbow Bursa and Ligament, Left/Right
Palmar ulnocarpal ligament ....use Wrist Bursa and Ligament, Left/Right
Patellar ligament....use Knee Bursa and Ligament, Left/Right
Pisohamate ligament ....use Hand Bursa and Ligament, Left/Right
Pisometacarpal ligament....use Hand Bursa and Ligament, Left/Right
Popliteal ligament....use Knee Bursa and Ligament, Left/Right
Posterior cruciate ligament (PCL) ....use Knee Bursa and Ligament, Left/Right
Prepatellar bursa....use Knee Bursa and Ligament, Left/Right
Pubofemoral ligament....use Hip Bursa and Ligament, Left/Right
Radial collateral carpal ligament ....use Wrist Bursa and Ligament, Left/Right
Radial collateral ligament....use Elbow Bursa and Ligament, Left/Right
Radiocarpal ligament ....use Wrist Bursa and Ligament, Left/Right
Radioulnar ligament ....use Wrist Bursa and Ligament, Left/Right
Sacrococcygeal ligament ....use Lower Spine Bursa and Ligament
Sacroiliac ligament ....use Lower Spine Bursa and Ligament
Sacrospinous ligament....use Lower Spine Bursa and Ligament
Sacrotuberous ligament....use Lower Spine Bursa and Ligament
Scapholunate ligament ....use Hand Bursa and Ligament, Left/Right
Scaphotrapezium ligament ....use Hand Bursa and Ligament, Left/Right
Sphenomandibular ligament....use Head and Neck Bursa and Ligament
Sternoclavicular ligament ....use Shoulder Bursa and Ligament, Left/Right
Sternocostal ligament ....use Sternum Bursa and Ligament
....use Rib(s) Bursa and Ligament
Stylomandibular ligament....use Head and Neck Bursa and Ligament
Subacromial bursa....use Shoulder Bursa and Ligament, Left/Right
Subtalar ligament ....use Foot Bursa and Ligament, Left/Right
Supraspinous ligament ....use Lower Spine/Upper Spine Bursa and Ligament
Talocalcaneal ligament ....use Foot Bursa and Ligament, Left/Right
Talocalcaneonavicular ligament ....use Foot Bursa and Ligament, Left/Right
Talofibular ligament ....use Ankle Bursa and Ligament, Left/Right
Tarsometatarsal ligament ....use Foot Bursa and Ligament, Left/Right
Transverse acetabular ligament....use Hip Bursa and Ligament, Left/Right
Transverse humeral ligament ....use Shoulder Bursa and Ligament, Left/Right
Transverse ligament of atlas ....use Head and Neck Bursa and Ligament
Transverse scapular ligament ....use Shoulder Bursa and Ligament, Left/Right
Trochanteric bursa ....use Hip Bursa and Ligament, Left/Right
Ulnar collateral carpal ligament ....use Wrist Bursa and Ligament, Left/Right
Ulnar collateral ligament ....use Elbow Bursa and Ligament, Left/Right

© 2018 Channel Publishing, Ltd.

Educational Annotations | M – Bursae and Ligaments

Device Key Listings of Bursae and Ligaments

See also Device Key in Appendix D

Autograft ....use Autologous Tissue Substitute
Tissue bank graft ....use Nonautologous Tissue Substitute

Device Aggregation Table Listings of Bursae and Ligaments

See also Device Aggregation Table in Appendix E

Specific Device	For Operation	In Body System	General Device
None Listed in Device Aggregation Table for this Body System			

Coding Notes of Bursae and Ligaments

Body System Relevant Coding Guidelines

General Guidelines

B2.1b

Where the general body part values "upper" and "lower" are provided as an option in the Upper Arteries, Lower Arteries, Upper Veins, Lower Veins, Muscles and Tendons body systems, "upper" or "lower "specifies body parts located above or below the diaphragm respectively.

Example: Vein body parts above the diaphragm are found in the Upper Veins body system; vein body parts below the diaphragm are found in the Lower Veins body system.

Tendons, ligaments, bursae and fascia near a joint

B4.5

Procedures performed on tendons, ligaments, bursae and fascia supporting a joint are coded to the body part in the respective body system that is the focus of the procedure. Procedures performed on joint structures themselves are coded to the body part in the joint body systems.

Examples: Repair of the anterior cruciate ligament of the knee is coded to the knee bursa and ligament body part in the bursae and ligaments body system.

Knee arthroscopy with shaving of articular cartilage is coded to the knee joint body part in the Lower Joints body system.

© 2018 Channel Publishing, Ltd.

1ST - 0 Medical and Surgical
2ND - M Bursae and Ligaments
3RD - 2 CHANGE

DEVICE GROUP: Change, Insertion, Removal, Replacement, Revision, Supplement
Root Operations that always involve a device.

CHANGE: Taking out or off a device from a body part and putting back an identical or similar device in or on the same body part without cutting or puncturing the skin or a mucous membrane.

Explanation: All CHANGE procedures are coded using the approach External
Examples: Exchange drain tube – CMS Ex: Urinary catheter change

Body Part – 4TH	Approach – 5TH	Device – 6TH	Qualifier – 7TH
X Upper Bursa and Ligament Y Lower Bursa and Ligament	X External	0 Drainage device Y Other device	Z No qualifier

1ST - 0 Medical and Surgical
2ND - M Bursae and Ligaments
3RD - 5 DESTRUCTION

EXCISION GROUP: Excision, Resection, Destruction, Extraction, (Detachment)
Root Operations that take out some or all of a body part.

DESTRUCTION: Physical eradication of all or a portion of a body part by the direct use of energy, force, or a destructive agent.

Explanation: None of the body part is physically taken out
Examples: Cryoablation ligament lesion – CMS Ex: Fulguration of rectal polyp

Body Part – 4TH	Approach – 5TH	Device – 6TH	Qualifier – 7TH
... Bursa and Ligament ... 0 Head and Neck ... 1 Shoulder ..., Right 2 Shoulder ..., Left 3 Elbow ..., Right 4 Elbow ..., Left 5 Wrist ..., Right 6 Wrist ..., Left 7 Hand ..., Right 8 Hand ..., Left 9 Upper Extremity ..., Right B Upper Extremity ..., Left C Upper Spine ... D Lower Spine ... F Sternum ... G Rib(s) ... H Abdomen ..., Right J Abdomen ..., Left K Perineum ... L Hip ..., Right M Hip ..., Left N Knee ..., Right P Knee ..., Left Q Ankle ..., Right R Ankle ..., Left S Foot ..., Right T Foot ..., Left V Lower Extremity ..., Right W Lower Extremity ..., Left	0 Open 3 Percutaneous 4 Percutaneous endoscopic	Z No device	Z No qualifier

1ST - 0 Medical and Surgical
2ND - M Bursae and Ligaments
3RD - 8 DIVISION

DIVISION GROUP: Division, Release
Root Operations involving cutting or separation only.

DIVISION: Cutting into a body part, without draining fluids and/or gases from the body part, in order to separate or transect a body part.

Explanation: All or a portion of the body part is separated into two or more portions
Examples: Ligament transection – CMS Ex: Spinal cordotomy

Body Part – 4TH	Approach – 5TH	Device – 6TH	Qualifier – 7TH
... Bursa and Ligament ... 0 Head and Neck ... 1 Shoulder ..., Right 2 Shoulder ..., Left 3 Elbow ..., Right 4 Elbow ..., Left 5 Wrist ..., Right 6 Wrist ..., Left 7 Hand ..., Right 8 Hand ..., Left 9 Upper Extremity ..., Right B Upper Extremity ..., Left C Upper Spine ... D Lower Spine ... F Sternum ... G Rib(s) ... H Abdomen ..., Right J Abdomen ..., Left K Perineum ... L Hip ..., Right M Hip ..., Left N Knee ..., Right P Knee ..., Left Q Ankle ..., Right R Ankle ..., Left S Foot ..., Right T Foot ..., Left V Lower Extremity ..., Right W Lower Extremity ..., Left	0 Open 3 Percutaneous 4 Percutaneous endoscopic	Z No device	Z No qualifier

© 2018 Channel Publishing, Ltd.

1ST - 0 Medical and Surgical
2ND - M Bursae and Ligaments
3RD - 9 DRAINAGE

DRAINAGE GROUP: Drainage, Extirpation, (Fragmentation)
Root Operations that take out solids/fluids/gases from a body part.

DRAINAGE: Taking or letting out fluids and/or gases from a body part.

Explanation: Qualifier "X Diagnostic" indicates drainage procedures that are biopsies
Examples: Aspiration prepatellar bursa fluid – CMS Ex: Thoracentesis

Body Part – 4TH	Approach – 5TH	Device – 6TH	Qualifier – 7TH
... Bursa and Ligament ... 0 Head and Neck ... 1 Shoulder ..., Right 2 Shoulder ..., Left 3 Elbow ..., Right 4 Elbow ..., Left 5 Wrist ..., Right 6 Wrist ..., Left 7 Hand ..., Right 8 Hand ..., Left 9 Upper Extremity ..., Right B Upper Extremity ..., Left C Upper Spine ... D Lower Spine ... F Sternum ... G Rib(s) ... H Abdomen ..., Right J Abdomen ..., Left K Perineum ... L Hip ..., Right M Hip ..., Left N Knee ..., Right P Knee ..., Left Q Ankle ..., Right R Ankle ..., Left S Foot ..., Right T Foot ..., Left V Lower Extremity ..., Right W Lower Extremity ..., Left	0 Open 3 Percutaneous 4 Percutaneous endoscopic	0 Drainage device	Z No qualifier
... Bursa and Ligament ... 0 Head and Neck ... 1 Shoulder ..., Right 2 Shoulder ..., Left 3 Elbow ..., Right 4 Elbow ..., Left 5 Wrist ..., Right 6 Wrist ..., Left 7 Hand ..., Right 8 Hand ..., Left 9 Upper Extremity ..., Right B Upper Extremity ..., Left C Upper Spine ... D Lower Spine ... F Sternum ... G Rib(s) ... H Abdomen ..., Right J Abdomen ..., Left K Perineum ... L Hip ..., Right M Hip ..., Left N Knee ..., Right P Knee ..., Left Q Ankle ..., Right R Ankle ..., Left S Foot ..., Right T Foot ..., Left V Lower Extremity ..., Right W Lower Extremity ..., Left	0 Open 3 Percutaneous 4 Percutaneous endoscopic	Z No device	X Diagnostic Z No qualifier

1ST - 0 Medical and Surgical
2ND - M Bursae and Ligaments
3RD - B EXCISION

EXCISION GROUP: Excision, Resection, Destruction, Extraction, (Detachment)
Root Operations that take out some or all of a body part.

EXCISION: Cutting out or off, without replacement, a portion of a body part.

Explanation: Qualifier "X Diagnostic" indicates excision procedures that are biopsies
Examples: Partial busrectomy elbow – CMS Ex: Liver biopsy

Body Part – 4TH	Approach – 5TH	Device – 6TH	Qualifier – 7TH
... Bursa and Ligament ... 0 Head and Neck ... 1 Shoulder ..., Right 2 Shoulder ..., Left 3 Elbow ..., Right 4 Elbow ..., Left 5 Wrist ..., Right 6 Wrist ..., Left 7 Hand ..., Right 8 Hand ..., Left 9 Upper Extremity ..., Right B Upper Extremity ..., Left C Upper Spine ... D Lower Spine ... F Sternum ... G Rib(s) ... H Abdomen ..., Right J Abdomen ..., Left K Perineum ... L Hip ..., Right M Hip ..., Left N Knee ..., Right P Knee ..., Left Q Ankle ..., Right R Ankle ..., Left S Foot ..., Right T Foot ..., Left V Lower Extremity ..., Right W Lower Extremity ..., Left	0 Open 3 Percutaneous 4 Percutaneous endoscopic	Z No device	X Diagnostic Z No qualifier

© 2018 Channel Publishing, Ltd.

1ST - 0 Medical and Surgical
2ND - M Bursae and Ligaments
3RD - C EXTIRPATION

DRAINAGE GROUP: Drainage, Extirpation, (Fragmentation)
Root Operations that take out solids/fluids/gases from a body part.

EXTIRPATION: Taking or cutting out solid matter from a body part.

Explanation: Abnormal byproduct or foreign body ...
Examples: Removal bursal calcification – CMS Ex: Thrombectomy

Body Part – 4TH	Approach – 5TH	Device – 6TH	Qualifier – 7TH
... Bursa and Ligament ... 0 Head and Neck ... 1 Shoulder ..., Right 2 Shoulder ..., Left 3 Elbow ..., Right 4 Elbow ..., Left 5 Wrist ..., Right 6 Wrist ..., Left 7 Hand ..., Right 8 Hand ..., Left 9 Upper Extremity ..., Right B Upper Extremity ..., Left C Upper Spine ... D Lower Spine ... F Sternum ... G Rib(s) ... H Abdomen ..., Right J Abdomen ..., Left K Perineum ... L Hip ..., Right M Hip ..., Left N Knee ..., Right P Knee ..., Left Q Ankle ..., Right R Ankle ..., Left S Foot ..., Right T Foot ..., Left V Lower Extremity ..., Right W Lower Extremity ..., Left	0 Open 3 Percutaneous 4 Percutaneous endoscopic	Z No device	Z No qualifier

1ST - 0 Medical and Surgical
2ND - M Bursae and Ligaments
3RD - D EXTRACTION

EXCISION GROUP: Excision, Resection, Destruction, Extraction, (Detachment)
Root Operations that take out some or all of a body part.

EXTRACTION: Pulling or stripping out or off all or a portion of a body part by the use of force.

Explanation: None for this Body System
Examples: Extraction bursal sac – CMS Ex: Dilation and curettage

Body Part – 4TH	Approach – 5TH	Device – 6TH	Qualifier – 7TH
... Bursa and Ligament ... 0 Head and Neck ... 1 Shoulder ..., Right 2 Shoulder ..., Left 3 Elbow ..., Right 4 Elbow ..., Left 5 Wrist ..., Right 6 Wrist ..., Left 7 Hand ..., Right 8 Hand ..., Left 9 Upper Extremity ..., Right B Upper Extremity ..., Left C Upper Spine ... D Lower Spine ... F Sternum ... G Rib(s) ... H Abdomen ..., Right J Abdomen ..., Left K Perineum ... L Hip ..., Right M Hip ..., Left N Knee ..., Right P Knee ..., Left Q Ankle ..., Right R Ankle ..., Left S Foot ..., Right T Foot ..., Left V Lower Extremity ..., Right W Lower Extremity ..., Left	0 Open 3 Percutaneous 4 Percutaneous endoscopic	Z No device	Z No qualifier

1ST - 0 Medical and Surgical
2ND - M Bursae and Ligaments
3RD - H INSERTION

DEVICE GROUP: Change, Insertion, Removal, Replacement, Revision, Supplement
Root Operations that always involve a device.

INSERTION: Putting in a nonbiological appliance that monitors, assists, performs, or prevents a physiological function but does not physically take the place of a body part.

Explanation: None
Examples: Insertion ligament device – CMS Ex: Insertion of central venous catheter

Body Part – 4TH	Approach – 5TH	Device – 6TH	Qualifier – 7TH
X Upper Bursa and Ligament Y Lower Bursa and Ligament	0 Open 3 Percutaneous 4 Percutaneous endoscopic	Y Other device	Z No qualifier

© 2018 Channel Publishing, Ltd.

1ST - 0 Medical and Surgical
2ND - M Bursae and Ligaments
3RD - J INSPECTION

EXAMINATION GROUP: Inspection, (Map)
Root Operations involving examination only.
INSPECTION: Visually and/or manually exploring a body part.

Explanation: Direct or instrumental visualization ...
Examples: Examination prepatellar bursa – CMS Ex: Exploratory laparotomy

Body Part – 4TH	Approach – 5TH	Device – 6TH	Qualifier – 7TH
X Upper Bursa and Ligament Y Lower Bursa and Ligament	0 Open 3 Percutaneous 4 Percutaneous endoscopic X External	Z No device	Z No qualifier

1ST - 0 Medical and Surgical
2ND - M Bursae and Ligaments
3RD - M REATTACHMENT

MOVE GROUP: Reattachment, Reposition, Transfer, (Transplantation)
Root Operations that put in/put back or move some/all of a body part.
REATTACHMENT: Putting back in or on all or a portion of a separated body part to its normal location or other suitable location.

Explanation: Vascular circulation and nervous pathways may or may not be reestablished
Examples: Reattachment torn ligament – CMS Ex: Reattachment of hand

Body Part – 4TH	Approach – 5TH	Device – 6TH	Qualifier – 7TH
... Bursa and Ligament ... 0 Head and Neck ... 1 Shoulder ..., Right 2 Shoulder ..., Left 3 Elbow ..., Right 4 Elbow ..., Left 5 Wrist ..., Right 6 Wrist ..., Left 7 Hand ..., Right 8 Hand ..., Left 9 Upper Extremity ..., Right B Upper Extremity ..., Left C Upper Spine ... D Lower Spine ... F Sternum ... G Rib(s) ... H Abdomen ..., Right J Abdomen ..., Left K Perineum ... L Hip ..., Right M Hip ..., Left N Knee ..., Right P Knee ..., Left Q Ankle ..., Right R Ankle ..., Left S Foot ..., Right T Foot ..., Left V Lower Extremity ..., Right W Lower Extremity ..., Left	0 Open 4 Percutaneous endoscopic	Z No device	Z No qualifier

1ST - 0 Medical and Surgical
2ND - M Bursae and Ligaments
3RD - N RELEASE

DIVISION GROUP: Division, Release
Root Operations involving cutting or separation only.
RELEASE: Freeing a body part from an abnormal physical constraint by cutting or by the use of force.

Explanation: Some of the restraining tissue may be taken out but none of the body part is taken out
Examples: Coracoacromial ligament release – CMS Ex: Carpal tunnel release

Body Part – 4TH	Approach – 5TH	Device – 6TH	Qualifier – 7TH
... Bursa and Ligament ... 0 Head and Neck ... 1 Shoulder ..., Right 2 Shoulder ..., Left 3 Elbow ..., Right 4 Elbow ..., Left 5 Wrist ..., Right 6 Wrist ..., Left 7 Hand ..., Right 8 Hand ..., Left 9 Upper Extremity ..., Right B Upper Extremity ..., Left C Upper Spine ... D Lower Spine ... F Sternum ... G Rib(s) ... H Abdomen ..., Right J Abdomen ..., Left K Perineum ... L Hip ..., Right M Hip ..., Left N Knee ..., Right P Knee ..., Left Q Ankle ..., Right R Ankle ..., Left S Foot ..., Right T Foot ..., Left V Lower Extremity ..., Right W Lower Extremity ..., Left	0 Open 3 Percutaneous 4 Percutaneous endoscopic X External	Z No device	Z No qualifier

© 2018 Channel Publishing, Ltd.

1ST - 0 Medical and Surgical
2ND - M Bursae and Ligaments
3RD - P REMOVAL

DEVICE GROUP: Change, Insertion, Removal, Replacement, Revision, Supplement
Root Operations that always involve a device.

REMOVAL: Taking out or off a device from a body part.

Explanation: Removal device without reinsertion ...
Examples: Removal drain tube – CMS Ex: Cardiac pacemaker removal

Body Part – 4TH	Approach – 5TH	Device – 6TH	Qualifier – 7TH
X Upper Bursa and Ligament Y Lower Bursa and Ligament	0 Open 3 Percutaneous 4 Percutaneous endoscopic	0 Drainage device 7 Autologous tissue substitute J Synthetic substitute K Nonautologous tissue substitute Y Other device	Z No qualifier
X Upper Bursa and Ligament Y Lower Bursa and Ligament	X External	0 Drainage device	Z No qualifier

1ST - 0 Medical and Surgical
2ND - M Bursae and Ligaments
3RD - Q REPAIR

OTHER REPAIRS GROUP: (Control), Repair
Root Operations that define other repairs.

REPAIR: Restoring, to the extent possible, a body part to its normal anatomic structure and function.

Explanation: Used only when the method to accomplish the repair is not one of the other root operations
Examples: Suture torn ligament – CMS Ex: Suture of laceration

Body Part – 4TH			Approach – 5TH	Device – 6TH	Qualifier – 7TH
... Bursa and Ligament ... 0 Head and Neck ... 1 Shoulder ..., Right 2 Shoulder ..., Left 3 Elbow ..., Right 4 Elbow ..., Left 5 Wrist ..., Right 6 Wrist ..., Left 7 Hand ..., Right 8 Hand ..., Left	9 Upper Extremity ..., Right B Upper Extremity ..., Left C Upper Spine ... D Lower Spine ... F Sternum ... G Rib(s) ... H Abdomen ..., Right J Abdomen ..., Left K Perineum ...	L Hip ..., Right M Hip ..., Left N Knee ..., Right P Knee ..., Left Q Ankle ..., Right R Ankle ..., Left S Foot ..., Right T Foot ..., Left V Lower Extremity ..., Right W Lower Extremity ..., Left	0 Open 3 Percutaneous 4 Percutaneous endoscopic	Z No device	Z No qualifier

1ST - 0 Medical and Surgical
2ND - M Bursae and Ligaments
3RD - R REPLACEMENT

DEVICE GROUP: Change, Insertion, Removal, Replacement, Revision, Supplement
Root Operations that always involve a device.

REPLACEMENT: Putting in or on biological or synthetic material that physically takes the place and/or function of all or a portion of a body part.

Explanation: Includes taking out or eradicating, or rendering non-functional, the body part ...
Examples: Ligament replacement with cadaver graft – CMS Ex: Total hip replacement

Body Part – 4TH			Approach – 5TH	Device – 6TH	Qualifier – 7TH
... Bursa and Ligament ... 0 Head and Neck ... 1 Shoulder ..., Right 2 Shoulder ..., Left 3 Elbow ..., Right 4 Elbow ..., Left 5 Wrist ..., Right 6 Wrist ..., Left 7 Hand ..., Right 8 Hand ..., Left	9 Upper Extremity ..., Right B Upper Extremity ..., Left C Upper Spine ... D Lower Spine ... F Sternum ... G Rib(s) ... H Abdomen ..., Right J Abdomen ..., Left K Perineum ...	L Hip ..., Right M Hip ..., Left N Knee ..., Right P Knee ..., Left Q Ankle ..., Right R Ankle ..., Left S Foot ..., Right T Foot ..., Left V Lower Extremity ..., Right W Lower Extremity ..., Left	0 Open 4 Percutaneous endoscopic	7 Autologous tissue substitute J Synthetic substitute K Nonautologous tissue substitute	Z No qualifier

© 2018 Channel Publishing, Ltd.

1ST - 0 Medical and Surgical
2ND - M Bursae and Ligaments
3RD - S REPOSITION

MOVE GROUP: Reattachment, Reposition, Transfer, (Transplantation)
Root Operations that put in/put back or move some/all of a body part.

REPOSITION: Moving to its normal location, or other suitable location, all or a portion of a body part.

Explanation: The body part may or may not be cut out or off to be moved to the new location ...
Examples: Reposition ACL ligament – CMS Ex: Fracture reduction

Body Part – 4TH			Approach – 5TH	Device – 6TH	Qualifier – 7TH
... Bursa and Ligament ... 0 Head and Neck ... 1 Shoulder ..., Right 2 Shoulder ..., Left 3 Elbow ..., Right 4 Elbow ..., Left 5 Wrist ..., Right 6 Wrist ..., Left 7 Hand ..., Right 8 Hand ..., Left	9 Upper Extremity ..., Right B Upper Extremity ..., Left C Upper Spine ... D Lower Spine ... F Sternum ... G Rib(s) ... H Abdomen ..., Right J Abdomen ..., Left K Perineum ...	L Hip ..., Right M Hip ..., Left N Knee ..., Right P Knee ..., Left Q Ankle ..., Right R Ankle ..., Left S Foot ..., Right T Foot ..., Left V Lower Extremity ..., Right W Lower Extremity ..., Left	0 Open 4 Percutaneous endoscopic	Z No device	Z No qualifier

1ST - 0 Medical and Surgical
2ND - M Bursae and Ligaments
3RD - T RESECTION

EXCISION GROUP: Excision, Resection, Destruction, Extraction, (Detachment)
Root Operations that take out some or all of a body part.

RESECTION: Cutting out or off, without replacement, all of a body part.

Explanation: None
Examples: Collateral ligament complete removal – CMS Ex: Total lobectomy of lung

Body Part – 4TH			Approach – 5TH	Device – 6TH	Qualifier – 7TH
... Bursa and Ligament ... 0 Head and Neck ... 1 Shoulder ..., Right 2 Shoulder ..., Left 3 Elbow ..., Right 4 Elbow ..., Left 5 Wrist ..., Right 6 Wrist ..., Left 7 Hand ..., Right 8 Hand ..., Left	9 Upper Extremity ..., Right B Upper Extremity ..., Left C Upper Spine ... D Lower Spine ... F Sternum ... G Rib(s) ... H Abdomen ..., Right J Abdomen ..., Left K Perineum ...	L Hip ..., Right M Hip ..., Left N Knee ..., Right P Knee ..., Left Q Ankle ..., Right R Ankle ..., Left S Foot ..., Right T Foot ..., Left V Lower Extremity ..., Right W Lower Extremity ..., Left	0 Open 4 Percutaneous endoscopic	Z No device	Z No qualifier

1ST - 0 Medical and Surgical
2ND - M Bursae and Ligaments
3RD - U SUPPLEMENT

DEVICE GROUP: Change, Insertion, Removal, Replacement, Revision, Supplement
Root Operations that always involve a device.

SUPPLEMENT: Putting in or on biological or synthetic material that physically reinforces and/or augments the function of a portion of a body part.

Explanation: Biological material is non-living, or is living and from the same individual ...
Examples: Augmentation ligamentoplasty – CMS Ex: Herniorrhaphy using mesh

Body Part – 4TH			Approach – 5TH	Device – 6TH	Qualifier – 7TH
... Bursa and Ligament ... 0 Head and Neck ... 1 Shoulder ..., Right 2 Shoulder ..., Left 3 Elbow ..., Right 4 Elbow ..., Left 5 Wrist ..., Right 6 Wrist ..., Left 7 Hand ..., Right 8 Hand ..., Left	9 Upper Extremity ..., Right B Upper Extremity ..., Left C Upper Spine ... D Lower Spine ... F Sternum ... G Rib(s) ... H Abdomen ..., Right J Abdomen ..., Left K Perineum ...	L Hip ..., Right M Hip ..., Left N Knee ..., Right P Knee ..., Left Q Ankle ..., Right R Ankle ..., Left S Foot ..., Right T Foot ..., Left V Lower Extremity ..., Right W Lower Extremity ..., Left	0 Open 4 Percutaneous endoscopic	7 Autologous tissue substitute J Synthetic substitute K Nonautologous tissue substitute	Z No qualifier

© 2018 Channel Publishing, Ltd.

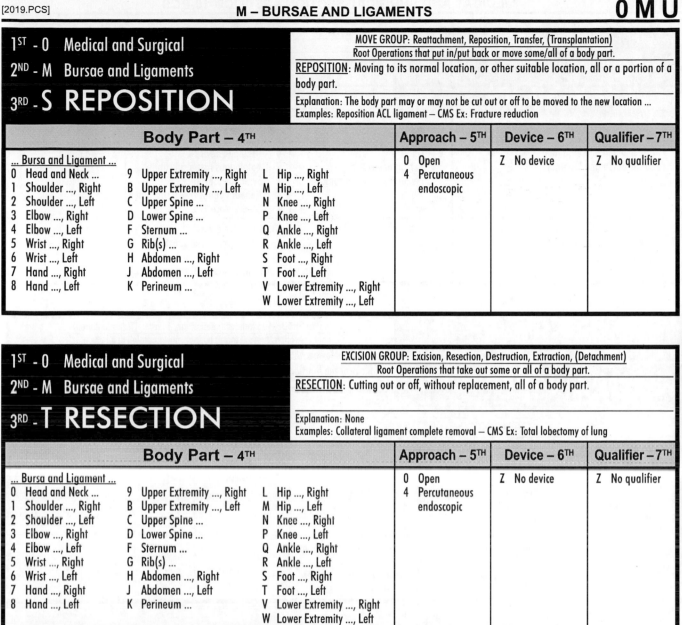

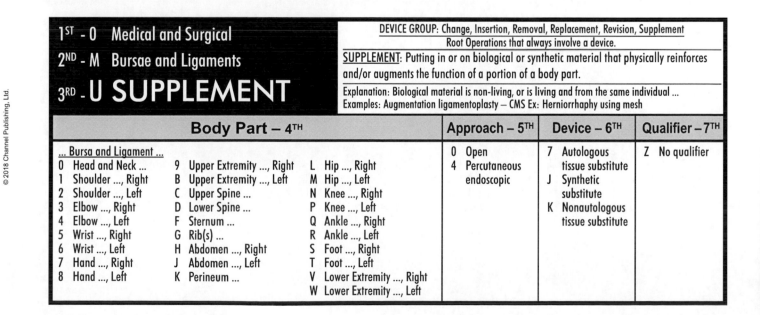

1ST - 0 Medical and Surgical
2ND - M Bursae and Ligaments
3RD - W REVISION

DEVICE GROUP: Change, Insertion, Removal, Replacement, Revision, Supplement
Root Operations that always involve a device.

REVISION: Correcting, to the extent possible, a portion of a malfunctioning device or the position of a displaced device.

Explanation: Correcting by taking out or putting in components of a device such as a screw or pin ...
Examples: Resuture ligament graft – CMS Ex: Recementing of hip prosthesis

Body Part – 4TH	Approach – 5TH	Device – 6TH	Qualifier – 7TH
X Upper Bursa and Ligament Y Lower Bursa and Ligament	0 Open 3 Percutaneous 4 Percutaneous endoscopic	0 Drainage device 7 Autologous tissue substitute J Synthetic substitute K Nonautologous tissue substitute Y Other device	Z No qualifier
X Upper Bursa and Ligament Y Lower Bursa and Ligament	X External	0 Drainage device 7 Autologous tissue substitute J Synthetic substitute K Nonautologous tissue substitute	Z No qualifier

1ST - 0 Medical and Surgical
2ND - M Bursae and Ligaments
3RD - X TRANSFER

MOVE GROUP: Reattachment, Reposition, Transfer, (Transplantation)
Root Operations that put in/put back or move some/all of a body part.

TRANSFER: Moving, without taking out, all or a portion of a body part to another location to take over the function of all or a portion of a body part.

Explanation: The body part transferred remains connected to its vascular and nervous supply
Examples: Carpal ligament transfer – CMS Ex: Tendon transfer

Body Part – 4TH			Approach – 5TH	Device – 6TH	Qualifier – 7TH
... Bursa and Ligament ... 0 Head and Neck ... 1 Shoulder ..., Right 2 Shoulder ..., Left 3 Elbow ..., Right 4 Elbow ..., Left 5 Wrist ..., Right 6 Wrist ..., Left 7 Hand ..., Right 8 Hand ..., Left	9 Upper Extremity ..., Right B Upper Extremity ..., Left C Upper Spine ... D Lower Spine ... F Sternum ... G Rib(s) ... H Abdomen ..., Right J Abdomen ..., Left K Perineum ...	L Hip ..., Right M Hip ..., Left N Knee ..., Right P Knee ..., Left Q Ankle ..., Right R Ankle ..., Left S Foot ..., Right T Foot ..., Left V Lower Extremity ..., Right W Lower Extremity ..., Left	0 Open 4 Percutaneous endoscopic	Z No device	Z No qualifier

© 2018 Channel Publishing, Ltd.

Educational Annotations | N – Head and Facial Bones

Body System Specific Educational Annotations for the Head and Facial Bones include:

- Anatomy and Physiology Review
- Anatomical Illustrations
- Definitions of Common Procedures
- AHA Coding Clinic® Reference Notations
- Body Part Key Listings
- Device Key Listings
- Device Aggregation Table Listings
- Coding Notes

Anatomy and Physiology Review of Head and Facial Bones

BODY PART VALUES – N - HEAD AND FACIAL BONES

Conchae Bone – The 2 small paired bones of the nasal cavity that are attached to the maxilla.
Ethmoid Bone – The single bone located between the orbits that forms the roof of the nasal cavity, part of the floor of the cranial cavity, and part of the orbit.
Facial Bone – Any one of the 14 bones of the facial area below the cranium (2 nasal bones, vomer, 2 conchae, 2 maxilla, mandible, 2 palatine bones, 2 zygomatic bones, 2 lacrimal bones).
Frontal Bone – The single bone in the front of the skull that also forms part of the roof of the nasal cavity and part of the orbit.
Hyoid Bone – The single horseshoe-shaped bone that lies in the front of the neck and just under the chin and aids in tongue movement and swallowing. It is not directly articulated with any other bone and not considered part of the skull.
Lacrimal Bone – The 2 small paired bones that form the medial side of the orbit and the nasolacrimal canal.
Mandible – The single horseshoe-shaped bone forming the lower jaw.
Maxilla – The 2 fused irregularly-shaped bones that form the upper jaw, the roof of the mouth, and a part of the orbit.
Nasal Bone – The 2 small paired bones that form the bridge of the nose.
Occipital Bone – The single bone of the base and back of the skull.
Orbit – The bones (7) which form the orbit (eye socket): Zygomatic, sphenoid, ethmoid, maxilla, lacrimal, palatine, and frontal.
Palatine Bone – The 2 small paired bones at the back of the nasal cavity that form the floor and lateral wall of the nasal cavity, part of the roof of the mouth, and part of the floor of the orbit.
Parietal Bone – The 2 paired bones that form the top and sides of the skull.
Skull – The skull consists of all (22) of the cranial and facial bones. Eight of these bones form the cranium (occipital bone, frontal bone, 2 temporal bones, 2 parietal bones, sphenoid bone, ethmoid bone), and 14 of these bones form the skull below the cranium (2 nasal bones, vomer, 2 conchae, 2 maxilla, mandible, 2 palatine bones, 2 zygomatic bones, 2 lacrimal bones).
Sphenoid Bone – The single winged-shaped bone of the skull floor that forms part of the base of the cranial cavity, sides of the skull, and part of the orbital floor and side.
Temporal Bone – The 2 paired bones that form the lower sides and base of the skull and contain the internal organs and structures of hearing.
Vomer Bone – The single bone of the inferior nasal septum.
Zygomatic Bone – The 2 paired quadrangular bones of the cheeks (also known as the malar bones) that form the cheek prominence and lower-outer part of the orbit.

Anatomical Illustrations of Head and Facial Bones

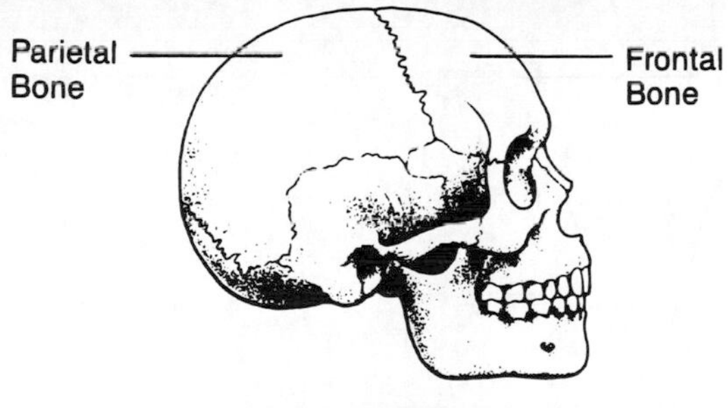

VAULT OF SKULL

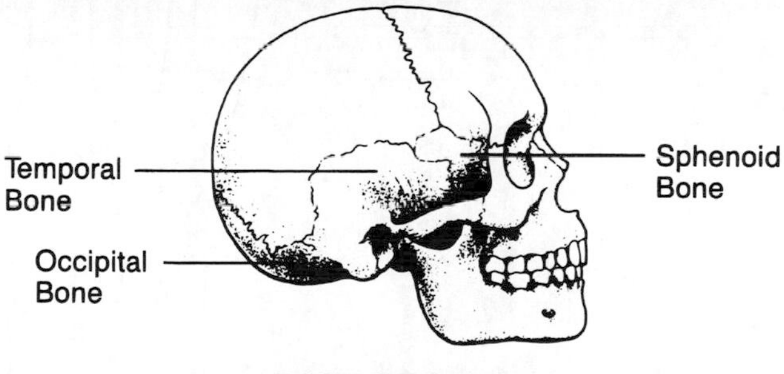

BASE OF SKULL

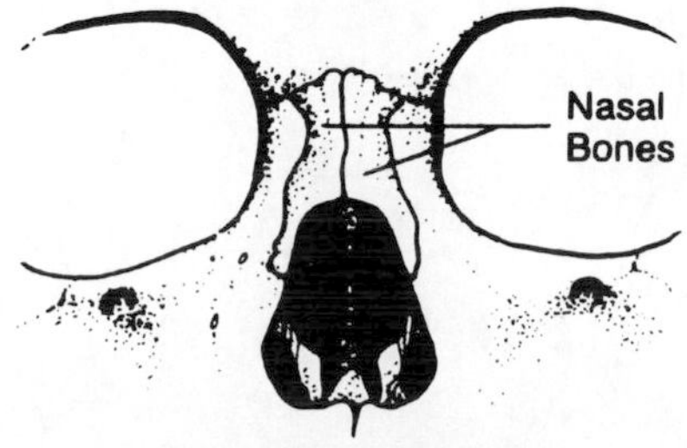

NASAL BONES

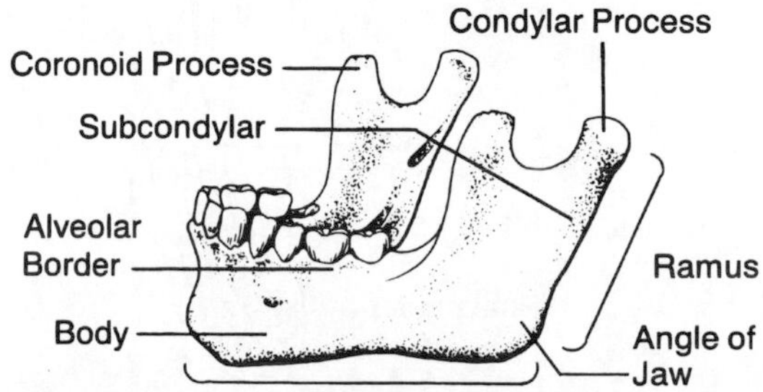

MANDIBLE

Continued on next page

© 2018 Channel Publishing, Ltd.

Educational Annotations | N – Head and Facial Bones

Anatomical Illustrations of Head and Facial Bones

Continued from previous page

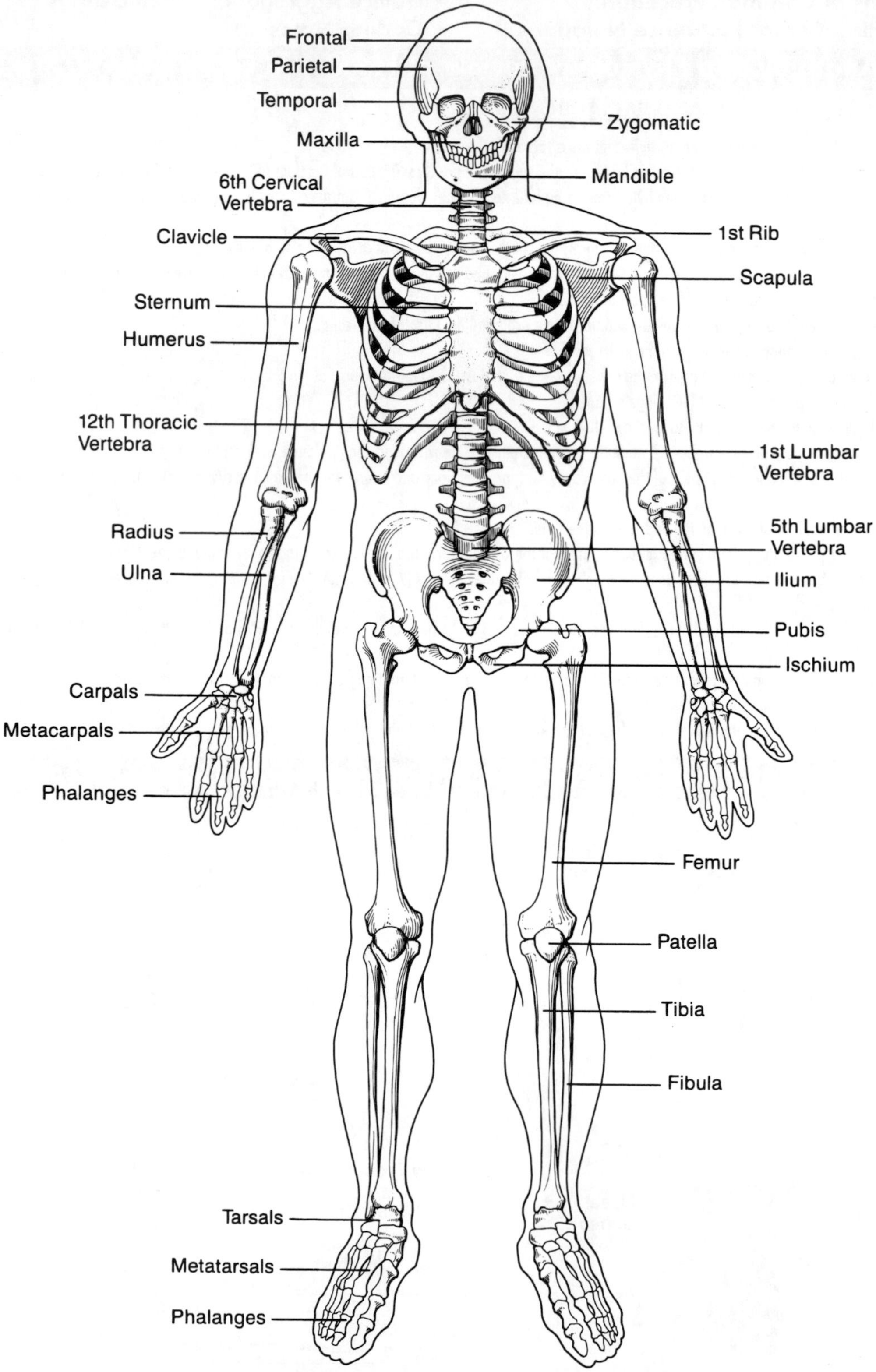

ANTERIOR VIEW OF HUMAN SKELETON

Continued on next page

© 2018 Channel Publishing, Ltd.

Educational Annotations | N – Head and Facial Bones

Anatomical Illustrations of Head and Facial Bones

Continued from previous page

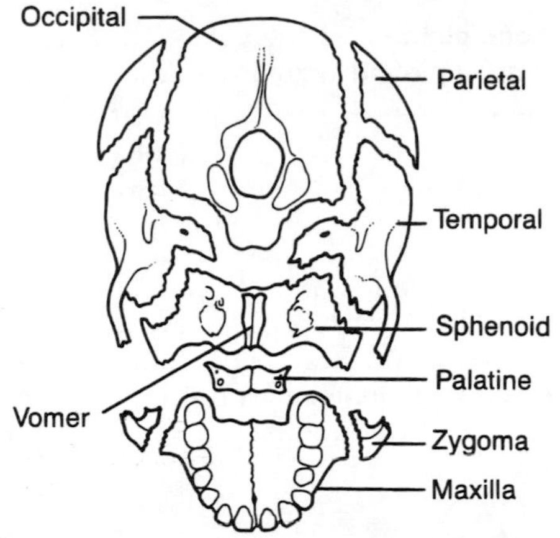

ORBITAL FLOOR AND MALAR BONES

Definitions of Common Procedures of Head and Facial Bones

Cranioplasty – The surgical repair of a skull defect or deformity using the previously excised skull segment, synthetic bone substitute, or synthetic (metal, plastic) plates.

Distraction osteogenesis for craniosynostosis – The surgical repair of prematurely fusing skull bone sutures using osteotomy, bone graft, plates, and an external fixation distractor device to move a portion of skull gradually into a more functional position.

Le Fort I osteotomy – The surgical sectioning (osteotomy) and repositioning of the maxilla along the Le Fort I fracture line to correct dentofacial anomalies of the maxilla.

Le Fort II osteotomy – The surgical sectioning (osteotomy) and repositioning of the maxilla along the Le Fort II fracture line to correct dentofacial anomalies and mid-face hypoplasia.

Le Fort III osteotomy – The surgical sectioning (osteotomy) and repositioning of the maxilla, nose, and cheek bones (zygoma) along the Le Fort III fracture line to correct dentofacial anomalies and mid-face hypoplasia.

Osteotomy – The surgical incision or division of a bone.

AHA Coding Clinic® Reference Notations of Head and Facial Bones

ROOT OPERATION SPECIFIC - N - HEAD AND FACIAL BONES

CHANGE - 2

DESTRUCTION - 5

DIVISION - 8

DRAINAGE - 9

EXCISION - B

- Harvesting of local bone for graft .... AHA 15:1Q:p30
- Nasal adhesion repair of cleft lip and palate .... AHA 17:1Q:p20
- Radical resection of eyelid and orbital tumor .... AHA 15:2Q:p12

EXTIRPATION - C

INSERTION - H

- Insertion of internal fixation device into skull .... AHA 15:3Q:p13

INSPECTION - J

RELEASE - N

REMOVAL - P

- Removal of internal fixation device from skull .... AHA 15:3Q:p13

REPAIR - Q

- Closure of patent alveolar cleft .... AHA 16:3Q:p29

Continued on next page

HEAD & FACIAL BONES 0 N

© 2018 Channel Publishing, Ltd.

Educational Annotations | N – Head and Facial Bones

AHA Coding Clinic® Reference Notations of Head and Facial Bones

ROOT OPERATION SPECIFIC - N - HEAD AND FACIAL BONES

Continued from previous page

REPLACEMENT - R

- Autologous bone graft and titanium bone plate .... AHA 17:1Q:p23
- Bone flap replacement using Lorenz cranial plating system .... AHA 17:3Q:p17
- Hemi-cranioplasty .... AHA 14:3Q:p7

REPOSITION - S

- Cranial vault reconstruction/reshaping .... AHA 15:3Q:p17
- Distraction osteogenesis for craniosynostosis .... AHA 13:3Q:p24
- Le Fort 1 osteotomy .... AHA 14:3Q:p23
- Nasal adhesion repair of cleft lip and palate .... AHA 17:1Q:p20
- Open reduction internal fixation of frontal bone fracture .... AHA 13:3Q:p25
- Raising of cranium .... AHA 15:3Q:p27
- Removal and placement of skull bone flap in abdominal wall .... AHA 16:2Q:p30
- Replacement of skull bone flap....... AHA 17:3Q:p22

RESECTION - T

SUPPLEMENT - U

- Dermal autograft closure of alveolar cleft .... AHA 16:3Q:p29
- Titanium plates to stabilize bone .... AHA 13:3Q:p 24

REVISION - W

Body Part Key Listings of Head and Facial Bones

See also Body Part Key in Appendix C

- Alveolar process of mandible .... use Mandible, Left/Right
- Alveolar process of maxilla .... use Maxilla
- Bony orbit .... use Orbit, Left/Right
- Condyloid process .... use Mandible, Left/Right
- Cribriform plate .... use Ethmoid Bone, Left/Right
- Foramen magnum .... use Occipital Bone
- Greater wing .... use Sphenoid Bone
- Lesser wing .... use Sphenoid Bone
- Mandibular notch .... use Mandible, Left/Right
- Mastoid process .... use Temporal Bone, Left/Right
- Mental foramen .... use Mandible, Left/Right
- Optic foramen .... use Sphenoid Bone
- Orbital portion of ethmoid bone .... use Orbit, Left/Right
- Orbital portion of frontal bone .... use Orbit, Left/Right
- Orbital portion of lacrimal bone .... use Orbit, Left/Right
- Orbital portion of maxilla .... use Orbit, Left/Right
- Orbital portion of palatine bone .... use Orbit, Left/Right
- Orbital portion of sphenoid bone .... use Orbit, Left/Right
- Orbital portion of zygomatic bone .... use Orbit, Left/Right
- Petrous part of temporal bone .... use Temporal Bone, Left/Right
- Pterygoid process .... use Sphenoid Bone
- Sella turcica .... use Sphenoid Bone
- Tympanic part of temporal bone .... use Temporal Bone, Left/Right
- Vomer of nasal septum .... use Nasal Bone
- Zygomatic process of frontal bone .... use Frontal Bone
- Zygomatic process of temporal bone .... use Temporal Bone, Left/Right

Device Key Listings of Head and Facial Bones

See also Device Key in Appendix D

- Autograft .... use Autologous Tissue Substitute
- Bone anchored hearing device .... use Hearing Device in Head and Facial Bones
- Bone bank bone graft .... use Nonautologous Tissue Substitute
- Bone screw (interlocking) (lag) (pedicle) (recessed) .... use Internal Fixation Device in Head and Facial Bones, Upper Bones, Lower Bones
- Electrical bone growth stimulator (EBGS) .... use Bone Growth Stimulator in Head and Facial Bones, Upper Bones, Lower Bones
- External fixator .... use External Fixation Device in Head and Facial Bones, Upper Bones, Lower Bones, Upper Joints, Lower Joints
- Kirschner wire (K-wire) .... use Internal Fixation Device in Head and Facial Bones, Upper Bones, Lower Bones, Upper Joints, Lower Joints
- Neutralization plate .... use Internal Fixation Device in Head and Facial Bones, Upper Bones, Lower Bones
- Polymethylmethacrylate (PMMA) .... use Synthetic Substitute
- RNS system neurostimulator generator .... use Neurostimulator Generator in Head and Facial Bones
- Tissue bank graft .... use Nonautologous Tissue Substitute
- Ultrasonic osteogenic stimulator .... use Bone Growth Stimulator in Head and Facial Bones, Upper Bones, Lower Bones
- Ultrasound bone healing system .... use Bone Growth Stimulator in Head and Facial Bones, Upper Bones, Lower Bones

© 2018 Channel Publishing, Ltd.

Educational Annotations | N – Head and Facial Bones

Device Aggregation Table Listings of Head and Facial Bones

See also Device Aggregation Table in Appendix E

Specific Device	For Operation	In Body System	General Device
None Listed in Device Aggregation Table for this Body System			

Coding Notes of Head and Facial Bones

Body System Relevant Coding Guidelines

Reposition for fracture treatment

B3.15

Reduction of a displaced fracture is coded to the root operation Reposition and the application of a cast or splint in conjunction with the Reposition procedure is not coded separately. Treatment of a nondisplaced fracture is coded to the procedure performed.

Examples: Casting of a nondisplaced fracture is coded to the root operation Immobilization in the Placement section.

Putting a pin in a nondisplaced fracture is coded to the root operation Insertion.

© 2018 Channel Publishing, Ltd.

1ST - 0 Medical and Surgical
2ND - N Head and Facial Bones
3RD - 2 CHANGE

DEVICE GROUP: Change, Insertion, Removal, Replacement, Revision, Supplement
Root Operations that always involve a device.

CHANGE: Taking out or off a device from a body part and putting back an identical or similar device in or on the same body part without cutting or puncturing the skin or a mucous membrane.

Explanation: All CHANGE procedures are coded using the approach External
Examples: Exchange drain tube – CMS Ex: Urinary catheter change

Body Part – 4TH	Approach – 5TH	Device – 6TH	Qualifier – 7TH
0 Skull B Nasal Bone W Facial Bone	X External	0 Drainage device Y Other device	Z No qualifier

1ST - 0 Medical and Surgical
2ND - N Head and Facial Bones
3RD - 5 DESTRUCTION

EXCISION GROUP: Excision, Resection, Destruction, Extraction, (Detachment)
Root Operations that take out some or all of a body part.

DESTRUCTION: Physical eradication of all or a portion of a body part by the direct use of energy, force, or a destructive agent.

Explanation: None of the body part is physically taken out
Examples: Cryoablation bone cyst – CMS Ex: Fulguration of rectal polyp

Body Part – 4TH			Approach – 5TH	Device – 6TH	Qualifier – 7TH
0 Skull 1 Frontal Bone 3 Parietal Bone, Right 4 Parietal Bone, Left 5 Temporal Bone, Right 6 Temporal Bone, Left 7 Occipital Bone B Nasal Bone	C Sphenoid Bone F Ethmoid Bone, Right G Ethmoid Bone, Left H Lacrimal Bone, Right J Lacrimal Bone, Left K Palatine Bone, Right L Palatine Bone, Left	M Zygomatic Bone, Right N Zygomatic Bone, Left P Orbit, Right Q Orbit, Left R Maxilla T Mandible, Right V Mandible, Left X Hyoid Bone	0 Open 3 Percutaneous 4 Percutaneous endoscopic	Z No device	Z No qualifier

HEAD & FACIAL BONES 0 N 2

1ST - 0 Medical and Surgical
2ND - N Head and Facial Bones
3RD - 8 DIVISION

DIVISION GROUP: Division, Release
Root Operations involving cutting or separation only.

DIVISION: Cutting into a body part, without draining fluids and/or gases from the body part, in order to separate or transect a body part.

Explanation: All or a portion of the body part is separated into two or more portions
Examples: Mandibular osteotomy – CMS Ex: Spinal cordotomy

Body Part – 4TH			Approach – 5TH	Device – 6TH	Qualifier – 7TH
0 Skull 1 Frontal Bone 3 Parietal Bone, Right 4 Parietal Bone, Left 5 Temporal Bone, Right 6 Temporal Bone, Left 7 Occipital Bone B Nasal Bone	C Sphenoid Bone F Ethmoid Bone, Right G Ethmoid Bone, Left H Lacrimal Bone, Right J Lacrimal Bone, Left K Palatine Bone, Right L Palatine Bone, Left	M Zygomatic Bone, Right N Zygomatic Bone, Left P Orbit, Right Q Orbit, Left R Maxilla T Mandible, Right V Mandible, Left X Hyoid Bone	0 Open 3 Percutaneous 4 Percutaneous endoscopic	Z No device	Z No qualifier

© 2018 Channel Publishing, Ltd.

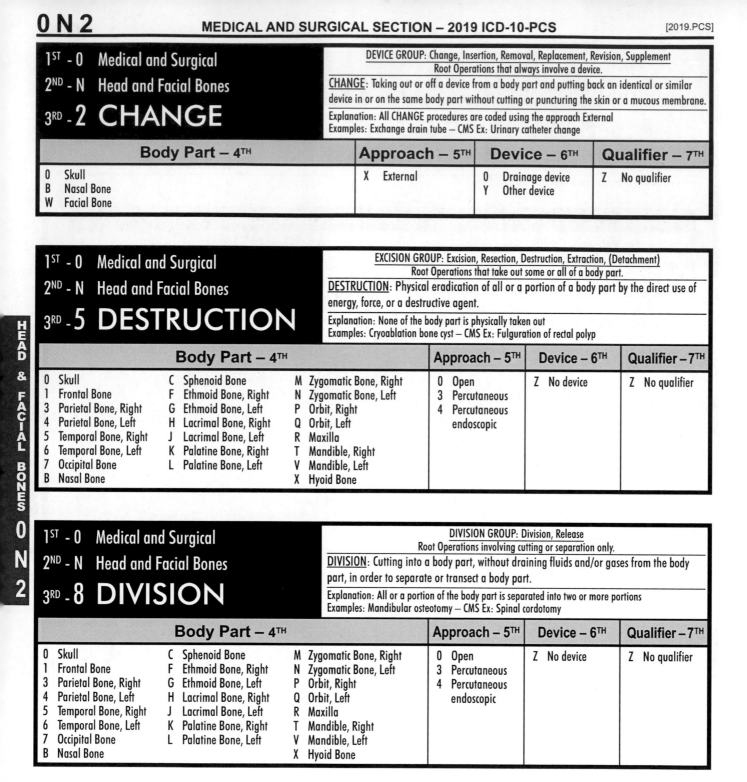

1ST - 0 Medical and Surgical
2ND - N Head and Facial Bones
3RD - 9 DRAINAGE

DRAINAGE GROUP: Drainage, Extirpation, (Fragmentation)
Root Operations that take out solids/fluids/gases from a body part.

DRAINAGE: Taking or letting out fluids and/or gases from a body part.

Explanation: Qualifier "X Diagnostic" indicates drainage procedures that are biopsies
Examples: Aspiration bone cyst – CMS Ex: Thoracentesis

Body Part – 4TH			Approach – 5TH	Device – 6TH	Qualifier – 7TH
0 Skull 1 Frontal Bone 3 Parietal Bone, Right 4 Parietal Bone, Left 5 Temporal Bone, Right 6 Temporal Bone, Left 7 Occipital Bone B Nasal Bone	C Sphenoid Bone F Ethmoid Bone, Right G Ethmoid Bone, Left H Lacrimal Bone, Right J Lacrimal Bone, Left K Palatine Bone, Right L Palatine Bone, Left	M Zygomatic Bone, Right N Zygomatic Bone, Left P Orbit, Right Q Orbit, Left R Maxilla T Mandible, Right V Mandible, Left X Hyoid Bone	0 Open 3 Percutaneous 4 Percutaneous endoscopic	0 Drainage device	Z No qualifier
0 Skull 1 Frontal Bone 3 Parietal Bone, Right 4 Parietal Bone, Left 5 Temporal Bone, Right 6 Temporal Bone, Left 7 Occipital Bone B Nasal Bone	C Sphenoid Bone F Ethmoid Bone, Right G Ethmoid Bone, Left H Lacrimal Bone, Right J Lacrimal Bone, Left K Palatine Bone, Right L Palatine Bone, Left	M Zygomatic Bone, Right N Zygomatic Bone, Left P Orbit, Right Q Orbit, Left R Maxilla T Mandible, Right V Mandible, Left X Hyoid Bone	0 Open 3 Percutaneous 4 Percutaneous endoscopic	Z No device	X Diagnostic Z No qualifier

1ST - 0 Medical and Surgical
2ND - N Head and Facial Bones
3RD - B EXCISION

EXCISION GROUP: Excision, Resection, Destruction, Extraction, (Detachment)
Root Operations that take out some or all of a body part.

EXCISION: Cutting out or off, without replacement, a portion of a body part.

Explanation: Qualifier "X Diagnostic" indicates excision procedures that are biopsies
Examples: Mandibular sequestrectomy – CMS Ex: Liver biopsy

Body Part – 4TH			Approach – 5TH	Device – 6TH	Qualifier – 7TH
0 Skull 1 Frontal Bone 3 Parietal Bone, Right 4 Parietal Bone, Left 5 Temporal Bone, Right 6 Temporal Bone, Left 7 Occipital Bone B Nasal Bone	C Sphenoid Bone F Ethmoid Bone, Right G Ethmoid Bone, Left H Lacrimal Bone, Right J Lacrimal Bone, Left K Palatine Bone, Right L Palatine Bone, Left	M Zygomatic Bone, Right N Zygomatic Bone, Left P Orbit, Right Q Orbit, Left R Maxilla T Mandible, Right V Mandible, Left X Hyoid Bone	0 Open 3 Percutaneous 4 Percutaneous endoscopic	Z No device	X Diagnostic Z No qualifier

1ST - 0 Medical and Surgical
2ND - N Head and Facial Bones
3RD - C EXTIRPATION

DRAINAGE GROUP: Drainage, Extirpation, (Fragmentation)
Root Operations that take out solids/fluids/gases from a body part.

EXTIRPATION: Taking or cutting out solid matter from a body part.

Explanation: Abnormal byproduct or foreign body ...
Examples: Removal foreign body – CMS Ex: Thrombectomy

Body Part – 4TH			Approach – 5TH	Device – 6TH	Qualifier – 7TH
1 Frontal Bone 3 Parietal Bone, Right 4 Parietal Bone, Left 5 Temporal Bone, Right 6 Temporal Bone, Left 7 Occipital Bone B Nasal Bone	C Sphenoid Bone F Ethmoid Bone, Right G Ethmoid Bone, Left H Lacrimal Bone, Right J Lacrimal Bone, Left K Palatine Bone, Right L Palatine Bone, Left	M Zygomatic Bone, Right N Zygomatic Bone, Left P Orbit, Right Q Orbit, Left R Maxilla T Mandible, Right V Mandible, Left X Hyoid Bone	0 Open 3 Percutaneous 4 Percutaneous endoscopic	Z No device	Z No qualifier

© 2018 Channel Publishing, Ltd.

1ST - 0 Medical and Surgical
2ND - N Head and Facial Bones
3RD - D EXTRACTION

EXCISION GROUP: Excision, Resection, Destruction, Extraction, (Detachment)
Root Operations that take out some or all of a body part.

EXTRACTION: Pulling or stripping out or off all or a portion of a body part by the use of force.

Explanation: None for this Body System
Examples: Non-excisional debridement – CMS Ex: Dilation and curettage

Body Part – 4TH			Approach – 5TH	Device – 6TH	Qualifier – 7TH
0 Skull 1 Frontal Bone 3 Parietal Bone, Right 4 Parietal Bone, Left 5 Temporal Bone, Right 6 Temporal Bone, Left 7 Occipital Bone B Nasal Bone	C Sphenoid Bone F Ethmoid Bone, Right G Ethmoid Bone, Left H Lacrimal Bone, Right J Lacrimal Bone, Left K Palatine Bone, Right L Palatine Bone, Left	M Zygomatic Bone, Right N Zygomatic Bone, Left P Orbit, Right Q Orbit, Left R Maxilla T Mandible, Right V Mandible, Left X Hyoid Bone	0 Open	Z No device	Z No qualifier

1ST - 0 Medical and Surgical
2ND - N Head and Facial Bones
3RD - H INSERTION

DEVICE GROUP: Change, Insertion, Removal, Replacement, Revision, Supplement
Root Operations that always involve a device.

INSERTION: Putting in a nonbiological appliance that monitors, assists, performs, or prevents a physiological function but does not physically take the place of a body part.

Explanation: None
Examples: Insertion bone growth stimulator – CMS Ex: Insertion of central venous catheter

Body Part – 4TH		Approach – 5TH	Device – 6TH	Qualifier – 7TH
0 Skull		0 Open	4 Internal fixation device 5 External fixation device M Bone growth stimulator N Neurostimulator generator	Z No qualifier
0 Skull		3 Percutaneous 4 Percutaneous endoscopic	4 Internal fixation device 5 External fixation device M Bone growth stimulator	Z No qualifier
1 Frontal Bone 3 Parietal Bone, Right 4 Parietal Bone, Left 7 Occipital Bone C Sphenoid Bone F Ethmoid Bone, Right G Ethmoid Bone, Left H Lacrimal Bone, Right	J Lacrimal Bone, Left K Palatine Bone, Right L Palatine Bone, Left M Zygomatic Bone, Right N Zygomatic Bone, Left P Orbit, Right Q Orbit, Left X Hyoid Bone	0 Open 3 Percutaneous 4 Percutaneous endoscopic	4 Internal fixation device	Z No qualifier
5 Temporal Bone, Right 6 Temporal Bone, Left		0 Open 3 Percutaneous 4 Percutaneous endoscopic	4 Internal fixation device S Hearing device	Z No qualifier
B Nasal Bone		0 Open 3 Percutaneous 4 Percutaneous endoscopic	4 Internal fixation device M Bone growth stimulator	Z No qualifier
R Maxilla T Mandible, Right V Mandible, Left		0 Open 3 Percutaneous 4 Percutaneous endoscopic	4 Internal fixation device 5 External fixation device	Z No qualifier
W Facial Bone		0 Open 3 Percutaneous 4 Percutaneous endoscopic	M Bone growth stimulator	Z No qualifier

© 2018 Channel Publishing, Ltd.

1ST - 0 Medical and Surgical
2ND - N Head and Facial Bones
3RD - J INSPECTION

EXAMINATION GROUP: Inspection, (Map)
Root Operations involving examination only.

INSPECTION: Visually and/or manually exploring a body part.

Explanation: Direct or instrumental visualization ...
Examples: Examination facial bones – CMS Ex: Exploratory laparotomy

Body Part – 4TH	Approach – 5TH	Device – 6TH	Qualifier – 7TH
0 Skull B Nasal Bone W Facial Bone	0 Open 3 Percutaneous 4 Percutaneous endoscopic X External	Z No device	Z No qualifier

1ST - 0 Medical and Surgical
2ND - N Head and Facial Bones
3RD - N RELEASE

DIVISION GROUP: Division, Release
Root Operations involving cutting or separation only.

RELEASE: Freeing a body part from an abnormal physical constraint by cutting or by the use of force.

Explanation: Some of the restraining tissue may be taken out but none of the body part is taken out
Examples: Extra-articular bone adhesiolysis – CMS Ex: Carpal tunnel release

Body Part – 4TH			Approach – 5TH	Device – 6TH	Qualifier – 7TH
1 Frontal Bone 3 Parietal Bone, Right 4 Parietal Bone, Left 5 Temporal Bone, Right 6 Temporal Bone, Left 7 Occipital Bone B Nasal Bone	C Sphenoid Bone F Ethmoid Bone, Right G Ethmoid Bone, Left H Lacrimal Bone, Right J Lacrimal Bone, Left K Palatine Bone, Right L Palatine Bone, Left	M Zygomatic Bone, Right N Zygomatic Bone, Left P Orbit, Right Q Orbit, Left R Maxilla T Mandible, Right V Mandible, Left X Hyoid Bone	0 Open 3 Percutaneous 4 Percutaneous endoscopic	Z No device	Z No qualifier

HEAD & FACIAL BONES 0 N N

© 2018 Channel Publishing, Ltd.

1ST - 0 Medical and Surgical
2ND - N Head and Facial Bones
3RD - P REMOVAL

DEVICE GROUP: Change, Insertion, Removal, Replacement, Revision, Supplement
Root Operations that always involve a device.

REMOVAL: Taking out or off a device from a body part.

Explanation: Removal device without reinsertion ...
Examples: Removal bone growth stimulator – CMS Ex: Cardiac pacemaker removal

Body Part – 4TH	Approach – 5TH	Device – 6TH	Qualifier – 7TH
0 Skull	0 Open	0 Drainage device 4 Internal fixation device 5 External fixation device 7 Autologous tissue substitute J Synthetic substitute K Nonautologous tissue substitute M Bone growth stimulator N Neurostimulator generator S Hearing device	Z No qualifier
0 Skull	3 Percutaneous 4 Percutaneous endoscopic	0 Drainage device 4 Internal fixation device 5 External fixation device 7 Autologous tissue substitute J Synthetic substitute K Nonautologous tissue substitute M Bone growth stimulator S Hearing device	Z No qualifier
0 Skull	X External	0 Drainage device 4 Internal fixation device 5 External fixation device M Bone growth stimulator S Hearing device	Z No qualifier
B Nasal Bone W Facial Bone	0 Open 3 Percutaneous 4 Percutaneous endoscopic	0 Drainage device 4 Internal fixation device 7 Autologous tissue substitute J Synthetic substitute K Nonautologous tissue substitute M Bone growth stimulator	Z No qualifier
B Nasal Bone W Facial Bone	X External	0 Drainage device 4 Internal fixation device M Bone growth stimulator	Z No qualifier

1ST - 0 Medical and Surgical
2ND - N Head and Facial Bones
3RD - Q REPAIR

OTHER REPAIRS GROUP: (Control), Repair
Root Operations that define other repairs.

REPAIR: Restoring, to the extent possible, a body part to its normal anatomic structure and function.

Explanation: Used only when the method to accomplish the repair is not one of the other root operations
Examples: Oribtal osteoplasty – CMS Ex: Suture of laceration

Body Part – 4TH			Approach – 5TH	Device – 6TH	Qualifier – 7TH
0 Skull 1 Frontal Bone 3 Parietal Bone, Right 4 Parietal Bone, Left 5 Temporal Bone, Right 6 Temporal Bone, Left 7 Occipital Bone B Nasal Bone	C Sphenoid Bone F Ethmoid Bone, Right G Ethmoid Bone, Left H Lacrimal Bone, Right J Lacrimal Bone, Left K Palatine Bone, Right L Palatine Bone, Left	M Zygomatic Bone, Right N Zygomatic Bone, Left P Orbit, Right Q Orbit, Left R Maxilla T Mandible, Right V Mandible, Left X Hyoid Bone	0 Open 3 Percutaneous 4 Percutaneous endoscopic X External	Z No device	Z No qualifier

HEAD & FACIAL BONES 0NP

© 2018 Channel Publishing, Ltd.

1ST - 0 Medical and Surgical
2ND - N Head and Facial Bones
3RD - R REPLACEMENT

DEVICE GROUP: Change, Insertion, Removal, Replacement, Revision, Supplement
Root Operations that always involve a device.

REPLACEMENT: Putting in or on biological or synthetic material that physically takes the place and/or function of all or a portion of a body part.

Explanation: Includes taking out or eradicating, or rendering non-functional, the body part ...
Examples: Hemi-cranioplasty defect repair with graft – CMS Ex: Total hip replacement

Body Part – 4TH			Approach – 5TH	Device – 6TH	Qualifier – 7TH
0 Skull 1 Frontal Bone 3 Parietal Bone, Right 4 Parietal Bone, Left 5 Temporal Bone, Right 6 Temporal Bone, Left 7 Occipital Bone B Nasal Bone	C Sphenoid Bone F Ethmoid Bone, Right G Ethmoid Bone, Left H Lacrimal Bone, Right J Lacrimal Bone, Left K Palatine Bone, Right L Palatine Bone, Left	M Zygomatic Bone, Right N Zygomatic Bone, Left P Orbit, Right Q Orbit, Left R Maxilla T Mandible, Right V Mandible, Left X Hyoid Bone	0 Open 3 Percutaneous 4 Percutaneous endoscopic	7 Autologous tissue substitute J Synthetic substitute K Nonautologous tissue substitute	Z No qualifier

1ST - 0 Medical and Surgical
2ND - N Head and Facial Bones
3RD - S REPOSITION

MOVE GROUP: (Reattachment), Reposition, (Transfer), (Transplantation)
Root Operations that put in/put back or move some/all of a body part.

REPOSITION: Moving to its normal location, or other suitable location, all or a portion of a body part.

Explanation: The body part may or may not be cut out or off to be moved to the new location ...
Examples: Le Fort 1 maxillary osteotomy – CMS Ex: Fracture reduction

Body Part – 4TH			Approach – 5TH	Device – 6TH	Qualifier – 7TH
0 Skull R Maxilla T Mandible, Right V Mandible, Left			0 Open 3 Percutaneous 4 Percutaneous endoscopic	4 Internal fixation device 5 External fixation device Z No device	Z No qualifier
0 Skull R Maxilla T Mandible, Right V Mandible, Left			X External	Z No device	Z No qualifier
1 Frontal Bone 3 Parietal Bone, Right 4 Parietal Bone, Left 5 Temporal Bone, Right 6 Temporal Bone, Left 7 Occipital Bone B Nasal Bone	C Sphenoid Bone F Ethmoid Bone, Right G Ethmoid Bone, Left H Lacrimal Bone, Right J Lacrimal Bone, Left K Palatine Bone, Right L Palatine Bone, Left	M Zygomatic Bone, Right N Zygomatic Bone, Left P Orbit, Right Q Orbit, Left X Hyoid Bone	0 Open 3 Percutaneous 4 Percutaneous endoscopic	4 Internal fixation device Z No device	Z No qualifier
1 Frontal Bone 3 Parietal Bone, Right 4 Parietal Bone, Left 5 Temporal Bone, Right 6 Temporal Bone, Left 7 Occipital Bone B Nasal Bone	C Sphenoid Bone F Ethmoid Bone, Right G Ethmoid Bone, Left H Lacrimal Bone, Right J Lacrimal Bone, Left K Palatine Bone, Right L Palatine Bone, Left	M Zygomatic Bone, Right N Zygomatic Bone, Left P Orbit, Right Q Orbit, Left X Hyoid Bone	X External	Z No device	Z No qualifier

© 2018 Channel Publishing, Ltd.

1ST - 0 Medical and Surgical
2ND - N Head and Facial Bones
3RD - T RESECTION

EXCISION GROUP: Excision, Resection, Destruction, Extraction, (Detachment)
Root Operations that take out some or all of a body part.

RESECTION: Cutting out or off, without replacement, all of a body part.

Explanation: None
Examples: Total removal hyoid bone – CMS Ex: Total lobectomy of lung

Body Part – 4TH			Approach – 5TH	Device – 6TH	Qualifier – 7TH
1 Frontal Bone 3 Parietal Bone, Right 4 Parietal Bone, Left 5 Temporal Bone, Right 6 Temporal Bone, Left 7 Occipital Bone B Nasal Bone	C Sphenoid Bone F Ethmoid Bone, Right G Ethmoid Bone, Left H Lacrimal Bone, Right J Lacrimal Bone, Left K Palatine Bone, Right L Palatine Bone, Left	M Zygomatic Bone, Right N Zygomatic Bone, Left P Orbit, Right Q Orbit, Left R Maxilla T Mandible, Right V Mandible, Left X Hyoid Bone	0 Open	Z No device	Z No qualifier

1ST - 0 Medical and Surgical
2ND - N Head and Facial Bones
3RD - U SUPPLEMENT

DEVICE GROUP: Change, Insertion, Removal, Replacement, Revision, Supplement
Root Operations that always involve a device.

SUPPLEMENT: Putting in or on biological or synthetic material that physically reinforces and/or augments the function of a portion of a body part.

Explanation: Biological material is non-living, or is living and from the same individual ...
Examples: Stabilizing plate for occipital bone defect – CMS Ex: Herniorrhaphy using mesh

Body Part – 4TH			Approach – 5TH	Device – 6TH	Qualifier – 7TH
0 Skull 1 Frontal Bone 3 Parietal Bone, Right 4 Parietal Bone, Left 5 Temporal Bone, Right 6 Temporal Bone, Left 7 Occipital Bone B Nasal Bone	C Sphenoid Bone F Ethmoid Bone, Right G Ethmoid Bone, Left H Lacrimal Bone, Right J Lacrimal Bone, Left K Palatine Bone, Right L Palatine Bone, Left	M Zygomatic Bone, Right N Zygomatic Bone, Left P Orbit, Right Q Orbit, Left R Maxilla T Mandible, Right V Mandible, Left X Hyoid Bone	0 Open 3 Percutaneous 4 Percutaneous endoscopic	7 Autologous tissue substitute J Synthetic substitute K Nonautologous tissue substitute	Z No qualifier

1ST - 0 Medical and Surgical
2ND - N Head and Facial Bones
3RD - W REVISION

DEVICE GROUP: Change, Insertion, Removal, Replacement, Revision, Supplement
Root Operations that always involve a device.

REVISION: Correcting, to the extent possible, a portion of a malfunctioning device or the position of a displaced device.

Explanation: Correcting by taking out or putting in components of a device such as a screw or pin ...
Examples: Reposition bone stimulator – CMS Ex: Recementing of hip prosthesis

Body Part – 4TH	Approach – 5TH	Device – 6TH	Qualifier – 7TH
0 Skull	0 Open	0 Drainage device 4 Internal fixation device 5 External fixation device 7 Autologous tissue substitute J Synthetic substitute K Nonautologous tissue substitute M Bone growth stimulator N Neurostimulator generator S Hearing device	Z No qualifier
0 Skull	3 Percutaneous 4 Percutaneous endoscopic X External	0 Drainage device 4 Internal fixation device 5 External fixation device 7 Autologous tissue substitute J Synthetic substitute K Nonautologous tissue substitute M Bone growth stimulator S Hearing device	Z No qualifier
B Nasal Bone W Facial Bone	0 Open 3 Percutaneous 4 Percutaneous endoscopic X External	0 Drainage device 4 Internal fixation device 7 Autologous tissue substitute J Synthetic substitute K Nonautologous tissue substitute M Bone growth stimulator	Z No qualifier

© 2018 Channel Publishing, Ltd.

Educational Annotations | P – Upper Bones

Body System Specific Educational Annotations for the Upper Bones include:

- Anatomy and Physiology Review
- Definitions of Common Procedures
- Anatomical Illustrations
- AHA Coding Clinic® Reference Notations
- Body Part Key Listings
- Device Key Listings
- Device Aggregation Table Listings
- Coding Notes

Anatomy and Physiology Review of Upper Bones

BODY PART VALUES – P - UPPER BONES

Carpal – The 8 compact bones of the wrist, forming 2 rows of 4 bones each. The proximal row contains the scaphoid, lunate, pisiform, and triquetrum. The distal row contains the trapezium, trapezoid, capitate, and hamate.
Cervical Vertebra – The cervical section of the spinal vertebral column comprised of 7 vertebra, C1-C7.
Clavicle – The paired, straightened S-shaped bones (also known as the collarbones) that connect the sternum with the scapula.
Finger Phalanx – The digital bones of the fingers. Each finger contains three bones: Proximal phalanx, intermediate (middle) phalanx, and distal phalanx.
Glenoid Cavity – The shallow, round depression of the scapula that articulates with the humeral head.
Humeral Head – The upper end of the humerus that is part of the shoulder joint.
Humeral Shaft – The middle, long portion of the humerus.
Humerus – The paired, long bones of the upper arm that articulate at the shoulder and the elbow. The capitulum of the humerus articulates with the head of the radius, and the trochlea of the humerus articulates with the trochlear notch of the ulna.
Metacarpal – One of the 5 cylindrical bones of the palm of the hand connecting the carpals to the phalanges of the hand.
Radius – The paired long bones of the forearms that are further away from the body than the ulnas.
Rib – The 12 paired arched bones of the rib cage that partially enclose and protect the chest cavity.
Scapula – The paired flat, triangular bones located in the upper back behind the shoulder (also called the shoulder blade).
Sternum – The long flat bone (also known as the breast bone) of the chest that connects to the clavicles and most of the ribs.
Thoracic Vertebra – The thoracic section of the spinal vertebral column comprised of 12 vertebra, T1-T12.
Thumb Phalanx – The digital bones of the thumb. The thumb contains two bones: Proximal phalanx and distal phalanx.
Ulna – The paired long bones of the forearms that are closer to the side of the body than the radii.
Upper Bone – Any of the bones designated in the Upper Bones PCS Body System.

Definitions of Common Procedures of Upper Bones

Laminectomy – The surgical excision of the lamina of a vertebra, usually to relieve spinal cord compression.
Open reduction, internal fixation of Colles' fracture – The open surgical repositioning of a fracture of the distal radius using internal fixation device(s) (plate, screws, pins).
Subacromial decompression (acromioplasty) – The surgical shaving of the undersurface of the acromial process of the scapula to create more space for the shoulder's soft tissue and reduce the pain of subacromial impingement syndrome.
Total claviculectomy – The surgical removal of the entire clavicle bone.
Vertebroplasty – The surgical injection of bone cement into a fractured vertebra.

Anatomical Illustrations of Upper Bones

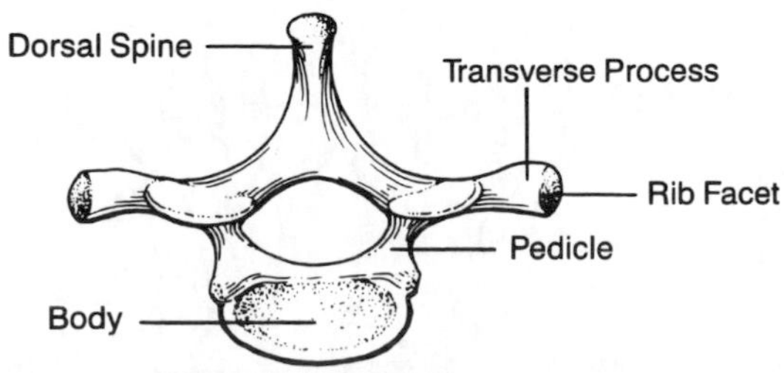

TYPICAL VERTEBRA — SUPERIOR VIEW

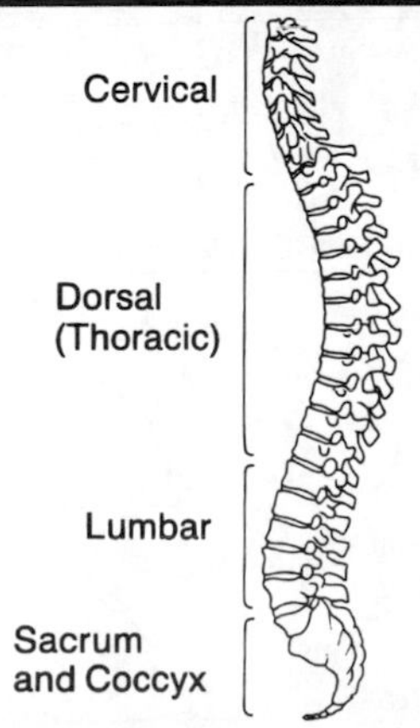

VERTEBRAL COLUMN

Continued on next page

© 2018 Channel Publishing, Ltd.

Educational Annotations | P – Upper Bones

Anatomical Illustrations of Upper Bones

Continued from previous page

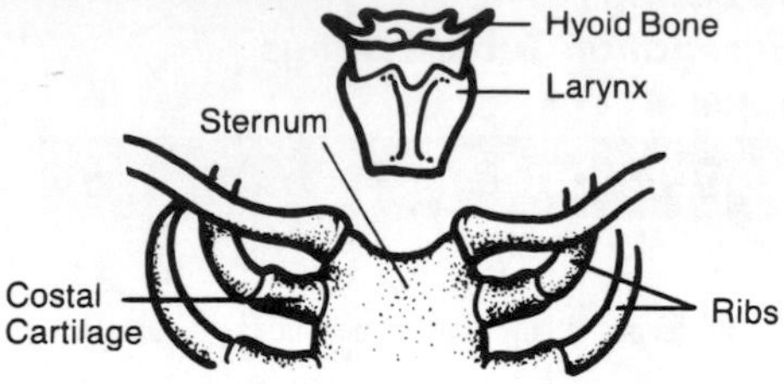

RIBS, STERNUM AND LARYNX

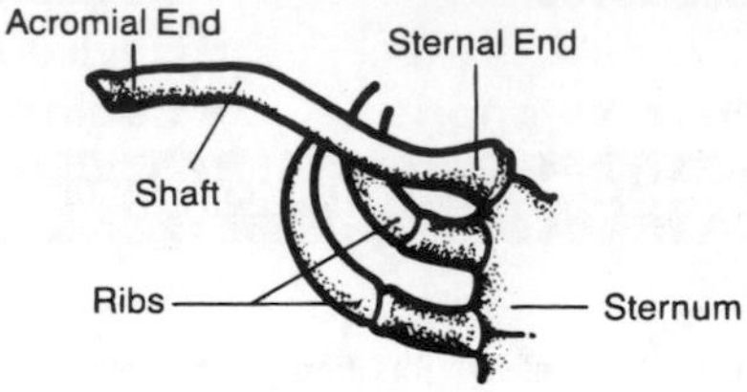

CLAVICLE

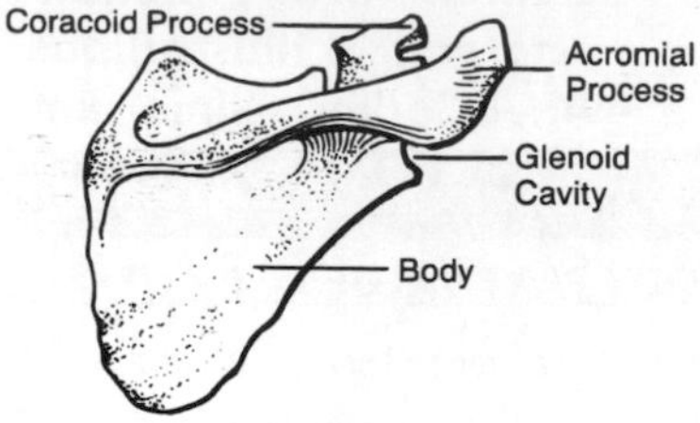

SCAPULA

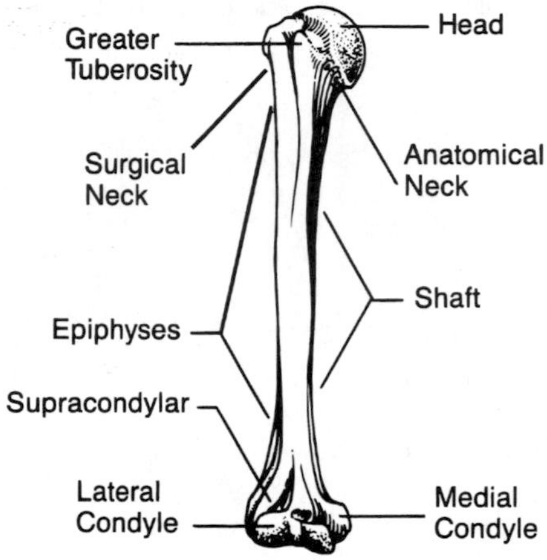

HUMERUS — ANTERIOR VIEW

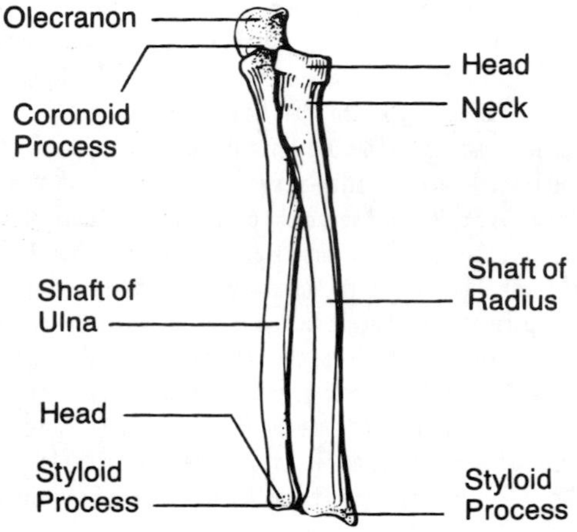

RADIUS AND ULNA — ANTERIOR VIEW

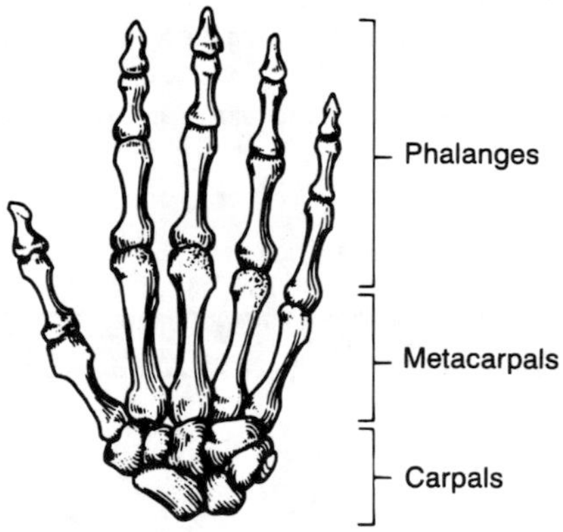

RIGHT HAND — DORSAL VIEW

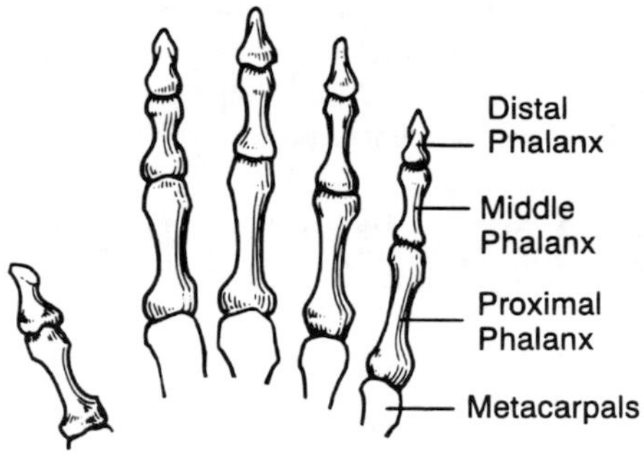

PHALANGES OF HAND

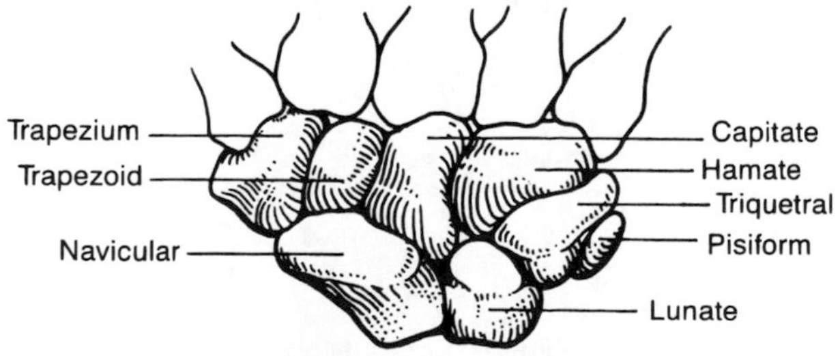

CARPAL BONES — DORSAL VIEW

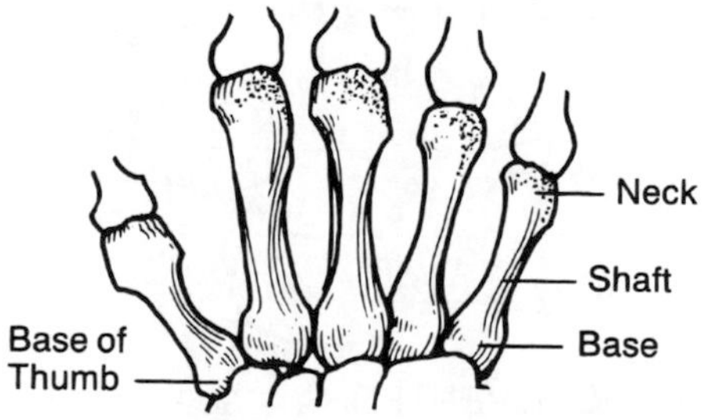

METACARPAL BONES

Continued on next page

UPPER BONES 0P

© 2018 Channel Publishing, Ltd.

Educational Annotations | P – Upper Bones

Anatomical Illustrations of Upper Bones

Continued from previous page

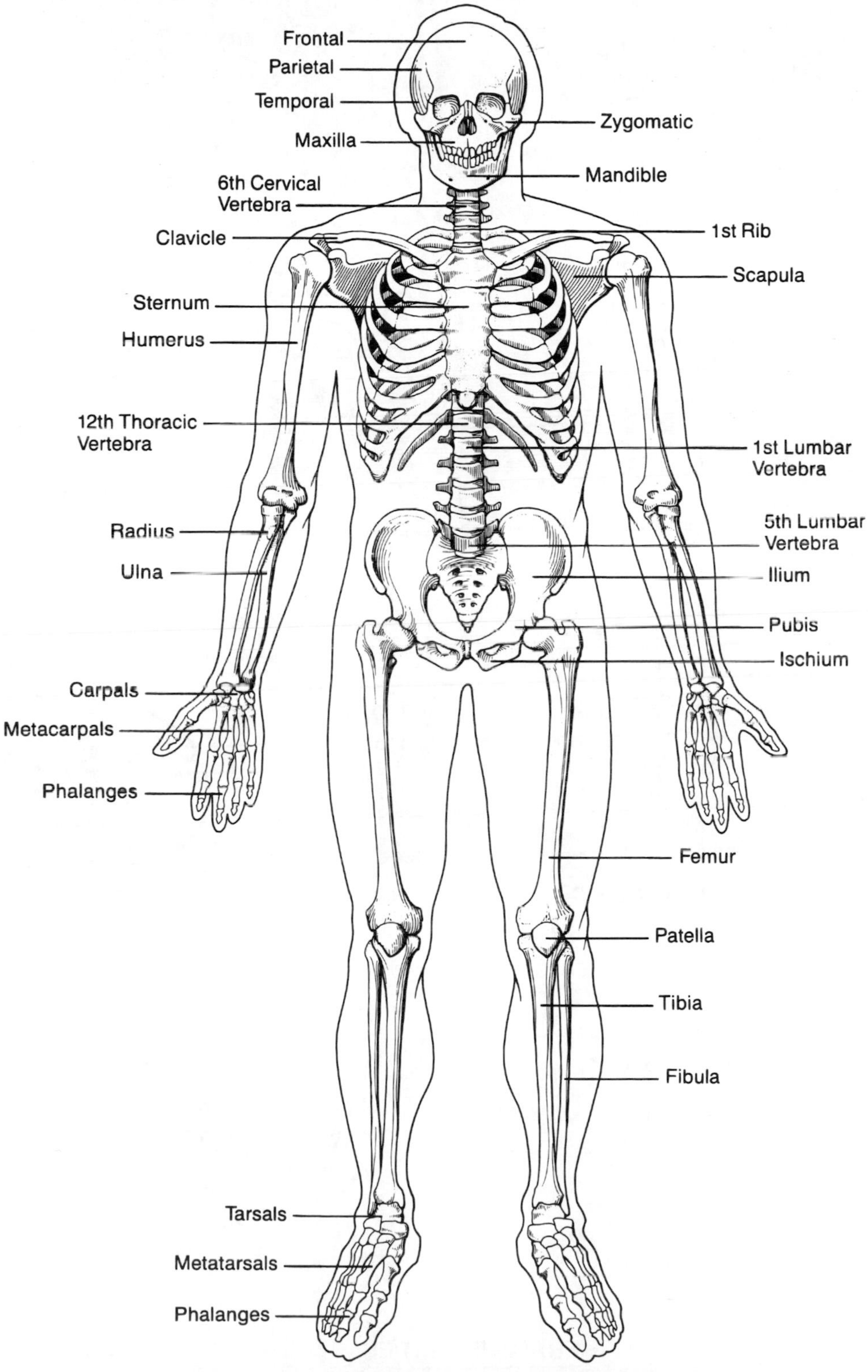

ANTERIOR VIEW OF HUMAN SKELETON

Continued on next page

© 2018 Channel Publishing, Ltd.

Educational Annotations | P – Upper Bones

Anatomical Illustrations of Upper Bones

Continued from previous page

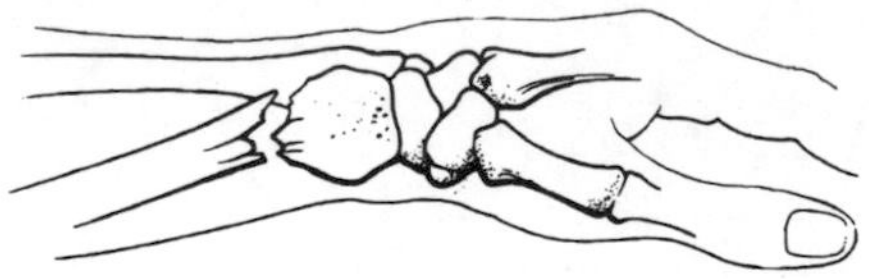

COLLES'

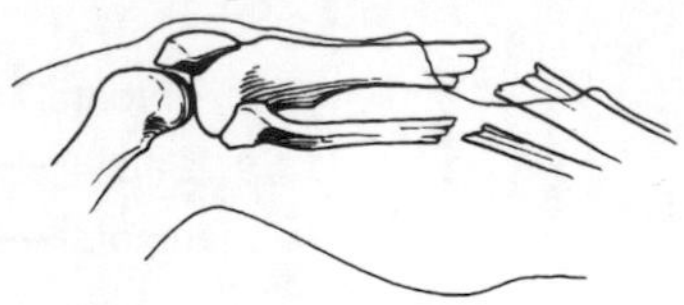

COMPOUND

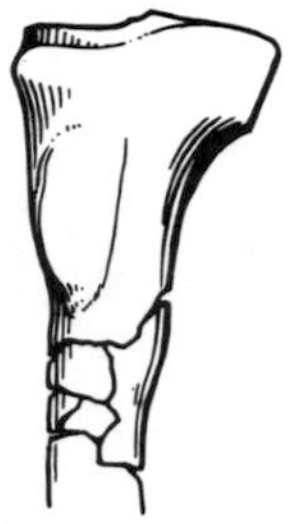

COMMINUTED

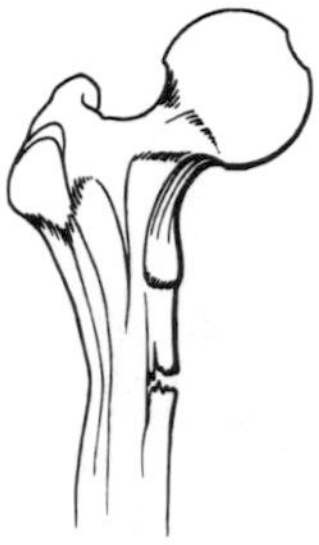

GREENSTICK

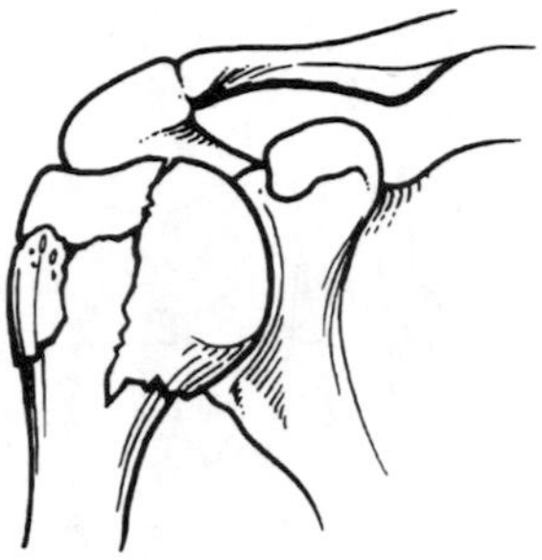

IMPACTED

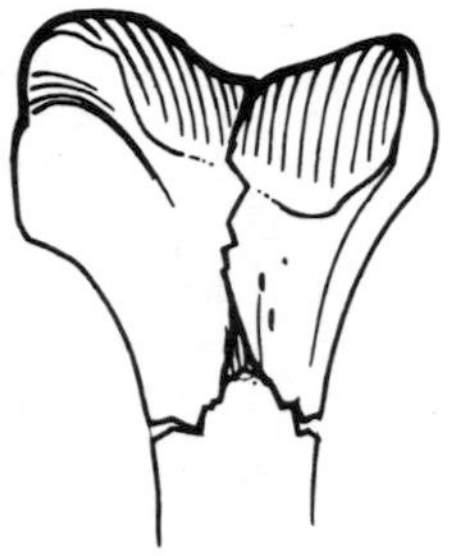

INTERCONDYLAR

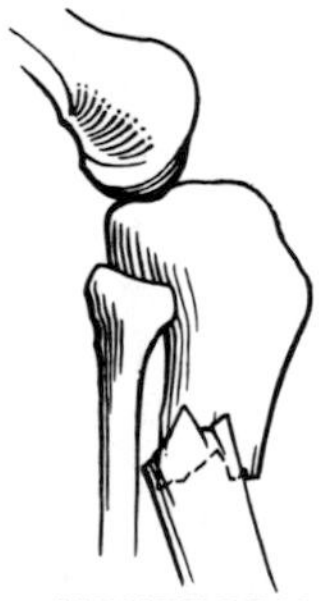

MONTEGGIA

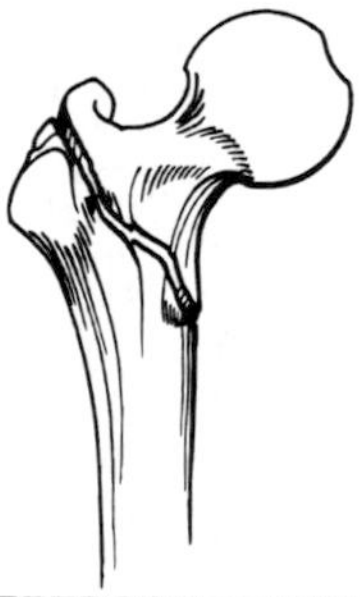

PERTROCHANTERIC

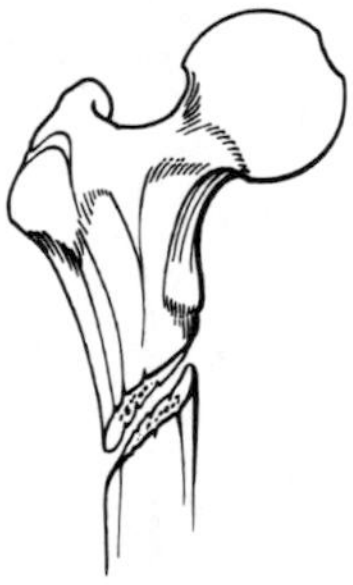

SPIRAL

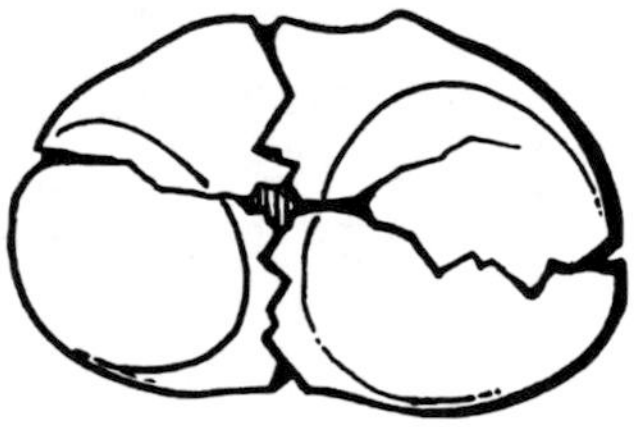

STELLATE

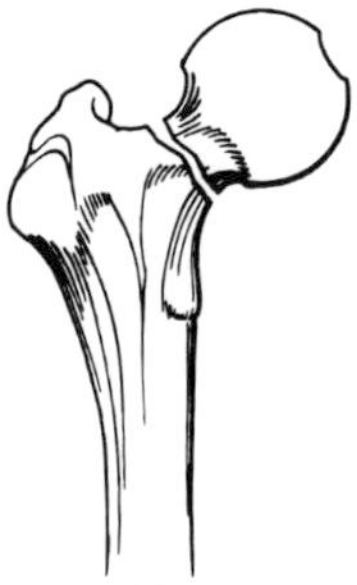

TRANSCERVICAL

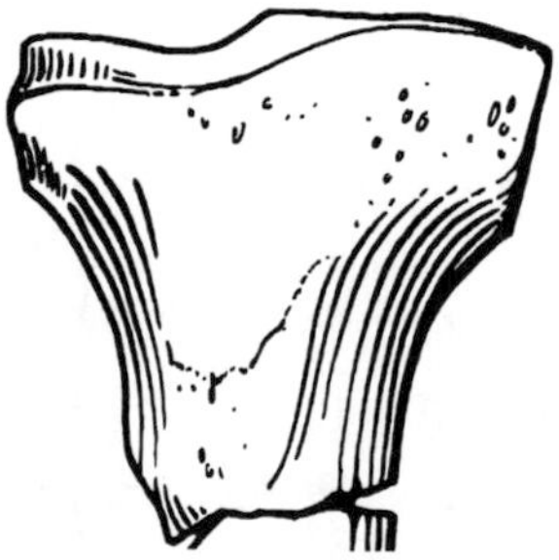

TRANSVERSE

FRACTURE TYPES

© 2018 Channel Publishing, Ltd.

Educational Annotations | P – Upper Bones

AHA Coding Clinic® Reference Notations of Upper Bones

ROOT OPERATION SPECIFIC - P - UPPER BONES

CHANGE - 2
DESTRUCTION - 5
DIVISION - 8
DRAINAGE - 9
EXCISION - B
- Harvesting of local bone for graft ....AHA 15:1Q:p30
- Resection of rib segment ....AHA 12:4Q:p101
- Spinal decompression meaning laminectomy ....AHA 13:4Q:p116
  - Official Clarification of 13:4Q:p116 ....AHA 15:2Q:p34
- Subacromial decompression....AHA 13:3Q:p20

EXTIRPATION - C
INSERTION - H
- Insertion/replacement of growing rods ....AHA 14:4Q:p28

INSPECTION - J
RELEASE - N
REMOVAL - P
- Removal/replacement of growing rods ....AHA 14:4Q:p28

REPAIR - Q
REPLACEMENT - R
REPOSITION - S
- Elongation derotation flexion cast change ....AHA 16:1Q:p21
- Open reduction internal fixation (ORIF) of forearm bones ....AHA 14:4Q:p32
- Open reduction internal fixation (ORIF) of rib fractures ....AHA 17:4Q:p53
- Placement of vertical expandable prosthetic titanium rib (VEPTR)....AHA 14:4Q:p26
- Ravitch procedure (removal of ends of the ribs and reposition of sternum)..AHA 15:4Q:p33
- Reposition of cervical vertebra fracture ....AHA 15:2Q:p34
- Reposition of healed distal radius fracture ....AHA 14:3Q:p33

RESECTION - T
- Resection of carpal bone with arthroplasty ....AHA 15:3Q:p26

SUPPLEMENT - U
- Laminoplasty with allograft ....AHA 15:2Q:p20
- Vertebroplasty with cement as a device value ....AHA 14:2Q:p12

REVISION - W
- Lengthening of growing rods ....AHA 14:4Q:p27
- Lengthening of vertical expandable prosthetic titanium rib (VEPTR) ....AHA 14:4Q:p26

Body Part Key Listings of Upper Bones

See also Body Part Key in Appendix C

Acromion (process) ....use Scapula, Left/Right
Capitate bone....use Carpal, Left/Right
Coracoid process....use Scapula, Left/Right
Dens ....use Cervical Vertebra
Distal humerus ....use Humeral Shaft, Left/Right
Glenoid fossa (of scapula) ....use Glenoid Cavity, Left/Right
Greater tuberosity ....use Humeral Head, Left/Right
Hamate bone....use Carpal, Left/Right
Humerus, distal ....use Humeral Shaft, Left/Right
Lateral epicondyle of humerus ....use Humeral Shaft, Left/Right
Lesser tuberosity ....use Humeral Head, Left/Right
Lunate bone....use Carpal, Left/Right
Manubrium ....use Sternum
Medial epicondyle of humerus....use Humeral Shaft, Left/Right
Neck of humerus (anatomical)
(surgical)....use Humeral Head, Left/Right
Odontoid process ....use Cervical Vertebra
Olecranon process ....use Ulna, Left/Right
Pisiform bone ....use Carpal, Left/Right
Radial notch....use Ulna, Left/Right
Scaphoid bone ....use Carpal, Left/Right
Spinous process ....use Cervical, Thoracic, Lumbar Vertebra
Suprasternal notch....use Sternum
Transverse foramen ....use Cervical Vertebra
Transverse process ....use Cervical, Thoracic, Lumbar Vertebra
Trapezium bone....use Carpal, Left/Right
Trapezoid bone ....use Carpal, Left/Right
Triquetral bone ....use Carpal, Left/Right
Ulnar notch ....use Radius, Left/Right
Vertebral arch ....use Cervical, Thoracic, Lumbar Vertebra
Vertebral body ....use Cervical, Thoracic, Lumbar Vertebra
Vertebral foramen ....use Cervical, Thoracic, Lumbar Vertebra
Vertebral lamina ....use Cervical, Thoracic, Lumbar Vertebra
Vertebral pedicle ....use Cervical, Thoracic, Lumbar Vertebra
Xiphoid process ....use Sternum

© 2018 Channel Publishing, Ltd.

Educational Annotations

P – Upper Bones

Device Key Listings of Upper Bones

See also Device Key in Appendix D

Autograft	use Autologous Tissue Substitute
Bone bank bone graft	use Nonautologous Tissue Substitute
Bone screw (interlocking) (lag) (pedicle) (recessed)	use Internal Fixation Device in Head and Facial Bones, Upper Bones, Lower Bones
Clamp and rod internal fixation system (CRIF)	use Internal Fixation Device in Upper Bones, Lower Bones
Delta frame external fixator	use External Fixation Device, Hybrid for Insertion in Upper Bones, Lower Bones
	use External Fixation Device, Hybrid for Reposition in Upper Bones, Lower Bones
Electrical bone growth stimulator (EBGS)	use Bone Growth Stimulator in Head and Facial Bones, Upper Bones, Lower Bones
External fixator	use External Fixation Device in Head and Facial Bones, Upper Bones, Lower Bones, Upper Joints, Lower Joints
Ilizarov external fixator	use External Fixation Device, Ring for Insertion in Upper Bones, Lower Bones
	use External Fixation Device, Ring for Reposition in Upper Bones, Lower Bones
Ilizarov-Vecklich device	use External Fixation Device, Limb Lengthening for Insertion in Upper Bones, Lower Bones
Intramedullary (IM) rod (nail)	use Internal Fixation Device, Intramedullary in Upper Bones, Lower Bones
Intramedullary skeletal kinetic distractor (ISKD)	use Internal Fixation Device, Intramedullary in Upper Bones, Lower Bones
Kirschner wire (K-wire)	use Internal Fixation Device in Head and Facial Bones, Upper Bones, Lower Bones, Upper Joints, Lower Joints
Kuntscher nail	use Internal Fixation Device, Intramedullary in Upper Bones, Lower Bones
Neutralization plate	use Internal Fixation Device in Head and Facial Bones, Upper Bones, Lower Bones
Polymethylmethacrylate (PMMA)	use Synthetic Substitute
Sheffield hybrid external fixator	use External Fixation Device, Hybrid for Insertion in Upper Bones, Lower Bones
	use External Fixation Device, Hybrid for Reposition in Upper Bones, Lower Bones
Sheffield ring external fixator	use External Fixation Device, Ring for Insertion in Upper Bones, Lower Bones
	use External Fixation Device, Ring for Reposition in Upper Bones, Lower Bones
Tissue bank graft	use Nonautologous Tissue Substitute
Titanium Sternal Fixation System (TSFS)	use Internal Fixation Device, Rigid Plate for Insertion in Upper Bones
	use Internal Fixation Device, Rigid Plate for Reposition in Upper Bones
Ultrasonic osteogenic stimulator	use Bone Growth Stimulator in Head and Facial Bones, Upper Bones, Lower Bones
Ultrasound bone healing system	use Bone Growth Stimulator in Head and Facial Bones, Upper Bones, Lower Bones
Uniplanar external fixator	use External Fixation Device, Monoplanar for Insertion in Upper Bones, Lower Bones
	use External Fixation Device, Monoplanar for Reposition in Upper Bones, Lower Bones

Device Aggregation Table Listings of Upper Bones

See also Device Aggregation Table in Appendix E

Specific Device	For Operation	In Body System	General Device
External Fixation Device, Hybrid	Insertion	Upper Bones	External Fixation Device
External Fixation Device, Hybrid	Reposition	Upper Bones	External Fixation Device
External Fixation Device, Limb Lengthening	Insertion	Upper Bones	External Fixation Device
External Fixation Device, Monoplanar	Insertion	Upper Bones	External Fixation Device
External Fixation Device, Monoplanar	Reposition	Upper Bones	External Fixation Device
External Fixation Device, Ring	Insertion	Upper Bones	External Fixation Device
External Fixation Device, Ring	Reposition	Upper Bones	External Fixation Device
Internal Fixation Device, Intramedullary	All applicable	Upper Bones	Internal Fixation Device
Internal Fixation Device, Rigid Plate	Insertion	Upper Bones	Internal Fixation Device
Internal Fixation Device, Rigid Plate	Reposition	Upper Bones	Internal Fixation Device

Coding Notes of Upper Bones

Body System Relevant Coding Guidelines

Reposition for fracture treatment

B3.15

Reduction of a displaced fracture is coded to the root operation Reposition and the application of a cast or splint in conjunction with the Reposition procedure is not coded separately. Treatment of a nondisplaced fracture is coded to the procedure performed.

Examples: Casting of a nondisplaced fracture is coded to the root operation Immobilization in the Placement section.

Putting a pin in a nondisplaced fracture is coded to the root operation Insertion.

© 2018 Channel Publishing, Ltd.

1ST - 0 Medical and Surgical
2ND - P Upper Bones
3RD - 2 CHANGE

DEVICE GROUP: Change, Insertion, Removal, Replacement, Revision, Supplement
Root Operations that always involve a device.

CHANGE: Taking out or off a device from a body part and putting back an identical or similar device in or on the same body part without cutting or puncturing the skin or a mucous membrane.

Explanation: All CHANGE procedures are coded using the approach External
Examples: Exchange drain tube – CMS Ex: Urinary catheter change

Body Part – 4TH	Approach – 5TH	Device – 6TH	Qualifier – 7TH
Y Upper Bone	X External	0 Drainage device Y Other device	Z No qualifier

1ST - 0 Medical and Surgical
2ND - P Upper Bones
3RD - 5 DESTRUCTION

EXCISION GROUP: Excision, Resection, Destruction, Extraction, (Detachment)
Root Operations that take out some or all of a body part.

DESTRUCTION: Physical eradication of all or a portion of a body part by the direct use of energy, force, or a destructive agent.

Explanation: None of the body part is physically taken out
Examples: Cryoablation bone cyst – CMS Ex: Fulguration of rectal polyp

Body Part – 4TH			Approach – 5TH	Device – 6TH	Qualifier – 7TH
0 Sternum 1 Ribs, 1 to 2 2 Ribs, 3 or more 3 Cervical Vertebra 4 Thoracic Vertebra 5 Scapula, Right 6 Scapula, Left 7 Glenoid Cavity, Right 8 Glenoid Cavity, Left	9 Clavicle, Right B Clavicle, Left C Humeral Head, Right D Humeral Head, Left F Humeral Shaft, Right G Humeral Shaft, Left H Radius, Right J Radius, Left K Ulna, Right	L Ulna, Left M Carpal, Right N Carpal, Left P Metacarpal, Right Q Metacarpal, Left R Thumb Phalanx, Right S Thumb Phalanx, Left T Finger Phalanx, Right V Finger Phalanx, Left	0 Open 3 Percutaneous 4 Percutaneous endoscopic	Z No device	Z No qualifier

1ST - 0 Medical and Surgical
2ND - P Upper Bones
3RD - 8 DIVISION

DIVISION GROUP: Division, Release
Root Operations involving cutting or separation only.

DIVISION: Cutting into a body part, without draining fluids and/or gases from the body part, in order to separate or transect a body part.

Explanation: All or a portion of the body part is separated into two or more portions
Examples: Carpal osteotomy – CMS Ex: Spinal cordotomy

Body Part – 4TH			Approach – 5TH	Device – 6TH	Qualifier – 7TH
0 Sternum 1 Ribs, 1 to 2 2 Ribs, 3 or more 3 Cervical Vertebra 4 Thoracic Vertebra 5 Scapula, Right 6 Scapula, Left 7 Glenoid Cavity, Right 8 Glenoid Cavity, Left	9 Clavicle, Right B Clavicle, Left C Humeral Head, Right D Humeral Head, Left F Humeral Shaft, Right G Humeral Shaft, Left H Radius, Right J Radius, Left K Ulna, Right	L Ulna, Left M Carpal, Right N Carpal, Left P Metacarpal, Right Q Metacarpal, Left R Thumb Phalanx, Right S Thumb Phalanx, Left T Finger Phalanx, Right V Finger Phalanx, Left	0 Open 3 Percutaneous 4 Percutaneous endoscopic	Z No device	Z No qualifier

© 2018 Channel Publishing, Ltd.

1ST - 0 Medical and Surgical
2ND - P Upper Bones
3RD - 9 DRAINAGE

DRAINAGE GROUP: Drainage, Extirpation, (Fragmentation)
Root Operations that take out solids/fluids/gases from a body part.

DRAINAGE: Taking or letting out fluids and/or gases from a body part.

Explanation: Qualifier "X Diagnostic" indicates drainage procedures that are biopsies
Examples: Aspiration bone cyst – CMS Ex: Thoracentesis

Body Part – 4TH			Approach – 5TH	Device – 6TH	Qualifier – 7TH
0 Sternum 1 Ribs, 1 to 2 2 Ribs, 3 or more 3 Cervical Vertebra 4 Thoracic Vertebra 5 Scapula, Right 6 Scapula, Left 7 Glenoid Cavity, Right 8 Glenoid Cavity, Left	9 Clavicle, Right B Clavicle, Left C Humeral Head, Right D Humeral Head, Left F Humeral Shaft, Right G Humeral Shaft, Left H Radius, Right J Radius, Left K Ulna, Right	L Ulna, Left M Carpal, Right N Carpal, Left P Metacarpal, Right Q Metacarpal, Left R Thumb Phalanx, Right S Thumb Phalanx, Left T Finger Phalanx, Right V Finger Phalanx, Left	0 Open 3 Percutaneous 4 Percutaneous endoscopic	0 Drainage device	Z No qualifier
0 Sternum 1 Ribs, 1 to 2 2 Ribs, 3 or more 3 Cervical Vertebra 4 Thoracic Vertebra 5 Scapula, Right 6 Scapula, Left 7 Glenoid Cavity, Right 8 Glenoid Cavity, Left	9 Clavicle, Right B Clavicle, Left C Humeral Head, Right D Humeral Head, Left F Humeral Shaft, Right G Humeral Shaft, Left H Radius, Right J Radius, Left K Ulna, Right	L Ulna, Left M Carpal, Right N Carpal, Left P Metacarpal, Right Q Metacarpal, Left R Thumb Phalanx, Right S Thumb Phalanx, Left T Finger Phalanx, Right V Finger Phalanx, Left	0 Open 3 Percutaneous 4 Percutaneous endoscopic	Z No device	X Diagnostic Z No qualifier

UPPER BONES 0P9

1ST - 0 Medical and Surgical
2ND - P Upper Bones
3RD - B EXCISION

EXCISION GROUP: Excision, Resection, Destruction, Extraction, (Detachment)
Root Operations that take out some or all of a body part.

EXCISION: Cutting out or off, without replacement, a portion of a body part.

Explanation: Qualifier "X Diagnostic" indicates excision procedures that are biopsies
Examples: Vertebral laminectomy – CMS Ex: Liver biopsy

Body Part – 4TH			Approach – 5TH	Device – 6TH	Qualifier – 7TH
0 Sternum 1 Ribs, 1 to 2 2 Ribs, 3 or more 3 Cervical Vertebra 4 Thoracic Vertebra 5 Scapula, Right 6 Scapula, Left 7 Glenoid Cavity, Right 8 Glenoid Cavity, Left	9 Clavicle, Right B Clavicle, Left C Humeral Head, Right D Humeral Head, Left F Humeral Shaft, Right G Humeral Shaft, Left H Radius, Right J Radius, Left K Ulna, Right	L Ulna, Left M Carpal, Right N Carpal, Left P Metacarpal, Right Q Metacarpal, Left R Thumb Phalanx, Right S Thumb Phalanx, Left T Finger Phalanx, Right V Finger Phalanx, Left	0 Open 3 Percutaneous 4 Percutaneous endoscopic	Z No device	X Diagnostic Z No qualifier

1ST - 0 Medical and Surgical
2ND - P Upper Bones
3RD - C EXTIRPATION

DRAINAGE GROUP: Drainage, Extirpation, (Fragmentation)
Root Operations that take out solids/fluids/gases from a body part.

EXTIRPATION: Taking or cutting out solid matter from a body part.

Explanation: Abnormal byproduct or foreign body ...
Examples: Removal foreign body – CMS Ex: Thrombectomy

Body Part – 4TH			Approach – 5TH	Device – 6TH	Qualifier – 7TH
0 Sternum 1 Ribs, 1 to 2 2 Ribs, 3 or more 3 Cervical Vertebra 4 Thoracic Vertebra 5 Scapula, Right 6 Scapula, Left 7 Glenoid Cavity, Right 8 Glenoid Cavity, Left	9 Clavicle, Right B Clavicle, Left C Humeral Head, Right D Humeral Head, Left F Humeral Shaft, Right G Humeral Shaft, Left H Radius, Right J Radius, Left K Ulna, Right	L Ulna, Left M Carpal, Right N Carpal, Left P Metacarpal, Right Q Metacarpal, Left R Thumb Phalanx, Right S Thumb Phalanx, Left T Finger Phalanx, Right V Finger Phalanx, Left	0 Open 3 Percutaneous 4 Percutaneous endoscopic	Z No device	Z No qualifier

© 2018 Channel Publishing, Ltd.

1ST - 0 Medical and Surgical
2ND - P Upper Bones
3RD - D EXTRACTION

EXCISION GROUP: Excision, Resection, Destruction, Extraction, (Detachment)
Root Operations that take out some or all of a body part.

EXTRACTION: Pulling or stripping out or off all or a portion of a body part by the use of force.

Explanation: None for this Body System
Examples: Non-excisional debridement – CMS Ex: Dilation and curettage

Body Part – 4TH			Approach – 5TH	Device – 6TH	Qualifier – 7TH
0 Sternum 1 Ribs, 1 to 2 2 Ribs, 3 or more 3 Cervical Vertebra 4 Thoracic Vertebra 5 Scapula, Right 6 Scapula, Left 7 Glenoid Cavity, Right 8 Glenoid Cavity, Left	9 Clavicle, Right B Clavicle, Left C Humeral Head, Right D Humeral Head, Left F Humeral Shaft, Right G Humeral Shaft, Left H Radius, Right J Radius, Left K Ulna, Right	L Ulna, Left M Carpal, Right N Carpal, Left P Metacarpal, Right Q Metacarpal, Left R Thumb Phalanx, Right S Thumb Phalanx, Left T Finger Phalanx, Right V Finger Phalanx, Left	0 Open	Z No device	Z No qualifier

1ST - 0 Medical and Surgical
2ND - P Upper Bones
3RD - H INSERTION

DEVICE GROUP: Change, Insertion, Removal, Replacement, Revision, Supplement
Root Operations that always involve a device.

INSERTION: Putting in a nonbiological appliance that monitors, assists, performs, or prevents a physiological function but does not physically take the place of a body part.

Explanation: None
Examples: Insertion external fixation pin – CMS Ex: Insertion of central venous catheter

Body Part – 4TH		Approach – 5TH	Device – 6TH	Qualifier – 7TH
0 Sternum		0 Open 3 Percutaneous 4 Percutaneous endoscopic	0 Internal fixation device, rigid plate 4 Internal fixation device	Z No qualifier
1 Ribs, 1 to 2 2 Ribs, 3 or more 3 Cervical Vertebra 4 Thoracic Vertebra 5 Scapula, Right	6 Scapula, Left 7 Glenoid Cavity, Right 8 Glenoid Cavity, Left 9 Clavicle, Right B Clavicle, Left	0 Open 3 Percutaneous 4 Percutaneous endoscopic	4 Internal fixation device	Z No qualifier
C Humeral Head, Right D Humeral Head, Left F Humeral Shaft, Right G Humeral Shaft, Left	H Radius, Right J Radius, Left K Ulna, Right L Ulna, Left	0 Open 3 Percutaneous 4 Percutaneous endoscopic	4 Internal fixation device 5 External fixation device 6 Internal fixation device, intramedullary 8 External fixation device, limb lengthening B External fixation device, monoplanar C External fixation device, ring D External fixation device, hybrid	Z No qualifier
M Carpal, Right N Carpal, Left P Metacarpal, Right Q Metacarpal, Left	R Thumb Phalanx, Right S Thumb Phalanx, Left T Finger Phalanx, Right V Finger Phalanx, Left	0 Open 3 Percutaneous 4 Percutaneous endoscopic	4 Internal fixation device 5 External fixation device	Z No qualifier
Y Upper Bone		0 Open 3 Percutaneous 4 Percutaneous endoscopic	M Bone growth stimulator	Z No qualifier

© 2018 Channel Publishing, Ltd.

1ST - 0 Medical and Surgical
2ND - P Upper Bones
3RD - J INSPECTION

EXAMINATION GROUP: Inspection, (Map)
Root Operations involving examination only.

INSPECTION: Visually and/or manually exploring a body part.

Explanation: Direct or instrumental visualization ...
Examples: Examination bone – CMS Ex: Exploratory laparotomy

Body Part – 4TH	Approach – 5TH	Device – 6TH	Qualifier – 7TH
Y Upper Bone	0 Open 3 Percutaneous 4 Percutaneous endoscopic X External	Z No device	Z No qualifier

1ST - 0 Medical and Surgical
2ND - P Upper Bones
3RD - N RELEASE

DIVISION GROUP: Division, Release
Root Operations involving cutting or separation only.

RELEASE: Freeing a body part from an abnormal physical constraint by cutting or by the use of force.

Explanation: Some of the restraining tissue may be taken out but none of the body part is taken out
Examples: Extra-articular bone adhesiolysis – CMS Ex: Carpal tunnel release

Body Part – 4TH			Approach – 5TH	Device – 6TH	Qualifier – 7TH
0 Sternum 1 Ribs, 1 to 2 2 Ribs, 3 or more 3 Cervical Vertebra 4 Thoracic Vertebra 5 Scapula, Right 6 Scapula, Left 7 Glenoid Cavity, Right 8 Glenoid Cavity, Left	9 Clavicle, Right B Clavicle, Left C Humeral Head, Right D Humeral Head, Left F Humeral Shaft, Right G Humeral Shaft, Left H Radius, Right J Radius, Left K Ulna, Right	L Ulna, Left M Carpal, Right N Carpal, Left P Metacarpal, Right Q Metacarpal, Left R Thumb Phalanx, Right S Thumb Phalanx, Left T Finger Phalanx, Right V Finger Phalanx, Left	0 Open 3 Percutaneous 4 Percutaneous endoscopic	Z No device	Z No qualifier

© 2018 Channel Publishing, Ltd.

1ST - 0 Medical and Surgical
2ND - P Upper Bones
3RD - P REMOVAL

DEVICE GROUP: Change, Insertion, Removal, Replacement, Revision, Supplement
Root Operations that always involve a device.

REMOVAL: Taking out or off a device from a body part.

Explanation: Removal device without reinsertion ...
Examples: Removal external fixation pin – CMS Ex: Cardiac pacemaker removal

Body Part – 4TH	Approach – 5TH	Device – 6TH	Qualifier – 7TH
0 Sternum 1 Ribs, 1 to 2 2 Ribs, 3 or more 3 Cervical Vertebra 4 Thoracic Vertebra 5 Scapula, Right 6 Scapula, Left 7 Glenoid Cavity, Right 8 Glenoid Cavity, Left 9 Clavicle, Right B Clavicle, Left	0 Open 3 Percutaneous 4 Percutaneous endoscopic	4 Internal fixation device 7 Autologous tissue substitute J Synthetic substitute K Nonautologous tissue substitute	Z No qualifier
0 Sternum 1 Ribs, 1 to 2 2 Ribs, 3 or more 3 Cervical Vertebra 4 Thoracic Vertebra 5 Scapula, Right 6 Scapula, Left 7 Glenoid Cavity, Right 8 Glenoid Cavity, Left 9 Clavicle, Right B Clavicle, Left	X External	4 Internal fixation device	Z No qualifier
C Humeral Head, Right D Humeral Head, Left F Humeral Shaft, Right G Humeral Shaft, Left H Radius, Right J Radius, Left K Ulna, Right L Ulna, Left M Carpal, Right N Carpal, Left P Metacarpal, Right Q Metacarpal, Left R Thumb Phalanx, Right S Thumb Phalanx, Left T Finger Phalanx, Right V Finger Phalanx, Left	0 Open 3 Percutaneous 4 Percutaneous endoscopic	4 Internal fixation device 5 External fixation device 7 Autologous tissue substitute J Synthetic substitute K Nonautologous tissue substitute	Z No qualifier
C Humeral Head, Right D Humeral Head, Left F Humeral Shaft, Right G Humeral Shaft, Left H Radius, Right J Radius, Left K Ulna, Right L Ulna, Left M Carpal, Right N Carpal, Left P Metacarpal, Right Q Metacarpal, Left R Thumb Phalanx, Right S Thumb Phalanx, Left T Finger Phalanx, Right V Finger Phalanx, Left	X External	4 Internal fixation device 5 External fixation device	Z No qualifier
Y Upper Bone	0 Open 3 Percutaneous 4 Percutaneous endoscopic X External	0 Drainage device M Bone growth stimulator	Z No qualifier

© 2018 Channel Publishing, Ltd.

1ST - 0 Medical and Surgical
2ND - P Upper Bones
3RD - Q REPAIR

OTHER REPAIRS GROUP: (Control), Repair
Root Operations that define other repairs.

REPAIR: Restoring, to the extent possible, a body part to its normal anatomic structure and function.

Explanation: Used only when the method to accomplish the repair is not one of the other root operations
Examples: Vertebral laminoplasty – CMS Ex: Suture of laceration

Body Part – 4TH			Approach – 5TH	Device – 6TH	Qualifier – 7TH
0 Sternum	9 Clavicle, Right	L Ulna, Left	0 Open	Z No device	Z No qualifier
1 Ribs, 1 to 2	B Clavicle, Left	M Carpal, Right	3 Percutaneous		
2 Ribs, 3 or more	C Humeral Head, Right	N Carpal, Left	4 Percutaneous endoscopic		
3 Cervical Vertebra	D Humeral Head, Left	P Metacarpal, Right	X External		
4 Thoracic Vertebra	F Humeral Shaft, Right	Q Metacarpal, Left			
5 Scapula, Right	G Humeral Shaft, Left	R Thumb Phalanx, Right			
6 Scapula, Left	H Radius, Right	S Thumb Phalanx, Left			
7 Glenoid Cavity, Right	J Radius, Left	T Finger Phalanx, Right			
8 Glenoid Cavity, Left	K Ulna, Right	V Finger Phalanx, Left			

1ST - 0 Medical and Surgical
2ND - P Upper Bones
3RD - R REPLACEMENT

DEVICE GROUP: Change, Insertion, Removal, Replacement, Revision, Supplement
Root Operations that always involve a device.

REPLACEMENT: Putting in or on biological or synthetic material that physically takes the place and/or function of all or a portion of a body part.

Explanation: Includes taking out or eradicating, or rendering non-functional, the body part ...
Examples: Humeral head replacement – CMS Ex: Total hip replacement

Body Part – 4TH			Approach – 5TH	Device – 6TH	Qualifier – 7TH
0 Sternum	9 Clavicle, Right	L Ulna, Left	0 Open	7 Autologous tissue substitute	Z No qualifier
1 Ribs, 1 to 2	B Clavicle, Left	M Carpal, Right	3 Percutaneous	J Synthetic substitute	
2 Ribs, 3 or more	C Humeral Head, Right	N Carpal, Left	4 Percutaneous endoscopic	K Nonautologous tissue substitute	
3 Cervical Vertebra	D Humeral Head, Left	P Metacarpal, Right			
4 Thoracic Vertebra	F Humeral Shaft, Right	Q Metacarpal, Left			
5 Scapula, Right	G Humeral Shaft, Left	R Thumb Phalanx, Right			
6 Scapula, Left	H Radius, Right	S Thumb Phalanx, Left			
7 Glenoid Cavity, Right	J Radius, Left	T Finger Phalanx, Right			
8 Glenoid Cavity, Left	K Ulna, Right	V Finger Phalanx, Left			

© 2018 Channel Publishing, Ltd.

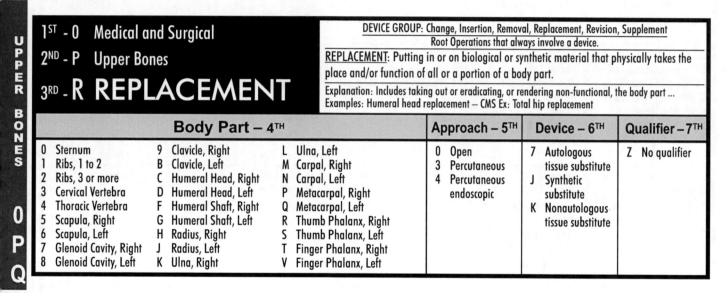

1ST - 0 Medical and Surgical 2ND - P Upper Bones 3RD - S REPOSITION	MOVE GROUP: (Reattachment), Reposition, (Transfer), (Transplantation) Root Operations that put in/put back or move some/all of a body part. REPOSITION: Moving to its normal location, or other suitable location, all or a portion of a body part. Explanation: The body part may or may not be cut out or off to be moved to the new location ... Examples: ORIF Colles' fracture – CMS Ex: Fracture reduction

Body Part – 4TH	Approach – 5TH	Device – 6TH	Qualifier – 7TH
0 Sternum	0 Open 3 Percutaneous 4 Percutaneous endoscopic	0 Internal fixation device, rigid plate 4 Internal fixation device Z No device	Z No qualifier
0 Sternum	X External	Z No device	Z No qualifier
1 Ribs, 1 to 2 2 Ribs, 3 or more 3 Cervical Vertebra 4 Thoracic Vertebra 5 Scapula, Right 6 Scapula, Left 7 Glenoid Cavity, Right 8 Glenoid Cavity, Left 9 Clavicle, Right B Clavicle, Left	0 Open 3 Percutaneous 4 Percutaneous endoscopic	4 Internal fixation device Z No device	Z No qualifier
1 Ribs, 1 to 2 2 Ribs, 3 or more 3 Cervical Vertebra 4 Thoracic Vertebra 5 Scapula, Right 6 Scapula, Left 7 Glenoid Cavity, Right 8 Glenoid Cavity, Left 9 Clavicle, Right B Clavicle, Left	X External	Z No device	Z No qualifier
C Humeral Head, Right D Humeral Head, Left F Humeral Shaft, Right G Humeral Shaft, Left H Radius, Right J Radius, Left K Ulna, Right L Ulna, Left	0 Open 3 Percutaneous 4 Percutaneous endoscopic	4 Internal fixation device 5 External fixation device 6 Internal fixation device, intramedullary B External fixation device, monoplanar C External fixation device, ring D External fixation device, hybrid Z No device	Z No qualifier
C Humeral Head, Right D Humeral Head, Left F Humeral Shaft, Right G Humeral Shaft, Left H Radius, Right J Radius, Left K Ulna, Right L Ulna, Left	X External	Z No device	Z No qualifier
M Carpal, Right N Carpal, Left P Metacarpal, Right Q Metacarpal, Left R Thumb Phalanx, Right S Thumb Phalanx, Left T Finger Phalanx, Right V Finger Phalanx, Left	0 Open 3 Percutaneous 4 Percutaneous endoscopic	4 Internal fixation device 5 External fixation device Z No device	Z No qualifier
M Carpal, Right N Carpal, Left P Metacarpal, Right Q Metacarpal, Left R Thumb Phalanx, Right S Thumb Phalanx, Left T Finger Phalanx, Right V Finger Phalanx, Left	X External	Z No device	Z No qualifier

1ST - 0 Medical and Surgical 2ND - P Upper Bones 3RD - T RESECTION	EXCISION GROUP: Excision, Resection, Destruction, Extraction, (Detachment) Root Operations that take out some or all of a body part. RESECTION: Cutting out or off, without replacement, all of a body part. Explanation: None Examples: Total claviculectomy – CMS Ex: Total lobectomy of lung

Body Part – 4TH	Approach – 5TH	Device – 6TH	Qualifier – 7TH
0 Sternum 1 Ribs, 1 to 2 2 Ribs, 3 or more 5 Scapula, Right 6 Scapula, Left 7 Glenoid Cavity, Right 8 Glenoid Cavity, Left 9 Clavicle, Right B Clavicle, Left C Humeral Head, Right D Humeral Head, Left F Humeral Shaft, Right G Humeral Shaft, Left H Radius, Right J Radius, Left K Ulna, Right L Ulna, Left M Carpal, Right N Carpal, Left P Metacarpal, Right Q Metacarpal, Left R Thumb Phalanx, Right S Thumb Phalanx, Left T Finger Phalanx, Right V Finger Phalanx, Left	0 Open	Z No device	Z No qualifier

© 2018 Channel Publishing, Ltd.

1ST - 0 Medical and Surgical
2ND - P Upper Bones
3RD - U SUPPLEMENT

DEVICE GROUP: Change, Insertion, Removal, Replacement, Revision, Supplement
Root Operations that always involve a device.

SUPPLEMENT: Putting in or on biological or synthetic material that physically reinforces and/or augments the function of a portion of a body part.

Explanation: Biological material is non-living, or is living and from the same individual ...
Examples: Application bone void filler – CMS Ex: Herniorrhaphy using mesh

Body Part – 4TH			Approach – 5TH	Device – 6TH	Qualifier – 7TH
0 Sternum 1 Ribs, 1 to 2 2 Ribs, 3 or more 3 Cervical Vertebra 4 Thoracic Vertebra 5 Scapula, Right 6 Scapula, Left 7 Glenoid Cavity, Right 8 Glenoid Cavity, Left	9 Clavicle, Right B Clavicle, Left C Humeral Head, Right D Humeral Head, Left F Humeral Shaft, Right G Humeral Shaft, Left H Radius, Right J Radius, Left K Ulna, Right	L Ulna, Left M Carpal, Right N Carpal, Left P Metacarpal, Right Q Metacarpal, Left R Thumb Phalanx, Right S Thumb Phalanx, Left T Finger Phalanx, Right V Finger Phalanx, Left	0 Open 3 Percutaneous 4 Percutaneous endoscopic	7 Autologous tissue substitute J Synthetic substitute K Nonautologous tissue substitute	Z No qualifier

1ST - 0 Medical and Surgical
2ND - P Upper Bones
3RD - W REVISION

DEVICE GROUP: Change, Insertion, Removal, Replacement, Revision, Supplement
Root Operations that always involve a device.

REVISION: Correcting, to the extent possible, a portion of a malfunctioning device or the position of a displaced device.

Explanation: Correcting by taking out or putting in components of a device such as a screw or pin ...
Examples: Adjustment bone lengthening growing rods – CMS Ex: Recementing of hip prosthesis

Body Part – 4TH		Approach – 5TH	Device – 6TH	Qualifier – 7TH
0 Sternum 1 Ribs, 1 to 2 2 Ribs, 3 or more 3 Cervical Vertebra 4 Thoracic Vertebra	5 Scapula, Right 6 Scapula, Left 7 Glenoid Cavity, Right 8 Glenoid Cavity, Left 9 Clavicle, Right B Clavicle, Left	0 Open 3 Percutaneous 4 Percutaneous endoscopic X External	4 Internal fixation device 7 Autologous tissue substitute J Synthetic substitute K Nonautologous tissue substitute	Z No qualifier
C Humeral Head, Right D Humeral Head, Left F Humeral Shaft, Right G Humeral Shaft, Left H Radius, Right J Radius, Left K Ulna, Right L Ulna, Left	M Carpal, Right N Carpal, Left P Metacarpal, Right Q Metacarpal, Left R Thumb Phalanx, Right S Thumb Phalanx, Left T Finger Phalanx, Right V Finger Phalanx, Left	0 Open 3 Percutaneous 4 Percutaneous endoscopic X External	4 Internal fixation device 5 External fixation device 7 Autologous tissue substitute J Synthetic substitute K Nonautologous tissue substitute	Z No qualifier
Y Upper Bone		0 Open 3 Percutaneous 4 Percutaneous endoscopic X External	0 Drainage device M Bone growth stimulator	Z No qualifier

© 2018 Channel Publishing, Ltd.

Educational Annotations | Q – Lower Bones

Body System Specific Educational Annotations for the Lower Bones include:

- Anatomy and Physiology Review
- Anatomical Illustrations
- Definitions of Common Procedures
- AHA Coding Clinic® Reference Notations
- Body Part Key Listings
- Device Key Listings
- Device Aggregation Table Listings
- Coding Notes

Anatomy and Physiology Review of Lower Bones

BODY PART VALUES – Q - LOWER BONES

Acetabulum – The round, concave depression in the pelvic bone that articulates with the femoral head forming the hip joint.
Coccyx – The small wedge-shaped bone (also known as the tailbone) at the end of the spinal column.
Femoral Shaft – The middle long portion of the femur.
Femur – The paired long bones (also known as the thigh bone) that articulate at the hip and the knee. It is the longest bone in the body.
Fibula – The paired long slender bones of the lower leg located toward the outside of the lower leg that articulate at the knee and the ankle.
Lower Bone – Any of the bones designated in the Lower Bones PCS Body System.
Lower Femur – The distal end of the femur that articulates with the knee joint.
Lumbar Vertebra – The lumbar section of the spinal vertebral column comprised of 5 vertebra, S1-S5.
Metatarsal – One of the 5 cylindrical bones connecting the tarsals and the phalanges of the foot.
Patella – The paired triangular-shaped bones situated at the front of the knee.
Pelvic Bone – Any of the three bones (ilium, ischium, pubis) that connect with the sacrum to form the pelvic girdle.
Sacrum – The large wedge-shaped vertebra at the lower end of the spine that connects with S5.
Tarsal – The seven bones of the foot (calcaneus, talus, cuboid, navicular, and the medial, intermediate, and lateral cuneiform bones) distal to the tibia and fibula and proximal to the metatarsal bones.
Tibia – The paired long bones of the lower leg (also known as the shin bone) that is the innermost bone of the lower leg supporting and articulating with the knee and with the ankle.
Toe Phalanx – The digital bones of the toes. Each toe contains three bones: Proximal phalanx, intermediate (middle) phalanx, and distal phalanx, except the great toe which only has proximal and distal phalanx bones.
Upper Femur – The proximal end of the femur (head) that articulates with the acetabulum to form the hip joint.

Anatomical Illustrations of Lower Bones

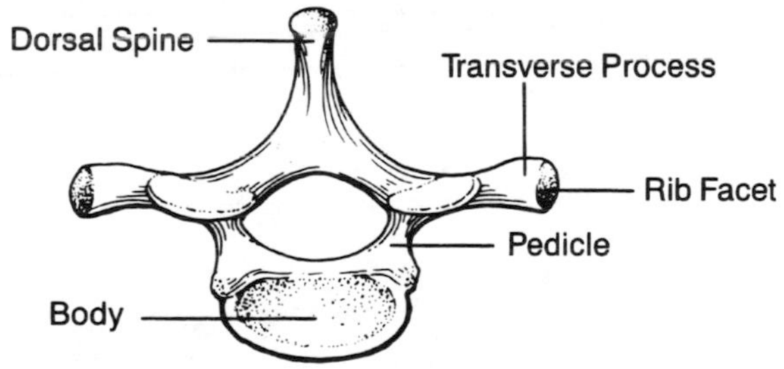

TYPICAL VERTEBRA — SUPERIOR VIEW

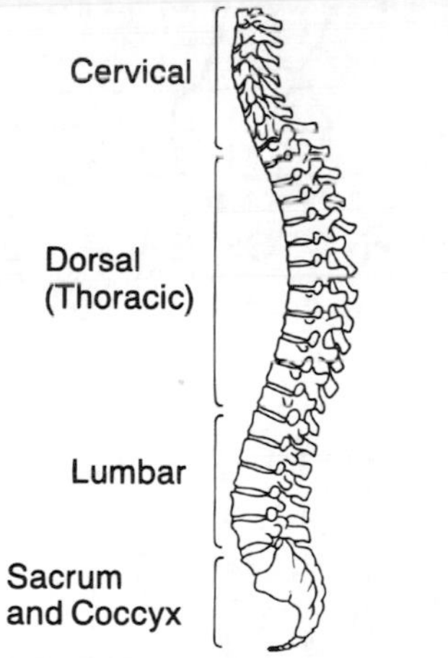

VERTEBRAL COLUMN

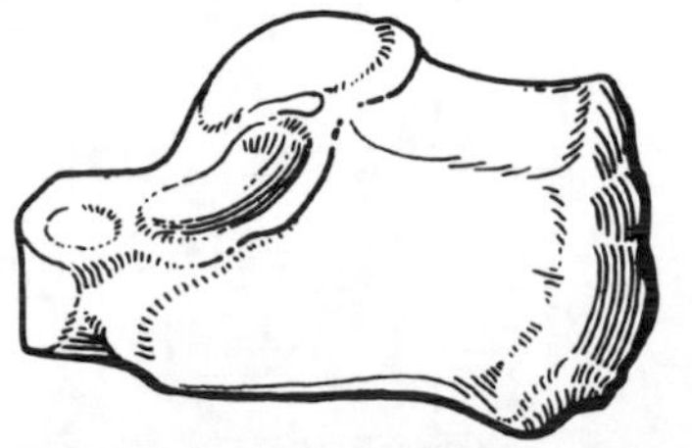

CALCANEUS — MEDIAL VIEW

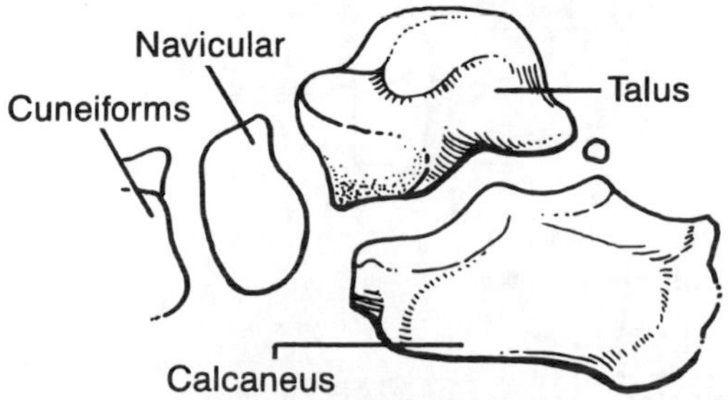

TARSAL BONES

Continued on next page

© 2018 Channel Publishing, Ltd.

Educational Annotations | Q – Lower Bones

Anatomical Illustrations of Lower Bones

Continued from previous page

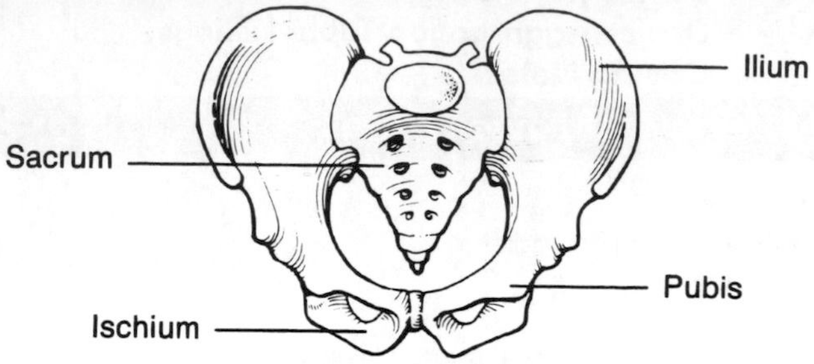

PELVIC BONES

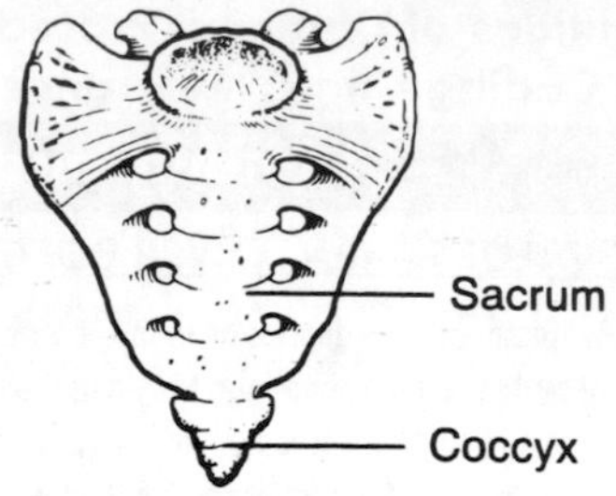

SACRUM AND COCCYX

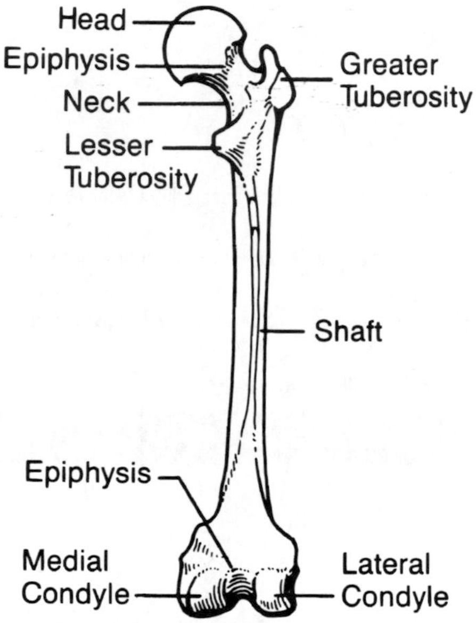

FEMUR — POSTERIOR VIEW

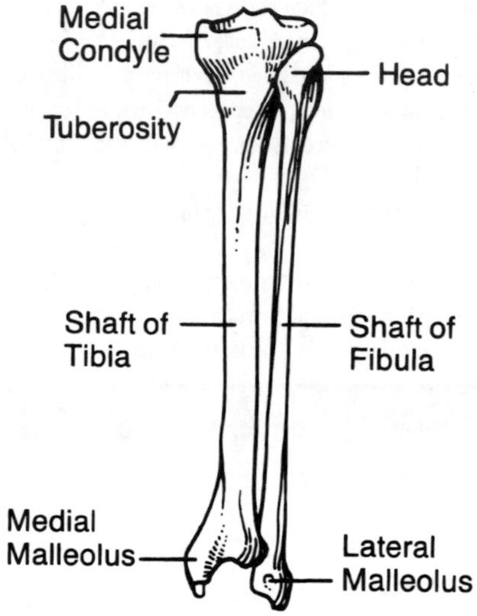

TIBIA AND FIBULA — POSTERIOR VIEW

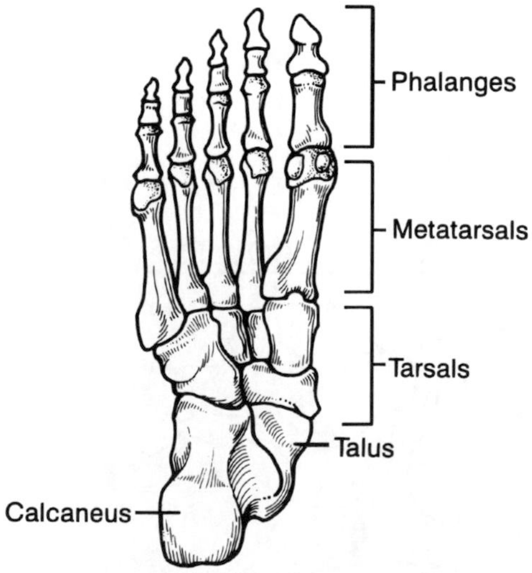

RIGHT FOOT — PLANTAR VIEW

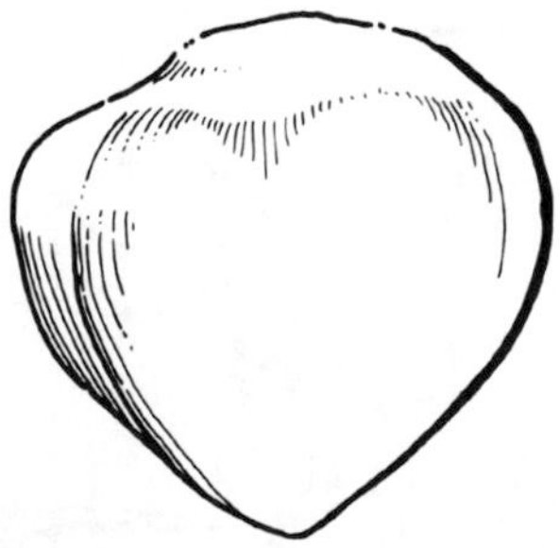

PATELLA — ANTERIOR VIEW

Continued on next page

© 2018 Channel Publishing, Ltd.

Educational Annotations | Q – Lower Bones

Anatomical Illustrations of Lower Bones

Continued from previous page

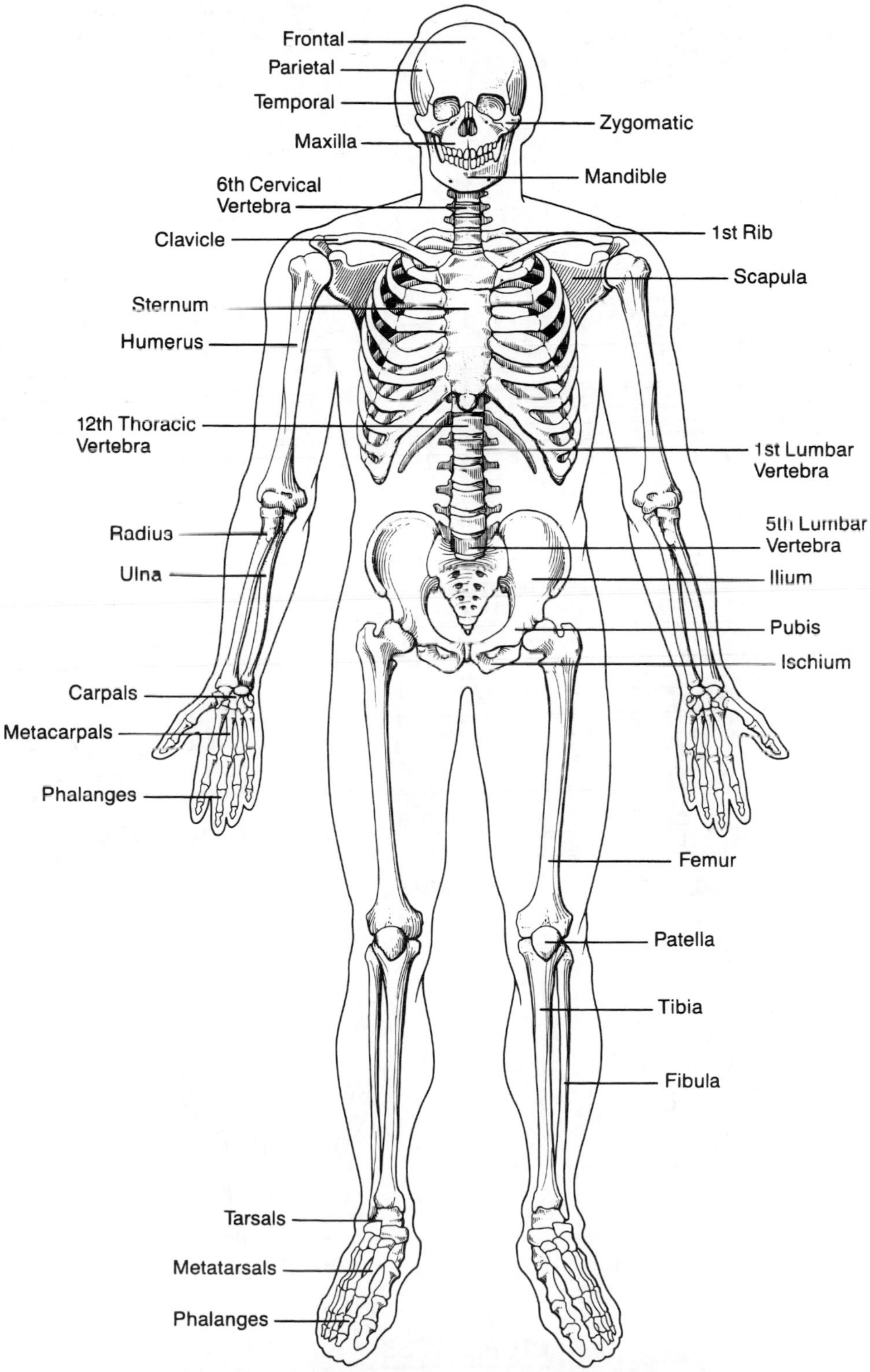

ANTERIOR VIEW OF HUMAN SKELETON

Continued on next page

© 2018 Channel Publishing, Ltd.

Educational Annotations | Q – Lower Bones

Anatomical Illustrations of Lower Bones

Continued from previous page

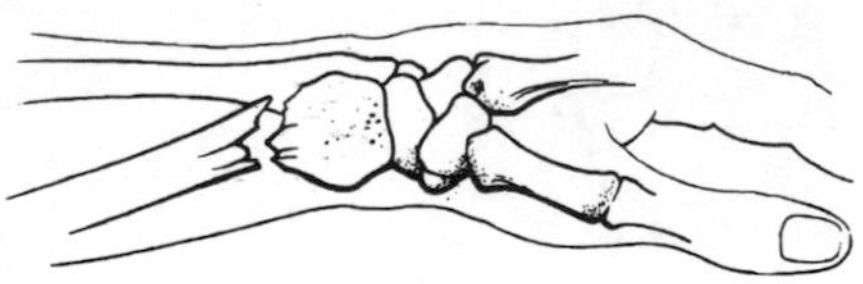

COLLES'

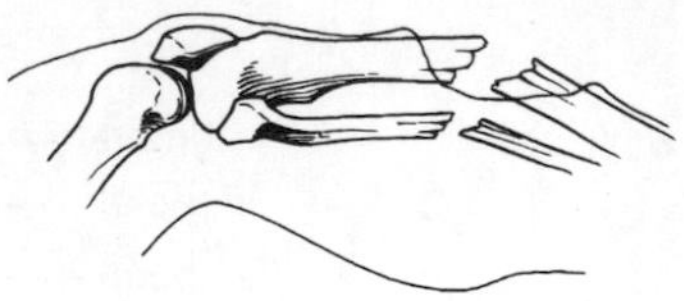

COMPOUND

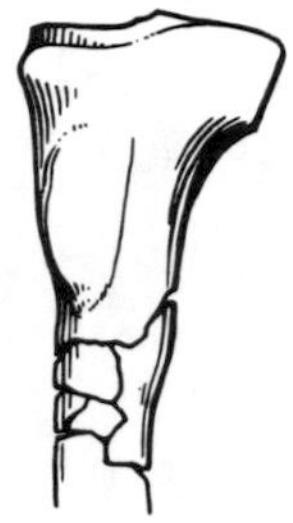

COMMINUTED

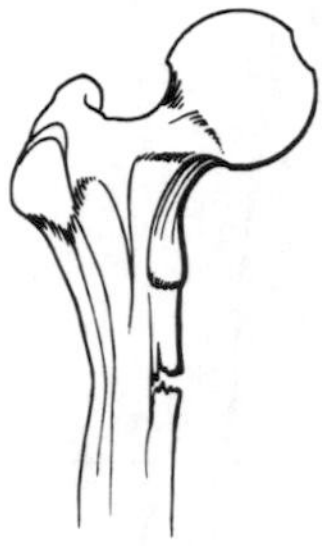

GREENSTICK

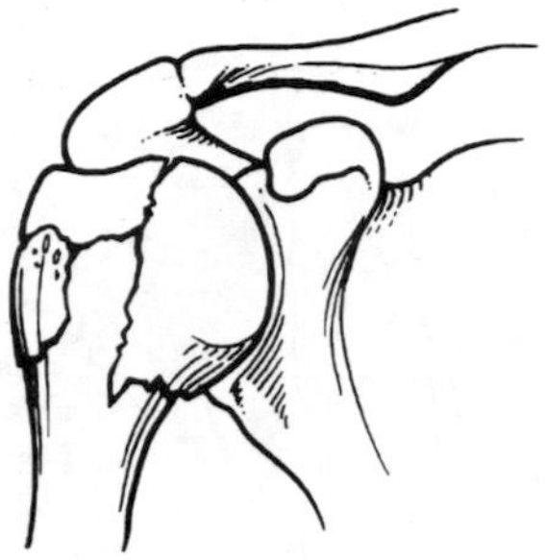

IMPACTED

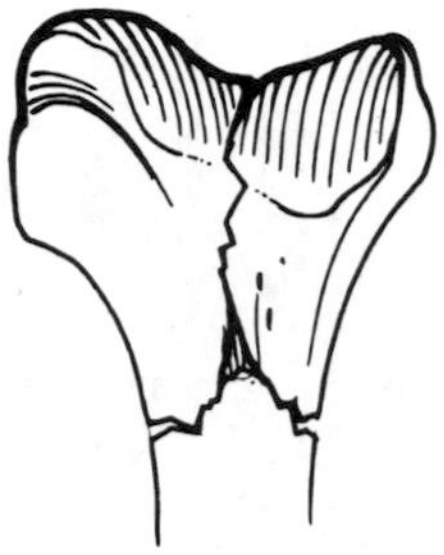

INTERCONDYLAR

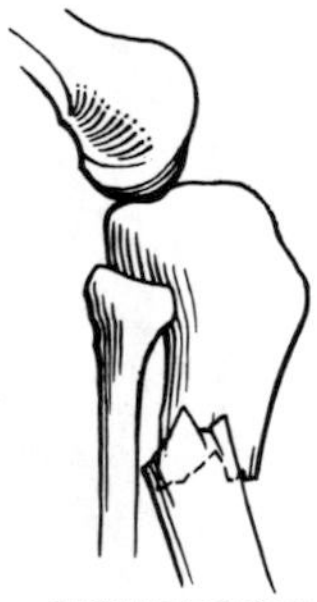

MONTEGGIA

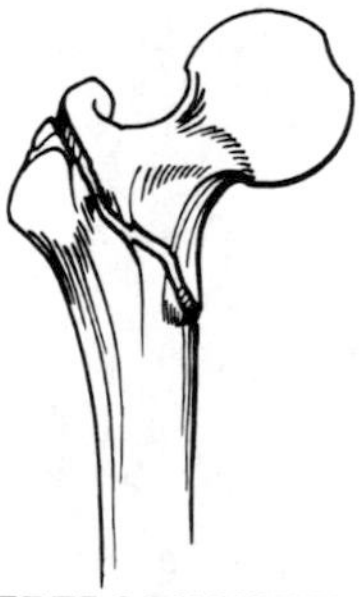

PERTROCHANTERIC

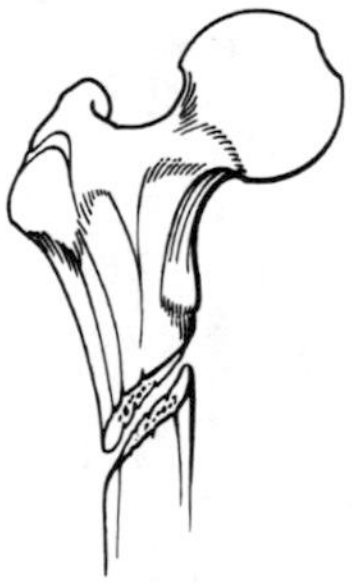

SPIRAL

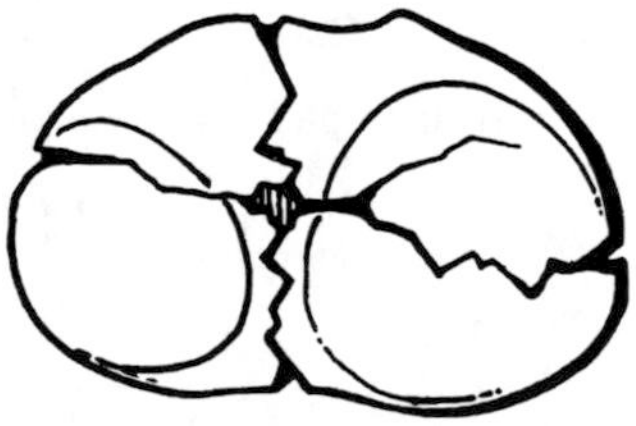

STELLATE

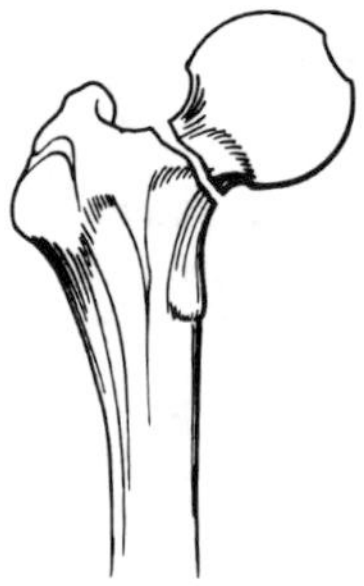

TRANSCERVICAL

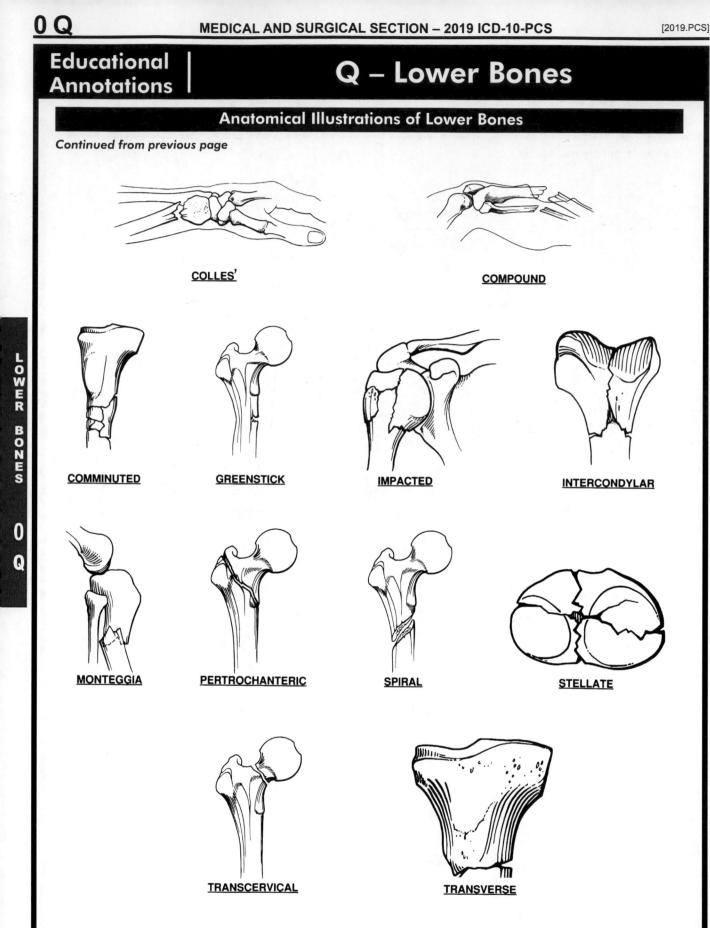

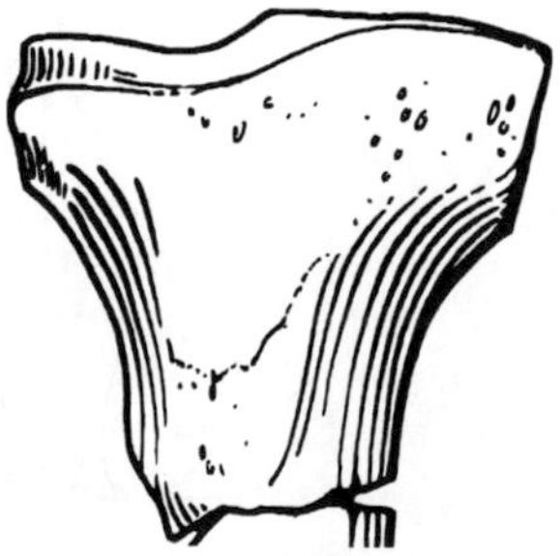

TRANSVERSE

FRACTURE TYPES

© 2018 Channel Publishing, Ltd.

Educational Annotations | Q – Lower Bones

Definitions of Common Procedures of Lower Bones

Bone void filler to iliac crest defect – The surgical placement of a bone void filler (usually synthetic bone material) to fill in a defect in the natural shape of the iliac crest and to enhance the stability and strength of the bone.

Distraction osteogenesis of femur – The surgical placement of a distractor limb lengthening system to lengthen the femur with gradual adjustments over time. The mid-femoral shaft is fractured (corticotomy) and external fixation pins are secured into both the proximal and distal femoral shaft and connected to the external distraction system, allowing new bone to grow and fill the gap.

Femoral head shaving – The surgical grinding down of the femoral head bone that is causing the pain and impaired range of motion (femoroacetabular impingement syndrome). Procedures on the joint tissues often accompany this procedure.

Harvest of bone for graft – The surgical removal of bone to be used as a graft in another location that is usually removed from the iliac crest. Other sites include the tibia, fibula, mandible, and sternum.

Implantable bone growth stimulator in lumbar spinal fusion – The surgical placement of electrical wires (cathodes) to each side of the fusion site that are connected to a subcutaneously placed direct electrical current generator. After the healing is accomplished, the subcutaneous generator can be surgically removed by detaching the cathodes from the generator leads and removing the generator and leads.

AHA Coding Clinic® Reference Notations of Lower Bones

ROOT OPERATION SPECIFIC - Q - LOWER BONES

CHANGE - 2

DESTRUCTION - 5

DIVISION - 8

- Periacetabular osteotomy .... AHA 16:2Q:p31
- Periacetabular osteotomy - Official Correction .... AHA 18:1Q:p25

DRAINAGE - 9

EXCISION - B

- Femoral shaving .... AHA 14:4Q:p25
- Harvesting of local bone for graft .... AHA 15:1Q:p30
- Harvesting of pelvic bone for spinal fusion .... AHA 14:2Q:p6
- Harvesting of fibula for bone graft .... AHA 13:2Q:p39
- Spinal decompression meaning laminectomy .... AHA 13:4Q:p116
  - Official Clarification of 13:4Q:p116 .... AHA 15:2Q:p34

EXTIRPATION - C

INSERTION - H

- Bilateral iliac fixation with spinal fusion .... AHA 17:1Q:p21

INSPECTION - J

RELEASE - N

REMOVAL - P

- Removal of internal fixation device .... AHA 15:2Q:p6

REPAIR - Q

- Pubic symphysis fusion .... AHA 18:1Q:p15
- Sacrum S1 laminoplasty .... AHA 14:3Q:p24

REPLACEMENT - R

REPOSITION - S

- Bilateral cuboid osteotomy .... AHA 18:1Q:p13
- Periacetabular osteotomy .... AHA 18:1Q:p25
- Realignment of femur with internal fixation .... AHA 14:4Q:p31
- Rotational osteosynthesis of tibia .... AHA 14:4Q:p29
- Tibia/fibula epiphysiodesis .... AHA 16:3Q:p34

RESECTION - T

- Femur resection arthroplasty .... AHA 16:3Q:p30
- Resection of femoral head and proximal femur .... AHA 15:3Q:p26
- Resection of lower femur and knee joint .... AHA 14:4Q:p29

SUPPLEMENT - U

- Application of bone graft matrix .... AHA 14:4Q:p31
- Bone void filler .... AHA 13:2Q:p35
- Hip replacement with acetabular reconstruction .... AHA 15:3Q:p18
- Vertebroplasty with cement as a device value .... AHA 14:2Q:p12

REVISION - W

- Reconnect loosened magnetic growth rod .... AHA 17:4Q:p75

© 2018 Channel Publishing, Ltd.

Educational Annotations | Q – Lower Bones

Body Part Key Listings of Lower Bones

See also Body Part Key in Appendix C

Body of femur ....use Femoral Shaft, Left/Right
Body of fibula ....use Fibula, Left/Right
Calcaneus....use Tarsal, Left/Right
Cuboid bone....use Tarsal, Left/Right
Femoral head ....use Upper Femur, Left/Right
Greater trochanter....use Upper Femur, Left/Right
Head of fibula ....use Fibula, Left/Right
Iliac crest ....use Pelvic Bone, Left/Right
Ilium ....use Pelvic Bone, Left/Right
Intermediate cuneiform bone ....use Tarsal, Left/Right
Ischium....use Pelvic Bone, Left/Right
Lateral condyle of femur ....use Lower Femur, Left/Right
Lateral condyle of tibia ....use Tibia, Left/Right
Lateral cuneiform bone ....use Tarsal, Left/Right
Lateral epicondyle of femur....use Lower Femur, Left/Right
Lateral malleolus....use Fibula, Left/Right
Lateral malleolus....use Fibula, Left/Right
Lesser trochanter ....use Upper Femur, Left/Right
Medial condyle of femur ....use Lower Femur, Left/Right
Medial condyle of tibia ....use Tibia, Left/Right
Medial cuneiform bone ....use Tarsal, Left/Right
Medial epicondyle of femur ....use Lower Femur, Left/Right
Medial malleolus ....use Tibia, Left/Right
Navicular bone....use Tarsal, Left/Right
Neck of femur ....use Upper Femur, Left/Right
Pubis ....use Pelvic Bone, Left/Right
Spinous process ....use Cervical, Thoracic, Lumbar Vertebra
Talus bone ....use Tarsal, Left/Right
Vertebral arch ....use Cervical, Thoracic, Lumbar Vertebra
Vertebral foramen ....use Cervical, Thoracic, Lumbar Vertebra
Vertebral lamina ....use Cervical, Thoracic, Lumbar Vertebra
Vertebral pedicle ....use Cervical, Thoracic, Lumbar Vertebra

Device Key Listings of Lower Bones

See also Device Key in Appendix D

Autograft....use Autologous Tissue Substitute
Bone bank bone graft....use Nonautologous Tissue Substitute
Bone screw (interlocking) (lag) (pedicle) (recessed) ....use Internal Fixation Device in Head and Facial Bones, Upper Bones, Lower Bones
Clamp and rod internal fixation system (CRIF) ....use Internal Fixation Device in Upper Bones, Lower Bones
Delta frame external fixator....use External Fixation Device, Hybrid for Insertion in Upper Bones, Lower Bones
....use External Fixation Device, Hybrid for Reposition in Upper Bones, Lower Bones
Electrical bone growth stimulator (EBGS) ....use Bone Growth Stimulator in Head and Facial Bones, Upper Bones, Lower Bones
External fixator....use External Fixation Device in Head and Facial Bones, Upper Bones, Lower Bones, Upper Joints, Lower Joints
Ilizarov external fixator ....use External Fixation Device, Ring for Insertion in Upper Bones, Lower Bones
....use External Fixation Device, Ring for Reposition in Upper Bones, Lower Bones
Ilizarov-Vecklich device....use External Fixation Device, Limb Lengthening for Insertion in Upper Bones, Lower Bones
Intramedullary (IM) rod (nail) ....use Internal Fixation Device, Intramedullary in Upper Bones, Lower Bones
Intramedullary skeletal kinetic distractor (ISKD)....use Internal Fixation Device, Intramedullary in Upper Bones, Lower Bones
Kirschner wire (K-wire)....use Internal Fixation Device in Head and Facial Bones, Upper Bones, Lower Bones, Upper Joints, Lower Joints
Kuntscher nail....use Internal Fixation Device, Intramedullary in Upper Bones, Lower Bones
Neutralization plate ....use Internal Fixation Device in Head and Facial Bones, Upper Bones, Lower Bones
Polymethylmethacrylate (PMMA)....use Synthetic Substitute
Sheffield hybrid external fixator....use External Fixation Device, Hybrid for Insertion in Upper Bones, Lower Bones
....use External Fixation Device, Hybrid for Reposition in Upper Bones, Lower Bones
Sheffield ring external fixator ....use External Fixation Device, Ring for Insertion in Upper Bones, Lower Bones
....use External Fixation Device, Ring for Reposition in Upper Bones, Lower Bones
Tissue bank graft ....use Nonautologous Tissue Substitute
Ultrasonic osteogenic stimulator....use Bone Growth Stimulator in Head and Facial Bones, Upper Bones, Lower Bones
Ultrasound bone healing system ....use Bone Growth Stimulator in Head and Facial Bones, Upper Bones, Lower Bones
Uniplanar external fixator ....use External Fixation Device, Monoplanar for Insertion in Upper Bones, Lower Bones
....use External Fixation Device, Monoplanar for Reposition in Upper Bones, Lower Bones

© 2018 Channel Publishing, Ltd.

Educational Annotations | Q – Lower Bones

Device Aggregation Table Listings of Lower Bones

See also Device Aggregation Table in Appendix E

Specific Device	For Operation	In Body System	General Device
External Fixation Device, Hybrid	Insertion	Lower Bones	External Fixation Device
External Fixation Device, Hybrid	Reposition	Lower Bones	External Fixation Device
External Fixation Device, Limb Lengthening	Insertion	Lower Bones	External Fixation Device
External Fixation Device, Monoplanar	Insertion	Lower Bones	External Fixation Device
External Fixation Device, Monoplanar	Reposition	Lower Bones	External Fixation Device
External Fixation Device, Ring	Insertion	Lower Bones	External Fixation Device
External Fixation Device, Ring	Reposition	Lower Bones	External Fixation Device
Internal Fixation Device, Intramedullary	All applicable	Lower Bones	Internal Fixation Device

Coding Notes of Lower Bones

Body System Relevant Coding Guidelines

Reposition for fracture treatment

B3.15

Reduction of a displaced fracture is coded to the root operation Reposition and the application of a cast or splint in conjunction with the Reposition procedure is not coded separately. Treatment of a nondisplaced fracture is coded to the procedure performed.

Examples: Casting of a nondisplaced fracture is coded to the root operation Immobilization in the Placement section.

Putting a pin in a nondisplaced fracture is coded to the root operation Insertion.

© 2018 Channel Publishing, Ltd.

1ST - 0 Medical and Surgical
2ND - Q Lower Bones
3RD - 2 CHANGE

DEVICE GROUP: Change, Insertion, Removal, Replacement, Revision, Supplement
Root Operations that always involve a device.

CHANGE: Taking out or off a device from a body part and putting back an identical or similar device in or on the same body part without cutting or puncturing the skin or a mucous membrane.

Explanation: All CHANGE procedures are coded using the approach External
Examples: Exchange drain tube – CMS Ex: Urinary catheter change

Body Part – 4TH	Approach – 5TH	Device – 6TH	Qualifier – 7TH
Y Lower Bone	X External	0 Drainage device Y Other device	Z No qualifier

1ST - 0 Medical and Surgical
2ND - Q Lower Bones
3RD - 5 DESTRUCTION

EXCISION GROUP: Excision, Resection, Destruction, Extraction, (Detachment)
Root Operations that take out some or all of a body part.

DESTRUCTION: Physical eradication of all or a portion of a body part by the direct use of energy, force, or a destructive agent.

Explanation: None of the body part is physically taken out
Examples: Cryoablation bone cyst – CMS Ex: Fulguration of rectal polyp

Body Part – 4TH			Approach – 5TH	Device – 6TH	Qualifier – 7TH
0 Lumbar Vertebra 1 Sacrum 2 Pelvic Bone, Right 3 Pelvic Bone, Left 4 Acetabulum, Right 5 Acetabulum, Left 6 Upper Femur, Right 7 Upper Femur, Left	8 Femoral Shaft, Right 9 Femoral Shaft, Left B Lower Femur, Right C Lower Femur, Left D Patella, Right F Patella, Left G Tibia, Right H Tibia, Left	J Fibula, Right K Fibula, Left L Tarsal, Right M Tarsal, Left N Metatarsal, Right P Metatarsal, Left Q Toe Phalanx, Right R Toe Phalanx, Left S Coccyx	0 Open 3 Percutaneous 4 Percutaneous endoscopic	Z No device	Z No qualifier

LOWER BONES 0Q2

1ST - 0 Medical and Surgical
2ND - Q Lower Bones
3RD - 8 DIVISION

DIVISION GROUP: Division, Release
Root Operations involving cutting or separation only.

DIVISION: Cutting into a body part, without draining fluids and/or gases from the body part, in order to separate or transect a body part.

Explanation: All or a portion of the body part is separated into two or more portions
Examples: Tarsal osteotomy – CMS Ex: Spinal cordotomy

Body Part – 4TH			Approach – 5TH	Device – 6TH	Qualifier – 7TH
0 Lumbar Vertebra 1 Sacrum 2 Pelvic Bone, Right 3 Pelvic Bone, Left 4 Acetabulum, Right 5 Acetabulum, Left 6 Upper Femur, Right 7 Upper Femur, Left	8 Femoral Shaft, Right 9 Femoral Shaft, Left B Lower Femur, Right C Lower Femur, Left D Patella, Right F Patella, Left G Tibia, Right H Tibia, Left	J Fibula, Right K Fibula, Left L Tarsal, Right M Tarsal, Left N Metatarsal, Right P Metatarsal, Left Q Toe Phalanx, Right R Toe Phalanx, Left S Coccyx	0 Open 3 Percutaneous 4 Percutaneous endoscopic	Z No device	Z No qualifier

© 2018 Channel Publishing, Ltd.

1ST - 0 Medical and Surgical
2ND - Q Lower Bones
3RD - 9 DRAINAGE

DRAINAGE GROUP: Drainage, Extirpation, (Fragmentation)
Root Operations that take out solids/fluids/gases from a body part.

DRAINAGE: Taking or letting out fluids and/or gases from a body part.

Explanation: Qualifier "X Diagnostic" indicates drainage procedures that are biopsies
Examples: Aspiration bone cyst – CMS Ex: Thoracentesis

Body Part – 4TH			Approach – 5TH	Device – 6TH	Qualifier – 7TH
0 Lumbar Vertebra 1 Sacrum 2 Pelvic Bone, Right 3 Pelvic Bone, Left 4 Acetabulum, Right 5 Acetabulum, Left 6 Upper Femur, Right 7 Upper Femur, Left	8 Femoral Shaft, Right 9 Femoral Shaft, Left B Lower Femur, Right C Lower Femur, Left D Patella, Right F Patella, Left G Tibia, Right H Tibia, Left	J Fibula, Right K Fibula, Left L Tarsal, Right M Tarsal, Left N Metatarsal, Right P Metatarsal, Left Q Toe Phalanx, Right R Toe Phalanx, Left S Coccyx	0 Open 3 Percutaneous 4 Percutaneous endoscopic	0 Drainage device	Z No qualifier
0 Lumbar Vertebra 1 Sacrum 2 Pelvic Bone, Right 3 Pelvic Bone, Left 4 Acetabulum, Right 5 Acetabulum, Left 6 Upper Femur, Right 7 Upper Femur, Left	8 Femoral Shaft, Right 9 Femoral Shaft, Left B Lower Femur, Right C Lower Femur, Left D Patella, Right F Patella, Left G Tibia, Right H Tibia, Left	J Fibula, Right K Fibula, Left L Tarsal, Right M Tarsal, Left N Metatarsal, Right P Metatarsal, Left Q Toe Phalanx, Right R Toe Phalanx, Left S Coccyx	0 Open 3 Percutaneous 4 Percutaneous endoscopic	Z No device	X Diagnostic Z No qualifier

1ST - 0 Medical and Surgical
2ND - Q Lower Bones
3RD - B EXCISION

EXCISION GROUP: Excision, Resection, Destruction, Extraction, (Detachment)
Root Operations that take out some or all of a body part.

EXCISION: Cutting out or off, without replacement, a portion of a body part.

Explanation: Qualifier "X Diagnostic" indicates excision procedures that are biopsies
Examples: Harvest bone for graft – CMS Ex: Liver biopsy

Body Part – 4TH			Approach – 5TH	Device – 6TH	Qualifier – 7TH
0 Lumbar Vertebra 1 Sacrum 2 Pelvic Bone, Right 3 Pelvic Bone, Left 4 Acetabulum, Right 5 Acetabulum, Left 6 Upper Femur, Right 7 Upper Femur, Left	8 Femoral Shaft, Right 9 Femoral Shaft, Left B Lower Femur, Right C Lower Femur, Left D Patella, Right F Patella, Left G Tibia, Right H Tibia, Left	J Fibula, Right K Fibula, Left L Tarsal, Right M Tarsal, Left N Metatarsal, Right P Metatarsal, Left Q Toe Phalanx, Right R Toe Phalanx, Left S Coccyx	0 Open 3 Percutaneous 4 Percutaneous endoscopic	Z No device	X Diagnostic Z No qualifier

1ST - 0 Medical and Surgical
2ND - Q Lower Bones
3RD - C EXTIRPATION

DRAINAGE GROUP: Drainage, Extirpation, (Fragmentation)
Root Operations that take out solids/fluids/gases from a body part.

EXTIRPATION: Taking or cutting out solid matter from a body part.

Explanation: Abnormal byproduct or foreign body ...
Examples: Removal foreign body – CMS Ex: Thrombectomy

Body Part – 4TH			Approach – 5TH	Device – 6TH	Qualifier – 7TH
0 Lumbar Vertebra 1 Sacrum 2 Pelvic Bone, Right 3 Pelvic Bone, Left 4 Acetabulum, Right 5 Acetabulum, Left 6 Upper Femur, Right 7 Upper Femur, Left	8 Femoral Shaft, Right 9 Femoral Shaft, Left B Lower Femur, Right C Lower Femur, Left D Patella, Right F Patella, Left G Tibia, Right H Tibia, Left	J Fibula, Right K Fibula, Left L Tarsal, Right M Tarsal, Left N Metatarsal, Right P Metatarsal, Left Q Toe Phalanx, Right R Toe Phalanx, Left S Coccyx	0 Open 3 Percutaneous 4 Percutaneous endoscopic	Z No device	Z No qualifier

© 2018 Channel Publishing, Ltd.

1ST - 0 Medical and Surgical
2ND - Q Lower Bones
3RD - D EXTRACTION

EXCISION GROUP: Excision, Resection, Destruction, Extraction, (Detachment)
Root Operations that take out some or all of a body part.

EXTRACTION: Pulling or stripping out or off all or a portion of a body part by the use of force.

Explanation: None for this Body System
Examples: Non-excisional debridement – CMS Ex: Dilation and curettage

Body Part – 4TH	Approach – 5TH	Device – 6TH	Qualifier – 7TH
0 Lumbar Vertebra 1 Sacrum 2 Pelvic Bone, Right 3 Pelvic Bone, Left 4 Acetabulum, Right 5 Acetabulum, Left 6 Upper Femur, Right 7 Upper Femur, Left 8 Femoral Shaft, Right 9 Femoral Shaft, Left B Lower Femur, Right C Lower Femur, Left D Patella, Right F Patella, Left G Tibia, Right H Tibia, Left J Fibula, Right K Fibula, Left L Tarsal, Right M Tarsal, Left N Metatarsal, Right P Metatarsal, Left Q Toe Phalanx, Right R Toe Phalanx, Left S Coccyx	0 Open	Z No device	Z No qualifier

1ST - 0 Medical and Surgical
2ND - Q Lower Bones
3RD - H INSERTION

DEVICE GROUP: Change, Insertion, Removal, Replacement, Revision, Supplement
Root Operations that always involve a device.

INSERTION: Putting in a nonbiological appliance that monitors, assists, performs, or prevents a physiological function but does not physically take the place of a body part.

Explanation: None
Examples: Insertion growing rods – CMS Ex: Insertion of central venous catheter

Body Part – 4TH	Approach – 5TH	Device – 6TH	Qualifier – 7TH
0 Lumbar Vertebra 1 Sacrum 2 Pelvic Bone, Right 3 Pelvic Bone, Left 4 Acetabulum, Right 5 Acetabulum, Left D Patella, Right F Patella, Left L Tarsal, Right M Tarsal, Left N Metatarsal, Right P Metatarsal, Left Q Toe Phalanx, Right R Toe Phalanx, Left S Coccyx	0 Open 3 Percutaneous 4 Percutaneous endoscopic	4 Internal fixation device 5 External fixation device	Z No qualifier
6 Upper Femur, Right 7 Upper Femur, Left 8 Femoral Shaft, Right 9 Femoral Shaft, Left B Lower Femur, Right C Lower Femur, Left G Tibia, Right H Tibia, Left J Fibula, Right K Fibula, Left	0 Open 3 Percutaneous 4 Percutaneous endoscopic	4 Internal fixation device 5 External fixation device 6 Internal fixation device, intramedullary 8 External fixation device, limb lengthening B External fixation device, monoplanar C External fixation device, ring D External fixation device, hybrid	Z No qualifier
Y Lower Bone	0 Open 3 Percutaneous 4 Percutaneous endoscopic	M Bone growth stimulator	Z No qualifier

1ST - 0 Medical and Surgical
2ND - Q Lower Bones
3RD - J INSPECTION

EXAMINATION GROUP: Inspection, (Map)
Root Operations involving examination only.

INSPECTION: Visually and/or manually exploring a body part.

Explanation: Direct or instrumental visualization ...
Examples: Examination bone – CMS Ex: Exploratory laparotomy

Body Part – 4TH	Approach – 5TH	Device – 6TH	Qualifier – 7TH
Y Lower Bone	0 Open 3 Percutaneous 4 Percutaneous endoscopic X External	Z No device	Z No qualifier

© 2018 Channel Publishing, Ltd.

1ST - 0 Medical and Surgical
2ND - Q Lower Bones
3RD - N RELEASE

DIVISION GROUP: Division, Release
Root Operations involving cutting or separation only.

RELEASE: Freeing a body part from an abnormal physical constraint by cutting or by the use of force.

Explanation: Some of the restraining tissue may be taken out but none of the body part is taken out
Examples: Extra-articular bone adhesiolysis – CMS Ex: Carpal tunnel release

Body Part – 4TH			Approach – 5TH	Device – 6TH	Qualifier – 7TH
0 Lumbar Vertebra 1 Sacrum 2 Pelvic Bone, Right 3 Pelvic Bone, Left 4 Acetabulum, Right 5 Acetabulum, Left 6 Upper Femur, Right 7 Upper Femur, Left	8 Femoral Shaft, Right 9 Femoral Shaft, Left B Lower Femur, Right C Lower Femur, Left D Patella, Right F Patella, Left G Tibia, Right H Tibia, Left	J Fibula, Right K Fibula, Left L Tarsal, Right M Tarsal, Left N Metatarsal, Right P Metatarsal, Left Q Toe Phalanx, Right R Toe Phalanx, Left S Coccyx	0 Open 3 Percutaneous 4 Percutaneous endoscopic	Z No device	Z No qualifier

1ST - 0 Medical and Surgical
2ND - Q Lower Bones
3RD - P REMOVAL

DEVICE GROUP: Change, Insertion, Removal, Replacement, Revision, Supplement
Root Operations that always involve a device.

REMOVAL: Taking out or off a device from a body part.

Explanation: Removal device without reinsertion ...
Examples: Removal bone lengthening growing rods – CMS Ex: Cardiac pacemaker removal

Body Part – 4TH			Approach – 5TH	Device – 6TH	Qualifier – 7TH
0 Lumbar Vertebra 1 Sacrum 4 Acetabulum, Right 5 Acetabulum, Left S Coccyx			0 Open 3 Percutaneous 4 Percutaneous endoscopic	4 Internal fixation device 7 Autologous tissue substitute J Synthetic substitute K Nonautologous tissue substitute	Z No qualifier
0 Lumbar Vertebra 1 Sacrum	4 Acetabulum, Right 5 Acetabulum, Left S Coccyx		X External	4 Internal fixation device	Z No qualifier
2 Pelvic Bone, Right 3 Pelvic Bone, Left 6 Upper Femur, Right 7 Upper Femur, Left 8 Femoral Shaft, Right 9 Femoral Shaft, Left B Lower Femur, Right C Lower Femur, Left	D Patella, Right F Patella, Left G Tibia, Right H Tibia, Left J Fibula, Right K Fibula, Left	L Tarsal, Right M Tarsal, Left N Metatarsal, Right P Metatarsal, Left Q Toe Phalanx, Right R Toe Phalanx, Left	0 Open 3 Percutaneous 4 Percutaneous endoscopic	4 Internal fixation device 5 External fixation device 7 Autologous tissue substitute J Synthetic substitute K Nonautologous tissue substitute	Z No qualifier
2 Pelvic Bone, Right 3 Pelvic Bone, Left 6 Upper Femur, Right 7 Upper Femur, Left 8 Femoral Shaft, Right 9 Femoral Shaft, Left B Lower Femur, Right C Lower Femur, Left	D Patella, Right F Patella, Left G Tibia, Right H Tibia, Left J Fibula, Right K Fibula, Left	L Tarsal, Right M Tarsal, Left N Metatarsal, Right P Metatarsal, Left Q Toe Phalanx, Right R Toe Phalanx, Left	X External	4 Internal fixation device 5 External fixation device	Z No qualifier
Y Lower Bone			0 Open 3 Percutaneous 4 Percutaneous endoscopic X External	0 Drainage device M Bone growth stimulator	Z No qualifier

© 2018 Channel Publishing, Ltd.

1ST - 0 Medical and Surgical
2ND - Q Lower Bones
3RD - Q REPAIR

OTHER REPAIRS GROUP: (Control), Repair
Root Operations that define other repairs.

REPAIR: Restoring, to the extent possible, a body part to its normal anatomic structure and function.

Explanation: Used only when the method to accomplish the repair is not one of the other root operations
Examples: Vertebral laminoplasty – CMS Ex: Suture of laceration

Body Part – 4TH			Approach – 5TH	Device – 6TH	Qualifier – 7TH
0 Lumbar Vertebra 1 Sacrum 2 Pelvic Bone, Right 3 Pelvic Bone, Left 4 Acetabulum, Right 5 Acetabulum, Left 6 Upper Femur, Right 7 Upper Femur, Left	8 Femoral Shaft, Right 9 Femoral Shaft, Left B Lower Femur, Right C Lower Femur, Left D Patella, Right F Patella, Left G Tibia, Right H Tibia, Left	J Fibula, Right K Fibula, Left L Tarsal, Right M Tarsal, Left N Metatarsal, Right P Metatarsal, Left Q Toe Phalanx, Right R Toe Phalanx, Left S Coccyx	0 Open 3 Percutaneous 4 Percutaneous endoscopic X External	Z No device	Z No qualifier

1ST - 0 Medical and Surgical
2ND - Q Lower Bones
3RD - R REPLACEMENT

DEVICE GROUP: Change, Insertion, Removal, Replacement, Revision, Supplement
Root Operations that always involve a device.

REPLACEMENT: Putting in or on biological or synthetic material that physically takes the place and/or function of all or a portion of a body part.

Explanation: Includes taking out or eradicating, or rendering non-functional, the body part ...
Examples: Patella replacement – CMS Ex: Total hip replacement

Body Part – 4TH			Approach – 5TH	Device – 6TH	Qualifier – 7TH
0 Lumbar Vertebra 1 Sacrum 2 Pelvic Bone, Right 3 Pelvic Bone, Left 4 Acetabulum, Right 5 Acetabulum, Left 6 Upper Femur, Right 7 Upper Femur, Left	8 Femoral Shaft, Right 9 Femoral Shaft, Left B Lower Femur, Right C Lower Femur, Left D Patella, Right F Patella, Left G Tibia, Right H Tibia, Left	J Fibula, Right K Fibula, Left L Tarsal, Right M Tarsal, Left N Metatarsal, Right P Metatarsal, Left Q Toe Phalanx, Right R Toe Phalanx, Left S Coccyx	0 Open 3 Percutaneous 4 Percutaneous endoscopic	7 Autologous tissue substitute J Synthetic substitute K Nonautologous tissue substitute	Z No qualifier

© 2018 Channel Publishing, Ltd.

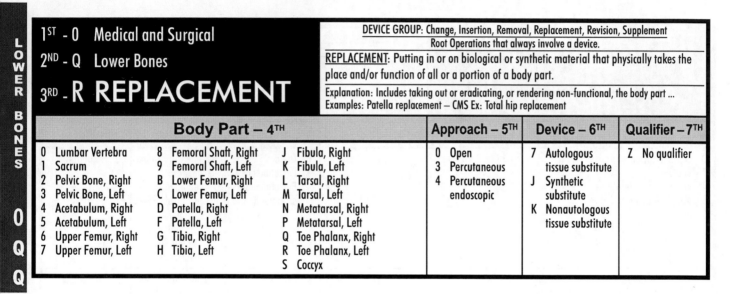

1ST - 0 Medical and Surgical
2ND - Q Lower Bones
3RD - S REPOSITION

MOVE GROUP: (Reattachment), Reposition, (Transfer), (Transplantation)
Root Operations that put in/put back or move some/all of a body part.

REPOSITION: Moving to its normal location, or other suitable location, all or a portion of a body part.

Explanation: The body part may or may not be cut out or off to be moved to the new location ...
Examples: Reduction with hybrid fixation device – CMS Ex: Fracture reduction

Body Part – 4TH	Approach – 5TH	Device – 6TH	Qualifier – 7TH
0 Lumbar Vertebra 1 Sacrum 4 Acetabulum, Right 5 Acetabulum, Left S Coccyx	0 Open 3 Percutaneous 4 Percutaneous endoscopic	4 Internal fixation device Z No device	Z No qualifier
0 Lumbar Vertebra 1 Sacrum 4 Acetabulum, Right 5 Acetabulum, Left S Coccyx	X External	Z No device	Z No qualifier
2 Pelvic Bone, Right 3 Pelvic Bone, Left D Patella, Right F Patella, Left L Tarsal, Right M Tarsal, Left Q Toe Phalanx, Right R Toe Phalanx, Left	0 Open 3 Percutaneous 4 Percutaneous endoscopic	4 Internal fixation device 5 External fixation device Z No device	Z No qualifier
2 Pelvic Bone, Right 3 Pelvic Bone, Left D Patella, Right F Patella, Left L Tarsal, Right M Tarsal, Left Q Toe Phalanx, Right R Toe Phalanx, Left	X External	Z No device	Z No qualifier
6 Upper Femur, Right 7 Upper Femur, Left 8 Femoral Shaft, Right 9 Femoral Shaft, Left B Lower Femur, Right C Lower Femur, Left G Tibia, Right H Tibia, Left J Fibula, Right K Fibula, Left	0 Open 3 Percutaneous 4 Percutaneous endoscopic	4 Internal fixation device 5 External fixation device 6 Internal fixation device, intramedullary B External fixation device, monoplanar C External fixation device, ring D External fixation device, hybrid Z No device	Z No qualifier
6 Upper Femur, Right 7 Upper Femur, Left 8 Femoral Shaft, Right 9 Femoral Shaft, Left B Lower Femur, Right C Lower Femur, Left G Tibia, Right H Tibia, Left J Fibula, Right K Fibula, Left	X External	Z No device	Z No qualifier
N Metatarsal, Right P Metatarsal, Left	0 Open 3 Percutaneous 4 Percutaneous endoscopic	4 Internal fixation device 5 External fixation device Z No device	2 Sesamoid Bone(s) 1st Toe Z No qualifier
N Metatarsal, Right P Metatarsal, Left	X External	Z No device	2 Sesamoid Bone(s) 1st Toe Z No qualifier

1ST - 0 Medical and Surgical
2ND - Q Lower Bones
3RD - T RESECTION

EXCISION GROUP: Excision, Resection, Destruction, Extraction, (Detachment)
Root Operations that take out some or all of a body part.

RESECTION: Cutting out or off, without replacement, all of a body part.

Explanation: None
Examples: Total patellectomy – CMS Ex: Total lobectomy of lung

Body Part – 4TH	Approach – 5TH	Device – 6TH	Qualifier – 7TH
2 Pelvic Bone, Right 3 Pelvic Bone, Left 4 Acetabulum, Right 5 Acetabulum, Left 6 Upper Femur, Right 7 Upper Femur, Left 8 Femoral Shaft, Right 9 Femoral Shaft, Left B Lower Femur, Right C Lower Femur, Left D Patella, Right F Patella, Left G Tibia, Right H Tibia, Left J Fibula, Right K Fibula, Left L Tarsal, Right M Tarsal, Left N Metatarsal, Right P Metatarsal, Left Q Toe Phalanx, Right R Toe Phalanx, Left S Coccyxt	0 Open	Z No device	Z No qualifier

© 2018 Channel Publishing, Ltd.

1ST - 0 Medical and Surgical
2ND - Q Lower Bones
3RD - U SUPPLEMENT

DEVICE GROUP: Change, Insertion, Removal, Replacement, Revision, Supplement
Root Operations that always involve a device.

SUPPLEMENT: Putting in or on biological or synthetic material that physically reinforces and/or augments the function of a portion of a body part.

Explanation: Biological material is non-living, or is living and from the same individual ...
Examples: Application bone void filler – CMS Ex: Herniorrhaphy using mesh

Body Part – 4TH			Approach – 5TH	Device – 6TH	Qualifier – 7TH
0 Lumbar Vertebra 1 Sacrum 2 Pelvic Bone, Right 3 Pelvic Bone, Left 4 Acetabulum, Right 5 Acetabulum, Left 6 Upper Femur, Right 7 Upper Femur, Left	8 Femoral Shaft, Right 9 Femoral Shaft, Left B Lower Femur, Right C Lower Femur, Left D Patella, Right F Patella, Left G Tibia, Right H Tibia, Left	J Fibula, Right K Fibula, Left L Tarsal, Right M Tarsal, Left N Metatarsal, Right P Metatarsal, Left Q Toe Phalanx, Right R Toe Phalanx, Left S Coccyx	0 Open 3 Percutaneous 4 Percutaneous endoscopic	7 Autologous tissue substitute J Synthetic substitute K Nonautologous tissue substitute	Z No qualifier

1ST - 0 Medical and Surgical
2ND - Q Lower Bones
3RD - W REVISION

DEVICE GROUP: Change, Insertion, Removal, Replacement, Revision, Supplement
Root Operations that always involve a device.

REVISION: Correcting, to the extent possible, a portion of a malfunctioning device or the position of a displaced device.

Explanation: Correcting by taking out or putting in components of a device such as a screw or pin ...
Examples: Adjustment bone lengthening growing rods – CMS Ex: Recementing of hip prosthesis

Body Part – 4TH			Approach – 5TH	Device – 6TH	Qualifier – 7TH
0 Lumbar Vertebra 1 Sacrum	4 Acetabulum, Right 5 Acetabulum, Left	S Coccyx	0 Open 3 Percutaneous 4 Percutaneous endoscopic X External	4 Internal fixation device 7 Autologous tissue substitute J Synthetic substitute K Nonautologous tissue substitute	Z No qualifier
2 Pelvic Bone, Right 3 Pelvic Bone, Left 6 Upper Femur, Right 7 Upper Femur, Left 8 Femoral Shaft, Right 9 Femoral Shaft, Left B Lower Femur, Right	C Lower Femur, Left D Patella, Right F Patella, Left G Tibia, Right H Tibia, Left J Fibula, Right K Fibula, Left	L Tarsal, Right M Tarsal, Left N Metatarsal, Right P Metatarsal, Left Q Toe Phalanx, Right R Toe Phalanx, Left	0 Open 3 Percutaneous 4 Percutaneous endoscopic X External	4 Internal fixation device 5 External fixation device 7 Autologous tissue substitute J Synthetic substitute K Nonautologous tissue substitute	Z No qualifier
Y Lower Bone			0 Open 3 Percutaneous 4 Percutaneous endoscopic X External	0 Drainage device M Bone growth stimulator	Z No qualifier

© 2018 Channel Publishing, Ltd.

Educational Annotations | R – Upper Joints

Body System Specific Educational Annotations for the Upper Joints include:

- Anatomy and Physiology Review
- Anatomical Illustrations
- Definitions of Common Procedures
- AHA Coding Clinic® Reference Notations
- Body Part Key Listings
- Device Key Listings
- Device Aggregation Table Listings
- Coding Notes

Anatomy and Physiology Review of Upper Joints

BODY PART VALUES – R - UPPER JOINTS

Acromioclavicular Joint – The joint formed between the acromion portion of the scapula and the distal end of the clavicle.
Carpal Joint – A complex collection of joints formed by the interconnection of the 8 carpal bones in the hand.
Cervical Vertebral Disc – The disc-shaped fibrocartilage pad between the cervical spine vertebral bodies comprised of a tough outer portion (annulus fibrosus) and a gel-like inner portion (nucleus pulposus).
Cervical Vertebral Joint – The synovial and cartilaginous joints connecting the vertebra of the cervical spine.
Cervicothoracic Vertebral Disc – The disc-shaped fibrocartilage pad between the C7 vertebral body of the cervical spine and the T1 vertebral body of the thoracic spine comprised of a tough outer portion (annulus fibrosus) and a gel-like inner portion (nucleus pulposus).
Cervicothoracic Vertebral Joint – The synovial and cartilaginous joints connecting the C7 vertebra of the cervical spine and the T1 vertebra of the thoracic spine.
Elbow Joint – A hinge joint between the humerus in the upper arm and the radius and ulna in the forearm.
Finger Phalangeal Joint – Any of 9 hinge joints in the fingers between the proximal and intermediate phalanges (PIP), and the intermediate and distal phalanges (DIP). The thumb has only two phalanges and therefore only one phalangeal joint.
Metacarpocarpal Joint – Any of the 5 joints in the hand that articulate the distal row of carpal bones and the proximal bases of the five metacarpal bones.
Metacarpophalangeal Joint – Any of 5 condyloid joints (except the hinge joint of the thumb) in the hand that articulate the distal heads of the five metacarpal bones and the proximal phalanx of each finger.
Occipital-cervical Joint – The joint formed between the C1 vertebra and the base of the skull (occipital bone).
Shoulder Joint – A multiaxial ball-and-socket joint (also known as the glenohumeral joint) between the head of the humerus and the rounded depression (glenoid fossa) of the scapula.
Sternoclavicular Joint – The joint formed between the upper portion of the sternum and the medial end of the clavicle.
Temporomandibular Joint – The joint formed between the mandible and temporal bone.
Thoracic Vertebral Disc – The disc-shaped fibrocartilage pad between the thoracic spine vertebral bodies comprised of a tough outer portion (annulus fibrosus) and a gel-like inner portion (nucleus pulposus).
Thoracic Vertebral Joint – The synovial and cartilaginous joints connecting the vertebra of the thoracic spine.
Thoracolumbar Vertebral Disc – The disc-shaped fibrocartilage pad between the T12 vertebral body of the thoracic spine and the L1 vertebral body of the lumbar spine comprised of a tough outer portion (annulus fibrosus) and a gel-like inner portion (nucleus pulposus).
Thoracolumbar Vertebral Joint – The synovial and cartilaginous joints connecting the T12 vertebra of the thoracic spine and the L1 vertebra of the lumbar spine.
Upper Joint – Any of the joints designated in the Upper Joints PCS Body System.
Wrist Joint – A pivot joint between the distal radius and the carpus.

Anatomical Illustrations of Upper Joints

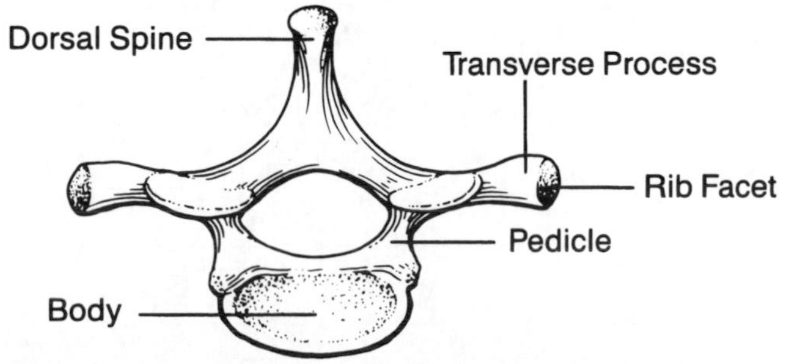

TYPICAL VERTEBRA — SUPERIOR VIEW

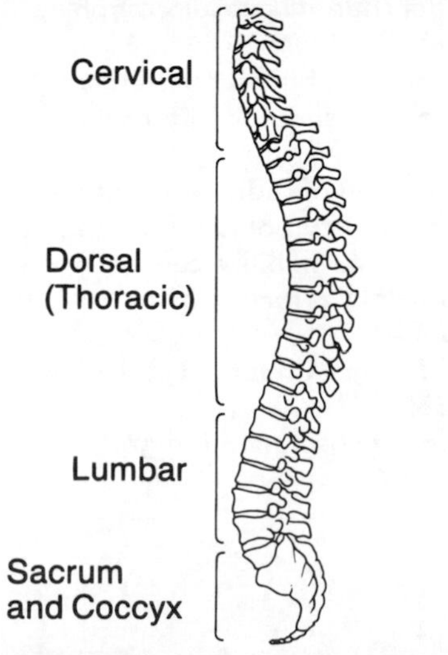

VERTEBRAL COLUMN

UPPER JOINTS 0 R

© 2018 Channel Publishing, Ltd.

Educational Annotations | R – Upper Joints

Definitions of Common Procedures of Upper Joints

Arthroscopy – The surgical visualization and examination of a joint using an endoscope and often the approach used for joint procedures.

Cervical interbody spinal fusion – The permanent surgical joining of two or more cervical vertebrae together using bone graft placed between the intervertebral space after the disc(s) have been removed and using metal or plastic cage to support the spine while the bone graft hardens.

Cervical spinal fusion – The permanent surgical joining of two or more cervical vertebrae together using a bone graft and immobilization by using plates, rods, screws, and/or wires.

Discectomy – The surgical removal of all (total) or a portion of an intervertebral disc.

Reverse total shoulder arthroplasty – The surgical replacement of the shoulder joint by reversing the cup and head replacement. The cup is placed onto the humerus and the ball is placed in the socket. This procedure is done for patients with severe rotator cuff damage.

Total shoulder arthroplasty – The surgical replacement of the shoulder joint socket (glenoid) cup and humeral head in the normal anatomical configuration.

Type 2 SLAP (superior labral tear from anterior to posterior) repair – The surgical repair of the glenoid labrum of the shoulder joint.

AHA Coding Clinic® Reference Notations of Upper Joints

ROOT OPERATION SPECIFIC - R - UPPER JOINTS

CHANGE - 2

DESTRUCTION - 5

DRAINAGE - 9

EXCISION - B

Spinal fusion with discectomy....AHA 14:2Q:p6

EXTIRPATION - C

FUSION - G

Components in fusion procedures included in Fusion root operation....AHA 14:3Q:p30

Fusion of cervicothoracic vertebral joint with interbody fusion device....AHA 13:1Q:p29

....AHA 14:2Q:p7

Fusion of interphalangeal joint....AHA 17:4Q:p62

Fusion of multiple vertebral joints....AHA 13:1Q:p21

INSERTION - H

Vertebral instrumentation without fusion....AHA 17:2Q:p23

Vertebral instrumentation without fusion - Official Clarification....AHA 18:1Q:p22

INSPECTION - J

RELEASE - N

Release of shoulder joint....AHA 15:2Q:p23

Rotator cuff repair with subacromial decompression....AHA 16:3Q:p32

Subacromial and rotator cuff decompression....AHA 15:2Q:p22

REMOVAL - P

REPAIR - Q

Shoulder thermal capsulorrhaphy....AHA 16:1Q:p30

REPLACEMENT - R

Replacement of fractured humeral head surface....AHA 15:3Q:p14

Reverse total shoulder arthroplasty....AHA 15:1Q:p27

REPOSITION - S

Manipulation of radioulnar joint dislocation....AHA 14:4Q:p32

Reposition of carpal joint....AHA 14:3Q:p33

Tongs used to stabilize cervical fracture....AHA 13:2Q:p39

Official Correction of 13:2Q:p39....AHA 15:2Q:p34

RESECTION - T

Spinal fusion with total discectomy....AHA 14:2Q:p7

SUPPLEMENT - U

Arthroplasty using tendon graft....AHA 15:3Q:p26

REVISION - W

© 2018 Channel Publishing, Ltd.

Educational Annotations | R – Upper Joints

Body Part Key Listings of Upper Joints

See also Body Part Key in Appendix C

Atlantoaxial joint .... use Cervical Vertebral Joint
Cervical facet joint .... use Cervical Vertebral Joint(s)
Cervicothoracic facet joint .... use Cervicothoracic Vertebral Joint
Costotransverse joint .... use Thoracic Vertebral Joint
Costovertebral joint .... use Thoracic Vertebral Joint
Distal humerus, involving joint .... use Elbow Joint, Left/Right
Distal radioulnar joint .... use Wrist Joint, Left/Right
Glenohumeral joint .... use Shoulder Joint, Left/Right
Glenoid ligament (labrum) .... use Shoulder Joint, Left/Right
Humeroradial joint .... use Elbow Joint, Left/Right
Humeroulnar joint .... use Elbow Joint, Left/Right
Intercarpal joint .... use Carpal Joint, Left/Right
Interphalangeal (IP) joint .... use Finger Phalangeal Joint, Left/Right
Midcarpal joint .... use Carpal Joint, Left/Right
Proximal radioulnar joint .... use Elbow Joint, Left/Right
Radiocarpal joint .... use Wrist Joint, Left/Right
Thoracic facet joint .... use Thoracic Vertebral Joint
Thoracolumbar facet joint .... use Thoracolumbar Vertebral Joint

Device Key Listings of Upper Joints

See also Device Key in Appendix D

Autograft .... use Autologous Tissue Substitute
BAK/C® Interbody Cervical Fusion System .... use Interbody Fusion Device in Upper Joints
BRYAN® Cervical Disc System .... use Synthetic Substitute
Delta III Reverse shoulder prosthesis .... use Synthetic Substitute, Reverse Ball and Socket for Replacement in Upper Joints
Dynesys® Dynamic Stabilization System .... use Spinal Stabilization Device, Pedicle-Based for Insertion in Upper Joints, Lower Joints
External fixator .... use External Fixation Device in Head and Facial Bones, Upper Bones, Lower Bones, Upper Joints, Lower Joints
Facet replacement spinal stabilization device .... use Spinal Stabilization Device, Facet Replacement for Insertion in Upper Joints, Lower Joints
Fusion screw (compression) (lag) (locking) .... use Internal Fixation Device in Upper Joints, Lower Joints
Interbody fusion (spine) cage .... use Interbody Fusion Device in Upper Joints, Lower Joints
Interspinous process spinal stabilization device .... use Spinal Stabilization Device, Interspinous Process for Insertion in Upper Joints, Lower Joints
Joint fixation plate .... use Internal Fixation Device in Upper Joints, Lower Joints
Joint spacer (antibiotic) .... use Spacer in Upper Joints, Lower Joints
Kirschner wire (K-wire) .... use Internal Fixation Device in Head and Facial Bones, Upper Bones, Lower Bones, Upper Joints, Lower Joints
Pedicle-based dynamic stabilization device .... use Spinal Stabilization Device, Pedicle-Based for Insertion in Upper Joints, Lower Joints
Polymethylmethacrylate (PMMA) .... use Synthetic Substitute
PRESTIGE® Cervical Disc .... use Synthetic Substitute
Prodisc-C .... use Synthetic Substitute
Reverse® Shoulder Prosthesis .... use Synthetic Substitute, Reverse Ball and Socket for Replacement in Upper Joints
Tissue bank graft .... use Nonautologous Tissue Substitute
X-STOP® Spacer .... use Spinal Stabilization Device, Interspinous Process for Insertion in Upper Joints, Lower Joints

Device Aggregation Table Listings of Upper Joints

See also Device Aggregation Table in Appendix E

Specific Device	For Operation	In Body System	General Device
Spinal Stabilization Device, Facet Replacement	Insertion	Upper Joints	Internal Fixation Device
Spinal Stabilization Device, Interspinous Process	Insertion	Upper Joints	Internal Fixation Device
Spinal Stabilization Device, Pedicle-Based	Insertion	Upper Joints	Internal Fixation Device

© 2018 Channel Publishing, Ltd.

Educational Annotations | R – Upper Joints

Coding Notes of Upper Joints

Body System Relevant Coding Guidelines

Fusion procedures of the spine

B3.10a

The body part coded for a spinal vertebral joint(s) rendered immobile by a spinal fusion procedure is classified by the level of the spine (e.g. thoracic). There are distinct body part values for a single vertebral joint and for multiple vertebral joints at each spinal level.

Example: Body part values specify Lumbar Vertebral Joint, Lumbar Vertebral Joints, 2 or More and Lumbosacral Vertebral Joint.

B3.10b

If multiple vertebral joints are fused, a separate procedure is coded for each vertebral joint that uses a different device and/or qualifier.

Example: Fusion of lumbar vertebral joint, posterior approach, anterior column and fusion of lumbar vertebral joint, posterior approach, posterior column are coded separately.

B3.10c

Combinations of devices and materials are often used on a vertebral joint to render the joint immobile. When combinations of devices are used on the same vertebral joint, the device value coded for the procedure is as follows:

- If an interbody fusion device is used to render the joint immobile (alone or containing other material like bone graft), the procedure is coded with the device value Interbody Fusion Device
- If bone graft is the only device used to render the joint immobile, the procedure is coded with the device value Nonautologous Tissue Substitute or Autologous Tissue Substitute
- If a mixture of autologous and nonautologous bone graft (with or without biological or synthetic extenders or binders) is used to render the joint immobile, code the procedure with the device value Autologous Tissue Substitute

Examples: Fusion of a vertebral joint using a cage style interbody fusion device containing morsellized bone graft is coded to the device Interbody Fusion Device.

Fusion of a vertebral joint using a bone dowel interbody fusion device made of cadaver bone and packed with a mixture of local morsellized bone and demineralized bone matrix is coded to the device Interbody Fusion Device.

Fusion of a vertebral joint using both autologous bone graft and bone bank bone graft is coded to the device Autologous Tissue Substitute.

Tendons, ligaments, bursae and fascia near a joint

B4.5

Procedures performed on tendons, ligaments, bursae and fascia supporting a joint are coded to the body part in the respective body system that is the focus of the procedure. Procedures performed on joint structures themselves are coded to the body part in the joint body systems.

Examples: Repair of the anterior cruciate ligament of the knee is coded to the knee bursa and ligament body part in the bursae and ligaments body system.

Knee arthroscopy with shaving of articular cartilage is coded to the knee joint body part in the Lower Joints body system.

© 2018 Channel Publishing, Ltd.

1ST - 0 Medical and Surgical
2ND - R Upper Joints
3RD - 2 CHANGE

DEVICE GROUP: Change, Insertion, Removal, Replacement, Revision, Supplement
Root Operations that always involve a device.

CHANGE: Taking out or off a device from a body part and putting back an identical or similar device in or on the same body part without cutting or puncturing the skin or a mucous membrane.

Explanation: All CHANGE procedures are coded using the approach External
Examples: Exchange drain tube – CMS Ex: Urinary catheter change

Body Part – 4TH	Approach – 5TH	Device – 6TH	Qualifier – 7TH
Y Upper Joint	X External	0 Drainage device Y Other device	Z No qualifier

1ST - 0 Medical and Surgical
2ND - R Upper Joints
3RD - 5 DESTRUCTION

EXCISION GROUP: Excision, Resection, Destruction, (Extraction), (Detachment)
Root Operations that take out some or all of a body part.

DESTRUCTION: Physical eradication of all or a portion of a body part by the direct use of energy, force, or a destructive agent.

Explanation: None of the body part is physically taken out
Examples: Radiofrequency ablation – CMS Ex: Fulguration of rectal polyp

Body Part – 4TH			Approach – 5TH	Device – 6TH	Qualifier–7TH
0 Occipital-cervical Joint 1 Cervical Vertebral Joint 3 Cervical Vertebral Disc 4 Cervicothoracic Vertebral Joint 5 Cervicothoracic Vertebral Disc 6 Thoracic Vertebral Joint 9 Thoracic Vertebral Disc A Thoracolumbar Vertebral Joint B Thoracolumbar Vertebral Disc C Temporomandibular Joint, Right D Temporomandibular Joint, Left	E Sternoclavicular Joint, Right F Sternoclavicular Joint, Left G Acromioclavicular Joint, Right H Acromioclavicular Joint, Left J Shoulder Joint, Right K Shoulder Joint, Left L Elbow Joint, Right M Elbow Joint, Left N Wrist Joint, Right P Wrist Joint, Left Q Carpal Joint, Right R Carpal Joint, Left	S Carpometacarpal Joint, Right T Carpometacarpal Joint, Left U Metacarpophalangeal Joint, Right V Metacarpophalangeal Joint, Left W Finger Phalangeal Joint, Right X Finger Phalangeal Joint, Left	0 Open 3 Percutaneous 4 Percutaneous endoscopic	Z No device	Z No qualifier

1ST - 0 Medical and Surgical
2ND - R Upper Joints
3RD - 9 DRAINAGE

DRAINAGE GROUP: Drainage, Extirpation, (Fragmentation)
Root Operations that take out solids/fluids/gases from a body part.

DRAINAGE: Taking or letting out fluids and/or gases from a body part.

Explanation: Qualifier "X Diagnostic" indicates drainage procedures that are biopsies
Examples: Aspiration fluid elbow joint – CMS Ex: Thoracentesis

Body Part – 4TH			Approach – 5TH	Device – 6TH	Qualifier–7TH
0 Occipital-cervical Joint 1 Cervical Vertebral Joint 3 Cervical Vertebral Disc 4 Cervicothoracic Vertebral Joint 5 Cervicothoracic Vertebral Disc 6 Thoracic Vertebral Joint 9 Thoracic Vertebral Disc A Thoracolumbar Vertebral Joint B Thoracolumbar Vertebral Disc C Temporomandibular Joint, Right D Temporomandibular Joint, Left	E Sternoclavicular Joint, Right F Sternoclavicular Joint, Left G Acromioclavicular Joint, Right H Acromioclavicular Joint, Left J Shoulder Joint, Right K Shoulder Joint, Left L Elbow Joint, Right M Elbow Joint, Left N Wrist Joint, Right P Wrist Joint, Left Q Carpal Joint, Right R Carpal Joint, Left	S Carpometacarpal Joint, Right T Carpometacarpal Joint, Left U Metacarpophalangeal Joint, Right V Metacarpophalangeal Joint, Left W Finger Phalangeal Joint, Right X Finger Phalangeal Joint, Left	0 Open 3 Percutaneous 4 Percutaneous endoscopic	0 Drainage device	Z No qualifier

continued ⇨

© 2018 Channel Publishing, Ltd.

0 R 9 DRAINAGE – *continued*

Body Part – 4TH	Approach – 5TH	Device – 6TH	Qualifier–7TH
0 Occipital-cervical Joint 1 Cervical Vertebral Joint 3 Cervical Vertebral Disc 4 Cervicothoracic Vertebral Joint 5 Cervicothoracic Vertebral Disc 6 Thoracic Vertebral Joint 9 Thoracic Vertebral Disc A Thoracolumbar Vertebral Joint B Thoracolumbar Vertebral Disc C Temporomandibular Joint, Right D Temporomandibular Joint, Left E Sternoclavicular Joint, Right F Sternoclavicular Joint, Left G Acromioclavicular Joint, Right H Acromioclavicular Joint, Left J Shoulder Joint, Right K Shoulder Joint, Left L Elbow Joint, Right M Elbow Joint, Left N Wrist Joint, Right P Wrist Joint, Left Q Carpal Joint, Right R Carpal Joint, Left S Carpometacarpal Joint, Right T Carpometacarpal Joint, Left U Metacarpophalangeal Joint, Right V Metacarpophalangeal Joint, Left W Finger Phalangeal Joint, Right X Finger Phalangeal Joint, Left	0 Open 3 Percutaneous 4 Percutaneous endoscopic	Z No device	X Diagnostic Z No qualifier

1ST - 0 Medical and Surgical

2ND - R Upper Joints

3RD - B EXCISION

EXCISION GROUP: Excision, Resection, Destruction, (Extraction), (Detachment)
Root Operations that take out some or all of a body part.

EXCISION: Cutting out or off, without replacement, a portion of a body part.

Explanation: Qualifier "X Diagnostic" indicates excision procedures that are biopsies
Examples: Partial cervical discectomy – CMS Ex: Liver biopsy

Body Part – 4TH	Approach – 5TH	Device – 6TH	Qualifier–7TH
0 Occipital-cervical Joint 1 Cervical Vertebral Joint 3 Cervical Vertebral Disc 4 Cervicothoracic Vertebral Joint 5 Cervicothoracic Vertebral Disc 6 Thoracic Vertebral Joint 9 Thoracic Vertebral Disc A Thoracolumbar Vertebral Joint B Thoracolumbar Vertebral Disc C Temporomandibular Joint, Right D Temporomandibular Joint, Left E Sternoclavicular Joint, Right F Sternoclavicular Joint, Left G Acromioclavicular Joint, Right H Acromioclavicular Joint, Left J Shoulder Joint, Right K Shoulder Joint, Left L Elbow Joint, Right M Elbow Joint, Left N Wrist Joint, Right P Wrist Joint, Left Q Carpal Joint, Right R Carpal Joint, Left S Carpometacarpal Joint, Right T Carpometacarpal Joint, Left U Metacarpophalangeal Joint, Right V Metacarpophalangeal Joint, Left W Finger Phalangeal Joint, Right X Finger Phalangeal Joint, Left	0 Open 3 Percutaneous 4 Percutaneous endoscopic	Z No device	X Diagnostic Z No qualifier

1ST - 0 Medical and Surgical

2ND - R Upper Joints

3RD - C EXTIRPATION

DRAINAGE GROUP: Drainage, Extirpation, (Fragmentation)
Root Operations that take out solids/fluids/gases from a body part.

EXTIRPATION: Taking or cutting out solid matter from a body part.

Explanation: Abnormal byproduct or foreign body ...
Examples: Removal loose bodies elbow – CMS Ex: Thrombectomy

Body Part – 4TH	Approach – 5TH	Device – 6TH	Qualifier–7TH
0 Occipital-cervical Joint 1 Cervical Vertebral Joint 3 Cervical Vertebral Disc 4 Cervicothoracic Vertebral Joint 5 Cervicothoracic Vertebral Disc 6 Thoracic Vertebral Joint 9 Thoracic Vertebral Disc A Thoracolumbar Vertebral Joint B Thoracolumbar Vertebral Disc C Temporomandibular Joint, Right D Temporomandibular Joint, Left E Sternoclavicular Joint, Right F Sternoclavicular Joint, Left G Acromioclavicular Joint, Right H Acromioclavicular Joint, Left J Shoulder Joint, Right K Shoulder Joint, Left L Elbow Joint, Right M Elbow Joint, Left N Wrist Joint, Right P Wrist Joint, Left Q Carpal Joint, Right R Carpal Joint, Left S Carpometacarpal Joint, Right T Carpometacarpal Joint, Left U Metacarpophalangeal Joint, Right V Metacarpophalangeal Joint, Left W Finger Phalangeal Joint, Right X Finger Phalangeal Joint, Left	0 Open 3 Percutaneous 4 Percutaneous endoscopic	Z No device	Z No qualifier

© 2018 Channel Publishing, Ltd.

1ST - 0 Medical and Surgical
2ND - R Upper Joints
3RD - G FUSION

OTHER OBJECTIVES GROUP: (Alteration), (Creation), Fusion
Root Operations that define other objectives.

FUSION: Joining together portions of an articular body part rendering the articular body part immobile.

Explanation: The body part is joined together by fixation device, bone graft, other means
Examples: Cervical spinal fusion – CMS Ex: Spinal fusion

Body Part – 4TH	Approach – 5TH	Device – 6TH	Qualifier – 7TH
0 Occipital-cervical Joint 1 Cervical Vertebral Joint 2 Cervical Vertebral Joints, 2 or more 4 Cervicothoracic Vertebral Joint 6 Thoracic Vertebral Joint 7 Thoracic Vertebral Joints, 2 to 7 8 Thoracic Vertebral Joints, 8 or more A Thoracolumbar Vertebral Joint	0 Open 3 Percutaneous 4 Percutaneous endoscopic	7 Autologous tissue substitute J Synthetic substitute K Nonautologous tissue substitute	0 Anterior approach, anterior column 1 Posterior approach, posterior column J Posterior approach, anterior column
0 Occipital-cervical Joint 1 Cervical Vertebral Joint 2 Cervical Vertebral Joints, 2 or more 4 Cervicothoracic Vertebral Joint 6 Thoracic Vertebral Joint 7 Thoracic Vertebral Joints, 2 to 7 8 Thoracic Vertebral Joints, 8 or more A Thoracolumbar Vertebral Joint	0 Open 3 Percutaneous 4 Percutaneous endoscopic	A Interbody fusion device	0 Anterior approach, anterior column J Posterior approach, anterior column
C Temporomandibular Joint, Right D Temporomandibular Joint, Left E Sternoclavicular Joint, Right F Sternoclavicular Joint, Left G Acromioclavicular Joint, Right H Acromioclavicular Joint, Left J Shoulder Joint, Right K Shoulder Joint, Left	0 Open 3 Percutaneous 4 Percutaneous endoscopic	4 Internal fixation device 7 Autologous tissue substitute J Synthetic substitute K Nonautologous tissue substitute	Z No qualifier
L Elbow Joint, Right M Elbow Joint, Left N Wrist Joint, Right P Wrist Joint, Left Q Carpal Joint, Right R Carpal Joint, Left S Carpometacarpal Joint, Right T Carpometacarpal Joint, Left U Metacarpophalangeal Joint, Right V Metacarpophalangeal Joint, Left W Finger Phalangeal Joint, Right X Finger Phalangeal Joint, Left	0 Open 3 Percutaneous 4 Percutaneous endoscopic	4 Internal fixation device 5 External fixation device 7 Autologous tissue substitute J Synthetic substitute K Nonautologous tissue substitute	Z No qualifier

© 2018 Channel Publishing, Ltd.

1ST - 0 Medical and Surgical
2ND - R Upper Joints
3RD - H INSERTION

DEVICE GROUP: Change, Insertion, Removal, Replacement, Revision, Supplement
Root Operations that always involve a device.

INSERTION: Putting in a nonbiological appliance that monitors, assists, performs, or prevents a physiological function but does not physically take the place of a body part.

Explanation: None
Examples: Implantation joint spacer – CMS Ex: Insertion of central venous catheter

Body Part – 4TH	Approach – 5TH	Device – 6TH	Qualifier – 7TH
0 Occipital-cervical Joint 1 Cervical Vertebral Joint 4 Cervicothoracic Vertebral Joint 6 Thoracic Vertebral Joint A Thoracolumbar Vertebral Joint	0 Open 3 Percutaneous 4 Percutaneous endoscopic	3 Infusion device 4 Internal fixation device 8 Spacer B Spinal stabilization device, interspinous process C Spinal stabilization device, pedicle-based D Spinal stabilization device, facet replacement	Z No qualifier
3 Cervical Vertebral Disc 5 Cervicothoracic Vertebral Disc 9 Thoracic Vertebral Disc B Thoracolumbar Vertebral Disc	0 Open 3 Percutaneous 4 Percutaneous endoscopic	3 Infusion device	Z No qualifier
C Temporomandibular Joint, Right D Temporomandibular Joint, Left E Sternoclavicular Joint, Right F Sternoclavicular Joint, Left G Acromioclavicular Joint, Right H Acromioclavicular Joint, Left J Shoulder Joint, Right K Shoulder Joint, Left	0 Open 3 Percutaneous 4 Percutaneous endoscopic	3 Infusion device 4 Internal fixation device 8 Spacer	Z No qualifier
L Elbow Joint, Right M Elbow Joint, Left N Wrist Joint, Right P Wrist Joint, Left Q Carpal Joint, Right R Carpal Joint, Left S Carpometacarpal Joint, Right T Carpometacarpal Joint, Left U Metacarpophalangeal Joint, Right V Metacarpophalangeal Joint, Left W Finger Phalangeal Joint, Right X Finger Phalangeal Joint, Left	0 Open 3 Percutaneous 4 Percutaneous endoscopic	3 Infusion device 4 Internal fixation device 5 External fixation device 8 Spacer	Z No qualifier

1ST - 0 Medical and Surgical
2ND - R Upper Joints
3RD - J INSPECTION

EXAMINATION GROUP: Inspection, (Map)
Root Operations involving examination only.

INSPECTION: Visually and/or manually exploring a body part.

Explanation: Direct or instrumental visualization ...
Examples: Diagnostic arthroscopy – CMS Ex: Exploratory laparotomy

Body Part – 4TH			Approach – 5TH	Device – 6TH	Qualifier–7TH
0 Occipital-cervical Joint 1 Cervical Vertebral Joint 3 Cervical Vertebral Disc 4 Cervicothoracic Vertebral Joint 5 Cervicothoracic Vertebral Disc 6 Thoracic Vertebral Joint 9 Thoracic Vertebral Disc A Thoracolumbar Vertebral Joint B Thoracolumbar Vertebral Disc C Temporomandibular Joint, Right D Temporomandibular Joint, Left	E Sternoclavicular Joint, Right F Sternoclavicular Joint, Left G Acromioclavicular Joint, Right H Acromioclavicular Joint, Left J Shoulder Joint, Right K Shoulder Joint, Left L Elbow Joint, Right M Elbow Joint, Left N Wrist Joint, Right P Wrist Joint, Left Q Carpal Joint, Right R Carpal Joint, Left	S Carpometacarpal Joint, Right T Carpometacarpal Joint, Left U Metacarpophalangeal Joint, Right V Metacarpophalangeal Joint, Left W Finger Phalangeal Joint, Right X Finger Phalangeal Joint, Left	0 Open 3 Percutaneous 4 Percutaneous endoscopic X External	Z No device	Z No qualifier

UPPER JOINTS 0RH

© 2018 Channel Publishing, Ltd.

1ST - 0 Medical and Surgical
2ND - R Upper Joints
3RD - N RELEASE

DIVISION GROUP: (Division), Release
Root Operations involving cutting or separation only.

RELEASE: Freeing a body part from an abnormal physical constraint by cutting or by the use of force.

Explanation: Some of the restraining tissue may be taken out but none of the body part is taken out
Examples: Manual rupture joint adhesions – CMS Ex: Carpal tunnel release

Body Part – 4TH			Approach – 5TH	Device – 6TH	Qualifier–7TH
0 Occipital-cervical Joint 1 Cervical Vertebral Joint 3 Cervical Vertebral Disc 4 Cervicothoracic Vertebral Joint 5 Cervicothoracic Vertebral Disc 6 Thoracic Vertebral Joint 9 Thoracic Vertebral Disc A Thoracolumbar Vertebral Joint B Thoracolumbar Vertebral Disc C Temporomandibular Joint, Right D Temporomandibular Joint, Left	E Sternoclavicular Joint, Right F Sternoclavicular Joint, Left G Acromioclavicular Joint, Right H Acromioclavicular Joint, Left J Shoulder Joint, Right K Shoulder Joint, Left L Elbow Joint, Right M Elbow Joint, Left N Wrist Joint, Right P Wrist Joint, Left Q Carpal Joint, Right R Carpal Joint, Left	S Carpometacarpal Joint, Right T Carpometacarpal Joint, Left U Metacarpophalangeal Joint, Right V Metacarpophalangeal Joint, Left W Finger Phalangeal Joint, Right X Finger Phalangeal Joint, Left	0 Open 3 Percutaneous 4 Percutaneous endoscopic X External	Z No device	Z No qualifier

1ST - 0 Medical and Surgical
2ND - R Upper Joints
3RD - P REMOVAL

DEVICE GROUP: Change, Insertion, Removal, Replacement, Revision, Supplement
Root Operations that always involve a device.

REMOVAL: Taking out or off a device from a body part.

Explanation: Removal device without reinsertion ...
Examples: Removal fixation device – CMS Ex: Cardiac pacemaker removal

Body Part – 4TH		Approach – 5TH	Device – 6TH	Qualifier – 7TH
0 Occipital-cervical Joint 1 Cervical Vertebral Joint 4 Cervicothoracic Vertebral Joint	6 Thoracic Vertebral Joint A Thoracolumbar Vertebral Joint	0 Open 3 Percutaneous 4 Percutaneous endoscopic	0 Drainage device 3 Infusion device 4 Internal fixation device 7 Autologous tissue substitute 8 Spacer A Interbody fusion device J Synthetic substitute K Nonautologous tissue substitute	Z No qualifier
0 Occipital-cervical Joint 1 Cervical Vertebral Joint 4 Cervicothoracic Vertebral Joint	6 Thoracic Vertebral Joint A Thoracolumbar Vertebral Joint	X External	0 Drainage device 3 Infusion device 4 Internal fixation device	Z No qualifier
3 Cervical Vertebral Disc 5 Cervicothoracic Vertebral Disc	9 Thoracic Vertebral Disc B Thoracolumbar Vertebral Disc	0 Open 3 Percutaneous 4 Percutaneous endoscopic	0 Drainage device 3 Infusion device 7 Autologous tissue substitute J Synthetic substitute K Nonautologous tissue substitute	Z No qualifier
3 Cervical Vertebral Disc 5 Cervicothoracic Vertebral Disc	9 Thoracic Vertebral Disc B Thoracolumbar Vertebral Disc	X External	0 Drainage device 3 Infusion device	Z No qualifier
C Temporomandibular Joint, Right D Temporomandibular Joint, Left E Sternoclavicular Joint, Right F Sternoclavicular Joint, Left	G Acromioclavicular Joint, Right H Acromioclavicular Joint, Left J Shoulder Joint, Right K Shoulder Joint, Left	0 Open 3 Percutaneous 4 Percutaneous endoscopic	0 Drainage device 3 Infusion device 4 Internal fixation device 7 Autologous tissue substitute 8 Spacer J Synthetic substitute K Nonautologous tissue substitute	Z No qualifier
C Temporomandibular Joint, Right D Temporomandibular Joint, Left E Sternoclavicular Joint, Right F Sternoclavicular Joint, Left	G Acromioclavicular Joint, Right H Acromioclavicular Joint, Left J Shoulder Joint, Right K Shoulder Joint, Left	X External	0 Drainage device 3 Infusion device 4 Internal fixation device	Z No qualifier

continued ⇨

© 2018 Channel Publishing, Ltd.

0 R P REMOVAL – *continued*

Body Part – 4TH	Approach - 5TH	Device – 6TH	Qualifier – 7TH
L Elbow Joint, Right M Elbow Joint, Left N Wrist Joint, Right P Wrist Joint, Left Q Carpal Joint, Right R Carpal Joint, Left S Carpometacarpal Joint, Right T Carpometacarpal Joint, Left U Metacarpophalangeal Joint, Right V Metacarpophalangeal Joint, Left W Finger Phalangeal Joint, Right X Finger Phalangeal Joint, Left	0 Open 3 Percutaneous 4 Percutaneous endoscopic	0 Drainage device 3 Infusion device 4 Internal fixation device 5 External fixation device 7 Autologous tissue substitute 8 Spacer J Synthetic dubstitute K Nonautologous tissue substitute	Z No qualifier
L Elbow Joint, Right M Elbow Joint, Left N Wrist Joint, Right P Wrist Joint, Left Q Carpal Joint, Right R Carpal Joint, Left S Carpometacarpal Joint, Right T Carpometacarpal Joint, Left U Metacarpophalangeal Joint, Right V Metacarpophalangeal Joint, Left W Finger Phalangeal Joint, Right X Finger Phalangeal Joint, Left	X External	0 Drainage device 3 Infusion device 4 Internal fixation device 5 External fixation device	Z No qualifier

UPPER JOINTS 0RP

1ST - 0 Medical and Surgical
2ND - R Upper Joints
3RD - Q REPAIR

OTHER REPAIRS GROUP: (Control), Repair
Root Operations that define other repairs.

REPAIR: Restoring, to the extent possible, a body part to its normal anatomic structure and function.

Explanation: Used only when the method to accomplish the repair is not one of the other root operations
Examples: Suture arthroplasty – CMS Ex: Suture of laceration

Body Part – 4TH	Approach – 5TH	Device – 6TH	Qualifier–7TH
0 Occipital-cervical Joint 1 Cervical Vertebral Joint 3 Cervical Vertebral Disc 4 Cervicothoracic Vertebral Joint 5 Cervicothoracic Vertebral Disc 6 Thoracic Vertebral Joint 9 Thoracic Vertebral Disc A Thoracolumbar Vertebral Joint B Thoracolumbar Vertebral Disc C Temporomandibular Joint, Right D Temporomandibular Joint, Left E Sternoclavicular Joint, Right F Sternoclavicular Joint, Left G Acromioclavicular Joint, Right H Acromioclavicular Joint, Left J Shoulder Joint, Right K Shoulder Joint, Left L Elbow Joint, Right M Elbow Joint, Left N Wrist Joint, Right P Wrist Joint, Left Q Carpal Joint, Right R Carpal Joint, Left S Carpometacarpal Joint, Right T Carpometacarpal Joint, Left U Metacarpophalangeal Joint, Right V Metacarpophalangeal Joint, Left W Finger Phalangeal Joint, Right X Finger Phalangeal Joint, Left	0 Open 3 Percutaneous 4 Percutaneous endoscopic X External	Z No device	Z No qualifier

1ST - 0 Medical and Surgical
2ND - R Upper Joints
3RD - R REPLACEMENT

DEVICE GROUP: Change, Insertion, Removal, Replacement, Revision, Supplement
Root Operations that always involve a device.

REPLACEMENT: Putting in or on biological or synthetic material that physically takes the place and/or function of all or a portion of a body part.

Explanation: Includes taking out or eradicating, or rendering non-functional, the body part ...
Examples: Reverse total shoulder arthroplasty – CMS Ex: Total hip replacement

Body Part – 4TH	Approach – 5TH	Device – 6TH	Qualifier–7TH
0 Occipital-cervical Joint 1 Cervical Vertebral Joint 3 Cervical Vertebral Disc 4 Cervicothoracic Vertebral Joint 5 Cervicothoracic Vertebral Disc 6 Thoracic Vertebral Joint 9 Thoracic Vertebral Disc A Thoracolumbar Vertebral Joint B Thoracolumbar Vertebral Disc C Temporomandibular Joint, Right D Temporomandibular Joint, Left E Sternoclavicular Joint, Right F Sternoclavicular Joint, Left G Acromioclavicular Joint, Right H Acromioclavicular Joint, Left L Elbow Joint, Right M Elbow Joint, Left N Wrist Joint, Right P Wrist Joint, Left Q Carpal Joint, Right R Carpal Joint, Left S Carpometacarpal Joint, Right T Carpometacarpal Joint, Left U Metacarpophalangeal Joint, Right V Metacarpophalangeal Joint, Left W Finger Phalangeal Joint, Right X Finger Phalangeal Joint, Left	0 Open	7 Autologous tissue substitute J Synthetic substitute K Nonautologous tissue substitute	Z No qualifier

continued ⇨

© 2018 Channel Publishing, Ltd.

0 R R REPLACEMENT – *continued*

Body Part – 4TH	Approach – 5TH	Device – 6TH	Qualifier – 7TH
J Shoulder Joint, Right K Shoulder Joint, Left	0 Open	0 Synthetic substitute, reverse ball and socket 7 Autologous tissue substitute K Nonautologous tissue substitute	Z No qualifier
J Shoulder Joint, Right K Shoulder Joint, Left	0 Open	J Synthetic substitute	6 Humeral Surface 7 Glenoid Surface Z No qualifier

1ST - 0 Medical and Surgical
2ND - R Upper Joints
3RD - S REPOSITION

MOVE GROUP: (Reattachment), Reposition, (Transfer), (Transplantation)
Root Operations that put in/put back or move some/all of a body part.

REPOSITION: Moving to its normal location, or other suitable location, all or a portion of a body part.

Explanation: The body part may or may not be cut out or off to be moved to the new location ...
Examples: Closed reduction elbow joint dislocation – CMS Ex: Fracture reduction

Body Part – 4TH		Approach – 5TH	Device – 6TH	Qualifier – 7TH
0 Occipital-cervical Joint 1 Cervical Vertebral Joint 4 Cervicothoracic Vertebral Joint 6 Thoracic Vertebral Joint A Thoracolumbar Vertebral Joint C Temporomandibular Joint, Right D Temporomandibular Joint, Left	E Sternoclavicular Joint, Right F Sternoclavicular Joint, Left G Acromioclavicular Joint, Right H Acromioclavicular Joint, Left J Shoulder Joint, Right K Shoulder Joint, Left	0 Open 3 Percutaneous 4 Percutaneous endoscopic X External	4 Internal fixation device Z No device	Z No qualifier
L Elbow Joint, Right M Elbow Joint, Left N Wrist Joint, Right P Wrist Joint, Left Q Carpal Joint, Right R Carpal Joint, Left	S Carpometacarpal Joint, Right T Carpometacarpal Joint, Left U Metacarpophalangeal Joint, Right V Metacarpophalangeal Joint, Left W Finger Phalangeal Joint, Right X Finger Phalangeal Joint, Left	0 Open 3 Percutaneous 4 Percutaneous endoscopic X External	4 Internal fixation device 5 External fixation device Z No device	Z No qualifier

1ST - 0 Medical and Surgical
2ND - R Upper Joints
3RD - T RESECTION

EXCISION GROUP: Excision, Resection, Destruction, (Extraction), (Detachment)
Root Operations that take out some or all of a body part.

RESECTION: Cutting out or off, without replacement, all of a body part.

Explanation: None
Examples: Total cervical discectomy – CMS Ex: Total lobectomy of lung

Body Part – 4TH			Approach – 5TH	Device – 6TH	Qualifier–7TH
3 Cervical Vertebral Disc 4 Cervicothoracic Vertebral Joint 5 Cervicothoracic Vertebral Disc 9 Thoracic Vertebral Disc B Thoracolumbar Vertebral Disc C Temporomandibular Joint, Right D Temporomandibular Joint, Left E Sternoclavicular Joint, Right F Sternoclavicular Joint, Left G Acromioclavicular Joint, Right H Acromioclavicular Joint, Left	J Shoulder Joint, Right K Shoulder Joint, Left L Elbow Joint, Right M Elbow Joint, Left N Wrist Joint, Right P Wrist Joint, Left Q Carpal Joint, Right R Carpal Joint, Left	S Carpometacarpal Joint, Right T Carpometacarpal Joint, Left U Metacarpophalangeal Joint, Right V Metacarpophalangeal Joint, Left W Finger Phalangeal Joint, Right X Finger Phalangeal Joint, Left	0 Open	Z No device	Z No qualifier

UPPER JOINTS 0RT

© 2018 Channel Publishing, Ltd.

1ST - 0 Medical and Surgical
2ND - R Upper Joints
3RD - U SUPPLEMENT

DEVICE GROUP: Change, Insertion, Removal, Replacement, Revision, Supplement
Root Operations that always involve a device.

SUPPLEMENT: Putting in or on biological or synthetic material that physically reinforces and/or augments the function of a portion of a body part.

Explanation: Biological material is non-living, or is living and from the same individual ...
Examples: Shoulder joint free graft – CMS Ex: Herniorrhaphy using mesh

Body Part – 4TH			Approach – 5TH	Device – 6TH	Qualifier–7TH
0 Occipital-cervical Joint 1 Cervical Vertebral Joint 3 Cervical Vertebral Disc 4 Cervicothoracic Vertebral Joint 5 Cervicothoracic Vertebral Disc 6 Thoracic Vertebral Joint 9 Thoracic Vertebral Disc A Thoracolumbar Vertebral Joint B Thoracolumbar Vertebral Disc C Temporomandibular Joint, Right D Temporomandibular Joint, Left	E Sternoclavicular Joint, Right F Sternoclavicular Joint, Left G Acromioclavicular Joint, Right H Acromioclavicular Joint, Left J Shoulder Joint, Right K Shoulder Joint, Left L Elbow Joint, Right M Elbow Joint, Left N Wrist Joint, Right P Wrist Joint, Left Q Carpal Joint, Right R Carpal Joint, Left	S Carpometacarpal Joint, Right T Carpometacarpal Joint, Left U Metacarpophalangeal Joint, Right V Metacarpophalangeal Joint, Left W Finger Phalangeal Joint, Right X Finger Phalangeal Joint, Left	0 Open 3 Percutaneous 4 Percutaneous endoscopic	7 Autologous tissue substitute J Synthetic substitute K Nonautologous tissue substitute	Z No qualifier

1ST - 0 Medical and Surgical
2ND - R Upper Joints
3RD - W REVISION

DEVICE GROUP: Change, Insertion, Removal, Replacement, Revision, Supplement
Root Operations that always involve a device.

REVISION: Correcting, to the extent possible, a portion of a malfunctioning device or the position of a displaced device.

Explanation: Correcting by taking out or putting in components of a device such as a screw or pin ...
Examples: Reposition joint spacer – CMS Ex: Recementing of hip prosthesis

Body Part – 4TH	Approach – 5TH	Device – 6TH	Qualifier – 7TH
0 Occipital-cervical Joint 1 Cervical Vertebral Joint 4 Cervicothoracic Vertebral Joint 6 Thoracic Vertebral Joint A Thoracolumbar Vertebral Joint	0 Open 3 Percutaneous 4 Percutaneous endoscopic X External	0 Drainage device 3 Infusion device 4 Internal fixation device 7 Autologous tissue substitute 8 Spacer A Interbody fusion device J Synthetic substitute K Nonautologous tissue substitute	Z No qualifier
3 Cervical Vertebral Disc 5 Cervicothoracic Vertebral Disc 9 Thoracic Vertebral Disc B Thoracolumbar Vertebral Disc	0 Open 3 Percutaneous 4 Percutaneous endoscopic X External	0 Drainage device 3 Infusion device 7 Autologous tissue substitute J Synthetic substitute K Nonautologous tissue substitute	Z No qualifier
C Temporomandibular Joint, Right D Temporomandibular Joint, Left E Sternoclavicular Joint, Right F Sternoclavicular Joint, Left G Acromioclavicular Joint, Right H Acromioclavicular Joint, Left J Shoulder Joint, Right K Shoulder Joint, Left	0 Open 3 Percutaneous 4 Percutaneous endoscopic X External	0 Drainage device 3 Infusion device 4 Internal fixation device 7 Autologous tissue substitute 8 Spacer J Synthetic substitute K Nonautologous tissue substitute	Z No qualifier
L Elbow Joint, Right M Elbow Joint, Left N Wrist Joint, Right P Wrist Joint, Left Q Carpal Joint, Right R Carpal Joint, Left S Carpometacarpal Joint, Right T Carpometacarpal Joint, Left U Metacarpophalangeal Joint, Right V Metacarpophalangeal Joint, Left W Finger Phalangeal Joint, Right X Finger Phalangeal Joint, Left	0 Open 3 Percutaneous 4 Percutaneous endoscopic X External	0 Drainage device 3 Infusion device 4 Internal fixation device 5 External fixation device 7 Autologous tissue substitute 8 Spacer J Synthetic substitute K Nonautologous tissue substitute	Z No qualifier

© 2018 Channel Publishing, Ltd.

Educational Annotations | S – Lower Joints

Body System Specific Educational Annotations for the Lower Joints include:

- Anatomy and Physiology Review
- Anatomical Illustrations
- Definitions of Common Procedures
- AHA Coding Clinic® Reference Notations
- Body Part Key Listings
- Device Key Listings
- Device Aggregation Table Listings
- Coding Notes

Anatomy and Physiology Review of Lower Joints

BODY PART VALUES – S - LOWER JOINTS

Ankle Joint – The hinge joint formed between the distal tibia and fibula and the talus.
Coccygeal Joint – The joints formed between the several (3-5) very small bones that make up the coccyx.
Hip Joint – A ball-and-socket joint between the head of the femur and the acetabulum of the pelvis.
Hip Joint, Acetabular Surface – The surface of the acetabulum of the pelvis.
Hip Joint, Femoral Surface – The surface of the femoral head.
Knee Joint – The large hinge joint between the femur and the tibia.
Knee Joint, Femoral Surface – The surface of the femoral condyles.
Knee Joint, Tibial Surface – The surface of the tibial head.
Lower Joint – Any of the joints designated in the Lower Joints PCS Body System.
Lumbar Vertebral Disc – The disc-shaped fibrocartilage pad between the lumbar spine vertebral bodies comprised of a tough outer portion (annulus fibrosus) and a gel-like inner portion (nucleus pulposus).
Lumbar Vertebral Joint – The synovial and cartilaginous joints connecting the vertebra of the lumbar spine.
Lumbosacral Disc – The disc-shaped fibrocartilage pad between the S5 vertebral body of the lumbar spine and the sacrum comprised of a tough outer portion (annulus fibrosus) and a gel-like inner portion (nucleus pulposus).
Lumbosacral Joint – The synovial and cartilaginous joints connecting the S5 vertebra of the thoracic spine and the sacrum.
Metatarsal-Phalangeal Joint – Any of 5 condyloid joints in the foot that articulate the distal heads of the five metatarsal bones and the proximal phalanx of each toe.
Metatarsal-Tarsal Joint – Any of the 5 joints in the foot that articulate the tarsal bones and the proximal bases of the five metatarsal bones.
Sacrococcygeal Joint – The joint formed between the sacrum and coccyx.
Sacroiliac Joint – The strong joint joining the sacrum to the ilium bones that form the rigid pelvis.
Tarsal Joint – A complex collection of joints formed by the interconnection of the 7 tarsal bones in the foot.
Toe Phalangeal Joint – Any of 9 hinge joints in the toes between the proximal and intermediate phalanges (PIP), and the intermediate and distal phalanges (DIP). The great toe has only two phalanges and therefore only one phalangeal joint.

Anatomical Illustrations of Lower Joints

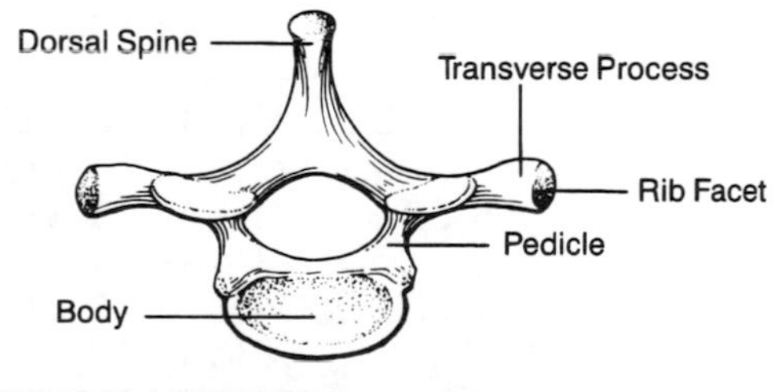

TYPICAL VERTEBRA — SUPERIOR VIEW

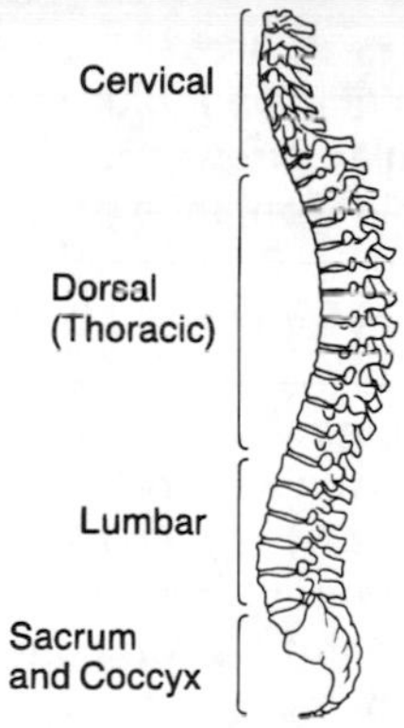

VERTEBRAL COLUMN

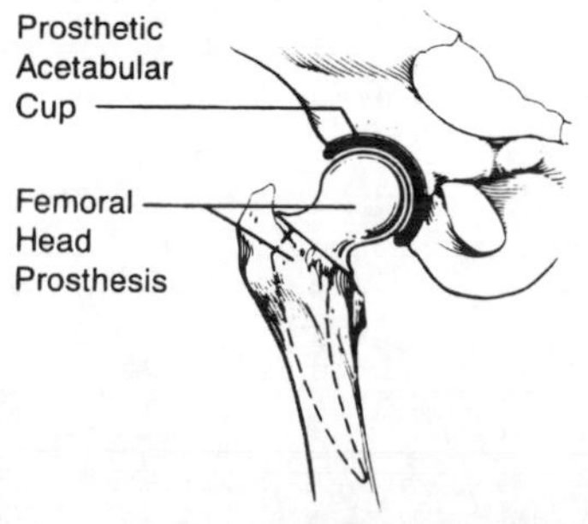

TOTAL HIP REPLACEMENT

LOWER JOINTS 0 S

© 2018 Channel Publishing, Ltd.

Educational Annotations | S – Lower Joints

Definitions of Common Procedures of Lower Joints

Arthroscopy – The surgical visualization and examination of a joint using an endoscope and often the approach used for joint procedures.
Discectomy – The surgical removal of all (total) or a portion of an intervertebral disc.
Interspinous process spacer – The surgical placement of a device between the spinous processes of vertebrae to relieve pressure on the spinal nerve roots.
Lumbar interbody spinal fusion – The permanent surgical joining of two or more lumbar vertebrae together using bone graft placed between the intervertebral space after the discs have been removed using metal or plastic cage to support the spine while the bone graft hardens.
Lumbar spinal fusion – The permanent surgical joining of two or more lumbar vertebrae together using a bone graft and immobilization by using plates, rods, screws, and/or wires.

AHA Coding Clinic® Reference Notations of Lower Joints

ROOT OPERATION SPECIFIC - S - LOWER JOINTS

CHANGE - 2
DESTRUCTION - 5
DRAINAGE - 9
Arthroscopic drainage of knee ....AHA 18:2Q:p17
EXCISION - B
Discectomy with decompressive foraminotomy/laminectomy ....AHA 16:2Q:p16
Menisectomy and abrasion chondroplasty with synovectomy ....AHA 15:1Q:p34
Spinal fusion with discectomy ....AHA 14:2Q:p6
EXTIRPATION - C
FUSION - G
360-degree spinal fusion ....AHA 13:3Q:p25
Ankle fusion with bone graft and internal fixation ....AHA 13:2Q:p39
Components in fusion procedures included in Fusion root operation ....AHA 14:3Q:p30
Fusion of multiple vertebral joints ....AHA 13:1Q:p21
Lumbar spinal fusion at two levels with pelvic bone graft ....AHA 14:2Q:p6
(*see also* AHA Correction Notice at 14:3Q:p36)
INSERTION - H
INSPECTION - J
Needle aspiration ankle joint with no fluid removed ....AHA 17:1Q:p50
RELEASE - N
REMOVAL - P
Removal of hip and knee devices ....AHA 16:4Q:p110
Removal of previous total knee replacement components ....AHA 15:2Q:p18
Removal of retained ankle screws ....AHA 13:2Q:p39
Removal of synthetic joint components ....AHA 15:2Q:p19
REPAIR - Q
Osteoplasty and labral refixation of hip joint ....AHA 14:4Q:p25
REPLACEMENT - R
Failed hip replacement, qualifier value selection ....AHA 16:3Q:p35
Hip replacement with acetabular reconstruction ....AHA 15:3Q:p18
Oxidized zirconium on polyethylene bearing surface ....AHA 17:4Q:p38
Partial (unicondylar) knee replacement ....AHA 16:4Q:p109
Replacement of femoral surface component ....AHA 15:2Q:p19
Replacement of hip joint liner ....AHA 18:2Q:p16
Replacement of patella in total knee joint replacement ....AHA 17:1Q:p22
Replacement of previous total knee replacement ....AHA 15:2Q:p18
REPOSITION - S
Periacetabular osteotomy ....AHA 16:2Q:p31
RESECTION - T
Metatarsophalangeal arthroplasty ....AHA 16:1Q:p20
Resection of lower femur and knee joint ....AHA 14:4Q:p29
Spinal fusion with total discectomy ....AHA 14:2Q:p7
SUPPLEMENT - U
Placement of new liner ....AHA 15:2Q:p19
REVISION - W
Revision of hip and knee devices ....AHA 16:4Q:p110
Revision of total ankle replacement ....AHA 17:4Q:p107

© 2018 Channel Publishing, Ltd.

Educational Annotations | S – Lower Joints

Body Part Key Listings of Lower Joints

See also Body Part Key in Appendix C

Acetabulofemoral joint	use Hip Joint, Left/Right
Calcaneocuboid joint	use Tarsal Joint, Left/Right
Cuboideonavicular joint	use Tarsal Joint, Left/Right
Cuneonavicular joint	use Tarsal Joint, Left/Right
Femoropatellar joint	use Knee Joint, Left/Right
	use Knee Joint, Femoral Surface, Left/Right
Femorotibial joint	use Knee Joint, Left/Right
	use Knee Joint, Tibial Surface, Left/Right
Inferior tibiofibular joint	use Ankle Joint, Left/Right
Intercuneiform joint	use Tarsal Joint, Left/Right
Interphalangeal (IP) joint	use Toe Phalangeal Joint, Left/Right
Lateral meniscus	use Knee Joint, Left/Right
Lumbar facet joint	use Lumbar Vertebral Joint
Lumbosacral facet joint	use Lumbosacral Joint
Medial meniscus	use Knee Joint, Left/Right
Metatarsophalangeal (MTP) joint	use Metatarsal-Phalangeal Joint, Left/Right
Patellofemoral joint	use Knee Joint, Left/Right
	use Knee Joint, Femoral Surface, Left/Right
Sacrococcygeal symphysis	use Sacrococcygeal Joint
Subtalar (talocalcaneal) joint	use Tarsal Joint, Left/Right
Talocalcaneal (subtalar) joint	use Tarsal Joint, Left/Right
Talocalcaneonavicular joint	use Tarsal Joint, Left/Right
Talocrural joint	use Ankle Joint, Left/Right
Tibiofemoral joint	use Knee Joint, Left/Right
	use Knee Joint, Tibial Surface, Left/Right

Device Key Listings of Lower Joints

See also Device Key in Appendix D

Acetabular cup	use Liner in Lower Joints
Autograft	use Autologous Tissue Substitute
Axial Lumbar Interbody Fusion System	use Interbody Fusion Device in Lower Joints
AxiaLIF® System	use Interbody Fusion Device in Lower Joints
Ceramic on ceramic bearing surface	use Synthetic Substitute, Ceramic for Replacement in Lower Joints
Cobalt/chromium head and polyethylene socket	use Synthetic Substitute, Metal on Polyethylene for Replacement in Lower Joints
Cobalt/chromium head and socket	use Synthetic Substitute, Ceramic for Replacement in Lower Joints
CONSERVE® PLUS Total Resurfacing Hip System	use Resurfacing Device in Lower Joints
Cormet Hip Resurfacing System	use Resurfacing Device in Lower Joints
CoRoent® XL	use Interbody Fusion Device in Lower Joints
Direct Lateral Interbody Fusion (DLIF) device	use Interbody Fusion Device in Lower Joints
Dynesys® Dynamic Stabilization System	use Spinal Stabilization Device, Pedicle-Based for Insertion in Upper Joints, Lower Joints
External fixator	use External Fixation Device in Head and Facial Bones, Upper Bones, Lower Bones, Upper Joints, Lower Joints
EXtreme Lateral Interbody Fusion (XLIF) device	use Interbody Fusion Device in Lower Joints
Facet replacement spinal stabilization device	use Spinal Stabilization Device, Facet Replacement for Insertion in Upper Joints, Lower Joints
Fusion screw (compression) (lag) (locking)	use Internal Fixation Device in Upper Joints, Lower Joints
Hip (joint) liner	use Liner in Lower Joints
Interbody fusion (spine) cage	use Interbody Fusion Device in Upper Joints, Lower Joints
Interspinous process spinal stabilization device	use Spinal Stabilization Device, Interspinous Process for Insertion in Upper Joints, Lower Joints
Joint fixation plate	use Internal Fixation Device in Upper Joints, Lower Joints
Joint liner (insert)	use Liner in Lower Joints
Joint spacer (antibiotic)	use Spacer in Upper Joints, Lower Joints
Kirschner wire (K-wire)	use Internal Fixation Device in Head and Facial Bones, Upper Bones, Lower Bones, Upper Joints, Lower Joints
Knee (implant) insert	use Liner in Lower Joints
Metal on metal bearing surface	use Synthetic Substitute, Metal for Replacement in Lower Joints
Novation® Ceramic AHS® (Articulation Hip System)	use Synthetic Substitute, Ceramic for Replacement in Lower Joints
OXINIUM	use Synthetic Substitute, Oxidized Zirconium on Polyethylene for Replacement in Lower Joints
Pedicle-based dynamic stabilization device	use Spinal Stabilization Device, Pedicle-Based for Insertion in Upper Joints, Lower Joints
Polyethylene socket	use Synthetic Substitute, Polyethylene for Replacement in Lower Joints
Polymethylmethacrylate (PMMA)	use Synthetic Substitute
Prodisc-L	use Synthetic Substitute
Tibial insert	use Liner in Lower Joints
Tissue bank graft	use Nonautologous Tissue Substitute
X-STOP® Spacer	use Spinal Stabilization Device, Interspinous Process for Insertion in Upper Joints, Lower Joints
XLIF® System	use Interbody Fusion Device in Lower Joints
Zimmer® NexGen® LPS Mobile Bearing Knee	use Synthetic Substitute
Zimmer® NexGen® LPS-Flex Mobile Knee	use Synthetic Substitute

© 2018 Channel Publishing, Ltd.

Educational Annotations

S – Lower Joints

Device Aggregation Table Listings of Lower Joints

See also Device Aggregation Table in Appendix E

Specific Device	For Operation	In Body System	General Device
Spinal Stabilization Device, Facet Replacement	Insertion	Lower Joints	Internal Fixation Device
Spinal Stabilization Device, Interspinous Process	Insertion	Lower Joints	Internal Fixation Device
Spinal Stabilization Device, Pedicle-Based	Insertion	Lower Joints	Internal Fixation Device
Synthetic Substitute, Ceramic	Replacement	Lower Joints	Synthetic Substitute
Synthetic Substitute, Ceramic on Polyethylene	Replacement	Lower Joints	Synthetic Substitute
Synthetic Substitute, Metal	Replacement	Lower Joints	Synthetic Substitute
Synthetic Substitute, Metal on Polyethylene	Replacement	Lower Joints	Synthetic Substitute
Synthetic Substitute, Oxidized Zirconium on Polyethylene	Replacement	Lower Joints	Synthetic Substitute
Synthetic Substitute, Polyethylene	Replacement	Lower Joints	Synthetic Substitute
Synthetic Substitute, Unicondylar	Replacement	Lower Joints	Synthetic Substitute

Coding Notes of Lower Joints

Body System Relevant Coding Guidelines

Fusion procedures of the spine

B3.10a

The body part coded for a spinal vertebral joint(s) rendered immobile by a spinal fusion procedure is classified by the level of the spine (e.g. thoracic). There are distinct body part values for a single vertebral joint and for multiple vertebral joints at each spinal level.
Example: Body part values specify Lumbar Vertebral Joint, Lumbar Vertebral Joints, 2 or More and Lumbosacral Vertebral Joint.

B3.10b

If multiple vertebral joints are fused, a separate procedure is coded for each vertebral joint that uses a different device and/or qualifier.
Example: Fusion of lumbar vertebral joint, posterior approach, anterior column and fusion of lumbar vertebral joint, posterior approach, posterior column are coded separately.

B3.10c

Combinations of devices and materials are often used on a vertebral joint to render the joint immobile. When combinations of devices are used on the same vertebral joint, the device value coded for the procedure is as follows:

- If an interbody fusion device is used to render the joint immobile (alone or containing other material like bone graft), the procedure is coded with the device value Interbody Fusion Device
- If bone graft is the only device used to render the joint immobile, the procedure is coded with the device value Nonautologous Tissue Substitute or Autologous Tissue Substitute
- If a mixture of autologous and nonautologous bone graft (with or without biological or synthetic extenders or binders) is used to render the joint immobile, code the procedure with the device value Autologous Tissue Substitute

Examples: Fusion of a vertebral joint using a cage style interbody fusion device containing morsellized bone graft is coded to the device Interbody Fusion Device.
Fusion of a vertebral joint using a bone dowel interbody fusion device made of cadaver bone and packed with a mixture of local morsellized bone and demineralized bone matrix is coded to the device Interbody Fusion Device.
Fusion of a vertebral joint using both autologous bone graft and bone bank bone graft is coded to the device Autologous Tissue Substitute.

Tendons, ligaments, bursae and fascia near a joint

B4.5

Procedures performed on tendons, ligaments, bursae and fascia supporting a joint are coded to the body part in the respective body system that is the focus of the procedure. Procedures performed on joint structures themselves are coded to the body part in the joint body systems.
Examples: Repair of the anterior cruciate ligament of the knee is coded to the knee bursa and ligament body part in the bursae and ligaments body system.
Knee arthroscopy with shaving of articular cartilage is coded to the knee joint body part in the Lower Joints body system.

© 2018 Channel Publishing, Ltd.

1ST - 0 Medical and Surgical
2ND - S Lower Joints
3RD - 2 CHANGE

DEVICE GROUP: Change, Insertion, Removal, Replacement, Revision, Supplement
Root Operations that always involve a device.

CHANGE: Taking out or off a device from a body part and putting back an identical or similar device in or on the same body part without cutting or puncturing the skin or a mucous membrane.

Explanation: All CHANGE procedures are coded using the approach External
Examples: Exchange drain tube – CMS Ex: Urinary catheter change

Body Part – 4TH	Approach – 5TH	Device – 6TH	Qualifier – 7TH
Y Lower Joint	X External	0 Drainage device Y Other device	Z No qualifier

1ST - 0 Medical and Surgical
2ND - S Lower Joints
3RD - 5 DESTRUCTION

EXCISION GROUP: Excision, Resection, Destruction, (Extraction), (Detachment)
Root Operations that take out some or all of a body part.

DESTRUCTION: Physical eradication of all or a portion of a body part by the direct use of energy, force, or a destructive agent.

Explanation: None of the body part is physically taken out
Examples: Radiofrequency ablation – CMS Ex: Fulguration of rectal polyp

Body Part – 4TH			Approach – 5TH	Device – 6TH	Qualifier–7TH
0 Lumbar Vertebral Joint 2 Lumbar Vertebral Disc 3 Lumbosacral Joint 4 Lumbosacral Disc 5 Sacrococcygeal Joint 6 Coccygeal Joint 7 Sacroiliac Joint, Right 8 Sacroiliac Joint, Left	9 Hip Joint, Right B Hip Joint, Left C Knee Joint, Right D Knee Joint, Left F Ankle Joint, Right G Ankle Joint, Left H Tarsal Joint, Right J Tarsal Joint, Left	K Tarsometatarsal Joint, Right L Tarsometatarsal Joint, Left M Metatarsal-Phalangeal Joint, Right N Metatarsal-Phalangeal Joint, Left P Toe Phalangeal Joint, Right Q Toe Phalangeal Joint, Left	0 Open 3 Percutaneous 4 Percutaneous endoscopic	Z No device	Z No qualifier

1ST - 0 Medical and Surgical
2ND - S Lower Joints
3RD - 9 DRAINAGE

DRAINAGE GROUP: Drainage, Extirpation, (Fragmentation)
Root Operations that take out solids/fluids/gases from a body part.

DRAINAGE: Taking or letting out fluids and/or gases from a body part.

Explanation: Qualifier "X Diagnostic" indicates drainage procedures that are biopsies
Examples: Aspiration fluid knee joint – CMS Ex: Thoracentesis

Body Part – 4TH			Approach – 5TH	Device – 6TH	Qualifier–7TH
0 Lumbar Vertebral Joint 2 Lumbar Vertebral Disc 3 Lumbosacral Joint 4 Lumbosacral Disc 5 Sacrococcygeal Joint 6 Coccygeal Joint 7 Sacroiliac Joint, Right 8 Sacroiliac Joint, Left	9 Hip Joint, Right B Hip Joint, Left C Knee Joint, Right D Knee Joint, Left F Ankle Joint, Right G Ankle Joint, Left H Tarsal Joint, Right J Tarsal Joint, Left	K Tarsometatarsal Joint, Right L Tarsometatarsal Joint, Left M Metatarsal-Phalangeal Joint, Right N Metatarsal-Phalangeal Joint, Left P Toe Phalangeal Joint, Right Q Toe Phalangeal Joint, Left	0 Open 3 Percutaneous 4 Percutaneous endoscopic	0 Drainage device	Z No qualifier
0 Lumbar Vertebral Joint 2 Lumbar Vertebral Disc 3 Lumbosacral Joint 4 Lumbosacral Disc 5 Sacrococcygeal Joint 6 Coccygeal Joint 7 Sacroiliac Joint, Right 8 Sacroiliac Joint, Left	9 Hip Joint, Right B Hip Joint, Left C Knee Joint, Right D Knee Joint, Left F Ankle Joint, Right G Ankle Joint, Left H Tarsal Joint, Right J Tarsal Joint, Left	K Tarsometatarsal Joint, Right L Tarsometatarsal Joint, Left M Metatarsal-Phalangeal Joint, Right N Metatarsal-Phalangeal Joint, Left P Toe Phalangeal Joint, Right Q Toe Phalangeal Joint, Left	0 Open 3 Percutaneous 4 Percutaneous endoscopic	Z No device	X Diagnostic Z No qualifier

LOWER JOINTS 0S9

© 2018 Channel Publishing, Ltd.

1ST - 0 Medical and Surgical
2ND - S Lower Joints
3RD - B EXCISION

EXCISION GROUP: Excision, Resection, Destruction, (Extraction), (Detachment)
Root Operations that take out some or all of a body part.

EXCISION: Cutting out or off, without replacement, a portion of a body part.

Explanation: Qualifier "X Diagnostic" indicates excision procedures that are biopsies
Examples: Partial medial menisectomy – CMS Ex: Liver biopsy

Body Part – 4TH			Approach – 5TH	Device – 6TH	Qualifier–7TH
0 Lumbar Vertebral Joint 2 Lumbar Vertebral Disc 3 Lumbosacral Joint 4 Lumbosacral Disc 5 Sacrococcygeal Joint 6 Coccygeal Joint 7 Sacroiliac Joint, Right 8 Sacroiliac Joint, Left	9 Hip Joint, Right B Hip Joint, Left C Knee Joint, Right D Knee Joint, Left F Ankle Joint, Right G Ankle Joint, Left H Tarsal Joint, Right J Tarsal Joint, Left	K Tarsometatarsal Joint, Right L Tarsometatarsal Joint, Left M Metatarsal-Phalangeal Joint, Right N Metatarsal-Phalangeal Joint, Left P Toe Phalangeal Joint, Right Q Toe Phalangeal Joint, Left	0 Open 3 Percutaneous 4 Percutaneous endoscopic	Z No device	X Diagnostic Z No qualifier

1ST - 0 Medical and Surgical
2ND - S Lower Joints
3RD - C EXTIRPATION

DRAINAGE GROUP: Drainage, Extirpation, (Fragmentation)
Root Operations that take out solids/fluids/gases from a body part.

EXTIRPATION: Taking or cutting out solid matter from a body part.

Explanation: Abnormal byproduct or foreign body ...
Examples: Removal loose bodies knee joint – CMS Ex: Thrombectomy

Body Part – 4TH			Approach – 5TH	Device – 6TH	Qualifier–7TH
0 Lumbar Vertebral Joint 2 Lumbar Vertebral Disc 3 Lumbosacral Joint 4 Lumbosacral Disc 5 Sacrococcygeal Joint 6 Coccygeal Joint 7 Sacroiliac Joint, Right 8 Sacroiliac Joint, Left	9 Hip Joint, Right B Hip Joint, Left C Knee Joint, Right D Knee Joint, Left F Ankle Joint, Right G Ankle Joint, Left H Tarsal Joint, Right J Tarsal Joint, Left	K Tarsometatarsal Joint, Right L Tarsometatarsal Joint, Left M Metatarsal-Phalangeal Joint, Right N Metatarsal-Phalangeal Joint, Left P Toe Phalangeal Joint, Right Q Toe Phalangeal Joint, Left	0 Open 3 Percutaneous 4 Percutaneous endoscopic	Z No device	Z No qualifier

1ST - 0 Medical and Surgical
2ND - S Lower Joints
3RD - G FUSION

OTHER OBJECTIVES GROUP: (Alteration), (Creation), Fusion
Root Operations that define other objectives.

FUSION: Joining together portions of an articular body part rendering the articular body part immobile.

Explanation: The body part is joined together by fixation device, bone graft, other means
Examples: Lumbosacral spinal fusion – CMS Ex: Spinal fusion

Body Part – 4TH	Approach - 5TH	Device – 6TH	Qualifier – 7TH
0 Lumbar Vertebral Joint 1 Lumbar Vertebral Joints, 2 or more 3 Lumbosacral Joint	0 Open 3 Percutaneous 4 Percutaneous endoscopic	7 Autologous tissue substitute J Synthetic substitute K Nonautologous tissue substitute	0 Anterior approach, anterior column 1 Posterior approach, posterior column J Posterior approach, anterior column
0 Lumbar Vertebral Joint 1 Lumbar Vertebral Joints, 2 or more 3 Lumbosacral Joint	0 Open 3 Percutaneous 4 Percutaneous endoscopic	A Interbody fusion device	0 Anterior approach, anterior column J Posterior approach, anterior column
5 Sacrococcygeal Joint 6 Coccygeal Joint 7 Sacroiliac Joint, Right 8 Sacroiliac Joint, Left	0 Open 3 Percutaneous 4 Percutaneous endoscopic	4 Internal fixation device 7 Autologous tissue substitute J Synthetic substitute K Nonautologous tissue substitute	Z No qualifier
9 Hip Joint, Right B Hip Joint, Left C Knee Joint, Right D Knee Joint, Left F Ankle Joint, Right G Ankle Joint, Left H Tarsal Joint, Right J Tarsal Joint, Left K Tarsometatarsal Joint, Right L Tarsometatarsal Joint, Left M Metatarsal-Phalangeal Joint, Right N Metatarsal-Phalangeal Joint, Left P Toe Phalangeal Joint, Right Q Toe Phalangeal Joint, Left	0 Open 3 Percutaneous 4 Percutaneous endoscopic	4 Internal fixation device 5 External fixation device 7 Autologous tissue substitute J Synthetic substitute K Nonautologous tissue substitute	Z No qualifier

© 2018 Channel Publishing, Ltd.

1ST - 0 Medical and Surgical
2ND - S Lower Joints
3RD - H INSERTION

DEVICE GROUP: Change, Insertion, Removal, Replacement, Revision, Supplement
Root Operations that always involve a device.

INSERTION: Putting in a nonbiological appliance that monitors, assists, performs, or prevents a physiological function but does not physically take the place of a body part.

Explanation: None
Examples: Implantation joint spacer – CMS Ex: Insertion of central venous catheter

Body Part – 4TH	Approach - 5TH	Device – 6TH	Qualifier - 7TH
0 Lumbar Vertebral Joint 3 Lumbosacral Joint	0 Open 3 Percutaneous 4 Percutaneous endoscopic	3 Infusion device 4 Internal fixation device 8 Spacer B Spinal stabilization device, interspinous process C Spinal stabilization device, pedicle-based D Spinal stabilization device, facet replacement	Z No qualifier
2 Lumbar Vertebral Disc 4 Lumbosacral Disc	0 Open 3 Percutaneous 4 Percutaneous endoscopic	3 Infusion device 8 Spacer	Z No qualifier
5 Sacrococcygeal Joint 6 Coccygeal Joint 7 Sacroiliac Joint, Right 8 Sacroiliac Joint, Left	0 Open 3 Percutaneous 4 Percutaneous endoscopic	3 Infusion device 4 Internal fixation device 8 Spacer	Z No qualifier
9 Hip Joint, Right B Hip Joint, Left C Knee Joint, Right D Knee Joint, Left F Ankle Joint, Right G Ankle Joint, Left H Tarsal Joint, Right J Tarsal Joint, Left K Tarsometatarsal Joint, Right L Tarsometatarsal Joint, Left M Metatarsal-Phalangeal Joint, Right N Metatarsal-Phalangeal Joint, Left P Toe Phalangeal Joint, Right Q Toe Phalangeal Joint, Left	0 Open 3 Percutaneous 4 Percutaneous endoscopic	3 Infusion device 4 Internal fixation device 5 External fixation device 8 Spacer	Z No qualifier

1ST - 0 Medical and Surgical
2ND - S Lower Joints
3RD - J INSPECTION

EXAMINATION GROUP: Inspection, (Map)
Root Operations involving examination only.

INSPECTION: Visually and/or manually exploring a body part.

Explanation: Direct or instrumental visualization ...
Examples: Diagnostic arthroscopy – CMS Ex: Exploratory laparotomy

Body Part – 4TH	Approach – 5TH	Device – 6TH	Qualifier–7TH
0 Lumbar Vertebral Joint 2 Lumbar Vertebral Disc 3 Lumbosacral Joint 4 Lumbosacral Disc 5 Sacrococcygeal Joint 6 Coccygeal Joint 7 Sacroiliac Joint, Right 8 Sacroiliac Joint, Left 9 Hip Joint, Right B Hip Joint, Left C Knee Joint, Right D Knee Joint, Left F Ankle Joint, Right G Ankle Joint, Left H Tarsal Joint, Right J Tarsal Joint, Left K Tarsometatarsal Joint, Right L Tarsometatarsal Joint, Left M Metatarsal-Phalangeal Joint, Right N Metatarsal-Phalangeal Joint, Left P Toe Phalangeal Joint, Right Q Toe Phalangeal Joint, Left	0 Open 3 Percutaneous 4 Percutaneous endoscopic X External	Z No device	Z No qualifier

1ST - 0 Medical and Surgical
2ND - S Lower Joints
3RD - N RELEASE

DIVISION GROUP: (Division), Release
Root Operations involving cutting or separation only.

RELEASE: Freeing a body part from an abnormal physical constraint by cutting or by the use of force.

Explanation: Some of the restraining tissue may be taken out but none of the body part is taken out
Examples: Manual rupture joint adhesions – CMS Ex: Carpal tunnel release

Body Part – 4TH	Approach – 5TH	Device – 6TH	Qualifier–7TH
0 Lumbar Vertebral Joint 2 Lumbar Vertebral Disc 3 Lumbosacral Joint 4 Lumbosacral Disc 5 Sacrococcygeal Joint 6 Coccygeal Joint 7 Sacroiliac Joint, Right 8 Sacroiliac Joint, Left 9 Hip Joint, Right B Hip Joint, Left C Knee Joint, Right D Knee Joint, Left F Ankle Joint, Right G Ankle Joint, Left H Tarsal Joint, Right J Tarsal Joint, Left K Tarsometatarsal Joint, Right L Tarsometatarsal Joint, Left M Metatarsal-Phalangeal Joint, Right N Metatarsal-Phalangeal Joint, Left P Toe Phalangeal Joint, Right Q Toe Phalangeal Joint, Left	0 Open 3 Percutaneous 4 Percutaneous endoscopic X External	Z No device	Z No qualifier

© 2018 Channel Publishing, Ltd.

1ST - 0 Medical and Surgical
2ND - S Lower Joints
3RD - P REMOVAL

DEVICE GROUP: Change, Insertion, Removal, Replacement, Revision, Supplement
Root Operations that always involve a device.

REMOVAL: Taking out or off a device from a body part.

Explanation: Removal device without reinsertion ...
Examples: Removal fixation device – CMS Ex: Cardiac pacemaker removal

Body Part – 4TH	Approach - 5TH	Device – 6TH	Qualifier - 7TH
0 Lumbar Vertebral Joint 3 Lumbosacral Joint	0 Open 3 Percutaneous 4 Percutaneous endoscopic	0 Drainage device 3 Infusion device 4 Internal fixation device 7 Autologous tissue substitute 8 Spacer A Interbody fusion device J Synthetic substitute K Nonautologous tissue substitute	Z No qualifier
0 Lumbar Vertebral Joint 3 Lumbosacral Joint	X External	0 Drainage device 3 Infusion device 4 Internal fixation device	Z No qualifier
2 Lumbar Vertebral Disc 4 Lumbosacral Disc	0 Open 3 Percutaneous 4 Percutaneous endoscopic	0 Drainage device 3 Infusion device 7 Autologous tissue substitute J Synthetic substitute K Nonautologous tissue substitute	Z No qualifier
2 Lumbar Vertebral Disc 4 Lumbosacral Disc	X External	0 Drainage device 3 Infusion device	Z No qualifier
5 Sacrococcygeal Joint 6 Coccygeal Joint 7 Sacroiliac Joint, Right 8 Sacroiliac Joint, Left	0 Open 3 Percutaneous 4 Percutaneous endoscopic	0 Drainage device 3 Infusion device 4 Internal fixation device 7 Autologous tissue substitute 8 Spacer J Synthetic substitute K Nonautologous tissue substitute	Z No qualifier
5 Sacrococcygeal Joint 6 Coccygeal Joint 7 Sacroiliac Joint, Right 8 Sacroiliac Joint, Left	X External	0 Drainage device 3 Infusion device 4 Internal fixation device	Z No qualifier
9 Hip Joint, Right B Hip Joint, Left	0 Open	0 Drainage device 3 Infusion device 4 Internal fixation device 5 External fixation device 7 Autologous tissue substitute 8 Spacer 9 Liner B Resurfacing device E Articulating spacer J Synthetic substitute K Nonautologous tissue substitute	Z No qualifier
9 Hip Joint, Right B Hip Joint, Left	3 Percutaneous 4 Percutaneous endoscopic	0 Drainage device 3 Infusion device 4 Internal fixation device 5 External fixation device 7 Autologous tissue substitute 8 Spacer J Synthetic substitute K Nonautologous tissue substitute	Z No qualifier
9 Hip Joint, Right B Hip Joint, Left	X External	0 Drainage device 3 Infusion device 4 Internal fixation device 5 External fixation device	Z No qualifier

continued ⇨

© 2018 Channel Publishing, Ltd.

0 S P REMOVAL – *continued*

Body Part – 4TH	Approach - 5TH	Device – 6TH	Qualifier - 7TH
A Hip Joint, Acetabular Surface, Right E Hip Joint, Acetabular Surface, Left R Hip Joint, Femoral Surface, Right S Hip Joint, Femoral Surface, Left T Knee Joint, Femoral Surface, Right U Knee Joint, Femoral Surface, Left V Knee Joint, Tibial Surface, Right W Knee Joint, Tibial Surface, Left	0 Open 3 Percutaneous 4 Percutaneous endoscopic	J Synthetic substitute	Z No qualifier
C Knee Joint, Right D Knee Joint, Left	0 Open	0 Drainage device 3 Infusion device 4 Internal fixation device 5 External fixation device 7 Autologous tissue substitute 8 Spacer 9 Liner E Articulating spacer K Nonautologous tissue substitute L Synthetic substitute, unicondylar medial M Synthetic substitute, unicondylar lateral N Synthetic substitute, patellofemoral	Z No qualifier
C Knee Joint, Right D Knee Joint, Left	0 Open	J Synthetic substitute	C Patellar surface Z No qualifier
C Knee Joint, Right D Knee Joint, Left	3 Percutaneous 4 Percutaneous endoscopic	0 Drainage device 3 Infusion device 4 Internal fixation device 5 External fixation device 7 Autologous tissue substitute 8 Spacer K Nonautologous tissue substitute L Synthetic substitute, unicondylar medial M Synthetic substitute, unicondylar lateral N Synthetic substitute, patellofemoral	Z No qualifier
C Knee Joint, Right D Knee Joint, Left	3 Percutaneous 4 Percutaneous endoscopic	J Synthetic substitute	C Patellar surface Z No qualifier
C Knee Joint, Right D Knee Joint, Left	X External	0 Drainage device 3 Infusion device 4 Internal fixation device 5 External fixation device	Z No qualifier
F Ankle Joint, Right G Ankle Joint, Left H Tarsal Joint, Right J Tarsal Joint, Left K Tarsometatarsal Joint, Right L Tarsometatarsal Joint, Left M Metatarsal-Phalangeal Joint, Right N Metatarsal-Phalangeal Joint, Left P Toe Phalangeal Joint, Right Q Toe Phalangeal Joint, Left	0 Open 3 Percutaneous 4 Percutaneous endoscopic	0 Drainage device 3 Infusion device 4 Internal fixation device 5 External fixation device 7 Autologous tissue substitute 8 Spacer J Synthetic substitute K Nonautologous tissue substitute	Z No qualifier
F Ankle Joint, Right G Ankle Joint, Left H Tarsal Joint, Right J Tarsal Joint, Left K Tarsometatarsal Joint, Right L Tarsometatarsal Joint, Left M Metatarsal-Phalangeal Joint, Right N Metatarsal-Phalangeal Joint, Left P Toe Phalangeal Joint, Right Q Toe Phalangeal Joint, Left	X External	0 Drainage device 3 Infusion device 4 Internal fixation device 5 External fixation device	Z No qualifier

© 2018 Channel Publishing, Ltd.

1ST - 0 Medical and Surgical
2ND - S Lower Joints
3RD - Q REPAIR

OTHER REPAIRS GROUP: (Control), Repair
Root Operations that define other repairs.

REPAIR: Restoring, to the extent possible, a body part to its normal anatomic structure and function.

Explanation: Used only when the method to accomplish the repair is not one of the other root operations
Examples: Suture arthroplasty – CMS Ex: Suture of laceration

Body Part – 4TH	Approach – 5TH	Device – 6TH	Qualifier–7TH
0 Lumbar Vertebral Joint 2 Lumbar Vertebral Disc 3 Lumbosacral Joint 4 Lumbosacral Disc 5 Sacrococcygeal Joint 6 Coccygeal Joint 7 Sacroiliac Joint, Right 8 Sacroiliac Joint, Left 9 Hip Joint, Right B Hip Joint, Left C Knee Joint, Right D Knee Joint, Left F Ankle Joint, Right G Ankle Joint, Left H Tarsal Joint, Right J Tarsal Joint, Left K Tarsometatarsal Joint, Right L Tarsometatarsal Joint, Left M Metatarsal-Phalangeal Joint, Right N Metatarsal-Phalangeal Joint, Left P Toe Phalangeal Joint, Right Q Toe Phalangeal Joint, Left	0 Open 3 Percutaneous 4 Percutaneous endoscopic X External	Z No device	Z No qualifier

1ST - 0 Medical and Surgical
2ND - S Lower Joints
3RD - R REPLACEMENT

DEVICE GROUP: Change, Insertion, Removal, Replacement, Revision, Supplement
Root Operations that always involve a device.

REPLACEMENT: Putting in or on biological or synthetic material that physically takes the place and/or function of all or a portion of a body part.

Explanation: Includes taking out or eradicating, or rendering non-functional, the body part ...
Examples: Total knee replacement – CMS Ex: Total hip replacement

Body Part – 4TH	Approach - 5TH	Device – 6TH	Qualifier - 7TH
0 Lumbar Vertebral Joint 2 Lumbar Vertebral Disc NC* 3 Lumbosacral Joint 4 Lumbosacral Disc NC* 5 Sacrococcygeal Joint 6 Coccygeal Joint 7 Sacroiliac Joint, Right 8 Sacroiliac Joint, Left H Tarsal Joint, Right J Tarsal Joint, Left K Tarsometatarsal Joint, Right L Tarsometatarsal Joint, Left M Metatarsal-Phalangeal Joint, Right N Metatarsal-Phalangeal Joint, Left P Toe Phalangeal Joint, Right Q Toe Phalangeal Joint, Left	0 Open	7 Autologous tissue substitute J Synthetic substitute K Nonautologous tissue substitute	Z No qualifier
9 Hip Joint, Right B Hip Joint, Left	0 Open	1 Synthetic substitute, metal 2 Synthetic substitute, metal on polyethylene 3 Synthetic substitute, ceramic 4 Synthetic substitute, ceramic on polyethylene 6 Synthetic substitute, oxidizedzirconium on polyethylene J Synthetic substitute	9 Cemented A Uncemented Z No qualifier
9 Hip Joint, Right B Hip Joint, Left	0 Open	7 Autologous tissue substitute E Articulating spacer K Nonautologous tissue substitute	Z No qualifier
A Hip Joint, Acetabular Surface, Right E Hip Joint, Acetabular Surface, Left	0 Open	0 Synthetic substitute, polyethylene 1 Synthetic substitute, metal 3 Synthetic substitute, ceramic J Synthetic substitute	9 Cemented A Uncemented Z No qualifier
A Hip Joint, Acetabular Surface, Right E Hip Joint, Acetabular Surface, Left	0 Open	7 Autologous tissue substitute K Nonautologous tissue substitute	Z No qualifier

NC* – Some procedures are considered non-covered by Medicare. See current Medicare Code Editor (patient over 60 years with Synthetic substitute) for details.

© 2018 Channel Publishing, Ltd.

continued ⇨

0 S R REPLACEMENT – *continued*

Body Part – 4TH	Approach - 5TH	Device – 6TH	Qualifier - 7TH
C Knee Joint, Right D Knee Joint, Left	0 Open	6 Synthetic substitute, oxidized zirconium on polyethylene J Synthetic substitute L Synthetic substitute, unicondylar medial M Synthetic substitute, unicondylar lateral N Synthetic substitute, patellofemoral	9 Cemented A Uncemented Z No qualifier
C Knee Joint, Right D Knee Joint, Left	0 Open	7 Autologous tissue substitute E Articulating spacer K Nonautologous tissue substitute	Z No qualifier
F Ankle Joint, Right G Ankle Joint, Left T Knee Joint, Femoral Surface, Right U Knee Joint, Femoral Surface, Left V Knee Joint, Tibial Surface, Right W Knee Joint, Tibial Surface, Left	0 Open	7 Autologous tissue substitute K Nonautologous tissue substitute	Z No qualifier
F Ankle Joint, Right G Ankle Joint, Left T Knee Joint, Femoral Surface, Right U Knee Joint, Femoral Surface, Left V Knee Joint, Tibial Surface, Right W Knee Joint, Tibial Surface, Left	0 Open	J Synthetic substitute	9 Cemented A Uncemented Z No qualifier
R Hip Joint, Femoral Surface, Right S Hip Joint, Femoral Surface, Left	0 Open	1 Synthetic substitute, metal 3 Synthetic substitute, ceramic J Synthetic substitute	9 Cemented A Uncemented Z No qualifier
R Hip Joint, Femoral Surface, Right S Hip Joint, Femoral Surface, Left	0 Open	7 Autologous tissue substitute K Nonautologous tissue substitute	Z No qualifier

1ST - 0 Medical and Surgical
2ND - S Lower Joints
3RD - S REPOSITION

MOVE GROUP: (Reattachment), Reposition, (Transfer), (Transplantation)
Root Operations that put in/put back or move some/all of a body part.

REPOSITION: Moving to its normal location, or other suitable location, all or a portion of a body part.

Explanation: The body part may or may not be cut out or off to be moved to the new location ...
Examples: Closed reduction hip joint dislocation – CMS Ex: Fracture reduction

Body Part – 4TH	Approach – 5TH	Device – 6TH	Qualifier – 7TH
0 Lumbar Vertebral Joint 3 Lumbosacral Joint 5 Sacrococcygeal Joint 6 Coccygeal Joint 7 Sacroiliac Joint, Right 8 Sacroiliac Joint, Left	0 Open 3 Percutaneous 4 Percutaneous endoscopic X External	4 Internal fixation device Z No device	Z No qualifier
9 Hip Joint, Right B Hip Joint, Left C Knee Joint, Right D Knee Joint, Left F Ankle Joint, Right G Ankle Joint, Left H Tarsal Joint, Right J Tarsal Joint, Left K Tarsometatarsal Joint, Right L Tarsometatarsal Joint, Left M Metatarsal-Phalangeal Joint, Right N Metatarsal-Phalangeal Joint, Left P Toe Phalangeal Joint, Right Q Toe Phalangeal Joint, Left	0 Open 3 Percutaneous 4 Percutaneous endoscopic X External	4 Internal fixation device 5 External fixation device Z No device	Z No qualifier

© 2018 Channel Publishing, Ltd.

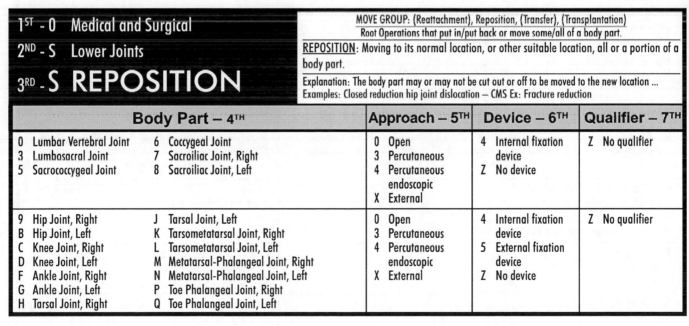

1ST - 0 Medical and Surgical
2ND - S Lower Joints
3RD - T RESECTION

EXCISION GROUP: Excision, Resection, Destruction, (Extraction), (Detachment)
Root Operations that take out some or all of a body part.

RESECTION: Cutting out or off, without replacement, all of a body part.

Explanation: None
Examples: Total lumbar discectomy – CMS Ex: Total lobectomy of lung

Body Part – 4TH	Approach – 5TH	Device – 6TH	Qualifier–7TH
2 Lumbar Vertebral Disc 4 Lumbosacral Disc 5 Sacrococcygeal Joint 6 Coccygeal Joint 7 Sacroiliac Joint, Right 8 Sacroiliac Joint, Left 9 Hip Joint, Right B Hip Joint, Left C Knee Joint, Right D Knee Joint, Left F Ankle Joint, Right G Ankle Joint, Left H Tarsal Joint, Right J Tarsal Joint, Left K Tarsometatarsal Joint, Right L Tarsometatarsal Joint, Left M Metatarsal-Phalangeal Joint, Right N Metatarsal-Phalangeal Joint, Left P Toe Phalangeal Joint, Right Q Toe Phalangeal Joint, Left	0 Open	Z No device	Z No qualifier

1ST - 0 Medical and Surgical
2ND - S Lower Joints
3RD - U SUPPLEMENT

DEVICE GROUP: Change, Insertion, Removal, Replacement, Revision, Supplement
Root Operations that always involve a device.

SUPPLEMENT: Putting in or on biological or synthetic material that physically reinforces and/or augments the function of a portion of a body part.

Explanation: Biological material is non-living, or is living and from the same individual ...
Examples: Placement patellar surface liner – CMS Ex: Herniorrhaphy using mesh

Body Part – 4TH	Approach – 5TH	Device – 6TH	Qualifier–7TH
0 Lumbar Vertebral Joint 2 Lumbar Vertebral Disc 3 Lumbosacral Joint 4 Lumbosacral Disc 5 Sacrococcygeal Joint 6 Coccygeal Joint 7 Sacroiliac Joint, Right 8 Sacroiliac Joint, Left F Ankle Joint, Right G Ankle Joint, Left H Tarsal Joint, Right J Tarsal Joint, Left K Tarsometatarsal Joint, Right L Tarsometatarsal Joint, Left M Metatarsal-Phalangeal Joint, Right N Metatarsal-Phalangeal Joint, Left P Toe Phalangeal Joint, Right Q Toe Phalangeal Joint, Left	0 Open 3 Percutaneous 4 Percutaneous endoscopic	7 Autologous tissue substitute J Synthetic substitute K Nonautologous tissue substitute	Z No qualifier
9 Hip Joint, Right B Hip Joint, Left	0 Open	7 Autologous tissue substitute 9 Liner B Resurfacing device J Synthetic substitute K Nonautologous tissue substitute	Z No qualifier
9 Hip Joint, Right B Hip Joint, Left	3 Percutaneous 4 Percutaneous endoscopic	7 Autologous tissue substitute J Synthetic substitute K Nonautologous tissue substitute	Z No qualifier
A Hip Joint, Acetabular Surface, Right E Hip Joint, Acetabular Surface, Left R Hip Joint, Femoral Surface, Right S Hip Joint, Femoral Surface, Left	0 Open	9 Liner B Resurfacing device	Z No qualifier
C Knee Joint, Right D Knee Joint, Left	0 Open	7 Autologous tissue substitute J Synthetic substitute K Nonautologous tissue substitute	Z No qualifier
C Knee Joint, Right D Knee Joint, Left	0 Open	9 Liner	C Patellar surface Z No qualifier
C Knee Joint, Right D Knee Joint, Left	3 Percutaneous 4 Percutaneous endoscopic	7 Autologous tissue substitute J Synthetic substitute K Nonautologous tissue substitute	Z No qualifier
T Knee Joint, Femoral Surface, Right U Knee Joint, Femoral Surface, Left V Knee Joint, Tibial Surface, Right W Knee Joint, Tibial Surface, Left	0 Open	9 Liner	Z No qualifier

© 2018 Channel Publishing, Ltd.

1ST - 0 Medical and Surgical
2ND - S Lower Joints
3RD - W REVISION

DEVICE GROUP: Change, Insertion, Removal, Replacement, Revision, Supplement
Root Operations that always involve a device.

REVISION: Correcting, to the extent possible, a portion of a malfunctioning device or the position of a displaced device.

Explanation: Correcting by taking out or putting in components of a device such as a screw or pin ...
Examples: Reposition joint spacer – CMS Ex: Recementing of hip prosthesis

Body Part – 4TH	Approach – 5TH	Device – 6TH	Qualifier–7TH
0 Lumbar Vertebral Joint 3 Lumbosacral Joint	0 Open 3 Percutaneous 4 Percutaneous endoscopic X External	0 Drainage device 3 Infusion device 4 Internal fixation device 7 Autologous tissue substitute 8 Spacer A Interbody infusion device J Synthetic substitute K Nonautologous tissue substitute	Z No qualifier
2 Lumbar Vertebral Disc 4 Lumbosacral Disc	0 Open 3 Percutaneous 4 Percutaneous endoscopic X External	0 Drainage device 3 Infusion device 7 Autologous tissue substitute J Synthetic substitute K Nonautologous tissue substitute	Z No qualifier
5 Sacrococcygeal Joint 6 Coccygeal Joint 7 Sacroiliac Joint, Right 8 Sacroiliac Joint, Left	0 Open 3 Percutaneous 4 Percutaneous endoscopic X External	0 Drainage device 3 Infusion device 4 Internal fixation device 7 Autologous tissue substitute 8 Spacer J Synthetic substitute K Nonautologous tissue substitute	Z No qualifier
9 Hip Joint, Right B Hip Joint, Left	0 Open	0 Drainage device 3 Infusion device 4 Internal fixation device 5 External fixation device 7 Autologous tissue substitute 8 Spacer 9 Liner B Resufacing device J Synthetic substitute K Nonautologous tissue substitute	Z No qualifier
9 Hip Joint, Right B Hip Joint, Left	3 Percutaneous 4 Percutaneous endoscopic X External	0 Drainage device 3 Infusion device 4 Internal fixation device 5 External fixation device 7 Autologous tissue substitute 8 Spacer J Synthetic substitute K Nonautologous tissue substitute	Z No qualifier
A Hip Joint, Acetabular Surface, Right E Hip Joint, Acetabular Surface, Left R Hip Joint, Femoral Surface, Right S Hip Joint, Femoral Surface, Left T Knee Joint, Femoral Surface, Right U Knee Joint, Femoral Surface, Left V Knee Joint, Tibial Surface, Right W Knee Joint, Tibial Surface, Left	0 Open 3 Percutaneous 4 Percutaneous endoscopic X External	J Synthetic substitute	Z No qualifier

continued ⇨

© 2018 Channel Publishing, Ltd.

0 S W REVISION – *continued*

Body Part – 4TH	Approach – 5TH	Device – 6TH	Qualifier–7TH
C Knee Joint, Right D Knee Joint, Left	0 Open	0 Drainage device 3 Infusion device 4 Internal fixation device 5 External fixation device 7 Autologous tissue substitute 8 Spacer 9 Liner K Nonautologous tissue substitute	Z No qualifier
C Knee Joint, Right D Knee Joint, Left	0 Open	J Synthetic substitute	C Patellar surface Z No qualifier
C Knee Joint, Right D Knee Joint, Left	3 Percutaneous 4 Percutaneous endoscopic X External	0 Drainage device 3 Infusion device 4 Internal fixation device 5 External fixation device 7 Autologous tissue substitute 8 Spacer K Nonautologous tissue substitute	Z No qualifier
C Knee Joint, Right D Knee Joint, Left	3 Percutaneous 4 Percutaneous endoscopic X External	J Synthetic substitute	C Patellar surface Z No qualifier
F Ankle Joint, Right G Ankle Joint, Left H Tarsal Joint, Right J Tarsal Joint, Left K Tarsometatarsal Joint, Right L Tarsometatarsal Joint, Left M Metatarsal-Phalangeal Joint, Right N Metatarsal-Phalangeal Joint, Left P Toe Phalangeal Joint, Right Q Toe Phalangeal Joint, Left	0 Open 3 Percutaneous 4 Percutaneous endoscopic X External	0 Drainage device 3 Infusion device 4 Internal fixation device 5 External fixation device 7 Autologous tissue substitute 8 Spacer J Synthetic substitute K Nonautologous tissue substitute	Z No qualifier

© 2018 Channel Publishing, Ltd.

Educational Annotations | T – Urinary System

Body System Specific Educational Annotations for the Urinary System include:

- Anatomy and Physiology Review
- Anatomical Illustrations
- Definitions of Common Procedures
- AHA Coding Clinic® Reference Notations
- Body Part Key Listings
- Device Key Listings
- Device Aggregation Table Listings
- Coding Notes

Anatomy and Physiology Review of Urinary System

BODY PART VALUES – T - URINARY SYSTEM

Bladder – ANATOMY – The urinary bladder is a hollow, collapsible musculomembranous organ located within the pelvic cavity behind the symphysis pubis. In the male, it lies against the rectum, and in the female it lies against the vagina and uterus. When filled it may contain 17 fluid ounces (500 ml) of urine and it pushes upward, indenting the abdominal cavity. The trigone area is the floor of the bladder formed by three points, the two ureteral orifices and the urethral orifice. The dome is the expandable superior surface of the bladder. The ureteric orifice is that area surrounding the ureteral openings. The urachus in the adult forms the middle umbilical ligament of the bladder. PHYSIOLOGY – The urinary bladder functions as a reservoir for the urine produced by the kidneys until the individual expels the urine (micturition). Micturition occurs when the bladder becomes distended with urine and stretch receptor nerves signal the micturition center in the sacral spinal cord. Parasympathetic nerve impulses start rhythmically contracting the bladder and the individual senses an urgency to urinate. Following the midbrain decision to urinate, the external urethral sphincter is relaxed, and urination begins as the bladder muscle contracts.

Bladder Neck – The bladder neck is that area surrounding the urethral orifice.

Kidney – ANATOMY – The kidneys are reddish-brown, bean-shaped organs about 4.7 inches (12 cm) long, 2.3 inches (6 cm) wide, and 1.2 inches (3 cm) thick, located on either side of the vertebral column in the retroperitoneal space. The kidneys are supplied with arterial blood from the renal arteries which branch off from the aorta, and are drained by the renal veins which connect with the inferior vena cava. PHYSIOLOGY – The kidneys function to remove metabolic wastes from the blood by transferring them into the urine. They also regulate red blood cell production, blood pressure, calcium absorption, and the pH level of the blood.

Kidney Pelvis – The kidney (renal) pelvis is the funnel-shaped urinary collecting system of the kidney at the upper end of the ureter.

Ureter – The ureter is the musculomembranous tube extending from the renal pelvis to the bladder that transports the urine from the kidney to the bladder using gravity and peristaltic contraction.

Urethra – The urethra is the musculomembranous tube which extends and carries urine from the bladder to the external urethral opening (meatus)

Anatomical Illustrations of Urinary System

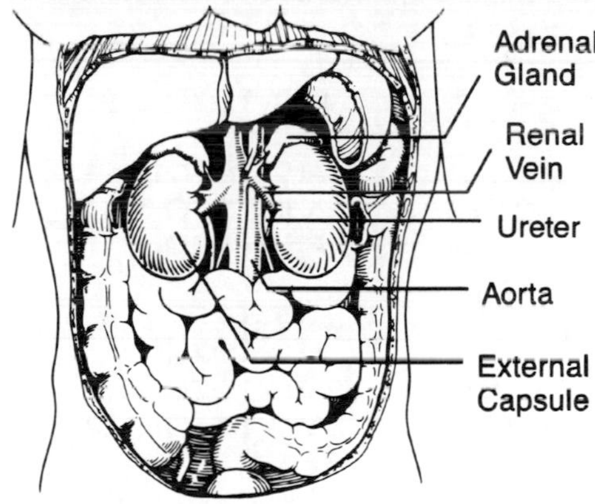

KIDNEY — ANTERIOR VIEW

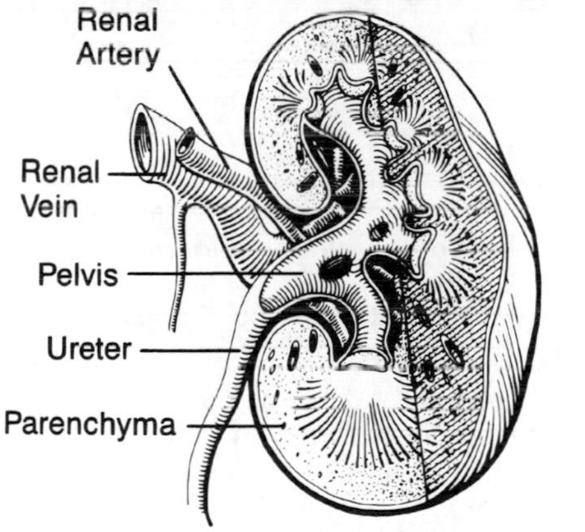

KIDNEY — (CUT AWAY VIEW)

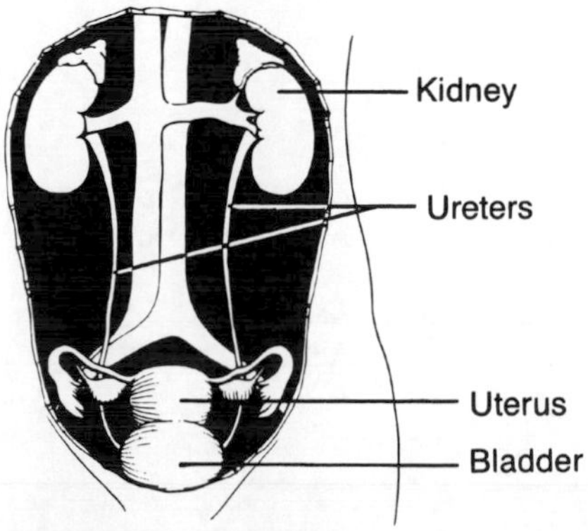

URINARY SYSTEM

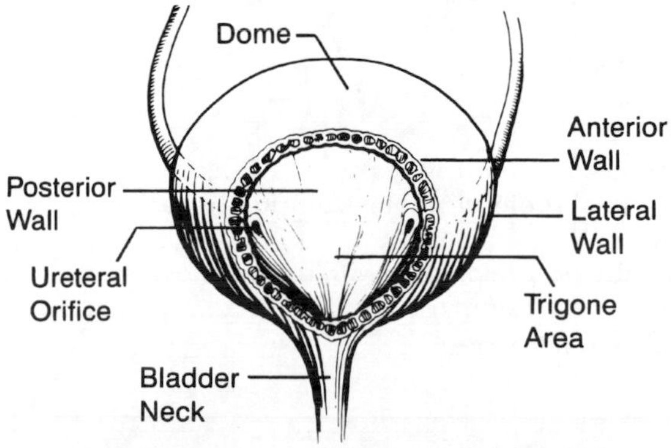

BLADDER — ANTERIOR (CUT-AWAY) VIEW

© 2018 Channel Publishing, Ltd.

URINARY 0 T

Educational Annotations | T – Urinary System

Definitions of Common Procedures of Urinary System

Bladder neck suspension – The surgical procedure to reposition and support the bladder neck using sutures or a sling of tissue that attaches each end of the sling to pelvic tissue (fascia) or the abdominal wall using stitches.

Cystoscopy – The insertion of an endoscope (cystoscope) through the urethra and into the bladder for visual examination and often to perform procedures on the bladder and urethra.

Extracorporeal shock wave lithotripsy (ESWL) on kidney stone – The breaking apart of kidney stones by using high-energy sound shock waves.

Kidney transplant – The surgical replacement of an end-stage diseased kidney using a donor kidney (living or non-living donor), and sometimes from a genetically identical twin (syngeneic).

Nephrectomy – The surgical removal of a kidney.

Nephropexy – The surgical fixation of a kidney to treat a floating kidney (nephroptosis).

Suprapubic cystostomy – The surgical bypass of the urine from the bladder to outside the body via an implanted catheter placed just above the pubic bone.

Transureteroureterostomy – The surgical anastomosis of one ureter to the other ureter across the midline to bypass distal ureteral obstruction.

Urethroplasty – The surgical repair of a birth defect (hypospadias) or damaged urethra using repositioning, anastomosis, onlay tissue graft, or forming a new urethral channel (Johanson's urethroplasty).

AHA Coding Clinic® Reference Notations of Urinary System

ROOT OPERATION SPECIFIC - T - URINARY SYSTEM

BYPASS - 1
- Colocutaneous Indiana pouch .... AHA 17:3Q:p21
- Rerouting of kinked ileal conduit .... AHA 15:3Q:p34
- Ureterocolonic anastomosis .... AHA 17:3Q:p20

CHANGE - 2

DESTRUCTION - 5

DILATION - 7
- Exchange of ureteral stents .... AHA 16:2Q:p27
- Exchange of ureteral stents - Official Correction .... AHA 17:4Q:p111
- Insertion (dilation) of ureteral stent........ AHA 15:2Q:p8
- Insertion of UroLift® System into prostate .... AHA 13:4Q:p123

DIVISION - 8

DRAINAGE - 9
- Urinary diversion by placing a ureteral stent........ AHA 17:3Q:p19

EXCISION - B
- Biopsy of neobladder .... AHA 16:1Q:p19
- Excision of Mitrofanoff channel (neo-urethra) polyps........ AHA 15:3Q:p34
- Polyp excision in ileal loop (neobladder) .... AHA 14:2Q:p8

EXTIRPATION - C
- Cystoscopy with removal of bladder stones........ AHA 16:3Q:p23
- Extirpation with fragmentation of renal pelvis stone .... AHA 15:2Q:p7
- Fragmentation and removal of kidney, ureteral, and bladder stones .... AHA 15:2Q:p8
- Ureteroscopic laser lithotripsy with removal of stone fragments........ AHA 13:4Q:p122

EXTRACTION - D

FRAGMENTATION - F
- Extracorporeal shock wave lithotripsy (ESWL) on kidney stone .... AHA 13:4Q:p122

INSERTION - H

INSPECTION - J

OCCLUSION - L

REATTACHMENT - M

RELEASE - N

REMOVAL - P
- Exchange of ureteral stents .... AHA 16:2Q:p27
- Exchange of ureteral stents - Official Correction .... AHA 17:4Q:p111

REPAIR - Q
- Dismembered pyeloplasty with ureter anastomosis - Official Correction .... AHA 18:2Q:p27
- Perineal urethrostomy .... AHA 17:1Q:p37

Continued on next page

© 2018 Channel Publishing, Ltd.

Educational Annotations | T – Urinary System

AHA Coding Clinic® Reference Notations of Urinary System

Continued from previous page

REPLACEMENT - R

Cystectomy with creation of Indiana pouch ....AHA 17:3Q:p20

REPOSITION - S

Dismembered pyeloplasty with ureter anastomosis ....AHA 17:1Q:p36

Dismembered pyeloplasty with ureter anastomosis - Official Correction ....AHA 18:2Q:p27

Pubovaginal sling placement ....AHA 16:1Q:p15

RESECTION - T

Complete nephroureterectomy....AHA 14:3Q:p16

SUPPLEMENT - U

Augmentation cystoplasty with Indiana pouch ....AHA 17:3Q:p21

RESTRICTION - V

Deflux injection into bladder at ureteral orifices ....AHA 15:2Q:p11

REVISION - W

TRANSPLANTATION - Y

Body Part Key Listings of Urinary System

See also Body Part Key in Appendix C

Bulbourethral (Cowper's) gland ....use Urethra
Cowper's (bulbourethral) gland....use Urethra
External urethral sphincter ....use Urethra
Internal urethral sphincter....use Urethra
Membranous urethra....use Urethra
Penile urethra ....use Urethra
Prostatic urethra ....use Urethra
Renal calyx ....use Kidney, Bilateral/Left/Right
Renal capsule....use Kidney, Bilateral/Left/Right
Renal cortex....use Kidney, Bilateral/Left/Right
Renal segment....use Kidney, Bilateral/Left/Right
Trigone of bladder ....use Bladder
Ureteral orifice....use Ureter, Bilateral/Left/Right
Ureteropelvic junction (UPJ) ....use Kidney Pelvis, Left/Right
Ureterovesical orifice ....use Ureter, Bilateral/Left/Right

Device Key Listings of Urinary System

See also Device Key in Appendix D

AMS 800® Urinary Control System ....use Artificial Sphincter in Urinary System
Artificial urinary sphincter (AUS)....use Artificial Sphincter in Urinary System
Autograft ....use Autologous Tissue Substitute
Cystostomy tube ....use Drainage Device
Foley catheter ....use Drainage Device
Percutaneous nephrostomy catheter ....use Drainage Device
Sacral nerve modulation (SNM) lead ....use Stimulator Lead in Urinary System
Sacral neuromodulation lead ....use Stimulator Lead in Urinary System
Stent, intraluminal (cardiovascular) ....use Intraluminal Device
(gastrointestinal) (hepatobiliary) (urinary) ....use Intraluminal Device
Tissue bank graft ....use Nonautologous Tissue Substitute
Urinary incontinence stimulator lead....use Stimulator Lead in Urinary System

Device Aggregation Table Listings of Urinary System

See also Device Aggregation Table in Appendix E

Specific Device	For Operation	In Body System	General Device
None Listed in Device Aggregation Table for this Body System			

Coding Notes of Urinary System

© 2018 Channel Publishing, Ltd.

URINARY 0T

1ST - 0 Medical and Surgical
2ND - T Urinary System
3RD - 1 BYPASS

TUBULAR GROUP: Bypass, Dilation, Occlusion, Restriction
Root Operations that alter the diameter/route of a tubular body part.

BYPASS: Altering the route of passage of the contents of a tubular body part.

Explanation: Rerouting contents to a downstream part ... with or without the use of a device ...
Examples: Ileal conduit urinary diversion – CMS Ex: Coronary artery bypass

Body Part – 4TH	Approach – 5TH	Device – 6TH	Qualifier – 7TH
3 Kidney Pelvis, Right 4 Kidney Pelvis, Left	0 Open 4 Percutaneous endoscopic	7 Autologous tissue substitute J Synthetic substitute K Nonautologous tissue substitute Z No device	3 Kidney Pelvis, Right 4 Kidney Pelvis, Left 6 Ureter, Right 7 Ureter, Left 8 Colon 9 Colocutaneous A Ileum B Bladder C Ileocutaneous D Cutaneous
3 Kidney Pelvis, Right 4 Kidney Pelvis, Left	3 Percutaneous	J Synthetic substitute	D Cutaneous
6 Ureter, Right 7 Ureter, Left 8 Ureters, Bilateral	0 Open 4 Percutaneous endoscopic	7 Autologous tissue substitute J Synthetic substitute K Nonautologous tissue substitute Z No device	6 Ureter, Right 7 Ureter, Left 8 Colon 9 Colocutaneous A Ileum B Bladder C Ileocutaneous D Cutaneous
6 Ureter, Right 7 Ureter, Left 8 Ureters, Bilateral	3 Percutaneous	J Synthetic substitute	D Cutaneous
B Bladder	0 Open 4 Percutaneous endoscopic	7 Autologous tissue substitute J Synthetic substitute K Nonautologous tissue substitute Z No device	9 Colocutaneous C Ileocutaneous D Cutaneous
B Bladder	3 Percutaneous	J Synthetic substitute	D Cutaneous

1ST - 0 Medical and Surgical
2ND - T Urinary System
3RD - 2 CHANGE

DEVICE GROUP: Change, Insertion, Removal, Replacement, Revision, Supplement
Root Operations that always involve a device.

CHANGE: Taking out or off a device from a body part and putting back an identical or similar device in or on the same body part without cutting or puncturing the skin or a mucous membrane.

Explanation: All CHANGE procedures are coded using the approach External
Examples: Exchange foley catheter – CMS Ex: Urinary catheter change

Body Part – 4TH		Approach – 5TH	Device – 6TH	Qualifier – 7TH
5 Kidney 9 Ureter	B Bladder D Urethra	X External	0 Drainage device Y Other device	Z No qualifier

© 2018 Channel Publishing, Ltd.

1ST - 0 Medical and Surgical
2ND - T Urinary System
3RD - 5 DESTRUCTION

EXCISION GROUP: Excision, Resection, Destruction, Extraction, (Detachment)
Root Operations that take out some or all of a body part.

DESTRUCTION: Physical eradication of all or a portion of a body part by the direct use of energy, force, or a destructive agent.

Explanation: None of the body part is physically taken out
Examples: Cystoscopic laser ablation – CMS Ex: Fulguration of rectal polyp

Body Part – 4TH		Approach – 5TH	Device – 6TH	Qualifier – 7TH
0 Kidney, Right 1 Kidney, Left 3 Kidney Pelvis, Right 4 Kidney Pelvis, Left	6 Ureter, Right 7 Ureter, Left B Bladder C Bladder Neck	0 Open 3 Percutaneous 4 Percutaneous endoscopic 7 Via natural or artificial opening 8 Via natural or artificial opening endoscopic	Z No device	Z No qualifier
D Urethra		0 Open 3 Percutaneous 4 Percutaneous endoscopic 7 Via natural or artificial opening 8 Via natural or artificial opening endoscopic X External	Z No device	Z No qualifier

1ST - 0 Medical and Surgical
2ND - T Urinary System
3RD - 7 DILATION

TUBULAR GROUP: Bypass, Dilation, Occlusion, Restriction
Root Operations that alter the diameter/route of a tubular body part.

DILATION: Expanding an orifice or the lumen of a tubular body part.

Explanation: Accomplished by stretching or cutting ... tubular body part or orifice ...
Examples: Urethral dilation – CMS Ex: Percutaneous transluminal angioplasty

Body Part – 4TH		Approach – 5TH	Device – 6TH	Qualifier – 7TH
3 Kidney Pelvis, Right 4 Kidney Pelvis, Left 6 Ureter, Right 7 Ureter, Left	8 Ureters, Bilateral B Bladder C Bladder Neck D Urethra	0 Open 3 Percutaneous 4 Percutaneous endoscopic 7 Via natural or artificial opening 8 Via natural or artificial opening endoscopic	D Intraluminal device Z No device	Z No qualifier

1ST - 0 Medical and Surgical
2ND - T Urinary System
3RD - 8 DIVISION

DIVISION GROUP: Division, Release
Root Operations involving cutting or separation only.

DIVISION: Cutting into a body part, without draining fluids and/or gases from the body part, in order to separate or transect a body part.

Explanation: All or a portion of the body part is separated into two or more portions
Examples: Division bladder neck – CMS Ex: Spinal cordotomy

Body Part – 4TH	Approach – 5TH	Device – 6TH	Qualifier – 7TH
2 Kidneys, Bilateral C Bladder Neck	0 Open 3 Percutaneous 4 Percutaneous endoscopic	Z No device	Z No qualifier

© 2018 Channel Publishing, Ltd.

1ST - 0 Medical and Surgical
2ND - T Urinary System
3RD - 9 DRAINAGE

DRAINAGE GROUP: Drainage, Extirpation, Fragmentation
Root Operations that take out solids/fluids/gases from a body part.

DRAINAGE: Taking or letting out fluids and/or gases from a body part.

Explanation: Qualifier "X Diagnostic" indicates drainage procedures that are biopsies
Examples: Foley catheter placement – CMS Ex: Thoracentesis

Body Part – 4TH		Approach – 5TH	Device – 6TH	Qualifier – 7TH
0 Kidney, Right 1 Kidney, Left 3 Kidney Pelvis, Right 4 Kidney Pelvis, Left	6 Ureter, Right 7 Ureter, Left 8 Ureters, Bilateral B Bladder C Bladder Neck	0 Open 3 Percutaneous 4 Percutaneous endoscopic 7 Via natural or artificial opening 8 Via natural or artificial opening endoscopic	0 Drainage device	Z No qualifier
0 Kidney, Right 1 Kidney, Left 3 Kidney Pelvis, Right 4 Kidney Pelvis, Left	6 Ureter, Right 7 Ureter, Left 8 Ureters, Bilateral B Bladder C Bladder Neck	0 Open 3 Percutaneous 4 Percutaneous endoscopic 7 Via natural or artificial opening 8 Via natural or artificial opening endoscopic	Z No device	X Diagnostic Z No qualifier
D Urethra		0 Open 3 Percutaneous 4 Percutaneous endoscopic 7 Via natural or artificial opening 8 Via natural or artificial opening endoscopic X External	0 Drainage device	Z No qualifier
D Urethra		0 Open 3 Percutaneous 4 Percutaneous endoscopic 7 Via natural or artificial opening 8 Via natural or artificial opening endoscopic X External	Z No device	X Diagnostic Z No qualifier

1ST - 0 Medical and Surgical
2ND - T Urinary System
3RD - B EXCISION

EXCISION GROUP: Excision, Resection, Destruction, Extraction, (Detachment)
Root Operations that take out some or all of a body part.

EXCISION: Cutting out or off, without replacement, a portion of a body part.

Explanation: Qualifier "X Diagnostic" indicates excision procedures that are biopsies
Examples: Needle core biopsy kidney – CMS Ex: Liver biopsy

Body Part – 4TH		Approach – 5TH	Device – 6TH	Qualifier – 7TH
0 Kidney, Right 1 Kidney, Left 3 Kidney Pelvis, Right 4 Kidney Pelvis, Left	6 Ureter, Right 7 Ureter, Left B Bladder C Bladder Neck	0 Open 3 Percutaneous 4 Percutaneous endoscopic 7 Via natural or artificial opening 8 Via natural or artificial opening endoscopic	Z No device	X Diagnostic Z No qualifier
D Urethra		0 Open 3 Percutaneous 4 Percutaneous endoscopic 7 Via natural or artificial opening 8 Via natural or artificial opening endoscopic X External	Z No device	X Diagnostic Z No qualifier

© 2018 Channel Publishing, Ltd.

1ST - 0 Medical and Surgical
2ND - T Urinary System
3RD - C EXTIRPATION

DRAINAGE GROUP: Drainage, Extirpation, Fragmentation
Root Operations that take out solids/fluids/gases from a body part.

EXTIRPATION: Taking or cutting out solid matter from a body part.

Explanation: Abnormal byproduct or foreign body ...
Examples: Removal bladder stone – CMS Ex: Thrombectomy

Body Part – 4TH	Approach – 5TH	Device – 6TH	Qualifier – 7TH
0 Kidney, Right 1 Kidney, Left 3 Kidney Pelvis, Right 4 Kidney Pelvis, Left 6 Ureter, Right 7 Ureter, Left B Bladder C Bladder Neck	0 Open 3 Percutaneous 4 Percutaneous endoscopic 7 Via natural or artificial opening 8 Via natural or artificial opening endoscopic	Z No device	Z No qualifier
D Urethra	0 Open 3 Percutaneous 4 Percutaneous endoscopic 7 Via natural or artificial opening 8 Via natural or artificial opening endoscopic X External	Z No device	Z No qualifier

1ST - 0 Medical and Surgical
2ND - T Urinary System
3RD - D EXTRACTION

EXCISION GROUP: Excision, Resection, Destruction, Extraction, (Detachment)
Root Operations that take out some or all of a body part.

EXTRACTION: Pulling or stripping out or off all or a portion of a body part by the use of force.

Explanation: None for this Body System
Examples: Kidney extraction – CMS Ex: Dilation and curettage

Body Part – 4TH	Approach – 5TH	Device – 6TH	Qualifier – 7TH
0 Kidney, Right 1 Kidney, Left	0 Open 3 Percutaneous 4 Percutaneous endoscopic	Z No device	Z No qualifier

1ST - 0 Medical and Surgical
2ND - T Urinary System
3RD - F FRAGMENTATION

DRAINAGE GROUP: Drainage, Extirpation, Fragmentation
Root Operations that take out solids/fluids/gases from a body part.

FRAGMENTATION: Breaking solid matter in a body part into pieces.

Explanation: Pieces are not taken out during the procedure ...
Examples: ESWL kidney pelvis stone – CMS Ex: Extracorporeal shockwave lithotripsy (ESWL)

Body Part – 4TH	Approach – 5TH	Device – 6TH	Qualifier – 7TH
3 Kidney Pelvis, Right 4 Kidney Pelvis, Left 6 Ureter, Right 7 Ureter, Left B Bladder C Bladder Neck D Urethra NC*	0 Open 3 Percutaneous 4 Percutaneous endoscopic 7 Via natural or artificial opening 8 Via natural or artificial opening endoscopic X External	Z No device	Z No qualifier

NC* – Some procedures are considered non-covered by Medicare. See current Medicare Code Editor for details.

© 2018 Channel Publishing, Ltd.

1ST - 0 Medical and Surgical
2ND - T Urinary System
3RD - H INSERTION

DEVICE GROUP: Change, Insertion, Removal, Replacement, Revision, Supplement
Root Operations that always involve a device.

INSERTION: Putting in a nonbiological appliance that monitors, assists, performs, or prevents a physiological function but does not physically take the place of a body part.

Explanation: None
Examples: Artificial bladder sphincter – CMS Ex: Insertion of central venous catheter

Body Part – 4TH	Approach – 5TH	Device – 6TH	Qualifier – 7TH
5 Kidney	0 Open 3 Percutaneous 4 Percutaneous endoscopic 7 Via natural or artificial opening 8 Via natural or artificial opening endoscopic	2 Monitoring device 3 Infusion device Y Other device	Z No qualifier
9 Ureter	0 Open 3 Percutaneous 4 Percutaneous endoscopic 7 Via natural or artificial opening 8 Via natural or artificial opening endoscopic	2 Monitoring device 3 Infusion device M Stimulator lead Y Other device	Z No qualifier
B Bladder	0 Open 3 Percutaneous 4 Percutaneous endoscopic 7 Via natural or artificial opening 8 Via natural or artificial opening endoscopic	2 Monitoring device 3 Infusion device L Artificial sphincter M Stimulator lead NC* Y Other device	Z No qualifier
C Bladder Neck	0 Open 3 Percutaneous 4 Percutaneous endoscopic 7 Via natural or artificial opening 8 Via natural or artificial opening endoscopic	L Artificial sphincter	Z No qualifier
D Urethra	0 Open 3 Percutaneous 4 Percutaneous endoscopic 7 Via natural or artificial opening 8 Via natural or artificial opening endoscopic	2 Monitoring device 3 Infusion device L Artificial sphincter Y Other device	Z No qualifier
D Urethra	X External	2 Monitoring device 3 Infusion device L Artificial sphincter	Z No qualifier

NC* – Non-covered by Medicare. See current Medicare Code Editor for details.

1ST - 0 Medical and Surgical
2ND - T Urinary System
3RD - J INSPECTION

EXAMINATION GROUP: Inspection, (Map)
Root Operations involving examination only.

INSPECTION: Visually and/or manually exploring a body part.

Explanation: Direct or instrumental visualization ...
Examples: Ureteroscopy – CMS Ex: Exploratory laparotomy

Body Part – 4TH	Approach – 5TH	Device – 6TH	Qualifier – 7TH
5 Kidney 9 Ureter B Bladder D Urethra	0 Open 3 Percutaneous 4 Percutaneous endoscopic 7 Via natural or artificial opening 8 Via natural or artificial opening endoscopic X External	Z No device	Z No qualifier

URINARY 0TH

© 2018 Channel Publishing, Ltd.

1ST - 0 Medical and Surgical
2ND - T Urinary System
3RD - L OCCLUSION

TUBULAR GROUP: Bypass, Dilation, Occlusion, Restriction
Root Operations that alter the diameter/route of a tubular body part.

OCCLUSION: Completely closing an orifice or the lumen of a tubular body part.

Explanation: The orifice can be a natural orifice or an artificially created orifice
Examples: Occlusion kidney pelvis – CMS Ex: Fallopian tube ligation

Body Part – 4TH	Approach – 5TH	Device – 6TH	Qualifier – 7TH
3 Kidney Pelvis, Right 4 Kidney Pelvis, Left 6 Ureter, Right 7 Ureter, Left B Bladder C Bladder Neck	0 Open 3 Percutaneous 4 Percutaneous endoscopic	C Extraluminal device D Intraluminal device Z No device	Z No qualifier
3 Kidney Pelvis, Right 4 Kidney Pelvis, Left 6 Ureter, Right 7 Ureter, Left B Bladder C Bladder Neck	7 Via natural or artificial opening 8 Via natural or artificial opening endoscopic	D Intraluminal device Z No device	Z No qualifier
D Urethra	0 Open 3 Percutaneous 4 Percutaneous endoscopic X External	C Extraluminal device D Intraluminal device Z No device	Z No qualifier
D Urethra	7 Via natural or artificial opening 8 Via natural or artificial opening endoscopic	D Intraluminal device Z No device	Z No qualifier

1ST - 0 Medical and Surgical
2ND - T Urinary System
3RD - M REATTACHMENT

MOVE GROUP: Reattachment, Reposition, (Transfer), Transplantation
Root Operations that put in/put back or move some/all of a body part.

REATTACHMENT: Putting back in or on all or a portion of a separated body part to its normal location or other suitable location.

Explanation: Vascular circulation and nervous pathways may or may not be reestablished
Examples: Replantation avulsed kidney – CMS Ex: Reattachment of hand

Body Part – 4TH	Approach – 5TH	Device – 6TH	Qualifier – 7TH
0 Kidney, Right 1 Kidney, Left 2 Kidneys, Bilateral 3 Kidney Pelvis, Right 4 Kidney Pelvis, Left 6 Ureter, Right 7 Ureter, Left 8 Ureters, Bilateral B Bladder C Bladder Neck D Urethra	0 Open 4 Percutaneous endoscopic	Z No device	Z No qualifier

1ST - 0 Medical and Surgical
2ND - T Urinary System
3RD - N RELEASE

DIVISION GROUP: Division, Release
Root Operations involving cutting or separation only.

RELEASE: Freeing a body part from an abnormal physical constraint by cutting or by the use of force.

Explanation: Some of the restraining tissue may be taken out but none of the body part is taken out
Examples: Adhesiolysis ureter – CMS Ex: Carpal tunnel release

Body Part – 4TH	Approach – 5TH	Device – 6TH	Qualifier – 7TH
0 Kidney, Right 1 Kidney, Left 3 Kidney Pelvis, Right 4 Kidney Pelvis, Left 6 Ureter, Right 7 Ureter, Left B Bladder C Bladder Neck	0 Open 3 Percutaneous 4 Percutaneous endoscopic 7 Via natural or artificial opening 8 Via natural or artificial opening endoscopic	Z No device	Z No qualifier
D Urethra	0 Open 3 Percutaneous 4 Percutaneous endoscopic 7 Via natural or artificial opening 8 Via natural or artificial opening endoscopic X External	Z No device	Z No qualifier

© 2018 Channel Publishing, Ltd.

1ST - 0 Medical and Surgical 2ND - T Urinary System 3RD - P REMOVAL	DEVICE GROUP: Change, Insertion, Removal, Replacement, Revision, Supplement Root Operations that always involve a device. REMOVAL: Taking out or off a device from a body part. Explanation: Removal device without reinsertion ... Examples: Removal ureteral stent – CMS Ex: Cardiac pacemaker removal

Body Part – 4TH	Approach – 5TH	Device – 6TH	Qualifier – 7TH
5 Kidney	0 Open 3 Percutaneous 4 Percutaneous endoscopic 7 Via natural or artificial opening 8 Via natural or artificial opening endoscopic	0 Drainage device 2 Monitoring device 3 Infusion device 7 Autologous tissue substitute C Extraluminal device D Intraluminal device J Synthetic substitute K Nonautologous tissue substitute Y Other device	Z No qualifier
5 Kidney	X External	0 Drainage device 2 Monitoring device 3 Infusion device D Intraluminal device	Z No qualifier
9 Ureter	0 Open 3 Percutaneous 4 Percutaneous endoscopic 7 Via natural or artificial opening 8 Via natural or artificial opening endoscopic	0 Drainage device 2 Monitoring device 3 Infusion device 7 Autologous tissue substitute C Extraluminal device D Intraluminal device J Synthetic substitute K Nonautologous tissue substitute M Stimulator lead Y Other device	Z No qualifier
9 Ureter	X External	0 Drainage device 2 Monitoring device 3 Infusion device D Intraluminal device M Stimulator lead	Z No qualifier
B Bladder	0 Open 3 Percutaneous 4 Percutaneous endoscopic 7 Via natural or artificial opening 8 Via natural or artificial opening endoscopic	0 Drainage device 2 Monitoring device 3 Infusion device 7 Autologous tissue substitute C Extraluminal device D Intraluminal device J Synthetic substitute K Nonautologous tissue substitute L Artificial sphincter M Stimulator lead NC* Y Other device	Z No qualifier
B Bladder	X External	0 Drainage device 2 Monitoring device 3 Infusion device D Intraluminal device L Artificial sphincter M Stimulator lead	Z No qualifier
D Urethra	0 Open 3 Percutaneous 4 Percutaneous endoscopic 7 Via natural or artificial opening 8 Via natural or artificial opening endoscopic	0 Drainage device 2 Monitoring device 3 Infusion device 7 Autologous tissue substitute C Extraluminal device D Intraluminal device J Synthetic substitute K Nonautologous tissue substitute L Artificial sphincter Y Other device	Z No qualifier
D Urethra	X External	0 Drainage device 2 Monitoring device 3 Infusion device D Intraluminal device L Artificial sphincter	Z No qualifier

NC* – Non-covered by Medicare. See current Medicare Code Editor for details.

© 2018 Channel Publishing, Ltd.

1ST - 0 Medical and Surgical
2ND - T Urinary System
3RD - Q REPAIR

OTHER REPAIRS GROUP: (Control), Repair
Root Operations that define other repairs.

REPAIR: Restoring, to the extent possible, a body part to its normal anatomic structure and function.

Explanation: Used only when the method to accomplish the repair is not one of the other root operations
Examples: Suture lacerated kidney – CMS Ex: Suture of laceration

Body Part – 4TH	Approach – 5TH	Device – 6TH	Qualifier – 7TH
0 Kidney, Right 1 Kidney, Left 3 Kidney Pelvis, Right 4 Kidney Pelvis, Left 6 Ureter, Right 7 Ureter, Left B Bladder C Bladder Neck	0 Open 3 Percutaneous 4 Percutaneous endoscopic 7 Via natural or artificial opening 8 Via natural or artificial opening endoscopic	Z No device	Z No qualifier
D Urethra	0 Open 3 Percutaneous 4 Percutaneous endoscopic 7 Via natural or artificial opening 8 Via natural or artificial opening endoscopic X External	Z No device	Z No qualifier

1ST - 0 Medical and Surgical
2ND - T Urinary System
3RD - R REPLACEMENT

DEVICE GROUP: Change, Insertion, Removal, Replacement, Revision, Supplement
Root Operations that always involve a device.

REPLACEMENT: Putting in or on biological or synthetic material that physically takes the place and/or function of all or a portion of a body part.

Explanation: Includes taking out or eradicating, or rendering non-functional, the body part ...
Examples: Segmental ureteral replacement – CMS Ex: Total hip replacement

Body Part – 4TH	Approach – 5TH	Device – 6TH	Qualifier – 7TH
3 Kidney Pelvis, Right 4 Kidney Pelvis, Left 6 Ureter, Right 7 Ureter, Left B Bladder C Bladder Neck	0 Open 4 Percutaneous endoscopic 7 Via natural or artificial opening 8 Via natural or artificial opening endoscopic	7 Autologous tissue substitute J Synthetic substitute K Nonautologous tissue substitute	Z No qualifier
D Urethra	0 Open 4 Percutaneous endoscopic 7 Via natural or artificial opening 8 Via natural or artificial opening endoscopic X External	7 Autologous tissue substitute J Synthetic substitute K Nonautologous tissue substitute	Z No qualifier

1ST - 0 Medical and Surgical
2ND - T Urinary System
3RD - S REPOSITION

MOVE GROUP: Reattachment, Reposition, (Transfer), Transplantation
Root Operations that put in/put back or move some/all of a body part.

REPOSITION: Moving to its normal location, or other suitable location, all or a portion of a body part.

Explanation: The body part may or may not be cut out or off to be moved to the new location ...
Examples: Bladder neck (sling) suspension – CMS Ex: Fracture reduction

Body Part – 4TH	Approach – 5TH	Device – 6TH	Qualifier – 7TH
0 Kidney, Right 1 Kidney, Left 2 Kidneys, Bilateral 3 Kidney Pelvis, Right 4 Kidney Pelvis, Left 6 Ureter, Right 7 Ureter, Left 8 Ureters, Bilateral B Bladder C Bladder Neck D Urethra	0 Open 4 Percutaneous endoscopic	Z No device	Z No qualifier

© 2018 Channel Publishing, Ltd.

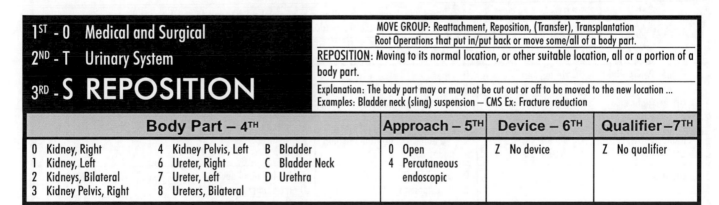

1ST - 0 Medical and Surgical
2ND - T Urinary System
3RD - T RESECTION

EXCISION GROUP: Excision, Resection, Destruction, Extraction, (Detachment)
Root Operations that take out some or all of a body part.

RESECTION: Cutting out or off, without replacement, all of a body part.

Explanation: None
Examples: Nephrectomy – CMS Ex: Total lobectomy of lung

Body Part – 4TH	Approach – 5TH	Device – 6TH	Qualifier – 7TH
0 Kidney, Right 1 Kidney, Left 2 Kidneys, Bilateral	0 Open 4 Percutaneous endoscopic	Z No device	Z No qualifier
3 Kidney Pelvis, Right 4 Kidney Pelvis, Left 6 Ureter, Right 7 Ureter, Left B Bladder C Bladder Neck D Urethra	0 Open 4 Percutaneous endoscopic 7 Via natural or artificial opening 8 Via natural or artificial opening endoscopic	Z No device	Z No qualifier

1ST - 0 Medical and Surgical
2ND - T Urinary System
3RD - U SUPPLEMENT

DEVICE GROUP: Change, Insertion, Removal, Replacement, Revision, Supplement
Root Operations that always involve a device.

SUPPLEMENT: Putting in or on biological or synthetic material that physically reinforces and/or augments the function of a portion of a body part.

Explanation: Biological material is non-living, or is living and from the same individual ...
Examples: Repair bladder neck defect with graft – CMS Ex: Herniorrhaphy using mesh

Body Part – 4TH	Approach – 5TH	Device – 6TH	Qualifier – 7TH
3 Kidney Pelvis, Right 4 Kidney Pelvis, Left 6 Ureter, Right 7 Ureter, Left B Bladder C Bladder Neck	0 Open 4 Percutaneous endoscopic 7 Via natural or artificial opening 8 Via natural or artificial opening endoscopic	7 Autologous tissue substitute J Synthetic substitute K Nonautologous tissue substitute	Z No qualifier
D Urethra	0 Open 4 Percutaneous endoscopic 7 Via natural or artificial opening 8 Via natural or artificial opening endoscopic X External	7 Autologous tissue substitute J Synthetic substitute K Nonautologous tissue substitute	Z No qualifier

1ST - 0 Medical and Surgical
2ND - T Urinary System
3RD - V RESTRICTION

TUBULAR GROUP: Bypass, Dilation, Occlusion, Restriction
Root Operations that alter the diameter/route of a tubular body part.

RESTRICTION: Partially closing an orifice or the lumen of a tubular body part.

Explanation: The orifice can be a natural orifice or an artificially created orifice.
Examples: Ureteral restrictive stent – CMS Ex: Cervical cerclage

Body Part – 4TH	Approach – 5TH	Device – 6TH	Qualifier – 7TH
3 Kidney Pelvis, Right 4 Kidney Pelvis, Left 6 Ureter, Right 7 Ureter, Left B Bladder C Bladder Neck	0 Open 3 Percutaneous 4 Percutaneous endoscopic	C Extraluminal device D Intraluminal device Z No device	Z No qualifier
3 Kidney Pelvis, Right 4 Kidney Pelvis, Left 6 Ureter, Right 7 Ureter, Left B Bladder C Bladder Neck	7 Via natural or artificial opening 8 Via natural or artificial opening endoscopic	D Intraluminal device Z No device	Z No qualifier
D Urethra	0 Open 3 Percutaneous 4 Percutaneous endoscopic	C Extraluminal device D Intraluminal device Z No device	Z No qualifier
D Urethra	7 Via natural or artificial opening 8 Via natural or artificial opening endoscopic	D Intraluminal device Z No device	Z No qualifier
D Urethra	X External	Z No device	Z No qualifier

© 2018 Channel Publishing, Ltd.

1ST - 0 Medical and Surgical
2ND - T Urinary System
3RD - W REVISION

DEVICE GROUP: Change, Insertion, Removal, Replacement, Revision, Supplement
Root Operations that always involve a device.

REVISION: Correcting, to the extent possible, a portion of a malfunctioning device or the position of a displaced device.

Explanation: Correcting by taking out or putting in components of a device such as a screw or pin ...
Examples: Reposition stimulator lead – CMS Ex: Recementing of hip prosthesis

Body Part – 4TH	Approach – 5TH	Device – 6TH	Qualifier – 7TH
5 Kidney	0 Open 3 Percutaneous 4 Percutaneous endoscopic 7 Via natural or artificial opening 8 Via natural or artificial opening endoscopic	0 Drainage device 2 Monitoring device 3 Infusion device 7 Autologous tissue substitute C Extraluminal device D Intraluminal device J Synthetic substitute K Nonautologous tissue substitute Y Other device	Z No qualifier
5 Kidney	X External	0 Drainage device 2 Monitoring device 3 Infusion device 7 Autologous tissue substitute C Extraluminal device D Intraluminal device J Synthetic substitute K Nonautologous tissue substitute	Z No qualifier
9 Ureter	0 Open 3 Percutaneous 4 Percutaneous endoscopic 7 Via natural or artificial opening 8 Via natural or artificial opening endoscopic	0 Drainage device 2 Monitoring device 3 Infusion device 7 Autologous tissue substitute C Extraluminal device D Intraluminal device J Synthetic substitute K Nonautologous tissue substitute M Stimulator lead Y Other device	Z No qualifier
9 Ureter	X External	0 Drainage device 2 Monitoring device 3 Infusion device 7 Autologous tissue substitute C Extraluminal device D Intraluminal device J Synthetic substitute K Nonautologous tissue substitute M Stimulator lead	Z No qualifier

continued ⇨

© 2018 Channel Publishing, Ltd.

0 T W REVISION – *continued*

Body Part – 4TH	Approach – 5TH	Device – 6TH	Qualifier – 7TH
B Bladder	0 Open 3 Percutaneous 4 Percutaneous endoscopic 7 Via natural or artificial opening 8 Via natural or artificial opening endoscopic	0 Drainage device 2 Monitoring device 3 Infusion device 7 Autologous tissue substitute C Extraluminal device D Intraluminal device J Synthetic substitute K Nonautologous tissue substitute L Artificial sphincter M Stimulator lead Y Other device	Z No qualifier
B Bladder	X External	0 Drainage device 2 Monitoring device 3 Infusion device 7 Autologous tissue substitute C Extraluminal device D Intraluminal device J Synthetic substitute K Nonautologous tissue substitute L Artificial sphincter M Stimulator lead	Z No qualifier
D Urethra	0 Open 3 Percutaneous 4 Percutaneous endoscopic 7 Via natural or artificial opening 8 Via natural or artificial opening endoscopic	0 Drainage device 2 Monitoring device 3 Infusion device 7 Autologous tissue substitute C Extraluminal device D Intraluminal device J Synthetic substitute K Nonautologous tissue substitute L Artificial sphincter Y Other device	Z No qualifier
D Urethra	X External	0 Drainage device 2 Monitoring device 3 Infusion device 7 Autologous tissue substitute C Extraluminal device D Intraluminal device J Synthetic substitute K Nonautologous tissue substitute L Artificial sphincter	Z No qualifier

1ST - 0 Medical and Surgical
2ND - T Urinary System
3RD - Y TRANSPLANTATION

MOVE GROUP: Reattachment, Reposition, (Transfer), Transplantation
Root Operations that put in/put back or move some/all of a body part.

TRANSPLANTATION: Putting in or on all or a portion of a living body part taken from another individual or animal to physically take the place and/or function of all or a portion of a similar body part.

Explanation: The native body part may or may not be taken out ...
Examples: Kidney transplant – CMS Ex: Kidney transplant

Body Part – 4TH	Approach – 5TH	Device – 6TH	Qualifier – 7TH
0 Kidney, Right NC*LC* 1 Kidney, Left NC*LC*	0 Open	Z No device	0 Allogeneic 1 Syngeneic 2 Zooplastic

NC*LC* – Some procedures are considered non-covered or limited coverage by Medicare. See current Medicare Code Editor for details.

© 2018 Channel Publishing, Ltd.

Educational Annotations | U – Female Reproductive System

Body System Specific Educational Annotations for the Female Reproductive System include:

- Anatomy and Physiology Review
- Definitions of Common Procedures
- Anatomical Illustrations
- AHA Coding Clinic® Reference Notations
- Body Part Key Listings
- Device Key Listings
- Device Aggregation Table Listings
- Coding Notes

Anatomy and Physiology Review of Female Reproductive System

BODY PART VALUES – U - FEMALE REPRODUCTIVE SYSTEM

Cervix – The cervix is the lower portion of the uterus that extends downward into the vagina.
Clitoris – ANATOMY – The highly innervated, sensitive female sex organ that is located above the urethral opening (meatus) and at the junction of the labia minora. PHYSIOLOGY – It is generally accepted as the primary anatomical source of female sexual pleasure.
Cul-de-sac – The deep peritoneal recess between the rectum and back wall of the uterus (also known as the pouch of Douglas and rectouterine pouch).
Endometrium – The mucous membrane interior lining of the uterus that lies upon the thick muscular myometrium of the body.
Fallopian Tube – ANATOMY – The fallopian tubes (also known as oviducts, uterine tubes, and salpinges) are the tubular canals from each side of the uterus to the area immediately next to each ovary (fimbriae). PHYSIOLOGY – The fallopian tubes serve to transport the ova to the uterus.
Hymen – The hymen is a membrane of tissue that surrounds or partially covers the vaginal opening.
Ova – The human reproductive egg(s).
Ovary – ANATOMY – The ovaries are the paired, flat, ovoid female reproductive glands located on each side of the uterus, attached to the broad ligament, and are approximately 1.4 inches (3.5 cm) in length and 0.8 inches (2 cm) in width. PHYSIOLOGY – The ovaries function to produce the human reproductive egg cell (ova, ovum), and to produce hormones. The ovaries secrete estrogen, testosterone, and progesterone.
Uterine Supporting Structure – The ligaments, fibromuscular bands, and connective tissue that support the uterus, ovaries, and fallopian tubes. The broad ligament is the double-layered fold of the peritoneum with the loose connective tissue between its layers, called the parametrium. The round ligaments are the fibromuscular bands attached to the uterus below the fallopian tube orifices and to the pelvic wall.
Uterus – ANATOMY – The uterus is the pear-shaped, hollow, muscular female reproductive organ that is about 2.8 inches (7 cm) in length and up to 2 inches (5 cm) in width, located within the pelvic cavity, and resting slightly above the bladder. The fallopian tubes enter into the upper portion. The cervix is the lower portion that extends downward into the vagina. The isthmus is the narrowed lower end of the body of the uterus. The body is the bulky upper portion with the dome above the fallopian tube orifices (also known as the fundus or corpus uteri). The endometrium is the mucous membrane interior lining lying upon the thick muscular myometrium of the body. The ovarian and uterine arteries supply blood to the uterus. PHYSIOLOGY – The uterus functions to receive the embryo, serve as attachment for the placenta, stretch and enlarge to allow for the fetus to grow, and to rhythmically contract for delivery of the fetus.
Vagina – ANATOMY – The vagina is the elastic, musculomembranous canal extending from the uterus to the vulva, passing in front of the rectum and behind the bladder, attached by loose connective tissue, and is approximately 3-4 inches (7.5-10 cm) in length. PHYSIOLOGY – The vagina functions to receive the penis and ejaculated sperm during intercourse, pass the fetus to birth during delivery, and convey the menstrual discharge out of the body.
Vestibular Gland – The vestibular glands (also known as paraurethral, Bartholin's, and Skene's glands) are small mucous-secreting glands that open on either side of the urethral orifice and vaginal opening.
Vulva – ANATOMY – The vulva is the group of external female genital organs comprising the labia majora, labia minora, clitoris, and vestibular glands. PHYSIOLOGY – The vulva functions to protect the genital organs at the entrance of the vagina, and aid in sexual stimulation and lubrication during intercourse.

Definitions of Common Procedures of Female Reproductive System

Cervical cerclage – The placement of an encircling suture in the cervix to prevent a miscarriage or premature birth.
Hysterectomy – The surgical removal of the uterus (subtotal) and often the cervix (total).
Oophorectomy – The surgical removal of one or both ovaries.
Ovarian cystectomy – The surgical removal of an ovarian cyst leaving the ovary intact.
Salpingectomy – The surgical removal of one or both fallopian tubes.
Vaginoplasty – The plastic surgical restoration of vaginal defects or deformities.

© 2018 Channel Publishing, Ltd.

Educational Annotations | U – Female Reproductive System

Anatomical Illustrations of Female Reproductive System

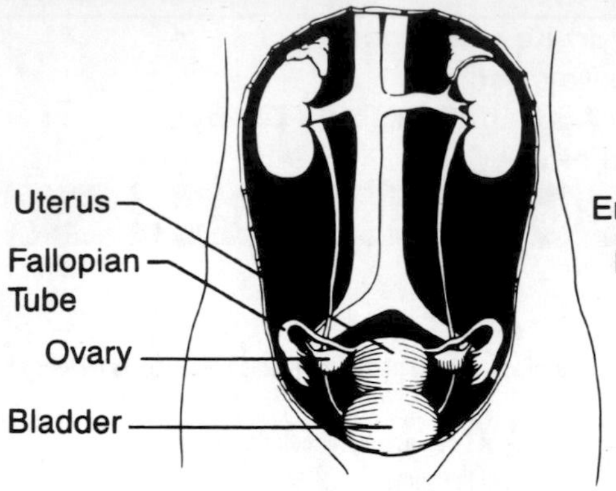

UTERUS AND ADNEXA

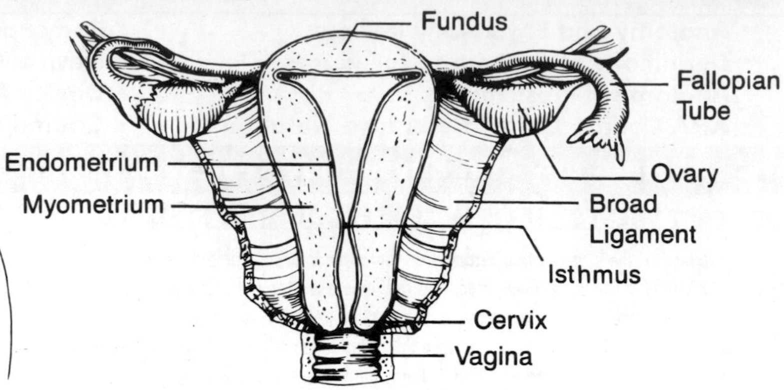

UTERUS AND ADNEXA — CUT-AWAY

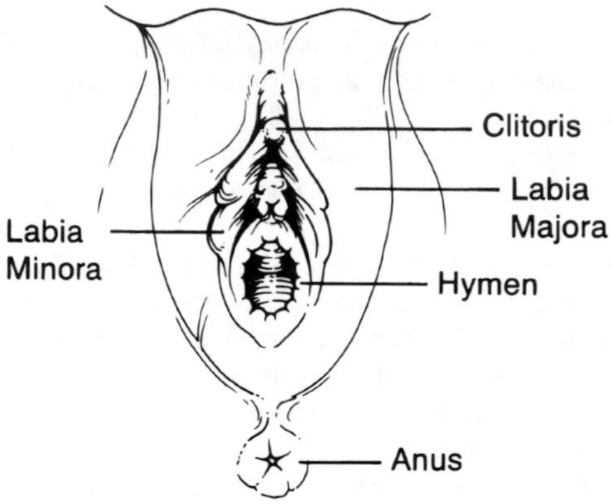

EXTERNAL FEMALE GENITALS

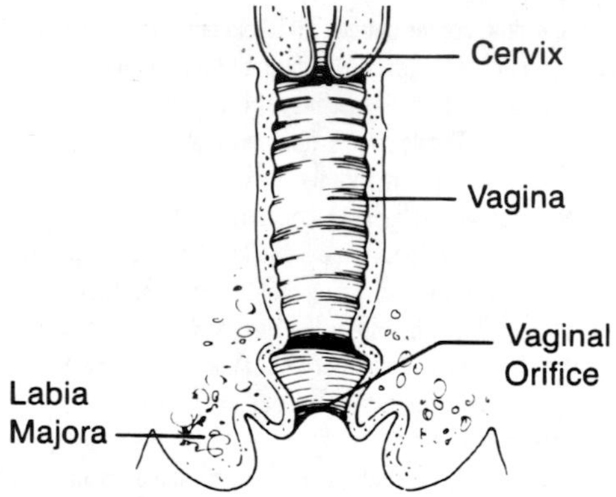

VAGINA — CUT-AWAY VIEW

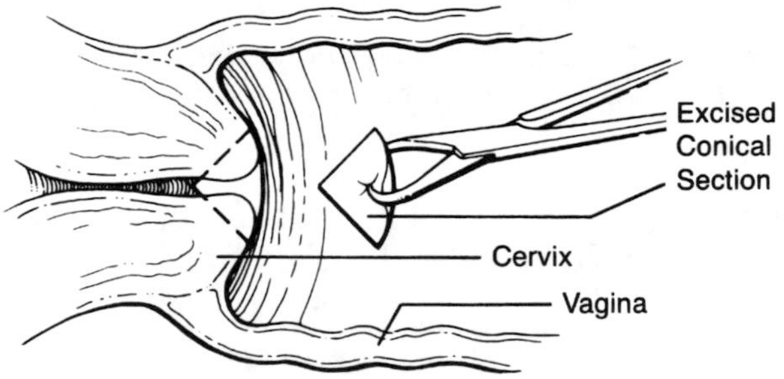

CONIZATION OF CERVIX

FEMALE 0 U

© 2018 Channel Publishing, Ltd.

Educational Annotations | U – Female Reproductive System

AHA Coding Clinic® Reference Notations of Female Reproductive System

ROOT OPERATION SPECIFIC - U - FEMALE REPRODUCTIVE SYSTEM

BYPASS - 1
CHANGE - 2
DESTRUCTION - 5
DILATION - 7
DIVISION - 8
DRAINAGE - 9
EXCISION - B

- Excision of labia majora skin tags ....AHA 14:3Q:p12
- Partial salpingectomy ....AHA 15:3Q:p31
- Partial salpingectomy - Official Clarification ....AHA 18:1Q:p23
- Segmental excision of fallopian tubes ....AHA 15:3Q:p31
- Uterine fibroids, multiple ....AHA 14:4Q:p16

EXTIRPATION - C

- Clot evacuation from uterus post delivery ....AHA 13:2Q:p38
- Removal of cervical cerclage ....AHA 15:3Q:p30x2

EXTRACTION - D
FRAGMENTATION - F
INSERTION - H

- IUD insertion during cesarean section ....AHA 13:2Q:p34
- Placement of tandem and ovoids into uterus and cervix-Official Correction ..AHA 18:1Q:p25

INSPECTION - J

- Laparoscopic procedure converted to open....AHA 15:1Q:p33

OCCLUSION - L
REATTACHMENT - M
RELEASE - N
REMOVAL - P
REPAIR - Q

- Periurethral obstetric laceration repair ....AHA 14:4Q:p18
- Repair of lacerated clitoris ....AHA 13:4Q:p120

REPOSITION - S

- Bimanual retroversion of pregnant uterus....AHA 16:1Q:p9

RESECTION - T

- Bilateral oophorectomy ....AHA 15:1Q:p33
- Bilateral salpingectomy ....AHA 15:1Q:p33
- Hysterectomy....AHA 15:1Q:p33
- Removal of cervix....AHA 15:1Q:p33
- Removal of remaining portion of ovary....AHA 13:1Q:p24
- Supracervical hysterectomy ....AHA 17:4Q:p68
- Total (open) hysterectomy....AHA 13:3Q:p28
- Total hysterectomy - Official Correction ....AHA 17:4Q:p68

SUPPLEMENT - U
RESTRICTION - V

- Cervical cerclage ....AHA 15:3Q:p30

REVISION - W
TRANSPLANTATION - Y

© 2018 Channel Publishing, Ltd.

Educational Annotations | U – Female Reproductive System

Body Part Key Listings of Female Reproductive System

See also Body Part Key in Appendix C

Bartholin's (greater vestibular) gland	use Vestibular Gland
Broad ligament	use Uterine Supporting Structure
Fundus uteri	use Uterus
Greater vestibular (Bartholin's) gland	use Vestibular Gland
Infundibulopelvic ligament	use Uterine Supporting Structure
Labia majora	use Vulva
Labia minora	use Vulva
Myometrium	use Uterus
Ovarian ligament	use Uterine Supporting Structure
Oviduct	use Fallopian Tube, Left/Right
Paraurethral (Skene's) gland	use Vestibular Gland
Perimetrium	use Uterus
Round ligament of uterus	use Uterine Supporting Structure
Salpinx	use Fallopian Tube, Left/Right
Skene's (paraurethral) gland	use Vestibular Gland
Uterine cornu	use Uterus
Uterine tube	use Fallopian Tube, Left/Right

Device Key Listings of Female Reproductive System

See also Device Key in Appendix D

Autograft	use Autologous Tissue Substitute
Brachytherapy seeds	use Radioactive Element
Cook Biodesign® Fistula Plug(s)	use Nonautologous Tissue Substitute
Intrauterine device (IUD)	use Contraceptive Device in Female Reproductive System
Pessary ring	use Intraluminal Device, Pessary in Female Reproductive System
Tissue bank graft	use Nonautologous Tissue Substitute
Vaginal pessary	use Intraluminal Device, Pessary in Female Reproductive System

Device Aggregation Table Listings of Female Reproductive System

See also Device Aggregation Table in Appendix E

Specific Device	For Operation	In Body System	General Device
Intraluminal Device, Pessary	All applicable	Female Reproductive System	Intraluminal Device

Coding Notes of Female Reproductive System

© 2018 Channel Publishing, Ltd.

1ST - 0 Medical and Surgical
2ND - U Female Reproductive System ♀
3RD - 1 BYPASS

TUBULAR GROUP: Bypass, Dilation, Occlusion, Restriction
Root Operations that alter the diameter/route of a tubular body part.

BYPASS: Altering the route of passage of the contents of a tubular body part.

Explanation: Rerouting contents to a downstream part ... with or without the use of a device ...
Examples: Fallopian tube bypass – CMS Ex: Coronary artery bypass

Body Part – 4TH	Approach – 5TH	Device – 6TH	Qualifier – 7TH
5 Fallopian Tube, Right 6 Fallopian Tube, Left	0 Open 4 Percutaneous endoscopic	7 Autologous tissue substitute J Synthetic substitute K Nonautologous tissue substitute Z No device	5 Fallopian Tube, Right 6 Fallopian Tube, Left 9 Uterus

1ST - 0 Medical and Surgical
2ND - U Female Reproductive System ♀
3RD - 2 CHANGE

DEVICE GROUP: Change, Insertion, Removal, (Replacement), Revision, Supplement
Root Operations that always involve a device.

CHANGE: Taking out or off a device from a body part and putting back an identical or similar device in or on the same body part without cutting or puncturing the skin or a mucous membrane.

Explanation: All CHANGE procedures are coded using the approach External
Examples: Exchange drain tube – CMS Ex: Urinary catheter change

Body Part – 4TH	Approach – 5TH	Device – 6TH	Qualifier – 7TH
3 Ovary 8 Fallopian Tube M Vulva	X External	0 Drainage device Y Other device	Z No qualifier
D Uterus and Cervix	X External	0 Drainage device H Contraceptive device Y Other device	Z No qualifier
H Vagina and Cul-de-sac	X External	0 Drainage device G Intraluminal device, pessary Y Other device	Z No qualifier

1ST - 0 Medical and Surgical
2ND - U Female Reproductive System ♀
3RD - 5 DESTRUCTION

EXCISION GROUP: Excision, Resection, Destruction, Extraction, (Detachment)
Root Operations that take out some or all of a body part.

DESTRUCTION: Physical eradication of all or a portion of a body part by the direct use of energy, force, or a destructive agent.

Explanation: None of the body part is physically taken out
Examples: Fulguration endometriosis – CMS Ex: Fulguration of rectal polyp

Body Part – 4TH	Approach – 5TH	Device – 6TH	Qualifier – 7TH
0 Ovary, Right 1 Ovary, Left 2 Ovaries, Bilateral 4 Uterine Supporting Structure	0 Open 3 Percutaneous 4 Percutaneous endoscopic 8 Via natural or artificial opening endoscopic	Z No device	Z No qualifier
5 Fallopian Tube, Right 6 Fallopian Tube, Left 7 Fallopian Tubes, Bilateral NC* 9 Uterus B Endometrium C Cervix F Cul-de-sac	0 Open 3 Percutaneous 4 Percutaneous endoscopic 7 Via natural or artificial opening 8 Via natural or artificial opening endoscopic	Z No device	Z No qualifier
G Vagina K Hymen	0 Open 3 Percutaneous 4 Percutaneous endoscopic 7 Via natural or artificial opening 8 Via natural or artificial opening endoscopic X External	Z No device	Z No qualifier
J Clitoris L Vestibular Gland M Vulva	0 Open X External	Z No device	Z No qualifier

NC* – Some procedures are considered non-covered by Medicare. See current Medicare Code Editor for details.

© 2018 Channel Publishing, Ltd.

1ST - 0 Medical and Surgical
2ND - U Female Reproductive System ♀
3RD - 7 DILATION

TUBULAR GROUP: Bypass, Dilation, Occlusion, Restriction
Root Operations that alter the diameter/route of a tubular body part.

DILATION: Expanding an orifice or the lumen of a tubular body part.

Explanation: Accomplished by stretching or cutting ... tubular body part or orifice ...
Examples: Dilation fallopian tubes – CMS Ex: Percutaneous transluminal angioplasty

Body Part – 4TH	Approach – 5TH	Device – 6TH	Qualifier – 7TH
5 Fallopian Tube, Right 6 Fallopian Tube, Left 7 Fallopian Tubes, Bilateral 9 Uterus C Cervix G Vagina	0 Open 3 Percutaneous 4 Percutaneous endoscopic 7 Via natural or artificial opening 8 Via natural or artificial opening endoscopic	D Intraluminal device Z No device	Z No qualifier
K Hymen	0 Open 3 Percutaneous 4 Percutaneous endoscopic 7 Via natural or artificial opening 8 Via natural or artificial opening endoscopic X External	D Intraluminal device Z No device	Z No qualifier

1ST - 0 Medical and Surgical
2ND - U Female Reproductive System ♀
3RD - 8 DIVISION

DIVISION GROUP: Division, Release
Root Operations involving cutting or separation only.

DIVISION: Cutting into a body part, without draining fluids and/or gases from the body part, in order to separate or transect a body part.

Explanation: All or a portion of the body part is separated into two or more portions
Examples: Hymenotomy – CMS Ex: Spinal cordotomy

Body Part – 4TH	Approach – 5TH	Device – 6TH	Qualifier – 7TH
0 Ovary, Right 1 Ovary, Left 2 Ovaries, Bilateral 4 Uterine Supporting Structure	0 Open 3 Percutaneous 4 Percutaneous endoscopic	Z No device	Z No qualifier
K Hymen	7 Via natural or artificial opening 8 Via natural or artificial opening endoscopic X External	Z No device	Z No qualifier

© 2018 Channel Publishing, Ltd.

1ST - 0 Medical and Surgical
2ND - U Female Reproductive System ♀
3RD - 9 DRAINAGE

DRAINAGE GROUP: Drainage, Extirpation, Fragmentation
Root Operations that take out solids/fluids/gases from a body part.

DRAINAGE: Taking or letting out fluids and/or gases from a body part.

Explanation: Qualifier "X Diagnostic" indicates drainage procedures that are biopsies
Examples: Aspiration draniage ovarian cyst – CMS Ex: Thoracentesis

Body Part – 4TH	Approach – 5TH	Device – 6TH	Qualifier – 7TH
0 Ovary, Right 1 Ovary, Left 2 Ovaries, Bilateral	0 Open 3 Percutaneous 4 Percutaneous endoscopic 8 Via natural or artificial opening endoscopic	0 Drainage device	Z No qualifier
0 Ovary, Right 1 Ovary, Left 2 Ovaries, Bilateral	0 Open 3 Percutaneous 4 Percutaneous endoscopic 8 Via natural or artificial opening endoscopic	Z No device	X Diagnostic Z No qualifier
0 Ovary, Right 1 Ovary, Left 2 Ovaries, Bilateral	X External	Z No device	Z No qualifier
4 Uterine Supporting Structure	0 Open 3 Percutaneous 4 Percutaneous endoscopic 8 Via natural or artificial opening endoscopic	0 Drainage device	Z No qualifier
4 Uterine Supporting Structure	0 Open 3 Percutaneous 4 Percutaneous endoscopic 8 Via natural or artificial opening endoscopic	Z No device	X Diagnostic Z No qualifier
5 Fallopian Tube, Right 6 Fallopian Tube, Left 7 Fallopian Tubes, Bilateral 9 Uterus C Cervix F Cul-de-sac	0 Open 3 Percutaneous 4 Percutaneous endoscopic 7 Via natural or artificial opening 8 Via natural or artificial opening endoscopic	0 Drainage device	Z No qualifier
5 Fallopian Tube, Right 6 Fallopian Tube, Left 7 Fallopian Tubes, Bilateral 9 Uterus C Cervix F Cul-de-sac	0 Open 3 Percutaneous 4 Percutaneous endoscopic 7 Via natural or artificial opening 8 Via natural or artificial opening endoscopic	Z No device	X Diagnostic Z No qualifier
G Vagina K Hymen	0 Open 3 Percutaneous 4 Percutaneous endoscopic 7 Via natural or artificial opening 8 Via natural or artificial opening endoscopic X External	0 Drainage device	Z No qualifier
G Vagina K Hymen	0 Open 3 Percutaneous 4 Percutaneous endoscopic 7 Via natural or artificial opening 8 Via natural or artificial opening endoscopic X External	Z No device	X Diagnostic Z No qualifier
J Clitoris L Vestibular Gland M Vulva	0 Open X External	0 Drainage device	Z No qualifier
J Clitoris L Vestibular Gland M Vulva	0 Open X External	Z No device	X Diagnostic Z No qualifier

© 2018 Channel Publishing, Ltd.

1ST - 0 Medical and Surgical
2ND - U Female Reproductive System ♀
3RD - B EXCISION

EXCISION GROUP: Excision, Resection, Destruction, Extraction, (Detachment)
Root Operations that take out some or all of a body part.

EXCISION: Cutting out or off, without replacement, a portion of a body part.

Explanation: Qualifier "X Diagnostic" indicates excision procedures that are biopsies
Examples: Excision uterine fibroids – CMS Ex: Liver biopsy

Body Part – 4TH	Approach – 5TH	Device – 6TH	Qualifier – 7TH
0 Ovary, Right 1 Ovary, Left 2 Ovaries, Bilateral 4 Uterine Supporting Structure 5 Fallopian Tube, Right 6 Fallopian Tube, Left 7 Fallopian Tubes, Bilateral 9 Uterus C Cervix F Cul-de-sac	0 Open 3 Percutaneous 4 Percutaneous endoscopic 7 Via natural or artificial opening 8 Via natural or artificial opening endoscopic	Z No device	X Diagnostic Z No qualifier
G Vagina K Hymen	0 Open 3 Percutaneous 4 Percutaneous endoscopic 7 Via natural or artificial opening 8 Via natural or artificial opening endoscopic X External	Z No device	X Diagnostic Z No qualifier
J Clitoris L Vestibular Gland M Vulva	0 Open X External	Z No device	X Diagnostic Z No qualifier

1ST - 0 Medical and Surgical
2ND - U Female Reproductive System ♀
3RD - C EXTIRPATION

DRAINAGE GROUP: Drainage, Extirpation, Fragmentation
Root Operations that take out solids/fluids/gases from a body part.

EXTIRPATION: Taking or cutting out solid matter from a body part.

Explanation: Abnormal byproduct or foreign body ...
Examples: Vaginal clot evacuation post delivery – CMS Ex: Thrombectomy

Body Part – 4TH	Approach – 5TH	Device – 6TH	Qualifier – 7TH
0 Ovary, Right 1 Ovary, Left 2 Ovaries, Bilateral 4 Uterine Supporting Structure	0 Open 3 Percutaneous 4 Percutaneous endoscopic 8 Via natural or artificial opening endoscopic	Z No device	Z No qualifier
5 Fallopian Tube, Right 6 Fallopian Tube, Left 7 Fallopian Tubes, Bilateral 9 Uterus B Endometrium C Cervix F Cul-de-sac	0 Open 3 Percutaneous 4 Percutaneous endoscopic 7 Via natural or artificial opening 8 Via natural or artificial opening endoscopic	Z No device	Z No qualifier
G Vagina K Hymen	0 Open 3 Percutaneous 4 Percutaneous endoscopic 7 Via natural or artificial opening 8 Via natural or artificial opening endoscopic X External	Z No device	Z No qualifier
J Clitoris L Vestibular Gland M Vulva	0 Open X External	Z No device	Z No qualifier

© 2018 Channel Publishing, Ltd.

1ST - 0 Medical and Surgical
2ND - U Female Reproductive System ♀
3RD - D EXTRACTION

EXCISION GROUP: Excision, Resection, Destruction, Extraction, (Detachment)
Root Operations that take out some or all of a body part.

EXTRACTION: Pulling or stripping out or off all or a portion of a body part by the use of force.

Explanation: Qualifier "X Diagnostic" indicates extraction procedures that are biopsies
Examples: Dilation and curettage – CMS Ex: Dilation and curettage

Body Part – 4TH	Approach – 5TH	Device – 6TH	Qualifier – 7TH
B Endometrium	7 Via natural or artificial opening 8 Via natural or artificial opening endoscopic	Z No device	X Diagnostic Z No qualifier
N Ova	0 Open 3 Percutaneous 4 Percutaneous endoscopic	Z No device	Z No qualifier

1ST - 0 Medical and Surgical
2ND - U Female Reproductive System ♀
3RD - F FRAGMENTATION

DRAINAGE GROUP: Drainage, Extirpation, Fragmentation
Root Operations that take out solids/fluids/gases from a body part.

FRAGMENTATION: Breaking solid matter in a body part into pieces.

Explanation: Pieces are not taken out during the procedure ...
Examples: Lithotripsy fallopian tube calcification – CMS Ex. Extracorporeal shockwave lithotripsy

Body Part – 4TH	Approach – 5TH	Device – 6TH	Qualifier – 7TH
5 Fallopian Tube, Right 6 Fallopian Tube, Left 7 Fallopian Tubes, Bilateral 9 Uterus	0 Open 3 Percutaneous 4 Percutaneous endoscopic 7 Via natural or artificial opening 8 Via natural or artificial opening endoscopic X External NC*	Z No device	Z No qualifier

NC* – Non-covered by Medicare. See current Medicare Code Editor for details.

© 2018 Channel Publishing, Ltd.

1ST - 0 Medical and Surgical
2ND - U Female Reproductive System ♀
3RD - H INSERTION

DEVICE GROUP: Change, Insertion, Removal, (Replacement), Revision, Supplement
Root Operations that always involve a device.

INSERTION: Putting in a nonbiological appliance that monitors, assists, performs, or prevents a physiological function but does not physically take the place of a body part.

Explanation: None
Examples: Insertion IUD – CMS Ex: Insertion of central venous catheter

Body Part – 4TH	Approach – 5TH	Device – 6TH	Qualifier – 7TH
3 Ovary	0 Open 3 Percutaneous 4 Percutaneous endoscopic	3 Infusion device Y Other device	Z No qualifier
3 Ovary	7 Via natural or artificial opening 8 Via natural or artificial opening endoscopic	Y Other device	Z No qualifier
8 Fallopian Tube D Uterus and Cervix H Vagina and Cul-de-sac	0 Open 3 Percutaneous 4 Percutaneous endoscopic 7 Via natural or artificial opening 8 Via natural or artificial opening endoscopic	3 Infusion device Y Other device	Z No qualifier
9 Uterus	0 Open 7 Via natural or artificial opening 8 Via natural or artificial opening endoscopic	H Contraceptive device	Z No qualifier
C Cervix	0 Open 3 Percutaneous 4 Percutaneous endoscopic	1 Radioactive element	Z No qualifier
C Cervix	7 Via natural or artificial opening 8 Via natural or artificial opening endoscopic	1 Radioactive element H Contraceptive device	Z No qualifier
F Cul-de-sac	7 Via natural or artificial opening 8 Via natural or artificial opening endoscopic	G Intraluminal device, pessary	Z No qualifier
G Vagina	0 Open 3 Percutaneous 4 Percutaneous endoscopic X External	1 Radioactive element	Z No qualifier
G Vagina	7 Via natural or artificial opening 8 Via natural or artificial opening endoscopic	1 Radioactive element G Intraluminal device, pessary	Z No qualifier

1ST - 0 Medical and Surgical
2ND - U Female Reproductive System ♀
3RD - J INSPECTION

EXAMINATION GROUP: Inspection, (Map)
Root Operations involving examination only.

INSPECTION: Visually and/or manually exploring a body part.

Explanation: Direct or instrumental visualization ...
Examples: Hysteroscopy – CMS Ex: Exploratory laparotomy

Body Part – 4TH	Approach – 5TH	Device – 6TH	Qualifier – 7TH
3 Ovary	0 Open 3 Percutaneous 4 Percutaneous endoscopic 8 Via natural or artificial opening endoscopic X External	Z No device	Z No qualifier
8 Fallopian Tube D Uterus and Cervix H Vagina and Cul-de-sac	0 Open 3 Percutaneous 4 Percutaneous endoscopic 7 Via natural or artificial opening 8 Via natural or artificial opening endoscopic X External	Z No device	Z No qualifier
M Vulva	0 Open X External	Z No device	Z No qualifier

© 2018 Channel Publishing, Ltd.

1ST - 0 Medical and Surgical
2ND - U Female Reproductive System ♀
3RD - L OCCLUSION

TUBULAR GROUP: Bypass, Dilation, Occlusion, Restriction
Root Operations that alter the diameter/route of a tubular body part.

OCCLUSION: Completely closing an orifice or the lumen of a tubular body part.

Explanation: The orifice can be a natural orifice or an artificially created orifice
Examples: Fallopian tube clipping – CMS Ex: Fallopian tube ligation

Body Part – 4TH	Approach – 5TH	Device – 6TH	Qualifier – 7TH
5 Fallopian Tube, Right 6 Fallopian Tube, Left 7 Fallopian Tubes, Bilateral NC*	0 Open 3 Percutaneous 4 Percutaneous endoscopic	C Extraluminal device D Intraluminal device Z No device	Z No qualifier
5 Fallopian Tube, Right 6 Fallopian Tube, Left 7 Fallopian Tubes, Bilateral NC*	7 Via natural or artificial opening 8 Via natural or artificial opening endoscopic	D Intraluminal device Z No device	Z No qualifier
F Cul-de-sac G Vagina	7 Via natural or artificial opening 8 Via natural or artificial opening endoscopic	D Intraluminal device Z No device	Z No qualifier

NC* – Some procedures are considered non-covered by Medicare. See current Medicare Code Editor for details.

1ST - 0 Medical and Surgical
2ND - U Female Reproductive System ♀
3RD - M REATTACHMENT

MOVE GROUP: Reattachment, Reposition, (Transfer), Transplantation
Root Operations that put in/put back or move some/all of a body part.

REATTACHMENT: Putting back in or on all or a portion of a separated body part to its normal location or other suitable location.

Explanation: Vascular circulation and nervous pathways may or may not be reestablished
Examples: Reattachment avulsed round ligament – CMS Ex: Reattachment of hand

Body Part – 4TH	Approach – 5TH	Device – 6TH	Qualifier – 7TH
0 Ovary, Right 1 Ovary, Left 2 Ovaries, Bilateral 4 Uterine Supporting Structure 5 Fallopian Tube, Right 6 Fallopian Tube, Left 7 Fallopian Tubes, Bilateral 9 Uterus C Cervix F Cul-de-sac G Vagina	0 Open 4 Percutaneous endoscopic	Z No device	Z No qualifier
J Clitoris M Vulva	X External	Z No device	Z No qualifier
K Hymen	0 Open 4 Percutaneous endoscopic X External	Z No device	Z No qualifier

FEMALE

0 U M

© 2018 Channel Publishing, Ltd.

1ST - 0 Medical and Surgical
2ND - U Female Reproductive System ♀
3RD - N RELEASE

DIVISION GROUP: Division, Release
Root Operations involving cutting or separation only.

RELEASE: Freeing a body part from an abnormal physical constraint by cutting or by the use of force.

Explanation: Some of the restraining tissue may be taken out but none of the body part is taken out
Examples: Adhesiolysis ovary and tube – CMS Ex: Carpal tunnel release

Body Part – 4TH	Approach – 5TH	Device – 6TH	Qualifier - 7TH
0 Ovary, Right 1 Ovary, Left 2 Ovaries, Bilateral 4 Uterine Supporting Structure	0 Open 3 Percutaneous 4 Percutaneous endoscopic 8 Via natural or artificial opening endoscopic	Z No device	Z No qualifier
5 Fallopian Tube, Right 6 Fallopian Tube, Left 7 Fallopian Tubes, Bilateral 9 Uterus C Cervix F Cul-de-sac	0 Open 3 Percutaneous 4 Percutaneous endoscopic 7 Via natural or artificial opening 8 Via natural or artificial opening endoscopic	Z No device	Z No qualifier
G Vagina K Hymen	0 Open 3 Percutaneous 4 Percutaneous endoscopic 7 Via natural or artificial opening 8 Via natural or artificial opening endoscopic X External	Z No device	Z No qualifier
J Clitoris L Vestibular Gland M Vulva	0 Open X External	Z No device	Z No qualifier

1ST - 0 Medical and Surgical
2ND - U Female Reproductive System ♀
3RD - P REMOVAL

DEVICE GROUP: Change, Insertion, Removal, (Replacement), Revision, Supplement
Root Operations that always involve a device.

REMOVAL: Taking out or off a device from a body part.

Explanation: Removal device without reinsertion ...
Examples: Removal IUD – CMS Ex: Cardiac pacemaker removal

Body Part – 4TH	Approach – 5TH	Device – 6TH	Qualifier – 7TH
3 Ovary	0 Open 3 Percutaneous 4 Percutaneous endoscopic	0 Drainage device 3 Infusion device Y Other device	Z No qualifier
3 Ovary	7 Via natural or artificial opening 8 Via natural or artificial opening endoscopic	Y Other device	Z No qualifier
3 Ovary	X External	0 Drainage device 3 Infusion device	Z No qualifier
8 Fallopian Tube	0 Open 3 Percutaneous 4 Percutaneous endoscopic 7 Via natural or artificial opening 8 Via natural or artificial opening endoscopic	0 Drainage device 3 Infusion device 7 Autologous tissue substitute C Extraluminal device D Intraluminal device J Synthetic substitute K Nonautologous tissue substitute Y Other device	Z No qualifier
8 Fallopian Tube	X External	0 Drainage device 3 Infusion device D Intraluminal device	Z No qualifier

continued ⇨

© 2018 Channel Publishing, Ltd.

0 U P REMOVAL – *continued*

Body Part – 4TH	Approach – 5TH	Device – 6TH	Qualifier – 7TH
D Uterus and Cervix	0 Open 3 Percutaneous 4 Percutaneous endoscopic 7 Via natural or artificial opening 8 Via natural or artificial opening endoscopic	0 Drainage device 1 Radioactive element 3 Infusion device 7 Autologous tissue substitute C Extraluminal device D Intraluminal device H Contraceptive device J Synthetic substitute K Nonautologous tissue substitute Y Other device	Z No qualifier
D Uterus and Cervix	X External	0 Drainage device 3 Infusion device D Intraluminal device H Contraceptive device	Z No qualifier
H Vagina and Cul-de-sac	0 Open 3 Percutaneous 4 Percutaneous endoscopic 7 Via natural or artificial opening 8 Via natural or artificial opening endoscopic	0 Drainage device 1 Radioactive element 3 Infusion device 7 Autologous tissue substitute D Intraluminal device J Synthetic substitute K Nonautologous tissue substitute Y Other device	Z No qualifier
H Vagina and Cul-de-sac	X External	0 Drainage device 1 Radioactive element 3 Infusion device D Intraluminal device	Z No qualifier
M Vulva	0 Open	0 Drainage device 7 Autologous tissue substitute J Synthetic substitute K Nonautologous tissue substitute	Z No qualifier
M Vulva	X External	0 Drainage device	Z No qualifier

1ST - 0 Medical and Surgical
2ND - U Female Reproductive System ♀
3RD - Q REPAIR

OTHER REPAIRS GROUP: (Control), Repair
Root Operations that define other repairs.

REPAIR: Restoring, to the extent possible, a body part to its normal anatomic structure and function.

Explanation: Used only when the method to accomplish the repair is not one of the other root operations
Examples: Repair vulvar laceration – CMS Ex: Suture of laceration

Body Part – 4TH	Approach – 5TH	Device – 6TH	Qualifier – 7TH
0 Ovary, Right 1 Ovary, Left 2 Ovaries, Bilateral 4 Uterine Supporting Structure	0 Open 3 Percutaneous 4 Percutaneous endoscopic 8 Via natural or artificial opening endoscopic	Z No device	Z No qualifier
5 Fallopian Tube, Right 6 Fallopian Tube, Left 7 Fallopian Tubes, Bilateral 9 Uterus C Cervix F Cul-de-sac	0 Open 3 Percutaneous 4 Percutaneous endoscopic 7 Via natural or artificial opening 8 Via natural or artificial opening endoscopic	Z No device	Z No qualifier
G Vagina K Hymen	0 Open 3 Percutaneous 4 Percutaneous endoscopic 7 Via natural or artificial opening 8 Via natural or artificial opening endoscopic X External	Z No device	Z No qualifier
J Clitoris L Vestibular Gland M Vulva	0 Open X External	Z No device	Z No qualifier

FEMALE 0UQ

© 2018 Channel Publishing, Ltd.

1ST - 0 Medical and Surgical
2ND - U Female Reproductive System ♀
3RD - S REPOSITION

MOVE GROUP: Reattachment, Reposition, (Transfer), Transplantation
Root Operations that put in/put back or move some/all of a body part.

REPOSITION: Moving to its normal location, or other suitable location, all or a portion of a body part.

Explanation: The body part may or may not be cut out or off to be moved to the new location ...
Examples: Relocation fallopian tube – CMS Ex: Fracture reduction

Body Part – 4TH	Approach – 5TH	Device – 6TH	Qualifier – 7TH
0 Ovary, Right 1 Ovary, Left 2 Ovaries, Bilateral 4 Uterine Supporting Structure 5 Fallopian Tube, Right 6 Fallopian Tube, Left 7 Fallopian Tubes, Bilateral C Cervix F Cul-de-sac	0 Open 4 Percutaneous endoscopic 8 Via natural or artificial opening endoscopic	Z No device	Z No qualifier
9 Uterus G Vagina	0 Open 4 Percutaneous endoscopic 7 Via natural or artificial opening 8 Via natural or artificial opening endoscopic X External	Z No device	Z No qualifier

1ST - 0 Medical and Surgical
2ND - U Female Reproductive System ♀
3RD - T RESECTION

EXCISION GROUP: Excision, Resection, Destruction, Extraction, (Detachment)
Root Operations that take out some or all of a body part.

RESECTION: Cutting out or off, without replacement, all of a body part.

Explanation: None
Examples: Bilateral oophorectomy – CMS Ex: Total lobectomy of lung

Body Part – 4TH	Approach – 5TH	Device – 6TH	Qualifier – 7TH
0 Ovary, Right 1 Ovary, Left 2 Ovaries, Bilateral 5 Fallopian Tube, Right 6 Fallopian Tube, Left 7 Fallopian Tubes, Bilateral	0 Open 4 Percutaneous endoscopic 7 Via natural or artificial opening 8 Via natural or artificial opening endoscopic F Via natural or artificial opening with percutaneous endoscopic assistance	Z No device	Z No qualifier
4 Uterine Supporting Structure C Cervix F Cul-de-sac G Vagina	0 Open 4 Percutaneous endoscopic 7 Via natural or artificial opening 8 Via natural or artificial opening endoscopic	Z No device	Z No qualifier
9 Uterus	0 Open 4 Percutaneous endoscopic 7 Via natural or artificial opening 8 Via natural or artificial opening endoscopic F Via natural or artificial opening with percutaneous endoscopic assistance	Z No device	L Supracervical Z No qualifier
J Clitoris L Vestibular Gland M Vulva	0 Open X External	Z No device	Z No qualifier
K Hymen	0 Open 4 Percutaneous endoscopic 7 Via natural or artificial opening 8 Via natural or artificial opening endoscopic X External	Z No device	Z No qualifier

© 2018 Channel Publishing, Ltd.

1ST - 0 Medical and Surgical
2ND - U Female Reproductive System ♀
3RD - U SUPPLEMENT

DEVICE GROUP: Change, Insertion, Removal, (Replacement), Revision, Supplement
Root Operations that always involve a device.

SUPPLEMENT: Putting in or on biological or synthetic material that physically reinforces and/or augments the function of a portion of a body part.

Explanation: Biological material is non-living, or is living and from the same individual ...
Examples: Colporrhaphy with mesh – CMS Ex: Herniorrhaphy using mesh

Body Part – 4TH	Approach – 5TH	Device – 6TH	Qualifier – 7TH
4 Uterine Supporting Structure	0 Open 4 Percutaneous endoscopic	7 Autologous tissue substitute J Synthetic substitute K Nonautologous tissue substitute	Z No qualifier
5 Fallopian Tube, Right 6 Fallopian Tube, Left 7 Fallopian Tubes, Bilateral F Cul-de-sac	0 Open 4 Percutaneous endoscopic 7 Via natural or artificial opening 8 Via natural or artificial opening endoscopic	7 Autologous tissue substitute J Synthetic substitute K Nonautologous tissue substitute	Z No qualifier
G Vagina K Hymen	0 Open 4 Percutaneous endoscopic 7 Via natural or artificial opening 8 Via natural or artificial opening endoscopic X External	7 Autologous tissue substitute J Synthetic substitute K Nonautologous tissue substitute	Z No qualifier
J Clitoris M Vulva	0 Open X External	7 Autologous tissue substitute J Synthetic substitute K Nonautologous tissue substitute	Z No qualifier

1ST - 0 Medical and Surgical
2ND - U Female Reproductive System ♀
3RD - V RESTRICTION

TUBULAR GROUP: Bypass, Dilation, Occlusion, Restriction
Root Operations that alter the diameter/route of a tubular body part.

RESTRICTION: Partially closing an orifice or the lumen of a tubular body part.

Explanation: The orifice can be a natural orifice or an artificially created orifice.
Examples: Cervical cerclage – CMS Ex: Cervical cerclage

Body Part – 4TH	Approach – 5TH	Device – 6TH	Qualifier – 7TH
C Cervix	0 Open 3 Percutaneous 4 Percutaneous endoscopic	C Extraluminal device D Intraluminal device Z No device	Z No qualifier
C Cervix	7 Via natural or artificial opening 8 Via natural or artificial opening endoscopic	D Intraluminal device Z No device	Z No qualifier

1ST - 0 Medical and Surgical
2ND - U Female Reproductive System ♀
3RD - W REVISION

DEVICE GROUP: Change, Insertion, Removal, (Replacement), Revision, Supplement
Root Operations that always involve a device.

REVISION: Correcting, to the extent possible, a portion of a malfunctioning device or the position of a displaced device.

Explanation: Correcting by taking out or putting in components of a device such as a screw or pin ...
Examples: Reposition intrauterine device – CMS Ex: Recementing of hip prosthesis

Body Part – 4TH	Approach – 5TH	Device – 6TH	Qualifier – 7TH
3 Ovary	0 Open 3 Percutaneous 4 Percutaneous endoscopic	0 Drainage device 3 Infusion device Y Other device	Z No qualifier
3 Ovary	7 Via natural or artificial opening 8 Via natural or artificial opening endoscopic	Y Other device	Z No qualifier
3 Ovary	X External	0 Drainage device 3 Infusion device	Z No qualifier
8 Fallopian Tube	0 Open 3 Percutaneous 4 Percutaneous endoscopic 7 Via natural or artificial opening 8 Via natural or artificial opening endoscopic	0 Drainage device 3 Infusion device 7 Autologous tissue substitute C Extraluminal device D Intraluminal device J Synthetic substitute K Nonautologous tissue substitute Y Other device	Z No qualifier

continued ⇨

FEMALE

0 U W

© 2018 Channel Publishing, Ltd.

0 U W REVISION – *continued*

Body Part – 4TH	Approach – 5TH	Device – 6TH	Qualifier – 7TH
8 Fallopian Tube	X External	0 Drainage device 3 Infusion device 7 Autologous tissue substitute C Extraluminal device D Intraluminal device J Synthetic substitute K Nonautologous tissue substitute	Z No qualifier
D Uterus and Cervix	0 Open 3 Percutaneous 4 Percutaneous endoscopic 7 Via natural or artificial opening 8 Via natural or artificial opening endoscopic	0 Drainage device 1 Radioactive element 3 Infusion device 7 Autologous tissue substitute C Extraluminal device D Intraluminal device H Contraceptive device J Synthetic substitute K Nonautologous tissue substitute Y Other device	Z No qualifier
D Uterus and Cervix	X External	0 Drainage device 3 Infusion device 7 Autologous tissue substitute C Extraluminal device D Intraluminal device H Contraceptive device J Synthetic substitute K Nonautologous tissue substitute	Z No qualifier
H Vagina and Cul-de-sac	0 Open 3 Percutaneous 4 Percutaneous endoscopic 7 Via natural or artificial opening 8 Via natural or artificial opening endoscopic	0 Drainage device 1 Radioactive element 3 Infusion device 7 Autologous tissue substitute D Intraluminal device J Synthetic substitute K Nonautologous tissue substitute Y Other device	Z No qualifier
H Vagina and Cul-de-sac	X External	0 Drainage device 3 Infusion device 7 Autologous tissue substitute D Intraluminal device J Synthetic substitute K Nonautologous tissue substitute	Z No qualifier
M Vulva	0 Open X External	0 Drainage device 7 Autologous tissue substitute J Synthetic substitute K Nonautologous tissue substitute	Z No qualifier

1ST - 0 Medical and Surgical
2ND - U Female Reproductive System ♀
3RD - Y TRANSPLANTATION

MOVE GROUP: Reattachment, Reposition, (Transfer), Transplantation
Root Operations that put in/put back or move some/all of a body part.

TRANSPLANTATION: Putting in or on all or a portion of a living body part taken from another individual or animal to physically take the place and/or function of all or a portion of a similar body part.

Explanation: The native body part may or may not be taken out ...
Examples: Ovary transplant – CMS Ex: Kidney transplant

Body Part – 4TH	Approach – 5TH	Device – 6TH	Qualifier – 7TH
0 Ovary, Right 1 Ovary, Left 9 Uterus	0 Open	Z No device	0 Allogeneic 1 Syngeneic 2 Zooplastic

© 2018 Channel Publishing, Ltd.

Educational Annotations | V – Male Reproductive System

Body System Specific Educational Annotations for the Male Reproductive System include:

- Anatomy and Physiology Review
- Definitions of Common Procedures
- Anatomical Illustrations
- AHA Coding Clinic® Reference Notations
- Body Part Key Listings
- Device Key Listings
- Device Aggregation Table Listings
- Coding Notes

Anatomy and Physiology Review of Male Reproductive System

BODY PART VALUES – V - MALE REPRODUCTIVE SYSTEM

Epididymis – ANATOMY – The epididymis is a tightly coiled, threadlike tube that is about 20 feet (6 m) long. It is connected to ducts within the testis and emerges from the top of the testis, descends along its posterior surface, and then courses upward to become the vas deferens. PHYSIOLOGY – The epididymis functions to store and mature sperm cells, and to transport the sperm from the testicular ducts to the vas deferens.

Penis – ANATOMY – The penis is the cylindrical male sexual organ which contains the urethra and is located at the base of the male perineum. The body (shaft) is composed of 3 columns of erectile tissue, including a pair of dorsally located corpora cavernosa and a single corpus spongiosum below. The corpus spongiosum, through which the urethra extends, is enlarged at its distal end to form a sensitive, cone-shaped glans penis. A loose fold of skin, called the prepuce (foreskin) covers the glans penis, unless removed by circumcision. PHYSIOLOGY – The penis functions as the specialized sexual organ in the male that when erect is inserted into the female vagina for sexual intercourse. It also functions to convey urine and seminal fluid through the urethra to the outside at the urethral opening (meatus). Erection is obtained by sexual excitement, stimulating parasympathetic nerve impulses causing blood engorgement of the corpora cavernosa and corpus spongiosum.

Prepuce – The loose fold of skin (foreskin) that covers the glans penis, unless removed by circumcision.

Prostate – ANATOMY – The walnut-shaped male reproductive organ that surrounds the urethra just below the bladder. PHYSIOLOGY – The prostate secretes a slightly alkaline fluid that constitutes approximately one-third of the volume of the semen. The alkalinity of semen helps neutralize the acidity of the vaginal tract, prolonging the lifespan of sperm.

Scrotum – ANATOMY – The scrotum is a pouch of skin, subcutaneous, and muscular tissue that hangs from the lower abdominal region behind the penis. PHYSIOLOGY – The scrotum protects the testis and spermatic cord by contracting and relaxing the dartos muscle.

Seminal Vesicle – ANATOMY – A pair of tubular male reproductive glands that are located above the prostate and below the bladder. They pass into the prostatic tissue and their excretory ducts open into the vas deferens and form the ejaculatory ducts. PHYSIOLOGY – The seminal vesicles secrete approximately two-thirds of the ejaculated semen volume. The nutrient-rich seminal fluid provides energy for the sperm cells.

Spermatic Cord – ANATOMY – The spermatic cord is a canal of peritoneal tissue about 18 inches (45 cm) long beginning at the testis and ending in the ejaculatory duct, and is externally contained along with the testis in the scrotum. PHYSIOLOGY – The spermatic cord contains and protects the vas deferens, arteries, nerves, and lymphatic vessels.

Testis – ANATOMY – The testes are the male reproductive organs that are ovoid structures in the scrotum, suspended by a spermatic cord, and approximately 2 inches (5 cm) in length and 1.2 inches (3 cm) in diameter. Each testis is enclosed by a tough, white fibrous capsule called the tunica albuginea. PHYSIOLOGY – The testes function to produce sperm cells for human reproduction and secrete male hormones, primarily testosterone.

Tunica Vaginalis – The serous membrane covering of the testes that is comprised of two layers, visceral and parietal.

Vas Deferens – ANATOMY – The vas deferens (ductus deferens) is a muscular tube that begins at the epididymis and ends at the union of the seminal vesicle and forms the ejaculatory duct within the prostatic tissue. PHYSIOLOGY – The vas deferens transports the sperm using peristalsis from the testis/epididymis to the ejaculatory duct.

Definitions of Common Procedures of Male Reproductive System

Orchiectomy – The surgical removal of one or both of the testicles.

Orchiopexy – The surgical procedure to move an undescended testicle into the scrotum and secure it in place.

Radical retropubic prostatectomy – The surgical removal of the entire prostate gland and some surrounding tissues that is performed through an open approach between the belly button and pubic bone.

TUNA (transurethral needle ablation of prostate) – The transurethral endoscopic destruction of prostate tissue using radiofrequency (RF) needles that delivers heat to reduce benign prostatic hyperplasia.

TURP (transurethral resection of prostate) – The surgical removal of part or all (total) of the prostate gland through an endoscopic approach.

Vasoepididymostomy – The microsurgical anastomosis of the epididymis to the vas deferens to reverse a vasectomy or to overcome an epididymal obstruction.

Vasovasostomy – The surgical re-anastomosis of the severed vas deferens to reverse a vasectomy.

MALE 0 V

© 2018 Channel Publishing, Ltd.

Educational Annotations | V – Male Reproductive System

Anatomical Illustrations of Male Reproductive System

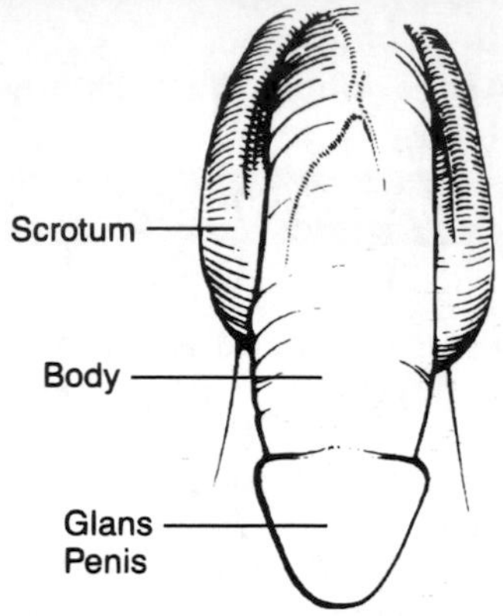

PENIS — FRONTAL VIEW

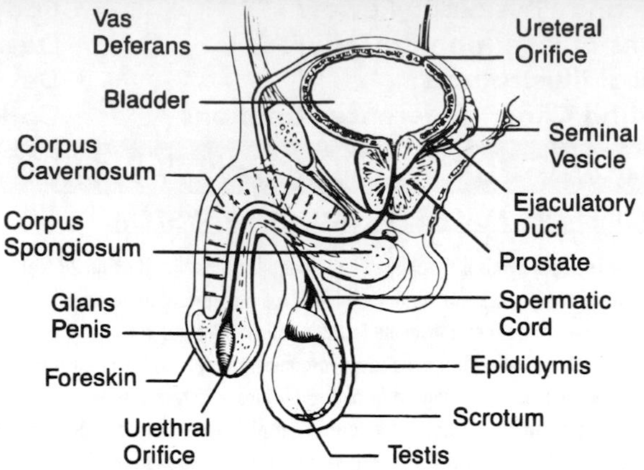

MALE GENITAL ORGANS — SAGITTAL VIEW

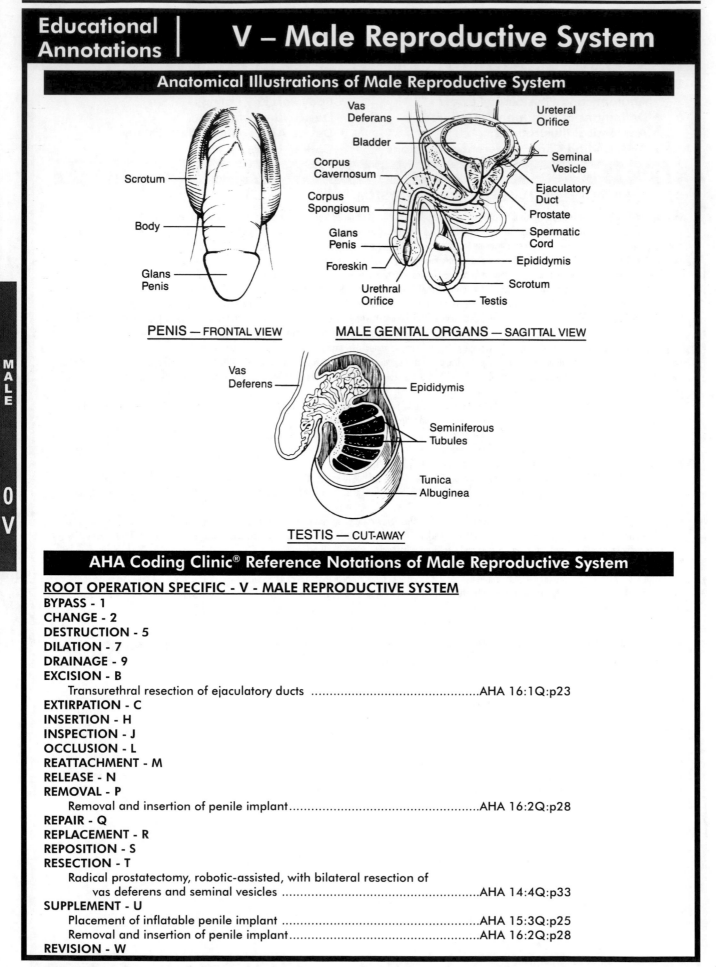

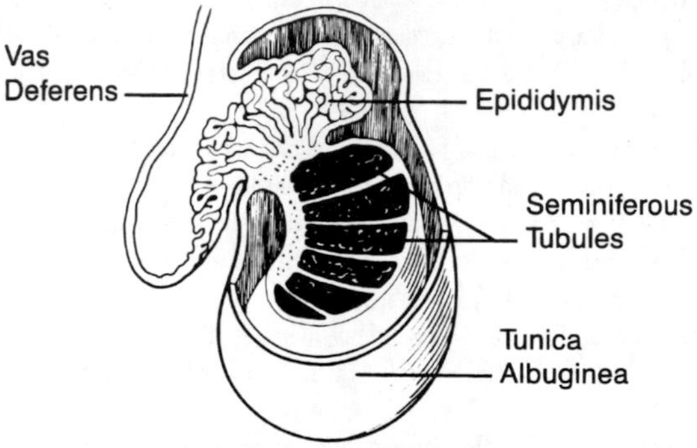

TESTIS — CUT-AWAY

AHA Coding Clinic® Reference Notations of Male Reproductive System

ROOT OPERATION SPECIFIC - V - MALE REPRODUCTIVE SYSTEM

BYPASS - 1
CHANGE - 2
DESTRUCTION - 5
DILATION - 7
DRAINAGE - 9
EXCISION - B
Transurethral resection of ejaculatory ducts ....AHA 16:1Q:p23
EXTIRPATION - C
INSERTION - H
INSPECTION - J
OCCLUSION - L
REATTACHMENT - M
RELEASE - N
REMOVAL - P
Removal and insertion of penile implant..AHA 16:2Q:p28
REPAIR - Q
REPLACEMENT - R
REPOSITION - S
RESECTION - T
Radical prostatectomy, robotic-assisted, with bilateral resection of vas deferens and seminal vesicles ....AHA 14:4Q:p33
SUPPLEMENT - U
Placement of inflatable penile implant ....AHA 15:3Q:p25
Removal and insertion of penile implant..AHA 16:2Q:p28
REVISION - W

MALE 0 V

© 2018 Channel Publishing, Ltd.

Educational Annotations | V – Male Reproductive System

Body Part Key Listings of Male Reproductive System

See also Body Part Key in Appendix C

Corpus cavernosum ....use Penis
Corpus spongiosum ....use Penis
Ductus deferens ....use Vas Deferens, Bilateral/Left/Right
Ejaculatory duct ....use Vas Deferens, Bilateral/Left/Right
Foreskin ....use Prepuce
Glans penis ....use Prepuce

Device Key Listings of Male Reproductive System

See also Device Key in Appendix D

Autograft ....use Autologous Tissue Substitute
Brachytherapy seeds ....use Radioactive Element
Cook Biodesign® Fistula Plug(s) ....use Nonautologous Tissue Substitute
Tissue bank graft ....use Nonautologous Tissue Substitute

Device Aggregation Table Listings of Male Reproductive System

See also Device Aggregation Table in Appendix E

Specific Device	For Operation	In Body System	General Device
None Listed in Device Aggregation Table for this Body System			

Coding Notes of Male Reproductive System

© 2018 Channel Publishing, Ltd.

1ST - 0 Medical and Surgical
2ND - V Male Reproductive System ♂
3RD - 1 BYPASS

TUBULAR GROUP: Bypass, Dilation, Occlusion, (Restriction)
Root Operations that alter the diameter/route of a tubular body part.

BYPASS: Altering the route of passage of the contents of a tubular body part.

Explanation: Rerouting contents to a downstream part ... with or without the use of a device ...
Examples: Vasoepididymostomy – CMS Ex: Coronary artery bypass

Body Part – 4TH	Approach – 5TH	Device – 6TH	Qualifier – 7TH
N Vas Deferens, Right P Vas Deferens, Left Q Vas Deferens, Bilateral	0 Open 4 Percutaneous endoscopic	7 Autologous tissue substitute J Synthetic substitute K Nonautologous tissue substitute Z No device	J Epididymis, Right K Epididymis, Left N Vas Deferens, Right P Vas Deferens, Left

1ST - 0 Medical and Surgical
2ND - V Male Reproductive System ♂
3RD - 2 CHANGE

DEVICE GROUP: Change, Insertion, Removal, Replacement, Revision, Supplement
Root Operations that always involve a device.

CHANGE: Taking out or off a device from a body part and putting back an identical or similar device in or on the same body part without cutting or puncturing the skin or a mucous membrane.

Explanation: All CHANGE procedures are coded using the approach External
Examples: Exchange drain tube – CMS Ex: Urinary catheter change

Body Part – 4TH	Approach – 5TH	Device – 6TH	Qualifier – 7TH
4 Prostate and Seminal Vesicles 8 Scrotum and Tunica Vaginalis D Testis M Epididymis and Spermatic Cord R Vas Deferens S Penis	X External	0 Drainage device Y Other device	Z No qualifier

1ST - 0 Medical and Surgical
2ND - V Male Reproductive System ♂
3RD - 5 DESTRUCTION

EXCISION GROUP: Excision, Resection, Destruction, (Extraction), (Detachment)
Root Operations that take out some or all of a body part.

DESTRUCTION: Physical eradication of all or a portion of a body part by the direct use of energy, force, or a destructive agent.

Explanation: None of the body part is physically taken out
Examples: Needle ablation (TUNA) prostate – CMS Ex: Fulguration of rectal polyp

Body Part – 4TH	Approach – 5TH	Device – 6TH	Qualifier – 7TH
0 Prostate	0 Open 3 Percutaneous 4 Percutaneous endoscopic 7 Via natural or artificial opening 8 Via natural or artificial opening endoscopic	Z No device	Z No qualifier
1 Seminal Vesicle, Right 2 Seminal Vesicle, Left 3 Seminal Vesicles, Bilateral 6 Tunica Vaginalis, Right 7 Tunica Vaginalis, Left 9 Testis, Right B Testis, Left C Testes, Bilateral	0 Open 3 Percutaneous 4 Percutaneous endoscopic	Z No device	Z No qualifier
5 Scrotum S Penis T Prepuce	0 Open 3 Percutaneous 4 Percutaneous endoscopic X External	Z No device	Z No qualifier
F Spermatic Cord, Right G Spermatic Cord, Left H Spermatic Cords, Bilateral J Epididymis, Right K Epididymis, Left L Epididymis, Bilateral N Vas Deferens, Right NC* P Vas Deferens, Left NC* Q Vas Deferens, Bilateral NC*	0 Open 3 Percutaneous 4 Percutaneous endoscopic 8 Via natural or artificial opening endoscopic	Z No device	Z No qualifier

NC* – Some procedures are considered non-covered by Medicare. See current Medicare Code Editor for details.

© 2018 Channel Publishing, Ltd.

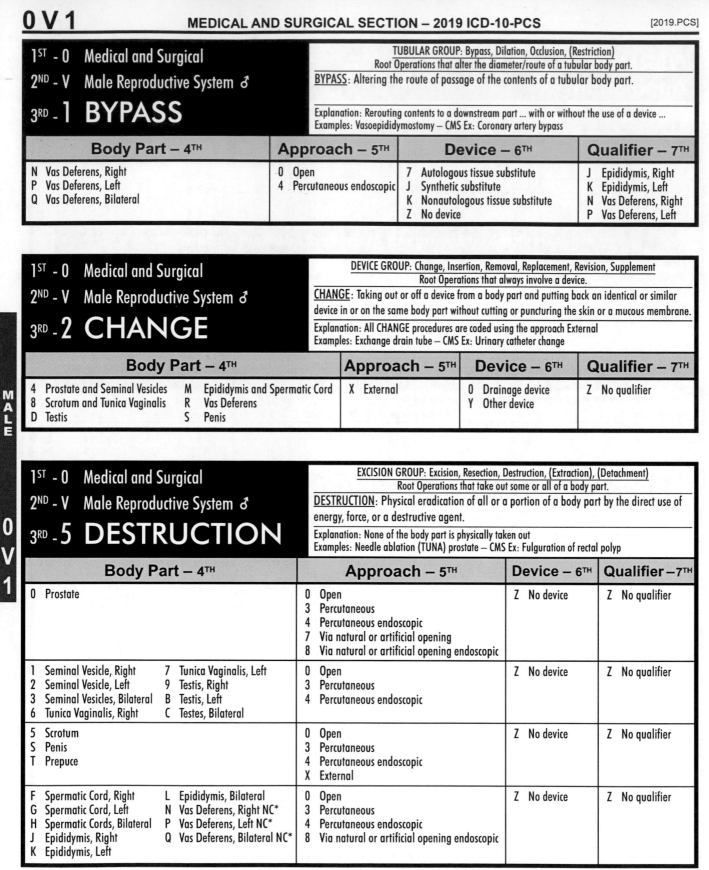

1ST - 0 Medical and Surgical
2ND - V Male Reproductive System ♂
3RD - 7 DILATION

TUBULAR GROUP: Bypass, Dilation, Occlusion, (Restriction)
Root Operations that alter the diameter/route of a tubular body part.

DILATION: Expanding an orifice or the lumen of a tubular body part.

Explanation: Accomplished by stretching or cutting ... tubular body part or orifice ...
Examples: Dilation vas deferens – CMS Ex: Percutaneous transluminal angioplasty

Body Part – 4TH	Approach – 5TH	Device – 6TH	Qualifier – 7TH
N Vas Deferens, Right P Vas Deferens, Left Q Vas Deferens, Bilateral	0 Open 3 Percutaneous 4 Percutaneous endoscopic	D Intraluminal device Z No device	Z No qualifier

1ST - 0 Medical and Surgical
2ND - V Male Reproductive System ♂
3RD - 9 DRAINAGE

DRAINAGE GROUP: Drainage, Extirpation, (Fragmentation)
Root Operations that take out solids/fluids/gases from a body part.

DRAINAGE: Taking or letting out fluids and/or gases from a body part.

Explanation: Qualifier "X Diagnostic" indicates drainage procedures that are biopsies
Examples: Drainage epididymal cyst – CMS Ex: Thoracentesis

Body Part – 4TH	Approach – 5TH	Device – 6TH	Qualifier – 7TH
0 Prostate	0 Open 3 Percutaneous 4 Percutaneous endoscopic 7 Via natural or artificial opening 8 Via natural or artificial opening endoscopic	0 Drainage device	Z No qualifier
0 Prostate	0 Open 3 Percutaneous 4 Percutaneous endoscopic 7 Via natural or artificial opening 8 Via natural or artificial opening endoscopic	Z No device	X Diagnostic Z No qualifier
1 Seminal Vesicle, Right 2 Seminal Vesicle, Left 3 Seminal Vesicles, Bilateral 6 Tunica Vaginalis, Right 7 Tunica Vaginalis, Left 9 Testis, Right B Testis, Left C Testes, Bilateral F Spermatic Cord, Right G Spermatic Cord, Left H Spermatic Cords, Bilateral J Epididymis, Right K Epididymis, Left L Epididymis, Bilateral N Vas Deferens, Right P Vas Deferens, Left Q Vas Deferens, Bilateral	0 Open 3 Percutaneous 4 Percutaneous endoscopic	0 Drainage device	Z No qualifier
1 Seminal Vesicle, Right 2 Seminal Vesicle, Left 3 Seminal Vesicles, Bilateral 6 Tunica Vaginalis, Right 7 Tunica Vaginalis, Left 9 Testis, Right B Testis, Left C Testes, Bilateral F Spermatic Cord, Right G Spermatic Cord, Left H Spermatic Cords, Bilateral J Epididymis, Right K Epididymis, Left L Epididymis, Bilateral N Vas Deferens, Right P Vas Deferens, Left Q Vas Deferens, Bilateral	0 Open 3 Percutaneous 4 Percutaneous endoscopic	Z No device	X Diagnostic Z No qualifier
5 Scrotum S Penis T Prepuce	0 Open 3 Percutaneous 4 Percutaneous endoscopic X External	0 Drainage device	Z No qualifier
5 Scrotum S Penis T Prepuce	0 Open 3 Percutaneous 4 Percutaneous endoscopic X External	Z No device	X Diagnostic Z No qualifier

© 2018 Channel Publishing, Ltd.

1ST - 0 Medical and Surgical 2ND - V Male Reproductive System ♂ 3RD - B EXCISION	EXCISION GROUP: Excision, Resection, Destruction, (Extraction), (Detachment) Root Operations that take out some or all of a body part. EXCISION: Cutting out or off, without replacement, a portion of a body part. Explanation: Qualifier "X Diagnostic" indicates excision procedures that are biopsies Examples: TURP (non-total) – CMS Ex: Liver biopsy		
Body Part – 4TH	**Approach – 5TH**	**Device – 6TH**	**Qualifier - 7TH**
0 Prostate	0 Open 3 Percutaneous 4 Percutaneous endoscopic 7 Via natural or artificial opening 8 Via natural or artificial opening endoscopic	Z No device	X Diagnostic Z No qualifier
1 Seminal Vesicle, Right 2 Seminal Vesicle, Left 3 Seminal Vesicles, Bilateral 6 Tunica Vaginalis, Right 7 Tunica Vaginalis, Left 9 Testis, Right B Testis, Left C Testes, Bilateral	0 Open 3 Percutaneous 4 Percutaneous endoscopic	Z No device	X Diagnostic Z No qualifier
5 Scrotum S Penis T Prepuce	0 Open 3 Percutaneous 4 Percutaneous endoscopic X External	Z No device	X Diagnostic Z No qualifier
F Spermatic Cord, Right G Spermatic Cord, Left H Spermatic Cords, Bilateral J Epididymis, Right K Epididymis, Left L Epididymis, Bilateral N Vas Deferens, Right NC* P Vas Deferens, Left NC* Q Vas Deferens, Bilateral NC*	0 Open 3 Percutaneous 4 Percutaneous endoscopic 8 Via natural or artificial opening endoscopic	Z No device	X Diagnostic Z No qualifier

NC* – Some procedures are considered non-covered by Medicare. See current Medicare Code Editor for details.

1ST - 0 Medical and Surgical 2ND - V Male Reproductive System ♂ 3RD - C EXTIRPATION	DRAINAGE GROUP: Drainage, Extirpation, (Fragmentation) Root Operations that take out solids/fluids/gases from a body part. EXTIRPATION: Taking or cutting out solid matter from a body part. Explanation: Abnormal byproduct or foreign body ... Examples: Removal foreign body – CMS Ex: Thrombectomy		
Body Part – 4TH	**Approach – 5TH**	**Device – 6TH**	**Qualifier - 7TH**
0 Prostate	0 Open 3 Percutaneous 4 Percutaneous endoscopic 7 Via natural or artificial opening 8 Via natural or artificial opening endoscopic	Z No device	Z No qualifier
1 Seminal Vesicle, Right 2 Seminal Vesicle, Left 3 Seminal Vesicles, Bilateral 6 Tunica Vaginalis, Right 7 Tunica Vaginalis, Left 9 Testis, Right B Testis, Left C Testes, Bilateral F Spermatic Cord, Right G Spermatic Cord, Left H Spermatic Cords, Bilateral J Epididymis, Right K Epididymis, Left L Epididymis, Bilateral N Vas Deferens, Right P Vas Deferens, Left Q Vas Deferens, Bilateral	0 Open 3 Percutaneous 4 Percutaneous endoscopic	Z No device	Z No qualifier
5 Scrotum S Penis T Prepuce	0 Open 3 Percutaneous 4 Percutaneous endoscopic X External	Z No device	Z No qualifier

© 2018 Channel Publishing, Ltd.

1ST - 0 Medical and Surgical
2ND - V Male Reproductive System ♂
3RD - H INSERTION

DEVICE GROUP: Change, Insertion, Removal, Replacement, Revision, Supplement
Root Operations that always involve a device.

INSERTION: Putting in a nonbiological appliance that monitors, assists, performs, or prevents a physiological function but does not physically take the place of a body part.

Explanation: None
Examples: Insertion radioactive element – CMS Ex: Insertion of central venous catheter

Body Part – 4TH	Approach – 5TH	Device – 6TH	Qualifier – 7TH
0 Prostate	0 Open 3 Percutaneous 4 Percutaneous endoscopic 7 Via natural or artificial opening 8 Via natural or artificial opening endoscopic	1 Radioactive element	Z No qualifier
4 Prostate and Seminal Vesicles 8 Scrotum and Tunica Vaginalis D Testis M Epididymis and Spermatic Cord R Vas Deferens	0 Open 3 Percutaneous 4 Percutaneous endoscopic 7 Via natural or artificial opening 8 Via natural or artificial opening endoscopic	3 Infusion device Y Other device	Z No qualifier
S Penis	0 Open 3 Percutaneous 4 Percutaneous endoscopic	3 Infusion device Y Other device	Z No qualifier
S Penis	7 Via natural or artificial opening 8 Via natural or artificial opening endoscopic	Y Other device	Z No qualifier
S Penis	X External	3 Infusion device	Z No qualifier

1ST - 0 Medical and Surgical
2ND - V Male Reproductive System ♂
3RD - J INSPECTION

EXAMINATION GROUP: Inspection, (Map)
Root Operations involving examination only.

INSPECTION: Visually and/or manually exploring a body part.

Explanation: Direct or instrumental visualization ...
Examples: Prostate exam – CMS Ex: Exploratory laparotomy

Body Part – 4TH	Approach – 5TH	Device – 6TH	Qualifier - 7TH
4 Prostate and Seminal Vesicles 8 Scrotum and Tunica Vaginalis D Testis M Epididymis and Spermatic Cord R Vas Deferens S Penis	0 Open 3 Percutaneous 4 Percutaneous endoscopic X External	Z No device	Z No qualifier

1ST - 0 Medical and Surgical
2ND - V Male Reproductive System ♂
3RD - L OCCLUSION

TUBULAR GROUP: Bypass, Dilation, Occlusion, (Restriction)
Root Operations that alter the diameter/route of a tubular body part.

OCCLUSION: Completely closing an orifice or the lumen of a tubular body part.

Explanation: The orifice can be a natural orifice or an artificially created orifice
Examples: Vasectomy – CMS Ex: Fallopian tube ligation

Body Part – 4TH	Approach – 5TH	Device – 6TH	Qualifier – 7TH
F Spermatic Cord, Right NC* G Spermatic Cord, Left NC* H Spermatic Cords, Bilateral NC* N Vas Deferens, Right NC* P Vas Deferens, Left NC* Q Vas Deferens, Bilateral NC*	0 Open 3 Percutaneous 4 Percutaneous endoscopic 8 Via natural or artificial opening endoscopic	C Extraluminal device D Intraluminal device Z No device	Z No qualifier

NC* – Some procedures are considered non-covered by Medicare. See current Medicare Code Editor for details.

© 2018 Channel Publishing, Ltd.

1ST - 0 Medical and Surgical
2ND - V Male Reproductive System ♂
3RD - M REATTACHMENT

MOVE GROUP: Reattachment, Reposition, Transfer, (Transplantation)
Root Operations that put in/put back or move some/all of a body part.

REATTACHMENT: Putting back in or on all or a portion of a separated body part to its normal location or other suitable location.

Explanation: Vascular circulation and nervous pathways may or may not be reestablished
Examples: Reattachment penis – CMS Ex: Reattachment of hand

Body Part – 4TH	Approach – 5TH	Device – 6TH	Qualifier – 7TH
5 Scrotum S Penis	X External	Z No device	Z No qualifier
6 Tunica Vaginalis, Right 7 Tunica Vaginalis, Left 9 Testis, Right B Testis, Left C Testes, Bilateral F Spermatic Cord, Right G Spermatic Cord, Left H Spermatic Cords, Bilateral	0 Open 4 Percutaneous endoscopic	Z No device	Z No qualifier

1ST - 0 Medical and Surgical
2ND - V Male Reproductive System ♂
3RD - N RELEASE

DIVISION GROUP: (Division), Release
Root Operations involving cutting or separation only.

RELEASE: Freeing a body part from an abnormal physical constraint by cutting or by the use of force.

Explanation: Some of the restraining tissue may be taken out but none of the body part is taken out
Examples: Adhesiolysis spermatic cord – CMS Ex: Carpal tunnel release

Body Part – 4TH	Approach – 5TH	Device – 6TH	Qualifier - 7TH
0 Prostate	0 Open 3 Percutaneous 4 Percutaneous endoscopic 7 Via natural or artificial opening 8 Via natural or artificial opening endoscopic	Z No device	Z No qualifier
1 Seminal Vesicle, Right 2 Seminal Vesicle, Left 3 Seminal Vesicles, Bilateral 6 Tunica Vaginalis, Right 7 Tunica Vaginalis, Left 9 Testis, Right B Testis, Left C Testes, Bilateral	0 Open 3 Percutaneous 4 Percutaneous endoscopic	Z No device	Z No qualifier
5 Scrotum S Penis T Prepuce	0 Open 3 Percutaneous 4 Percutaneous endoscopic X External	Z No device	Z No qualifier
F Spermatic Cord, Right G Spermatic Cord, Left H Spermatic Cords, Bilateral J Epididymis, Right K Epididymis, Left L Epididymis, Bilateral N Vas Deferens, Right P Vas Deferens, Left Q Vas Deferens, Bilateral	0 Open 3 Percutaneous 4 Percutaneous endoscopic 8 Via natural or artificial opening endoscopic	Z No device	Z No qualifier

© 2018 Channel Publishing, Ltd.

1ST - 0 Medical and Surgical
2ND - V Male Reproductive System ♂
3RD - P REMOVAL

DEVICE GROUP: Change, Insertion, Removal, Replacement, Revision, Supplement
Root Operations that always involve a device.

REMOVAL: Taking out or off a device from a body part.

Explanation: Removal device without reinsertion ...
Examples: Removal drain tube – CMS Ex: Cardiac pacemaker removal

Body Part – 4TH	Approach – 5TH	Device – 6TH	Qualifier – 7TH
4 Prostate and Seminal Vesicles	0 Open 3 Percutaneous 4 Percutaneous endoscopic 7 Via natural or artificial opening 8 Via natural or artificial opening endoscopic	0 Drainage device 1 Radioactive element 3 Infusion device 7 Autologous tissue substitute J Synthetic substitute K Nonautologous tissue substitute Y Other device	Z No qualifier
4 Prostate and Seminal Vesicles	X External	0 Drainage device 1 Radioactive element 3 Infusion device	Z No qualifier
8 Scrotum and Tunica Vaginalis D Testis S Penis	0 Open 3 Percutaneous 4 Percutaneous endoscopic 7 Via natural or artificial opening 8 Via natural or artificial opening endoscopic	0 Drainage device 3 Infusion device 7 Autologous tissue substitute J Synthetic substitute K Nonautologous tissue substitute Y Other device	Z No qualifier
8 Scrotum and Tunica Vaginalis D Testis S Penis	X External	0 Drainage device 3 Infusion device	Z No qualifier
M Epididymis and Spermatic Cord	0 Open 3 Percutaneous 4 Percutaneous endoscopic 7 Via natural or artificial opening 8 Via natural or artificial opening endoscopic	0 Drainage device 3 Infusion device 7 Autologous tissue substitute C Extraluminal device J Synthetic substitute K Nonautologous tissue substitute Y Other device	Z No qualifier
M Epididymis and Spermatic Cord	X External	0 Drainage device 3 Infusion device	Z No qualifier
R Vas Deferens	0 Open 3 Percutaneous 4 Percutaneous endoscopic 7 Via natural or artificial opening 8 Via natural or artificial opening endoscopic	0 Drainage device 3 Infusion device 7 Autologous tissue substitute C Extraluminal device D Intraluminal device J Synthetic substitute K Nonautologous tissue substitute Y Other device	Z No qualifier
R Vas Deferens	X External	0 Drainage device 3 Infusion device D Intraluminal device	Z No qualifier

© 2018 Channel Publishing, Ltd.

1ST - 0 Medical and Surgical
2ND - V Male Reproductive System ♂
3RD - Q REPAIR

OTHER REPAIRS GROUP: (Control), Repair
Root Operations that define other repairs.

REPAIR: Restoring, to the extent possible, a body part to its normal anatomic structure and function.

Explanation: Used only when the method to accomplish the repair is not one of the other root operations
Examples: Repair lacerated scrotum – CMS Ex: Suture of laceration

Body Part – 4TH	Approach – 5TH	Device – 6TH	Qualifier - 7TH
0 Prostate	0 Open 3 Percutaneous 4 Percutaneous endoscopic 7 Via natural or artificial opening 8 Via natural or artificial opening endoscopic	Z No device	Z No qualifier
1 Seminal Vesicle, Right 2 Seminal Vesicle, Left 3 Seminal Vesicles, Bilateral 6 Tunica Vaginalis, Right 7 Tunica Vaginalis, Left 9 Testis, Right B Testis, Left C Testes, Bilateral	0 Open 3 Percutaneous 4 Percutaneous endoscopic	Z No device	Z No qualifier
5 Scrotum S Penis T Prepuce	0 Open 3 Percutaneous 4 Percutaneous endoscopic X External	Z No device	Z No qualifier
F Spermatic Cord, Right G Spermatic Cord, Left H Spermatic Cords, Bilateral J Epididymis, Right K Epididymis, Left L Epididymis, Bilateral N Vas Deferens, Right P Vas Deferens, Left Q Vas Deferens, Bilateral	0 Open 3 Percutaneous 4 Percutaneous endoscopic 8 Via natural or artificial opening endoscopic	Z No device	Z No qualifier

1ST - 0 Medical and Surgical
2ND - V Male Reproductive System ♂
3RD - R REPLACEMENT

DEVICE GROUP: Change, Insertion, Removal, Replacement, Revision, Supplement
Root Operations that always involve a device.

REPLACEMENT: Putting in or on biological or synthetic material that physically takes the place and/or function of all or a portion of a body part.

Explanation: Includes taking out or eradicating, or rendering non-functional, the body part ...
Examples: Testis removal with replacement – CMS Ex: Total hip replacement

Body Part – 4TH	Approach – 5TH	Device – 6TH	Qualifier – 7TH
9 Testis, Right B Testis, Left C Testes, Bilateral	0 Open	J Synthetic substitute	Z No qualifier

1ST - 0 Medical and Surgical
2ND - V Male Reproductive System ♂
3RD - S REPOSITION

MOVE GROUP: Reattachment, Reposition, Transfer, (Transplantation)
Root Operations that put in/put back or move some/all of a body part.

REPOSITION: Moving to its normal location, or other suitable location, all or a portion of a body part.

Explanation: The body part may or may not be cut out or off to be moved to the new location ...
Examples: Relocation undescended testis – CMS Ex: Fracture reduction

Body Part – 4TH	Approach – 5TH	Device – 6TH	Qualifier - 7TH
9 Testis, Right B Testis, Left C Testes, Bilateral F Spermatic Cord, Right G Spermatic Cord, Left H Spermatic Cords, Bilateral	0 Open 3 Percutaneous 4 Percutaneous endoscopic 8 Via natural or artificial opening endoscopic	Z No device	Z No qualifier

© 2018 Channel Publishing, Ltd.

1ST - 0 Medical and Surgical 2ND - V Male Reproductive System ♂ 3RD - T RESECTION	EXCISION GROUP: Excision, Resection, Destruction, (Extraction), (Detachment) Root Operations that take out some or all of a body part. RESECTION: Cutting out or off, without replacement, all of a body part. Explanation: None Examples: Total retropubic prostatectomy – CMS Ex: Total lobectomy of lung		
Body Part – 4TH	**Approach – 5TH**	**Device – 6TH**	**Qualifier - 7TH**
0 Prostate	0 Open 4 Percutaneous endoscopic 7 Via natural or artificial opening 8 Via natural or artificial opening endoscopic	Z No device	Z No qualifier
1 Seminal Vesicle, Right 2 Seminal Vesicle, Left 3 Seminal Vesicles, Bilateral 6 Tunica Vaginalis, Right 7 Tunica Vaginalis, Left 9 Testis, Right B Testis, Left C Testes, Bilateral F Spermatic Cord, Right G Spermatic Cord, Left H Spermatic Cords, Bilateral J Epididymis, Right K Epididymis, Left L Epididymis, Bilateral N Vas Deferens, Right NC* P Vas Deferens, Left NC* Q Vas Deferens, Bilateral NC*	0 Open 4 Percutaneous endoscopic	Z No device	Z No qualifier
5 Scrotum S Penis T Prepuce	0 Open 4 Percutaneous endoscopic X External	Z No device	Z No qualifier

NC* – Some procedures are considered non-covered by Medicare. See current Medicare Code Editor for details.

1ST - 0 Medical and Surgical 2ND - V Male Reproductive System ♂ 3RD - U SUPPLEMENT	DEVICE GROUP: Change, Insertion, Removal, Replacement, Revision, Supplement Root Operations that always involve a device. SUPPLEMENT: Putting in or on biological or synthetic material that physically reinforces and/or augments the function of a portion of a body part. Explanation: Biological material is non-living, or is living and from the same individual ... Examples: Tunica vaginalis repair with graft – CMS Ex: Herniorrhaphy using mesh		
Body Part – 4TH	**Approach – 5TH**	**Device – 6TH**	**Qualifier – 7TH**
1 Seminal Vesicle, Right 2 Seminal Vesicle, Left 3 Seminal Vesicles, Bilateral 6 Tunica Vaginalis, Right 7 Tunica Vaginalis, Left F Spermatic Cord, Right G Spermatic Cord, Left H Spermatic Cords, Bilateral J Epididymis, Right K Epididymis, Left L Epididymis, Bilateral N Vas Deferens, Right P Vas Deferens, Left Q Vas Deferens, Bilateral	0 Open 4 Percutaneous endoscopic 8 Via natural or artificial opening endoscopic	7 Autologous tissue substitute J Synthetic substitute K Nonautologous tissue substitute	Z No qualifier
5 Scrotum S Penis T Prepuce	0 Open 4 Percutaneous endoscopic X External	7 Autologous tissue substitute J Synthetic substitute K Nonautologous tissue substitute	Z No qualifier
9 Testis, Right B Testis, Left C Testes, Bilateral	0 Open	7 Autologous tissue substitute J Synthetic substitute K Nonautologous tissue substitute	Z No qualifier

© 2018 Channel Publishing, Ltd.

1ST - 0 Medical and Surgical
2ND - V Male Reproductive System ♂
3RD - W REVISION

DEVICE GROUP: Change, Insertion, Removal, Replacement, Revision, Supplement
Root Operations that always involve a device.

REVISION: Correcting, to the extent possible, a portion of a malfunctioning device or the position of a displaced device.

Explanation: Correcting by taking out or putting in components of a device such as a screw or pin ...
Examples: Reposition drain tube – CMS Ex: Recementing of hip prosthesis

Body Part – 4TH	Approach – 5TH	Device – 6TH	Qualifier – 7TH
4 Prostate and Seminal Vesicles 8 Scrotum and Tunica Vaginalis D Testis S Penis	0 Open 3 Percutaneous 4 Percutaneous endoscopic 7 Via natural or artificial opening 8 Via natural or artificial opening endoscopic	0 Drainage device 3 Infusion device 7 Autologous tissue substitute J Synthetic substitute K Nonautologous tissue substitute Y Other device	Z No qualifier
4 Prostate and Seminal Vesicles 8 Scrotum and Tunica Vaginalis D Testis S Penis	X External	0 Drainage device 3 Infusion device 7 Autologous tissue substitute J Synthetic substitute K Nonautologous tissue substitute	Z No qualifier
M Epididymis and Spermatic Cord	0 Open 3 Percutaneous 4 Percutaneous endoscopic 7 Via natural or artificial opening 8 Via natural or artificial opening endoscopic	0 Drainage device 3 Infusion device 7 Autologous tissue substitute C Extraluminal device J Synthetic substitute K Nonautologous tissue substitute Y Other device	Z No qualifier
M Epididymis and Spermatic Cord	X External	0 Drainage device 3 Infusion device 7 Autologous tissue substitute C Extraluminal device J Synthetic substitute K Nonautologous tissue substitute	Z No qualifier
R Vas Deferens	0 Open 3 Percutaneous 4 Percutaneous endoscopic 7 Via natural or artificial opening 8 Via natural or artificial opening endoscopic	0 Drainage device 3 Infusion device 7 Autologous tissue substitute C Extraluminal device D Intraluminal device J Synthetic substitute K Nonautologous tissue substitute Y Other device	Z No qualifier
R Vas Deferens	X External	0 Drainage device 3 Infusion device 7 Autologous tissue substitute C Extraluminal device D Intraluminal device J Synthetic substitute K Nonautologous tissue substitute	Z No qualifier

1ST - 0 Medical and Surgical
2ND - V Male Reproductive System ♂
3RD - X TRANSFER

MOVE GROUP: Reattachment, Reposition, Transfer, (Transplantation)
Root Operations that put in/put back or move some/all of a body part.

TRANSFER: Moving, without taking out, all or a portion of a body part to another location to take over the function of all or a portion of a body part.

Explanation: The body part transferred remains connected to its vascular and nervous supply
Examples: Foreskin urethroplasty – CMS Ex: Tendon transfer

Body Part – 4TH	Approach – 5TH	Device – 6TH	Qualifier – 7TH
T Prepuce	0 Open X External	Z No device	D Urethra S Penis

© 2018 Channel Publishing, Ltd.

Educational Annotations | W – Anatomical Regions, General

Body System Specific Educational Annotations for the Anatomical Regions, General include:

- Anatomy and Physiology Review
- Anatomical Illustrations
- Definitions of Common Procedures
- AHA Coding Clinic® Reference Notations
- Body Part Key Listings
- Device Key Listings
- Device Aggregation Table Listings
- Coding Notes

Anatomy and Physiology Review of Anatomical Regions, General

BODY PART VALUES – W - ANATOMICAL REGIONS, GENERAL

Coding Guideline B2.1a - Body System, General Guideline – The procedure codes in the general anatomical regions body systems can be used when the procedure is performed on an anatomical region rather than a specific body part (e.g., root operations Control and Detachment, Drainage of a body cavity) or on the rare occasion when no information is available to support assignment of a code to a specific body part.
Examples: Control of postoperative hemorrhage is coded to the root operation Control found in the general anatomical regions body systems. Chest tube drainage of the pleural cavity is coded to the root operation Drainage found in the general anatomical regions body systems. Suture repair of the abdominal wall is coded to the root operation Repair in the general anatomical regions body system.

Abdominal Wall – The multi-tissue-layered covering of the abdominal and pelvic portions of the trunk.
Back – The multi-tissue-layered covering of the back portion of the trunk.
Chest Wall – The multi-tissue-layered covering of the thoracic portion of the trunk.
Cranial Cavity – The space inside the skull.
Face – The multi-tissue-layered covering of the anterior portion of the head.
Gastrointestinal Tract – The alimentary tract from the esophagus to the anus.
Genitourinary Tract – The organs and structures of the urinary and reproductive systems.
Head – The portion of the human body above the neck.
Jaw – The anterior, lower, movable, articulated portion of the head.
Mediastinum – The central portion of the thoracic cavity that lies between the right pleura, left pleura, sternum, and vertebral column and contains the heart, great vessels, esophagus, bronchi, and thymus.
Neck – The portion of the human body above the trunk and below the head.
Oral Cavity and Throat – The space formed by the mouth, pharynx, and larynx.
Pelvic Cavity – The lower abdominal space containing the rectum, bladder, and reproductive organs.
Pericardial Cavity – The thoracic, fluid-filled space formed by the double-walled peritoneal sac that contains the heart.
Perineum, Female – The multi-tissue-layered area between the vulva and the anus.
Perineum, Male – The multi-tissue-layered area between the scrotum and the anus.
Peritoneal Cavity – The abdominal space between the parietal peritoneum and visceral peritoneum.
Pleural Cavity – The thoracic, fluid-filled space between the visceral pleura and parietal pleura.
Respiratory Tract – The organs and structures involved in respiration.
Retroperitoneum – The space behind the peritoneum that borders the deep muscles of the back and contains the kidneys, adrenals, most of the duodenum, ascending and descending colon, and the pancreas.

Anatomical Illustrations of Anatomical Regions, General

None for the Anatomical Regions, General Body System

Definitions of Common Procedures of Anatomical Regions, General

Abdominoplasty (tummy tuck) – The cosmetic plastic surgical procedure to remove excess fat and skin from the abdominal wall area.
Chest tube for pneumothorax – The surgical insertion of a plastic tube through the chest wall and into the pleural space to remove the air of a pneumothorax.
Episiotomy – The surgical incision of the perineum (with subsequent closure) to expand the opening of the vagina and prevent tearing of the perineal tissues during delivery.
Face lift (rhytidectomy) – The cosmetic plastic surgical procedure to remove the visible signs of aging in the face and neck including removing excess skin and fat with resulting tightening of the facial skin. The procedure often includes a cosmetic blepharoplasty of the eyelids.
Paracentesis – The procedural insertion of a needle or catheter through the abdominal wall and into the peritoneal cavity to drain excess fluid.
Pleuroperitoneal shunt – The shunting redirection of excessive pleural fluid by placing a catheter into the pleural space and tunneling it into the peritoneal cavity.
Thoracentesis – The procedural insertion of a needle or catheter through the chest wall and into the pleural space to drain fluid (pleural effusion, empyema, blood, chyle).

© 2018 Channel Publishing, Ltd.

Educational Annotations | W – Anatomical Regions, General

AHA Coding Clinic® Reference Notations of Anatomical Regions, General

ROOT OPERATION SPECIFIC - W - ANATOMICAL REGIONS, GENERAL

ALTERATION - 0
- Browpexy ....AHA 15:1Q:p31

BYPASS - 1
- Creation of percutaneous cutaneoperitoneal fistula for peritoneal dialysis ....AHA 13:4Q:p126
  - Official Correction of 13:4Q:p126 & 127 ....AHA 15:2Q:p36
- Creation of percutaneous cutaneoperitoneal fistula laparoscopically for peritoneal dialysis ....AHA 13:4Q:p127
  - Official Correction of 13:4Q:p126 & 127 ....AHA 15:2Q:p36

CHANGE - 2

CONTROL - 3
- Ablation of duodenal vascular lesions ....AHA 18:1Q:p19
- Control of bleeding ....AHA 16:4Q:p99
- Control of duodenal ulcer bleeding ....AHA 17:4Q:p105
- Control of post vaginal delivery bleeding ....AHA 14:4Q:p44

CREATION - 4

DIVISION - 8

DRAINAGE - 9
- Diagnostic and therapeutic paracentesis ....AHA 17:3Q:p12
- Drainage of abscess of floor of mouth ....AHA 17:2Q:p16

EXCISION - B
- Excision of inclusion cyst of perineum ....AHA 13:4Q:p119
- Excision of urachal mass ....AHA 16:1Q:p21

EXTIRPATION - C

FRAGMENTATION - F

INSERTION - H
- Peritoneal port-a-cath insertion ....AHA 16:2Q:p14
- Placement of peritoneal dialysis device ....AHA 15:2Q:p36

INSPECTION - J
- Ventriculoperitoneal (VP) shunt with laparoscopic assistance ....AHA 13:2Q:p36

REATTACHMENT - M

REMOVAL - P

REPAIR - Q
- Abdominoplasty of ventral hernia ....AHA 14:4Q:p38
- Parastomal hernia repair ....AHA 14:3Q:p28
- Removal of silo and closure of abdominal wall defect ....AHA 17:3Q:p8

SUPPLEMENT - U
- Mobilized flap omentoplasty ....AHA 16:3Q:p40
- Protective silo around the intestine outside the abdomen ....AHA 17:3Q:p8
- Reconstruction of chest wall using Marlex overlay plate ....AHA 12:4Q:p101
- Repair of incisional hernia with component release and mesh ....AHA 14:4Q:p39

REVISION - W
- Replacement of disconnected abdominal portion of VP shunt ....AHA 15:2Q:p9

Body Part Key Listings of Anatomical Regions, General

See also Body Part Key in Appendix C

Retroperitoneal space ....use Retroperitoneum
Retropubic space ....use Pelvic Cavity

© 2018 Channel Publishing, Ltd.

Educational Annotations | W – Anatomical Regions, General

Device Key Listings of Anatomical Regions, General

See also Device Key in Appendix D

Autograft	use Autologous Tissue Substitute
Bard® Composix® Kugel® patch	use Synthetic Substitute
Bard® Ventralex™ hernia patch	use Synthetic Substitute
Bard® Composix® (E/X)(LP) mesh	use Synthetic Substitute
Bard® Dulex™ mesh	use Synthetic Substitute
Brachytherapy seeds	use Radioactive Element
Cook Biodesign® Hernia Graft(s)	use Nonautologous Tissue Substitute
Cook Biodesign® Layered Graft(s)	use Nonautologous Tissue Substitute
Cook Zenapro™ Layered Graft(s)	use Nonautologous Tissue Substitute
Flexible Composite Mesh	use Synthetic Substitute
GORE® DUALMESH®	use Synthetic Substitute
Nitinol framed polymer mesh	use Synthetic Substitute
Partially absorbable mesh	use Synthetic Substitute
PHYSIOMESH™ Flexible Composite Mesh	use Synthetic Substitute
Polypropylene mesh	use Synthetic Substitute
PROCEED™ Ventral Patch	use Synthetic Substitute
PROLENE Polypropylene Hernia System (PHS)	use Synthetic Substitute
Rebound HRD® (Hernia Repair Device)	use Synthetic Substitute
Thoracostomy tube	use Drainage Device
Tissue bank graft	use Nonautologous Tissue Substitute
ULTRAPRO Hernia System (UHS)	use Synthetic Substitute
ULTRAPRO Partially Absorbable Lightweight Mesh	use Synthetic Substitute
ULTRAPRO Plug	use Synthetic Substitute
Ventrio™ Hernia Patch	use Synthetic Substitute

Aggregation Key Listings of Anatomical Regions, General

See also Device Aggregation Table in Appendix E

Specific Device	For Operation	In Body System	General Device
None Listed in Device Aggregation Table for this Body System			

Coding Notes of Anatomical Regions, General

Body System Relevant Coding Guidelines

General Guidelines

B2.1a

The procedure codes in the general anatomical regions body systems can be used when the procedure is performed on an anatomical region rather than a specific body part (e.g., root operations Control and Detachment, Drainage of a body cavity) or on the rare occasion when no information is available to support assignment of a code to a specific body part.

Examples: Control of postoperative hemorrhage is coded to the root operation Control found in the general anatomical regions body systems.

Chest tube drainage of the pleural cavity is coded to the root operation Drainage found in the general anatomical regions body systems. Suture repair of the abdominal wall is coded to the root operation Repair in the general anatomical regions body system.

Control vs. more definitive root operations

B3.7

The root operation Control is defined as, "Stopping, or attempting to stop, postprocedural or other acute bleeding." If an attempt to stop postprocedural or other acute bleeding is unsuccessful, and to stop the bleeding requires performing a more definitive root operation, such as Bypass, Detachment, Excision, Extraction, Reposition, Replacement, or Resection, then the more definitive root operation is coded instead of Control.

Example: Resection of spleen to stop bleeding is coded to Resection instead of Control.

© 2018 Channel Publishing, Ltd.

1ST - 0 Medical and Surgical
2ND - W Anatomical Regions, General
3RD - 0 ALTERATION

OTHER OBJECTIVES GROUP: Alteration, Creation, (Fusion)
Root Operations that define other objectives.

ALTERATION: Modifying the anatomic structure of a body part without affecting the function of the body part.

Explanation: Principal purpose is to improve appearance
Examples: Abdominoplasty (tummy tuck) – CMS Ex: Face lift

Body Part – 4TH			Approach – 5TH	Device – 6TH	Qualifier – 7TH
0 Head 2 Face 4 Upper Jaw 5 Lower Jaw	6 Neck 8 Chest Wall F Abdominal Wall K Upper Back	L Lower Back M Perineum, Male ♂ N Perineum, Female ♀	0 Open 3 Percutaneous 4 Percutaneous endoscopic	7 Autologous tissue substitute J Synthetic substitute K Nonautologous tissue substitute Z No device	Z No qualifier

1ST - 0 Medical and Surgical
2ND - W Anatomical Regions, General
3RD - 1 BYPASS

TUBULAR GROUP: Bypass, (Dilation), (Occlusion), (Restriction)
Root Operations that alter the diameter/route of a tubular body part.

BYPASS: Altering the route of passage of the contents of a tubular body part.

Explanation: Rerouting contents to a downstream part ... with or without the use of a device ...
Examples: Pleuroperitoneal shunt – CMS Ex: Coronary artery bypass

Body Part – 4TH	Approach – 5TH	Device – 6TH	Qualifier – 7TH
1 Cranial Cavity	0 Open	J Synthetic substitute	9 Pleural Cavity, Right B Pleural Cavity, Left G Peritoneal Cavity J Pelvic Cavity
9 Pleural Cavity, Right B Pleural Cavity, Left G Peritoneal Cavity J Pelvic Cavity	0 Open 3 Percutaneous 4 Percutaneous endoscopic	J Synthetic substitute	4 Cutaneous 9 Pleural Cavity, Right B Pleural Cavity, Left G Peritoneal Cavity J Pelvic Cavity W Upper Vein Y Lower Vein

1ST - 0 Medical and Surgical
2ND - W Anatomical Regions, General
3RD - 2 CHANGE

DEVICE GROUP: Change, Insertion, Removal, (Replacement), Revision, Supplement
Root Operations that always involve a device.

CHANGE: Taking out or off a device from a body part and putting back an identical or similar device in or on the same body part without cutting or puncturing the skin or a mucous membrane.

Explanation: All CHANGE procedures are coded using the approach External
Examples: Exchange chest tube – CMS Ex: Urinary catheter change

Body Part – 4TH			Approach – 5TH	Device – 6TH	Qualifier – 7TH
0 Head 1 Cranial Cavity 2 Face 4 Upper Jaw 5 Lower Jaw 6 Neck 8 Chest Wall	9 Pleural Cavity, Right B Pleural Cavity, Left C Mediastinum D Pericardial Cavity F Abdominal Wall G Peritoneal Cavity	H Retroperitoneum J Pelvic Cavity K Upper Back L Lower Back M Perineum, Male ♂ N Perineum, Female ♀	X External	0 Drainage device Y Other device	Z No qualifier

© 2018 Channel Publishing, Ltd.

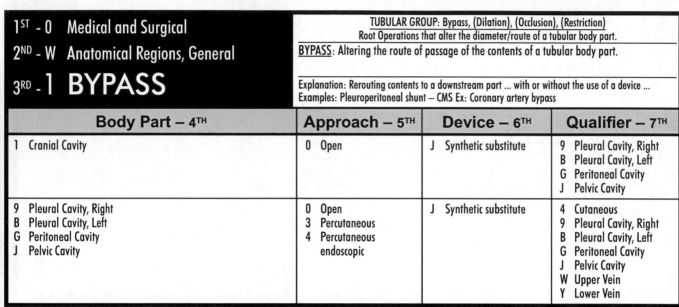

1ST - 0 Medical and Surgical
2ND - W Anatomical Regions, General
3RD - 3 CONTROL

OTHER REPAIRS GROUP: Control, Repair
Root Operations that define other repairs.

CONTROL: Stopping, or attempting to stop, postprocedural or other acute bleeding.

Explanation: The site of the bleeding is coded as an anatomical region and not to a specific body part
Examples: Cautery post-op oozing – CMS Ex: Control of bleeding duodenal ulcer

Body Part – 4TH	Approach – 5TH	Device – 6TH	Qualifier – 7TH
0 Head 1 Cranial Cavity 2 Face 4 Upper Jaw 5 Lower Jaw 6 Neck 8 Chest Wall 9 Pleural Cavity, Right B Pleural Cavity, Left C Mediastinum D Pericardial Cavity F Abdominal Wall G Peritoneal Cavity H Retroperitoneum J Pelvic Cavity K Upper Back L Lower Back M Perineum, Male ♂ N Perineum, Female ♀	0 Open 3 Percutaneous 4 Percutaneous endoscopic	Z No device	Z No qualifier
3 Oral Cavity and Throat	0 Open 3 Percutaneous 4 Percutaneous endoscopic 7 Via natural or artificial opening 8 Via natural or artificial opening endoscopic X External	Z No device	Z No qualifier
P Gastrointestinal Tract Q Respiratory Tract R Genitourinary Tract	0 Open 3 Percutaneous 4 Percutaneous endoscopic 7 Via natural or artificial opening 8 Via natural or artificial opening endoscopic	Z No device	Z No qualifier

1ST - 0 Medical and Surgical
2ND - W Anatomical Regions, General
3RD - 4 CREATION

OTHER OBJECTIVES GROUP: Alteration, Creation, (Fusion)
Root Operations that define other objectives.

CREATION: Putting in or on biological or synthetic material to form a new body part that to the extent possible replicates the anatomic structure or function of an absent body part.

Explanation: Gender reassignment surgery and corrective procedures for congenital anomalies
Examples: Creation penis in female – CMS Ex: Creation of vagina in male

Body Part – 4TH	Approach – 5TH	Device – 6TH	Qualifier – 7TH
M Perineum, Male ♂	0 Open	7 Autologous tissue substitute J Synthetic substitute K Nonautologous tissue substitute	0 Vagina
N Perineum, Female ♀	0 Open	7 Autologous tissue substitute J Synthetic substitute K Nonautologous tissue substitute	1 Penis

1ST - 0 Medical and Surgical
2ND - W Anatomical Regions, General
3RD - 8 DIVISION

DIVISION GROUP: Division, (Release)
Root Operations involving cutting or separation only.

DIVISION: Cutting into a body part, without draining fluids and/or gases from the body part, in order to separate or transect a body part.

Explanation: All or a portion of the body part is separated into two or more portions
Examples: Episiotomy – CMS Ex: Spinal cordotomy

Body Part – 4TH	Approach – 5TH	Device – 6TH	Qualifier – 7TH
N Perineum, Female ♀	X External	Z No device	Z No qualifier

© 2018 Channel Publishing, Ltd.

1ST - 0 Medical and Surgical
2ND - W Anatomical Regions, General
3RD - 9 DRAINAGE

DRAINAGE GROUP: Drainage, Extirpation, Fragmentation
Root Operations that take out solids/fluids/gases from a body part.

DRAINAGE: Taking or letting out fluids and/or gases from a body part.

Explanation: Qualifier "X Diagnostic" indicates drainage procedures that are biopsies
Examples: Paracentesis for ascites – CMS Ex: Thoracentesis

Body Part – 4TH	Approach – 5TH	Device – 6TH	Qualifier - 7TH
0 Head 1 Cranial Cavity 2 Face 3 Oral Cavity and Throat 4 Upper Jaw 5 Lower Jaw 6 Neck 8 Chest Wall 9 Pleural Cavity, Right B Pleural Cavity, Left C Mediastinum D Pericardial Cavity F Abdominal Wall G Peritoneal Cavity H Retroperitoneum J Pelvic Cavity K Upper Back L Lower Back M Perineum, Male ♂ N Perineum, Female ♀	0 Open 3 Percutaneous 4 Percutaneous endoscopic	0 Drainage device	Z No qualifier
0 Head 1 Cranial Cavity 2 Face 3 Oral Cavity and Throat 4 Upper Jaw 5 Lower Jaw 6 Neck 8 Chest Wall 9 Pleural Cavity, Right B Pleural Cavity, Left C Mediastinum D Pericardial Cavity F Abdominal Wall G Peritoneal Cavity H Retroperitoneum J Pelvic Cavity K Upper Back L Lower Back M Perineum, Male ♂ N Perineum, Female ♀	0 Open 3 Percutaneous 4 Percutaneous endoscopic	Z No device	X Diagnostic Z No qualifier

1ST - 0 Medical and Surgical
2ND - W Anatomical Regions, General
3RD - B EXCISION

EXCISION GROUP: Excision, (Resection), (Destruction), (Extraction), (Detachment)
Root Operations that take out some or all of a body part.

EXCISION: Cutting out or off, without replacement, a portion of a body part.

Explanation: Qualifier "X Diagnostic" indicates excision procedures that are biopsies
Examples: Excision perineal inclusion cyst – CMS Ex: Liver biopsy

Body Part – 4TH	Approach – 5TH	Device – 6TH	Qualifier - 7TH
0 Head 2 Face 3 Oral Cavity and Throat 4 Upper Jaw 5 Lower Jaw 8 Chest Wall K Upper Back L Lower Back M Perineum, Male ♂ N Perineum, Female ♀	0 Open 3 Percutaneous 4 Percutaneous endoscopic X External	Z No device	X Diagnostic Z No qualifier
6 Neck F Abdominal Wall	0 Open 3 Percutaneous 4 Percutaneous endoscopic	Z No device	X Diagnostic Z No qualifier
6 Neck F Abdominal Wall	X External	Z No device	2 Stoma X Diagnostic Z No qualifier
C Mediastinum H Retroperitoneum	0 Open 3 Percutaneous 4 Percutaneous endoscopic	Z No device	X Diagnostic Z No qualifier

© 2018 Channel Publishing, Ltd.

1ST - 0 Medical and Surgical
2ND - W Anatomical Regions, General
3RD - C EXTIRPATION

DRAINAGE GROUP: Drainage, Extirpation, Fragmentation
Root Operations that take out solids/fluids/gases from a body part.
EXTIRPATION: Taking or cutting out solid matter from a body part.

Explanation: Abnormal byproduct or foreign body ...
Examples: Evacuation cranial cavity clot – CMS Ex: Thrombectomy

Body Part – 4TH		Approach – 5TH	Device – 6TH	Qualifier – 7TH
1 Cranial Cavity 3 Oral Cavity and Throat 9 Pleural Cavity, Right B Pleural Cavity, Left	C Mediastinum D Pericardial Cavity G Peritoneal Cavity H Retroperitoneum J Pelvic Cavity	0 Open 3 Percutaneous 4 Percutaneous endoscopic X External	Z No device	Z No qualifier
P Gastrointestinal Tract Q Respiratory Tract R Genitourinary Tract		0 Open 3 Percutaneous 4 Percutaneous endoscopic 7 Via natural or artificial opening 8 Via natural or artificial opening endoscopic X External	Z No device	Z No qualifier

1ST - 0 Medical and Surgical
2ND - W Anatomical Regions, General
3RD - F FRAGMENTATION

DRAINAGE GROUP: Drainage, Extirpation, Fragmentation
Root Operations that take out solids/fluids/gases from a body part.
FRAGMENTATION: Breaking solid matter in a body part into pieces.

Explanation: Pieces are not taken out during the procedure ...
Examples: Lithotripsy pericardial cavity – CMS Ex: Extracorporeal shockwave lithotripsy

Body Part – 4TH		Approach – 5TH	Device – 6TH	Qualifier – 7TH
1 Cranial Cavity 3 Oral Cavity and Throat 9 Pleural Cavity, Right B Pleural Cavity, Left	C Mediastinum D Pericardial Cavity G Peritoneal Cavity J Pelvic Cavity	0 Open 3 Percutaneous 4 Percutaneous endoscopic X External NC*	Z No device	Z No qualifier
P Gastrointestinal Tract Q Respiratory Tract R Genitourinary Tract		0 Open 3 Percutaneous 4 Percutaneous endoscopic 7 Via natural or artificial opening 8 Via natural or artificial opening endoscopic X External NC*	Z No device	Z No qualifier

NC* – Some procedures are considered non-covered by Medicare. See current Medicare Code Editor for details.

1ST - 0 Medical and Surgical
2ND - W Anatomical Regions, General
3RD - H INSERTION

DEVICE GROUP: Change, Insertion, Removal, (Replacement), Revision, Supplement
Root Operations that always involve a device.
INSERTION: Putting in a nonbiological appliance that monitors, assists, performs, or prevents a physiological function but does not physically take the place of a body part.
Explanation: None
Examples: Implantation infusion pump – CMS Ex: Insertion of central venous catheter

Body Part – 4TH		Approach – 5TH	Device – 6TH	Qualifier – 7TH
0 Head 1 Cranial Cavity 2 Face 3 Oral Cavity and Throat 4 Upper Jaw 5 Lower Jaw 6 Neck 8 Chest Wall 9 Pleural Cavity, Right B Pleural Cavity, Left	C Mediastinum D Pericardial Cavity F Abdominal Wall G Peritoneal Cavity H Retroperitoneum J Pelvic Cavity K Upper Back L Lower Back M Perineum, Male ♂ N Perineum, Female ♀	0 Open 3 Percutaneous 4 Percutaneous endoscopic	1 Radioactive element 3 Infusion device Y Other device	Z No qualifier
P Gastrointestinal Tract Q Respiratory Tract R Genitourinary Tract		0 Open 3 Percutaneous 4 Percutaneous endoscopic 7 Via natural or artificial opening 8 Via natural or artificial opening endoscopic	1 Radioactive element 3 Infusion device Y Other device	Z No qualifier

© 2018 Channel Publishing, Ltd.

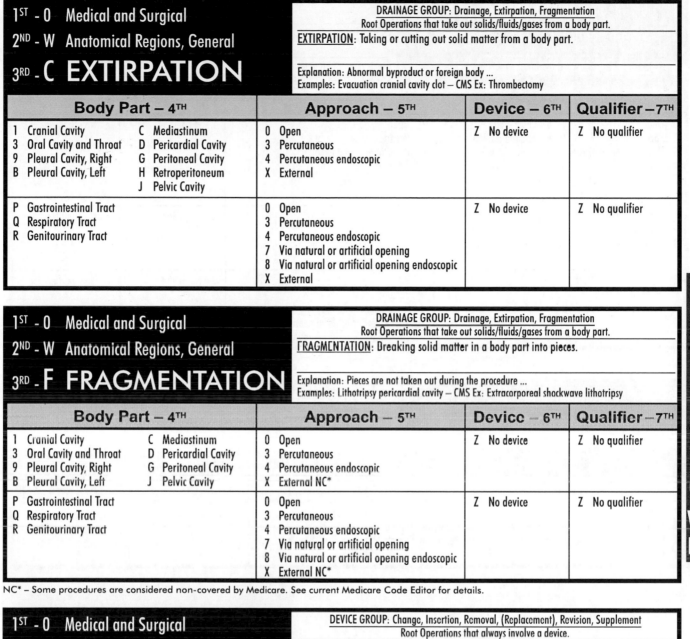

1ST - 0 Medical and Surgical
2ND - W Anatomical Regions, General
3RD - J INSPECTION

EXAMINATION GROUP: Inspection, (Map)
Root Operations involving examination only.

INSPECTION: Visually and/or manually exploring a body part.

Explanation: Direct or instrumental visualization ...
Examples: Exploration peritoneal cavity – CMS Ex: Exploratory laparotomy

Body Part – 4TH	Approach – 5TH	Device – 6TH	Qualifier – 7TH
0 Head 2 Face 3 Oral Cavity and Throat 4 Upper Jaw 5 Lower Jaw 6 Neck 8 Chest Wall F Abdominal Wall K Upper Back L Lower Back M Perineum, Male ♂ N Perineum, Female ♀	0 Open 3 Percutaneous 4 Percutaneous endoscopic X External	Z No device	Z No qualifier
1 Cranial Cavity 9 Pleural Cavity, Right B Pleural Cavity, Left C Mediastinum D Pericardial Cavity G Peritoneal Cavity H Retroperitoneum J Pelvic Cavity	0 Open 3 Percutaneous 4 Percutaneous endoscopic	Z No device	Z No qualifier
P Gastrointestinal Tract Q Respiratory Tract R Genitourinary Tract	0 Open 3 Percutaneous 4 Percutaneous endoscopic 7 Via natural or artificial opening 8 Via natural or artificial opening endoscopic	Z No device	Z No qualifier

1ST - 0 Medical and Surgical
2ND - W Anatomical Regions, General
3RD - M REATTACHMENT

MOVE GROUP: Reattachment, (Reposition), (Transfer), Transplantation
Root Operations that put in/put back or move some/all of a body part.

REATTACHMENT: Putting back in or on all or a portion of a separated body part to its normal location or other suitable location.

Explanation: Vascular circulation and nervous pathways may or may not be reestablished
Examples: Replantation avulsed perineum – CMS Ex: Reattachment of hand

Body Part – 4TH	Approach – 5TH	Device – 6TH	Qualifier – 7TH
2 Face 4 Upper Jaw 5 Lower Jaw 6 Neck 8 Chest Wall F Abdominal Wall K Upper Back L Lower Back M Perineum, Male ♂ N Perineum, Female ♀	0 Open	Z No device	Z No qualifier

© 2018 Channel Publishing, Ltd.

1ST - 0 Medical and Surgical
2ND - W Anatomical Regions, General
3RD - P REMOVAL

DEVICE GROUP: Change, Insertion, Removal, (Replacement), Revision, Supplement
Root Operations that always involve a device.

REMOVAL: Taking out or off a device from a body part.

Explanation: Removal device without reinsertion ...
Examples: Removal infusion pump – CMS Ex: Cardiac pacemaker removal

Body Part – 4TH	Approach – 5TH	Device – 6TH	Qualifier – 7TH
0 Head 2 Face 4 Upper Jaw 5 Lower Jaw 6 Neck 8 Chest Wall C Mediastinum F Abdominal Wall K Upper Back L Lower Back M Perineum, Male ♂ N Perineum, Female ♀	0 Open 3 Percutaneous 4 Percutaneous endoscopic X External	0 Drainage device 1 Radioactive element 3 Infusion device 7 Autologous tissue substitute J Synthetic substitute K Nonautologous tissue substitute Y Other device	Z No qualifier
1 Cranial Cavity 9 Pleural Cavity, Right B Pleural Cavity, Left G Peritoneal Cavity J Pelvic Cavity	0 Open 3 Percutaneous 4 Percutaneous endoscopic	0 Drainage device 1 Radioactive element 3 Infusion device J Synthetic substitute Y Other device	Z No qualifier
1 Cranial Cavity 9 Pleural Cavity, Right B Pleural Cavity, Left G Peritoneal Cavity J Pelvic Cavity	X External	0 Drainage device 1 Radioactive element 3 Infusion device	Z No qualifier
D Pericardial Cavity H Retroperitoneum	0 Open 3 Percutaneous 4 Percutaneous endoscopic	0 Drainage device 1 Radioactive element 3 Infusion device Y Other device	Z No qualifier
D Pericardial Cavity H Retroperitoneum	X External	0 Drainage device 1 Radioactive element 3 Infusion device	Z No qualifier
P Gastrointestinal Tract Q Respiratory Tract R Genitourinary Tract	0 Open 3 Percutaneous 4 Percutaneous endoscopic 7 Via natural or artificial opening 8 Via natural or artificial opening endoscopic X External	1 Radioactive element 3 Infusion device Y Other device	Z No qualifier

1ST - 0 Medical and Surgical
2ND - W Anatomical Regions, General
3RD - Q REPAIR

OTHER REPAIRS GROUP: Control, Repair
Root Operations that define other repairs.

REPAIR: Restoring, to the extent possible, a body part to its normal anatomic structure and function.

Explanation: Used only when the method to accomplish the repair is not one of the other root operations
Examples: Parastomal hernia repair – CMS Ex: Suture of laceration

Body Part – 4TH	Approach – 5TH	Device – 6TH	Qualifier - 7TH
0 Head 2 Face 3 Oral Cavity and Throat 4 Upper Jaw 5 Lower Jaw 8 Chest Wall K Upper Back L Lower Back M Perineum, Male ♂ N Perineum, Female ♀	0 Open 3 Percutaneous 4 Percutaneous endoscopic X External	Z No device	Z No qualifier
6 Neck F Abdominal Wall	0 Open 3 Percutaneous 4 Percutaneous endoscopic	Z No device	Z No qualifier
6 Neck F Abdominal Wall	X External	Z No device	2 Stoma Z No qualifier
C Mediastinum	0 Open 3 Percutaneous 4 Percutaneous endoscopic	Z No device	Z No qualifier

REGIONS GENERAL 0WQ

© 2018 Channel Publishing, Ltd.

1ST - 0 Medical and Surgical
2ND - W Anatomical Regions, General
3RD - U SUPPLEMENT

DEVICE GROUP: Change, Insertion, Removal, (Replacement), Revision, Supplement
Root Operations that always involve a device.

SUPPLEMENT: Putting in or on biological or synthetic material that physically reinforces and/or augments the function of a portion of a body part.

Explanation: Biological material is non-living, or is living and from the same individual ...
Examples: Parastomal hernia repair with graft – CMS Ex: Herniorrhaphy using mesh

Body Part – 4TH	Approach – 5TH	Device – 6TH	Qualifier - 7TH
0 Head 2 Face 4 Upper Jaw 5 Lower Jaw 6 Neck 8 Chest Wall C Mediastinum F Abdominal Wall K Upper Back L Lower Back M Perineum, Male ♂ N Perineum, Female ♀	0 Open 4 Percutaneous endoscopic	7 Autologous tissue substitute J Synthetic substitute K Nonautologous tissue substitute	Z No qualifier

1ST - 0 Medical and Surgical
2ND - W Anatomical Regions, General
3RD - W REVISION

DEVICE GROUP: Change, Insertion, Removal, (Replacement), Revision, Supplement
Root Operations that always involve a device.

REVISION: Correcting, to the extent possible, a portion of a malfunctioning device or the position of a displaced device.

Explanation: Correcting by taking out or putting in components of a device such as a screw or pin ...
Examples: Reposition infusion pump – CMS Ex: Recementing of hip prosthesis

Body Part – 4TH	Approach – 5TH	Device – 6TH	Qualifier-7TH
0 Head 2 Face 4 Upper Jaw 5 Lower Jaw 6 Neck 8 Chest Wall C Mediastinum F Abdominal Wall K Upper Back L Lower Back M Perineum, Male ♂ N Perineum, Female ♀	0 Open 3 Percutaneous 4 Percutaneous endoscopic X External	0 Drainage device 1 Radioactive element 3 Infusion device 7 Autologous tissue substitute J Synthetic substitute K Nonautologous tissue substitute Y Other device	Z No qualifier
1 Cranial Cavity 9 Pleural Cavity, Right B Pleural Cavity, Left G Peritoneal Cavity J Pelvic Cavity	0 Open 3 Percutaneous 4 Percutaneous endoscopic X External	0 Drainage device 1 Radioactive element 3 Infusion device J Synthetic substitute Y Other device	Z No qualifier
D Pericardial Cavity H Retroperitoneum	0 Open 3 Percutaneous 4 Percutaneous endoscopic X External	0 Drainage device 1 Radioactive element 3 Infusion device Y Other device	Z No qualifier
P Gastrointestinal Tract Q Respiratory Tract R Genitourinary Tract	0 Open 3 Percutaneous 4 Percutaneous endoscopic 7 Via natural or artificial opening 8 Via natural or artificial opening endoscopic X External	1 Radioactive element 3 Infusion device Y Other device	Z No qualifier

1ST - 0 Medical and Surgical
2ND - W Anatomical Regions, General
3RD - Y TRANSPLANTATION

MOVE GROUP: Reattachment, (Reposition), (Transfer), Transplantation
Root Operations that put in/put back or move some/all of a body part.

TRANSPLANTATION: Putting in or on all or a portion of a living body part taken from another individual or animal to physically take the place and/or function of all or a portion of a similar body part.

Explanation: The native body part may or may not be taken out ...
Examples: Face transplant – CMS Ex: Kidney transplant

Body Part – 4TH	Approach – 5TH	Device – 6TH	Qualifier – 7TH
2 Face	0 Open	Z No device	0 Allogeneic 1 Syngeneic

© 2018 Channel Publishing, Ltd.

Educational Annotations | X – Anatomical Regions, Upper Extremities

Body System Specific Educational Annotations for the Anatomical Regions, Upper Extremities include:

- Anatomy and Physiology Review
- Anatomical Illustrations
- Definitions of Common Procedures
- AHA Coding Clinic® Reference Notations
- Body Part Key Listings
- Device Key Listings
- Device Aggregation Table Listings
- Coding Notes

Anatomy and Physiology Review of Anatomical Regions, Upper Extremities

BODY PART VALUES – X - ANATOMICAL REGIONS, UPPER EXTREMITIES

Coding Guideline B2.1a - Body System, General Guideline – The procedure codes in the general anatomical regions body systems can be used when the procedure is performed on an anatomical region rather than a specific body part (e.g., root operations Control and Detachment, Drainage of a body cavity) or on the rare occasion when no information is available to support assignment of a code to a specific body part.
Examples: Control of postoperative hemorrhage is coded to the root operation Control found in the general anatomical regions body systems. Chest tube drainage of the pleural cavity is coded to the root operation Drainage found in the general anatomical regions body systems. Suture repair of the abdominal wall is coded to the root operation Repair in the general anatomical regions body system.

1st Ray – The first digit of the hand and its associated first metacarpal bone.
2nd Ray – The second digit of the hand and its associated second metacarpal bone.
3rd Ray – The third digit of the hand and its associated third metacarpal bone.
4th Ray – The fourth digit of the hand and its associated fourth metacarpal bone.
5th Ray – The fifth digit of the hand and its associated fifth metacarpal bone.
Axilla – The multi-tissue-layered area at the junction of the arm and trunk on the underside of the shoulder joint.
Elbow Region – The multi-tissue-layered elbow joint area.
Forequarter – The portion of the body including the upper extremity, scapula, and clavicle.
Hand – The portion of the upper extermity distal to the forearm.
Index Finger – The second digit of the hand.
Little Finger – The fifth digit of the hand.
Lower Arm – The portion of the upper extermity distal to the elbow.
Middle Finger – The third digit of the hand.
Ring Finger – The fourth digit of the hand.
Shoulder Region – The multi-tissue-layered shoulder joint area.
Thumb – The first digit of the hand.
Upper Arm – The portion of the upper extermity distal to the shoulder and proximal to the elbow.
Upper Extremity – The entire upper extremity (arm).
Wrist Region – The multi-tissue-layered wrist joint area.

Anatomical Illustrations of Anatomical Regions, Upper Extremities

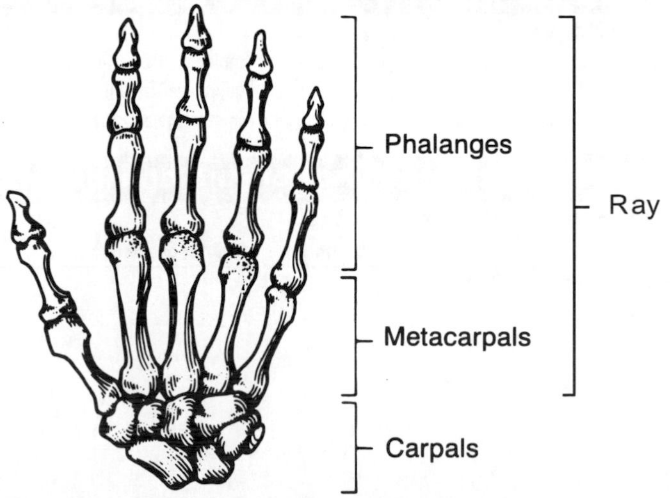

RIGHT HAND — DORSAL VIEW

© 2018 Channel Publishing, Ltd.

Educational Annotations | X – Anatomical Regions, Upper Extremities

Definitions of Common Procedures of Anatomical Regions, Upper Extremities

Amputation through elbow – The surgical detachment and removal of the lower arm including the entire radius and ulna that is performed through the elbow joint.
Forequarter amputation – The surgical detachment and removal of the entire arm including part or all of the scapula and clavicle.
Reattachment of severed thumb – The surgical reconnection of a thumb that has been traumatically amputated.
Transfer of index finger to thumb – The surgical dissection and migration of the index finger, including division of the metacarpal index ray bone that is positioned to function as the thumb.
Transplantation of toe to thumb – The surgical detachment of the great toe or second toe and microsurgical connection at the thumb site to function as the thumb.

AHA Coding Clinic® Reference Notations of Anatomical Regions, Upper Extremities

ROOT OPERATION SPECIFIC - X - ANATOMICAL REGIONS, UPPER EXTREMITIES
ALTERATION - 0
CHANGE - 2
CONTROL - 3
Control of bleeding ....AHA 16:4Q:p99
Control of post arterial bypass bleeding ....AHA 15:1Q:p35
DETACHMENT - 6
Detachment qualifiers defined ....AHA 17:2Q:p3
Excision of supernumerary digit ....AHA 17:2Q:p18
Higher level surgical amputation of traumatic amputation site ....AHA 16:3Q:p33
Official Correction to 2016:3Q:p33........AHA 17:1Q:p52
DRAINAGE - 9
EXCISION - B
INSERTION - H
Insertion of antibiotic-impregnated spacer ....AHA 17:2Q:p20
INSPECTION - J
REATTACHMENT - M
REMOVAL - P
REPAIR - Q
REPLACEMENT - R
SUPPLEMENT - U
REVISION - W
TRANSFER - X

Body Part Key Listings of Anatomical Regions, Upper Extremities

See also Body Part Key in Appendix C
None for the Anatomical Regions, Upper Extremities Body System

Device Key Listings of Anatomical Regions, Upper Extremities

See also Device Key in Appendix D
Autograft ....use Autologous Tissue Substitute
Brachytherapy seeds ....use Radioactive Element
Tissue bank graft ....use Nonautologous Tissue Substitute

Device Aggregation Table Listings of Anatomical Regions, Upper Extremities

See also Device Aggregation Table in Appendix E

Specific Device	For Operation	In Body System	General Device
None Listed in Device Aggregation Table for this Body System			

© 2018 Channel Publishing, Ltd.

Educational Annotations | X – Anatomical Regions, Upper Extremities

Coding Notes of Anatomical Regions, Upper Extremities

Body System Relevant Coding Guidelines

General Guidelines

B2.1a

The procedure codes in the general anatomical regions body systems can be used when the procedure is performed on an anatomical region rather than a specific body part (e.g., root operations Control and Detachment, Drainage of a body cavity) or on the rare occasion when no information is available to support assignment of a code to a specific body part.

Examples: Control of postoperative hemorrhage is coded to the root operation Control found in the general anatomical regions body systems.

Chest tube drainage of the pleural cavity is coded to the root operation Drainage found in the general anatomical regions body systems. Suture repair of the abdominal wall is coded to the root operation Repair in the general anatomical regions body system.

Control vs. more definitive root operations

B3.7

The root operation Control is defined as, "Stopping, or attempting to stop, postprocedural or other acute bleeding." If an attempt to stop postprocedural or other acute bleeding is unsuccessful, and to stop the bleeding requires performing a more definitive root operation, such as Bypass, Detachment, Excision, Extraction, Reposition, Replacement, or Resection, then the more definitive root operation is coded instead of Control.

Example: Resection of spleen to stop bleeding is coded to Resection instead of Control.

© 2018 Channel Publishing, Ltd.

1ST - 0 Medical and Surgical
2ND - X Anatomical Regions, Upper Extremities
3RD - 0 ALTERATION

OTHER OBJECTIVES GROUP: Alteration, (Creation), (Fusion)
Root Operations that define other objectives.

ALTERATION: Modifying the anatomic structure of a body part without affecting the function of the body part.

Explanation: Principal purpose is to improve appearance
Examples: Cosmetic shoulder augmentation – CMS Ex: Face lift

Body Part – 4TH		Approach - 5TH	Device – 6TH	Qualifier – 7TH
2 Shoulder Region, Right	9 Upper Arm, Left	0 Open	7 Autologous tissue substitute	Z No qualifier
3 Shoulder Region, Left	B Elbow Region, Right	3 Percutaneous	J Synthetic substitute	
4 Axilla, Right	C Elbow Region, Left	4 Percutaneous endoscopic	K Nonautologous tissue substitute	
5 Axilla, Left	D Lower Arm, Right		Z No device	
6 Upper Extremity, Right	F Lower Arm, Left			
7 Upper Extremity, Left	G Wrist Region, Right			
8 Upper Arm, Right	H Wrist Region, Left			

1ST - 0 Medical and Surgical
2ND - X Anatomical Regions, Upper Extremities
3RD - 2 CHANGE

DEVICE GROUP: Change, Insertion, Removal, Replacement, Revision, Supplement
Root Operations that always involve a device.

CHANGE: Taking out or off a device from a body part and putting back an identical or similar device in or on the same body part without cutting or puncturing the skin or a mucous membrane.

Explanation: All CHANGE procedures are coded using the approach External
Examples: Exchange drain tube – CMS Ex: Urinary catheter change

Body Part – 4TH	Approach – 5TH	Device – 6TH	Qualifier – 7TH
6 Upper Extremity, Right	X External	0 Drainage device	Z No qualifier
7 Upper Extremity, Left		Y Other device	

1ST - 0 Medical and Surgical
2ND - E System
3RD - 3 CONTROL

OTHER REPAIRS GROUP: Control, Repair
Root Operations that define other repairs.

CONTROL: Stopping, or attempting to stop, postprocedural or other acute bleeding.

Explanation: The site of the bleeding is coded as an anatomical region and not to a specific body part
Examples: Ligation post-op bleeder – CMS Ex: Control of bleeding duodenal ulcer

Body Part – 4TH		Approach – 5TH	Device – 6TH	Qualifier – 7TH
2 Shoulder Region, Right	B Elbow Region, Right	0 Open	Z No device	Z No qualifier
3 Shoulder Region, Left	C Elbow Region, Left	3 Percutaneous		
4 Axilla, Right	D Lower Arm, Right	4 Percutaneous endoscopic		
5 Axilla, Left	F Lower Arm, Left			
6 Upper Extremity, Right	G Wrist Region, Right			
7 Upper Extremity, Left	H Wrist Region, Left			
8 Upper Arm, Right	J Hand, Right			
9 Upper Arm, Left	K Hand, Left			

© 2018 Channel Publishing, Ltd.

1ST - 0 Medical and Surgical
2ND - X Anatomical Regions, Upper Extremities
3RD - 6 DETACHMENT

EXCISION GROUP: Excision, (Resection), (Destruction), (Extraction), Detachment
Root Operations that take out some or all of a body part.

DETACHMENT: Cutting off all or a portion of the upper or lower extremities.

Explanation: The body part value is the site of the detachment ... qualifier may specify level ...
Examples: Amputation hand – CMS Ex: Below knee amputation

Body Part – 4TH	Approach – 5TH	Device – 6TH	Qualifier – 7TH
0 Forequarter, Right 1 Forequarter, Left 2 Shoulder Region, Right 3 Shoulder Region, Left B Elbow Region, Right C Elbow Region, Left	0 Open	Z No device	Z No qualifier
8 Upper Arm, Right 9 Upper Arm, Left D Lower Arm, Right F Lower Arm, Left	0 Open	Z No device	1 High 2 Mid 3 Low
J Hand, Right K Hand, Left	0 Open	Z No device	0 Complete 4 Complete 1st Ray 5 Complete 2nd Ray 6 Complete 3rd Ray 7 Complete 4th Ray 8 Complete 5th Ray 9 Partial 1st Ray B Partial 2nd Ray C Partial 3rd Ray D Partial 4th Ray F Partial 5th Ray
L Thumb, Right M Thumb, Left N Index Finger, Right P Index Finger, Left Q Middle Finger, Right R Middle Finger, Left S Ring Finger, Right T Ring Finger, Left V Little Finger, Right W Little Finger, Left	0 Open	Z No device	0 Complete 1 High 2 Mid 3 Low

1ST - 0 Medical and Surgical
2ND - X Anatomical Regions, Upper Extremities
3RD - 9 DRAINAGE

DRAINAGE GROUP: Drainage, (Extirpation), (Fragmentation)
Root Operations that take out solids/fluids/gases from a body part.

DRAINAGE: Taking or letting out fluids and/or gases from a body part.

Explanation: Qualifier "X Diagnostic" indicates drainage procedures that are biopsies
Examples: Incision and drainage deep wound infection forearm – CMS Ex: Thoracentesis

Body Part – 4TH	Approach – 5TH	Device – 6TH	Qualifier – 7TH
2 Shoulder Region, Right 3 Shoulder Region, Left 4 Axilla, Right 5 Axilla, Left 6 Upper Extremity, Right 7 Upper Extremity, Left 8 Upper Arm, Right 9 Upper Arm, Left B Elbow Region, Right C Elbow Region, Left D Lower Arm, Right F Lower Arm, Left G Wrist Region, Right H Wrist Region, Left J Hand, Right K Hand, Left	0 Open 3 Percutaneous 4 Percutaneous endoscopic	0 Drainage device	Z No qualifier
2 Shoulder Region, Right 3 Shoulder Region, Left 4 Axilla, Right 5 Axilla, Left 6 Upper Extremity, Right 7 Upper Extremity, Left 8 Upper Arm, Right 9 Upper Arm, Left B Elbow Region, Right C Elbow Region, Left D Lower Arm, Right F Lower Arm, Left G Wrist Region, Right H Wrist Region, Left J Hand, Right K Hand, Left	0 Open 3 Percutaneous 4 Percutaneous endoscopic	Z No device	X Diagnostic Z No qualifier

© 2018 Channel Publishing, Ltd.

1ST - 0 Medical and Surgical
2ND - X Anatomical Regions, Upper Extremities
3RD - B EXCISION

EXCISION GROUP: Excision, (Resection), (Destruction), (Extraction), Detachment
Root Operations that take out some or all of a body part.

EXCISION: Cutting out or off, without replacement, a portion of a body part.

Explanation: Qualifier "X Diagnostic" indicates excision procedures that are biopsies
Examples: Excision tumor axilla region – CMS Ex: Liver biopsy

Body Part – 4TH			Approach – 5TH	Device – 6TH	Qualifier – 7TH
2 Shoulder Region, Right	8 Upper Arm, Right	G Wrist Region, Right	0 Open	Z No device	X Diagnostic
3 Shoulder Region, Left	9 Upper Arm, Left	H Wrist Region, Left	3 Percutaneous		Z No qualifier
4 Axilla, Right	B Elbow Region, Right	J Hand, Right	4 Percutaneous endoscopic		
5 Axilla, Left	C Elbow Region, Left	K Hand, Left			
6 Upper Extremity, Right	D Lower Arm, Right				
7 Upper Extremity, Left	F Lower Arm, Left				

1ST - 0 Medical and Surgical
2ND - X Anatomical Regions, Upper Extremities
3RD - H INSERTION

DEVICE GROUP: Change, Insertion, Removal, Replacement, Revision, Supplement
Root Operations that always involve a device.

INSERTION: Putting in a nonbiological appliance that monitors, assists, performs, or prevents a physiological function but does not physically take the place of a body part.

Explanation: None
Examples: Implantation infusion device – CMS Ex: Insertion of central venous catheter

Body Part – 4TH			Approach – 5TH	Device – 6TH	Qualifier – 7TH
2 Shoulder Region, Right	8 Upper Arm, Right	G Wrist Region, Right	0 Open	1 Radioactive element	Z No qualifier
3 Shoulder Region, Left	9 Upper Arm, Left	H Wrist Region, Left	3 Percutaneous	3 Infusion device	
4 Axilla, Right	B Elbow Region, Right	J Hand, Right	4 Percutaneous endoscopic	Y Other device	
5 Axilla, Left	C Elbow Region, Left	K Hand, Left			
6 Upper Extremity, Right	D Lower Arm, Right				
7 Upper Extremity, Left	F Lower Arm, Left				

1ST - 0 Medical and Surgical
2ND - X Anatomical Regions, Upper Extremities
3RD - J INSPECTION

EXAMINATION GROUP: Inspection, (Map)
Root Operations involving examination only.

INSPECTION: Visually and/or manually exploring a body part.

Explanation: Direct or instrumental visualization ...
Examples: Exploration axilla region – CMS Ex: Exploratory laparotomy

Body Part – 4TH			Approach – 5TH	Device – 6TH	Qualifier – 7TH
2 Shoulder Region, Right	8 Upper Arm, Right	G Wrist Region, Right	0 Open	Z No device	Z No qualifier
3 Shoulder Region, Left	9 Upper Arm, Left	H Wrist Region, Left	3 Percutaneous		
4 Axilla, Right	B Elbow Region, Right	J Hand, Right	4 Percutaneous endoscopic		
5 Axilla, Left	C Elbow Region, Left	K Hand, Left	X External		
6 Upper Extremity, Right	D Lower Arm, Right				
7 Upper Extremity, Left	F Lower Arm, Left				

1ST - 0 Medical and Surgical
2ND - X Anatomical Regions, Upper Extremities
3RD - M REATTACHMENT

MOVE GROUP: Reattachment, (Reposition), Transfer, Transplantation
Root Operations that put in/put back or move some/all of a body part.

REATTACHMENT: Putting back in or on all or a portion of a separated body part to its normal location or other suitable location.

Explanation: Vascular circulation and nervous pathways may or may not be reestablished
Examples: Reattachment severed thumb – CMS Ex: Reattachment of hand

Body Part – 4TH			Approach – 5TH	Device – 6TH	Qualifier – 7TH
0 Forequarter, Right	B Elbow Region, Right	N Index Finger, Right	0 Open	Z No device	Z No qualifier
1 Forequarter, Left	C Elbow Region, Left	P Index Finger, Left			
2 Shoulder Region, Right	D Lower Arm, Right	Q Middle Finger, Right			
3 Shoulder Region, Left	F Lower Arm, Left	R Middle Finger, Left			
4 Axilla, Right	G Wrist Region, Right	S Ring Finger, Right			
5 Axilla, Left	H Wrist Region, Left	T Ring Finger, Left			
6 Upper Extremity, Right	J Hand, Right	V Little Finger, Right			
7 Upper Extremity, Left	K Hand, Left	W Little Finger, Left			
8 Upper Arm, Right	L Thumb, Right				
9 Upper Arm, Left	M Thumb, Left				

© 2018 Channel Publishing, Ltd.

1ST - 0 Medical and Surgical
2ND - X Anatomical Regions, Upper Extremities
3RD - P REMOVAL

DEVICE GROUP: Change, Insertion, Removal, Replacement, Revision, Supplement
Root Operations that always involve a device.

REMOVAL: Taking out or off a device from a body part.

Explanation: Removal device without reinsertion ...
Examples: Removal drain tube – CMS Ex: Cardiac pacemaker removal

Body Part – 4TH	Approach – 5TH	Device – 6TH	Qualifier – 7TH
6 Upper Extremity, Right 7 Upper Extremity, Left	0 Open 3 Percutaneous 4 Percutaneous endoscopic X External	0 Drainage device 1 Radioactive element 3 Infusion device 7 Autologous tissue substitute J Synthetic substitute K Nonautologous tissue substitute Y Other device	Z No qualifier

1ST - 0 Medical and Surgical
2ND - X Anatomical Regions, Upper Extremities
3RD - Q REPAIR

OTHER REPAIRS GROUP: Control, Repair
Root Operations that define other repairs.

REPAIR: Restoring, to the extent possible, a body part to its normal anatomic structure and function.

Explanation: Used only when the method to accomplish the repair is not one of the other root operations
Examples: Repair forearm – CMS Ex: Suture of laceration

Body Part – 4TH			Approach – 5TH	Device – 6TH	Qualifier – 7TH
2 Shoulder Region, Right 3 Shoulder Region, Left 4 Axilla, Right 5 Axilla, Left 6 Upper Extremity, Right 7 Upper Extremity, Left 8 Upper Arm, Right 9 Upper Arm, Left B Elbow Region, Right C Elbow Region, Left	D Lower Arm, Right F Lower Arm, Left G Wrist Region, Right H Wrist Region, Left J Hand, Right K Hand, Left L Thumb, Right M Thumb, Left	N Index Finger, Right P Index Finger, Left Q Middle Finger, Right R Middle Finger, Left S Ring Finger, Right T Ring Finger, Left V Little Finger, Right W Little Finger, Left	0 Open 3 Percutaneous 4 Percutaneous endoscopic X External	Z No device	Z No qualifier

1ST - 0 Medical and Surgical
2ND - X Anatomical Regions, Upper Extremities
3RD - R REPLACEMENT

DEVICE GROUP: Change, Insertion, Removal, Replacement, Revision, Supplement
Root Operations that always involve a device.

REPLACEMENT: Putting in or on biological or synthetic material that physically takes the place and/or function of all or a portion of a body part.

Explanation: Includes taking out or eradicating, or rendering non-functional, the body part ...
Examples: Replacement thumb with toe – CMS Ex: Total hip replacement

Body Part – 4TH	Approach – 5TH	Device – 6TH	Qualifier – 7TH
L Thumb, Right M Thumb, Left	0 Open 4 Percutaneous endoscopic	7 Autologous tissue substitute	N Toe, Right P Toe, Left

© 2018 Channel Publishing, Ltd.

1ST - 0 Medical and Surgical
2ND - X Anatomical Regions, Upper Extremities
3RD - U SUPPLEMENT

DEVICE GROUP: Change, Insertion, Removal, Replacement, Revision, Supplement
Root Operations that always involve a device.

SUPPLEMENT: Putting in or on biological or synthetic material that physically reinforces and/or augments the function of a portion of a body part.

Explanation: Biological material is non-living, or is living and from the same individual ...
Examples: Augmentation graft axilla – CMS Ex: Herniorrhaphy using mesh

Body Part – 4TH			Approach – 5TH	Device – 6TH	Qualifier – 7TH
2 Shoulder Region, Right 3 Shoulder Region, Left 4 Axilla, Right 5 Axilla, Left 6 Upper Extremity, Right 7 Upper Extremity, Left 8 Upper Arm, Right 9 Upper Arm, Left B Elbow Region, Right C Elbow Region, Left	D Lower Arm, Right F Lower Arm, Left G Wrist Region, Right H Wrist Region, Left J Hand, Right K Hand, Left L Thumb, Right M Thumb, Left	N Index Finger, Right P Index Finger, Left Q Middle Finger, Right R Middle Finger, Left S Ring Finger, Right T Ring Finger, Left V Little Finger, Right W Little Finger, Left	0 Open 4 Percutaneous endoscopic	7 Autologous tissue substitute J Synthetic substitute K Nonautologous tissue substitute	Z No qualifier

1ST - 0 Medical and Surgical
2ND - X Anatomical Regions, Upper Extremities
3RD - W REVISION

DEVICE GROUP: Change, Insertion, Removal, Replacement, Revision, Supplement
Root Operations that always involve a device.

REVISION: Correcting, to the extent possible, a portion of a malfunctioning device or the position of a displaced device.

Explanation: Correcting by taking out or putting in components of a device such as a screw or pin ...
Examples: Reposition drain tube – CMS Ex: Recementing of hip prosthesis

Body Part – 4TH	Approach – 5TH	Device – 6TH	Qualifier – 7TH
6 Upper Extremity, Right 7 Upper Extremity, Left	0 Open 3 Percutaneous 4 Percutaneous endoscopic X External	0 Drainage device 3 Infusion device 7 Autologous tissue substitute J Synthetic substitute K Nonautologous tissue substitute Y Other device	Z No qualifier

1ST - 0 Medical and Surgical
2ND - X Anatomical Regions, Upper Extremities
3RD - X TRANSFER

MOVE GROUP: Reattachment, (Reposition), Transfer, Transplantation
Root Operations that put in/put back or move some/all of a body part.

TRANSFER: Moving, without taking out, all or a portion of a body part to another location to take over the function of all or a portion of a body part.

Explanation: The body part transferred remains connected to its vascular and nervous supply
Examples: Transfer index finger to thumb – CMS Ex: Tendon transfer

Body Part – 4TH	Approach – 5TH	Device – 6TH	Qualifier – 7TH
N Index Finger, Right	0 Open	Z No device	L Thumb, Right
P Index Finger, Left	0 Open	Z No device	M Thumb, Left

1ST - 0 Medical and Surgical
2ND - X Anatomical Regions, Upper Extremities
3RD - Y TRANSPLANTATION

MOVE GROUP: Reattachment, (Reposition), Transfer, Transplantation
Root Operations that put in/put back or move some/all of a body part.

TRANSPLANTATION: Putting in or on all or a portion of a living body part taken from another individual or animal to physically take the place and/or function of all or a portion of a similar body part.

Explanation: The native body part may or may not be taken out ...
Examples: Hand transplantation – CMS Ex: Kidney transplant

Body Part – 4TH	Approach – 5TH	Device – 6TH	Qualifier – 7TH
J Hand, Right K Hand, Left	0 Open	Z No device	0 Allogeneic 1 Syngeneic

© 2018 Channel Publishing, Ltd.

Educational Annotations | Y – Anatomical Regions, Lower Extremities

Body System Specific Educational Annotations for the Anatomical Regions, Lower Extremities include:

- Anatomy and Physiology Review
- Anatomical Illustrations
- Definitions of Common Procedures
- AHA Coding Clinic® Reference Notations
- Body Part Key Listings
- Device Key Listings
- Device Aggregation Table Listings
- Coding Notes

Anatomy and Physiology Review of Anatomical Regions, Lower Extremities

BODY PART VALUES – Y - ANATOMICAL REGIONS, LOWER EXTREMITIES

Coding Guideline B2.1a - Body System, General Guideline – The procedure codes in the general anatomical regions body systems can be used when the procedure is performed on an anatomical region rather than a specific body part (e.g., root operations Control and Detachment, Drainage of a body cavity) or on the rare occasion when no information is available to support assignment of a code to a specific body part.
Examples: Control of postoperative hemorrhage is coded to the root operation Control found in the general anatomical regions body systems. Chest tube drainage of the pleural cavity is coded to the root operation Drainage found in the general anatomical regions body systems. Suture repair of the abdominal wall is coded to the root operation Repair in the general anatomical regions body system.

1st Ray – The first digit of the foot and its associated first metatarsal bone.
2nd Ray – The second digit of the foot and its associated second metatarsal bone.
3rd Ray – The third digit of the foot and its associated third metatarsal bone.
4th Ray – The fourth digit of the foot and its associated fourth metatarsal bone.
5th Ray – The fifth digit of the foot and its associated fifth metatarsal bone.
1st Toe – The first digit of the foot.
2nd Toe – The second digit of the foot.
3rd Toe – The third digit of the foot.
4th Toe – The fourth digit of the foot.
5th Toe – The fifth digit of the foot.
Ankle Region – The multi-tissue-layered ankle joint area.
Buttock – The rounded lower portions of the posterior trunk including the gluteus muscles.
Femoral Region – The multi-tissue-layered area of the anterior upper inner portion of the thigh (also known as the femoral triangle). See also the body part "Upper Leg."
Foot – The portion of the lower extermity distal to the lower end of the tibia and fibula.
Hindquarter – The portion of the body including the lower extremity, buttock, and pelvis.
Inguinal Region – The multi-tissue-layered area between the lower abdomen, thigh, and pubic bone.
Knee Region – The multi-tissue-layered knee joint area.
Lower Extremity – The entire lower extremity (leg).
Lower Leg – The portion of the lower extermity distal to the knee.
Upper Leg – The portion of the lower extermity distal to the hip and proximal to the knee.

Anatomical Illustrations of Anatomical Regions, Lower Extremities

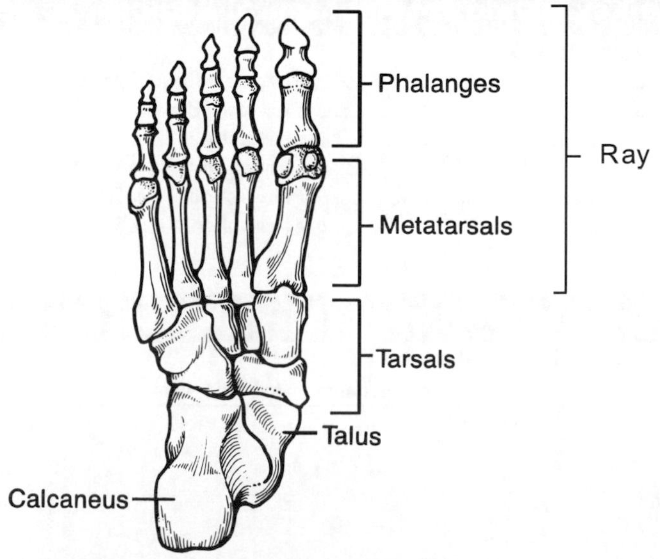

RIGHT FOOT — PLANTAR VIEW

© 2018 Channel Publishing, Ltd.

Educational Annotations | Y – Anatomical Regions, Lower Extremities

Definitions of Common Procedures of Anatomical Regions, Lower Extremities

Buttock implants – The plastic surgical enhancement of the buttocks usually using solid silicone implants or by fat transfers.
Hindquarter amputation – The surgical detachment and removal of the entire leg including part or all of the buttock and pelvis.
Midfoot amputation – The surgical detachment and removal of the distal foot that is performed through the tarsal-metatarsal joints.

AHA Coding Clinic® Reference Notations of Anatomical Regions, Lower Extremities

ROOT OPERATION SPECIFIC - Y - ANATOMICAL REGIONS, LOWER EXTREMITIES

ALTERATION - 0
CHANGE - 2
CONTROL - 3
- Control of bleeding .... AHA 16:4Q:p99

DETACHMENT - 6
- Amputation of 1st toe at the interphalangeal joint .... AHA 15:2Q:p2
- Chopart amputation of foot .... AHA 17:1Q:p22
- Detachment qualifiers defined .... AHA 17:2Q:p3
- Midfoot amputation .... AHA 15:1Q:p28

DRAINAGE - 9
- Incision and drainage of femoral region wound infection .... AHA 15:1Q:p22
- Incision and drainage of inguinal region wound infection .... AHA 15:1Q:p22

EXCISION - B
INSERTION - H
INSPECTION - J
REATTACHMENT - M
REMOVAL - P
REPAIR - Q
SUPPLEMENT - U
REVISION - W

Body Part Key Listings of Anatomical Regions, Lower Extremities

See also Body Part Key in Appendix C

Hallux .... use 1st Toe, Left/Right
Inguinal canal .... use Inguinal Region, Bilateral/Left/Right
Inguinal triangle .... use Inguinal Region, Bilateral/Left/Right

Device Key Listings of Anatomical Regions, Lower Extremities

See also Device Key in Appendix D

Autograft .... use Autologous Tissue Substitute
Brachytherapy seeds .... use Radioactive Element
Cook Biodesign® Hernia Graft(s) .... use Nonautologous Tissue Substitute
Cook Biodesign® Layered Graft(s) .... use Nonautologous Tissue Substitute
Cook Zenapro™ Layered Graft(s) .... use Nonautologous Tissue Substitute
Tissue bank graft .... use Nonautologous Tissue Substitute

Device Aggregation Table Listings of Anatomical Regions, Lower Extremities

See also Device Aggregation Table in Appendix E

Specific Device	For Operation	In Body System	General Device
None Listed in Device Aggregation Table for this Body System			

© 2018 Channel Publishing, Ltd.

Educational Annotations | Y – Anatomical Regions, Lower Extremities

Coding Notes of Anatomical Regions, Lower Extremities

Body System Relevant Coding Guidelines

General Guidelines

B2.1a

The procedure codes in the general anatomical regions body systems can be used when the procedure is performed on an anatomical region rather than a specific body part (e.g., root operations Control and Detachment, Drainage of a body cavity) or on the rare occasion when no information is available to support assignment of a code to a specific body part.

Examples: Control of postoperative hemorrhage is coded to the root operation Control found in the general anatomical regions body systems.

Chest tube drainage of the pleural cavity is coded to the root operation Drainage found in the general anatomical regions body systems. Suture repair of the abdominal wall is coded to the root operation Repair in the general anatomical regions body system.

Control vs. more definitive root operations

B3.7

The root operation Control is defined as, "Stopping, or attempting to stop, postprocedural or other acute bleeding." If an attempt to stop postprocedural or other acute bleeding is unsuccessful, and to stop the bleeding requires performing a more definitive root operation, such as Bypass, Detachment, Excision, Extraction, Reposition, Replacement, or Resection, then the more definitive root operation is coded instead of Control.

Example: Resection of spleen to stop bleeding is coded to Resection instead of Control.

© 2018 Channel Publishing, Ltd.

1ST - 0 Medical and Surgical
2ND - Y Anatomical Regions, Lower Extremities
3RD - 0 ALTERATION

OTHER OBJECTIVES GROUP: Alteration, (Creation), (Fusion)
Root Operations that define other objectives.

ALTERATION: Modifying the anatomic structure of a body part without affecting the function of the body part.

Explanation: Principal purpose is to improve appearance
Examples: Cosmetic buttock augmentation – CMS Ex: Face lift

Body Part – 4TH		Approach – 5TH	Device – 6TH	Qualifier – 7TH
0 Buttock, Right 1 Buttock, Left 9 Lower Extremity, Right B Lower Extremity, Left C Upper Leg, Right D Upper Leg, Left	F Knee Region, Right G Knee Region, Left H Lower Leg, Right J Lower Leg, Left K Ankle Region, Right L Ankle Region, Left	0 Open 3 Percutaneous 4 Percutaneous endoscopic	7 Autologous tissue substitute J Synthetic substitute K Nonautologous tissue substitute Z No device	Z No qualifier

1ST - 0 Medical and Surgical
2ND - Y Anatomical Regions, Lower Extremities
3RD - 2 CHANGE

DEVICE GROUP: Change, Insertion, Removal, (Replacement), Revision, Supplement
Root Operations that always involve a device.

CHANGE: Taking out or off a device from a body part and putting back an identical or similar device in or on the same body part without cutting or puncturing the skin or a mucous membrane.

Explanation: All CHANGE procedures are coded using the approach External
Examples: Exchange drain tube – CMS Ex: Urinary catheter change

Body Part – 4TH	Approach – 5TH	Device – 6TH	Qualifier – 7TH
9 Lower Extremity, Right B Lower Extremity, Left	X External	0 Drainage device Y Other device	Z No qualifier

1ST - 0 Medical and Surgical
2ND - Y Anatomical Regions, Lower Extremities
3RD - 3 CONTROL

OTHER REPAIRS GROUP: Control, Repair
Root Operations that define other repairs.

CONTROL: Stopping, or attempting to stop, postprocedural or other acute bleeding.

Explanation: The site of the bleeding is coded as an anatomical region and not to a specific body part
Examples: Ligation post-op bleeder – CMS Ex: Control of bleeding duodenal ulcer

Body Part – 4TH			Approach – 5TH	Device – 6TH	Qualifier – 7TH
0 Buttock, Right 1 Buttock, Left 5 Inguinal Region, Right 6 Inguinal Region, Left 7 Femoral Region, Right 8 Femoral Region, Left	9 Lower Extremity, Right B Lower Extremity, Left C Upper Leg, Right D Upper Leg, Left F Knee Region, Right G Knee Region, Left	H Lower Leg, Right J Lower Leg, Left K Ankle Region, Right L Ankle Region, Left M Foot, Right N Foot, Left	0 Open 3 Percutaneous 4 Percutaneous endoscopic	Z No device	Z No qualifier

© 2018 Channel Publishing, Ltd.

1ST - 0 Medical and Surgical
2ND - Y Anatomical Regions, Lower Extremities
3RD - 6 DETACHMENT

EXCISION GROUP: Excision, (Resection), (Destruction), (Extraction), Detachment
Root Operations that take out some or all of a body part.

DETACHMENT: Cutting off all or a portion of the upper or lower extremities.

Explanation: The body part value is the site of the detachment ... qualifier may specify level ...
Examples: Below knee amputation – CMS Ex: Below knee amputation

Body Part – 4TH	Approach – 5TH	Device – 6TH	Qualifier – 7TH
2 Hindquarter, Right 3 Hindquarter, Left 4 Hindquarter, Bilateral 7 Femoral Region, Right 8 Femoral Region, Left F Knee Region, Right G Knee Region, Left	0 Open	Z No device	Z No qualifier
C Upper Leg, Right D Upper Leg, Left H Lower Leg, Right J Lower Leg, Left	0 Open	Z No device	1 High 2 Mid 3 Low
M Foot, Right N Foot, Left	0 Open	Z No device	0 Complete 4 Complete 1st Ray 5 Complete 2nd Ray 6 Complete 3rd Ray 7 Complete 4th Ray 8 Complete 5th Ray 9 Partial 1st Ray B Partial 2nd Ray C Partial 3rd Ray D Partial 4th Ray F Partial 5th Ray
P 1st Toe, Right Q 1st Toe, Left R 2nd Toe, Right S 2nd Toe, Left T 3rd Toe, Right U 3rd Toe, Left V 4th Toe, Right W 4th Toe, Left X 5th Toe, Right Y 5th Toe, Left	0 Open	Z No device	0 Complete 1 High 2 Mid 3 Low

1ST - 0 Medical and Surgical
2ND - Y Anatomical Regions, Lower Extremities
3RD - 9 DRAINAGE

DRAINAGE GROUP: Drainage, (Extirpation), (Fragmentation)
Root Operations that take out solids/fluids/gases from a body part.

DRAINAGE: Taking or letting out fluids and/or gases from a body part.

Explanation: Qualifier "X Diagnostic" indicates drainage procedures that are biopsies
Examples: Incision and drainage deep wound infection – CMS Ex: Thoracentesis

Body Part – 4TH	Approach – 5TH	Device – 6TH	Qualifier – 7TH
0 Buttock, Right 1 Buttock, Left 5 Inguinal Region, Right 6 Inguinal Region, Left 7 Femoral Region, Right 8 Femoral Region, Left 9 Lower Extremity, Right B Lower Extremity, Left C Upper Leg, Right D Upper Leg, Left F Knee Region, Right G Knee Region, Left H Lower Leg, Right J Lower Leg, Left K Ankle Region, Right L Ankle Region, Left M Foot, Right N Foot, Left	0 Open 3 Percutaneous 4 Percutaneous endoscopic	0 Drainage device	Z No qualifier
0 Buttock, Right 1 Buttock, Left 5 Inguinal Region, Right 6 Inguinal Region, Left 7 Femoral Region, Right 8 Femoral Region, Left 9 Lower Extremity, Right B Lower Extremity, Left C Upper Leg, Right D Upper Leg, Left F Knee Region, Right G Knee Region, Left H Lower Leg, Right J Lower Leg, Left K Ankle Region, Right L Ankle Region, Left M Foot, Right N Foot, Left	0 Open 3 Percutaneous 4 Percutaneous endoscopic	Z No device	X Diagnostic Z No qualifier

© 2018 Channel Publishing, Ltd.

1ST - 0 Medical and Surgical
2ND - Y Anatomical Regions, Lower Extremities
3RD - B EXCISION

EXCISION GROUP: Excision, (Resection), (Destruction), (Extraction), Detachment
Root Operations that take out some or all of a body part.

EXCISION: Cutting out or off, without replacement, a portion of a body part.

Explanation: Qualifier "X Diagnostic" indicates excision procedures that are biopsies
Examples: Excision tumor inguinal region – CMS Ex: Liver biopsy

Body Part – 4TH			Approach – 5TH	Device – 6TH	Qualifier – 7TH
0 Buttock, Right	9 Lower Extremity, Right	H Lower Leg, Right	0 Open	Z No device	X Diagnostic
1 Buttock, Left	B Lower Extremity, Left	J Lower Leg, Left	3 Percutaneous		Z No qualifier
5 Inguinal Region, Right	C Upper Leg, Right	K Ankle Region, Right	4 Percutaneous endoscopic		
6 Inguinal Region, Left	D Upper Leg, Left	L Ankle Region, Left			
7 Femoral Region, Right	F Knee Region, Right	M Foot, Right			
8 Femoral Region, Left	G Knee Region, Left	N Foot, Left			

1ST - 0 Medical and Surgical
2ND - Y Anatomical Regions, Lower Extremities
3RD - H INSERTION

DEVICE GROUP: Change, Insertion, Removal, (Replacement), Revision, Supplement
Root Operations that always involve a device.

INSERTION: Putting in a nonbiological appliance that monitors, assists, performs, or prevents a physiological function but does not physically take the place of a body part.

Explanation: None
Examples: Implantation infusion device – CMS Ex: Insertion of central venous catheter

Body Part – 4TH			Approach – 5TH	Device – 6TH	Qualifier – 7TH
0 Buttock, Right	9 Lower Extremity, Right	H Lower Leg, Right	0 Open	1 Radioactive element	Z No qualifier
1 Buttock, Left	B Lower Extremity, Left	J Lower Leg, Left	3 Percutaneous	3 Infusion device	
5 Inguinal Region, Right	C Upper Leg, Right	K Ankle Region, Right	4 Percutaneous endoscopic	Y Other device	
6 Inguinal Region, Left	D Upper Leg, Left	L Ankle Region, Left			
7 Femoral Region, Right	F Knee Region, Right	M Foot, Right			
8 Femoral Region, Left	G Knee Region, Left	N Foot, Left			

1ST - 0 Medical and Surgical
2ND - Y Anatomical Regions, Lower Extremities
3RD - J INSPECTION

EXAMINATION GROUP: Inspection, (Map)
Root Operations involving examination only.

INSPECTION: Visually and/or manually exploring a body part.

Explanation: Direct or instrumental visualization ...
Examples: Exploration femoral region – CMS Ex: Exploratory laparotomy

Body Part – 4TH			Approach – 5TH	Device – 6TH	Qualifier – 7TH
0 Buttock, Right	A Inguinal Region, Bilateral	F Knee Region, Right	0 Open	Z No device	Z No qualifier
1 Buttock, Left	B Lower Extremity, Left	G Knee Region, Left	3 Percutaneous		
5 Inguinal Region, Right	C Upper Leg, Right	H Lower Leg, Right	4 Percutaneous endoscopic		
6 Inguinal Region, Left	D Upper Leg, Left	J Lower Leg, Left	X External		
7 Femoral Region, Right	E Femoral Region, Bilateral	K Ankle Region, Right			
8 Femoral Region, Left		L Ankle Region, Left			
9 Lower Extremity, Right		M Foot, Right			
		N Foot, Left			

© 2018 Channel Publishing, Ltd.

1ST - 0 Medical and Surgical
2ND - Y Anatomical Regions, Lower Extremities
3RD - M REATTACHMENT

MOVE GROUP: Reattachment, (Reposition), (Transfer), (Transplantation)
Root Operations that put in/put back or move some/all of a body part.

REATTACHMENT: Putting back in or on all or a portion of a separated body part to its normal location or other suitable location.

Explanation: Vascular circulation and nervous pathways may or may not be reestablished
Examples: Reattachment severed 1st toe – CMS Ex: Reattachment of hand

Body Part – 4TH			Approach – 5TH	Device – 6TH	Qualifier – 7TH
0 Buttock, Right	C Upper Leg, Right	P 1st Toe, Right	0 Open	Z No device	Z No qualifier
1 Buttock, Left	D Upper Leg, Left	Q 1st Toe, Left			
2 Hindquarter, Right	F Knee Region, Right	R 2nd Toe, Right			
3 Hindquarter, Left	G Knee Region, Left	S 2nd Toe, Left			
4 Hindquarter, Bilateral	H Lower Leg, Right	T 3rd Toe, Right			
5 Inguinal Region, Right	J Lower Leg, Left	U 3rd Toe, Left			
6 Inguinal Region, Left	K Ankle Region, Right	V 4th Toe, Right			
7 Femoral Region, Right	L Ankle Region, Left	W 4th Toe, Left			
8 Femoral Region, Left	M Foot, Right	X 5th Toe, Right			
9 Lower Extremity, Right	N Foot, Left	Y 5th Toe, Left			
B Lower Extremity, Left					

1ST - 0 Medical and Surgical
2ND - Y Anatomical Regions, Lower Extremities
3RD - P REMOVAL

DEVICE GROUP: Change, Insertion, Removal, (Replacement), Revision, Supplement
Root Operations that always involve a device.

REMOVAL: Taking out or off a device from a body part.

Explanation: Removal device without reinsertion ...
Examples: Removal drain tube – CMS Ex: Cardiac pacemaker removal

Body Part – 4TH	Approach – 5TH	Device – 6TH	Qualifier – 7TH
9 Lower Extremity, Right	0 Open	0 Drainage device	Z No qualifier
B Lower Extremity, Left	3 Percutaneous	1 Radioactive element	
	4 Percutaneous endoscopic	3 Infusion device	
	X External	7 Autologous tissue substitute	
		J Synthetic substitute	
		K Nonautologous tissue substitute	
		Y Other device	

1ST - 0 Medical and Surgical
2ND - Y Anatomical Regions, Lower Extremities
3RD - Q REPAIR

OTHER REPAIRS GROUP: Control, Repair
Root Operations that define other repairs.

REPAIR: Restoring, to the extent possible, a body part to its normal anatomic structure and function.

Explanation: Used only when the method to accomplish the repair is not one of the other root operations
Examples: Inguinal hernia repair using sutures – CMS Ex: Suture of laceration

Body Part – 4TH			Approach – 5TH	Device – 6TH	Qualifier – 7TH
0 Buttock, Right	D Upper Leg, Left	P 1st Toe, Right	0 Open	Z No device	Z No qualifier
1 Buttock, Left	E Femoral Region, Bilateral	Q 1st Toe, Left	3 Percutaneous		
5 Inguinal Region, Right	F Knee Region, Right	R 2nd Toe, Right	4 Percutaneous endoscopic		
6 Inguinal Region, Left	G Knee Region, Left	S 2nd Toe, Left	X External		
7 Femoral Region, Right	H Lower Leg, Right	T 3rd Toe, Right			
8 Femoral Region, Left	J Lower Leg, Left	U 3rd Toe, Left			
9 Lower Extremity, Right	K Ankle Region, Right	V 4th Toe, Right			
A Inguinal Region, Bilateral	L Ankle Region, Left	W 4th Toe, Left			
B Lower Extremity, Left	M Foot, Right	X 5th Toe, Right			
C Upper Leg, Right	N Foot, Left	Y 5th Toe, Left			

REGIONS LOWER EXT 0 Y Q

© 2018 Channel Publishing, Ltd.

1ST - 0 Medical and Surgical
2ND - Y Anatomical Regions, Lower Extremities
3RD - U SUPPLEMENT

DEVICE GROUP: Change, Insertion, Removal, (Replacement), Revision, Supplement
Root Operations that always involve a device.

SUPPLEMENT: Putting in or on biological or synthetic material that physically reinforces and/or augments the function of a portion of a body part.

Explanation: Biological material is non-living, or is living and from the same individual ...
Examples: Inguinal hernia repair with mesh – CMS Ex: Herniorrhaphy using mesh

Body Part – 4TH			Approach – 5TH	Device – 6TH	Qualifier – 7TH
0 Buttock, Right 1 Buttock, Left 5 Inguinal Region, Right 6 Inguinal Region, Left 7 Femoral Region, Right 8 Femoral Region, Left 9 Lower Extremity, Right A Inguinal Region, Bilateral B Lower Extremity, Left C Upper Leg, Right	D Upper Leg, Left E Femoral Region, Bilateral F Knee Region, Right G Knee Region, Left H Lower Leg, Right J Lower Leg, Left K Ankle Region, Right L Ankle Region, Left M Foot, Right N Foot, Left	P 1st Toe, Right Q 1st Toe, Left R 2nd Toe, Right S 2nd Toe, Left T 3rd Toe, Right U 3rd Toe, Left V 4th Toe, Right W 4th Toe, Left X 5th Toe, Right Y 5th Toe, Left	0 Open 4 Percutaneous endoscopic	7 Autologous tissue substitute J Synthetic substitute K Nonautologous tissue substitute	Z No qualifier

1ST - 0 Medical and Surgical
2ND - Y Anatomical Regions, Lower Extremities
3RD - W REVISION

DEVICE GROUP: Change, Insertion, Removal, (Replacement), Revision, Supplement
Root Operations that always involve a device.

REVISION: Correcting, to the extent possible, a portion of a malfunctioning device or the position of a displaced device.

Explanation: Correcting by taking out or putting in components of a device such as a screw or pin ...
Examples: Reposition drain tube – CMS Ex: Recementing of hip prosthesis

Body Part – 4TH	Approach – 5TH	Device – 6TH	Qualifier – 7TH
9 Lower Extremity, Right B Lower Extremity, Left	0 Open 3 Percutaneous 4 Percutaneous endoscopic X External	0 Drainage device 3 Infusion device 7 Autologous tissue substitute J Synthetic substitute K Nonautologous tissue substitute Y Other device	Z No qualifier

© 2018 Channel Publishing, Ltd.

Educational Annotations

Section 1 – Obstetrics

Section Specific Educational Annotations for the Obstetrics Section include:

- Anatomy and Physiology Review
- Anatomical Illustrations
- AHA Coding Clinic® Reference Notations
- Definitions of Common Procedures
- Body Part Key Listings
- Device Key Listings
- Device Aggregation Table Listings
- Coding Notes

Anatomy and Physiology Review of Obstetrics

BODY PART VALUES – 0 - Obstetrics

Products of Conception – The fetus, placenta, and other tissue derived from a fertilized gestation.
Products of Conception, Ectopic – Products of conception that develop outside the uterus.
Products of Conception, Retained – Products of conception that remain in the uterus following delivery, termination of pregnancy, or miscarriage.

Anatomical Illustrations of Obstetrics

None for the Obstetrics Section

AHA Coding Clinic® Reference Notations of Obstetrics

ROOT OPERATION SPECIFIC - OBSTETRICS - Section 1

MISC
- Induction of labor, IV oxytocin, peripheral vein ....AHA 14:4Q:p17
- Induction of labor with Cervidil dinoprostone vaginal tampon ....AHA 14:2Q:p8
- Pitocin to augment active labor ....AHA 14:2Q:p9

CHANGE - 2

DRAINAGE - 9
- Artificial rupture of membranes ....AHA 14:2Q:p9
- Laser microseptostomy for twin-twin transfusion syndrome ....AHA 14:3Q:p12

ABORTION - A

EXTRACTION - D
- Cesarean section with vacuum assistance ....AHA 14:4Q:p43
- High transverse cesarean delivery ....AHA 18:2Q:p17
- Vacuum assisted low forceps delivery ....AHA 16:1Q:p9
- Vacuum D&C for blighted ovum ....AHA 14:4Q:p43

DELIVERY - E
- Assisted vaginal delivery ....AHA 14:2Q:p9
- Delivery of placenta after birth outside hospital ....AHA 17:3Q:p5
- Manually assisted vaginal delivery ....AHA 16:2Q:p34

INSERTION - H
- Intrauterine pressure monitoring during labor ....AHA 13:2Q:p36

INSPECTION - J

REMOVAL - P

REPAIR - Q
- Fetoscopic laser photocoagulation of vascular connections ....AHA 14:3Q:p12

REPOSITION - S

RESECTION - T
- Excision/removal of fallopian tube ectopic pregnancy ....AHA 15:3Q:p31

TRANSPLANTATION - Y

OBSTETRICS 1

© 2018 Channel Publishing, Ltd.

Educational Annotations | Section 1 – Obstetrics

Definitions of Common Procedures of Obstetrics

Amniocentesis – The medical procedure of inserting a needle with ultrasound guidance through the abdominal wall and uterine wall, and then puncturing the amniotic sac to withdraw a small amount of amniotic fluid that is used for testing for fetal abnormalities, usually done early in the second trimester.

Amnioscopy – The instrumental visualization of the fetus and lower amniotic sac by using an amnioscope that is inserted into the vaginal canal and used in late pregnancy or during labor.

Cesarean section (C-section) – The surgical delivery of the fetus through an incision in the uterine wall. The classical c-section incision is a vertical incision in the abdomen and in the mid to upper portion of the uterus. The low cervical c-section incision is a transverse (horizontal) or vertical incision in the abdomen just above the pubis and in the lower portion of the uterus just above the cervix.

Forceps-assisted vaginal delivery – The use of special tools that are curved and shallow cup-shaped to assist delivering a fetus that is having difficulty passing through the birth canal. The descriptions of low, mid, or high forceps are based on the stage of fetal head engagement and station of progress entering and passing through the birth canal.

Removal of tubal pregnancy – The open or laparoscopic-approach surgical removal of an ectopic pregnancy (embryo attaches outside the uterus) that is attached in a fallopian tube. The fallopian tube may be incised (salpingostomy) or a segment may need to be excised (salpingectomy).

Vacuum-assisted vaginal delivery – The use of a special vacuum extractor with a soft plastic cup that attaches to the fetal head with suction to help deliver the fetus through the birth canal.

Body Part Key Listings of Obstetrics

None for the Obstetrics Section

Device Key Listings of Obstetrics

None for the Obstetrics Section

Device Aggregation Table Listings of Obstetrics

None for the Obstetrics Section

Coding Notes of Obstetrics

Body System Relevant Coding Guidelines

C. Obstetrics Section

Products of conception

C1

Procedures performed on the products of conception are coded to the Obstetrics section. Procedures performed on the pregnant female other than the products of conception are coded to the appropriate root operation in the Medical and Surgical section.

Examples: Amniocentesis is coded to the products of conception body part in the Obstetrics section.
Repair of obstetric urethral laceration is coded to the urethra body part in the Medical and Surgical section.

Procedures following delivery or abortion

C2

Procedures performed following a delivery or abortion for curettage of the endometrium or evacuation of retained products of conception are all coded in the Obstetrics section, to the root operation Extraction and the body part Products of Conception, Retained. Diagnostic or therapeutic dilation and curettage performed during times other than the postpartum or post-abortion period are all coded in the Medical and Surgical section, to the root operation Extraction and the body part Endometrium.

© 2018 Channel Publishing, Ltd.

1ST - 1 Obstetrics
2ND - 0 Pregnancy ♀
3RD - 2 CHANGE

OBSTETRICS SECTION: Change, Drainage, Abortion, Extraction, Delivery, Insertion, Inspection, Removal, Repair, Reposition, Resection, Transplantation
Root Operations that are performed on the products of conception.

CHANGE: Taking out or off a device from a body part and putting back an identical or similar device in or on the same body part without cutting or puncturing the skin or a mucous membrane.

Explanation: None Example: Exchanging intrauterine pressure monitor

Body Part – 4TH	Approach – 5TH	Device – 6TH	Qualifier – 7TH
0 Products of Conception	7 Via natural or artificial opening	3 Monitoring electrode Y Other device	Z No qualifier

1ST - 1 Obstetrics
2ND - 0 Pregnancy ♀
3RD - 9 DRAINAGE

OBSTETRICS SECTION: Change, Drainage, Abortion, Extraction, Delivery, Insertion, Inspection, Removal, Repair, Reposition, Resection, Transplantation
Root Operations that are performed on the products of conception.

DRAINAGE: Taking or letting out fluids and/or gases from a body part.

Explanation: Qualifier identifies type of fluid Example: Amniocentesis

Body Part – 4TH	Approach – 5TH	Device – 6TH	Qualifier – 7TH
0 Products of Conception	0 Open 3 Percutaneous 4 Percutaneous endoscopic 7 Via natural or artificial opening 8 Via natural or artificial opening endoscopic	Z No device	9 Fetal blood A Fetal cerebrospinal fluid B Fetal fluid, other C Amniotic fluid, therapeutic D Fluid, other U Amniotic fluid, diagnostic

1ST - 1 Obstetrics
2ND - 0 Pregnancy ♀
3RD - A ABORTION

OBSTETRICS SECTION: Change, Drainage, Abortion, Extraction, Delivery, Insertion, Inspection, Removal, Repair, Reposition, Resection, Transplantation
Root Operations that are performed on the products of conception.

ABORTION: Artificially terminating a pregnancy.

Explanation: None Example: Therapeutic abortion

Body Part – 4TH	Approach – 5TH	Device – 6TH	Qualifier – 7TH
0 Products of Conception	0 Open 3 Percutaneous 4 Percutaneous endoscopic 8 Via natural or artificial opening endoscopic	Z No device	Z No qualifier
0 Products of Conception	7 Via natural or artificial opening	Z No device	6 Vacuum W Laminaria X Abortifacient Z No qualifier

© 2018 Channel Publishing, Ltd.

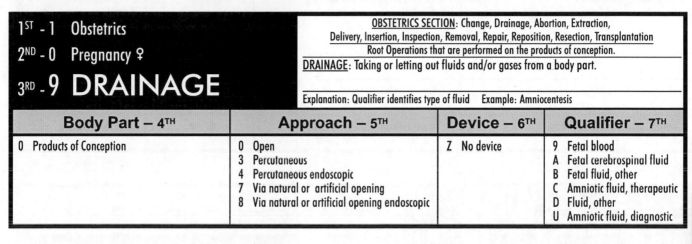

1ST - 1 Obstetrics
2ND - 0 Pregnancy ♀
3RD - D EXTRACTION

OBSTETRICS SECTION: Change, Drainage, Abortion, Extraction, Delivery, Insertion, Inspection, Removal, Repair, Reposition, Resection, Transplantation Root Operations that are performed on the products of conception.

EXTRACTION: Pulling or stripping out or off all or a portion of a body part by the use of force.

Explanation: Qualifier identifies type of instrumentation/assistance Example: Cesarean delivery

Body Part – 4TH	Approach – 5TH	Device – 6TH	Qualifier – 7TH
0 Products of Conception	0 Open	Z No device	0 High 1 Low 2 Extraperitoneal
0 Products of Conception	7 Via natural or artificial opening	Z No device	3 Low forceps 4 Mid forceps 5 High forceps 6 Vacuum 7 Internal version 8 Other
1 Products of Conception, Retained	7 Via natural or artificial opening 8 Via natural or artificial opening endoscopic	Z No device	9 Manual Z No qualifier
2 Products of Conception, Ectopic	7 Via natural or artificial opening 8 Via natural or artificial opening endoscopic	Z No device	Z No qualifier

1ST - 1 Obstetrics
2ND - 0 Pregnancy ♀
3RD - E DELIVERY

OBSTETRICS SECTION: Change, Drainage, Abortion, Extraction, Delivery, Insertion, Inspection, Removal, Repair, Reposition, Resection, Transplantation Root Operations that are performed on the products of conception.

DELIVERY: Assisting the passage of the products of conception from the genital canal.

Explanation: Manually assisted delivery without instruments Example: Vaginal delivery

Body Part – 4TH	Approach – 5TH	Device – 6TH	Qualifier – 7TH
0 Products of Conception	X External	Z No device	Z No qualifier

1ST - 1 Obstetrics
2ND - 0 Pregnancy ♀
3RD - H INSERTION

OBSTETRICS SECTION: Change, Drainage, Abortion, Extraction, Delivery, Insertion, Inspection, Removal, Repair, Reposition, Resection, Transplantation Root Operations that are performed on the products of conception.

INSERTION: Putting in a nonbiological appliance that monitors, assists, performs, or prevents a physiological function but does not physically take the place of a body part.

Explanation: None Example: Insertion intrauterine pressure monitor

Body Part – 4TH	Approach – 5TH	Device – 6TH	Qualifier – 7TH
0 Products of Conception	0 Open 7 Via natural or artificial opening	3 Monitoring electrode Y Other device	Z No qualifier

1ST - 1 Obstetrics
2ND - 0 Pregnancy ♀
3RD - J INSPECTION

OBSTETRICS SECTION: Change, Drainage, Abortion, Extraction, Delivery, Insertion, Inspection, Removal, Repair, Reposition, Resection, Transplantation Root Operations that are performed on the products of conception.

INSPECTION: Visually and/or manually exploring a body part.

Explanation: Direct or instrumental visualization ... Example: Bimanual pregnancy exam

Body Part – 4TH	Approach – 5TH	Device – 6TH	Qualifier – 7TH
0 Products of Conception 1 Products of Conception, Retained 2 Products of Conception, Ectopic	0 Open 3 Percutaneous 4 Percutaneous endoscopic 7 Via natural or artificial opening 8 Via natural or artificial opening endoscopic X External	Z No device	Z No qualifier

© 2018 Channel Publishing, Ltd.

1ST - 1 Obstetrics
2ND - 0 Pregnancy ♀
3RD - P REMOVAL

OBSTETRICS SECTION: Change, Drainage, Abortion, Extraction, Delivery, Insertion, Inspection, Removal, Repair, Reposition, Resection, Transplantation
Root Operations that are performed on the products of conception.

REMOVAL: Taking out or off a device from a body part, region or orifice.

Explanation: Removal device without reinsertion ... Example: Removal fetal monitoring electrode

Body Part – 4TH	Approach – 5TH	Device – 6TH	Qualifier – 7TH
0 Products of Conception	0 Open 7 Via natural or artificial opening	3 Monitoring electrode Y Other device	Z No qualifier

1ST - 1 Obstetrics
2ND - 0 Pregnancy ♀
3RD - Q REPAIR

OBSTETRICS SECTION: Change, Drainage, Abortion, Extraction, Delivery, Insertion, Inspection, Removal, Repair, Reposition, Resection, Transplantation
Root Operations that are performed on the products of conception.

REPAIR: Restoring, to the extent possible, a body part to its normal anatomic structure and function.

Explanation: Only when no other root operation applies ... Example: In utero repair fetal hernia

Body Part – 4TH	Approach – 5TH	Device – 6TH	Qualifier – 7TH
0 Products of Conception	0 Open 3 Percutaneous 4 Percutaneous endoscopic 7 Via natural or artificial opening 8 Via natural or artificial opening endoscopic	Y Other device Z No device	E Nervous System F Cardiovascular System G Lymphatics and Hemic H Eye J Ear, Nose and Sinus K Respiratory System L Mouth and Throat M Gastrointestinal System N Hepatobiliary and Pancreas P Endocrine System Q Skin R Musculoskeletal System S Urinary System T Female Reproductive System V Male Reproductive System Y Other Body System

1ST - 1 Obstetrics
2ND - 0 Pregnancy ♀
3RD - S REPOSITION

OBSTETRICS SECTION: Change, Drainage, Abortion, Extraction, Delivery, Insertion, Inspection, Removal, Repair, Reposition, Resection, Transplantation
Root Operations that are performed on the products of conception.

REPOSITION: Moving to its normal location, or other suitable location, all or a portion of a body part.

Explanation: May or may not be cut out to be moved ... Example: Manual external version fetus

Body Part – 4TH	Approach – 5TH	Device – 6TH	Qualifier – 7TH
0 Products of Conception	7 Via natural or artificial opening X External	Z No device	Z No qualifier
2 Products of Conception, Ectopic	0 Open 3 Percutaneous 4 Percutaneous endoscopic 7 Via natural or artificial opening 8 Via natural or artificial opening endoscopic	Z No device	Z No qualifier

© 2018 Channel Publishing, Ltd.

1ST - 1 Obstetrics
2ND - 0 Pregnancy ♀
3RD - T RESECTION

OBSTETRICS SECTION: Change, Drainage, Abortion, Extraction, Delivery, Insertion, Inspection, Removal, Repair, Reposition, Resection, Transplantation
Root Operations that are performed on the products of conception.

RESECTION: Cutting out or off, without replacement, all of a body part.

Explanation: None Example: Surgical removal ectopic pregnancy

Body Part – 4TH	Approach – 5TH	Device – 6TH	Qualifier – 7TH
2 Products of Conception, Ectopic	0 Open 3 Percutaneous 4 Percutaneous endoscopic 7 Via natural or artificial opening 8 Via natural or artificial opening endoscopic	Z No device	Z No qualifier

1ST - 1 Obstetrics
2ND - 0 Pregnancy ♀
3RD - Y TRANSPLANTATION

OBSTETRICS SECTION: Change, Drainage, Abortion, Extraction, Delivery, Insertion, Inspection, Removal, Repair, Reposition, Resection, Transplantation
Root Operations that are performed on the products of conception.

TRANSPLANTATION: Putting in or on all or a portion of a living body part taken from another individual or animal to physically take the place and/or function of all or a portion of a similar body part.

Explanation: The native body part may or may not be taken out ... Example: Fetal kidney transplant

Body Part – 4TH	Approach – 5TH	Device – 6TH	Qualifier – 7TH
0 Products of Conception	3 Percutaneous 4 Percutaneous endoscopic 7 Via natural or artificial opening	Z No device	E Nervous System F Cardiovascular System G Lymphatics and Hemic H Eye J Ear, Nose and Sinus K Respiratory System L Mouth and Throat M Gastrointestinal System N Hepatobiliary and Pancreas P Endocrine System Q Skin R Musculoskeletal System S Urinary System T Female Reproductive System V Male Reproductive System Y Other Body System

© 2018 Channel Publishing, Ltd.

Educational Annotations | Section 2 – Placement

Section Specific Educational Annotations for the Placement Section include:

- Anatomy and Physiology Review
- Anatomical Illustrations
- AHA Coding Clinic® Reference Notations
- Body Part Key Listings
- Device Key Listings
- Device Aggregation Table Listings
- Coding Notes

Anatomy and Physiology Review of Placement

BODY REGION VALUES - 2 - Placement

Abdominal Wall – The multi-tissue-layered covering of the abdominal and pelvic portions of the trunk.
Anorectal – The multi-tissue-layered area containing the anus and rectum.
Back – The multi-tissue-layered covering of the back portion of the trunk.
Chest Wall – The multi-tissue-layered covering of the thoracic portion of the trunk.
Ear – The organ of hearing comprised of the external ear (auricle or pinna), middle ear (malleus, incus, and stapes bones), and inner ear (cochlea).
Face – The multi-tissue-layered covering of the anterior portion of the head.
Female Genital Tract – The organs and structures of the reproductive systems.
Finger – A digit of the hand.
Foot – The portion of the lower extermity distal to the lower end of the tibia and fibula.
Hand – The portion of the upper extermity distal to the forearm.
Head – The portion of the human body above the neck.
Inguinal Region – The multi-tissue-layered area between the lower abdomen, thigh, and pubic bone.
Lower Arm – The portion of the upper extermity distal to the elbow.
Lower Extremity – The entire lower extremity (leg).
Lower Leg – The portion of the lower extermity distal to the knee.
Mouth and Pharynx – The portion of the head formed by the oral cavity and pharynx.
Nasal – The multi-tissue-layered area of the nose in the anterior portion of the head.
Neck – The portion of the human body above the trunk and below the head.
Thumb – The first digit of the hand.
Toe – A digit of the foot.
Upper Arm – The portion of the upper extermity distal to the shoulder and proximal to the elbow.
Upper Extremity – The entire upper extremity (arm).
Upper Leg – The portion of the lower extermity distal to the hip and proximal to the knee.
Urethra – The urethra is the musculomembranous tube which extends and carries urine from the bladder to the external urethral opening (meatus).

Anatomical Illustrations of Placement

None for the Placement Section

AHA Coding Clinic® Reference Notations of Placement

ROOT OPERATION SPECIFIC - PLACEMENT - Section 2

CHANGE - 0
COMPRESSION - 1
DRESSING - 2
IMMOBILIZATION - 3
PACKING - 4
Nasal tampon to stop nasal bleeding ....AHA 17:4Q:p106
REMOVAL - 5
TRACTION - 6
Tongs used to stabilize cervical fracture ....AHA 13:2Q:p39

PLACEMENT 2

© 2018 Channel Publishing, Ltd.

Educational Annotations

Section 2 – Placement

Body Part Key Listings of Placement

See also Body Part Key in Appendix C

Hallux ....use 1st Toe, Left/Right
Inguinal canal ....use Inguinal Region, Bilateral/Left/Right
Inguinal triangle ....use Inguinal Region, Bilateral/Left/Right

Device Key Listings of Placement

None for the Placement Section

Device Aggregation Table Listings of Placement

None for the Placement Section

Coding Notes of Placement

© 2018 Channel Publishing, Ltd.

1ST - 2 Placement
2ND - W Anatomical Regions
3RD - 0 CHANGE

PLACEMENT SECTION: Change, Compression, Dressing, Immobilization, Packing, Removal, Traction Root Operations include only those that are performed without an incision or a puncture.

CHANGE: Taking out or off a device from a body part and putting back an identical or similar device in or on the same body part without cutting or puncturing the skin or a mucous membrane.

Explanation: Performed without an incision or puncture ...
Example: Changing a cast

Body Part – 4TH			Approach-5TH	Device – 6TH	Qualifier-7TH
0 Head 2 Neck 3 Abdominal Wall 4 Chest Wall 5 Back 6 Inguinal Region, Right 7 Inguinal Region, Left 8 Upper Extremity, Right 9 Upper Extremity, Left	A Upper Arm, Right B Upper Arm, Left C Lower Arm, Right D Lower Arm, Left E Hand, Right F Hand, Left G Thumb, Right H Thumb, Left J Finger, Right K Finger, Left	L Lower Extremity, Right M Lower Extremity, Left N Upper Leg, Right P Upper Leg, Left Q Lower Leg, Right R Lower Leg, Left S Foot, Right T Foot, Left U Toe, Right V Toe, Left	X External	0 Traction apparatus 1 Splint 2 Cast 3 Brace 4 Bandage 5 Packing material 6 Pressure dressing 7 Intermittent pressure device Y Other device	Z No qualifier
1 Face			X External	0 Traction apparatus 1 Splint 2 Cast 3 Brace 4 Bandage 5 Packing material 6 Pressure dressing 7 Intermittent pressure device 9 Wire Y Other device	Z No qualifier

1ST - 2 Placement
2ND - W Anatomical Regions
3RD - 1 COMPRESSION

PLACEMENT SECTION: Change, Compression, Dressing, Immobilization, Packing, Removal, Traction Root Operations include only those that are performed without an incision or a puncture.

COMPRESSION: Putting pressure on a body region.

Explanation: Performed without an incision or puncture ...
Example: Application of pressure dressing

Body Part – 4TH			Approach-5TH	Device – 6TH	Qualifier-7TH
0 Head 1 Face 2 Neck 3 Abdominal Wall 4 Chest Wall 5 Back 6 Inguinal Region, Right 7 Inguinal Region, Left 8 Upper Extremity, Right 9 Upper Extremity, Left	A Upper Arm, Right B Upper Arm, Left C Lower Arm, Right D Lower Arm, Left E Hand, Right F Hand, Left G Thumb, Right H Thumb, Left J Finger, Right K Finger, Left	L Lower Extremity, Right M Lower Extremity, Left N Upper Leg, Right P Upper Leg, Left Q Lower Leg, Right R Lower Leg, Left S Foot, Right T Foot, Left U Toe, Right V Toe, Left	X External	6 Pressure dressing 7 Intermittent pressure device	Z No qualifier

© 2018 Channel Publishing, Ltd.

1ST - 2 Placement
2ND - W Anatomical Regions
3RD - 2 DRESSING

PLACEMENT SECTION: Change, Compression, Dressing, Immobilization, Packing, Removal, Traction
Root Operations include only those that are performed without an incision or a puncture.
DRESSING: Putting material on a body region for protection.

Explanation: Performed without an incision or puncture ...
Example: Bandage-type dressing

Body Part – 4TH			Approach-5TH	Device – 6TH	Qualifier-7TH
0 Head 1 Face 2 Neck 3 Abdominal Wall 4 Chest Wall 5 Back 6 Inguinal Region, Right 7 Inguinal Region, Left 8 Upper Extremity, Right 9 Upper Extremity, Left	A Upper Arm, Right B Upper Arm, Left C Lower Arm, Right D Lower Arm, Left E Hand, Right F Hand, Left G Thumb, Right H Thumb, Left J Finger, Right K Finger, Left	L Lower Extremity, Right M Lower Extremity, Left N Upper Leg, Right P Upper Leg, Left Q Lower Leg, Right R Lower Leg, Left S Foot, Right T Foot, Left U Toe, Right V Toe, Left	X External	4 Bandage	Z No qualifier

1ST - 2 Placement
2ND - W Anatomical Regions
3RD - 3 IMMOBILIZATION

PLACEMENT SECTION: Change, Compression, Dressing, Immobilization, Packing, Removal, Traction
Root Operations include only those that are performed without an incision or a puncture.
IMMOBILIZATION: Limiting or preventing motion of a body region.

Explanation: Performed without an incision or puncture ...
Example: Application of brace or splint

Body Part – 4TH			Approach-5TH	Device – 6TH	Qualifier-7TH
0 Head 2 Neck 3 Abdominal Wall 4 Chest Wall 5 Back 6 Inguinal Region, Right 7 Inguinal Region, Left 8 Upper Extremity, Right 9 Upper Extremity, Left	A Upper Arm, Right B Upper Arm, Left C Lower Arm, Right D Lower Arm, Left E Hand, Right F Hand, Left G Thumb, Right H Thumb, Left J Finger, Right K Finger, Left	L Lower Extremity, Right M Lower Extremity, Left N Upper Leg, Right P Upper Leg, Left Q Lower Leg, Right R Lower Leg, Left S Foot, Right T Foot, Left U Toe, Right V Toe, Left	X External	1 Splint 2 Cast 3 Brace Y Other device	Z No qualifier
1 Face			X External	1 Splint 2 Cast 3 Brace 9 Wire Y Other device	Z No qualifier

1ST - 2 Placement
2ND - W Anatomical Regions
3RD - 4 PACKING

PLACEMENT SECTION: Change, Compression, Dressing, Immobilization, Packing, Removal, Traction
Root Operations include only those that are performed without an incision or a puncture.
PACKING: Putting material in a body region or orifice.

Explanation: Performed without an incision or puncture ...
Example: Open wound packing

Body Part – 4TH			Approach-5TH	Device – 6TH	Qualifier-7TH
0 Head 1 Face 2 Neck 3 Abdominal Wall 4 Chest Wall 5 Back 6 Inguinal Region, Right 7 Inguinal Region, Left 8 Upper Extremity, Right 9 Upper Extremity, Left	A Upper Arm, Right B Upper Arm, Left C Lower Arm, Right D Lower Arm, Left E Hand, Right F Hand, Left G Thumb, Right H Thumb, Left J Finger, Right K Finger, Left	L Lower Extremity, Right M Lower Extremity, Left N Upper Leg, Right P Upper Leg, Left Q Lower Leg, Right R Lower Leg, Left S Foot, Right T Foot, Left U Toe, Right V Toe, Left	X External	5 Packing material	Z No qualifier

© 2018 Channel Publishing, Ltd.

1ST - 2 Placement
2ND - W Anatomical Regions
3RD - 5 REMOVAL

PLACEMENT SECTION: Change, Compression, Dressing, Immobilization, Packing, Removal, Traction Root Operations include only those that are performed without an incision or a puncture.

REMOVAL: Taking out or off a device from a body part.

Explanation: Performed without an incision or puncture ...
Example: Cast removal

Body Part – 4TH			Approach-5TH	Device – 6TH	Qualifier-7TH
0 Head 2 Neck 3 Abdominal Wall 4 Chest Wall 5 Back 6 Inguinal Region, Right 7 Inguinal Region, Left 8 Upper Extremity, Right 9 Upper Extremity, Left	A Upper Arm, Right B Upper Arm, Left C Lower Arm, Right D Lower Arm, Left E Hand, Right F Hand, Left G Thumb, Right H Thumb, Left J Finger, Right K Finger, Left	L Lower Extremity, Right M Lower Extremity, Left N Upper Leg, Right P Upper Leg, Left Q Lower Leg, Right R Lower Leg, Left S Foot, Right T Foot, Left U Toe, Right V Toe, Left	X External	0 Traction apparatus 1 Splint 2 Cast 3 Brace 4 Bandage 5 Packing material 6 Pressure dressing 7 Intermittent pressure device Y Other device	Z No qualifier
1 Face			X External	0 Traction apparatus 1 Splint 2 Cast 3 Brace 4 Bandage 5 Packing material 6 Pressure dressing 7 Intermittent pressure device 9 Wire Y Other device	Z No qualifier

1ST - 2 Placement
2ND - W Anatomical Regions
3RD - 6 TRACTION

PLACEMENT SECTION: Change, Compression, Dressing, Immobilization, Packing, Removal, Traction Root Operations include only those that are performed without an incision or a puncture.

TRACTION: Exerting a pulling force on a body region in a distal direction.

Explanation: Performed without an incision or puncture ...
Example: Lumbar traction using traction table

Body Part – 4TH			Approach-5TH	Device – 6TH	Qualifier-7TH
0 Head 1 Face 2 Neck 3 Abdominal Wall 4 Chest Wall 5 Back 6 Inguinal Region, Right 7 Inguinal Region, Left 8 Upper Extremity, Right 9 Upper Extremity, Left	A Upper Arm, Right B Upper Arm, Left C Lower Arm, Right D Lower Arm, Left E Hand, Right F Hand, Left G Thumb, Right H Thumb, Left J Finger, Right K Finger, Left	L Lower Extremity, Right M Lower Extremity, Left N Upper Leg, Right P Upper Leg, Left Q Lower Leg, Right R Lower Leg, Left S Foot, Right T Foot, Left U Toe, Right V Toe, Left	X External	0 Traction apparatus Z No device	Z No qualifier

© 2018 Channel Publishing, Ltd.

1ST - 2 Placement
2ND - Y Anatomical Orifices
3RD - 0 CHANGE

PLACEMENT SECTION: Change, Compression, Dressing, Immobilization, Packing, Removal, Traction
Root Operations include only those that are performed without an incision or a puncture.

CHANGE: Taking out or off a device from a body part and putting back an identical or similar device in or on the same body part without cutting or puncturing the skin or a mucous membrane.

Explanation: Performed without an incision or puncture ...
Example: Replacing nasal packing

Body Part – 4TH	Approach – 5TH	Device – 6TH	Qualifier – 7TH
0 Mouth and Pharynx 1 Nasal 2 Ear 3 Anorectal 4 Female Genital Tract ♀ 5 Urethra	X External	5 Packing material	Z No qualifier

1ST - 2 Placement
2ND - Y Anatomical Orifices
3RD - 4 PACKING

PLACEMENT SECTION: Change, Compression, Dressing, Immobilization, Packing, Removal, Traction
Root Operations include only those that are performed without an incision or a puncture.

PACKING: Putting material in a body region or orifice.

Explanation: Performed without an incision or puncture ...
Example: Insertion nasal packing

Body Part – 4TH	Approach – 5TH	Device – 6TH	Qualifier – 7TH
0 Mouth and Pharynx 1 Nasal 2 Ear 3 Anorectal 4 Female Genital Tract ♀ 5 Urethra	X External	5 Packing material	Z No qualifier

1ST - 2 Placement
2ND - Y Anatomical Orifices
3RD - 5 REMOVAL

PLACEMENT SECTION: Change, Compression, Dressing, Immobilization, Packing, Removal, Traction
Root Operations include only those that are performed without an incision or a puncture.

REMOVAL: Taking out or off a device from a body part.

Explanation: Performed without an incision or puncture ...
Example: Removal nasal packing

Body Part – 4TH	Approach – 5TH	Device – 6TH	Qualifier – 7TH
0 Mouth and Pharynx 1 Nasal 2 Ear 3 Anorectal 4 Female Genital Tract ♀ 5 Urethra	X External	5 Packing material	Z No qualifier

© 2018 Channel Publishing, Ltd.

Educational Annotations | Section 3 – Administration

Section Specific Educational Annotations for the Administration Section include:

- **AHA Coding Clinic® Reference Notations**
- **Coding Notes**

AHA Coding Clinic® Reference Notations of Administration

ROOT OPERATION SPECIFIC - ADMINISTRATION - Section 3

INTRODUCTION - 0

Bone morphogenic protein graft .... AHA 16:3Q:p29
Chemoembolization of hepatic artery .... AHA 15:1Q:p38
EGD with epinephrine injection .... AHA 15:3Q:p24
Fibrin injection into enterocutaneous fistula tract .... AHA 17:1Q:p37
Glucagon to flush bile duct stones .... AHA 14:3Q:p11
Imaging report to identify the body part of an infusion device .... AHA 14:3Q:p5
Immune globulin (Rh-D, anti-D), injection, intramuscular .... AHA 14:4Q:p16
Induction of labor, IV oxytocin, peripheral vein .... AHA 14:4Q:p17
Induction of labor with Cervidil dinoprostone vaginal tampon .... AHA 14:2Q:p8
Infusion of thrombolytic therapy .... AHA 14:4Q:p19
Infusion of tPA into the pleural cavity .... AHA 17:2Q:p14
Injection of combination of drugs .... AHA 14:4Q:p45
Injection of intrathecal chemotherapy .... AHA 15:1Q:p31
Injection of Ovation® (extracellular matrix) into amputation wound .... AHA 15:2Q:p27
Injection of sclerosing agent into an esophageal varix .... AHA 13:1Q:p27
Injection of substances with vitrectomy .... AHA 15:2Q:p24
Injection of talc in pleura for pleurodesis .... AHA 15:2Q:p31
Instillation of saline and Seprafilm solution .... AHA 14:4Q:p38
Intraoperative (open) placement of chemotherapy wafers .... AHA 14:4Q:p34
Nasogastric (NG) tube used for both drainage and feeding .... AHA 15:2Q:p29
Neulasta injection to prevent infection .... AHA 14:2Q:p10
Placement of bone morphogenetic protein (BMP) .... AHA 18:1Q:p8
Placement of chemotherapy wafers into cranial cavity .... AHA 16:4Q:p113
Seprafilm use during procedures .... AHA 15:3Q:p29
tPA administration .... AHA 13:4Q:p124

IRRIGATION - 1

TRANSFUSION - 2

ADMINISTRATION 3

Coding Notes of Administration

© 2018 Channel Publishing, Ltd.

1ST - 3 Administration
2ND - 0 Circulatory
3RD - 2 TRANSFUSION

ADMINISTRATION SECTION: Introduction, Irrigation, Transfusion
Root Operations that define procedures where a diagnostic or therapeutic substance is given to the patient.
TRANSFUSION: Putting in blood or blood products.

Explanation: Blood products, bone marrow, and stem cells
Example: Whole blood transfusion

Body Part/Region - 4TH	Approach – 5TH	Substance – 6TH	Qualifier – 7TH
3 Peripheral Vein 4 Central Vein	0 Open 3 Percutaneous	A Stem cells, embryonic NC*	Z No qualifier
3 Peripheral Vein 4 Central Vein	0 Open 3 Percutaneous	G Bone marrow NC* X Stem cells, cord blood Y Stem cells, hematopoietic NC*	0 Autologous 2 Allogeneic, related 3 Allogeneic, unrelated 4 Allogeneic, unspecified
3 Peripheral Vein 4 Central Vein	0 Open 3 Percutaneous	H Whole blood J Serum albumin K Frozen plasma L Fresh plasma M Plasma cryoprecipitate N Red blood cells P Frozen red cells Q White cells R Platelets S Globulin T Fibrinogen V Antihemophilic factors W Factor IX	0 Autologous 1 Nonautologous
5 Peripheral Artery 6 Central Artery	0 Open 3 Percutaneous	G Bone marrow NC* H Whole blood J Serum albumin K Frozen plasma L Fresh plasma M Plasma cryoprecipitate N Red blood cells P Frozen red cells Q White cells R Platelets S Globulin T Fibrinogen V Antihemophilic factors W Factor IX X Stem cells, cord blood Y Stem cells, hematopoietic NC*	0 Autologous 1 Nonautologous
7 Products of Conception, Circulatory ♀	3 Percutaneous 7 Via natural or artificial opening	H Whole blood J Serum albumin K Frozen plasma L Fresh plasma M Plasma cryoprecipitate N Red blood cells P Frozen red cells Q White cells R Platelets S Globulin T Fibrinogen V Antihemophilic factors W Factor IX	1 Nonautologous
8 Vein	0 Open 3 Percutaneous	B 4-Factor prothrombin complex concentrate	1 Nonautologous

NC* – Some procedures are considered non-covered by Medicare. See current Medicare Code Editor for details.

1ST - 3 Administration
2ND - C Indwelling Device
3RD - 1 IRRIGATION

ADMINISTRATION SECTION: Introduction, Irrigation, Transfusion
Root Operations that define procedures where a diagnostic or therapeutic substance is given to the patient.
IRRIGATION: Putting in or on a cleansing substance.

Explanation: Cleansing substance
Example: Irrigation catheter port

Body Part/Region - 4TH	Approach – 5TH	Substance – 6TH	Qualifier – 7TH
Z None	X External	8 Irrigating substance	Z No qualifier

© 2018 Channel Publishing, Ltd.

1ST - 3 Administration
2ND - E Physiological Systems and Anatomical Regions
3RD - 0 INTRODUCTION

ADMINISTRATION SECTION: Introduction, Irrigation, Transfusion
Root Operations that define procedures where a diagnostic or therapeutic substance is given to the patient.

INTRODUCTION: Putting in or on a therapeutic, diagnostic, nutritional, physiological, or prophylactic substance except blood or blood products.

Explanation: Substances other than blood and cleansing
Example: Infusion chemotherapy agent

Body Part/Region - 4TH	Approach – 5TH	Substance – 6TH	Qualifier – 7TH
0 Skin and Mucous Membranes	X External	0 Antineoplastic	5 Other antineoplastic M Monoclonal antibody
0 Skin and Mucous Membranes	X External	2 Anti-infective	8 Oxazolidinones 9 Other anti-infective
0 Skin and Mucous Membranes	X External	3 Anti-inflammatory 4 Serum, toxoid and vaccine B Anesthetic agent K Other diagnostic substance M Pigment N Analgesics, hypnotics, sedatives T Destructive agent	Z No qualifier
0 Skin and Mucous Membranes	X External	G Other therapeutic substance	C Other substance
1 Subcutaneous Tissue	0 Open	2 Anti-infective	A Anti-infective envelope
1 Subcutaneous Tissue	3 Percutaneous	0 Antineoplastic	5 Other antineoplastic M Monoclonal antibody
1 Subcutaneous Tissue	3 Percutaneous	2 Anti-infective	8 Oxazolidinones 9 Other anti-infective A Anti-infective envelope
1 Subcutaneous Tissue	3 Percutaneous	3 Anti-inflammatory 6 Nutritional substance 7 Electrolytic and water balance substance B Local anesthetic H Radioactive substance K Other diagnostic substance N Analgesics, hypnotics, sedatives T Destructive agent	Z No qualifier
1 Subcutaneous Tissue	3 Percutaneous	4 Serum, toxoid and vaccine	0 Influenza vaccine Z No qualifier
1 Subcutaneous Tissue	3 Percutaneous	G Other therapeutic substance	C Other substance
1 Subcutaneous Tissue	3 Percutaneous	V Hormone	G Insulin J Other hormone
2 Muscle	3 Percutaneous	0 Antineoplastic	5 Other antineoplastic M Monoclonal antibody
2 Muscle	3 Percutaneous	2 Anti-infective	8 Oxazolidinones 9 Other anti-infective
2 Muscle	3 Percutaneous	3 Anti-inflammatory 6 Nutritional substance 7 Electrolytic and water balance substance B Anesthetic agent H Radioactive substance K Other diagnostic substance N Analgesics, hypnotics, sedatives T Destructive agent	Z No qualifier
2 Muscle	3 Percutaneous	4 Serum, toxoid and vaccine	0 Influenza vaccine Z No qualifier
2 Muscle	3 Percutaneous	G Other therapeutic substance	C Other substance

continued ⇨

© 2018 Channel Publishing, Ltd.

3 E 0 INTRODUCTION—*continued*

Body Part/Region - 4TH	Approach – 5TH	Substance – 6TH	Qualifier – 7TH
3 Peripheral Vein	0 Open	0 Antineoplastic	2 High-dose interleukin-2 3 Low-dose interleukin-2 5 Other antineoplastic M Monoclonal antibody P Clofarabine
3 Peripheral Vein	0 Open	1 Thrombolytic	6 Recombinant human-activated protein C 7 Other thrombolytic
3 Peripheral Vein	0 Open	2 Anti-infective	8 Oxazolidinones 9 Other anti-infective
3 Peripheral Vein	0 Open	3 Anti-inflammatory 4 Serum, toxoid and vaccine 6 Nutritional substance 7 Electrolytic and water balance substance F Intracirculatory anesthetic H Radioactive substance K Other diagnostic substance N Analgesics, hypnotics, sedatives P Platelet inhibitor R Antiarrhythmic T Destructive agent X Vasopressor	Z No qualifier
3 Peripheral Vein	0 Open	G Other therapeutic substance	C Other substance N Blood brain barrier disruption
3 Peripheral Vein	0 Open	U Pancreatic islet cells	0 Autologous 1 Nonautologous
3 Peripheral Vein	0 Open	V Hormone	G Insulin H Human B-type natriuretic peptide J Other hormone
3 Peripheral Vein	0 Open	W Immunotherapeutic	K Immunostimulator L Immunosuppressive
3 Peripheral Vein	3 Percutaneous	0 Antineoplastic	2 High-dose interleukin-2 3 Low-dose interleukin-2 5 Other antineoplastic M Monoclonal antibody P Clofarabine
3 Peripheral Vein	3 Percutaneous	1 Thrombolytic	6 Recombinant human-activated protein C 7 Other thrombolytic
3 Peripheral Vein	3 Percutaneous	2 Anti-infective	8 Oxazolidinones 9 Other anti-infective
3 Peripheral Vein	3 Percutaneous	3 Anti-inflammatory 4 Serum, toxoid and vaccine 6 Nutritional substance 7 Electrolytic and water balance substance F Intracirculatory anesthetic H Radioactive substance K Other diagnostic substance N Analgesics, hypnotics, sedatives P Platelet inhibitor R Antiarrhythmic T Destructive agent X Vasopressor	Z No qualifier

continued ⇨

© 2018 Channel Publishing, Ltd.

3 E 0 INTRODUCTION—*continued*

Body Part/Region - 4TH	Approach – 5TH	Substance – 6TH	Qualifier – 7TH
3 Peripheral Vein	3 Percutaneous	G Other therapeutic substance	C Other substance N Blood brain barrier disruption Q Glucarpidase
3 Peripheral Vein	3 Percutaneous	U Pancreatic islet cells	0 Autologous 1 Nonautologous
3 Peripheral Vein	3 Percutaneous	V Hormone	G Insulin H Human B-type natriuretic peptide J Other hormone
3 Peripheral Vein	3 Percutaneous	W Immunotherapeutic	K Immunostimulator L Immunosuppressive
4 Central Vein	0 Open	0 Antineoplastic	2 High-dose interleukin-2 3 Low-dose interleukin-2 5 Other antineoplastic M Monoclonal antibody P Clofarabine
4 Central Vein	0 Open	1 Thrombolytic	6 Recombinant human-activated protein C 7 Other thrombolytic
4 Central Vein	0 Open	2 Anti-infective	8 Oxazolidinones 9 Other anti-infective
4 Central Vein	0 Open	3 Anti-inflammatory 4 Serum, toxoid and vaccine 6 Nutritional substance 7 Electrolytic and water balance substance F Intracirculatory anesthetic H Radioactive substance K Other diagnostic substance N Analgesics, hypnotics, sedatives P Platelet inhibitor R Antiarrhythmic T Destructive agent X Vasopressor	Z No qualifier
4 Central Vein	0 Open	G Other therapeutic substance	C Other substance N Blood brain barrier disruption
4 Central Vein	0 Open	V Hormone	G Insulin H Human B-type natriuretic peptide J Other hormone
4 Central Vein	0 Open	W Immunotherapeutic	K Immunostimulator L Immunosuppressive
4 Central Vein	3 Percutaneous	0 Antineoplastic	2 High-dose interleukin-2 3 Low-dose interleukin-2 5 Other antineoplastic M Monoclonal antibody P Clofarabine
4 Central Vein	3 Percutaneous	1 Thrombolytic	6 Recombinant human-activated protein C 7 Other thrombolytic

continued ⇨

ADMINISTRATION 3 E 0

© 2018 Channel Publishing, Ltd.

3 E 0 INTRODUCTION—*continued*

Body Part/Region - 4TH	Approach – 5TH	Substance – 6TH	Qualifier – 7TH
4 Central Vein	3 Percutaneous	2 Anti-infective	8 Oxazolidinones 9 Other anti-infective
4 Central Vein	3 Percutaneous	3 Anti-inflammatory 4 Serum, toxoid and vaccine 6 Nutritional substance 7 Electrolytic and water balance substance F Intracirculatory anesthetic H Radioactive substance K Other diagnostic substance N Analgesics, hypnotics, sedatives P Platelet inhibitor R Antiarrhythmic T Destructive agent X Vasopressor	Z No qualifier
4 Central Vein	3 Percutaneous	G Other therapeutic substance	C Other substance N Blood brain barrier disruption Q Glucarpidase
4 Central Vein	3 Percutaneous	V Hormone	G Insulin H Human B-type natriuretic peptide J Other hormone
4 Central Vein	3 Percutaneous	W Immunotherapeutic	K Immunostimulator L Immunosuppressive
5 Peripheral Artery 6 Central Artery	0 Open 3 Percutaneous	0 Antineoplastic	2 High-dose interleukin-2 3 Low-dose interleukin-2 5 Other antineoplastic M Monoclonal antibody P Clofarabine
5 Peripheral Artery 6 Central Artery	0 Open 3 Percutaneous	1 Thrombolytic	6 Recombinant human-activated protein C 7 Other thrombolytic
5 Peripheral Artery 6 Central Artery	0 Open 3 Percutaneous	2 Anti-infective	8 Oxazolidinones 9 Other anti-infective
5 Peripheral Artery 6 Central Artery	0 Open 3 Percutaneous	3 Anti-inflammatory 4 Serum, toxoid and vaccine 6 Nutritional substance 7 Electrolytic and water balance substance F Intracirculatory anesthetic H Radioactive substance K Other diagnostic substance N Analgesics, hypnotics, sedatives P Platelet inhibitor R Antiarrhythmic T Destructive agent X Vasopressor	Z No qualifier
5 Peripheral Artery 6 Central Artery	0 Open 3 Percutaneous	G Other therapeutic substance	C Other substance N Blood brain barrier disruption
5 Peripheral Artery 6 Central Artery	0 Open 3 Percutaneous	V Hormone	G Insulin H Human B-type natriuretic peptide J Other hormone

continued ⇨

© 2018 Channel Publishing, Ltd.

3 E 0 INTRODUCTION—*continued*

Body Part/Region - 4TH	Approach – 5TH	Substance – 6TH	Qualifier – 7TH
5 Peripheral Artery 6 Central Artery	0 Open 3 Percutaneous	W Immunotherapeutic	K Immunostimulator L Immunosuppressive
7 Coronary Artery 8 Heart	0 Open 3 Percutaneous	1 Thrombolytic	6 Recombinant human-activated protein C 7 Other thrombolytic
7 Coronary Artery 8 Heart	0 Open 3 Percutaneous	G Other therapeutic substance	C Other substance
7 Coronary Artery 8 Heart	0 Open 3 Percutaneous	K Other diagnostic substance P Platelet inhibitor	Z No qualifier
7 Coronary Artery 8 Heart	4 Percutaneous endoscopic	G Other therapeutic substance	C Other substance
9 Nose	3 Percutaneous 7 Via natural or artificial opening X External	0 Antineoplastic	5 Other antineoplastic M Monoclonal antibody
9 Nose	3 Percutaneous 7 Via natural or artificial opening X External	2 Anti-infective	8 Oxazolidinones 9 Other anti-infective
9 Nose	3 Percutaneous 7 Via natural or artificial opening X External	3 Anti-inflammatory 4 Serum, toxoid and vaccine B Anesthetic agent H Radioactive substance K Other diagnostic substance N Analgesics, hypnotics, sedatives T Destructive agent	Z No qualifier
9 Nose	3 Percutaneous 7 Via natural or artificial opening X External	G Other therapeutic substance	C Other substance
A Bone Marrow	3 Percutaneous	0 Antineoplastic	5 Other antineoplastic M Monoclonal antibody
A Bone Marrow	3 Percutaneous	G Other therapeutic substance	C Other substance
B Ear	3 Percutaneous 7 Via natural or artificial opening X External	0 Antineoplastic	4 Liquid brachytherapy radioisotope 5 Other antineoplastic M Monoclonal antibody
B Ear	3 Percutaneous 7 Via natural or artificial opening X External	2 Anti-infective	8 Oxazolidinones 9 Other anti-infective
B Ear	3 Percutaneous 7 Via natural or artificial opening X External	3 Anti-inflammatory B Anesthetic agent H Radioactive substance K Other diagnostic substance N Analgesics, hypnotics, sedatives T Destructive agent	Z No qualifier
B Ear	3 Percutaneous 7 Via natural or artificial opening X External	G Other therapeutic substance	C Other substance
C Eye	3 Percutaneous 7 Via natural or artificial opening X External	0 Antineoplastic	4 Liquid brachytherapy radioisotope 5 Other antineoplastic M Monoclonal antibody

continued ⇨

© 2018 Channel Publishing, Ltd.

3 E 0 INTRODUCTION—*continued*

Body Part/Region - 4TH	Approach – 5TH	Substance – 6TH	Qualifier – 7TH
C Eye	3 Percutaneous 7 Via natural or artificial opening X External	2 Anti-infective	8 Oxazolidinones 9 Other anti-infective
C Eye	3 Percutaneous 7 Via natural or artificial opening X External	3 Anti-inflammatory B Anesthetic agent H Radioactive substance K Other diagnostic substance M Pigment N Analgesics, hypnotics, sedatives T Destructive agent	Z No qualifier
C Eye	3 Percutaneous 7 Via natural or artificial opening X External	G Other therapeutic substance	C Other substance
C Eye	3 Percutaneous 7 Via natural or artificial opening X External	S Gas	F Other gas
D Mouth and Pharynx	3 Percutaneous 7 Via natural or artificial opening X External	0 Antineoplastic	4 Liquid brachytherapy radioisotope 5 Other antineoplastic M Monoclonal antibody
D Mouth and Pharynx	3 Percutaneous 7 Via natural or artificial opening X External	2 Anti-infective	8 Oxazolidinones 9 Other anti-infective
D Mouth and Pharynx	3 Percutaneous 7 Via natural or artificial opening X External	3 Anti-inflammatory 4 Serum, toxoid and vaccine 6 Nutritional substance 7 Electrolytic and water balance substance B Anesthetic agent H Radioactive substance K Other diagnostic substance N Analgesics, hypnotics, sedatives R Antiarrhythmic T Destructive agent	Z No qualifier
D Mouth and Pharynx	3 Percutaneous 7 Via natural or artificial opening X External	G Other therapeutic substance	C Other substance
E Products of Conception ♀ G Upper GI H Lower GI K Genitourinary Tract N Male Reproductive ♂	3 Percutaneous 7 Via natural or artificial opening 8 Via natural or artificial opening endoscopic	0 Antineoplastic	4 Liquid brachytherapy radioisotope 5 Other antineoplastic M Monoclonal antibody
E Products of Conception ♀ G Upper GI H Lower GI K Genitourinary Tract N Male Reproductive ♂	3 Percutaneous 7 Via natural or artificial opening 8 Via natural or artificial opening endoscopic	2 Anti-infective	8 Oxazolidinones 9 Other anti-infective
E Products of Conception ♀ G Upper GI H Lower GI K Genitourinary Tract N Male Reproductive ♂	3 Percutaneous 7 Via natural or artificial opening 8 Via natural or artificial opening endoscopic	3 Anti-inflammatory 6 Nutritional substance 7 Electrolytic and water balance substance B Anesthetic agent H Radioactive substance K Other diagnostic substance N Analgesics, hypnotics, sedatives T Destructive agent	Z No qualifier

continued ⇨

© 2018 Channel Publishing, Ltd.

3 E 0 INTRODUCTION—*continued*

Body Part/Region - 4TH	Approach – 5TH	Substance – 6TH	Qualifier – 7TH
E Products of Conception ♀ G Upper GI H Lower GI K Genitourinary Tract N Male Reproductive ♂	3 Percutaneous 7 Via natural or artificial opening 8 Via natural or artificial opening endoscopic	G Other therapeutic substance	C Other substance
E Products of Conception ♀ G Upper GI H Lower GI K Genitourinary Tract N Male Reproductive ♂	3 Percutaneous 7 Via natural or artificial opening 8 Via natural or artificial opening endoscopic	S Gas	F Other gas
E Products of Conception ♀ G Upper GI H Lower GI K Genitourinary Tract N Male Reproductive ♂	4 Percutaneous endoscopic	G Other therapeutic substance	C Other substance
F Respiratory Tract	3 Percutaneous 7 Via natural or artificial opening 8 Via natural or artificial opening endoscopic	0 Antineoplastic	4 Liquid brachytherapy radioisotope 5 Other antineoplastic M Monoclonal antibody
F Respiratory Tract	3 Percutaneous 7 Via natural or artificial opening 8 Via natural or artificial opening endoscopic	2 Anti-infective	8 Oxazolidinones 9 Other anti-infective
F Respiratory Tract	3 Percutaneous 7 Via natural or artificial opening 8 Via natural or artificial opening endoscopic	3 Anti-inflammatory 6 Nutritional substance 7 Electrolytic and water balance substance B Anesthetic agent H Radioactive substance K Other diagnostic substance N Analgesics, hypnotics, sedatives T Destructive agent	Z No qualifier
F Respiratory Tract	3 Percutaneous 7 Via natural or artificial opening 8 Via natural or artificial opening endoscopic	G Other therapeutic substance	C Other substance
F Respiratory Tract	3 Percutaneous 7 Via natural or artificial opening 8 Via natural or artificial opening endoscopic	S Gas	D Nitric oxide F Other gas
F Respiratory Tract	4 Percutaneous endoscopic	G Other therapeutic substance	C Other substance
J Biliary and Pancreatic Tract	3 Percutaneous 7 Via natural or artificial opening 8 Via natural or artificial opening endoscopic	0 Antineoplastic	4 Liquid brachytherapy radioisotope 5 Other antineoplastic M Monoclonal antibody
J Biliary and Pancreatic Tract	3 Percutaneous 7 Via natural or artificial opening 8 Via natural or artificial opening endoscopic	2 Anti-infective	8 Oxazolidinones 9 Other anti-infective
J Biliary and Pancreatic Tract	3 Percutaneous 7 Via natural or artificial opening 8 Via natural or artificial opening endoscopic	3 Anti-inflammatory 6 Nutritional substance 7 Electrolytic and water balance substance B Anesthetic agent H Radioactive substance K Other diagnostic substance N Analgesics, hypnotics, sedatives T Destructive agent	Z No qualifier

continued ⇨

© 2018 Channel Publishing, Ltd.

3 E 0 INTRODUCTION—*continued*

Body Part/Region - 4TH	Approach – 5TH	Substance – 6TH	Qualifier – 7TH
J Biliary and Pancreatic Tract	3 Percutaneous 7 Via natural or artificial opening 8 Via natural or artificial opening endoscopic	G Other therapeutic substance	C Other substance
J Biliary and Pancreatic Tract	3 Percutaneous 7 Via natural or artificial opening 8 Via natural or artificial opening endoscopic	S Gas	F Other gas
J Biliary and Pancreatic Tract	3 Percutaneous 7 Via natural or artificial opening 8 Via natural or artificial opening endoscopic	U Pancreatic islet cells	0 Autologous 1 Nonautologous
J Biliary and Pancreatic Tract	4 Percutaneous endoscopic	G Other therapeutic substance	C Other substance
L Pleural Cavity M Peritoneal Cavity	0 Open	5 Adhesion barrier	Z No qualifier
L Pleural Cavity M Peritoneal Cavity	3 Percutaneous	0 Antineoplastic	4 Liquid brachytherapy radioisotope 5 Other antineoplastic M Monoclonal antibody
L Pleural Cavity M Peritoneal Cavity	3 Percutaneous	2 Anti-infective	8 Oxazolidinones 9 Other anti-infective
L Pleural Cavity M Peritoneal Cavity	3 Percutaneous	3 Anti-inflammatory 5 Adhesion barrier 6 Nutritional substance 7 Electrolytic and water balance substance B Anesthetic agent H Radioactive substance K Other diagnostic substance N Analgesics, hypnotics, sedatives T Destructive agent	Z No qualifier
L Pleural Cavity M Peritoneal Cavity	3 Percutaneous	G Other therapeutic substance	C Other substance
L Pleural Cavity M Peritoneal Cavity	3 Percutaneous	S Gas	F Other gas
L Pleural Cavity M Peritoneal Cavity	4 Percutaneous endoscopic	5 Adhesion barrier	Z No qualifier
L Pleural Cavity M Peritoneal Cavity	4 Percutaneous endoscopic	G Other therapeutic substance	C Other substance
L Pleural Cavity M Peritoneal Cavity	7 Via natural or artificial opening	0 Antineoplastic	4 Liquid brachytherapy radioisotope 5 Other antineoplastic M Monoclonal antibody
L Pleural Cavity M Peritoneal Cavity	7 Via natural or artificial opening	S Gas	F Other gas
P Female Reproductive ♀	0 Open	5 Adhesion barrier	Z No qualifier
P Female Reproductive ♀	3 Percutaneous	0 Antineoplastic	4 Liquid brachytherapy radioisotope 5 Other antineoplastic M Monoclonal antibody
P Female Reproductive ♀	3 Percutaneous	2 Anti-infective	8 Oxazolidinones 9 Other anti-infective

continued ⇨

© 2018 Channel Publishing, Ltd.

3 E 0 INTRODUCTION—*continued*

Body Part/Region - 4TH	Approach – 5TH	Substance – 6TH	Qualifier – 7TH
P Female Reproductive ♀	3 Percutaneous	3 Anti-inflammatory 5 Adhesion barrier 6 Nutritional substance 7 Electrolytic and water balance substance B Anesthetic agent H Radioactive substance K Other diagnostic substance L Sperm N Analgesics, hypnotics, sedatives T Destructive agent V Hormone	Z No qualifier
P Female Reproductive ♀	3 Percutaneous	G Other therapeutic substance	C Other substance
P Female Reproductive ♀	3 Percutaneous	Q Fertilized ovum	0 Autologous 1 Nonautologous
P Female Reproductive ♀	3 Percutaneous	S Gas	F Other gas
P Female Reproductive ♀	4 Percutaneous endoscopic	5 Adhesion barrier	Z No qualifier
P Female Reproductive ♀	4 Percutaneous endoscopic	G Other therapeutic substance	C Other substance
P Female Reproductive ♀	7 Via natural or artificial opening	0 Antineoplastic	4 Liquid brachytherapy radioisotope 5 Other antineoplastic M Monoclonal antibody
P Female Reproductive ♀	7 Via natural or artificial opening	2 Anti-infective	8 Oxazolidinones 9 Other anti-infective
P Female Reproductive ♀	7 Via natural or artificial opening	3 Anti-inflammatory 6 Nutritional substance 7 Electrolytic and water balance substance B Anesthetic agent H Radioactive substance K Other diagnostic substance L Sperm N Analgesics, hypnotics, sedatives T Destructive agent V Hormone	Z No qualifier
P Female Reproductive ♀	7 Via natural or artificial opening	G Other therapeutic substance	C Other substance
P Female Reproductive ♀	7 Via natural or artificial opening	Q Fertilized ovum	0 Autologous 1 Nonautologous
P Female Reproductive ♀	7 Via natural or artificial opening	S Gas	F Other gas
P Female Reproductive ♀	8 Via natural or artificial opening endoscopic	0 Antineoplastic	4 Liquid brachytherapy radioisotope 5 Other antineoplastic M Monoclonal antibody
P Female Reproductive ♀	8 Via natural or artificial opening endoscopic	2 Anti-infective	8 Oxazolidinones 9 Other anti-infective
P Female Reproductive ♀	8 Via natural or artificial opening endoscopic	3 Anti-inflammatory 6 Nutritional substance 7 Electrolytic and water balance substance B Anesthetic agent H Radioactive substance K Other diagnostic substance N Analgesics, hypnotics, sedatives T Destructive agent	Z No qualifier

continued ⇨

© 2018 Channel Publishing, Ltd.

3 E 0 INTRODUCTION—*continued*

Body Part/Region - 4TH	Approach – 5TH	Substance – 6TH	Qualifier – 7TH
P Female Reproductive ♀	8 Via natural or artificial opening endoscopic	G Other therapeutic substance	C Other substance
P Female Reproductive ♀	8 Via natural or artificial opening endoscopic	S Gas	F Other gas
Q Cranial Cavity and Brain	0 Open 3 Percutaneous	0 Antineoplastic	4 Liquid brachytherapy radioisotope 5 Other antineoplastic M Monoclonal antibody
Q Cranial Cavity and Brain	0 Open 3 Percutaneous	2 Anti-infective	8 Oxazolidinones 9 Other anti-infective
Q Cranial Cavity and Brain	0 Open 3 Percutaneous	3 Anti-inflammatory 6 Nutritional substance 7 Electrolytic and water balance substance A Stem cells, embryonic B Anesthetic agent H Radioactive substance K Other diagnostic substance N Analgesics, hypnotics, sedatives T Destructive agent	Z No qualifier
Q Cranial Cavity and Brain	0 Open 3 Percutaneous	E Stem cells, somatic	0 Autologous 1 Nonautologous
Q Cranial Cavity and Brain	0 Open 3 Percutaneous	G Other therapeutic substance	C Other substance
Q Cranial Cavity and Brain	0 Open 3 Percutaneous	S Gas	F Other gas
Q Cranial Cavity and Brain	7 Via natural or artificial opening	0 Antineoplastic	4 Liquid brachytherapy radioisotope 5 Other antineoplastic M Monoclonal antibody
Q Cranial Cavity and Brain	7 Via natural or artificial opening	S Gas	F Other gas
R Spinal Canal	0 Open	A Stem cells, embryonic	Z No qualifier
R Spinal Canal	0 Open	E Stem cells, somatic	0 Autologous 1 Nonautologous
R Spinal Canal	3 Percutaneous	0 Antineoplastic	2 High-dose Interleukin-2 3 Low-dose Interleukin-2 4 Liquid brachytherapy radioisotope 5 Other antineoplastic M Monoclonal antibody
R Spinal Canal	3 Percutaneous	2 Anti-infective	8 Oxazolidinones 9 Other anti-infective
R Spinal Canal	3 Percutaneous	3 Anti-inflammatory 6 Nutritional substance 7 Electrolytic and water balance substance A Stem cells, embryonic B Anesthetic agent H Radioactive substance K Other diagnostic substance N Analgesics, hypnotics, sedatives T Destructive agent	Z No qualifier
R Spinal Canal	3 Percutaneous	E Stem cells, somatic	0 Autologous 1 Nonautologous

continued ⇨

© 2018 Channel Publishing, Ltd.

3 E 0 INTRODUCTION—*continued*

Body Part/Region - 4TH	Approach – 5TH	Substance – 6TH	Qualifier – 7TH
R Spinal Canal	3 Percutaneous	G Other therapeutic substance	C Other substance
R Spinal Canal	3 Percutaneous	S Gas	F Other gas
R Spinal Canal	7 Via natural or artificial opening	S Gas	F Other gas
S Epidural Space	3 Percutaneous	0 Antineoplastic	2 High-dose Interleukin-2 3 Low-dose Interleukin-2 4 Liquid brachytherapy radioisotope 5 Other antineoplastic M Monoclonal antibody
S Epidural Space	3 Percutaneous	2 Anti-infective	8 Oxazolidinones 9 Other anti-infective
S Epidural Space	3 Percutaneous	3 Anti-inflammatory 6 Nutritional substance 7 Electrolytic and water balance substance B Anesthetic agent H Radioactive substance K Other diagnostic substance N Analgesics, hypnotics, sedatives T Destructive agent	Z No qualifier
S Epidural Space	3 Percutaneous	G Other therapeutic substance	C Other substance
S Epidural Space	3 Percutaneous	S Gas	F Other gas
S Epidural Space	7 Via natural or artificial opening	S Gas	F Other gas
T Peripheral Nerves and Plexi X Cranial Nerves	3 Percutaneous	3 Anti-inflammatory B Anesthetic agent T Destructive agent	Z No qualifier
T Peripheral Nerves and Plexi X Cranial Nerves	3 Percutaneous	G Other therapeutic substance	C Other substance
U Joints	0 Open	2 Anti-infective	8 Oxazolidinones 9 Other anti-infective
U Joints	0 Open	G Other therapeutic substance	B Recombinant bone morphogenetic protein
U Joints	3 Percutaneous	0 Antineoplastic	4 Liquid brachytherapy radioisotope 5 Other antineoplastic M Monoclonal antibody
U Joints	3 Percutaneous	2 Anti-infective	8 Oxazolidinones 9 Other anti-infective
U Joints	3 Percutaneous	3 Anti-inflammatory 6 Nutritional substance 7 Electrolytic and water balance substance B Anesthetic agent H Radioactive substance K Other diagnostic substance N Analgesics, hypnotics, sedatives T Destructive agent	Z No qualifier
U Joints	3 Percutaneous	G Other therapeutic substance	B Recombinant bone morphogenetic protein C Other substance

continued ⇨

© 2018 Channel Publishing, Ltd.

3 E 0 INTRODUCTION—*continued*

Body Part/Region - 4TH	Approach – 5TH	Substance – 6TH	Qualifier – 7TH
U Joints	3 Percutaneous	S Gas	F Other gas
U Joints	4 Percutaneous endoscopic	G Other therapeutic substance	C Other substance
V Bones	0 Open	G Other therapeutic substance	B Recombinant bone morphogenetic protein
V Bones	3 Percutaneous	0 Antineoplastic	5 Other antineoplastic M Monoclonal antibody
V Bones	3 Percutaneous	2 Anti-infective	8 Oxazolidinones 9 Other anti-infective
V Bones	3 Percutaneous	3 Anti-inflammatory 6 Nutritional substance 7 Electrolytic and water balance substance B Anesthetic agent H Radioactive substance K Other diagnostic substance N Analgesics, hypnotics, sedatives T Destructive agent	Z No qualifier
V Bones	3 Percutaneous	G Other therapeutic substance	B Recombinant bone morphogenetic protein C Other substance
W Lymphatics	3 Percutaneous	0 Antineoplastic	5 Other antineoplastic M Monoclonal antibody
W Lymphatics	3 Percutaneous	2 Anti-infective	8 Oxazolidinones 9 Other anti-infective
W Lymphatics	3 Percutaneous	3 Anti-inflammatory 6 Nutritional substance 7 Electrolytic and water balance substance B Anesthetic agent H Radioactive substance K Other diagnostic substance N Analgesics, hypnotics, sedatives T Destructive agent	Z No qualifier
W Lymphatics	3 Percutaneous	G Other therapeutic substance	C Other substance
Y Pericardial Cavity	3 Percutaneous	0 Antineoplastic	4 Liquid brachytherapy radioisotope 5 Other antineoplastic M Monoclonal antibody
Y Pericardial Cavity	3 Percutaneous	2 Anti-infective	8 Oxazolidinones 9 Other anti-infective
Y Pericardial Cavity	3 Percutaneous	3 Anti-inflammatory 6 Nutritional substance 7 Electrolytic and water balance substance B Anesthetic agent H Radioactive substance K Other diagnostic substance N Analgesics, hypnotics, sedatives T Destructive agent	Z No qualifier
Y Pericardial Cavity	3 Percutaneous	G Other therapeutic substance	C Other substance
Y Pericardial Cavity	3 Percutaneous	S Gas	F Other gas

continued ⇨

© 2018 Channel Publishing, Ltd.

3 E 0 INTRODUCTION—*continued*

Body Part/Region - 4TH	Approach – 5TH	Substance – 6TH	Qualifier – 7TH
Y Pericardial Cavity	4 Percutaneous endoscopic	G Other therapeutic substance	C Other substance
Y Pericardial Cavity	7 Via natural or artificial opening	0 Antineoplastic	4 Liquid brachytherapy radioisotope 5 Other antineoplastic M Monoclonal antibody
Y Pericardial Cavity	7 Via natural or artificial opening	S Gas	F Other gas

1ST - 3 Administration
2ND - E Physiological Systems and Anatomical Regions
3RD - 1 IRRIGATION

ADMINISTRATION SECTION: Introduction, Irrigation, Transfusion
Root Operations that define procedures where a diagnostic or therapeutic substance is given to the patient.
IRRIGATION: Putting in or on a cleansing substance.

Explanation: Cleansing substance or dialysate
Example: Flushing eye

Body Part – 4TH	Approach – 5TH	Device – 6TH	Qualifier – 7TH
0 Skin and Mucous Membranes C Eye	3 Percutaneous X External	8 Irrigating substance	X Diagnostic Z No qualifier
9 Nose B Ear F Respiratory Tract G Upper GI H Lower GI J Biliary and Pancreatic Tract K Genitourinary Tract N Male Reproductive ♂ P Female Reproductive ♀	3 Percutaneous 7 Via natural or artificial opening 8 Via natural or artificial opening endoscopic	8 Irrigating substance	X Diagnostic Z No qualifier
L Pleural Cavity Q Cranial Cavity and Brain R Spinal Canal S Epidural Space U Joints Y Pericardial Cavity	3 Percutaneous	8 Irrigating substance	X Diagnostic Z No qualifier
M Peritoneal Cavity	3 Percutaneous	8 Irrigating substance	X Diagnostic Z No qualifier
M Peritoneal Cavity	3 Percutaneous	9 Dialysate	Z No qualifier

© 2018 Channel Publishing, Ltd.

NOTES

© 2018 Channel Publishing, Ltd.

Educational Annotations | Section 4 – Measurement and Monitoring

Section Specific Educational Annotations for the Measurement and Monitoring Section include:

- **AHA Coding Clinic® Reference Notations**
- **Coding Notes**

AHA Coding Clinic® Reference Notations of Measurement and Monitoring

ROOT OPERATION SPECIFIC - MEASUREMENT AND MONITORING - Section 4

MEASUREMENT - 0

Left heart cardiac catheterization .... AHA 13:3Q:p26
Measurement of cardiac sampling and pressure with right and left heart cathetization .... AHA 18:1Q:p12
Myocardial Fractional Flow Reserve (FFR) measurement .... AHA 16:3Q:p37

MONITORING - 1

Continuous arterial pressure monitoring........ AHA 16:2Q:p33
EMG monitoring during surgery .... AHA 15:2Q:p14
Intraoperative neuromonitoring .... AHA 14:4Q:p28
.... AHA 15:1Q:p26
Monitoring using fluorescence vascular angiography .... AHA 16:4Q:p114

Coding Notes of Measurement and Monitoring

MEASUREMENT 4

© 2018 Channel Publishing, Ltd.

1ST - 4 Measurement and Monitoring
2ND - A Physiological Systems
3RD - 0 MEASUREMENT

MEASUREMENT AND MONITORING SECTION: Measurement, Monitoring
Root Operations that define one procedure/level and a series of procedures/levels obtained at intervals.
MEASUREMENT: Determining the level of a physiological or physical function at a point in time.

Explanation: Describes a single measurement
Example: EKG (single electrocardiogram)

Body System – 4TH	Approach – 5TH	Function/Device – 6TH	Qualifier – 7TH
0 Central Nervous	0 Open	2 Conductivity 4 Electrical activity B Pressure	Z No qualifier
0 Central Nervous	3 Percutaneous 7 Via natural or artificial opening 8 Via natural or artificial opening endoscopic	4 Electrical activity	Z No qualifier
0 Central Nervous	3 Percutaneous 7 Via natural or artificial opening 8 Via natural or artificial opening endoscopic	B Pressure K Temperature R Saturation	D Intracranial
0 Central Nervous	X External	2 Conductivity 4 Electrical activity	Z No qualifier
1 Peripheral Nervous	0 Open 3 Percutaneous 7 Via natural or artificial opening 8 Via natural or artificial opening endoscopic X External	2 Conductivity	9 Sensory B Motor
1 Peripheral Nervous	0 Open 3 Percutaneous 7 Via natural or artificial opening 8 Via natural or artificial opening endoscopic X External	4 Electrical activity	Z No qualifier
2 Cardiac	0 Open 3 Percutaneous 7 Via natural or artificial opening 8 Via natural or artificial opening endoscopic	4 Electrical activity 9 Output C Rate F Rhythm H Sound P Action currents	Z No qualifier
2 Cardiac	0 Open 3 Percutaneous 7 Via natural or artificial opening 8 Via natural or artificial opening endoscopic	N Sampling and pressure	6 Right heart 7 Left heart 8 Bilateral
2 Cardiac	X External	4 Electrical activity	A Guidance Z No qualifier
2 Cardiac	X External	9 Output C Rate F Rhythm H Sound P Action currents	Z No qualifier
2 Cardiac	X External	M Total activity	4 Stress
3 Arterial	0 Open 3 Percutaneous	5 Flow J Pulse	1 Peripheral 3 Pulmonary C Coronary
3 Arterial	0 Open 3 Percutaneous	B Pressure	1 Peripheral 3 Pulmonary C Coronary F Other Thoracic
3 Arterial	0 Open 3 Percutaneous	H Sound R Saturation	1 Peripheral

continued ⇨

© 2018 Channel Publishing, Ltd.

4 A 0 MEASUREMENT – *continued*

Body System – 4TH	Approach – 5TH	Function/Device – 6TH	Qualifier – 7TH
3 Arterial	X External	5 Flow B Pressure H Sound J Pulse R Saturation	1 Peripheral
4 Venous	0 Open 3 Percutaneous	5 Flow B Pressure J Pulse	0 Central 1 Peripheral 2 Portal 3 Pulmonary
4 Venous	0 Open 3 Percutaneous	R Saturation	1 Peripheral
4 Venous	X External	5 Flow B Pressure J Pulse R Saturation	1 Peripheral
5 Circulatory	X External	L Volume	Z No qualifier
6 Lymphatic	0 Open 3 Percutaneous 7 Via natural or artificial opening 8 Via natural or artificial opening endoscopic	5 Flow B Pressure	Z No qualifier
7 Visual	X External	0 Acuity 7 Mobility B Pressure	Z No qualifier
8 Olfactory	X External	0 Acuity	Z No qualifier
9 Respiratory	7 Via natural or artificial opening 8 Via natural or artificial opening endoscopic X External	1 Capacity 5 Flow C Rate D Resistance L Volume M Total activity	Z No qualifier
B Gastrointestinal	7 Via natural or artificial opening 8 Via natural or artificial opening endoscopic	0 Motility B Pressure G Secretion	Z No qualifier
C Biliary	3 Percutaneous 4 Percutaneous endoscopic 7 Via natural or artificial opening 8 Via natural or artificial opening endoscopic	5 Flow B Pressure	Z No qualifier
D Urinary	7 Via natural or artificial opening 8 Via natural or artificial opening endoscopic	3 Contractility 5 Flow B Pressure D Resistance L Volume	Z No qualifier
F Musculoskeletal	3 Percutaneous X External	3 Contractility	Z No qualifier
H Products of Conception, Cardiac ♀	7 Via natural or artificial opening 8 Via natural or artificial opening endoscopic X External	4 Electrical activity C Rate F Rhythm H Sound	Z No qualifier
J Products of Conception, Nervous ♀	7 Via natural or artificial opening 8 Via natural or artificial opening endoscopic X External	2 Conductivity 4 Electrical activity B Pressure	Z No qualifier
Z None	7 Via natural or artificial opening	6 Metabolism K Temperature	Z No qualifier
Z None	X External	6 Metabolism K Temperature Q Sleep	Z No qualifier

© 2018 Channel Publishing, Ltd.

1ST - 4 Measurement and Monitoring
2ND - A Physiological Systems
3RD - 1 MONITORING

MEASUREMENT AND MONITORING SECTION: Measurement, Monitoring
Root Operations that define one procedure/level and a series of procedures/levels obtained at intervals.
MONITORING: Determining the level of a physiological or physical function repetitively over a period of time.
Explanation: Describes a series of measurements
Example: Holter monitor

Body System – 4TH	Approach – 5TH	Function/Device – 6TH	Qualifier – 7TH
0 Central Nervous	0 Open	2 Conductivity B Pressure	Z No qualifier
0 Central Nervous	0 Open	4 Electrical activity	G Intraoperative Z No qualifier
0 Central Nervous	3 Percutaneous 7 Via natural or artificial opening 8 Via natural or artificial opening endoscopic	4 Electrical activity	G Intraoperative Z No qualifier
0 Central Nervous	3 Percutaneous 7 Via natural or artificial opening 8 Via natural or artificial opening endoscopic	B Pressure K Temperature R Saturation	D Intracranial
0 Central Nervous	X External	2 Conductivity	Z No qualifier
0 Central Nervous	X External	4 Electrical activity	G Intraoperative Z No qualifier
1 Peripheral Nervous	0 Open 3 Percutaneous 7 Via natural or artificial opening 8 Via natural or artificial opening endoscopic X External	2 Conductivity	9 Sensory B Motor
1 Peripheral Nervous	0 Open 3 Percutaneous 7 Via natural or artificial opening 8 Via natural or artificial opening endoscopic X External	4 Electrical activity	G Intraoperative Z No qualifier
2 Cardiac	0 Open 3 Percutaneous 7 Via natural or artificial opening 8 Via natural or artificial opening endoscopic	4 Electrical activity 9 Output C Rate F Rhythm H Sound	Z No qualifier
2 Cardiac	X External	4 Electrical activity	5 Ambulatory Z No qualifier
2 Cardiac	X External	9 Output C Rate F Rhythm H Sound	Z No qualifier
2 Cardiac	X External	M Total activity	4 Stress
2 Cardiac	X External	S Vascular perfusion	H Indocyanine green dye
3 Arterial	0 Open 3 Percutaneous	5 Flow B Pressure J Pulse	1 Peripheral 3 Pulmonary C Coronary
3 Arterial	0 Open 3 Percutaneous	H Sound R Saturation	1 Peripheral
3 Arterial	X External	5 Flow B Pressure H Sound J Pulse R Saturation	1 Peripheral

continued ⇨

© 2018 Channel Publishing, Ltd.

4 A 1 MONITORING—continued

Body System – 4TH	Approach – 5TH	Function/Device – 6TH	Qualifier – 7TH
4 Venous	0 Open 3 Percutaneous	5 Flow B Pressure J Pulse	0 Central 1 Peripheral 2 Portal 3 Pulmonary
4 Venous	0 Open 3 Percutaneous	R Saturation	0 Central 2 Portal 3 Pulmonary
4 Venous	X External	5 Flow B Pressure J Pulse	1 Peripheral
6 Lymphatic	0 Open 3 Percutaneous 7 Via natural or artificial opening 8 Via natural or artificial opening endoscopic	5 Flow B Pressure	Z No qualifier
9 Respiratory	7 Via natural or artificial opening X External	1 Capacity 5 Flow C Rate D Resistance L Volume	Z No qualifier
B Gastrointestinal	7 Via natural or artificial opening 8 Via natural or artificial opening endoscopic	8 Motility B Pressure G Secretion	Z No qualifier
B Gastrointestinal	X External	S Vascular perfusion	H Indocyanine green dye
D Urinary	7 Via natural or artificial opening 8 Via natural or artificial opening endoscopic	3 Contractility 5 Flow B Pressure D Resistance L Volume	Z No qualifier
G Skin and Breast	X External	S Vascular perfusion	H Indocyanine green dye
H Products of Conception, Cardiac ♀	7 Via natural or artificial opening 8 Via natural or artificial opening endoscopic X External	4 Electrical activity C Rate F Rhythm H Sound	Z No qualifier
J Products of Conception, Nervous ♀	7 Via natural or artificial opening 8 Via natural or artificial opening endoscopic X External	2 Conductivity 4 Electrical activity B Pressure	Z No qualifier
Z None	7 Via natural or artificial opening	K Temperature	Z No qualifier
Z None	X External	K Temperature Q Sleep	Z No qualifier

© 2018 Channel Publishing, Ltd.

1ST - 4 Measurement and Monitoring
2ND - B Physiological Devices
3RD - 0 MEASUREMENT

MEASUREMENT AND MONITORING SECTION: Measurement, Monitoring
Root Operations that define one procedure/level and a series of procedures/levels obtained at intervals.
MEASUREMENT: Determining the level of a physiological or physical function at a point in time.
Explanation: Describes a single measurement
Example: Pacemaker rate check

Body Part – 4TH	Approach – 5TH	Device – 6TH	Qualifier – 7TH
0 Central Nervous 1 Peripheral Nervous F Musculoskeletal	X External	V Stimulator	Z No qualifier
2 Cardiac	X External	S Pacemaker T Defibrillator	Z No qualifier
9 Respiratory	X External	S Pacemaker	Z No qualifier

© 2018 Channel Publishing, Ltd.

Educational Annotations | Section 5 – Extracorporeal or Systemic Assistance and Performance

Section Specific Educational Annotations for the Extracorporeal or Systemic Assistance and Performance Section include:

- **AHA Coding Clinic® Reference Notations**
- **Coding Notes**

AHA Coding Clinic® Reference Notations of Extracoporeal or Systemic Assistance and Performance

ROOT OPERATION SPECIFIC - EXTRACORPOREAL OR SYSTEMIC ASSISTANCE AND PERFORMANCE - Section 5

ASSISTANCE - 0

Assistance with cardiac output using impeller pump ....AHA 17:1Q:p10-12
BiPAP ventilatory support system................................AHA 14:4Q:p9
Extracorporeal carbon dioxide removal (ECCO2R) ....AHA 17:4Q:p71
Impella assistance/support................................AHA 14:3Q:p19
Intra-aortic balloon pump ....AHA 13:3Q:p18
Intra-aortic balloon pump - Official Advice Superceded ....AHA 18:2Q:p3
Intra-aortic balloon pump (IABP) ....AHA 18:2Q:p3
Noninvasive ventilation (NIV) performed on newborns ....AHA 17:1Q:p29
Positive pressure ventilation (PPV) for newborn resuscitation ....AHA 17:1Q:p29

PERFORMANCE - 1

Cardiopulmonary bypass ....AHA 14:3Q:p17,20
................................AHA 14:1Q:P10
................................AHA 13:3Q:p18
Continuous cardiac pacing................................AHA 13:3Q:p18
Extracoporeal liver assist device (ELAD) filtration................................AHA 16:1Q:p28
Hemodialysis and renal replacement therapy ....AHA 17:4Q:p71
Hemodialysis treatments, multiple ....AHA 16:1Q:p29
Mechanical ventilation ....AHA 14:4Q:p3
Mechanical ventilation, at night for sleep apnea................................AHA 14:4Q:p11
Ventilator assistance in hospital using patient's home ventilator ....AHA 18:1Q:p13

RESTORATION - 2

Coding Notes of Extracoporeal or Systemic Assistance and Performance

EXTRA ASSISTANCE 5

1ST - 5 Extracorporeal or Systemic Assistance and Performance
2ND - A Physiological Systems
3RD - 0 **ASSISTANCE**

EXTRACORPOREAL OR SYSTEMIC ASSISTANCE AND PERFORMANCE SECTION: Assistance, Performance, Restoration
Root Operations that use equipment to support a physiological function in some manner.
ASSISTANCE: Taking over a portion of a physiological function by extracorporeal means.

Explanation: Supports, but does not take over function
Example: Intra-aortic balloon pump

Body System – 4TH	Duration – 5TH	Function – 6TH	Qualifier – 7TH
2 Cardiac	1 Intermittent 2 Continuous	1 Output	0 Balloon pump 5 Pulsatile compression 6 Other pump D Impeller pump
5 Circulatory	1 Intermittent 2 Continuous	2 Oxygenation	1 Hyperbaric C Supersaturated
9 Respiratory	2 Continuous	0 Filtration	Z No qualifier
9 Respiratory	3 Less than 24 consecutive hours 4 24-96 consecutive hours 5 Greater than 96 consecutive hours	5 Ventilation	7 Continuous positive airway pressure 8 Intermittent positive airway pressure 9 Continuous negative airway pressure B Intermittent negative airway pressure Z No qualifier

© 2018 Channel Publishing, Ltd.

1ST - 5 Extracorporeal or Systemic Assistance and Performance
2ND - A Physiological Systems
3RD - 1 PERFORMANCE

EXTRACORPOREAL OR SYSTEMIC ASSISTANCE AND PERFORMANCE SECTION: Assistance, Performance, Restoration
Root Operations that use equipment to support a physiological function in some manner.
PERFORMANCE: Completely taking over a physiological function by extracorporeal means.

Explanation: Completely takes over function ...
Example: Cardiopulmonary bypass in CABG

Body System – 4TH	Duration – 5TH	Function – 6TH	Qualifier – 7TH
2 Cardiac	0 Single	1 Output	2 Manual
2 Cardiac	1 Intermittent	3 Pacing	Z No qualifier
2 Cardiac	2 Continuous	1 Output 3 Pacing	Z No qualifier
5 Circulatory	2 Continuous	2 Oxygenation	F Membrane, central G Membrane, peripheral veno-arterial H Membrane, peripheral veno-venous
9 Respiratory	0 Single	5 Ventilation	4 Nonmechanical
9 Respiratory	3 Less than 24 consecutive hours 4 24-96 consecutive hours 5 Greater than 96 consecutive hours LOS*	5 Ventilation	Z No qualifier
C Biliary	0 Single 6 Multiple	0 Filtration	Z No qualifier
D Urinary	7 Intermittent, less than 6 hours per day 8 Prolonged intermittent, 6-18 hours per day 9 Continuous, greater than 18 hours per day	0 Filtration	Z No qualifier

LOS* – Procedure Inconsistent with LOS Edit – Code only when the respiratory ventilation is provided for greater than four consecutive days during the length of stay. See current Medicare Code Editor for details.

1ST - 5 Extracorporeal or Systemic Assistance and Performance
2ND - A Physiological Systems
3RD - 2 RESTORATION

EXTRACORPOREAL OR SYSTEMIC ASSISTANCE AND PERFORMANCE SECTION: Assistance, Performance, Restoration
Root Operations that use equipment to support a physiological function in some manner.
RESTORATION: Returning, or attempting to return, a physiological function to its original state by extracorporeal means.

Explanation: Defibrillation and cardioversion only ...
Example: Cardiac defibrillation

Body System – 4TH	Duration – 5TH	Function – 6TH	Qualifier – 7TH
2 Cardiac	0 Single	4 Rhythm	Z No qualifier

© 2018 Channel Publishing, Ltd.

Educational Annotations | Section 6 – Extracorporeal or Systemic Therapies

Section Specific Educational Annotations for the Extracorporeal or Systemic Therapies Section include:
- **AHA Coding Clinic® Reference Notations**
- **Coding Notes**

AHA Coding Clinic® Reference Notations of Extracorporeal or Systemic Therapies

ROOT OPERATION SPECIFIC - EXTRACORPOREAL THERAPIES - Section 6
ATMOSPHERIC CONTROL - 0
DECOMPRESSION - 1
ELECTROMAGNETIC THERAPY - 2
HYPERTHERMIA - 3
HYPOTHERMIA - 4
PHERESIS - 5
PHOTOTHERAPY - 6
ULTRASOUND THERAPY - 7
Ultrasound accelerated thrombolysis ....AHA 14:4Q:p19
ULTRVIOLET LIGHT THERAPY - 8
SHOCK WAVE THERAPY - 9

Coding Notes of Extracorporeal or Systemic Therapies

© 2018 Channel Publishing, Ltd.

1ST - 6 Extracorporeal or Systemic Therapies
2ND - A Physiological Systems
3RD - 0 ATMOSPHERIC CONTROL

EXTRACORPOREAL OR SYSTEMIC THERAPIES SECTION: Atmospheric Control, Decompression, Electromagnetic Therapy, Hyperthermia, Hypothermia, Pheresis, Phototherapy, Ultrasound Therapy, Ultraviolet Light Therapy, Shock Wave Therapy, Perfusion
Root Operations that describe other extracorporeal procedures that are not defined in Section 5.
ATMOSPHERIC CONTROL: Extracorporeal control of atmospheric pressure and composition.
Explanation: Control air composition and pressure ... Example: Antigen-free air conditioning

Body System – 4TH	Duration – 5TH	Qualifier – 6TH	Qualifier – 7TH
Z None	0 Single 1 Multiple	Z No qualifier	Z No qualifier

1ST - 6 Extracorporeal or Systemic Therapies
2ND - A Physiological Systems
3RD - 1 DECOMPRESSION

EXTRACORPOREAL OR SYSTEMIC THERAPIES SECTION: Atmospheric Control, Decompression, Electromagnetic Therapy, Hyperthermia, Hypothermia, Pheresis, Phototherapy, Ultrasound Therapy, Ultraviolet Light Therapy, Shock Wave Therapy, Perfusion
Root Operations that describe other extracorporeal procedures that are not defined in Section 5.
DECOMPRESSION: Extracorporeal elimination of undisolved gas from body fluids.
Explanation: Used to treat the "bends" ... Example: Decompression chamber treatment

Body System – 4TH	Duration – 5TH	Qualifier – 6TH	Qualifier – 7TH
5 Circulatory	0 Single 1 Multiple	Z No qualifier	Z No qualifier

1ST - 6 Extracorporeal or Systemic Therapies
2ND - A Physiological Systems
3RD - 2 ELECTROMAGNETIC THERAPY

EXTRACORPOREAL OR SYSTEMIC THERAPIES SECTION: Atmospheric Control, Decompression, Electromagnetic Therapy, Hyperthermia, Hypothermia, Pheresis, Phototherapy, Ultrasound Therapy, Ultraviolet Light Therapy, Shock Wave Therapy, Perfusion
Root Operations that describe other extracorporeal procedures that are not defined in Section 5.
ELECTROMAGNETIC THERAPY: Extracorporeal treatment by electromagnetic rays.
Explanation: EM energy to stimulate cells ... Example: Transcranial magnetic stimulation (TMS)

Body System – 4TH	Duration – 5TH	Qualifier – 6TH	Qualifier – 7TH
1 Urinary 2 Central Nervous	0 Single 1 Multiple	Z No qualifier	Z No qualifier

1ST - 6 Extracorporeal or Systemic Therapies
2ND - A Physiological Systems
3RD - 3 HYPERTHERMIA

EXTRACORPOREAL OR SYSTEMIC THERAPIES SECTION: Atmospheric Control, Decompression, Electromagnetic Therapy, Hyperthermia, Hypothermia, Pheresis, Phototherapy, Ultrasound Therapy, Ultraviolet Light Therapy, Shock Wave Therapy, Perfusion
Root Operations that describe other extracorporeal procedures that are not defined in Section 5.
HYPERTHERMIA: Extracorporeal raising of body temperature.
Explanation: Used to treat temperature imbalance ... Example: Whole body hyperthermia

Body System – 4TH	Duration – 5TH	Qualifier – 6TH	Qualifier – 7TH
Z None	0 Single 1 Multiple	Z No qualifier	Z No qualifier

© 2018 Channel Publishing, Ltd.

1ST - 6 Extracorporeal or Systemic Therapies
2ND - A Physiological Systems
3RD - 4 HYPOTHERMIA

EXTRACORPOREAL OR SYSTEMIC THERAPIES SECTION: Atmospheric Control, Decompression, Electromagnetic Therapy, Hyperthermia, Hypothermia, Pheresis, Phototherapy, Ultrasound Therapy, Ultraviolet Light Therapy, Shock Wave Therapy, Perfusion
Root Operations that describe other extracorporeal procedures that are not defined in Section 5.

HYPOTHERMIA: Extracorporeal lowering of body temperature.

Explanation: Used to treat temperature imbalance ... Example: Whole body hypothermia

Body System – 4TH	Duration – 5TH	Qualifier – 6TH	Qualifier – 7TH
Z None	0 Single 1 Multiple	Z No qualifier	Z No qualifier

1ST - 6 Extracorporeal or Systemic Therapies
2ND - A Physiological Systems
3RD - 5 PHERESIS

EXTRACORPOREAL OR SYSTEMIC THERAPIES SECTION: Atmospheric Control, Decompression, Electromagnetic Therapy, Hyperthermia, Hypothermia, Pheresis, Phototherapy, Ultrasound Therapy, Ultraviolet Light Therapy, Shock Wave Therapy, Perfusion
Root Operations that describe other extracorporeal procedures that are not defined in Section 5.

PHERESIS: Extracorporeal separation of blood products.

Explanation: Used to separate and remove blood products ... Example: Therapeutic leukapheresis

Body System – 4TH	Duration – 5TH	Qualifier – 6TH	Qualifier – 7TH
5 Circulatory	0 Single 1 Multiple	Z No qualifier	0 Erythrocytes 1 Leukocytes 2 Platelets 3 Plasma T Stem cells, cord blood V Stem cells, hematopoietic

1ST - 6 Extracorporeal or Systemic Therapies
2ND - A Physiological Systems
3RD - 6 PHOTOTHERAPY

EXTRACORPOREAL OR SYSTEMIC THERAPIES SECTION: Atmospheric Control, Decompression, Electromagnetic Therapy, Hyperthermia, Hypothermia, Pheresis, Phototherapy, Ultrasound Therapy, Ultraviolet Light Therapy, Shock Wave Therapy, Perfusion
Root Operations that describe other extracorporeal procedures that are not defined in Section 5.

PHOTOTHERAPY: Extracorporeal treatment by light rays.

Explanation: Uses light rays for treatment ... Example: Phototherapy of circulatory system

Body System – 4TH	Duration – 5TH	Qualifier – 6TH	Qualifier – 7TH
0 Skin 5 Circulatory	0 Single 1 Multiple	Z No qualifier	Z No qualifier

1ST - 6 Extracorporeal or Systemic Therapies
2ND - A Physiological Systems
3RD - 7 ULTRASOUND THERAPY

EXTRACORPOREAL OR SYSTEMIC THERAPIES SECTION: Atmospheric Control, Decompression, Electromagnetic Therapy, Hyperthermia, Hypothermia, Pheresis, Phototherapy, Ultrasound Therapy, Ultraviolet Light Therapy, Shock Wave Therapy, Perfusion
Root Operations that describe other extracorporeal procedures that are not defined in Section 5.

ULTRASOUND THERAPY: Extracorporeal treatment by ultrasound.

Explanation: Therapeutic use of ultrasound waves ... Example: Therapeutic ultrasound of vessels

Body System – 4TH	Duration – 5TH	Qualifier – 6TH	Qualifier – 7TH
5 Circulatory	0 Single 1 Multiple	Z No qualifier	4 Head and Neck Vessels 5 Heart 6 Peripheral Vessels 7 Other Vessels Z No qualifier

© 2018 Channel Publishing, Ltd.

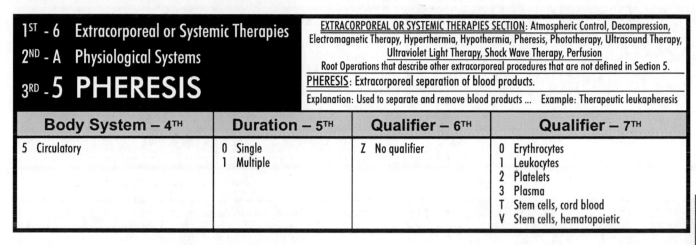

1ST - 6 Extracorporeal or Systemic Therapies
2ND - A Physiological Systems
3RD - 8 ULTRAVIOLET LIGHT THERAPY

EXTRACORPOREAL OR SYSTEMIC THERAPIES SECTION: Atmospheric Control, Decompression, Electromagnetic Therapy, Hyperthermia, Hypothermia, Pheresis, Phototherapy, Ultrasound Therapy, Ultraviolet Light Therapy, Shock Wave Therapy, Perfusion
Root Operations that describe other extracorporeal procedures that are not defined in Section 5.
ULTRAVIOLET LIGHT THERAPY: Extracorporeal treatment by ultraviolet light.
Explanation: Ultraviolet for treatment ... Example: Ultraviolet light therapy of newborns

Body System – 4TH	Duration – 5TH	Qualifier – 6TH	Qualifier – 7TH
0 Skin	0 Single 1 Multiple	Z No qualifier	Z No qualifier

1ST - 6 Extracorporeal or Systemic Therapies
2ND - A Physiological Systems
3RD - 9 SHOCK WAVE THERAPY

EXTRACORPOREAL OR SYSTEMIC THERAPIES SECTION: Atmospheric Control, Decompression, Electromagnetic Therapy, Hyperthermia, Hypothermia, Pheresis, Phototherapy, Ultrasound Therapy, Ultraviolet Light Therapy, Shock Wave Therapy, Perfusion
Root Operations that describe other extracorporeal procedures that are not defined in Section 5.
SHOCK WAVE THERAPY: Extracorporeal treatment by shock waves.
Explanation: Uses pulses of sound waves for treatment ... Example: Shock wave treatment of fascia

Body System – 4TH	Duration – 5TH	Qualifier – 6TH	Qualifier – 7TH
3 Musculoskeletal	0 Single 1 Multiple	Z No qualifier	Z No qualifier

1ST - 6 Extracorporeal or Systemic Therapies
2ND - A Physiological Systems
3RD - B PERFUSION

EXTRACORPOREAL OR SYSTEMIC THERAPIES SECTION: Atmospheric Control, Decompression, Electromagnetic Therapy, Hyperthermia, Hypothermia, Pheresis, Phototherapy, Ultrasound Therapy, Ultraviolet Light Therapy, Shock Wave Therapy, Perfusion
Root Operations that describe other extracorporeal procedures that are not defined in Section 5.
PERFUSION: Extracorporeal treatment by diffusion of therapeutic fluid.
Explanation: Perfusion of donor organ Example: Perfusion of donor organ

Body System – 4TH	Duration – 5TH	Qualifier – 6TH	Qualifier – 7TH
5 Circulatory B Respiratory System F Hepatobiliary System and Pancreas T Urinary System	0 Single	B Donor organ	Z No qualifier

© 2018 Channel Publishing, Ltd.

Educational Annotations | Section 7 – Osteopathic

Section Specific Educational Annotations for the Osteopathic Section include:

- AHA Coding Clinic® Reference Notations
- Coding Notes

AHA Coding Clinic® Reference Notations of Osteopathic

ROOT OPERATION SPECIFIC - OSTEOPATHIC - Section 7

TREATMENT - 0

Coding Notes of Osteopathic

1ST - 7 Osteopathic

2ND - W Anatomical Regions

3RD - 0 TREATMENT

OSTEOPATHIC SECTION: Treatment
Root Operation that defines osteopathic treatment.

TREATMENT: Manual treatment to eliminate or alleviate somatic dysfunction and related disorders.

Explanation: Uses only osteopathic methods and treatments
Example: Articulopathy osteopathic treatment

Body Region – 4TH	Approach – 5TH	Method – 6TH	Qualifier – 7TH
0 Head	X External	0 Articulatory-raising	Z None
1 Cervical		1 Fascial release	
2 Thoracic		2 General mobilization	
3 Lumbar		3 High velocity-low amplitude	
4 Sacrum		4 Indirect	
5 Pelvis		5 Low velocity-high amplitude	
6 Lower Extremities		6 Lymphatic pump	
7 Upper Extremities		7 Muscle energy-isometric	
8 Rib Cage		8 Muscle energy-isotonic	
9 Abdomen		9 Other method	

© 2018 Channel Publishing, Ltd.

NOTES

© 2018 Channel Publishing, Ltd.

Educational Annotations | Section 8 – Other Procedures

Section Specific Educational Annotations for the Other Procedures Section include:

- AHA Coding Clinic® Reference Notations
- Coding Notes

AHA Coding Clinic® Reference Notations of Other Procedures

ROOT OPERATION SPECIFIC - OTHER PROCEDURES - Section 8
COLLECTION - 6
NEAR INFRARED SPECTROSCOPY - D
COMPUTER ASSISTED PROCEDURE - B
ROBOTIC ASSISTED PROCEDURE - C
Radical prostatectomy, robotic-assisted, with bilateral resection of vas deferens and seminal vesicles ....AHA 14:4Q:p33
Robotic assisted procedure ....AHA 15:1Q:p33
ACUPUNCTURE - 0
THERAPEUTIC MASSAGE - 1
OTHER METHOD - Y

Coding Notes of Other Procedures

1ST - 8 Other Procedures
2ND - C Indwelling Device
3RD - 0 OTHER PROCEDURES

OTHER PROCEDURES SECTION: Other Procedures
Root Operation that defines procedures not included in the Medical and Medical/Surgical related sections.
OTHER PROCEDURES: Methodologies which attempt to remediate or cure a disorder or disease.
Explanation: Procedures not included elsewhere
Example: None

Body Region – 4TH	Approach – 5TH	Method – 6TH	Qualifier – 7TH
1 Nervous System	X External	6 Collection	J Cerebrospinal fluid L Other fluid
2 Circulatory System	X External	6 Collection	K Blood L Other fluid

© 2018 Channel Publishing, Ltd.

1ST - 8 Other Procedures
2ND - E Physiological Systems and Anatomical Regions
3RD - 0 OTHER PROCEDURES

OTHER PROCEDURES SECTION: Other Procedures
Root Operation that defines procedures not included in the Medical and Medical/Surgical related sections.
OTHER PROCEDURES: Methodologies which attempt to remediate or cure a disorder or disease.
Explanation: Procedures not included elsewhere
Example: Suture removal

Body Region – 4TH	Approach – 5TH	Method – 6TH	Qualifier – 7TH
1 Nervous System U Female Reproductive System ♀	X External	Y Other method	7 Examination
2 Circulatory System	3 Percutaneous	D Near infrared spectroscopy	Z No qualifier
9 Head and Neck Region W Trunk Region	0 Open 3 Percutaneous 4 Percutaneous endoscopic 7 Via natural or artificial opening 8 Via natural or artificial opening endoscopic	C Robotic assisted procedure	Z No qualifier
9 Head and Neck Region W Trunk Region	X External	B Computer assisted procedure	F With fluoroscopy G With computerized tomography H With magnetic resonance imaging Z No qualifier
9 Head and Neck Region W Trunk Region	X External	C Robotic assisted procedure	Z No qualifier
9 Head and Neck Region W Trunk Region	X External	Y Other method	8 Suture removal
H Integumentary System and Breast	3 Percutaneous	0 Acupuncture	0 Anesthesia Z No qualifier
H Integumentary System and Breast ♀	X External	6 Collection	2 Breast milk
H Integumentary System and Breast	X External	Y Other method	9 Piercing
K Musculoskeletal System	X External	1 Therapeutic massage	Z No qualifier
K Musculoskeletal System	X External	Y Other method	7 Examination
V Male Reproductive System	X External	1 Therapeutic massage	C Prostate ♂ D Rectum
V Male Reproductive System ♂	X External	6 Collection	3 Sperm
X Upper Extremity Y Lower Extremity	0 Open 3 Percutaneous 4 Percutaneous endoscopic	C Robotic assisted procedure	Z No qualifier
X Upper Extremity Y Lower Extremity	X External	B Computer assisted procedure	F With fluoroscopy G With computerized tomography H With magnetic resonance imaging Z No qualifier
X Upper Extremity Y Lower Extremity	X External	C Robotic assisted procedure	Z No qualifier
X Upper Extremity Y Lower Extremity	X External	Y Other method	8 Suture removal
Z None	X External	Y Other method	1 In vitro fertilization 4 Yoga therapy 5 Meditation 6 Isolation

© 2018 Channel Publishing, Ltd.

Educational Annotations | Section 9 – Chiropractic

Section Specific Educational Annotations for the Chiropractic Section include:

- **AHA Coding Clinic® Reference Notations**
- **Coding Notes**

AHA Coding Clinic® Reference Notations of Chiropractic

ROOT OPERATION SPECIFIC - CHIROPRACTIC - Section 9

MANIPULATION - B

Coding Notes of Chiropractic

1ST - 9 Chiropractic
2ND - W Anatomical Regions
3RD - B MANIPULATION

CHIROPRACTIC SECTION: Treatment
Root Operation that defines chiropractic treatment.

MANIPULATION: Manual procedure that involves a directed thrust to move a joint past the physiological range of motion, without exceeding the anatomical limit.

Explanation: None
Example: Chiropractic manipulation of spine

Body Region – 4TH	Approach – 5TH	Method – 6TH	Qualifier – 7TH
0 Head 1 Cervical 2 Thoracic 3 Lumbar 4 Sacrum 5 Pelvis 6 Lower Extremities 7 Upper Extremities 8 Rib Cage 9 Abdomen	X External	B Non-manual C Indirect visceral D Extra-articular F Direct visceral G Long lever specific contact H Short lever specific contact J Long and short lever specific contact K Mechanically assisted L Other method	Z None

© 2018 Channel Publishing, Ltd.

NOTES

© 2018 Channel Publishing, Ltd.

Educational Annotations | Section B – Imaging

Section Specific Educational Annotations for the Imaging Section include:

- AHA Coding Clinic® Reference Notations
- Coding Notes

AHA Coding Clinic® Reference Notations of Imaging

ROOT TYPE SPECIFIC - IMAGING - Section B

PLAIN RADIOGRAPHY - 0

FLUOROSCOPY - 1

Fluoroscopic guidance of central venous catheter ....AHA 15:4Q:p30

Nonionic iso-osmolar contrast ....AHA 16:3Q:p36

COMPUTERIZED TOMOGRAPHY (CT SCAN) - 2

MAGNETIC RESONANCE IMAGING (MRI) - 3

ULTRASONOGRAPHY - 4

Ultrasonic guidance during ERCP ....AHA 14:3Q:p15

Coding Notes of Imaging

© 2018 Channel Publishing, Ltd.

1ST - B Imaging
2ND - 0 Central Nervous System
3RD - 0 PLAIN RADIOGRAPHY

PLAIN RADIOGRAPHY: Planar display of an image developed from the capture of external ionizing radiation on photographic or photoconductive plate.

Example: Chest X-ray

Body Part – 4TH	Contrast – 5TH	Qualifier – 6TH	Qualifier – 7TH
B Spinal Cord	0 High osmolar 1 Low osmolar Y Other contrast Z None	Z None	Z None

1ST - B Imaging
2ND - 0 Central Nervous System
3RD - 1 FLUOROSCOPY

FLUOROSCOPY: Single plane or bi-plane real time display of an image developed from the capture of external ionizing radiation on a fluorescent screen. The image may also be stored by either digital or analog means.

Example: Fluoroscopic guidance

Body Part – 4TH	Contrast – 5TH	Qualifier – 6TH	Qualifier – 7TH
B Spinal Cord	0 High osmolar 1 Low osmolar Y Other contrast Z None	Z None	Z None

1ST - B Imaging
2ND - 0 Central Nervous System
3RD - 2 COMPUTERIZED TOMOGRAPHY (CT Scan)

COMPUTERIZED TOMOGRAPHY (CT Scan): Computer reformatted digital display of multiplanar images developed from the capture of multiple exposures of external ionizing radiation.

Example: CT Scan of head

Body Part – 4TH	Contrast – 5TH	Qualifier – 6TH	Qualifier – 7TH
0 Brain 7 Cisterna 8 Cerebral Ventricle(s) 9 Sella Turcica/Pituitary Gland B Spinal Cord	0 High osmolar 1 Low osmolar Y Other contrast	0 Unenhanced and enhanced Z None	Z None
0 Brain 7 Cisterna 8 Cerebral Ventricle(s) 9 Sella Turcica/Pituitary Gland B Spinal Cord	Z None	Z None	Z None

1ST - B Imaging
2ND - 0 Central Nervous System
3RD - 3 MAGNETIC RESONANCE IMAGING (MRI)

MAGNETIC RESONANCE IMAGING (MRI): Computer reformatted digital display of multiplanar images developed from the capture of radiofrequency signals emitted by nuclei in a body site excited within a magnetic field.

Example: MRI of knee

Body Part – 4TH	Contrast – 5TH	Qualifier – 6TH	Qualifier – 7TH
0 Brain 9 Sella Turcica/Pituitary Gland B Spinal Cord C Acoustic Nerves	Y Other contrast	0 Unenhanced and enhanced Z None	Z None
0 Brain 9 Sella Turcica/Pituitary Gland B Spinal Cord C Acoustic Nerves	Z None	Z None	Z None

1ST - B Imaging
2ND - 0 Central Nervous System
3RD - 4 ULTRASONOGRAPHY

ULTRASONOGRAPHY: Real time display of images of anatomy or flow information developed from the capture of reflected and attenuated high frequency sound waves.

Example: Abdominal ultrasound

Body Part – 4TH	Contrast – 5TH	Qualifier – 6TH	Qualifier – 7TH
0 Brain B Spinal Cord	Z None	Z None	Z None

© 2018 Channel Publishing, Ltd.

1ST - B Imaging
2ND - 2 Heart
3RD - 0 PLAIN RADIOGRAPHY

PLAIN RADIOGRAPHY: Planar display of an image developed from the capture of external ionizing radiation on photographic or photoconductive plate.

Example: Chest X-ray

Body Part – 4TH		Contrast – 5TH	Qualifier – 6TH	Qualifier – 7TH
0 Coronary Artery, Single 1 Coronary Arteries, Multiple 2 Coronary Artery Bypass Graft, Single 3 Coronary Artery Bypass Grafts, Multiple 4 Heart, Right	5 Heart, Left 6 Heart, Right and Left 7 Internal Mammary Bypass Graft, Right 8 Internal Mammary Bypass Graft, Left F Bypass Graft, Other	0 High osmolar 1 Low osmolar Y Other contrast	Z None	Z None

1ST - B Imaging
2ND - 2 Heart
3RD - 1 FLUOROSCOPY

FLUOROSCOPY: Single plane or bi-plane real time display of an image developed from the capture of external ionizing radiation on a fluorescent screen. The image may also be stored by either digital or analog means.

Example: Fluoroscopic guidance

Body Part – 4TH		Contrast – 5TH	Qualifier – 6TH	Qualifier – 7TH
0 Coronary Artery, Single 1 Coronary Arteries, Multiple	2 Coronary Artery Bypass Graft, Single 3 Coronary Artery Bypass Grafts, Multiple	0 High osmolar 1 Low osmolar Y Other contrast	1 Laser	0 Intraoperative
0 Coronary Artery, Single 1 Coronary Arteries, Multiple	2 Coronary Artery Bypass Graft, Single 3 Coronary Artery Bypass Grafts, Multiple	0 High osmolar 1 Low osmolar Y Other contrast	Z None	Z None
4 Heart, Right 5 Heart, Left 6 Heart, Right and Left	7 Internal Mammary Bypass Graft, Right 8 Internal Mammary Bypass Graft, Left F Bypass Graft, Other	0 High osmolar 1 Low osmolar Y Other contrast	Z None	Z None

1ST - B Imaging
2ND - 2 Heart
3RD - 2 COMPUTERIZED TOMOGRAPHY (CT Scan)

COMPUTERIZED TOMOGRAPHY (CT Scan): Computer reformatted digital display of multiplanar images developed from the capture of multiple exposures of external ionizing radiation.

Example: CT Scan of head

Body Part – 4TH	Contrast – 5TH	Qualifier – 6TH	Qualifier – 7TH
1 Coronary Arteries, Multiple 3 Coronary Artery Bypass Grafts, Multiple 6 Heart, Right and Left	0 High osmolar 1 Low osmolar Y Other contrast	0 Unenhanced and enhanced Z None	Z None
1 Coronary Arteries, Multiple 3 Coronary Artery Bypass Grafts, Multiple 6 Heart, Right and Left	Z None	2 Intravascular optical coherence Z None	Z None

1ST - B Imaging
2ND - 2 Heart
3RD - 3 MAGNETIC RESONANCE IMAGING (MRI)

MAGNETIC RESONANCE IMAGING (MRI): Computer reformatted digital display of multiplanar images developed from the capture of radiofrequency signals emitted by nuclei in a body site excited within a magnetic field.

Example: MRI of knee

Body Part – 4TH	Contrast – 5TH	Qualifier – 6TH	Qualifier – 7TH
1 Coronary Arteries, Multiple 3 Coronary Artery Bypass Grafts, Multiple 6 Heart, Right and Left	Y Other contrast	0 Unenhanced and enhanced Z None	Z None
1 Coronary Arteries, Multiple 3 Coronary Artery Bypass Grafts, Multiple 6 Heart, Right and Left	Z None	Z None	Z None

© 2018 Channel Publishing, Ltd.

1ST - B Imaging
2ND - 2 Heart
3RD - 4 ULTRASONOGRAPHY

ULTRASONOGRAPHY: Real time display of images of anatomy or flow information developed from the capture of reflected and attenuated high frequency sound waves.

Example: Abdominal ultrasound

Body Part – 4TH		Contrast – 5TH	Qualifier – 6TH	Qualifier – 7TH
0 Coronary Artery, Single 1 Coronary Arteries, Multiple 4 Heart, Right 5 Heart, Left	6 Heart, Right and Left B Heart with Aorta C Pericardium D Pediatric Heart	Y Other contrast	Z None	Z None
0 Coronary Artery, Single 1 Coronary Arteries, Multiple 4 Heart, Right 5 Heart, Left	6 Heart, Right and Left B Heart with Aorta C Pericardium D Pediatric Heart	Z None	Z None	3 Intravascular 4 Transesophageal Z None

1ST - B Imaging
2ND - 3 Upper Arteries
3RD - 0 PLAIN RADIOGRAPHY

PLAIN RADIOGRAPHY: Planar display of an image developed from the capture of external ionizing radiation on photographic or photoconductive plate.

Example: Chest X-ray

Body Part – 4TH		Contrast – 5TH	Qualifier – 6TH	Qualifier – 7TH
0 Thoracic Aorta 1 Brachiocephalic-Subclavian Artery, Right 2 Subclavian Artery, Left 3 Common Carotid Artery, Right 4 Common Carotid Artery, Left 5 Common Carotid Arteries, Bilateral 6 Internal Carotid Artery, Right 7 Internal Carotid Artery, Left 8 Internal Carotid Arteries, Bilateral 9 External Carotid Artery, Right B External Carotid Artery, Left C External Carotid Arteries, Bilateral D Vertebral Artery, Right	F Vertebral Artery, Left G Vertebral Arteries, Bilateral H Upper Extremity Arteries, Right J Upper Extremity Arteries, Left K Upper Extremity Arteries, Bilateral L Intercostal and Bronchial Arteries M Spinal Arteries N Upper Arteries, Other P Thoraco-Abdominal Aorta Q Cervico-Cerebral Arch R Intracranial Arteries S Pulmonary Artery, Right T Pulmonary Artery, Left	0 High osmolar 1 Low osmolar Y Other contrast Z None	Z None	Z None

1ST - B Imaging
2ND - 3 Upper Arteries
3RD - 1 FLUOROSCOPY

FLUOROSCOPY: Single plane or bi-plane real time display of an image developed from the capture of external ionizing radiation on a fluorescent screen. The image may also be stored by either digital or analog means.

Example: Fluoroscopic guidance

Body Part – 4TH		Contrast – 5TH	Qualifier – 6TH	Qualifier – 7TH
0 Thoracic Aorta 1 Brachiocephalic-Subclavian Artery, Right 2 Subclavian Artery, Left 3 Common Carotid Artery, Right 4 Common Carotid Artery, Left 5 Common Carotid Arteries, Bilateral 6 Internal Carotid Artery, Right 7 Internal Carotid Artery, Left 8 Internal Carotid Arteries, Bilateral 9 External Carotid Artery, Right B External Carotid Artery, Left C External Carotid Arteries, Bilateral D Vertebral Artery, Right	F Vertebral Artery, Left G Vertebral Arteries, Bilateral H Upper Extremity Arteries, Right J Upper Extremity Arteries, Left K Upper Extremity Arteries, Bilateral L Intercostal and Bronchial Arteries M Spinal Arteries N Upper Arteries, Other P Thoraco-Abdominal Aorta Q Cervico-Cerebral Arch R Intracranial Arteries S Pulmonary Artery, Right T Pulmonary Artery, Left U Pulmonary Artery, Trunk	0 High osmolar 1 Low osmolar Y Other contrast	1 Laser	0 Intraoperative

continued ⇨

© 2018 Channel Publishing, Ltd.

B 3 1 FLUOROSCOPY—*continued*

Body Part – 4TH		Contrast – 5TH	Qualifier – 6TH	Qualifier – 7TH
0 Thoracic Aorta 1 Brachiocephalic-Subclavian Artery, Right 2 Subclavian Artery, Left 3 Common Carotid Artery, Right 4 Common Carotid Artery, Left 5 Common Carotid Arteries, Bilateral 6 Internal Carotid Artery, Right 7 Internal Carotid Artery, Left 8 Internal Carotid Arteries, Bilateral 9 External Carotid Artery, Right B External Carotid Artery, Left C External Carotid Arteries, Bilateral D Vertebral Artery, Right	F Vertebral Artery, Left G Vertebral Arteries, Bilateral H Upper Extremity Arteries, Right J Upper Extremity Arteries, Left K Upper Extremity Arteries, Bilateral L Intercostal and Bronchial Arteries M Spinal Arteries N Upper Arteries, Other P Thoraco-Abdominal Aorta Q Cervico-Cerebral Arch R Intracranial Arteries S Pulmonary Artery, Right T Pulmonary Artery, Left U Pulmonary Artery, Trunk	0 High osmolar 1 Low osmolar Y Other contrast	Z None	Z None
0 Thoracic Aorta 1 Brachiocephalic-Subclavian Artery, Right 2 Subclavian Artery, Left 3 Common Carotid Artery, Right 4 Common Carotid Artery, Left 5 Common Carotid Arteries, Bilateral 6 Internal Carotid Artery, Right 7 Internal Carotid Artery, Left 8 Internal Carotid Arteries, Bilateral 9 External Carotid Artery, Right B External Carotid Artery, Left C External Carotid Arteries, Bilateral D Vertebral Artery, Right	F Vertebral Artery, Left G Vertebral Arteries, Bilateral H Upper Extremity Arteries, Right J Upper Extremity Arteries, Left K Upper Extremity Arteries, Bilateral L Intercostal and Bronchial Arteries M Spinal Arteries N Upper Arteries, Other P Thoraco-Abdominal Aorta Q Cervico-Cerebral Arch R Intracranial Arteries S Pulmonary Artery, Right T Pulmonary Artery, Left U Pulmonary Artery, Trunk	Z None	Z None	Z None

1ST - B Imaging
2ND - 3 Upper Arteries
3RD - 2 COMPUTERIZED TOMOGRAPHY (CT Scan)

COMPUTERIZED TOMOGRAPHY (CT Scan): Computer reformatted digital display of multiplanar images developed from the capture of multiple exposures of external ionizing radiation.

Example: CT Scan of head

Body Part – 4TH		Contrast – 5TH	Qualifier – 6TH	Qualifier – 7TH
0 Thoracic Aorta 5 Common Carotid Arteries, Bilateral 8 Internal Carotid Arteries, Bilateral G Vertebral Arteries, Bilateral	R Intracranial Arteries S Pulmonary Artery, Right T Pulmonary Artery, Left	0 High osmolar 1 Low osmolar Y Other contrast	Z None	Z None
0 Thoracic Aorta 5 Common Carotid Arteries, Bilateral 8 Internal Carotid Arteries, Bilateral G Vertebral Arteries, Bilateral	R Intracranial Arteries S Pulmonary Artery, Right T Pulmonary Artery, Left	Z None	2 Intravascular optical coherence Z None	Z None

© 2018 Channel Publishing, Ltd.

1ST - B Imaging
2ND - 3 Upper Arteries
3RD - 3 MAGNETIC RESONANCE IMAGING (MRI)

MAGNETIC RESONANCE IMAGING (MRI): Computer reformatted digital display of multiplanar images developed from the capture of radiofrequency signals emitted by nuclei in a body site excited within a magnetic field.

Example: MRI of knee

Body Part – 4TH	Contrast – 5TH	Qualifier – 6TH	Qualifier – 7TH
0 Thoracic Aorta 5 Common Carotid Arteries, Bilateral 8 Internal Carotid Arteries, Bilateral G Vertebral Arteries, Bilateral H Upper Extremity Arteries, Right J Upper Extremity Arteries, Left K Upper Extremity Arteries, Bilateral M Spinal Arteries Q Cervico-Cerebral Arch R Intracranial Arteries	Y Other contrast	0 Unenhanced and enhanced Z None	Z None
0 Thoracic Aorta 5 Common Carotid Arteries, Bilateral 8 Internal Carotid Arteries, Bilateral G Vertebral Arteries, Bilateral H Upper Extremity Arteries, Right J Upper Extremity Arteries, Left K Upper Extremity Arteries, Bilateral M Spinal Arteries Q Cervico-Cerebral Arch R Intracranial Arteries	Z None	Z None	Z None

1ST - B Imaging
2ND - 3 Upper Arteries
3RD - 4 ULTRASONOGRAPHY

ULTRASONOGRAPHY: Real time display of images of anatomy or flow information developed from the capture of reflected and attenuated high frequency sound waves.

Example: Abdominal ultrasound

Body Part – 4TH	Contrast – 5TH	Qualifier – 6TH	Qualifier – 7TH
0 Thoracic Aorta 1 Brachiocephalic-Subclavian Artery, Right 2 Subclavian Artery, Left 3 Common Carotid Artery, Right 4 Common Carotid Artery, Left 5 Common Carotid Arteries, Bilateral 6 Internal Carotid Artery, Right 7 Internal Carotid Artery, Left 8 Internal Carotid Arteries, Bilateral H Upper Extremity Arteries, Right J Upper Extremity Arteries, Left K Upper Extremity Arteries, Bilateral R Intracranial Arteries S Pulmonary Artery, Right T Pulmonary Artery, Left V Ophthalmic Arteries	Z None	Z None	3 Intravascular Z None

1ST - B Imaging
2ND - 4 Lower Arteries
3RD - 0 PLAIN RADIOGRAPHY

PLAIN RADIOGRAPHY: Planar display of an image developed from the capture of external ionizing radiation on photographic or photoconductive plate.

Example: Chest X-ray

Body Part – 4TH	Contrast – 5TH	Qualifier – 6TH	Qualifier – 7TH
0 Abdominal Aorta 2 Hepatic Artery 3 Splenic Arteries 4 Superior Mesenteric Artery 5 Inferior Mesenteric Artery 6 Renal Artery, Right 7 Renal Artery, Left 8 Renal Arteries, Bilateral 9 Lumbar Arteries B Intra-Abdominal Arteries, Other C Pelvic Arteries D Aorta and Bilateral Lower Extremity Arteries F Lower Extremity Arteries, Right G Lower Extremity Arteries, Left J Lower Arteries, Other M Renal Artery Transplant	0 High osmolar 1 Low osmolar Y Other contrast	Z None	Z None

© 2018 Channel Publishing, Ltd.

1ST - B Imaging
2ND - 4 Lower Arteries
3RD - 1 FLUOROSCOPY

FLUOROSCOPY: Single plane or bi-plane real time display of an image developed from the capture of external ionizing radiation on a fluorescent screen. The image may also be stored by either digital or analog means.

Example: Fluoroscopic guidance

Body Part – 4TH		Contrast – 5TH	Qualifier – 6TH	Qualifier – 7TH
0 Abdominal Aorta 2 Hepatic Artery 3 Splenic Arteries 4 Superior Mesenteric Artery 5 Inferior Mesenteric Artery 6 Renal Artery, Right 7 Renal Artery, Left 8 Renal Arteries, Bilateral	9 Lumbar Arteries B Intra-Abdominal Arteries, Other C Pelvic Arteries D Aorta and Bilateral Lower Extremity Arteries F Lower Extremity Arteries, Right G Lower Extremity Arteries, Left J Lower Arteries, Other	0 High osmolar 1 Low osmolar Y Other contrast	1 Laser	0 Intraoperative
0 Abdominal Aorta 2 Hepatic Artery 3 Splenic Arteries 4 Superior Mesenteric Artery 5 Inferior Mesenteric Artery 6 Renal Artery, Right 7 Renal Artery, Left 8 Renal Arteries, Bilateral	9 Lumbar Arteries B Intra-Abdominal Arteries, Other C Pelvic Arteries D Aorta and Bilateral Lower Extremity Arteries F Lower Extremity Arteries, Right G Lower Extremity Arteries, Left J Lower Arteries, Other	0 High osmolar 1 Low osmolar Y Other contrast	Z None	Z None
0 Abdominal Aorta 2 Hepatic Artery 3 Splenic Arteries 4 Superior Mesenteric Artery 5 Inferior Mesenteric Artery 6 Renal Artery, Right 7 Renal Artery, Left 8 Renal Arteries, Bilateral	9 Lumbar Arteries B Intra-Abdominal Arteries, Other C Pelvic Arteries D Aorta and Bilateral Lower Extremity Arteries F Lower Extremity Arteries, Right G Lower Extremity Arteries, Left J Lower Arteries, Other	Z None	Z None	Z None

1ST - B Imaging
2ND - 4 Lower Arteries
3RD - 2 COMPUTERIZED TOMOGRAPHY (CT Scan)

COMPUTERIZED TOMOGRAPHY (CT Scan): Computer reformatted digital display of multiplanar images developed from the capture of multiple exposures of external ionizing radiation.

Example: CT Scan of head

Body Part – 4TH		Contrast – 5TH	Qualifier – 6TH	Qualifier – 7TH
0 Abdominal Aorta 1 Celiac Artery 4 Superior Mesenteric Artery 8 Renal Arteries, Bilateral C Pelvic Arteries	F Lower Extremity Arteries, Right G Lower Extremity Arteries, Left H Lower Extremity Arteries, Bilateral M Renal Artery Transplant	0 High osmolar 1 Low osmolar Y Other contrast	Z None	Z None
0 Abdominal Aorta 1 Celiac Artery 4 Superior Mesenteric Artery 8 Renal Arteries, Bilateral C Pelvic Arteries	F Lower Extremity Arteries, Right G Lower Extremity Arteries, Left H Lower Extremity Arteries, Bilateral M Renal Artery Transplant	Z None	2 Intravascular optical coherence Z None	Z None

© 2018 Channel Publishing, Ltd.

1ST - B Imaging
2ND - 4 Lower Arteries
3RD - 3 MAGNETIC RESONANCE IMAGING (MRI)

MAGNETIC RESONANCE IMAGING (MRI): Computer reformatted digital display of multiplanar images developed from the capture of radiofrequency signals emitted by nuclei in a body site excited within a magnetic field.

Example: MRI of knee

Body Part – 4TH	Contrast – 5TH	Qualifier – 6TH	Qualifier – 7TH
0 Abdominal Aorta 1 Celiac Artery 4 Superior Mesenteric Artery 8 Renal Arteries, Bilateral C Pelvic Arteries F Lower Extremity Arteries, Right G Lower Extremity Arteries, Left H Lower Extremity Arteries, Bilateral	Y Other contrast	0 Unenhanced and enhanced Z None	Z None
0 Abdominal Aorta 1 Celiac Artery 4 Superior Mesenteric Artery 8 Renal Arteries, Bilateral C Pelvic Arteries F Lower Extremity Arteries, Right G Lower Extremity Arteries, Left H Lower Extremity Arteries, Bilateral	Z None	Z None	Z None

1ST - B Imaging
2ND - 4 Lower Arteries
3RD - 4 ULTRASONOGRAPHY

ULTRASONOGRAPHY: Real time display of images of anatomy or flow information developed from the capture of reflected and attenuated high frequency sound waves.

Example: Abdominal ultrasound

Body Part – 4TH	Contrast – 5TH	Qualifier – 6TH	Qualifier – 7TH
0 Abdominal Aorta 4 Superior Mesenteric Artery 5 Inferior Mesenteric Artery 6 Renal Artery, Right 7 Renal Artery, Left 8 Renal Arteries, Bilateral B Intra-Abdominal Arteries, Other F Lower Extremity Arteries, Right G Lower Extremity Arteries, Left H Lower Extremity Arteries, Bilateral K Celiac and Mesenteric Arteries L Femoral Artery N Penile Arteries	Z None	Z None	3 Intravascular Z None

1ST - B Imaging
2ND - 5 Veins
3RD - 0 PLAIN RADIOGRAPHY

PLAIN RADIOGRAPHY: Planar display of an image developed from the capture of external ionizing radiation on photographic or photoconductive plate.

Example: Chest X-ray

Body Part – 4TH	Contrast – 5TH	Qualifier – 6TH	Qualifier – 7TH
0 Epidural Veins 1 Cerebral and Cerebellar Veins 2 Intracranial Sinuses 3 Jugular Veins, Right 4 Jugular Veins, Left 5 Jugular Veins, Bilateral 6 Subclavian Vein, Right 7 Subclavian Vein, Left 8 Superior Vena Cava 9 Inferior Vena Cava B Lower Extremity Veins, Right C Lower Extremity Veins, Left D Lower Extremity Veins, Bilateral F Pelvic (Iliac) Veins, Right G Pelvic (Iliac) Veins, Left H Pelvic (Iliac) Veins, Bilateral J Renal Vein, Right K Renal Vein, Left L Renal Veins, Bilateral M Upper Extremity Veins, Right N Upper Extremity Veins, Left P Upper Extremity Veins, Bilateral Q Pulmonary Vein, Right R Pulmonary Vein, Left S Pulmonary Veins, Bilateral T Portal and Splanchnic Veins V Veins, Other W Dialysis Shunt/Fistula	0 High osmolar 1 Low osmolar Y Other contrast	Z None	Z None

© 2018 Channel Publishing, Ltd.

1ST - B Imaging
2ND - 5 Veins
3RD - 1 FLUOROSCOPY

FLUOROSCOPY: Single plane or bi-plane real time display of an image developed from the capture of external ionizing radiation on a fluorescent screen. The image may also be stored by either digital or analog means.

Example: Fluoroscopic guidance

Body Part – 4TH		Contrast – 5TH	Qualifier – 6TH	Qualifier – 7TH
0 Epidural Veins 1 Cerebral and Cerebellar Veins 2 Intracranial Sinuses 3 Jugular Veins, Right 4 Jugular Veins, Left 5 Jugular Veins, Bilateral 6 Subclavian Vein, Right 7 Subclavian Vein, Left 8 Superior Vena Cava 9 Inferior Vena Cava B Lower Extremity Veins, Right C Lower Extremity Veins, Left D Lower Extremity Veins, Bilateral F Pelvic (Iliac) Veins, Right	G Pelvic (Iliac) Veins, Left H Pelvic (Iliac) Veins, Bilateral J Renal Vein, Right K Renal Vein, Left L Renal Veins, Bilateral M Upper Extremity Veins, Right N Upper Extremity Veins, Left P Upper Extremity Veins, Bilateral Q Pulmonary Vein, Right R Pulmonary Vein, Left S Pulmonary Veins, Bilateral T Portal and Splanchnic Veins V Veins, Other W Dialysis Shunt/Fistula	0 High osmolar 1 Low osmolar Y Other contrast Z None	Z None	A Guidance Z None

1ST - B Imaging
2ND - 5 Veins
3RD - 2 COMPUTERIZED TOMOGRAPHY (CT Scan)

COMPUTERIZED TOMOGRAPHY (CT Scan): Computer reformatted digital display of multiplanar images developed from the capture of multiple exposures of external ionizing radiation.

Example: CT Scan of head

Body Part – 4TH			Contrast – 5TH	Qualifier – 6TH	Qualifier – 7TH
2 Intracranial Sinuses 8 Superior Vena Cava 9 Inferior Vena Cava F Pelvic (Iliac) Veins, Right G Pelvic (Iliac) Veins, Left	H Pelvic (Iliac) Veins, Bilateral J Renal Vein, Right K Renal Vein, Left L Renal Veins, Bilateral	Q Pulmonary Vein, Right R Pulmonary Vein, Left S Pulmonary Veins, Bilateral T Portal and Splanchnic Veins	0 High osmolar 1 Low osmolar Y Other contrast	0 Unenhanced and enhanced Z None	Z None
2 Intracranial Sinuses 8 Superior Vena Cava 9 Inferior Vena Cava F Pelvic (Iliac) Veins, Right G Pelvic (Iliac) Veins, Left	H Pelvic (Iliac) Veins, Bilateral J Renal Vein, Right K Renal Vein, Left L Renal Veins, Bilateral	Q Pulmonary Vein, Right R Pulmonary Vein, Left S Pulmonary Veins, Bilateral T Portal and Splanchnic Veins	Z None	2 Intravascular optical coherence Z None	Z None

1ST - B Imaging
2ND - 5 Veins
3RD - 3 MAGNETIC RESONANCE IMAGING (MRI)

MAGNETIC RESONANCE IMAGING (MRI): Computer reformatted digital display of multiplanar images developed from the capture of radiofrequency signals emitted by nuclei in a body site excited within a magnetic field.

Example: MRI of knee

Body Part – 4TH		Contrast – 5TH	Qualifier – 6TH	Qualifier – 7TH
1 Cerebral and Cerebellar Veins 2 Intracranial Sinuses 5 Jugular Veins, Bilateral 8 Superior Vena Cava 9 Inferior Vena Cava B Lower Extremity Veins, Right C Lower Extremity Veins, Left D Lower Extremity Veins, Bilateral	H Pelvic (Iliac) Veins, Bilateral L Renal Veins, Bilateral M Upper Extremity Veins, Right N Upper Extremity Veins, Left P Upper Extremity Veins, Bilateral S Pulmonary Veins, Bilateral T Portal and Splanchnic Veins V Veins, Other	Y Other contrast	0 Unenhanced and enhanced Z None	Z None
1 Cerebral and Cerebellar Veins 2 Intracranial Sinuses 5 Jugular Veins, Bilateral 8 Superior Vena Cava 9 Inferior Vena Cava B Lower Extremity Veins, Right C Lower Extremity Veins, Left D Lower Extremity Veins, Bilateral	H Pelvic (Iliac) Veins, Bilateral L Renal Veins, Bilateral M Upper Extremity Veins, Right N Upper Extremity Veins, Left P Upper Extremity Veins, Bilateral S Pulmonary Veins, Bilateral T Portal and Splanchnic Veins V Veins, Other	Z None	Z None	Z None

© 2018 Channel Publishing, Ltd.

1ST - B Imaging
2ND - 5 Veins
3RD - 4 ULTRASONOGRAPHY

ULTRASONOGRAPHY: Real time display of images of anatomy or flow information developed from the capture of reflected and attenuated high frequency sound waves.

Example: Abdominal ultrasound

Body Part – 4TH		Contrast – 5TH	Qualifier – 6TH	Qualifier – 7TH
3 Jugular Veins, Right 4 Jugular Veins, Left 6 Subclavian Vein, Right 7 Subclavian Vein, Left 8 Superior Vena Cava 9 Inferior Vena Cava B Lower Extremity Veins, Right C Lower Extremity Veins, Left	D Lower Extremity Veins, Bilateral J Renal Vein, Right K Renal Vein, Left L Renal Veins, Bilateral M Upper Extremity Veins, Right N Upper Extremity Veins, Left P Upper Extremity Veins, Bilateral T Portal and Splanchnic Veins	Z None	Z None	3 Intravascular A Guidance Z None

1ST - B Imaging
2ND - 7 Lymphatic System
3RD - 0 PLAIN RADIOGRAPHY

PLAIN RADIOGRAPHY: Planar display of an image developed from the capture of external ionizing radiation on photographic or photoconductive plate.

Example: Chest X-ray

Body Part – 4TH		Contrast – 5TH	Qualifier – 6TH	Qualifier – 7TH
0 Abdominal/Retroperitoneal Lymphatics, Unilateral 1 Abdominal/Retroperitoneal Lymphatics, Bilateral 4 Lymphatics, Head and Neck 5 Upper Extremity Lymphatics, Right 6 Upper Extremity Lymphatics, Left	7 Upper Extremity Lymphatics, Bilateral 8 Lower Extremity Lymphatics, Right 9 Lower Extremity Lymphatics, Left B Lower Extremity Lymphatics, Bilateral C Lymphatics, Pelvic	0 High osmolar 1 Low osmolar Y Other contrast	Z None	Z None

1ST - B Imaging
2ND - 8 Eye
3RD - 0 PLAIN RADIOGRAPHY

PLAIN RADIOGRAPHY: Planar display of an image developed from the capture of external ionizing radiation on photographic or photoconductive plate.

Example: Chest X-ray

Body Part – 4TH	Contrast – 5TH	Qualifier – 6TH	Qualifier – 7TH
0 Lacrimal Duct, Right 1 Lacrimal Duct, Left 2 Lacrimal Ducts, Bilateral	0 High osmolar 1 Low osmolar Y Other contrast	Z None	Z None
3 Optic Foramina, Right 4 Optic Foramina, Left 5 Eye, Right 6 Eye, Left 7 Eyes, Bilateral	Z None	Z None	Z None

1ST - B Imaging
2ND - 8 Eye
3RD - 2 COMPUTERIZED TOMOGRAPHY (CT Scan)

COMPUTERIZED TOMOGRAPHY (CT Scan): Computer reformatted digital display of multiplanar images developed from the capture of multiple exposures of external ionizing radiation.

Example: CT Scan of head

Body Part – 4TH	Contrast – 5TH	Qualifier – 6TH	Qualifier – 7TH
5 Eye, Right 6 Eye, Left 7 Eyes, Bilateral	0 High osmolar 1 Low osmolar Y Other contrast	0 Unenhanced and enhanced Z None	Z None
5 Eye, Right 6 Eye, Left 7 Eyes, Bilateral	Z None	Z None	Z None

© 2018 Channel Publishing, Ltd.

1ST - B Imaging
2ND - 8 Eye
3RD - 3 MAGNETIC RESONANCE IMAGING (MRI)

MAGNETIC RESONANCE IMAGING (MRI): Computer reformatted digital display of multiplanar images developed from the capture of radiofrequency signals emitted by nuclei in a body site excited within a magnetic field.

Example: MRI of knee

Body Part – 4TH	Contrast – 5TH	Qualifier – 6TH	Qualifier – 7TH
5 Eye, Right 6 Eye, Left 7 Eyes, Bilateral	Y Other contrast	0 Unenhanced and enhanced Z None	Z None
5 Eye, Right 6 Eye, Left 7 Eyes, Bilateral	Z None	Z None	Z None

1ST - B Imaging
2ND - 8 Eye
3RD - 4 ULTRASONOGRAPHY

ULTRASONOGRAPHY: Real time display of images of anatomy or flow information developed from the capture of reflected and attenuated high frequency sound waves.

Example: Abdominal ultrasound

Body Part – 4TH	Contrast – 5TH	Qualifier – 6TH	Qualifier – 7TH
5 Eye, Right 6 Eye, Left 7 Eyes, Bilateral	Z None	Z None	Z None

1ST - B Imaging
2ND - 9 Ear, Nose, Mouth and Throat
3RD - 0 PLAIN RADIOGRAPHY

PLAIN RADIOGRAPHY: Planar display of an image developed from the capture of external ionizing radiation on photographic or photoconductive plate.

Example: Chest X-ray

Body Part – 4TH	Contrast – 5TH	Qualifier – 6TH	Qualifier – 7TH
2 Paranasal Sinuses F Nasopharynx/Oropharynx H Mastoids	Z None	Z None	Z None
4 Parotid Gland, Right 5 Parotid Gland, Left 6 Parotid Glands, Bilateral 7 Submandibular Gland, Right 8 Submandibular Gland, Left 9 Submandibular Glands, Bilateral B Salivary Gland, Right C Salivary Gland, Left D Salivary Glands, Bilateral	0 High osmolar 1 Low osmolar Y Other contrast	Z None	Z None

1ST - B Imaging
2ND - 9 Ear, Nose, Mouth and Throat
3RD - 1 FLUOROSCOPY

FLUOROSCOPY: Single plane or bi-plane real time display of an image developed from the capture of external ionizing radiation on a fluorescent screen. The image may also be stored by either digital or analog means.

Example: Fluoroscopic guidance

Body Part – 4TH	Contrast – 5TH	Qualifier – 6TH	Qualifier – 7TH
G Pharynx and Epiglottis J Larynx	Y Other contrast Z None	Z None	Z None

1ST - B Imaging
2ND - 9 Ear, Nose, Mouth and Throat
3RD - 2 COMPUTERIZED TOMOGRAPHY (CT Scan)

COMPUTERIZED TOMOGRAPHY (CT Scan): Computer reformatted digital display of multiplanar images developed from the capture of multiple exposures of external ionizing radiation.

Example: CT Scan of head

Body Part – 4TH	Contrast – 5TH	Qualifier – 6TH	Qualifier – 7TH
0 Ear 2 Paranasal Sinuses 6 Parotid Glands, Bilateral 9 Submandibular Glands, Bilateral D Salivary Glands, Bilateral F Nasopharynx/ Oropharynx J Larynx	0 High osmolar 1 Low osmolar Y Other contrast	0 Unenhanced and enhanced Z None	Z None
0 Ear 2 Paranasal Sinuses 6 Parotid Glands, Bilateral 9 Submandibular Glands, Bilateral D Salivary Glands, Bilateral F Nasopharynx/ Oropharynx J Larynx	Z None	Z None	Z None

© 2018 Channel Publishing, Ltd.

1ST - B Imaging
2ND - 9 Ear, Nose, Mouth and Throat
3RD - 3 MAGNETIC RESONANCE IMAGING (MRI)

MAGNETIC RESONANCE IMAGING (MRI): Computer reformatted digital display of multiplanar images developed from the capture of radiofrequency signals emitted by nuclei in a body site excited within a magnetic field.

Example: MRI of knee

Body Part – 4TH	Contrast – 5TH	Qualifier – 6TH	Qualifier – 7TH
0 Ear 2 Paranasal Sinuses 6 Parotid Glands, Bilateral 9 Submandibular Glands, Bilateral D Salivary Glands, Bilateral F Nasopharynx/ Oropharynx J Larynx	Y Other contrast	0 Unenhanced and enhanced Z None	Z None
0 Ear 2 Paranasal Sinuses 6 Parotid Glands, Bilateral 9 Submandibular Glands, Bilateral D Salivary Glands, Bilateral F Nasopharynx/ Oropharynx J Larynx	Z None	Z None	Z None

1ST - B Imaging
2ND - B Respiratory System
3RD - 0 PLAIN RADIOGRAPHY

PLAIN RADIOGRAPHY: Planar display of an image developed from the capture of external ionizing radiation on photographic or photoconductive plate.

Example: Chest X-ray

Body Part – 4TH	Contrast – 5TH	Qualifier – 6TH	Qualifier – 7TH
7 Tracheobronchial Tree, Right 8 Tracheobronchial Tree, Left 9 Tracheobronchial Trees, Bilateral	Y Other contrast	Z None	Z None
D Upper Airways	Z None	Z None	Z None

1ST - B Imaging
2ND - B Respiratory System
3RD - 1 FLUOROSCOPY

FLUOROSCOPY: Single plane or bi-plane real time display of an image developed from the capture of external ionizing radiation on a fluorescent screen. The image may also be stored by either digital or analog means.

Example: Fluoroscopic guidance

Body Part – 4TH	Contrast – 5TH	Qualifier – 6TH	Qualifier – 7TH
2 Lung, Right 3 Lung, Left 4 Lungs, Bilateral 6 Diaphragm C Mediastinum D Upper Airways	Z None	Z None	Z None
7 Tracheobronchial Tree, Right 8 Tracheobronchial Tree, Left 9 Tracheobronchial Trees, Bilateral	Y Other contrast	Z None	Z None

1ST - B Imaging
2ND - B Respiratory System
3RD - 2 COMPUTERIZED TOMOGRAPHY (CT Scan)

COMPUTERIZED TOMOGRAPHY (CT Scan): Computer reformatted digital display of multiplanar images developed from the capture of multiple exposures of external ionizing radiation.

Example: CT Scan of head

Body Part – 4TH	Contrast – 5TH	Qualifier – 6TH	Qualifier – 7TH
4 Lungs, Bilateral 7 Tracheobronchial Tree, Right 8 Tracheobronchial Tree, Left 9 Tracheobronchial Trees, Bilateral F Trachea/Airways	0 High osmolar 1 Low osmolar Y Other contrast	0 Unenhanced and enhanced Z None	Z None
4 Lungs, Bilateral 7 Tracheobronchial Tree, Right 8 Tracheobronchial Tree, Left 9 Tracheobronchial Trees, Bilateral F Trachea/Airways	Z None	Z None	Z None

© 2018 Channel Publishing, Ltd.

1ST - B Imaging
2ND - B Respiratory System
3RD - 3 MAGNETIC RESONANCE IMAGING (MRI)

MAGNETIC RESONANCE IMAGING (MRI): Computer reformatted digital display of multiplanar images developed from the capture of radiofrequency signals emitted by nuclei in a body site excited within a magnetic field.

Example: MRI of knee

Body Part – 4TH	Contrast – 5TH	Qualifier – 6TH	Qualifier – 7TH
G Lung Apices	Y Other contrast	0 Unenhanced and enhanced Z None	Z None
G Lung Apices	Z None	Z None	Z None

1ST - B Imaging
2ND - B Respiratory System
3RD - 4 ULTRASONOGRAPHY

ULTRASONOGRAPHY: Real time display of images of anatomy or flow information developed from the capture of reflected and attenuated high frequency sound waves.

Example: Abdominal ultrasound

Body Part – 4TH	Contrast – 5TH	Qualifier – 6TH	Qualifier – 7TH
B Pleura C Mediastinum	Z None	Z None	Z None

1ST - B Imaging
2ND - D Gastrointestinal System
3RD - 1 FLUOROSCOPY

FLUOROSCOPY: Single plane or bi-plane real time display of an image developed from the capture of external ionizing radiation on a fluorescent screen. The image may also be stored by either digital or analog means.

Example: Fluoroscopic guidance

Body Part – 4TH	Contrast – 5TH	Qualifier – 6TH	Qualifier – 7TH
1 Esophagus 2 Stomach 3 Small Bowel 4 Colon 5 Upper GI 6 Upper GI and Small Bowel 9 Duodenum B Mouth/Oropharynx	Y Other contrast Z None	Z None	Z None

1ST - B Imaging
2ND - D Gastrointestinal System
3RD - 2 COMPUTERIZED TOMOGRAPHY (CT Scan)

COMPUTERIZED TOMOGRAPHY (CT Scan): Computer reformatted digital display of multiplanar images developed from the capture of multiple exposures of external ionizing radiation.

Example: CT Scan of head

Body Part – 4TH	Contrast – 5TH	Qualifier – 6TH	Qualifier – 7TH
4 Colon	0 High osmolar 1 Low osmolar Y Other contrast	0 Unenhanced and enhanced Z None	Z None
4 Colon	Z None	Z None	Z None

1ST - B Imaging
2ND - D Gastrointestinal System
3RD - 4 ULTRASONOGRAPHY

ULTRASONOGRAPHY: Real time display of images of anatomy or flow information developed from the capture of reflected and attenuated high frequency sound waves.

Example: Abdominal ultrasound

Body Part – 4TH	Contrast – 5TH	Qualifier – 6TH	Qualifier – 7TH
1 Esophagus 2 Stomach 7 Gastrointestinal Tract 8 Appendix 9 Duodenum C Rectum	Z None	Z None	Z None

© 2018 Channel Publishing, Ltd.

1ST - B Imaging
2ND - F Hepatobiliary System and Pancreas
3RD - 0 PLAIN RADIOGRAPHY

PLAIN RADIOGRAPHY: Planar display of an image developed from the capture of external ionizing radiation on photographic or photoconductive plate.

Example: Chest X-ray

Body Part – 4TH	Contrast – 5TH	Qualifier – 6TH	Qualifier – 7TH
0 Bile Ducts 3 Gallbladder and Bile Ducts C Hepatobiliary System, All	0 High osmolar 1 Low osmolar Y Other contrast	Z None	Z None

1ST - B Imaging
2ND - F Hepatobiliary System and Pancreas
3RD - 1 FLUOROSCOPY

FLUOROSCOPY: Single plane or bi-plane real time display of an image developed from the capture of external ionizing radiation on a fluorescent screen. The image may also be stored by either digital or analog means.

Example: Fluoroscopic guidance

Body Part – 4TH	Contrast – 5TH	Qualifier – 6TH	Qualifier – 7TH
0 Bile Ducts 1 Biliary and Pancreatic Ducts 2 Gallbladder 3 Gallbladder and Bile Ducts 4 Gallbladder, Bile Ducts and Pancreatic Ducts 8 Pancreatic Ducts	0 High osmolar 1 Low osmolar Y Other contrast	Z None	Z None

1ST - B Imaging
2ND - F Hepatobiliary System and Pancreas
3RD - 2 COMPUTERIZED TOMOGRAPHY (CT Scan)

COMPUTERIZED TOMOGRAPHY (CT Scan): Computer reformatted digital display of multiplanar images developed from the capture of multiple exposures of external ionizing radiation.

Example: CT Scan of head

Body Part – 4TH	Contrast – 5TH	Qualifier – 6TH	Qualifier – 7TH
5 Liver 6 Liver and Spleen 7 Pancreas C Hepatobiliary System, All	0 High osmolar 1 Low osmolar Y Other contrast	0 Unenhanced and enhanced Z None	Z None
5 Liver 6 Liver and Spleen 7 Pancreas C Hepatobiliary System, All	Z None	Z None	Z None

1ST - B Imaging
2ND - F Hepatobiliary System and Pancreas
3RD - 3 MAGNETIC RESONANCE IMAGING (MRI)

MAGNETIC RESONANCE IMAGING (MRI): Computer reformatted digital display of multiplanar images developed from the capture of radiofrequency signals emitted by nuclei in a body site excited within a magnetic field.

Example: MRI of knee

Body Part – 4TH	Contrast – 5TH	Qualifier – 6TH	Qualifier – 7TH
5 Liver 6 Liver and Spleen 7 Pancreas	Y Other contrast	0 Unenhanced and enhanced Z None	Z None
5 Liver 6 Liver and Spleen 7 Pancreas	Z None	Z None	Z None

1ST - B Imaging
2ND - F Hepatobiliary System and Pancreas
3RD - 4 ULTRASONOGRAPHY

ULTRASONOGRAPHY: Real time display of images of anatomy or flow information developed from the capture of reflected and attenuated high frequency sound waves.

Example: Abdominal ultrasound

Body Part – 4TH	Contrast – 5TH	Qualifier – 6TH	Qualifier – 7TH
0 Bile Ducts 2 Gallbladder 3 Gallbladder and Bile Ducts 5 Liver 6 Liver and Spleen 7 Pancreas C Hepatobiliary System, All	Z None	Z None	Z None

© 2018 Channel Publishing, Ltd.

1ST - B Imaging
2ND - G Endocrine System
3RD - 2 COMPUTERIZED TOMOGRAPHY (CT Scan)

COMPUTERIZED TOMOGRAPHY (CT Scan): Computer reformatted digital display of multiplanar images developed from the capture of multiple exposures of external ionizing radiation.

Example: CT Scan of head

Body Part – 4TH	Contrast – 5TH	Qualifier – 6TH	Qualifier – 7TH
2 Adrenal Glands, Bilateral 3 Parathyroid Glands 4 Thyroid Gland	0 High osmolar 1 Low osmolar Y Other contrast	0 Unenhanced and enhanced Z None	Z None
2 Adrenal Glands, Bilateral 3 Parathyroid Glands 4 Thyroid Gland	Z None	Z None	Z None

1ST - B Imaging
2ND - G Endocrine System
3RD - 3 MAGNETIC RESONANCE IMAGING (MRI)

MAGNETIC RESONANCE IMAGING (MRI): Computer reformatted digital display of multiplanar images developed from the capture of radiofrequency signals emitted by nuclei in a body site excited within a magnetic field.

Example: MRI of knee

Body Part – 4TH	Contrast – 5TH	Qualifier – 6TH	Qualifier – 7TH
2 Adrenal Glands, Bilateral 3 Parathyroid Glands 4 Thyroid Gland	Y Other contrast	0 Unenhanced and enhanced Z None	Z None
2 Adrenal Glands, Bilateral 3 Parathyroid Glands 4 Thyroid Gland	Z None	Z None	Z None

1ST - B Imaging
2ND - G Endocrine System
3RD - 4 ULTRASONOGRAPHY

ULTRASONOGRAPHY: Real time display of images of anatomy or flow information developed from the capture of reflected and attenuated high frequency sound waves.

Example: Abdominal ultrasound

Body Part – 4TH	Contrast – 5TH	Qualifier – 6TH	Qualifier – 7TH
0 Adrenal Gland, Right 1 Adrenal Gland, Left 2 Adrenal Glands, Bilateral 3 Parathyroid Glands 4 Thyroid Gland	Z None	Z None	Z None

1ST - B Imaging
2ND - H Skin, Subcutaneous Tissue and Breast
3RD - 0 PLAIN RADIOGRAPHY

PLAIN RADIOGRAPHY: Planar display of an image developed from the capture of external ionizing radiation on photographic or photoconductive plate.

Example: Chest X-ray

Body Part – 4TH	Contrast – 5TH	Qualifier – 6TH	Qualifier – 7TH
0 Breast, Right 1 Breast, Left 2 Breasts, Bilateral	Z None	Z None	Z None
3 Single Mammary Duct, Right 4 Single Mammary Duct, Left 5 Multiple Mammary Ducts, Right 6 Multiple Mammary Ducts, Left	0 High osmolar 1 Low osmolar Y Other contrast Z None	Z None	Z None

© 2018 Channel Publishing, Ltd.

1ST - B Imaging
2ND - H Skin, Subcutaneous Tissue and Breast
3RD - 3 MAGNETIC RESONANCE IMAGING (MRI)

MAGNETIC RESONANCE IMAGING (MRI): Computer reformatted digital display of multiplanar images developed from the capture of radiofrequency signals emitted by nuclei in a body site excited within a magnetic field.

Example: MRI of knee

Body Part – 4TH	Contrast – 5TH	Qualifier – 6TH	Qualifier – 7TH
0 Breast, Right 1 Breast, Left 2 Breasts, Bilateral D Subcutaneous Tissue, Head/Neck F Subcutaneous Tissue, Upper Extremity G Subcutaneous Tissue, Thorax H Subcutaneous Tissue, Abdomen and Pelvis J Subcutaneous Tissue, Lower Extremity	Y Other contrast	0 Unenhanced and enhanced Z None	Z None
0 Breast, Right 1 Breast, Left 2 Breasts, Bilateral D Subcutaneous Tissue, Head/Neck F Subcutaneous Tissue, Upper Extremity G Subcutaneous Tissue, Thorax H Subcutaneous Tissue, Abdomen and Pelvis J Subcutaneous Tissue, Lower Extremity	Z None	Z None	Z None

1ST - B Imaging
2ND - H Skin, Subcutaneous Tissue and Breast
3RD - 4 ULTRASONOGRAPHY

ULTRASONOGRAPHY: Real time display of images of anatomy or flow information developed from the capture of reflected and attenuated high frequency sound waves.

Example: Abdominal ultrasound

Body Part – 4TH	Contrast – 5TH	Qualifier – 6TH	Qualifier – 7TH
0 Breast, Right 1 Breast, Left 2 Breasts, Bilateral 7 Extremity, Upper 8 Extremity, Lower 9 Abdominal Wall B Chest Wall C Head and Neck	Z None	Z None	Z None

1ST - B Imaging
2ND - L Connective Tissue
3RD - 3 MAGNETIC RESONANCE IMAGING (MRI)

MAGNETIC RESONANCE IMAGING (MRI): Computer reformatted digital display of multiplanar images developed from the capture of radiofrequency signals emitted by nuclei in a body site excited within a magnetic field.

Example: MRI of knee

Body Part – 4TH	Contrast – 5TH	Qualifier – 6TH	Qualifier – 7TH
0 Connective Tissue, Upper Extremity 1 Connective Tissue, Lower Extremity 2 Tendons, Upper Extremity 3 Tendons, Lower Extremity	Y Other contrast	0 Unenhanced and enhanced Z None	Z None
0 Connective Tissue, Upper Extremity 1 Connective Tissue, Lower Extremity 2 Tendons, Upper Extremity 3 Tendons, Lower Extremity	Z None	Z None	Z None

1ST - B Imaging
2ND - L Connective Tissue
3RD - 4 ULTRASONOGRAPHY

ULTRASONOGRAPHY: Real time display of images of anatomy or flow information developed from the capture of reflected and attenuated high frequency sound waves.

Example: Abdominal ultrasound

Body Part – 4TH	Contrast – 5TH	Qualifier – 6TH	Qualifier – 7TH
0 Connective Tissue, Upper Extremity 1 Connective Tissue, Lower Extremity 2 Tendons, Upper Extremity 3 Tendons, Lower Extremity	Z None	Z None	Z None

© 2018 Channel Publishing, Ltd.

1ST - B Imaging
2ND - N Skull and Facial Bones
3RD - 0 PLAIN RADIOGRAPHY

PLAIN RADIOGRAPHY: Planar display of an image developed from the capture of external ionizing radiation on photographic or photoconductive plate.

Example: Chest X-ray

Body Part – 4TH	Contrast – 5TH	Qualifier – 6TH	Qualifier – 7TH
0 Skull 1 Orbit, Right 2 Orbit, Left 3 Orbits, Bilateral 4 Nasal Bones 5 Facial Bones 6 Mandible B Zygomatic Arch, Right C Zygomatic Arch, Left D Zygomatic Arches, Bilateral G Tooth, Single H Teeth, Multiple J Teeth, All	Z None	Z None	Z None
7 Temporomandibular Joint, Right 8 Temporomandibular Joint, Left 9 Temporomandibular Joints, Bilateral	0 High osmolar 1 Low osmolar Y Other contrast Z None	Z None	Z None

1ST - B Imaging
2ND - N Skull and Facial Bones
3RD - 1 FLUOROSCOPY

FLUOROSCOPY: Single plane or bi-plane real time display of an image developed from the capture of external ionizing radiation on a fluorescent screen. The image may also be stored by either digital or analog means.

Example: Fluoroscopic guidance

Body Part – 4TH	Contrast – 5TH	Qualifier – 6TH	Qualifier – 7TH
7 Temporomandibular Joint, Right 8 Temporomandibular Joint, Left 9 Temporomandibular Joints, Bilateral	0 High osmolar 1 Low osmolar Y Other contrast Z None	Z None	Z None

1ST - B Imaging
2ND - N Skull and Facial Bones
3RD - 2 COMPUTERIZED TOMOGRAPHY (CT Scan)

COMPUTERIZED TOMOGRAPHY (CT Scan): Computer reformatted digital display of multiplanar images developed from the capture of multiple exposures of external ionizing radiation.

Example: CT Scan of head

Body Part – 4TH	Contrast – 5TH	Qualifier – 6TH	Qualifier – 7TH
0 Skull 3 Orbits, Bilateral 5 Facial Bones 6 Mandible 9 Temporomandibular Joints, Bilateral F Temporal Bones	0 High osmolar 1 Low osmolar Y Other contrast Z None	Z None	Z None

1ST - B Imaging
2ND - N Skull and Facial Bones
3RD - 3 MAGNETIC RESONANCE IMAGING (MRI)

MAGNETIC RESONANCE IMAGING (MRI): Computer reformatted digital display of multiplanar images developed from the capture of radiofrequency signals emitted by nuclei in a body site excited within a magnetic field.

Example: MRI of knee

Body Part – 4TH	Contrast – 5TH	Qualifier – 6TH	Qualifier – 7TH
9 Temporomandibular Joints, Bilateral	Y Other contrast Z None	Z None	Z None

© 2018 Channel Publishing, Ltd.

1ST - B Imaging
2ND - P Non-Axial Upper Bones
3RD - 0 PLAIN RADIOGRAPHY

PLAIN RADIOGRAPHY: Planar display of an image developed from the capture of external ionizing radiation on photographic or photoconductive plate.

Example: Chest X-ray

Body Part – 4TH	Contrast – 5TH	Qualifier – 6TH	Qualifier – 7TH
0 Sternoclavicular Joint, Right 1 Sternoclavicular Joint, Left 2 Sternoclavicular Joints, Bilateral 3 Acromioclavicular Joints, Bilateral 4 Clavicle, Right 5 Clavicle, Left 6 Scapula, Right 7 Scapula, Left A Humerus, Right B Humerus, Left E Upper Arm, Right F Upper Arm, Left J Forearm, Right K Forearm, Left N Hand, Right P Hand, Left R Finger(s), Right S Finger(s), Left X Ribs, Right Y Ribs, Left	Z None	Z None	Z None
8 Shoulder, Right 9 Shoulder, Left C Hand/Finger Joint, Right D Hand/Finger Joint, Left G Elbow, Right H Elbow, Left L Wrist, Right M Wrist, Left	0 High osmolar 1 Low osmolar Y Other contrast Z None	Z None	Z None

1ST - B Imaging
2ND - P Non-Axial Upper Bones
3RD - 1 FLUOROSCOPY

FLUOROSCOPY: Single plane or bi-plane real time display of an image developed from the capture of external ionizing radiation on a fluorescent screen. The image may also be stored by either digital or analog means.

Example: Fluoroscopic guidance

Body Part – 4TH	Contrast – 5TH	Qualifier – 6TH	Qualifier – 7TH
0 Sternoclavicular Joint, Right 1 Sternoclavicular Joint, Left 2 Sternoclavicular Joints, Bilateral 3 Acromioclavicular Joints, Bilateral 4 Clavicle, Right 5 Clavicle, Left 6 Scapula, Right 7 Scapula, Left A Humerus, Right B Humerus, Left E Upper Arm, Right F Upper Arm, Left J Forearm, Right K Forearm, Left N Hand, Right P Hand, Left R Finger(s), Right S Finger(s), Left X Ribs, Right Y Ribs, Left	Z None	Z None	Z None
8 Shoulder, Right 9 Shoulder, Left L Wrist, Right M Wrist, Left	0 High osmolar 1 Low osmolar Y Other contrast Z None	Z None	Z None
C Hand/Finger Joint, Right D Hand/Finger Joint, Left G Elbow, Right H Elbow, Left	0 High osmolar 1 Low osmolar Y Other contrast	Z None	Z None

1ST - B Imaging
2ND - P Non-Axial Upper Bones
3RD - 2 COMPUTERIZED TOMOGRAPHY (CT Scan)

COMPUTERIZED TOMOGRAPHY (CT Scan): Computer reformatted digital display of multiplanar images developed from the capture of multiple exposures of external ionizing radiation.

Example: CT Scan of head

Body Part – 4TH	Contrast – 5TH	Qualifier – 6TH	Qualifier – 7TH
0 Sternoclavicular Joint, Right 1 Sternoclavicular Joint, Left W Thorax	0 High osmolar 1 Low osmolar Y Other contrast	Z None	Z None
2 Sternoclavicular Joints, Bilateral 3 Acromioclavicular Joints, Bilateral 4 Clavicle, Right 5 Clavicle, Left 6 Scapula, Right 7 Scapula, Left 8 Shoulder, Right 9 Shoulder, Left A Humerus, Right B Humerus, Left E Upper Arm, Right F Upper Arm, Left G Elbow, Right H Elbow, Left J Forearm, Right K Forearm, Left L Wrist, Right M Wrist, Left N Hand, Right P Hand, Left Q Hands and Wrists, Bilateral R Finger(s), Right S Finger(s), Left T Upper Extremity, Right U Upper Extremity, Left V Upper Extremities, Bilateral X Ribs, Right Y Ribs, Left	0 High osmolar 1 Low osmolar Y Other contrast Z None	Z None	Z None
C Hand/Finger Joint, Right D Hand/Finger Joint, Left	Z None	Z None	Z None

© 2018 Channel Publishing, Ltd.

1ST - B Imaging
2ND - P Non-Axial Upper Bones
3RD - 3 MAGNETIC RESONANCE IMAGING (MRI)

MAGNETIC RESONANCE IMAGING (MRI): Computer reformatted digital display of multiplanar images developed from the capture of radiofrequency signals emitted by nuclei in a body site excited within a magnetic field.

Example: MRI of knee

Body Part – 4TH	Contrast – 5TH	Qualifier – 6TH	Qualifier – 7TH
8 Shoulder, Right 9 Shoulder, Left C Hand/Finger Joint, Right D Hand/Finger Joint, Left E Upper Arm, Right F Upper Arm, Left G Elbow, Right H Elbow, Left J Forearm, Right K Forearm, Left L Wrist, Right M Wrist, Left	Y Other contrast	0 Unenhanced and enhanced Z None	Z None
8 Shoulder, Right 9 Shoulder, Left C Hand/Finger Joint, Right D Hand/Finger Joint, Left E Upper Arm, Right F Upper Arm, Left G Elbow, Right H Elbow, Left J Forearm, Right K Forearm, Left L Wrist, Right M Wrist, Left	Z None	Z None	Z None

1ST - B Imaging
2ND - P Non-Axial Upper Bones
3RD - 4 ULTRASONOGRAPHY

ULTRASONOGRAPHY: Real time display of images of anatomy or flow information developed from the capture of reflected and attenuated high frequency sound waves.

Example: Abdominal ultrasound

Body Part – 4TH	Contrast – 5TH	Qualifier – 6TH	Qualifier – 7TH
8 Shoulder, Right 9 Shoulder, Left G Elbow, Right H Elbow, Left L Wrist, Right M Wrist, Left N Hand, Right P Hand, Left	Z None	Z None	1 Densitometry Z None

1ST - B Imaging
2ND - Q Non-Axial Lower Bones
3RD - 0 PLAIN RADIOGRAPHY

PLAIN RADIOGRAPHY: Planar display of an image developed from the capture of external ionizing radiation on photographic or photoconductive plate.

Example: Chest X-ray

Body Part – 4TH	Contrast – 5TH	Qualifier – 6TH	Qualifier – 7TH
0 Hip, Right 1 Hip, Left	0 High osmolar 1 Low osmolar Y Other contrast	Z None	Z None
0 Hip, Right 1 Hip, Left	Z None	Z None	1 Densitometry Z None
3 Femur, Right 4 Femur, Left	Z None	Z None	1 Densitometry Z None
7 Knee, Right 8 Knee, Left G Ankle, Right H Ankle, Left	0 High osmolar 1 Low osmolar Y Other contrast Z None	Z None	Z None
D Lower Leg, Right F Lower Leg, Left J Calcaneus, Right K Calcaneus, Left L Foot, Right M Foot, Left P Toe(s), Right Q Toe(s), Left V Patella, Right W Patella, Left	Z None	Z None	Z None
X Foot/Toe Joint, Right Y Foot/Toe Joint, Left	0 High osmolar 1 Low osmolar Y Other contrast	Z None	Z None

© 2018 Channel Publishing, Ltd.

1ST - B Imaging
2ND - Q Non-Axial Lower Bones
3RD - 1 FLUOROSCOPY

FLUOROSCOPY: Single plane or bi-plane real time display of an image developed from the capture of external ionizing radiation on a fluorescent screen. The image may also be stored by either digital or analog means.

Example: Fluoroscopic guidance

Body Part – 4TH	Contrast – 5TH	Qualifier – 6TH	Qualifier – 7TH
0 Hip, Right 1 Hip, Left 7 Knee, Right 8 Knee, Left G Ankle, Right H Ankle, Left X Foot/Toe Joint, Right Y Foot/Toe Joint, Left	0 High osmolar 1 Low osmolar Y Other contrast Z None	Z None	Z None
3 Femur, Right 4 Femur, Left D Lower Leg, Right F Lower Leg, Left J Calcaneus, Right K Calcaneus, Left L Foot, Right M Foot, Left P Toe(s), Right Q Toe(s), Left V Patella, Right W Patella, Left	Z None	Z None	Z None

1ST - B Imaging
2ND - Q Non-Axial Lower Bones
3RD - 2 COMPUTERIZED TOMOGRAPHY (CT Scan)

COMPUTERIZED TOMOGRAPHY (CT Scan): Computer reformatted digital display of multiplanar images developed from the capture of multiple exposures of external ionizing radiation.

Example: CT Scan of head

Body Part – 4TH	Contrast – 5TH	Qualifier – 6TH	Qualifier – 7TH
0 Hip, Right 1 Hip, Left 3 Femur, Right 4 Femur, Left 7 Knee, Right 8 Knee, Left D Lower Leg, Right F Lower Leg, Left G Ankle, Right H Ankle, Left J Calcaneus, Right K Calcaneus, Left L Foot, Right M Foot, Left P Toe(s), Right Q Toe(s), Left R Lower Extremity, Right S Lower Extremity, Left V Patella, Right W Patella, Left X Foot/Toe Joint, Right Y Foot/Toe Joint, Left	0 High osmolar 1 Low osmolar Y Other contrast Z None	Z None	Z None
B Tibia/Fibula, Right C Tibia/Fibula, Left	0 High osmolar 1 Low osmolar Y Other contrast	Z None	Z None

1ST - B Imaging
2ND - Q Non-Axial Lower Bones
3RD - 3 MAGNETIC RESONANCE IMAGING (MRI)

MAGNETIC RESONANCE IMAGING (MRI): Computer reformatted digital display of multiplanar images developed from the capture of radiofrequency signals emitted by nuclei in a body site excited within a magnetic field.

Example: MRI of knee

Body Part – 4TH	Contrast – 5TH	Qualifier – 6TH	Qualifier – 7TH
0 Hip, Right 1 Hip, Left 3 Femur, Right 4 Femur, Left 7 Knee, Right 8 Knee, Left D Lower Leg, Right F Lower Leg, Left G Ankle, Right H Ankle, Left J Calcaneus, Right K Calcaneus, Left L Foot, Right M Foot, Left P Toe(s), Right Q Toe(s), Left V Patella, Right W Patella, Left	Y Other contrast	0 Unenhanced and enhanced Z None	Z None
0 Hip, Right 1 Hip, Left 3 Femur, Right 4 Femur, Left 7 Knee, Right 8 Knee, Left D Lower Leg, Right F Lower Leg, Left G Ankle, Right H Ankle, Left J Calcaneus, Right K Calcaneus, Left L Foot, Right M Foot, Left P Toe(s), Right Q Toe(s), Left V Patella, Right W Patella, Left	Z None	Z None	Z None

© 2018 Channel Publishing, Ltd.

1ST - B Imaging
2ND - Q Non-Axial Lower Bones
3RD - 4 ULTRASONOGRAPHY

ULTRASONOGRAPHY: Real time display of images of anatomy or flow information developed from the capture of reflected and attenuated high frequency sound waves.

Example: Abdominal ultrasound

Body Part – 4TH		Contrast – 5TH	Qualifier – 6TH	Qualifier – 7TH
0 Hip, Right 1 Hip, Left 2 Hips, Bilateral	7 Knee, Right 8 Knee, Left 9 Knees, Bilateral	Z None	Z None	Z None

1ST - B Imaging
2ND - R Axial Skeleton, Except Skull and Facial Bones
3RD - 0 PLAIN RADIOGRAPHY

PLAIN RADIOGRAPHY: Planar display of an image developed from the capture of external ionizing radiation on photographic or photoconductive plate.

Example: Chest X-ray

Body Part – 4TH			Contrast – 5TH	Qualifier – 6TH	Qualifier – 7TH
0 Cervical Spine 7 Thoracic Spine	9 Lumbar Spine G Whole Spine		Z None	Z None	1 Densitometry Z None
1 Cervical Disc(s) 2 Thoracic Disc(s) 3 Lumbar Disc(s)	4 Cervical Facet Joint(s) 5 Thoracic Facet Joint(s) 6 Lumbar Facet Joint(s) D Sacroiliac Joints		0 High osmolar 1 Low osmolar Y Other contrast Z None	Z None	Z None
8 Thoracolumbar Joint B Lumbosacral Joint	C Pelvis F Sacrum and Coccyx	H Sternum	Z None	Z None	Z None

1ST - B Imaging
2ND - R Axial Skeleton, Except Skull and Facial Bones
3RD - 1 FLUOROSCOPY

FLUOROSCOPY: Single plane or bi-plane real time display of an image developed from the capture of external ionizing radiation on a fluorescent screen. The image may also be stored by either digital or analog means.

Example: Fluoroscopic guidance

Body Part – 4TH			Contrast – 5TH	Qualifier – 6TH	Qualifier – 7TH
0 Cervical Spine 1 Cervical Disc(s) 2 Thoracic Disc(s) 3 Lumbar Disc(s)	4 Cervical Facet Joint(s) 5 Thoracic Facet Joint(s) 6 Lumbar Facet Joint(s) 7 Thoracic Spine 8 Thoracolumbar Joint 9 Lumbar Spine	B Lumbosacral Joint C Pelvis D Sacroiliac Joints F Sacrum and Coccyx G Whole Spine H Sternum	0 High osmolar 1 Low osmolar Y Other contrast Z None	Z None	Z None

1ST - B Imaging
2ND - R Axial Skeleton, Except Skull and Facial Bones
3RD - 2 COMPUTERIZED TOMOGRAPHY (CT Scan)

COMPUTERIZED TOMOGRAPHY (CT Scan): Computer reformatted digital display of multiplanar images developed from the capture of multiple exposures of external ionizing radiation.

Example: CT Scan of head

Body Part – 4TH		Contrast – 5TH	Qualifier – 6TH	Qualifier – 7TH
0 Cervical Spine 7 Thoracic Spine 9 Lumbar Spine	C Pelvis D Sacroiliac Joints F Sacrum and Coccyx	0 High osmolar 1 Low osmolar Y Other contrast Z None	Z None	Z None

© 2018 Channel Publishing, Ltd.

1ST - B Imaging
2ND - R Axial Skeleton, Except Skull and Facial Bones
3RD - 3 MAGNETIC RESONANCE IMAGING (MRI)

MAGNETIC RESONANCE IMAGING (MRI): Computer reformatted digital display of multiplanar images developed from the capture of radiofrequency signals emitted by nuclei in a body site excited within a magnetic field.

Example: MRI of knee

Body Part – 4TH	Contrast – 5TH	Qualifier – 6TH	Qualifier – 7TH
0 Cervical Spine 1 Cervical Disc(s) 2 Thoracic Disc(s) 3 Lumbar Disc(s) 7 Thoracic Spine 9 Lumbar Spine C Pelvis F Sacrum and Coccyx	Y Other contrast	0 Unenhanced and enhanced Z None	Z None
0 Cervical Spine 1 Cervical Disc(s) 2 Thoracic Disc(s) 3 Lumbar Disc(s) 7 Thoracic Spine 9 Lumbar Spine C Pelvis F Sacrum and Coccyx	Z None	Z None	Z None

1ST - B Imaging
2ND - R Axial Skeleton, Except Skull and Facial Bones
3RD - 4 ULTRASONOGRAPHY

ULTRASONOGRAPHY: Real time display of images of anatomy or flow information developed from the capture of reflected and attenuated high frequency sound waves.

Example: Abdominal ultrasound

Body Part – 4TH	Contrast – 5TH	Qualifier – 6TH	Qualifier – 7TH
0 Cervical Spine 7 Thoracic Spine 9 Lumbar Spine F Sacrum and Coccyx	Z None	Z None	Z None

1ST - B Imaging
2ND - T Urinary System
3RD - 0 PLAIN RADIOGRAPHY

PLAIN RADIOGRAPHY: Planar display of an image developed from the capture of external ionizing radiation on photographic or photoconductive plate.

Example: Chest X-ray

Body Part – 4TH	Contrast – 5TH	Qualifier – 6TH	Qualifier – 7TH
0 Bladder 1 Kidney, Right 2 Kidney, Left 3 Kidneys, Bilateral 4 Kidneys, Ureters and Bladder 5 Urethra 6 Ureter, Right 7 Ureter, Left 8 Ureters, Bilateral B Bladder and Urethra C Ileal Diversion Loop	0 High osmolar 1 Low osmolar Y Other contrast Z None	Z None	Z None

1ST - B Imaging
2ND - T Urinary System
3RD - 1 FLUOROSCOPY

FLUOROSCOPY: Single plane or bi-plane real time display of an image developed from the capture of external ionizing radiation on a fluorescent screen. The image may also be stored by either digital or analog means.

Example: Fluoroscopic guidance

Body Part – 4TH	Contrast – 5TH	Qualifier – 6TH	Qualifier – 7TH
0 Bladder 1 Kidney, Right 2 Kidney, Left 3 Kidneys, Bilateral 4 Kidneys, Ureters and Bladder 5 Urethra 6 Ureter, Right 7 Ureter, Left B Bladder and Urethra C Ileal Diversion Loop D Kidney, Ureter and Bladder, Right F Kidney, Ureter and Bladder, Left G Ileal Loop, Ureters and Kidneys	0 High osmolar 1 Low osmolar Y Other contrast Z None	Z None	Z None

1ST - B Imaging
2ND - T Urinary System
3RD - 2 COMPUTERIZED TOMOGRAPHY (CT Scan)

COMPUTERIZED TOMOGRAPHY (CT Scan): Computer reformatted digital display of multiplanar images developed from the capture of multiple exposures of external ionizing radiation.

Example: CT Scan of head

Body Part – 4TH	Contrast – 5TH	Qualifier – 6TH	Qualifier – 7TH
0 Bladder 1 Kidney, Right 2 Kidney, Left 3 Kidneys, Bilateral 9 Kidney Transplant	0 High osmolar 1 Low osmolar Y Other contrast	0 Unenhanced and enhanced Z None	Z None
0 Bladder 1 Kidney, Right 2 Kidney, Left 3 Kidneys, Bilateral 9 Kidney Transplant	Z None	Z None	Z None

IMAGING BR3

© 2018 Channel Publishing, Ltd.

1ST - B Imaging
2ND - T Urinary System
3RD - 3 MAGNETIC RESONANCE IMAGING (MRI)

MAGNETIC RESONANCE IMAGING (MRI): Computer reformatted digital display of multiplanar images developed from the capture of radiofrequency signals emitted by nuclei in a body site excited within a magnetic field.

Example: MRI of knee

Body Part – 4TH	Contrast – 5TH	Qualifier – 6TH	Qualifier – 7TH
0 Bladder 1 Kidney, Right 2 Kidney, Left 3 Kidneys, Bilateral 9 Kidney Transplant	Y Other contrast	0 Unenhanced and enhanced Z None	Z None
0 Bladder 1 Kidney, Right 2 Kidney, Left 3 Kidneys, Bilateral 9 Kidney Transplant	Z None	Z None	Z None

1ST - B Imaging
2ND - T Urinary System
3RD - 4 ULTRASONOGRAPHY

ULTRASONOGRAPHY: Real time display of images of anatomy or flow information developed from the capture of reflected and attenuated high frequency sound waves.

Example: Abdominal ultrasound

Body Part – 4TH	Contrast – 5TH	Qualifier – 6TH	Qualifier – 7TH
0 Bladder 1 Kidney, Right 2 Kidney, Left 3 Kidneys, Bilateral 5 Urethra 6 Ureter, Right 7 Ureter, Left 8 Ureters, Bilateral 9 Kidney Transplant J Kidneys and Bladder	Z None	Z None	Z None

1ST - B Imaging
2ND - U Female Reproductive System ♀
3RD - 0 PLAIN RADIOGRAPHY

PLAIN RADIOGRAPHY: Planar display of an image developed from the capture of external ionizing radiation on photographic or photoconductive plate.

Example: Chest X-ray

Body Part – 4TH	Contrast – 5TH	Qualifier – 6TH	Qualifier – 7TH
0 Fallopian Tube, Right 1 Fallopian Tube, Left 2 Fallopian Tubes, Bilateral 6 Uterus 8 Uterus and Fallopian Tubes 9 Vagina	0 High osmolar 1 Low osmolar Y Other contrast	Z None	Z None

1ST - B Imaging
2ND - U Female Reproductive System ♀
3RD - 1 FLUOROSCOPY

FLUOROSCOPY: Single plane or bi-plane real time display of an image developed from the capture of external ionizing radiation on a fluorescent screen. The image may also be stored by either digital or analog means.

Example: Fluoroscopic guidance

Body Part – 4TH	Contrast – 5TH	Qualifier – 6TH	Qualifier – 7TH
0 Fallopian Tube, Right 1 Fallopian Tube, Left 2 Fallopian Tubes, Bilateral 6 Uterus 8 Uterus and Fallopian Tubes 9 Vagina	0 High osmolar 1 Low osmolar Y Other contrast Z None	Z None	Z None

1ST - B Imaging
2ND - U Female Reproductive System ♀
3RD - 3 MAGNETIC RESONANCE IMAGING (MRI)

MAGNETIC RESONANCE IMAGING (MRI): Computer reformatted digital display of multiplanar images developed from the capture of radiofrequency signals emitted by nuclei in a body site excited within a magnetic field.

Example: MRI of knee

Body Part – 4TH	Contrast – 5TH	Qualifier – 6TH	Qualifier – 7TH
3 Ovary, Right 4 Ovary, Left 5 Ovaries, Bilateral 6 Uterus 9 Vagina B Pregnant Uterus C Uterus and Ovaries	Y Other contrast	0 Unenhanced and enhanced Z None	Z None
3 Ovary, Right 4 Ovary, Left 5 Ovaries, Bilateral 6 Uterus 9 Vagina B Pregnant Uterus C Uterus and Ovaries	Z None	Z None	Z None

© 2018 Channel Publishing, Ltd.

1ST - B Imaging
2ND - U Female Reproductive System ♀
3RD - 4 ULTRASONOGRAPHY

ULTRASONOGRAPHY: Real time display of images of anatomy or flow information developed from the capture of reflected and attenuated high frequency sound waves.

Example: Abdominal ultrasound

Body Part – 4TH			Contrast – 5TH	Qualifier – 6TH	Qualifier – 7TH
0 Fallopian Tube, Right 1 Fallopian Tube, Left 2 Fallopian Tubes, Bilateral	3 Ovary, Right 4 Ovary, Left 5 Ovaries, Bilateral	6 Uterus C Uterus and Ovaries	Y Other contrast Z None	Z None	Z None

1ST - B Imaging
2ND - V Male Reproductive System ♂
3RD - 0 PLAIN RADIOGRAPHY

PLAIN RADIOGRAPHY: Planar display of an image developed from the capture of external ionizing radiation on photographic or photoconductive plate.

Example: Chest X-ray

Body Part – 4TH			Contrast – 5TH	Qualifier – 6TH	Qualifier – 7TH
0 Corpora Cavernosa 1 Epididymis, Right 2 Epididymis, Left	3 Prostate 5 Testicle, Right 6 Testicle, Left	8 Vasa Vasorum	0 High osmolar 1 Low osmolar Y Other contrast	Z None	Z None

1ST - B Imaging
2ND - V Male Reproductive System ♂
3RD - 1 FLUOROSCOPY

FLUOROSCOPY: Single plane or bi-plane real time display of an image developed from the capture of external ionizing radiation on a fluorescent screen. The image may also be stored by either digital or analog means.

Example: Fluoroscopic guidance

Body Part – 4TH	Contrast – 5TH		Qualifier – 6TH	Qualifier – 7TH
0 Corpora Cavernosa 8 Vasa Vasorum	0 High osmolar 1 Low osmolar	Y Other contrast Z None	Z None	Z None

1ST - B Imaging
2ND - V Male Reproductive System ♂
3RD - 2 COMPUTERIZED TOMOGRAPHY (CT Scan)

COMPUTERIZED TOMOGRAPHY (CT Scan): Computer reformatted digital display of multiplanar images developed from the capture of multiple exposures of external ionizing radiation.

Example: CT Scan of head

Body Part – 4TH	Contrast – 5TH		Qualifier – 6TH	Qualifier – 7TH
3 Prostate	0 High osmolar 1 Low osmolar	Y Other contrast	0 Unenhanced and enhanced Z None	Z None
3 Prostate	Z None		Z None	Z None

1ST - B Imaging
2ND - V Male Reproductive System ♂
3RD - 3 MAGNETIC RESONANCE IMAGING (MRI)

MAGNETIC RESONANCE IMAGING (MRI): Computer reformatted digital display of multiplanar images developed from the capture of radiofrequency signals emitted by nuclei in a body site excited within a magnetic field.

Example: MRI of knee

Body Part – 4TH			Contrast – 5TH	Qualifier – 6TH	Qualifier – 7TH
0 Corpora Cavernosa 3 Prostate	4 Scrotum 5 Testicle, Right	6 Testicle, Left 7 Testicles, Bilateral	Y Other contrast	0 Unenhanced and enhanced Z None	Z None
0 Corpora Cavernosa 3 Prostate	4 Scrotum 5 Testicle, Right	6 Testicle, Left 7 Testicles, Bilateral	Z None	Z None	Z None

© 2018 Channel Publishing, Ltd.

1ST - B Imaging
2ND - V Male Reproductive System ♂
3RD - 4 ULTRASONOGRAPHY

ULTRASONOGRAPHY: Real time display of images of anatomy or flow information developed from the capture of reflected and attenuated high frequency sound waves.

Example: Abdominal ultrasound

Body Part – 4TH	Contrast – 5TH	Qualifier – 6TH	Qualifier – 7TH
4 Scrotum 9 Prostate and Seminal Vesicles B Penis	Z None	Z None	Z None

1ST - B Imaging
2ND - W Anatomical Regions
3RD - 0 PLAIN RADIOGRAPHY

PLAIN RADIOGRAPHY: Planar display of an image developed from the capture of external ionizing radiation on photographic or photoconductive plate.

Example: Chest X-ray

Body Part – 4TH	Contrast – 5TH	Qualifier – 6TH	Qualifier – 7TH
0 Abdomen 1 Abdomen and Pelvis 3 Chest B Long Bones, All C Lower Extremity J Upper Extremity K Whole Body L Whole Skeleton M Whole Body, Infant	Z None	Z None	Z None

1ST - B Imaging
2ND - W Anatomical Regions
3RD - 1 FLUOROSCOPY

FLUOROSCOPY: Single plane or bi-plane real time display of an image developed from the capture of external ionizing radiation on a fluorescent screen. The image may also be stored by either digital or analog means.

Example: Fluoroscopic guidance

Body Part – 4TH	Contrast – 5TH	Qualifier – 6TH	Qualifier – 7TH
1 Abdomen and Pelvis 9 Head and Neck C Lower Extremity J Upper Extremity	0 High osmolar 1 Low osmolar Y Other contrast Z None	Z None	Z None

1ST - B Imaging
2ND - W Anatomical Regions
3RD - 2 COMPUTERIZED TOMOGRAPHY (CT Scan)

COMPUTERIZED TOMOGRAPHY (CT Scan): Computer reformatted digital display of multiplanar images developed from the capture of multiple exposures of external ionizing radiation.

Example: CT Scan of head

Body Part – 4TH	Contrast – 5TH	Qualifier – 6TH	Qualifier – 7TH
0 Abdomen 1 Abdomen and Pelvis 4 Chest and Abdomen 5 Chest, Abdomen and Pelvis 8 Head 9 Head and Neck F Neck G Pelvic Region	0 High osmolar 1 Low osmolar Y Other contrast	0 Unenhanced and enhanced Z None	Z None
0 Abdomen 1 Abdomen and Pelvis 4 Chest and Abdomen 5 Chest, Abdomen and Pelvis 8 Head 9 Head and Neck F Neck G Pelvic Region	Z None	Z None	Z None

1ST - B Imaging
2ND - W Anatomical Regions
3RD - 3 MAGNETIC RESONANCE IMAGING (MRI)

MAGNETIC RESONANCE IMAGING (MRI): Computer reformatted digital display of multiplanar images developed from the capture of radiofrequency signals emitted by nuclei in a body site excited within a magnetic field.

Example: MRI of knee

Body Part – 4TH	Contrast – 5TH	Qualifier – 6TH	Qualifier – 7TH
0 Abdomen 8 Head F Neck G Pelvic Region H Retroperitoneum P Brachial Plexus	Y Other contrast	0 Unenhanced and enhanced Z None	Z None
0 Abdomen 8 Head F Neck G Pelvic Region H Retroperitoneum P Brachial Plexus	Z None	Z None	Z None
3 Chest	Y Other contrast	0 Unenhanced and enhanced Z None	Z None

© 2018 Channel Publishing, Ltd.

1ST - B Imaging 2ND - W Anatomical Regions 3RD - 4 ULTRASONOGRAPHY	ULTRASONOGRAPHY: Real time display of images of anatomy or flow information developed from the capture of reflected and attenuated high frequency sound waves. Example: Abdominal ultrasound		
Body Part – 4TH	**Contrast – 5TH**	**Qualifier – 6TH**	**Qualifier – 7TH**
0 Abdomen 1 Abdomen and Pelvis F Neck G Pelvic Region	Z None	Z None	Z None

1ST - B Imaging 2ND - Y Fetus and Obstetrical ♀ 3RD - 3 MAGNETIC RESONANCE IMAGING (MRI)	MAGNETIC RESONANCE IMAGING (MRI): Computer reformatted digital display of multiplanar images developed from the capture of radiofrequency signals emitted by nuclei in a body site excited within a magnetic field. Example: MRI of knee		
Body Part – 4TH	**Contrast – 5TH**	**Qualifier – 6TH**	**Qualifier – 7TH**
0 Fetal Head 1 Fetal Heart 2 Fetal Thorax 3 Fetal Abdomen 4 Fetal Spine 5 Fetal Extremities 6 Whole Fetus	Y Other contrast	0 Unenhanced and enhanced Z None	Z None
0 Fetal Head 1 Fetal Heart 2 Fetal Thorax 3 Fetal Abdomen 4 Fetal Spine 5 Fetal Extremities 6 Whole Fetus	Z None	Z None	Z None

1ST - B Imaging 2ND - Y Fetus and Obstetrical ♀ 3RD - 4 ULTRASONOGRAPHY	ULTRASONOGRAPHY: Real time display of images of anatomy or flow information developed from the capture of reflected and attenuated high frequency sound waves. Example: Abdominal ultrasound		
Body Part – 4TH	**Contrast – 5TH**	**Qualifier – 6TH**	**Qualifier – 7TH**
7 Fetal Umbilical Cord 8 Placenta 9 First Trimester, Single Fetus B First Trimester, Multiple Gestation C Second Trimester, Single Fetus D Second Trimester, Multiple Gestation F Third Trimester, Single Fetus G Third Trimester, Multiple Gestation	Z None	Z None	Z None

© 2018 Channel Publishing, Ltd.

Educational Annotations | Section C – Nuclear Medicine

Section Specific Educational Annotations for the Nuclear Medicine Section include:

- AHA Coding Clinic® Reference Notations
- Coding Notes

AHA Coding Clinic® Reference Notations of Nuclear Medicine

ROOT TYPE SPECIFIC - NUCLEAR MEDICINE - Section C
PLANAR NUCLEAR MEDICINE IMAGING - 1
TOMOGRAPHIC (TOMO) NUCLEAR MEDICINE IMAGING - 2
POSITRON EMMISION TOMOGRAPHY (PET) - 3
NONIMAGING NUCLEAR MEDICINE UPTAKE - 4
NONIMAGING NUCLEAR MEDICINE PROBE - 5
NONIMAGING NUCLEAR MEDICINE ASSAY - 6
SYSTEMIC NUCLEAR MEDICINE THERAPY - 7

Coding Notes of Nuclear Medicine

© 2018 Channel Publishing, Ltd.

1ST - C Nuclear Medicine
2ND - 0 Central Nervous System
3RD - 1 PLANAR NUCLEAR MEDICINE IMAGING

PLANAR NUCLEAR MEDICINE IMAGING: Introduction of radioactive materials into the body for single plane display of images developed from the capture of radioactive emissions.

Example: Gallium scan, single plane image

Body Part – 4TH	Radionuclide – 5TH	Qualifier – 6TH	Qualifier – 7TH
0 Brain	1 Technetium 99m (Tc-99m) Y Other radionuclide	Z None	Z None
5 Cerebrospinal Fluid	D Indium 111 (In-111) Y Other radionuclide	Z None	Z None
Y Central Nervous System	Y Other radionuclide	Z None	Z None

1ST - C Nuclear Medicine
2ND - 0 Central Nervous System
3RD - 2 TOMOGRAPHIC (TOMO) NUCLEAR MEDICINE IMAGING

TOMOGRAPHIC (TOMO) NUCLEAR MEDICINE IMAGING: Introduction of radioactive materials into the body for three dimensional display of images developed from the capture of radioactive emissions.

Example: Tomo scan of breast

Body Part – 4TH	Radionuclide – 5TH	Qualifier – 6TH	Qualifier – 7TH
0 Brain	1 Technetium 99m (Tc-99m) F Iodine 123 (I-123) S Thallium 201 (Tl-201) Y Other radionuclide	Z None	Z None
5 Cerebrospinal Fluid	D Indium 111 (In-111) Y Other radionuclide	Z None	Z None
Y Central Nervous System	Y Other radionuclide	Z None	Z None

1ST - C Nuclear Medicine
2ND - 0 Central Nervous System
3RD - 3 POSITRON EMISSION TOMOGRAPHIC (PET) IMAGING

POSITRON EMISSION TOMOGRAPHIC (PET) IMAGING: Introduction of radioactive materials into the body for three dimensional display of images developed from the simultaneous capture, 180 degrees apart, of radioactive emissions.

Example: PET scan of brain

Body Part – 4TH	Radionuclide – 5TH	Qualifier – 6TH	Qualifier – 7TH
0 Brain	B Carbon 11 (C-11) K Fluorine 18 (F-18) M Oxygen 15 (O-15) Y Other radionuclide	Z None	Z None
Y Central Nervous System	Y Other radionuclide	Z None	Z None

1ST - C Nuclear Medicine
2ND - 0 Central Nervous System
3RD - 5 NONIMAGING NUCLEAR MEDICINE PROBE

NONIMAGING NUCLEAR MEDICINE PROBE: Introduction of radioactive materials into the body for the study of distribution and fate of certain substances by the detection of radioactive emissions; or, alternatively, measurement of absorption of radioactive emissions from an external source.

Example: Xenon gas nonimaging probe of brain

Body Part – 4TH	Radionuclide – 5TH	Qualifier – 6TH	Qualifier – 7TH
0 Brain	V Xenon 133 (Xe-133) Y Other radionuclide	Z None	Z None
Y Central Nervous System	Y Other radionuclide	Z None	Z None

1ST - C Nuclear Medicine
2ND - 2 Heart
3RD - 1 PLANAR NUCLEAR MEDICINE IMAGING

PLANAR NUCLEAR MEDICINE IMAGING: Introduction of radioactive materials into the body for single plane display of images developed from the capture of radioactive emissions.

Example: Gallium scan, single plane image

Body Part – 4TH	Radionuclide – 5TH	Qualifier – 6TH	Qualifier – 7TH
6 Heart, Right and Left	1 Technetium 99m (Tc-99m) Y Other radionuclide	Z None	Z None
G Myocardium	1 Technetium 99m (Tc-99m) D Indium 111 (In-111) S Thallium 201 (Tl-201) Y Other radionuclide Z None	Z None	Z None
Y Heart	Y Other radionuclide	Z None	Z None

© 2018 Channel Publishing, Ltd.

1ST - C Nuclear Medicine
2ND - 2 Heart
3RD - 2 TOMOGRAPHIC (TOMO) NUCLEAR MEDICINE IMAGING

TOMOGRAPHIC (TOMO) NUCLEAR MEDICINE IMAGING: Introduction of radioactive materials into the body for three dimensional display of images developed from the capture of radioactive emissions.

Example: Tomo scan of breast

Body Part – 4TH	Radionuclide – 5TH	Qualifier – 6TH	Qualifier – 7TH
6 Heart, Right and Left	1 Technetium 99m (Tc-99m) Y Other radionuclide	Z None	Z None
G Myocardium	1 Technetium 99m (Tc-99m) D Indium 111 (In-111) K Fluorine 18 (F-18) S Thallium 201 (Tl-201) Y Other radionuclide Z None	Z None	Z None
Y Heart	Y Other radionuclide	Z None	Z None

1ST - C Nuclear Medicine
2ND - 2 Heart
3RD - 3 POSITRON EMISSION TOMOGRAPHIC (PET) IMAGING

POSITRON EMISSION TOMOGRAPHIC (PET) IMAGING: Introduction of radioactive materials into the body for three dimensional display of images developed from the simultaneous capture, 180 degrees apart, of radioactive emissions.

Example: PET scan of brain

Body Part – 4TH	Radionuclide – 5TH	Qualifier – 6TH	Qualifier – 7TH
G Myocardium	K Fluorine 18 (F-18) M Oxygon 15 (O 15) Q Rubidium 82 (Rb-82) R Nitrogen 13 (N-13) Y Other radionuclide	Z None	Z None
Y Heart	Y Other radionuclide	Z None	Z None

1ST - C Nuclear Medicine
2ND - 2 Heart
3RD - 5 NONIMAGING NUCLEAR MEDICINE PROBE

NONIMAGING NUCLEAR MEDICINE PROBE: Introduction of radioactive materials into the body for the study of distribution and fate of certain substances by the detection of radioactive emissions; or, alternatively, measurement of absorption of radioactive emissions from an external source.

Example: Xenon gas nonimaging probe of brain

Body Part – 4TH	Radionuclide – 5TH	Qualifier – 6TH	Qualifier – 7TH
6 Heart, Right and Left	1 Technetium 99m (Tc-99m) Y Other radionuclide	Z None	Z None
Y Heart	Y Other radionuclide	Z None	Z None

1ST - C Nuclear Medicine
2ND - 5 Veins
3RD - 1 PLANAR NUCLEAR MEDICINE IMAGING

PLANAR NUCLEAR MEDICINE IMAGING: Introduction of radioactive materials into the body for single plane display of images developed from the capture of radioactive emissions.

Example: Gallium scan, single plane image

Body Part – 4TH	Radionuclide – 5TH	Qualifier – 6TH	Qualifier – 7TH
B Lower Extremity Veins, Right C Lower Extremity Veins, Left D Lower Extremity Veins, Bilateral N Upper Extremity Veins, Right P Upper Extremity Veins, Left Q Upper Extremity Veins, Bilateral R Central Veins	1 Technetium 99m (Tc-99m) Y Other radionuclide	Z None	Z None
Y Veins	Y Other radionuclide	Z None	Z None

NUCLEAR MEDICINE C 5 1

© 2018 Channel Publishing, Ltd.

1ST - C Nuclear Medicine
2ND - 7 Lymphatic and Hematologic System
3RD - 1 PLANAR NUCLEAR MEDICINE IMAGING

PLANAR NUCLEAR MEDICINE IMAGING: Introduction of radioactive materials into the body for single plane display of images developed from the capture of radioactive emissions.

Example: Gallium scan, single plane image

Body Part – 4TH	Radionuclide – 5TH	Qualifier – 6TH	Qualifier – 7TH
0 Bone Marrow	1 Technetium 99m (Tc-99m) D Indium 111 (In-111) Y Other radionuclide	Z None	Z None
2 Spleen 5 Lymphatics, Head and Neck D Lymphatics, Pelvic J Lymphatics, Head K Lymphatics, Neck L Lymphatics, Upper Chest M Lymphatics, Trunk N Lymphatics, Upper Extremity P Lymphatics, Lower Extremity	1 Technetium 99m (Tc-99m) Y Other radionuclide	Z None	Z None
3 Blood	D Indium 111 (In-111) Y Other radionuclide	Z None	Z None
Y Lymphatic and Hematologic System	Y Other radionuclide	Z None	Z None

1ST - C Nuclear Medicine
2ND - 7 Lymphatic and Hematologic System
3RD - 2 TOMOGRAPHIC (TOMO) NUCLEAR MEDICINE IMAGING

TOMOGRAPHIC (TOMO) NUCLEAR MEDICINE IMAGING: Introduction of radioactive materials into the body for three dimensional display of images developed from the capture of radioactive emissions.

Example: Tomo scan of breast

Body Part – 4TH	Radionuclide – 5TH	Qualifier – 6TH	Qualifier – 7TH
2 Spleen	1 Technetium 99m (Tc-99m) Y Other radionuclide	Z None	Z None
Y Lymphatic and Hematologic System	Y Other radionuclide	Z None	Z None

1ST - C Nuclear Medicine
2ND - 7 Lymphatic and Hematologic System
3RD - 5 NONIMAGING NUCLEAR MEDICINE PROBE

NONIMAGING NUCLEAR MEDICINE PROBE: Introduction of radioactive materials into the body for the study of distribution and fate of certain substances by the detection of radioactive emissions; or, alternatively, measurement of absorption of radioactive emissions from an external source.

Example: Xenon gas nonimaging probe of brain

Body Part – 4TH	Radionuclide – 5TH	Qualifier – 6TH	Qualifier – 7TH
5 Lymphatics, Head and Neck D Lymphatics, Pelvic J Lymphatics, Head K Lymphatics, Neck L Lymphatics, Upper Chest M Lymphatics, Trunk N Lymphatics, Upper Extremity P Lymphatics, Lower Extremity	1 Technetium 99m (Tc-99m) Y Other radionuclide	Z None	Z None
Y Lymphatic and Hematologic System	Y Other radionuclide	Z None	Z None

1ST - C Nuclear Medicine
2ND - 7 Lymphatic and Hematologic System
3RD - 6 NONIMAGING NUCLEAR MEDICINE ASSAY

NONIMAGING NUCLEAR MEDICINE ASSAY: Introduction of radioactive materials into the body for the study of body fluids and blood elements, by the detection of radioactive emissions.

Example: Technetium assay of kidneys

Body Part – 4TH	Radionuclide – 5TH	Qualifier – 6TH	Qualifier – 7TH
3 Blood	1 Technetium 99m (Tc-99m) 7 Cobalt 58 (Co-58) C Cobalt 57 (Co-57) D Indium 111 (In-111) H Iodine 125 (I-125) W Chromium (Cr-51) Y Other radionuclide	Z None	Z None
Y Lymphatic and Hematologic System	Y Other radionuclide	Z None	Z None

© 2018 Channel Publishing, Ltd.

1ST - C Nuclear Medicine
2ND - 8 Eye
3RD - 1 PLANAR NUCLEAR MEDICINE IMAGING

PLANAR NUCLEAR MEDICINE IMAGING: Introduction of radioactive materials into the body for single plane display of images developed from the capture of radioactive emissions.

Example: Gallium scan, single plane image

Body Part – 4TH	Radionuclide – 5TH	Qualifier – 6TH	Qualifier – 7TH
9 Lacrimal Ducts, Bilateral	1 Technetium 99m (Tc-99m) Y Other radionuclide	Z None	Z None
Y Eye	Y Other radionuclide	Z None	Z None

1ST - C Nuclear Medicine
2ND - 9 Ear, Nose, Mouth and Throat
3RD - 1 PLANAR NUCLEAR MEDICINE IMAGING

PLANAR NUCLEAR MEDICINE IMAGING: Introduction of radioactive materials into the body for single plane display of images developed from the capture of radioactive emissions.

Example: Gallium scan, single plane image

Body Part – 4TH	Radionuclide – 5TH	Qualifier – 6TH	Qualifier – 7TH
B Salivary Glands, Bilateral	1 Technetium 99m (Tc-99m) Y Other radionuclide	Z None	Z None
Y Ear, Nose, Mouth and Throat	Y Other radionuclide	Z None	Z None

1ST - C Nuclear Medicine
2ND - B Respiratory System
3RD - 1 PLANAR NUCLEAR MEDICINE IMAGING

PLANAR NUCLEAR MEDICINE IMAGING: Introduction of radioactive materials into the body for single plane display of images developed from the capture of radioactive emissions.

Example: Gallium scan, single plane image

Body Part – 4TH	Radionuclide – 5TH	Qualifier – 6TH	Qualifier – 7TH
2 Lungs and Bronchi	1 Technetium 99m (Tc-99m) 9 Krypton (Kr-81m) T Xenon 127 (Xe-127) V Xenon 133 (Xe-133) Y Other radionuclide	Z None	Z None
Y Respiratory System	Y Other radionuclide	Z None	Z None

1ST - C Nuclear Medicine
2ND - B Respiratory System
3RD - 2 TOMOGRAPHIC (TOMO) NUCLEAR MEDICINE IMAGING

TOMOGRAPHIC (TOMO) NUCLEAR MEDICINE IMAGING: Introduction of radioactive materials into the body for three dimensional display of images developed from the capture of radioactive emissions.

Example: Tomo scan of breast

Body Part – 4TH	Radionuclide – 5TH	Qualifier – 6TH	Qualifier – 7TH
2 Lungs and Bronchi	1 Technetium 99m (Tc-99m) 9 Krypton (Kr-81m) Y Other radionuclide	Z None	Z None
Y Respiratory System	Y Other radionuclide	Z None	Z None

1ST - C Nuclear Medicine
2ND - B Respiratory System
3RD - 3 POSITRON EMISSION TOMOGRAPHIC (PET) IMAGING

POSITRON EMISSION TOMOGRAPHIC (PET) IMAGING: Introduction of radioactive materials into the body for three dimensional display of images developed from the simultaneous capture, 180 degrees apart, of radioactive emissions.

Example: PET scan of brain

Body Part – 4TH	Radionuclide – 5TH	Qualifier – 6TH	Qualifier – 7TH
2 Lungs and Bronchi	K Fluorine 18 (F-18) Y Other radionuclide	Z None	Z None
Y Respiratory System	Y Other radionuclide	Z None	Z None

© 2018 Channel Publishing, Ltd.

1ST - C Nuclear Medicine
2ND - D Gastrointestinal System
3RD - 1 PLANAR NUCLEAR MEDICINE IMAGING

PLANAR NUCLEAR MEDICINE IMAGING: Introduction of radioactive materials into the body for single plane display of images developed from the capture of radioactive emissions.

Example: Gallium scan, single plane image

Body Part – 4TH	Radionuclide – 5TH	Qualifier – 6TH	Qualifier – 7TH
5 Upper Gastrointestinal Tract 7 Gastrointestinal Tract	1 Technetium 99m (Tc-99m) D Indium 111 (In-111) Y Other radionuclide	Z None	Z None
Y Digestive System	Y Other radionuclide	Z None	Z None

1ST - C Nuclear Medicine
2ND - D Gastrointestinal System
3RD - 2 TOMOGRAPHIC (TOMO) NUCLEAR MEDICINE IMAGING

TOMOGRAPHIC (TOMO) NUCLEAR MEDICINE IMAGING: Introduction of radioactive materials into the body for three dimensional display of images developed from the capture of radioactive emissions.

Example: Tomo scan of breast

Body Part – 4TH	Radionuclide – 5TH	Qualifier – 6TH	Qualifier – 7TH
7 Gastrointestinal Tract	1 Technetium 99m (Tc-99m) D Indium 111 (In-111) Y Other radionuclide	Z None	Z None
Y Digestive System	Y Other radionuclide	Z None	Z None

1ST - C Nuclear Medicine
2ND - F Hepatobiliary System and Pancreas
3RD - 1 PLANAR NUCLEAR MEDICINE IMAGING

PLANAR NUCLEAR MEDICINE IMAGING: Introduction of radioactive materials into the body for single plane display of images developed from the capture of radioactive emissions.

Example: Gallium scan, single plane image

Body Part – 4TH	Radionuclide – 5TH	Qualifier – 6TH	Qualifier – 7TH
4 Gallbladder 5 Liver 6 Liver and Spleen C Hepatobiliary System, All	1 Technetium 99m (Tc-99m) Y Other radionuclide	Z None	Z None
Y Hepatobiliary System and Pancreas	Y Other radionuclide	Z None	Z None

1ST - C Nuclear Medicine
2ND - F Hepatobiliary System and Pancreas
3RD - 2 TOMOGRAPHIC (TOMO) NUCLEAR MEDICINE IMAGING

TOMOGRAPHIC (TOMO) NUCLEAR MEDICINE IMAGING: Introduction of radioactive materials into the body for three dimensional display of images developed from the capture of radioactive emissions.

Example: Tomo scan of breast

Body Part – 4TH	Radionuclide – 5TH	Qualifier – 6TH	Qualifier – 7TH
4 Gallbladder 5 Liver 6 Liver and Spleen	1 Technetium 99m (Tc-99m) Y Other radionuclide	Z None	Z None
Y Hepatobiliary System and Pancreas	Y Other radionuclide	Z None	Z None

1ST - C Nuclear Medicine
2ND - G Endocrine System
3RD - 1 PLANAR NUCLEAR MEDICINE IMAGING

PLANAR NUCLEAR MEDICINE IMAGING: Introduction of radioactive materials into the body for single plane display of images developed from the capture of radioactive emissions.

Example: Gallium scan, single plane image

Body Part – 4TH	Radionuclide – 5TH	Qualifier – 6TH	Qualifier – 7TH
1 Parathyroid Glands	1 Technetium 99m (Tc-99m) S Thallium 201 (Tl-201) Y Other radionuclide	Z None	Z None
2 Thyroid Gland	1 Technetium 99m (Tc-99m) F Iodine 123 (I-123) G Iodine 131 (I-131) Y Other radionuclide	Z None	Z None
4 Adrenal Glands, Bilateral	G Iodine 131 (I-131) Y Other radionuclide	Z None	Z None
Y Endocrine System	Y Other radionuclide	Z None	Z None

© 2018 Channel Publishing, Ltd.

1ST - C Nuclear Medicine
2ND - G Endocrine System
3RD - 2 TOMOGRAPHIC (TOMO) NUCLEAR MEDICINE IMAGING

TOMOGRAPHIC (TOMO) NUCLEAR MEDICINE IMAGING: Introduction of radioactive materials into the body for three dimensional display of images developed from the capture of radioactive emissions.

Example: Tomo scan of breast

Body Part – 4TH	Radionuclide – 5TH	Qualifier – 6TH	Qualifier – 7TH
1 Parathyroid Glands	1 Technetium 99m (Tc-99m) S Thallium 201 (Tl-201) Y Other radionuclide	Z None	Z None
Y Endocrine System	Y Other radionuclide	Z None	Z None

1ST - C Nuclear Medicine
2ND - G Endocrine System
3RD - 4 NONIMAGING NUCLEAR MEDICINE UPTAKE

NONIMAGING NUCLEAR MEDICINE UPTAKE: Introduction of radioactive materials into the body for measurements of organ function, from the detection of radioactive emissions.

Example: Iodine uptake test of thyroid

Body Part – 4TH	Radionuclide – 5TH	Qualifier – 6TH	Qualifier – 7TH
2 Thyroid Gland	1 Technetium 99m (Tc-99m) F Iodine 123 (I-123) G Iodine 131 (I-131) Y Other radionuclide	Z None	Z None
Y Endocrine System	Y Other radionuclide	Z None	Z None

1ST - C Nuclear Medicine
2ND - H Skin, Subcutaneous Tissue and Breast
3RD - 1 PLANAR NUCLEAR MEDICINE IMAGING

PLANAR NUCLEAR MEDICINE IMAGING: Introduction of radioactive materials into the body for single plane display of images developed from the capture of radioactive emissions.

Example: Gallium scan, single plane image

Body Part – 4TH	Radionuclide – 5TH	Qualifier – 6TH	Qualifier – 7TH
0 Breast, Right 1 Breast, Left 2 Breasts, Bilateral	1 Technetium 99m (Tc-99m) S Thallium 201 (Tl-201) Y Other radionuclide	Z None	Z None
Y Skin, Subcutaneous Tissue and Breast	Y Other radionuclide	Z None	Z None

1ST - C Nuclear Medicine
2ND - H Skin, Subcutaneous Tissue and Breast
3RD - 2 TOMOGRAPHIC (TOMO) NUCLEAR MEDICINE IMAGING

TOMOGRAPHIC (TOMO) NUCLEAR MEDICINE IMAGING: Introduction of radioactive materials into the body for three dimensional display of images developed from the capture of radioactive emissions.

Example: Tomo scan of breast

Body Part – 4TH	Radionuclide – 5TH	Qualifier – 6TH	Qualifier – 7TH
0 Breast, Right 1 Breast, Left 2 Breasts, Bilateral	1 Technetium 99m (Tc-99m) S Thallium 201 (Tl-201) Y Other radionuclide	Z None	Z None
Y Skin, Subcutaneous Tissue and Breast	Y Other radionuclide	Z None	Z None

1ST - C Nuclear Medicine
2ND - P Musculoskeletal System
3RD - 1 PLANAR NUCLEAR MEDICINE IMAGING

PLANAR NUCLEAR MEDICINE IMAGING: Introduction of radioactive materials into the body for single plane display of images developed from the capture of radioactive emissions.

Example: Gallium scan, single plane image

Body Part – 4TH	Radionuclide – 5TH	Qualifier – 6TH	Qualifier – 7TH
1 Skull 4 Thorax 5 Spine 6 Pelvis 7 Spine and Pelvis 8 Upper Extremity, Right 9 Upper Extremity, Left B Upper Extremities, Bilateral C Lower Extremity, Right D Lower Extremity, Left F Lower Extremities, Bilateral Z Musculoskeletal System, All	1 Technetium 99m (Tc-99m) Y Other radionuclide	Z None	Z None
Y Musculoskeletal System, Other	Y Other radionuclide	Z None	Z None

NUCLEAR MEDICINE CP1

© 2018 Channel Publishing, Ltd.

1ST - C Nuclear Medicine 2ND - P Musculoskeletal System 3RD - 2 TOMOGRAPHIC (TOMO) NUCLEAR MEDICINE IMAGING	TOMOGRAPHIC (TOMO) NUCLEAR MEDICINE IMAGING: Introduction of radioactive materials into the body for three dimensional display of images developed from the capture of radioactive emissions. Example: Tomo scan of breast		
Body Part – 4TH	**Radionuclide – 5TH**	**Qualifier – 6TH**	**Qualifier – 7TH**
1 Skull 2 Cervical Spine 3 Skull and Cervical Spine 4 Thorax 6 Pelvis 7 Spine and Pelvis 8 Upper Extremity, Right 9 Upper Extremity, Left B Upper Extremities, Bilateral C Lower Extremity, Right D Lower Extremity, Left F Lower Extremities, Bilateral G Thoracic Spine H Lumbar Spine J Thoracolumbar Spine	1 Technetium 99m (Tc-99m) Y Other radionuclide	Z None	Z None
Y Musculoskeletal System, Other	Y Other radionuclide	Z None	Z None

1ST - C Nuclear Medicine 2ND - P Musculoskeletal System 3RD - 5 NONIMAGING NUCLEAR MEDICINE PROBE	NONIMAGING NUCLEAR MEDICINE PROBE: Introduction of radioactive materials into the body for the study of distribution and fate of certain substances by the detection of radioactive emissions; or, alternatively, measurement of absorption of radioactive emissions from an external source. Example: Xenon gas nonimaging probe of brain		
Body Part – 4TH	**Radionuclide – 5TH**	**Qualifier – 6TH**	**Qualifier – 7TH**
5 Spine N Upper Extremities P Lower Extremities	Z None	Z None	Z None
Y Musculoskeletal System, Other	Y Other radionuclide	Z None	Z None

1ST - C Nuclear Medicine 2ND - T Urinary System 3RD - 1 PLANAR NUCLEAR MEDICINE IMAGING	PLANAR NUCLEAR MEDICINE IMAGING: Introduction of radioactive materials into the body for single plane display of images developed from the capture of radioactive emissions. Example: Gallium scan, single plane image		
Body Part – 4TH	**Radionuclide – 5TH**	**Qualifier – 6TH**	**Qualifier – 7TH**
3 Kidneys, Ureters and Bladder	1 Technetium 99m (Tc-99m) F Iodine 123 (I-123) G Iodine 131 (I-131) Y Other radionuclide	Z None	Z None
H Bladder and Ureters	1 Technetium 99m (Tc-99m) Y Other radionuclide	Z None	Z None
Y Urinary System	Y Other radionuclide	Z None	Z None

1ST - C Nuclear Medicine 2ND - T Urinary System 3RD - 2 TOMOGRAPHIC (TOMO) NUCLEAR MEDICINE IMAGING	TOMOGRAPHIC (TOMO) NUCLEAR MEDICINE IMAGING: Introduction of radioactive materials into the body for three dimensional display of images developed from the capture of radioactive emissions. Example: Tomo scan of breast		
Body Part – 4TH	**Radionuclide – 5TH**	**Qualifier – 6TH**	**Qualifier – 7TH**
3 Kidneys, Ureters and Bladder	1 Technetium 99m (Tc-99m) Y Other radionuclide	Z None	Z None
Y Urinary System	Y Other radionuclide	Z None	Z None

1ST - C Nuclear Medicine 2ND - T Urinary System 3RD - 6 NONIMAGING NUCLEAR MEDICINE ASSAY	NONIMAGING NUCLEAR MEDICINE ASSAY: Introduction of radioactive materials into the body for the study of body fluids and blood elements, by the detection of radioactive emissions. Example: Technetium assay of kidneys		
Body Part – 4TH	**Radionuclide – 5TH**	**Qualifier – 6TH**	**Qualifier – 7TH**
3 Kidneys, Ureters and Bladder	1 Technetium 99m (Tc-99m) F Iodine 123 (I-123) G Iodine 131 (I-131) H Iodine 125 (I-125) Y Other radionuclide	Z None	Z None
Y Urinary System	Y Other radionuclide	Z None	Z None

© 2018 Channel Publishing, Ltd.

1ST - C Nuclear Medicine 2ND - V Male Reproductive System 3RD - 1 PLANAR NUCLEAR MEDICINE IMAGING	PLANAR NUCLEAR MEDICINE IMAGING: Introduction of radioactive materials into the body for single plane display of images developed from the capture of radioactive emissions. Example: Gallium scan, single plane image		
Body Part – 4TH	**Radionuclide – 5TH**	**Qualifier – 6TH**	**Qualifier – 7TH**
9 Testicles, Bilateral ♂	1 Technetium 99m (Tc-99m) Y Other radionuclide	Z None	Z None
Y Male Reproductive System ♂	Y Other radionuclide	Z None	Z None

1ST - C Nuclear Medicine 2ND - W Anatomical Regions 3RD - 1 PLANAR NUCLEAR MEDICINE IMAGING	PLANAR NUCLEAR MEDICINE IMAGING: Introduction of radioactive materials into the body for single plane display of images developed from the capture of radioactive emissions. Example: Gallium scan, single plane image		
Body Part – 4TH	**Radionuclide – 5TH**	**Qualifier – 6TH**	**Qualifier – 7TH**
0 Abdomen 1 Abdomen and Pelvis 4 Chest and Abdomen 6 Chest and Neck B Head and Neck D Lower Extremity J Pelvic Region M Upper Extremity N Whole Body	1 Technetium 99m (Tc-99m) D Indium 111 (In-111) F Iodine 123 (I-123) G Iodine 131 (I-131) L Gallium 67 (Ga-67) S Thallium 201 (Tl-201) Y Other radionuclide	Z None	Z None
3 Chest	1 Technetium 99m (Tc-99m) D Indium 111 (In-111) F Iodine 123 (I-123) G Iodine 131 (I-131) K Fluorine 18 (F-18) L Gallium 67 (Ga-67) S Thallium 201 (Tl-201) Y Other radionuclide	Z None	Z None
Y Anatomical Regions, Multiple	Y Other radionuclide	Z None	Z None
Z Anatomical Region, Other	Z None	Z None	Z None

1ST - C Nuclear Medicine 2ND - W Anatomical Regions 3RD - 2 TOMOGRAPHIC (TOMO) NUCLEAR MEDICINE IMAGING	TOMOGRAPHIC (TOMO) NUCLEAR MEDICINE IMAGING: Introduction of radioactive materials into the body for three dimensional display of images developed from the capture of radioactive emissions. Example: Tomo scan of breast		
Body Part – 4TH	**Radionuclide – 5TH**	**Qualifier – 6TH**	**Qualifier – 7TH**
0 Abdomen 1 Abdomen and Pelvis 3 Chest 4 Chest and Abdomen 6 Chest and Neck B Head and Neck D Lower Extremity J Pelvic Region M Upper Extremity	1 Technetium 99m (Tc-99m) D Indium 111 (In-111) F Iodine 123 (I-123) G Iodine 131 (I-131) K Fluorine 18 (F-18) L Gallium 67 (Ga-67) S Thallium 201 (Tl-201) Y Other radionuclide	Z None	Z None
Y Anatomical Regions, Multiple	Y Other radionuclide	Z None	Z None

1ST - C Nuclear Medicine 2ND - W Anatomical Regions 3RD - 3 POSITRON EMISSION TOMOGRAPHIC (PET) IMAGING	POSITRON EMISSION TOMOGRAPHIC (PET) IMAGING: Introduction of radioactive materials into the body for three dimensional display of images developed from the simultaneous capture, 180 degrees apart, of radioactive emissions. Example: PET scan of brain		
Body Part – 4TH	**Radionuclide – 5TH**	**Qualifier – 6TH**	**Qualifier – 7TH**
N Whole Body	Y Other radionuclide	Z None	Z None

© 2018 Channel Publishing, Ltd.

1ST - C Nuclear Medicine
2ND - W Anatomical Regions
3RD - 5 NONIMAGING NUCLEAR MEDICINE PROBE

NONIMAGING NUCLEAR MEDICINE PROBE: Introduction of radioactive materials into the body for the study of distribution and fate of certain substances by the detection of radioactive emissions; or, alternatively, measurement of absorption of radioactive emissions from an external source.

Example: Xenon gas nonimaging probe of brain

Body Part – 4TH	Radionuclide – 5TH	Qualifier – 6TH	Qualifier – 7TH
0 Abdomen 1 Abdomen and Pelvis 3 Chest 4 Chest and Abdomen 6 Chest and Neck B Head and Neck D Lower Extremity J Pelvic Region M Upper Extremity	1 Technetium 99m (Tc-99m) D Indium 111 (In-111) Y Other radionuclide	Z None	Z None

1ST - C Nuclear Medicine
2ND - W Anatomical Regions
3RD - 7 SYSTEMIC NUCLEAR MEDICINE THERAPY

SYSTEMIC NUCLEAR MEDICINE THERAPY: Introduction of unsealed radioactive materials into the body for treatment.

Example: Radioactive substance combined with a specific antibody into blood stream

Body Part – 4TH	Radionuclide – 5TH	Qualifier – 6TH	Qualifier – 7TH
0 Abdomen 3 Chest	N Phosphorus 32 (P-32) Y Other radionuclide	Z None	Z None
G Thyroid	G Iodine 131 (I-131) Y Other radionuclide	Z None	Z None
N Whole Body	8 Samarium 153 (Sm-153) G Iodine 131 (I-131) N Phosphorus 32 (P-32) P Strontium 89 (Sr-89) Y Other radionuclide	Z None	Z None
Y Anatomical Regions, Multiple	Y Other radionuclide	Z None	Z None

© 2018 Channel Publishing, Ltd.

Educational Annotations | Section D – Radiation Therapy

Section Specific Educational Annotations for the Radiation Therapy Section include:

- AHA Coding Clinic® Reference Notations
- Coding Notes

AHA Coding Clinic® Reference Notations of Radiation Therapy

ROOT TYPE SPECIFIC - RADIATION THERAPY - Section D
BEAM RADIATION - 0
BRACHYTHERAPY - 1
STEREOTACTIC RADIOSURGERY - 3
OTHER RADIATION - Y

Coding Notes of Radiation Therapy

© 2018 Channel Publishing, Ltd.

1ST - D Radiation Therapy
2ND - 0 Central and Peripheral Nervous System
3RD - 0 **BEAM RADIATION**

MODALITY: BEAM RADIATION

Example: External beam radiation

Treatment Site – 4TH	Modality Qualifier – 5TH	Isotope – 6TH	Qualifier – 7TH
0 Brain 1 Brain Stem 6 Spinal Cord 7 Peripheral Nerve	0 Photons <1 MeV 1 Photons 1 - 10 MeV 2 Photons >10 MeV 4 Heavy particles (protons, ions) 5 Neutrons 6 Neutron capture	Z None	Z None
0 Brain 1 Brain Stem 6 Spinal Cord 7 Peripheral Nerve	3 Electrons	Z None	0 Intraoperative Z None

1ST - D Radiation Therapy
2ND - 0 Central and Peripheral Nervous System
3RD - 1 **BRACHYTHERAPY**

MODALITY: BRACHYTHERAPY

Example: Insertion of radioactive material

Treatment Site – 4TH	Modality Qualifier – 5TH	Isotope – 6TH	Qualifier – 7TH
0 Brain 1 Brain Stem 6 Spinal Cord 7 Peripheral Nerve	9 High dose rate (HDR) B Low dose rate (LDR)	7 Cesium 137 (Cs-137) 8 Iridium 192 (Ir-192) 9 Iodine 125 (I-125) B Palladium 103 (Pd-103) C Californium 252 (Cf-252) Y Other isotope	Z None

1ST - D Radiation Therapy
2ND - 0 Central and Peripheral Nervous System
3RD - 2 **STEREOTACTIC RADIOSURGERY**

MODALITY: STEREOTACTIC RADIOSURGERY

Example: Particulate stereotactic radiosurgery

Treatment Site – 4TH	Modality Qualifier – 5TH	Isotope – 6TH	Qualifier – 7TH
0 Brain 1 Brain Stem 6 Spinal Cord 7 Peripheral Nerve	D Stereotactic other photon radiosurgery H Stereotactic particulate radiosurgery J Stereotactic gamma beam radiosurgery	Z None	Z None

1ST - D Radiation Therapy
2ND - 0 Central and Peripheral Nervous System
3RD - Y **OTHER RADIATION**

MODALITY: OTHER RADIATION

Example: Laser interstitial thermal therapy

Treatment Site – 4TH	Modality Qualifier – 5TH	Isotope – 6TH	Qualifier – 7TH
0 Brain 1 Brain Stem 6 Spinal Cord 7 Peripheral Nerve	7 Contact radiation 8 Hyperthermia F Plaque radiation K Laser interstitial thermal therapy	Z None	Z None

1ST - D Radiation Therapy
2ND - 7 Lymphatic and Hematologic System
3RD - 0 **BEAM RADIATION**

MODALITY: BEAM RADIATION

Example: External beam radiation

Treatment Site – 4TH	Modality Qualifier – 5TH	Isotope – 6TH	Qualifier – 7TH
0 Bone Marrow 1 Thymus 2 Spleen 3 Lymphatics, Neck 4 Lymphatics, Axillary 5 Lymphatics, Thorax 6 Lymphatics, Abdomen 7 Lymphatics, Pelvis 8 Lymphatics, Inguinal	0 Photons <1 MeV 1 Photons 1 - 10 MeV 2 Photons >10 MeV 4 Heavy particles (protons, ions) 5 Neutrons 6 Neutron capture	Z None	Z None
0 Bone Marrow 1 Thymus 2 Spleen 3 Lymphatics, Neck 4 Lymphatics, Axillary 5 Lymphatics, Thorax 6 Lymphatics, Abdomen 7 Lymphatics, Pelvis 8 Lymphatics, Inguinal	3 Electrons	Z None	0 Intraoperative Z None

© 2018 Channel Publishing, Ltd.

1ST - D Radiation Therapy
2ND - 7 Lymphatic and Hematologic System
3RD - 1 BRACHYTHERAPY

MODALITY: BRACHYTHERAPY

Example: Insertion of radioactive material

Treatment Site – 4TH	Modality Qualifier – 5TH	Isotope – 6TH	Qualifier – 7TH
0 Bone Marrow 1 Thymus 2 Spleen 3 Lymphatics, Neck 4 Lymphatics, Axillary 5 Lymphatics, Thorax 6 Lymphatics, Abdomen 7 Lymphatics, Pelvis 8 Lymphatics, Inguinal	9 High dose rate (HDR) B Low dose rate (LDR)	7 Cesium 137 (Cs-137) 8 Iridium 192 (Ir-192) 9 Iodine 125 (I-125) B Palladium 103 (Pd-103) C Californium 252 (Cf-252) Y Other isotope	Z None

1ST - D Radiation Therapy
2ND - 7 Lymphatic and Hematologic System
3RD - 2 STEREOTACTIC RADIOSURGERY

MODALITY: STEREOTACTIC RADIOSURGERY

Example: Particulate stereotactic radiosurgery

Treatment Site – 4TH	Modality Qualifier – 5TH	Isotope – 6TH	Qualifier – 7TH
0 Bone Marrow 1 Thymus 2 Spleen 3 Lymphatics, Neck 4 Lymphatics, Axillary 5 Lymphatics, Thorax 6 Lymphatics, Abdomen 7 Lymphatics, Pelvis 8 Lymphatics, Inguinal	D Stereotactic other photon radiosurgery H Stereotactic particulate radiosurgery J Stereotactic gamma beam radiosurgery	Z None	Z None

1ST - D Radiation Therapy
2ND - 7 Lymphatic and Hematologic System
3RD - Y OTHER RADIATION

MODALITY: OTHER RADIATION

Example: Laser interstitial thermal therapy

Treatment Site – 4TH	Modality Qualifier – 5TH	Isotope – 6TH	Qualifier – 7TH
0 Bone Marrow 1 Thymus 2 Spleen 3 Lymphatics, Neck 4 Lymphatics, Axillary 5 Lymphatics, Thorax 6 Lymphatics, Abdomen 7 Lymphatics, Pelvis 8 Lymphatics, Inguinal	8 Hyperthermia F Plaque radiation	Z None	Z None

1ST - D Radiation Therapy
2ND - 8 Eye
3RD - 0 BEAM RADIATION

MODALITY: BEAM RADIATION

Example: External beam radiation

Treatment Site – 4TH	Modality Qualifier – 5TH	Isotope – 6TH	Qualifier – 7TH
0 Eye	0 Photons <1 MeV 1 Photons 1 - 10 MeV 2 Photons >10 MeV 4 Heavy particles (protons, ions) 5 Neutrons 6 Neutron capture	Z None	Z None
0 Eye	3 Electrons	Z None	0 Intraoperative Z None

1ST - D Radiation Therapy
2ND - 8 Eye
3RD - 1 BRACHYTHERAPY

MODALITY: BRACHYTHERAPY

Example: Insertion of radioactive material

Treatment Site – 4TH	Modality Qualifier – 5TH	Isotope – 6TH	Qualifier – 7TH
0 Eye	9 High dose rate (HDR) B Low dose rate (LDR)	7 Cesium 137 (Cs-137) 8 Iridium 192 (Ir-192) 9 Iodine 125 (I-125) B Palladium 103 (Pd-103) C Californium 252 (Cf-252) Y Other isotope	Z None

© 2018 Channel Publishing, Ltd.

1ST - D Radiation Therapy
2ND - 8 Eye
3RD - 2 STEREOTACTIC RADIOSURGERY

MODALITY: STEREOTACTIC RADIOSURGERY

Example: Particulate stereotactic radiosurgery

Treatment Site – 4TH	Modality Qualifier – 5TH	Isotope – 6TH	Qualifier – 7TH
0 Eye	D Stereotactic other photon radiosurgery H Stereotactic particulate radiosurgery J Stereotactic gamma beam radiosurgery	Z None	Z None

1ST - D Radiation Therapy
2ND - 8 Eye
3RD - Y OTHER RADIATION

MODALITY: OTHER RADIATION

Example: Laser interstitial thermal therapy

Treatment Site – 4TH	Modality Qualifier – 5TH	Isotope – 6TH	Qualifier – 7TH
0 Eye	7 Contact radiation 8 Hyperthermia F Plaque radiation	Z None	Z None

1ST - D Radiation Therapy
2ND - 9 Ear, Nose, Mouth and Throat
3RD - 0 BEAM RADIATION

MODALITY: BEAM RADIATION

Example: External beam radiation

Treatment Site – 4TH	Modality Qualifier – 5TH	Isotope – 6TH	Qualifier – 7TH
0 Ear 1 Nose 3 Hypopharynx 4 Mouth 5 Tongue 6 Salivary Glands 7 Sinuses 8 Hard Palate 9 Soft Palate B Larynx D Nasopharynx F Oropharynx	0 Photons <1 MeV 1 Photons 1 - 10 MeV 2 Photons >10 MeV 4 Heavy particles (protons, ions) 5 Neutrons 6 Neutron capture	Z None	Z None
0 Ear 1 Nose 3 Hypopharynx 4 Mouth 5 Tongue 6 Salivary Glands 7 Sinuses 8 Hard Palate 9 Soft Palate B Larynx D Nasopharynx F Oropharynx	3 Electrons	Z None	0 Intra-operative Z None

1ST - D Radiation Therapy
2ND - 9 Ear, Nose, Mouth and Throat
3RD - 1 BRACHYTHERAPY

MODALITY: BRACHYTHERAPY

Example: Insertion of radioactive material

Treatment Site – 4TH	Modality Qualifier – 5TH	Isotope – 6TH	Qualifier – 7TH
0 Ear 1 Nose 3 Hypopharynx 4 Mouth 5 Tongue 6 Salivary Glands 7 Sinuses 8 Hard Palate 9 Soft Palate B Larynx D Nasopharynx F Oropharynx	9 High dose rate (HDR) B Low dose rate (LDR)	7 Cesium 137 (Cs-137) 8 Iridium 192 (Ir-192) 9 Iodine 125 (I-125) B Palladium 103 (Pd-103) C Californium 252 (Cf-252) Y Other isotope	Z None

1ST - D Radiation Therapy
2ND - 9 Ear, Nose, Mouth and Throat
3RD - 2 STEREOTACTIC RADIOSURGERY

MODALITY: STEREOTACTIC RADIOSURGERY

Example: Particulate stereotactic radiosurgery

Treatment Site – 4TH	Modality Qualifier – 5TH	Isotope – 6TH	Qualifier – 7TH
0 Ear 1 Nose 4 Mouth 5 Tongue 6 Salivary Glands 7 Sinuses 8 Hard Palate 9 Soft Palate B Larynx C Pharynx D Nasopharynx	D Stereotactic other photon radiosurgery H Stereotactic particulate radiosurgery J Stereotactic gamma beam radiosurgery	Z None	Z None

© 2018 Channel Publishing, Ltd.

1ST - D Radiation Therapy
2ND - 9 Ear, Nose, Mouth and Throat
3RD - Y OTHER RADIATION

MODALITY: OTHER RADIATION

Example: Laser interstitial thermal therapy

Treatment Site – 4TH	Modality Qualifier – 5TH	Isotope – 6TH	Qualifier – 7TH
0 Ear 1 Nose 5 Tongue 6 Salivary Glands 7 Sinuses 8 Hard Palate 9 Soft Palate	7 Contact radiation 8 Hyperthermia F Plaque radiation	Z None	Z None
3 Hypopharynx F Oropharynx	7 Contact radiation 8 Hyperthermia	Z None	Z None
4 Mouth B Larynx D Nasopharynx	7 Contact radiation 8 Hyperthermia C Intraoperative radiation therapy (IORT) F Plaque radiation	Z None	Z None
C Pharynx	C Intraoperative radiation therapy (IORT) F Plaque radiation	Z None	Z None

1ST - D Radiation Therapy
2ND - B Respiratory System
3RD - 0 BEAM RADIATION

MODALITY: BEAM RADIATION

Example: External beam radiation

Treatment Site – 4TH	Modality Qualifier – 5TH	Isotope – 6TH	Qualifier – 7TH
0 Trachea 1 Bronchus 2 Lung 5 Pleura 6 Mediastinum 7 Chest Wall 8 Diaphragm	0 Photons <1 MeV 1 Photons 1 - 10 MeV 2 Photons >10 MeV 4 Heavy particles (protons, ions) 5 Neutrons 6 Neutron capture	Z None	Z None
0 Trachea 1 Bronchus 2 Lung 5 Pleura 6 Mediastinum 7 Chest Wall 8 Diaphragm	3 Electrons	Z None	0 Intraoperative Z None

1ST - D Radiation Therapy
2ND - B Respiratory System
3RD - 1 BRACHYTHERAPY

MODALITY: BRACHYTHERAPY

Example: Insertion of radioactive material

Treatment Site – 4TH	Modality Qualifier – 5TH	Isotope – 6TH	Qualifier – 7TH
0 Trachea 1 Bronchus 2 Lung 5 Pleura 6 Mediastinum 7 Chest Wall 8 Diaphragm	9 High dose rate (HDR) B Low dose rate (LDR)	7 Cesium 137 (Cs-137) 8 Iridium 192 (Ir-192) 9 Iodine 125 (I-125) B Palladium 103 (Pd-103) C Californium 252 (Cf-252) Y Other isotope	Z None

1ST - D Radiation Therapy
2ND - B Respiratory System
3RD - 2 STEREOTACTIC RADIOSURGERY

MODALITY: STEREOTACTIC RADIOSURGERY

Example: Particulate stereotactic radiosurgery

Treatment Site – 4TH	Modality Qualifier – 5TH	Isotope – 6TH	Qualifier – 7TH
0 Trachea 1 Bronchus 2 Lung 5 Pleura 6 Mediastinum 7 Chest Wall 8 Diaphragm	D Stereotactic other photon radiosurgery H Stereotactic particulate radiosurgery J Stereotactic gamma beam radiosurgery	Z None	Z None

© 2018 Channel Publishing, Ltd.

1ST - D Radiation Therapy
2ND - B Respiratory System
3RD - Y OTHER RADIATION

MODALITY: OTHER RADIATION

Example: Laser interstitial thermal therapy

Treatment Site – 4TH	Modality Qualifier – 5TH	Isotope – 6TH	Qualifier – 7TH
0 Trachea 1 Bronchus 2 Lung 5 Pleura 6 Mediastinum 7 Chest Wall 8 Diaphragm	7 Contact radiation 8 Hyperthermia F Plaque radiation K Laser interstitial thermal therapy	Z None	Z None

1ST - D Radiation Therapy
2ND - D Gastrointestinal System
3RD - 0 BEAM RADIATION

MODALITY: BEAM RADIATION

Example: External beam radiation

Treatment Site – 4TH	Modality Qualifier – 5TH	Isotope – 6TH	Qualifier – 7TH
0 Esophagus 1 Stomach 2 Duodenum 3 Jejunum 4 Ileum 5 Colon 7 Rectum	0 Photons <1 MeV 1 Photons 1 - 10 MeV 2 Photons >10 MeV 4 Heavy particles (protons, ions) 5 Neutrons 6 Neutron capture	Z None	Z None
0 Esophagus 1 Stomach 2 Duodenum 3 Jejunum 4 Ileum 5 Colon 7 Rectum	3 Electrons	Z None	0 Intraoperative Z None

1ST - D Radiation Therapy
2ND - D Gastrointestinal System
3RD - 1 BRACHYTHERAPY

MODALITY: BRACHYTHERAPY

Example: Insertion of radioactive material

Treatment Site – 4TH	Modality Qualifier – 5TH	Isotope – 6TH	Qualifier – 7TH
0 Esophagus 1 Stomach 2 Duodenum 3 Jejunum 4 Ileum 5 Colon 7 Rectum	9 High dose rate (HDR) B Low dose rate (LDR)	7 Cesium 137 (Cs-137) 8 Iridium 192 (Ir-192) 9 Iodine 125 (I-125) B Palladium 103 (Pd-103) C Californium 252 (Cf-252) Y Other isotope	Z None

1ST - D Radiation Therapy
2ND - D Gastrointestinal System
3RD - 2 STEREOTACTIC RADIOSURGERY

MODALITY: STEREOTACTIC RADIOSURGERY

Example: Particulate stereotactic radiosurgery

Treatment Site – 4TH	Modality Qualifier – 5TH	Isotope – 6TH	Qualifier – 7TH
0 Esophagus 1 Stomach 2 Duodenum 3 Jejunum 4 Ileum 5 Colon 7 Rectum	D Stereotactic other photon radiosurgery H Stereotactic particulate radiosurgery J Stereotactic gamma beam radiosurgery	Z None	Z None

© 2018 Channel Publishing, Ltd.

1ST - D Radiation Therapy
2ND - D Gastrointestinal System
3RD - Y OTHER RADIATION

MODALITY: OTHER RADIATION

Example: Laser interstitial thermal therapy

Treatment Site – 4TH	Modality Qualifier – 5TH	Isotope – 6TH	Qualifier – 7TH
0 Esophagus	7 Contact radiation 8 Hyperthermia F Plaque radiation K Laser interstitial thermal therapy	Z None	Z None
1 Stomach 2 Duodenum 3 Jejunum 4 Ileum 5 Colon 7 Rectum	7 Contact radiation 8 Hyperthermia C Intraoperative radiation therapy (IORT) F Plaque radiation K Laser interstitial thermal therapy	Z None	Z None
8 Anus	C Intraoperative radiation therapy (IORT) F Plaque radiation K Laser interstitial thermal therapy	Z None	Z None

1ST - D Radiation Therapy
2ND - F Hepatobiliary System and Pancreas
3RD - 0 BEAM RADIATION

MODALITY: BEAM RADIATION

Example: External beam radiation

Treatment Site – 4TH	Modality Qualifier – 5TH	Isotope – 6TH	Qualifier – 7TH
0 Liver 1 Gallbladder 2 Bile Ducts 3 Pancreas	0 Photons <1 MeV 1 Photons 1 - 10 MeV 2 Photons >10 MeV 4 Heavy particles (protons, ions) 5 Neutrons 6 Neutron capture	Z None	Z None
0 Liver 1 Gallbladder 2 Bile Ducts 3 Pancreas	3 Electrons	Z None	0 Intraoperative Z None

1ST - D Radiation Therapy
2ND - F Hepatobiliary System and Pancreas
3RD - 1 BRACHYTHERAPY

MODALITY: BRACHYTHERAPY

Example: Insertion of radioactive material

Treatment Site – 4TH	Modality Qualifier – 5TH	Isotope – 6TH	Qualifier – 7TH
0 Liver 1 Gallbladder 2 Bile Ducts 3 Pancreas	9 High dose rate (HDR) B Low dose rate (LDR)	7 Cesium 137 (Cs-137) 8 Iridium 192 (Ir-192) 9 Iodine 125 (I-125) B Palladium 103 (Pd-103) C Californium 252 (Cf-252) Y Other isotope	Z None

1ST - D Radiation Therapy
2ND - F Hepatobiliary System and Pancreas
3RD - 2 STEREOTACTIC RADIOSURGERY

MODALITY: STEREOTACTIC RADIOSURGERY

Example: Particulate stereotactic radiosurgery

Treatment Site – 4TH	Modality Qualifier – 5TH	Isotope – 6TH	Qualifier – 7TH
0 Liver 1 Gallbladder 2 Bile Ducts 3 Pancreas	D Stereotactic other photon radiosurgery H Stereotactic particulate radiosurgery J Stereotactic gamma beam radiosurgery	Z None	Z None

1ST - D Radiation Therapy
2ND - F Hepatobiliary System and Pancreas
3RD - Y OTHER RADIATION

MODALITY: OTHER RADIATION

Example: Laser interstitial thermal therapy

Treatment Site – 4TH	Modality Qualifier – 5TH	Isotope – 6TH	Qualifier – 7TH
0 Liver 1 Gallbladder 2 Bile Ducts 3 Pancreas	7 Contact radiation 8 Hyperthermia C Intraoperative radiation therapy (IORT) F Plaque radiation K Laser interstitial thermal therapy	Z None	Z None

© 2018 Channel Publishing, Ltd.

1ST - D Radiation Therapy
2ND - G Endocrine System
3RD - 0 BEAM RADIATION

MODALITY: BEAM RADIATION

Example: External beam radiation

Treatment Site – 4TH	Modality Qualifier – 5TH	Isotope – 6TH	Qualifier – 7TH
0 Pituitary Gland 1 Pineal Body 2 Adrenal Glands 4 Parathyroid Glands 5 Thyroid	0 Photons <1 MeV 1 Photons 1 - 10 MeV 2 Photons >10 MeV 5 Neutrons 6 Neutron capture	Z None	Z None
0 Pituitary Gland 1 Pineal Body 2 Adrenal Glands 4 Parathyroid Glands 5 Thyroid	3 Electrons	Z None	0 Intraoperative Z None

1ST - D Radiation Therapy
2ND - G Endocrine System
3RD - 1 BRACHYTHERAPY

MODALITY: BRACHYTHERAPY

Example: Insertion of radioactive material

Treatment Site – 4TH	Modality Qualifier – 5TH	Isotope – 6TH	Qualifier – 7TH
0 Pituitary Gland 1 Pineal Body 2 Adrenal Glands 4 Parathyroid Glands 5 Thyroid	9 High dose rate (HDR) B Low dose rate (LDR)	7 Cesium 137 (Cs-137) 8 Iridium 192 (Ir-192) 9 Iodine 125 (I-125) B Palladium 103 (Pd-103) C Californium 252 (Cf-252) Y Other isotope	Z None

1ST - D Radiation Therapy
2ND - G Endocrine System
3RD - 2 STEREOTACTIC RADIOSURGERY

MODALITY: STEREOTACTIC RADIOSURGERY

Example: Particulate stereotactic radiosurgery

Treatment Site – 4TH	Modality Qualifier – 5TH	Isotope – 6TH	Qualifier – 7TH
0 Pituitary Gland 1 Pineal Body 2 Adrenal Glands 4 Parathyroid Glands 5 Thyroid	D Stereotactic other photon radiosurgery H Stereotactic particulate radiosurgery J Stereotactic gamma beam radiosurgery	Z None	Z None

1ST - D Radiation Therapy
2ND - G Endocrine System
3RD - Y OTHER RADIATION

MODALITY: OTHER RADIATION

Example: Laser interstitial thermal therapy

Treatment Site – 4TH	Modality Qualifier – 5TH	Isotope – 6TH	Qualifier – 7TH
0 Pituitary Gland 1 Pineal Body 2 Adrenal Glands 4 Parathyroid Glands 5 Thyroid	7 Contact radiation 8 Hyperthermia F Plaque radiation K Laser interstitial thermal therapy	Z None	Z None

1ST - D Radiation Therapy
2ND - H Skin
3RD - 0 BEAM RADIATION

MODALITY: BEAM RADIATION

Example: External beam radiation

Treatment Site – 4TH	Modality Qualifier – 5TH	Isotope – 6TH	Qualifier – 7TH
2 Skin, Face 3 Skin, Neck 4 Skin, Arm 6 Skin, Chest 7 Skin, Back 8 Skin, Abdomen 9 Skin, Buttock B Skin, Leg	0 Photons <1 MeV 1 Photons 1 - 10 MeV 2 Photons >10 MeV 4 Heavy particles (protons, ions) 5 Neutrons 6 Neutron capture	Z None	Z None
2 Skin, Face 3 Skin, Neck 4 Skin, Arm 6 Skin, Chest 7 Skin, Back 8 Skin, Abdomen 9 Skin, Buttock B Skin, Leg	3 Electrons	Z None	0 Intraoperative Z None

RADIATION THERAPY D G 0

© 2018 Channel Publishing, Ltd.

1ST - D Radiation Therapy
2ND - H Skin
3RD - Y OTHER RADIATION

MODALITY: OTHER RADIATION

Example: Laser interstitial thermal therapy

Treatment Site – 4TH	Modality Qualifier – 5TH	Isotope – 6TH	Qualifier – 7TH
2 Skin, Face 3 Skin, Neck 4 Skin, Arm 6 Skin, Chest 7 Skin, Back 8 Skin, Abdomen 9 Skin, Buttock B Skin, Leg	7 Contact radiation 8 Hyperthermia F Plaque radiation	Z None	Z None
5 Skin, Hand C Skin, Foot	F Plaque radiation	Z None	Z None

1ST - D Radiation Therapy
2ND - M Breast
3RD - 0 BEAM RADIATION

MODALITY: BEAM RADIATION

Example: External beam radiation

Treatment Site – 4TH	Modality Qualifier – 5TH	Isotope – 6TH	Qualifier – 7TH
0 Breast, Left 1 Breast, Right	0 Photons <1 MeV 1 Photons 1 - 10 MeV 2 Photons >10 MeV 4 Heavy particles (protons, ions) 5 Neutrons 6 Neutron capture	Z None	Z None
0 Breast, Left 1 Breast, Right	3 Electrons	Z None	0 Intraoperative Z None

1ST - D Radiation Therapy
2ND - M Breast
3RD - 1 BRACHYTHERAPY

MODALITY: BRACHYTHERAPY

Example: Insertion of radioactive material

Treatment Site – 4TH	Modality Qualifier – 5TH	Isotope – 6TH	Qualifier – 7TH
0 Breast, Left 1 Breast, Right	9 High dose rate (HDR) B Low dose rate (LDR)	7 Cesium 137 (Cs-137) 8 Iridium 192 (Ir-192) 9 Iodine 125 (I-125) B Palladium 103 (Pd-103) C Californium 252 (Cf-252) Y Other isotope	Z None

1ST - D Radiation Therapy
2ND - M Breast
3RD - 2 STEREOTACTIC RADIOSURGERY

MODALITY: STEREOTACTIC RADIOSURGERY

Example: Particulate stereotactic radiosurgery

Treatment Site – 4TH	Modality Qualifier – 5TH	Isotope – 6TH	Qualifier – 7TH
0 Breast, Left 1 Breast, Right	D Stereotactic other photon radiosurgery H Stereotactic particulate radiosurgery J Stereotactic gamma beam radiosurgery	Z None	Z None

1ST - D Radiation Therapy
2ND - M Breast
3RD - Y OTHER RADIATION

MODALITY: OTHER RADIATION

Example: Laser interstitial thermal therapy

Treatment Site – 4TH	Modality Qualifier – 5TH	Isotope – 6TH	Qualifier – 7TH
0 Breast, Left 1 Breast, Right	7 Contact radiation 8 Hyperthermia F Plaque radiation K Laser interstitial thermal therapy	Z None	Z None

© 2018 Channel Publishing, Ltd.

1ST - D Radiation Therapy
2ND - P Musculoskeletal System
3RD - 0 BEAM RADIATION

MODALITY: BEAM RADIATION

Example: External beam radiation

Treatment Site – 4TH	Modality Qualifier – 5TH	Isotope – 6TH	Qualifier – 7TH
0 Skull 2 Maxilla 3 Mandible 4 Sternum 5 Rib(s) 6 Humerus 7 Radius/Ulna 8 Pelvic Bones 9 Femur B Tibia/Fibula C Other Bone	0 Photons <1 MeV 1 Photons 1 - 10 MeV 2 Photons >10 MeV 4 Heavy particles (protons, ions) 5 Neutrons 6 Neutron capture	Z None	Z None
0 Skull 2 Maxilla 3 Mandible 4 Sternum 5 Rib(s) 6 Humerus 7 Radius/Ulna 8 Pelvic Bones 9 Femur B Tibia/Fibula C Other Bone	3 Electrons	Z None	0 Intra-operative Z None

1ST - D Radiation Therapy
2ND - P Musculoskeletal System
3RD - Y OTHER RADIATION

MODALITY: OTHER RADIATION

Example: Laser interstitial thermal therapy

Treatment Site – 4TH	Modality Qualifier – 5TH	Isotope – 6TH	Qualifier – 7TH
0 Skull 2 Maxilla 3 Mandible 4 Sternum 5 Rib(s) 6 Humerus 7 Radius/Ulna 8 Pelvic Bones 9 Femur B Tibia/Fibula C Other Bone	7 Contact radiation 8 Hyperthermia F Plaque radiation	Z None	Z None

1ST - D Radiation Therapy
2ND - T Urinary System
3RD - 0 BEAM RADIATION

MODALITY: BEAM RADIATION

Example: External beam radiation

Treatment Site – 4TH	Modality Qualifier – 5TH	Isotope – 6TH	Qualifier – 7TH
0 Kidney 1 Ureter 2 Bladder 3 Urethra	0 Photons <1 MeV 1 Photons 1 - 10 MeV 2 Photons >10 MeV 4 Heavy particles (protons, ions) 5 Neutrons 6 Neutron capture	Z None	Z None
0 Kidney 1 Ureter 2 Bladder 3 Urethra	3 Electrons	Z None	0 Intraoperative Z None

1ST - D Radiation Therapy
2ND - T Urinary System
3RD - 1 BRACHYTHERAPY

MODALITY: BRACHYTHERAPY

Example: Insertion of radioactive material

Treatment Site – 4TH	Modality Qualifier – 5TH	Isotope – 6TH	Qualifier – 7TH
0 Kidney 1 Ureter 2 Bladder 3 Urethra	9 High dose rate (HDR) B Low dose rate (LDR)	7 Cesium 137 (Cs-137) 8 Iridium 192 (Ir-192) 9 Iodine 125 (I-125) B Palladium 103 (Pd-103) C Californium 252 (Cf-252) Y Other isotope	Z None

© 2018 Channel Publishing, Ltd.

1ST - D Radiation Therapy
2ND - T Urinary System
3RD - 2 STEREOTACTIC RADIOSURGERY

MODALITY: STEREOTACTIC RADIOSURGERY

Example: Particulate stereotactic radiosurgery

Treatment Site – 4TH	Modality Qualifier – 5TH	Isotope – 6TH	Qualifier – 7TH
0 Kidney 1 Ureter 2 Bladder 3 Urethra	D Stereotactic other photon radiosurgery H Stereotactic particulate radiosurgery J Stereotactic gamma beam radiosurgery	Z None	Z None

1ST - D Radiation Therapy
2ND - T Urinary System
3RD - Y OTHER RADIATION

MODALITY: OTHER RADIATION

Example: Laser interstitial thermal therapy

Treatment Site – 4TH	Modality Qualifier – 5TH	Isotope – 6TH	Qualifier – 7TH
0 Kidney 1 Ureter 2 Bladder 3 Urethra	7 Contact radiation 8 Hyperthermia C Intraoperative radiation therapy (IORT) F Plaque radiation	Z None	Z None

1ST - D Radiation Therapy
2ND - U Female Reproductive System ♀
3RD - 0 BEAM RADIATION

MODALITY: BEAM RADIATION

Example: External beam radiation

Treatment Site – 4TH	Modality Qualifier – 5TH	Isotope – 6TH	Qualifier – 7TH
0 Ovary 1 Cervix 2 Uterus	0 Photons <1 MeV 1 Photons 1 - 10 MeV 2 Photons >10 MeV 4 Heavy particles (protons, ions) 5 Neutrons 6 Neutron capture	Z None	Z None
0 Ovary 1 Cervix 2 Uterus	3 Electrons	Z None	0 Intraoperative Z None

1ST - D Radiation Therapy
2ND - U Female Reproductive System ♀
3RD - 1 BRACHYTHERAPY

MODALITY: BRACHYTHERAPY

Example: Insertion of radioactive material

Treatment Site – 4TH	Modality Qualifier – 5TH	Isotope – 6TH	Qualifier – 7TH
0 Ovary 1 Cervix 2 Uterus	9 High dose rate (HDR) B Low dose rate (LDR)	7 Cesium 137 (Cs-137) 8 Iridium 192 (Ir-192) 9 Iodine 125 (I-125) B Palladium 103 (Pd-103) C Californium 252 (Cf-252) Y Other isotope	Z None

1ST - D Radiation Therapy
2ND - U Female Reproductive System ♀
3RD - 2 STEREOTACTIC RADIOSURGERY

MODALITY: STEREOTACTIC RADIOSURGERY

Example: Particulate stereotactic radiosurgery

Treatment Site – 4TH	Modality Qualifier – 5TH	Isotope – 6TH	Qualifier – 7TH
0 Ovary 1 Cervix 2 Uterus	D Stereotactic other photon radiosurgery H Stereotactic particulate radiosurgery J Stereotactic gamma beam radiosurgery	Z None	Z None

© 2018 Channel Publishing, Ltd.

1ST - D Radiation Therapy
2ND - U Female Reproductive System ♀
3RD - Y OTHER RADIATION

MODALITY: OTHER RADIATION

Example: Laser interstitial thermal therapy

Treatment Site – 4TH	Modality Qualifier – 5TH	Isotope – 6TH	Qualifier – 7TH
0 Ovary 1 Cervix 2 Uterus	7 Contact radiation 8 Hyperthermia C Intraoperative radiation therapy (IORT) F Plaque radiation	Z None	Z None

1ST - D Radiation Therapy
2ND - V Male Reproductive System ♂
3RD - 0 BEAM RADIATION

MODALITY: BEAM RADIATION

Example: External beam radiation

Treatment Site – 4TH	Modality Qualifier – 5TH	Isotope – 6TH	Qualifier – 7TH
0 Prostate 1 Testis	0 Photons <1 MeV 1 Photons 1 - 10 MeV 2 Photons >10 MeV 4 Heavy particles (protons, ions) 5 Neutrons 6 Neutron capture	Z None	Z None
0 Prostate 1 Testis	3 Electrons	Z None	0 Intraoperative Z None

1ST - D Radiation Therapy
2ND - V Male Reproductive System ♂
3RD - 1 BRACHYTHERAPY

MODALITY: BRACHYTHERAPY

Example: Insertion of radioactive material

Treatment Site – 4TH	Modality Qualifier – 5TH	Isotope – 6TH	Qualifier – 7TH
0 Prostate 1 Testis	9 High dose rate (HDR) B Low dose rate (LDR)	7 Cesium 137 (Cs-137) 8 Iridium 192 (Ir-192) 9 Iodine 125 (I-125) B Palladium 103 (Pd-103) C Californium 252 (Cf-252) Y Other isotope	Z None

1ST - D Radiation Therapy
2ND - V Male Reproductive System ♂
3RD - 2 STEREOTACTIC RADIOSURGERY

MODALITY: STEREOTACTIC RADIOSURGERY

Example: Particulate stereotactic radiosurgery

Treatment Site – 4TH	Modality Qualifier – 5TH	Isotope – 6TH	Qualifier – 7TH
0 Prostate 1 Testis	D Stereotactic other photon radiosurgery H Stereotactic particulate radiosurgery J Stereotactic gamma beam radiosurgery	Z None	Z None

© 2018 Channel Publishing, Ltd.

1ST - D Radiation Therapy
2ND - V Male Reproductive System ♂
3RD - Y OTHER RADIATION

MODALITY: OTHER RADIATION

Example: Laser interstitial thermal therapy

Treatment Site – 4TH	Modality Qualifier – 5TH	Isotope – 6TH	Qualifier – 7TH
0 Prostate	7 Contact radiation 8 Hyperthermia C Intraoperative radiation therapy (IORT) F Plaque radiation K Laser interstitial thermal therapy	Z None	Z None
1 Testis	7 Contact radiation 8 Hyperthermia F Plaque radiation	Z None	Z None

1ST - D Radiation Therapy
2ND - W Anatomical Regions
3RD - 0 BEAM RADIATION

MODALITY: BEAM RADIATION

Example: External beam radiation

Treatment Site – 4TH	Modality Qualifier – 5TH	Isotope – 6TH	Qualifier – 7TH
1 Head and Neck 2 Chest 3 Abdomen 4 Hemibody 5 Whole Body 6 Pelvic Region	0 Photons <1 MeV 1 Photons 1 - 10 MeV 2 Photons >10 MeV 4 Heavy particles (protons, ions) 5 Neutrons 6 Neutron capture	Z None	Z None
1 Head and Neck 2 Chest 3 Abdomen 4 Hemibody 5 Whole Body 6 Pelvic Region	3 Electrons	Z None	0 Intra-operative Z None

1ST - D Radiation Therapy
2ND - W Anatomical Regions
3RD - 1 BRACHYTHERAPY

MODALITY: BRACHYTHERAPY

Example: Insertion of radioactive material

Treatment Site – 4TH	Modality Qualifier – 5TH	Isotope – 6TH	Qualifier – 7TH
1 Head and Neck 2 Chest 3 Abdomen 6 Pelvic Region	9 High dose rate (HDR) B Low dose rate (LDR)	7 Cesium 137 (Cs-137) 8 Iridium 192 (Ir-192) 9 Iodine 125 (I-125) B Palladium 103 (Pd-103) C Californium 252 (Cf-252) Y Other isotope	Z None

1ST - D Radiation Therapy
2ND - W Anatomical Regions
3RD - 2 STEREOTACTIC RADIOSURGERY

MODALITY: STEREOTACTIC RADIOSURGERY

Example: Particulate stereotactic radiosurgery

Treatment Site – 4TH	Modality Qualifier – 5TH	Isotope – 6TH	Qualifier – 7TH
1 Head and Neck 2 Chest 3 Abdomen 6 Pelvic Region	D Stereotactic other photon radiosurgery H Stereotactic particulate radiosurgery J Stereotactic gamma beam radiosurgery	Z None	Z None

© 2018 Channel Publishing, Ltd.

1ST - D Radiation Therapy
2ND - W Anatomical Regions
3RD - Y OTHER RADIATION

MODALITY: OTHER RADIATION

Example: Laser interstitial thermal therapy

Treatment Site – 4TH	Modality Qualifier – 5TH	Isotope – 6TH	Qualifier – 7TH
1 Head and Neck 2 Chest 3 Abdomen 4 Hemibody 6 Pelvic Region	7 Contact radiation 8 Hyperthermia F Plaque radiation	Z None	Z None
5 Whole Body	7 Contact radiation 8 Hyperthermia F Plaque radiation	Z None	Z None
5 Whole Body	G Isotope administration	D Iodine 131 (I-131) F Phosphorus 32 (P-32) G Strontium 89 (Sr-89) H Strontium 90 (Sr-90) Y Other isotope	Z None

© 2018 Channel Publishing, Ltd.

Educational Annotations | Section F – Physical Rehabilitation and Diagnostic Audiology

Section Specific Educational Annotations for the Physical Rehabilitation and Diagnostic Audiology Section include:

- AHA Coding Clinic® Reference Notations
- Coding Notes

AHA Coding Clinic® Reference Notations of Physical Rehabilitation and Diagnostic Audiology

ROOT TYPE SPECIFIC - PHYSICAL REHABILITATION AND DIAGNOSTIC AUDIOLOGY - Section F

SPEECH ASSESSMENT - 0
MOTOR AND/OR NERVE FUNCTION ASSESSMENT - 1
ACTIVITIES OF DAILY LIVING ASSESSMENT - 2
HEARING ASSESSMENT - 3
HEARING AID ASSESSMENT - 4
VESTIBULAR ASSESSMENT - 5
SPEECH TREATMENT - 6
MOTOR TREATMENT - 7
ACTIVITIES OF DAILY LIVING TREATMENT - 8
HEARING TREATMENT - 9
COCHLEAR IMPLANT TREATMENT - B
VESTIBULAR TREATMENT - C
DEVICE FITTING - D
CAREGIVER TRAINING - F

Coding Notes of Physical Rehabilitation and Diagnostic Audiology

© 2018 Channel Publishing, Ltd.

1ST - F Physical Rehabilitation and Diagnostic Audiology
2ND - 0 Rehabilitation
3RD - 0 SPEECH ASSESSMENT

SPEECH ASSESSMENT: Measurement of speech and related functions.

Body System/ Region – 4TH	Type Qualifier – 5TH	Equipment – 6TH	Qualifier – 7TH
3 Neurological System - Whole Body	G Communicative/cognitive integration skills	K Audiovisual M Augmentative/ alternative communication P Computer Y Other equipment Z None	Z None
Z None	0 Filtered speech 3 Staggered spondaic word Q Performance intensity phonetically balanced speech discrimination R Brief tone stimuli S Distorted speech T Dichotic stimuli V Temporal ordering of stimuli W Masking patterns	1 Audiometer 2 Sound field/booth K Audiovisual Z None	Z None
Z None	1 Speech threshold 2 Speech/word recognition	1 Audiometer 2 Sound field/booth 9 Cochlear implant K Audiovisual Z None	Z None
Z None	4 Sensorineural acuity level	1 Audiometer 2 Sound field/booth Z None	Z None
Z None	5 Synthetic sentence identification	1 Audiometer 2 Sound field/booth 9 Cochlear implant K Audiovisual	Z None
Z None	6 Speech and/or language screening 7 Nonspoken language 8 Receptive/expressive language C Aphasia G Communicative/cognitive integration skills L Augmentative/alternative communication system	K Audiovisual M Augmentative/ alternative communication P Computer Y Other equipment Z None	Z None
Z None	9 Articulation/phonology	K Audiovisual P Computer Q Speech analysis Y Other equipment Z None	Z None
Z None	B Motor speech	K Audiovisual N Biosensory feedback P Computer Q Speech analysis T Aerodynamic function Y Other equipment Z None	Z None
Z None	D Fluency	K Audiovisual N Biosensory feedback P Computer Q Speech analysis S Voice analysis T Aerodynamic function Y Other equipment Z None	Z None
Z None	F Voice	K Audiovisual N Biosensory feedback P Computer S Voice analysis T Aerodynamic function Y Other equipment Z None	Z None
Z None	H Bedside swallowing and oral function P Oral peripheral mechanism	Y Other equipment Z None	Z None
Z None	J Instrumental swallowing and oral function	T Aerodynamic function W Swallowing Y Other equipment	Z None
Z None	K Orofacial myofunctional	K Audiovisual P Computer Y Other equipment Z None	Z None
Z None	M Voice prosthetic	K Audiovisual P Computer S Voice analysis V Speech prosthesis Y Other equipment Z None	Z None
Z None	N Non-invasive instrumental status	N Biosensory feedback P Computer Q Speech analysis S Voice analysis T Aerodynamic function Y Other equipment	Z None
Z None	X Other specified central auditory processing	Z None	Z None

© 2018 Channel Publishing, Ltd.

1ST - F Physical Rehabilitation and Diagnostic Audiology
2ND - 0 Rehabilitation
3RD - 1 MOTOR AND/OR NERVE FUNCTION ASSESSMENT

MOTOR AND/OR NERVE FUNCTION ASSESSMENT: Measurement of motor, nerve, and related functions.

Body System/Region – 4TH	Type Qualifier – 5TH	Equipment – 6TH	Qualifier – 7TH
0 Neurological System - Head and Neck 1 Neurological System - Upper Back/Upper Extremity 2 Neurological System - Lower Back/Lower Extremity 3 Neurological System - Whole Body	0 Muscle performance	E Orthosis F Assistive, adaptive, supportive or protective U Prosthesis Y Other equipment Z None	Z None
0 Neurological System - Head and Neck 1 Neurological System - Upper Back/Upper Extremity 2 Neurological System - Lower Back/Lower Extremity 3 Neurological System - Whole Body	1 Integumentary integrity 3 Coordination/dexterity 4 Motor function G Reflex integrity	Z None	Z None
0 Neurological System - Head and Neck 1 Neurological System - Upper Back/Upper Extremity 2 Neurological System - Lower Back/Lower Extremity 3 Neurological System - Whole Body	5 Range of motion and joint integrity 6 Sensory awareness/processing/ integrity	Y Other equipment Z None	Z None
D Integumentary System - Head and Neck F Integumentary System - Upper Back/Upper Extremity G Integumentary System- Lower Back/Lower Extremity H Integumentary System - Whole Body J Musculoskeletal System - Head and Neck K Musculoskeletal System - Upper Back/Upper Extremity L Musculoskeletal System Lower Back/Lower Extremity M Musculoskeletal System - Whole Body	0 Muscle performance	E Orthosis F Assistive, adaptive, supportive or protective U Prosthesis Y Other equipment Z None	Z None
D Integumentary System - Head and Neck F Integumentary System - Upper Back/Upper Extremity G Integumentary System - Lower Back/Lower Extremity H Integumentary System - Whole Body J Musculoskeletal System - Head and Neck K Musculoskeletal System - Upper Back/Upper Extremity L Musculoskeletal System - Lower Back/Lower Extremity M Musculoskeletal System - Whole Body	1 Integumentary integrity	Z None	Z None
D Integumentary System - Head and Neck F Integumentary System - Upper Back/Upper Extremity G Integumentary System - Lower Back/Lower Extremity H Integumentary System - Whole Body J Musculoskeletal System - Head and Neck K Musculoskeletal System - Upper Back/Upper Extremity L Musculoskeletal System - Lower Back/Lower Extremity M Musculoskeletal System - Whole Body	5 Range of motion and joint integrity 6 Sensory awareness/processing/ integrity	Y Other equipment Z None	Z None
N Genitourinary System	0 Muscle performance	E Orthosis F Assistive, adaptive, supportive or protective U Prosthesis Y Other equipment Z None	Z None
Z None	2 Visual motor integration	K Audiovisual M Augmentative/alternative communication N Biosensory feedback P Computer Q Speech analysis S Voice analysis Y Other equipment Z None	Z None

continued ⇨

© 2018 Channel Publishing, Ltd.

F 0 1 MOTOR AND/OR NERVE FUNCTION ASSESSMENT –*continued*

Body System/Region – 4TH	Type Qualifier – 5TH	Equipment – 6TH	Qualifier – 7TH
Z None	7 Facial nerve function	7 Electrophysiologic	Z None
Z None	9 Somatosensory evoked potentials	J Somatosensory	Z None
Z None	B Bed Mobility C Transfer F Wheelchair mobility	E Orthosis F Assistive, adaptive, supportive or protective U Prosthesis Z None	Z None
Z None	D Gait and/or balance	E Orthosis F Assistive, adaptive, supportive or protective U Prosthesis Y Other equipment Z None	Z None

1ST - F Physical Rehabilitation and Diagnostic Audiology
2ND - 0 Rehabilitation
3RD - 2 ACTIVITIES OF DAILY LIVING ASSESSMENT

ACTIVITIES OF DAILY LIVING ASSESSMENT: Measurement of functional level for activities of daily living.

Body System/Region – 4TH	Type Qualifier – 5TH	Equipment – 6TH	Qualifier – 7TH
0 Neurological System - Head and Neck	9 Cranial nerve integrity D Neuromotor development	Y Other equipment Z None	Z None
1 Neurological System - Upper Back/Upper Extremity 2 Neurological System - Lower Back/Lower Extremity 3 Neurological System - Whole Body	D Neuromotor development	Y Other equipment Z None	Z None
4 Circulatory System - Head and Neck 5 Circulatory System - Upper Back/Upper Extremity 6 Circulatory System - Lower Back/Lower Extremity 8 Respiratory System - Head and Neck 9 Respiratory System - Upper Back/Upper Extremity B Respiratory System - Lower Back/Lower Extremity	G Ventilation, respiration and circulation	C Mechanical G Aerobic endurance and conditioning Y Other equipment Z None	Z None
7 Circulatory System - Whole Body C Respiratory System - Whole Body	7 Aerobic capacity and endurance	E Orthosis G Aerobic endurance and conditioning U Prosthesis Y Other equipment Z None	Z None
7 Circulatory System - Whole Body C Respiratory System - Whole Body	G Ventilation, respiration and circulation	C Mechanical G Aerobic endurance and conditioning Y Other equipment Z None	Z None
Z None	0 Bathing/showering 1 Dressing 3 Grooming/personal hygiene 4 Home management	E Orthosis F Assistive, adaptive, supportive or protective U Prosthesis Z None	Z None
Z None	2 Feeding/eating 8 Anthropometric characteristics F Pain	Y Other equipment Z None	Z None

continued ⇨

© 2018 Channel Publishing, Ltd.

F 0 2 ACTIVITIES OF DAILY LIVING ASSESSMENT –*continued*

Body System/ Region – 4TH	Type Qualifier – 5TH	Equipment – 6TH	Qualifier – 7TH
Z None	5 Perceptual processing	K Audiovisual M Augmentative/alternative communication N Biosensory feedback P Computer Q Speech analysis S Voice analysis Y Other equipment Z None	Z None
Z None	6 Psychosocial skills	Z None	Z None
Z None	B Environmental, home and work barriers C Ergonomics and body mechanics	E Orthosis F Assistive, adaptive, supportive or protective U Prosthesis Y Other equipment Z None	Z None
Z None	H Vocational activities and functional community or work reintegration skills	E Orthosis F Assistive, adaptive, supportive or protective G Aerobic endurance and conditioning U Prosthesis Y Other equipment Z None	Z None

1ST - F Physical Rehabilitation and Diagnostic Audiology
2ND - 0 Rehabilitation
3RD - 6 SPEECH TREATMENT

SPEECH TREATMENT: Application of techniques to improve, augment, or compensate for speech and related functional impairment.

Body System/ Region – 4TH	Type Qualifier – 5TH	Equipment – 6TH	Qualifier – 7TH
3 Neurological System - Whole Body	6 Communicative/cognitive integration skills	K Audiovisual M Augmentative/alternative communication P Computer Y Other equipment Z None	Z None
Z None	0 Nonspoken language 3 Aphasia 6 Communicative/cognitive integration skills	K Audiovisual M Augmentative/alternative communication P Computer Y Other equipment Z None	Z None
Z None	1 Speech-language pathology and related disorders counseling 2 Speech-language pathology and related disorders prevention	K Audiovisual Z None	Z None
Z None	4 Articulation/phonology	K Audiovisual P Computer Q Speech analysis T Aerodynamic function Y Other equipment Z None	Z None
Z None	5 Aural rehabilitation	K Audiovisual L Assistive listening M Augmentative/alternative communication N Biosensory feedback P Computer Q Speech analysis S Voice analysis Y Other equipment Z None	Z None
Z None	7 Fluency	4 Electroacoustic immitance/acoustic reflex K Audiovisual N Biosensory feedback Q Speech analysis S Voice analysis T Aerodynamic function Y Other equipment Z None	Z None
Z None	8 Motor speech	K Audiovisual N Biosensory feedback P Computer Q Speech analysis S Voice analysis T Aerodynamic function Y Other equipment Z None	Z None
Z None	9 Orofacial myofunctional	K Audiovisual P Computer Y Other equipment Z None	Z None

continued ⇨

© 2018 Channel Publishing, Ltd.

F 0 6 SPEECH TREATMENT —*continued*

Body System/ Region – 4TH	Type Qualifier – 5TH	Equipment – 6TH	Qualifier – 7TH
Z None	B Receptive/expressive language	K Audiovisual L Assistive listening M Augmentative/alternative communication P Computer Y Other equipment Z None	Z None
Z None	C Voice	K Audiovisual N Biosensory feedback P Computer S Voice analysis T Aerodynamic function V Speech prosthesis Y Other equipment Z None	Z None
Z None	D Swallowing dysfunction	M Augmentative/alternative communication T Aerodynamic function V Speech prosthesis Y Other equipment Z None	Z None

1ST - F Physical Rehabilitation and Diagnostic Audiology
2ND - 0 Rehabilitation
3RD - 7 MOTOR TREATMENT

<u>MOTOR TREATMENT</u>: Exercise or activities to increase or facilitate motor function.

Body System/Region – 4TH	Type Qualifier – 5TH	Equipment – 6TH	Qualifier – 7TH
0 Neurological System - Head and Neck 1 Neurological System - Upper Back/Upper Extremity 2 Neurological System - Lower Back/Lower Extremity 3 Neurological System - Whole Body D Integumentary System - Head and Neck F Integumentary System - Upper Back/Upper Extremity G Integumentary System - Lower Back/Lower Extremity H Integumentary System - Whole Body J Musculoskeletal System - Head and Neck K Musculoskeletal System - Upper Back/Upper Extremity L Musculoskeletal System - Lower Back/Lower Extremity M Musculoskeletal System - Whole Body	0 Range of motion and joint mobility 1 Muscle performance 2 Coordination/dexterity 3 Motor function	E Orthosis F Assistive, adaptive, supportive or protective U Prosthesis Y Other equipment Z None	Z None
0 Neurological System - Head and Neck 1 Neurological System - Upper Back/Upper Extremity 2 Neurological System - Lower Back/Lower Extremity 3 Neurological System - Whole Body D Integumentary System - Head and Neck F Integumentary System - Upper Back/Upper Extremity G Integumentary System - Lower Back/Lower Extremity H Integumentary System - Whole Body J Musculoskeletal System - Head and Neck K Musculoskeletal System - Upper Back/Upper Extremity L Musculoskeletal System - Lower Back/Lower Extremity M Musculoskeletal System - Whole Body	6 Therapeutic exercise	B Physical Agents C Mechanical D Electrotherapeutic E Orthosis F Assistive, adaptive, supportive or protective G Aerobic endurance and conditioning H Mechanical or electromechanical U Prosthesis Y Other equipment Z None	Z None
0 Neurological System - Head and Neck 1 Neurological System - Upper Back/Upper Extremity 2 Neurological System - Lower Back/Lower Extremity 3 Neurological System - Whole Body D Integumentary System - Head and Neck F Integumentary System - Upper Back/Upper Extremity G Integumentary System - Lower Back/Lower Extremity H Integumentary System - Whole Body J Musculoskeletal System - Head and Neck K Musculoskeletal System - Upper Back/Upper Extremity L Musculoskeletal System - Lower Back/Lower Extremity M Musculoskeletal System - Whole Body	7 Manual therapy techniques	Z None	Z None

continued ⇨

© 2018 Channel Publishing, Ltd.

F 0 7 MOTOR TREATMENT – *continued*

Body System/Region – 4TH	Type Qualifier – 5TH	Equipment – 6TH	Qualifier – 7TH
4 Circulatory System - Head and Neck 5 Circulatory System - Upper Back/Upper Extremity 6 Circulatory System - Lower Back/Lower Extremity 7 Circulatory System - Whole Body 8 Respiratory System - Head and Neck 9 Respiratory System - Upper Back/Upper Extremity B Respiratory System - Lower Back/Lower Extremity C Respiratory System - Whole Body	6 Therapeutic exercise	B Physical Agents C Mechanical D Electrotherapeutic E Orthosis F Assistive, adaptive, supportive or protective G Aerobic endurance and conditioning H Mechanical or electromechanical U Prosthesis Y Other equipment Z None	Z None
N Genitourinary System	1 Muscle performance	E Orthosis F Assistive, adaptive, supportive or protective U Prosthesis Y Other equipment Z None	Z None
N Genitourinary System	6 Therapeutic exercise	B Physical Agents C Mechanical D Electrotherapeutic E Orthosis F Assistive, adaptive, supportive or protective G Aerobic endurance and conditioning H Mechanical or electromechanical U Prosthesis Y Other equipment Z None	Z None
Z None	4 Wheelchair mobility	D Electrotherapeutic E Orthosis F Assistive, adaptive, supportive or protective U Prosthesis Y Other equipment Z None	Z None
Z None	5 Bed mobility	C Mechanical E Orthosis F Assistive, adaptive, supportive or protective U Prosthesis Y Other equipment Z None	Z None
Z None	8 Transfer training	C Mechanical D Electrotherapeutic E Orthosis F Assistive, adaptive, supportive or protective U Prosthesis Y Other equipment Z None	Z None
Z None	9 Gait training/ functional ambulation	C Mechanical D Electrotherapeutic E Orthosis F Assistive, adaptive, supportive or protective G Aerobic endurance and conditioning U Prosthesis Y Other equipment Z None	Z None

1ST - F Physical Rehabilitation and Diagnostic Audiology
2ND - 0 Rehabilitation
3RD - 8 ACTIVITIES OF DAILY LIVING TREATMENT

ACTIVITIES OF DAILY LIVING TREATMENT: Exercise or activities to facilitate functional competence for activities of daily living.

Body System/Region – 4TH	Type Qualifier – 5TH	Equipment – 6TH	Qualifier – 7TH
D Integumentary System - Head and Neck F Integumentary System - Upper Back/Upper Extremity G Integumentary System- Lower Back/Lower Extremity H Integumentary System - Whole Body J Musculoskeletal System - Head and Neck K Musculoskeletal System - Upper Back/Upper Extremity L Musculoskeletal System - Lower Back/Lower Extremity M Musculoskeletal System - Whole Body	5 Wound Management	B Physical Agents C Mechanical D Electrotherapeutic E Orthosis F Assistive, adaptive, supportive or protective U Prosthesis Y Other equipment Z None	Z None

continued ⇨

© 2018 Channel Publishing, Ltd.

F 0 8 ACTIVITIES OF DAILY LIVING TREATMENT –*continued*

Body System/Region – 4TH	Type Qualifier – 5TH	Equipment – 6TH	Qualifier – 7TH
Z None	0 Bathing/showering techniques 1 Dressing techniques 2 Grooming/personal hygiene	E Orthosis F Assistive, adaptive, supportive or protective U Prosthesis Y Other equipment Z None	Z None
Z None	3 Feeding/eating	C Mechanical D Electrotherapeutic E Orthosis F Assistive, adaptive, supportive or protective U Prosthesis Y Other equipment Z None	Z None
Z None	4 Home management	D Electrotherapeutic E Orthosis F Assistive, adaptive, supportive or protective U Prosthesis Y Other equipment Z None	Z None
Z None	6 Psychosocial skills	Z None	Z None
Z None	7 Vocational activities and functional community or work reintegration skills	B Physical Agents C Mechanical D Electrotherapeutic E Orthosis F Assistive, adaptive, supportive or protective G Aerobic endurance and conditioning U Prosthesis Y Other equipment Z None	Z None

1ST - F Physical Rehabilitation and Diagnostic Audiology
2ND - 0 Rehabilitation
3RD - 9 HEARING TREATMENT

HEARING TREATMENT: Application of techniques to improve, augment, or compensate for hearing and related functional impairment.

Body System/ Region – 4TH	Type Qualifier – 5TH	Equipment – 6TH	Qualifier – 7TH
Z None	0 Hearing and related disorders counseling 1 Hearing and related disorders prevention	K Audiovisual Z None	Z None
Z None	2 Auditory processing	K Audiovisual L Assistive listening P Computer Y Other equipment Z None	Z None
Z None	3 Cerumen management	X Cerumen management Z None	Z None

1ST - F Physical Rehabilitation and Diagnostic Audiology
2ND - 0 Rehabilitation
3RD - B COCHLEAR IMPLANT TREATMENT

COCHLEAR IMPLANT TREATMENT: Application of techniques to improve communication abilities of individuals with cochlear implant.

Body System/ Region – 4TH	Type Qualifier – 5TH	Equipment – 6TH	Qualifier – 7TH
Z None	0 Cochlear implant rehabilitation	1 Audiometer 2 Sound field/booth 9 Cochlear implant K Audiovisual P Computer Y Other equipment	Z None

© 2018 Channel Publishing, Ltd.

1ST - F Physical Rehabilitation and Diagnostic Audiology
2ND - 0 Rehabilitation
3RD - C VESTIBULAR TREATMENT

VESTIBULAR TREATMENT: Application of techniques to improve, augment, or compensate for vestibular and related functional impairment.

Body System/Region – 4TH	Type Qualifier – 5TH	Equipment – 6TH	Qualifier – 7TH
3 Neurological System - Whole Body H Integumentary System - Whole Body M Musculoskeletal System - Whole Body	3 Postural control	E Orthosis F Assistive, adaptive, supportive or protective U Prosthesis Y Other equipment Z None	Z None
Z None	0 Vestibular	8 Vestibular/balance Z None	Z None
Z None	1 Perceptual processing 2 Visual motor integration	K Audiovisual L Assistive listening N Biosensory feedback P Computer Q Speech analysis S Voice analysis T Aerodynamic function Y Other equipment Z None	Z None

1ST - F Physical Rehabilitation and Diagnostic Audiology
2ND - 0 Rehabilitation
3RD - D DEVICE FITTING

DEVICE FITTING: Fitting of a device designed to facilitate or support achievement of a higher level of function.

Body System/Region – 4TH	Type Qualifier – 5TH	Equipment – 6TH	Qualifier – 7TH
Z None	0 Tinnitus masker	5 Hearing aid selection/fitting/test Z None	Z None
Z None	1 Monaural hearing aid 2 Binaural hearing aid 5 Assistive listening device	1 Audiometer 2 Sound field/booth 5 Hearing aid selection/fitting/test K Audiovisual L Assistive listening Z None	Z None
Z None	3 Augmentative/alternative communication system	M Augmentative/alternative communication	Z None
Z None	4 Voice prosthetic	S Voice analysis V Speech prosthesis	Z None
Z None	6 Dynamic orthosis 7 Static orthosis 8 Prosthesis 9 Assistive, adaptive, supportive or protective devices	E Orthosis F Assistive, adaptive, supportive or protective U Prosthesis Z None	Z None

1ST - F Physical Rehabilitation and Diagnostic Audiology
2ND - 0 Rehabilitation
3RD - F CAREGIVER TRAINING

CAREGIVER TRAINING: Training in activities to support patient's optimal level of function.

Body System/Region – 4TH	Type Qualifier – 5TH	Equipment – 6TH	Qualifier – 7TH
Z None	0 Bathing/showering technique 1 Dressing 2 Feeding and eating 3 Grooming/personal hygiene 4 Bed mobility 5 Transfer 6 Wheelchair mobility 7 Therapeutic exercise 8 Airway clearance techniques 9 Wound management B Vocational activities and functional community or work reintegration skills C Gait training/functional ambulation D Application, proper use and care of devices F Application, proper use and care of orthoses G Application, proper use and care of prosthesis H Home management	E Orthosis F Assistive, adaptive, supportive or protective U Prosthesis Z None	Z None
Z None	J Communication skills	K Audiovisual L Assistive Listening M Augmentative/alternative communication P Computer Z None	Z None

© 2018 Channel Publishing, Ltd.

1ST - F Physical Rehabilitation and Diagnostic Audiology
2ND - 1 Diagnostic Audiology
3RD - 3 HEARING ASSESSMENT

HEARING ASSESSMENT: Measurement of hearing and related functions.

Body System/ Region – 4TH	Type Qualifier – 5TH	Equipment – 6TH	Qualifier – 7TH
Z None	0 Hearing screening	0 Occupational hearing 1 Audiometer 2 Sound field/booth 3 Tympanometer 8 Vestibular/balance 9 Cochlear implant Z None	Z None
Z None	1 Pure tone audiometry, air 2 Pure tone audiometry, air and bone	0 Occupational hearing 1 Audiometer 2 Sound field/booth Z None	Z None
Z None	3 Bekesy audiometry 6 Visual reinforcement audiometry 9 Short increment sensitivity index B Stenger C Pure tone stenger	1 Audiometer 2 Sound field/booth Z None	Z None
Z None	4 Conditioned play audiometry 5 Select picture audiometry	1 Audiometer 2 Sound field/booth K Audiovisual Z None	Z None
Z None	7 Alternate binaural or monaural loudness balance	1 Audiometer K Audiovisual Z None	Z None
Z None	8 Tone decay D Tympanometry F Eustachian tube function G Acoustic reflex patterns H Acoustic reflex threshold J Acoustic reflex decay	3 Tympanometer 4 Electroacoustic immitance/acoustic reflex Z None	Z None
Z None	K Electrocochleography L Auditory evoked potentials	7 Electrophysiologic Z None	Z None
Z None	M Evoked otoacoustic emissions, screening N Evoked otoacoustic emissions, diagnostic	6 Otoacoustic emission (OAE) Z None	Z None
Z None	P Aural rehabilitation status	1 Audiometer 2 Sound field/booth 4 Electroacoustic immitance/ acoustic reflex 9 Cochlear implant K Audiovisual L Assistive listening P Computer Z None	Z None
Z None	Q Auditory processing	K Audiovisual P Computer Y Other equipment Z None	Z None

© 2018 Channel Publishing, Ltd.

1ST - F Physical Rehabilitation and Diagnostic Audiology
2ND - 1 Diagnostic Audiology
3RD - 4 HEARING AID ASSESSMENT

HEARING AID ASSESSMENT: Measurement of the appropriateness and/or effectiveness of a hearing device.

Body System/ Region – 4TH	Type Qualifier – 5TH	Equipment – 6TH	Qualifier – 7TH
Z None	0 Cochlear implant	1 Audiometer 2 Sound field/booth 3 Tympanometer 4 Electroacoustic immitance/ acoustic reflex 5 Hearing Aid Selection/fitting/test 7 Electrophysiologic 9 Cochlear implant K Audiovisual L Assistive listening P Computer Y Other equipment Z None	Z None
Z None	1 Ear canal probe microphone 6 Binaural electroacoustic hearing aid check 8 Monaural electroacoustic hearing aid check	5 Hearing Aid Selection/fitting/test Z None	Z None
Z None	2 Monaural hearing aid 3 Binaural hearing aid	1 Audiometer 2 Sound field/booth 3 Tympanometer 4 Electroacoustic immitance/ acoustic reflex 5 Hearing Aid Selection/fitting/test K Audiovisual L Assistive listening P Computer Z None	Z None
Z None	4 Assistive listening system/device selection	1 Audiometer 2 Sound field/booth 3 Tympanometer 4 Electroacoustic immitance/acoustic reflex K Audiovisual L Assistive listening Z None	Z None
Z None	5 Sensory aids	1 Audiometer 2 Sound field/booth 3 Tympanometer 4 Electroacoustic immitance/ acoustic reflex 5 Hearing Aid Selection/fitting/test K Audiovisual L Assistive listening Z None	Z None
Z None	7 Ear protector attentuation	0 Occupational hearing Z None	Z None

1ST - F Physical Rehabilitation and Diagnostic Audiology
2ND - 1 Diagnostic Audiology
3RD - 5 VESTIBULAR ASSESSMENT

VESTIBULAR ASSESSMENT: Measurement of the vestibular system and related functions.

Body System/ Region – 4TH	Type Qualifier – 5TH	Equipment – 6TH	Qualifier – 7TH
Z None	0 Bithermal, binaural caloric irrigation 1 Bithermal, monaural caloric irrigation 2 Unithermal binaural screen 3 Oscillating tracking 4 Sinusoidal vertical axis rotational 5 Dix-Hallpike dynamic 6 Computerized dynamic posturography	8 Vestibular/balance Z None	Z None
Z None	7 Tinnitus masker	5 Hearing aid selection/fitting/test Z None	Z None

REHAB & AUDIOLOGY F15

© 2018 Channel Publishing, Ltd.

NOTES

© 2018 Channel Publishing, Ltd.

Educational Annotations | Section G – Mental Health

Section Specific Educational Annotations for the Mental Health Section include:

- **AHA Coding Clinic® Reference Notations**
- **Coding Notes**

AHA Coding Clinic® Reference Notations of Mental Health

ROOT TYPE SPECIFIC - MENTAL HEALTH - Section G
PSYCHOLOGICAL TESTS - 1
CRISIS INTERVENTION - 2
INDIVIDUAL PSYCHOTHERAPY - 5
COUNSELING - 6
FAMILY PSYCHOTHERAPY - 7
ELECTROCONVULSIVE THERAPY - B
BIOFEEDBACK - C
HYPNOSIS - F
NARCOSYNTHESIS - G
GROUP THERAPY - H
LIGHT THERAPY - J

Coding Notes of Mental Health

© 2018 Channel Publishing, Ltd.

1ST - G Mental Health
2ND - Z None
3RD - 1 PSYCHOLOGICAL TESTS

PSYCHOLOGICAL TESTS: The administration and interpretation of standardized psychological tests and measurement instruments for the assessment of psychological function.

Explanation/Includes/Examples: None

Qualifier – 4TH	Qualifier – 5TH	Qualifier – 7TH	Qualifier – 7TH
0 Developmental 1 Personality and behavioral 2 Intellectual and psychoeducational 3 Neuropsychological 4 Neurobehavioral and cognitive status	Z None	Z None	Z None

1ST - G Mental Health
2ND - Z None
3RD - 2 CRISIS INTERVENTION

CRISIS INTERVENTION: Treatment of a traumatized, acutely disturbed or distressed individual for the purpose of short-term stabilization.

Includes/Examples: Includes defusing, debriefing, counseling, psychotherapy and/or coordination of care with other providers or agencies.

Qualifier – 4TH	Qualifier – 5TH	Qualifier – 7TH	Qualifier – 7TH
Z None	Z None	Z None	Z None

1ST - G Mental Health
2ND - Z None
3RD - 3 MEDICATION MANAGEMENT

MEDICATION MANAGEMENT: Monitoring and adjusting the use of medications for the treatment of a mental health disorder.

Explanation/Includes/Examples: None

Qualifier – 4TH	Qualifier – 5TH	Qualifier – 7TH	Qualifier – 7TH
Z None	Z None	Z None	Z None

1ST - G Mental Health
2ND - Z None
3RD - 5 INDIVIDUAL PSYCHOTHERAPY

INDIVIDUAL PSYCHOTHERAPY: Treatment of an individual with a mental health disorder by behavioral, cognitive, psychoanalytic, psychodynamic or psychophysiological means to improve functioning or well-being.

Explanation/Includes/Examples: None

Qualifier – 4TH	Qualifier – 5TH	Qualifier – 7TH	Qualifier – 7TH
0 Interactive 1 Behavioral 2 Cognitive 3 Interpersonal 4 Psychoanalysis 5 Psychodynamic 6 Supportive 8 Cognitive-Behavioral 9 Psychophysiological	Z None	Z None	Z None

1ST - G Mental Health
2ND - Z None
3RD - 6 COUNSELING

COUNSELING: The application of psychological methods to treat an individual with normal developmental issues and psychological problems in order to increase function, improve well-being, alleviate distress, maladjustment or resolve crises.

Explanation/Includes/Examples: None

Qualifier – 4TH	Qualifier – 5TH	Qualifier – 7TH	Qualifier – 7TH
0 Educational 1 Vocational 3 Other counseling	Z None	Z None	Z None

© 2018 Channel Publishing, Ltd.

1ST - G Mental Health
2ND - Z None
3RD - 7 FAMILY PSYCHOTHERAPY

FAMILY PSYCHOTHERAPY: Treatment that includes one or more family members of an individual with a mental health disorder by behavioral, cognitive, psychoanalytic, psychodynamic or psychophysiological means to improve functioning or well-being.

Explanation: Remediation of emotional or behavioral problems presented by one or more family members in cases where psychotherapy with more than one family member is indicated.

Qualifier – 4TH	Qualifier – 5TH	Qualifier – 7TH	Qualifier – 7TH
2 Other family psychotherapy	Z None	Z None	Z None

1ST - G Mental Health
2ND - Z None
3RD - B ELECTROCONVULSIVE THERAPY

ELECTROCONVULSIVE THERAPY: The application of controlled electrical voltages to treat a mental health disorder.

Includes/Examples: Includes appropriate sedation and other preparation of the individual.

Qualifier – 4TH	Qualifier – 5TH	Qualifier – 7TH	Qualifier – 7TH
0 Unilateral-single seizure 1 Unilateral-multiple seizure 2 Bilateral-single seizure 3 Bilateral-multiple seizure 4 Other electroconvulsive therapy	Z None	Z None	Z None

1ST - G Mental Health
2ND - Z None
3RD - C BIOFEEDBACK

BIOFEEDBACK: Provision of information from the monitoring and regulating of physiological processes in conjunction with cognitive-behavioral techniques to improve patient functioning or well-being.

Includes/Examples: Includes EEG, blood pressure, skin temperature or peripheral blood flow, ECG, electrooculogram, EMG, respirometry or capnometry, GSR/EDR, perineometry to monitor/regulate bowel/bladder activity, electrogastrogram to monitor/regulate gastric motility.

Qualifier – 4TH	Qualifier – 5TH	Qualifier – 7TH	Qualifier – 7TH
9 Other biofeedback	Z None	Z None	Z None

1ST - G Mental Health
2ND - Z None
3RD - F HYPNOSIS

HYPNOSIS: Induction of a state of heightened suggestibility by auditory, visual and tactile techniques to elicit an emotional or behavioral response.

Explanation/Includes/Examples: None

Qualifier – 4TH	Qualifier – 5TH	Qualifier – 7TH	Qualifier – 7TH
Z None	Z None	Z None	Z None

1ST - G Mental Health
2ND - Z None
3RD - G NARCOSYNTHESIS

NARCOSYNTHESIS: Administration of intravenous barbiturates in order to release suppressed or repressed thoughts.

Explanation/Includes/Examples: None

Qualifier – 4TH	Qualifier – 5TH	Qualifier – 7TH	Qualifier – 7TH
Z None	Z None	Z None	Z None

© 2018 Channel Publishing, Ltd.

1ST - G Mental Health 2ND - Z None 3RD - H GROUP PSYCHOTHERAPY	GROUP PSYCHOTHERAPY: Treatment of two or more individuals with a mental health disorder by behavioral, cognitive, psychoanalytic, psychodynamic or psychophysiological means to improve functioning or well-being. Explanation/Includes/Examples: None		
Qualifier – 4TH	Qualifier – 5TH	Qualifier – 7TH	Qualifier – 7TH
Z None	Z None	Z None	Z None

1ST - G Mental Health 2ND - Z None 3RD - J LIGHT THERAPY	LIGHT THERAPY: Application of specialized light treatments to improve functioning or well-being. Explanation/Includes/Examples: None		
Qualifier – 4TH	Qualifier – 5TH	Qualifier – 7TH	Qualifier – 7TH
Z None	Z None	Z None	Z None

© 2018 Channel Publishing, Ltd.

Educational Annotations | Section H – Substance Abuse

Section Specific Educational Annotations for the Substance Abuse Section include:

- AHA Coding Clinic® Reference Notations
- Coding Notes

AHA Coding Clinic® Reference Notations of Substance Abuse

ROOT TYPE SPECIFIC - SUBSTANCE ABUSE TREATMENT - Section H

DETOXIFICATION SERVICES - 2
INDIVIDUAL COUNSELING - 3
GROUP COUNSELING - 4
INDIVIDUAL PSYCHOTHERAPY - 5
FAMILY COUNSELING - 6
MEDICATION MANAGEMENT - 8
PHARMACOTHERAPY - 9

Coding Notes of Substance Abuse

1ST - H Substance Abuse Treatment
2ND - Z None
3RD - 2 DETOXIFICATION SERVICES

DETOXIFICATION SERVICES: Detoxification from alcohol and/or drugs.

Explanation: Not a treatment modality, but helps the patient stabilize physically and psychologically until the body becomes free of drugs and the effects of alcohol.

Qualifier – 4TH	Qualifier – 5TH	Qualifier – 7TH	Qualifier – 7TH
Z None	Z None	Z None	Z None

1ST - H Substance Abuse Treatment
2ND - Z None
3RD - 3 INDIVIDUAL COUNSELING

INDIVIDUAL COUNSELING: The application of psychological methods to treat an individual with addictive behavior.

Explanation: Comprised of several different techniques, which apply various strategies to address drug addiction.

Qualifier – 4TH	Qualifier – 5TH	Qualifier – 7TH	Qualifier – 7TH
0 Cognitive 1 Behavioral 2 Cognitive-behavioral 3 12-Step 4 Interpersonal 5 Vocational 6 Psychoeducation 7 Motivational enhancement 8 Confrontational 9 Continuing care B Spiritual C Pre/post-test infectious disease	Z None	Z None	Z None

© 2018 Channel Publishing, Ltd.

1ST - H Substance Abuse Treatment
2ND - Z None
3RD - 4 GROUP COUNSELING

GROUP COUNSELING: The application of psychological methods to treat two or more individuals with addictive behavior.

Explanation: Provides structured group counseling sessions and healing power through the connection with others.

Qualifier – 4TH	Qualifier – 5TH	Qualifier – 7TH	Qualifier – 7TH
0 Cognitive 1 Behavioral 2 Cognitive-behavioral 3 12-Step 4 Interpersonal 5 Vocational 6 Psychoeducation 7 Motivational enhancement 8 Confrontational 9 Continuing care B Spiritual C Pre/post-test infectious disease	Z None	Z None	Z None

1ST - H Substance Abuse Treatment
2ND - Z None
3RD - 5 INDIVIDUAL PSYCHOTHERAPY

INDIVIDUAL PSYCHOTHERAPY: Treatment of an individual with addictive behavior by behavioral, cognitive, psychoanalytic, psychodynamic or psychophysiological means.

Explanation: None

Qualifier – 4TH	Qualifier – 5TH	Qualifier – 7TH	Qualifier – 7TH
0 Cognitive 1 Behavioral 2 Cognitive-behavioral 3 12-Step 4 Interpersonal 5 Interactive 6 Psychoeducation 7 Motivational enhancement 8 Confrontational 9 Supportive B Psychoanalysis C Psychodynamic D Psychophysiological	Z None	Z None	Z None

1ST - H Substance Abuse Treatment
2ND - Z None
3RD - 6 FAMILY COUNSELING

FAMILY COUNSELING: The application of psychological methods that includes one or more family members to treat an individual with addictive behavior.

Explanation: Provides support and education for family members of addicted individuals. Family member participation is seen as a critical area of substance abuse treatment.

Qualifier – 4TH	Qualifier – 5TH	Qualifier – 7TH	Qualifier – 7TH
3 Other family counseling	Z None	Z None	Z None

1ST - H Substance Abuse Treatment
2ND - Z None
3RD - 8 MEDICATION MANAGEMENT

MEDICATION MANAGEMENT: Monitoring and adjusting the use of replacement medications for the treatment of addiction.

Explanation: None

Qualifier – 4TH	Qualifier – 5TH	Qualifier – 7TH	Qualifier – 7TH
0 Nicotine replacement 1 Methadone maintenance 2 Levo-alpha-acetyl-methadol (LAAM) 3 Antabuse 4 Naltrexone 5 Naloxone 6 Clonidine 7 Bupropion 8 Psychiatric medication 9 Other replacement medication	Z None	Z None	Z None

1ST - H Substance Abuse Treatment
2ND - Z None
3RD - 9 PHARMACOTHERAPY

PHARMACOTHERAPY: The use of replacement medications for the treatment of addiction.

Explanation: None

Qualifier – 4TH	Qualifier – 5TH	Qualifier – 7TH	Qualifier – 7TH
0 Nicotine replacement 1 Methadone maintenance 2 Levo-alpha-acetyl-methadol (LAAM) 3 Antabuse 4 Naltrexone 5 Naloxone 6 Clonidine 7 Bupropion 8 Psychiatric medication 9 Other replacement medication	Z None	Z None	Z None

© 2018 Channel Publishing, Ltd.

Educational Annotations | Section X – New Technology

Section Specific Educational Annotations for the New Technology Section include:

- AHA Coding Clinic® Reference Notations
- Coding Notes
- Device Key Listings

NEW TECHNOLOGY – SECTION X

Section X New Technology is the section in ICD-10-PCS for codes that uniquely identify procedures requested via the New Technology Application Process, and for codes that capture new technologies not currently classified in ICD-10-PCS.

This section may include codes for medical and surgical procedures, medical and surgical-related procedures, or ancillary procedures designated as new technology.

In section X, the seven characters are defined as follows:

- First character: section (X)
- Second character: body system
- Third character: operation
- Fourth character: body part
- Fifth character: approach
- Sixth character: device/substance/technology
- Seventh character: new technology group

The New Technology section includes infusions of new technology drugs, and can potentially include a wide range of other new technology medical, surgical, and ancillary procedures. The example below is for infusion of a new technology drug.

Coding Note: Seventh Character New Technology Group
In ICD-10-PCS, the type of information specified in the seventh character is called the qualifier, and the information specified depends on the section. In this section, the seventh character is used exclusively to indicate the new technology group.

The New Technology Group is a number or letter that changes each year that new technology codes are added to the system. For example, Section X codes added for the first year have the seventh character value 1, New Technology Group 1, and the next year that Section X codes are added have the seventh character value 2 New Technology Group 2, and so on.

Changing the seventh character New Technology Group to a unique value every year that there are new codes in this section allows the ICD-10-PCS to "recycle" the values in the third, fourth, and sixth characters as needed. This avoids the creation of duplicate codes, because the root operation, body part, and device/substance/technology values can specify a different meaning with every new technology group, if needed. Having a unique value for the New Technology Group maximizes the flexibility and capacity of section X over its lifespan, and allows it to evolve as medical technology evolves.

Body System Values
Second character body systems in this section do not change from year to year. They are a fixed set of values that combine the uses of body system, body region, and physiological system as specified in other sections in ICD-10-PCS. As a result, the second character body system values are broader values. This allows body part values to be as general or specific as they need to be to efficiently represent the body part applicable to a new technology.

Root Operations
Third character root operations in this section use the same root operation values as their counterparts in other sections of ICD-10-PCS. The example above uses the root operation value Introduction. This root operation has the same definition as its counterpart in section 3 of ICD-10-PCS, as given below.

- 0 – Introduction: Putting in or on a therapeutic, diagnostic, nutritional, physiological, or prophylactic substance except blood or blood products

Body Part Values
Fourth character body part values in this section use the same body part values as their closest counterparts in other sections of ICD-10-PCS. The example above uses the body part value 4 Central Vein. This is its closest counterpart in section 3 of ICD-10-PCS.

Device/Substance/Technology Values
In this section, the sixth character contains a general description of the key feature of the new technology. The example above uses the device/substance/technology value 2 Ceftazidime-Avibactam Anti-infective.

© 2018 Channel Publishing, Ltd.

Educational Annotations | Section X – New Technology

AHA Coding Clinic® Reference Notations of New Technology

ROOT OPERATION SPECIFIC - NEW TECHNOLOGY - Section X

ASSISTANCE - A

Cerebral embolic filtration during cardiac procedures ....AHA 16:4Q:p115

EXTIRPATION - C

Orbital atherectomy and drug-eluting balloon angioplasty of coronary artery ....AHA 15:4Q:p13

FUSION - G

Lumbar fusion using COALESCE radiolucent porous interbody device ....AHA 17:4Q:p76

INTRODUCTION - 0

Blincyto infusion (blinatumomab) ....AHA 15:4Q:p14

Concentrated bone marrow aspirate ....AHA 17:4Q:p74

Intraoperative treatment of vein grafts ....AHA 17:4Q:p78

Introduction of idarucizumab prior to surgery ....AHA 15:4Q:p13

MISC

REPLACEMENT - R

Aortic valve rapid deployment ....AHA 16:4Q:p116

Application of biologic wound matrix ....AHA 16:4Q:p116

REPOSITION - S

Placement of magnetic growth rods ....AHA 16:4Q:p117

Replacement of magnetic growth rod ....AHA 17:4Q:p75

Device Key Listings of New Technology

See also Device Key in Appendix D

COALESCE® Radiolucent interbody fusion device ....use Interbody Fusion Device, Radiolucent Porous

COHERE® Radiolucent interbody fusion device ....use Interbody Fusion Device, Radiolucent Porous

EDWARDS INTUITY Elite valve system ....use Zooplastic Tisssue, Rapid Deployment Technique

INTUITY Elite valve system, EDWARDS ....use Zooplastic Tisssue, Rapid Deployment Technique

MAGEC® Spinal Bracing and Distraction System ....use Magnetically Controlled Growth Rod(s)

MICRODERM™ Biologic Wound Matrix ....use Skin Substitute, Porcine Liver Derived

nanoLOCK™ interbody fusion device ....use Interbody Fusion Device, Nanotextured Surface

Perceval sutureless valve ....use Zooplastic Tisssue, Rapid Deployment Technique

Spiral growth rod(s), magnetically controlled ....use Magnetically Controlled Growth Rod(s)

Sutureless valve, Perceval ....use Zooplastic Tisssue, Rapid Deployment Technique

Coding Notes of New Technology

Body System Relevant Coding Guidelines

D. New Technology Section – Section X

General guidelines

D1

Section X codes are standalone codes. They are not supplemental codes. Section X codes fully represent the specific procedure described in the code title, and do not require any additional codes from other sections of ICD-10-PCS. When section X contains a code title which describes a specific new technology procedure, only that X code is reported for the procedure. There is no need to report a broader, non-specific code in another section of ICD-10-PCS.

Example: XW04321 Introduction of Ceftazidime-Avibactam Anti-infective into Central Vein, Percutaneous Approach, New Technology Group 1, can be coded to indicate that Ceftazidime-Avibactam Anti-infective was administered via a central vein. A separate code from table 3E0 in the Administration section of ICD-10-PCS is not coded in addition to this code.

© 2018 Channel Publishing, Ltd.

1ST - X New Technology
2ND - 2 Cardiovascular System
3RD - A ASSISTANCE

ASSISTANCE: Taking over a portion of a physiological function by extracorporeal means.

Explanation: Supports, but does not take over function ...
Examples: Cerebral embolic filtration – CMS Ex: None

Body Part – 4TH	Approach – 5TH	Device/Substance/ Technology – 6TH	Qualifier – 7TH
5 Innominate Artery and Left Common Carotid Artery	3 Percutaneous	1 Cerebral embolic filtration, dual filter	2 New Technology Group 2

1ST - X New Technology
2ND - 2 Cardiovascular System
3RD - C EXTIRPATION

EXTIRPATION: Taking or cutting out solid matter from a body part.

Explanation: Abnormal byproduct or foreign body ...
Examples: Removal coronary artery plaque – CMS Ex: Thrombectomy

Body Part – 4TH	Approach – 5TH	Device/Substance/ Technology – 6TH	Qualifier – 7TH
0 Coronary Artery, One Artery 1 Coronary Artery, Two Arteries 2 Coronary Artery, Three Arteries 3 Coronary Artery, Four or More Arteries	3 Percutaneous	6 Orbital atherectomy technology	1 New Technology Group 1

1ST - X New Technology
2ND - 2 Cardiovascular System
3RD - R REPLACEMENT

REPLACEMENT: Putting in or on biological or synthetic material that physically takes the place and/or function of all or a portion of a body part.

Explanation: Includes taking out or eradicating, or rendering non-functional, the body part ...
Examples: Rapid deployment technique aortic valve replacement – CMS Ex: Total hip replacement

Body Part – 4TH	Approach – 5TH	Device/Substance/ Technology – 6TH	Qualifier – 7TH
F Aortic Valve	0 Open 3 Percutaneous 4 Percutaneous endoscopic	3 Zooplastic tissue, rapid deployment technique	2 New Technology Group 2

1ST - X New Technology
2ND - H Skin, Subcutaneous Tissue, Fascia, and Breast
3RD - R REPLACEMENT

REPLACEMENT: Putting in or on biological or synthetic material that physically takes the place and/or function of all or a portion of a body part.

Explanation: Includes taking out or eradicating, or rendering non-functional, the body part ...
Examples: Porcine liver derived skin substitute – CMS Ex: Total hip replacement

Body Part – 4TH	Approach – 5TH	Device/Substance/ Technology – 6TH	Qualifier – 7TH
P Skin	X External	L Skin substitute, porcine liver derived	2 New Technology Group 2

1ST - X New Technology
2ND - K Muscles, Tendons, Bursae, and Ligaments
3RD - 0 INTRODUCTION

INTRODUCTION: Putting in or on a therapeutic, diagnostic, nutritional, physiological, or prophylactic substance except blood or blood products.

Explanation: Substances other than blood and cleansing
Example: Infusion substance

Body Part – 4TH	Approach – 5TH	Device/Substance/ Technology – 6TH	Qualifier – 7TH
2 Muscle	3 Percutaneous	0 Concentrated bone marrow aspirate	3 New Technology Group 3

© 2018 Channel Publishing, Ltd.

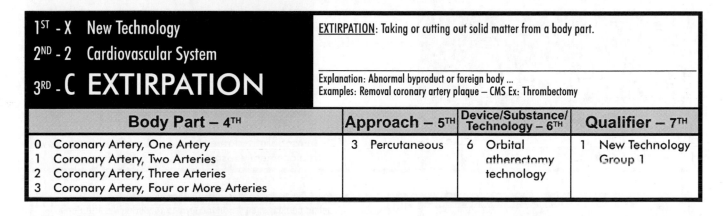

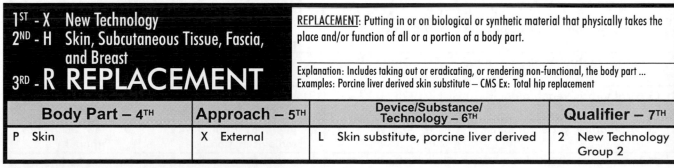

1ST - X New Technology
2ND - N Bones
3RD - S REPOSITION

REPOSITION: Moving to its normal location, or other suitable location, all or a portion of a body part.

Explanation: The body part may or may not be cut out or off to be moved to the new location ...
Examples: Adjusting magnetically controlled growth rod(s) – CMS Ex: Fracture reduction

Body Part – 4TH	Approach – 5TH	Device/Substance/ Technology – 6TH	Qualifier – 7TH
0 Lumbar Vertebra 3 Cervical Vertebra 4 Thoracic Vertebra	0 Open 3 Percutaneous	3 Magnetically controlled growth rod(s)	2 New Technology Group 2

1ST - X New Technology
2ND - R Joints
3RD - 2 MONITORING

MONITORING: Determining the level of a physiological or physical function repetitively over a period of time.

Explanation: Describes a series of measurements
Example: Intraoperative knee replacement sensor

Body Part – 4TH	Approach – 5TH	Device/Substance/ Technology – 6TH	Qualifier – 7TH
G Knee Joint, Right H Knee Joint, Left	0 Open	2 Intraoperative knee replacement sensor	1 New Technology Group 1

1ST - X New Technology
2ND - R Joints
3RD - G FUSION

FUSION: Joining together portions of an articular body part rendering the articular body part immobile.

Explanation: The body part is joined together by fixation device, bone graft, other means
Examples: Nontextured surface interbody fusion device – CMS Ex: Spinal fusion

Body Part – 4TH	Approach – 5TH	Device/Substance/ Technology – 6TH	Qualifier – 7TH
0 Occipital-cervical Joint	0 Open	9 Interbody fusion device, nanotextured surface	2 New Technology Group 2
0 Occipital-cervical Joint	0 Open	F Interbody fusion device, radiolucent porous	3 New Technology Group 3
1 Cervical Vertebral Joint	0 Open	9 Interbody fusion device, nanotextured surface	2 New Technology Group 2
1 Cervical Vertebral Joint	0 Open	F Interbody fusion device, radiolucent porous	3 New Technology Group 3
2 Cervical Vertebral Joints, 2 or more	0 Open	9 Interbody fusion device, nanotextured surface	2 New Technology Group 2
2 Cervical Vertebral Joints, 2 or more	0 Open	F Interbody fusion device, radiolucent porous	3 New Technology Group 3
4 Cervicothoracic Vertebral Joint	0 Open	9 Interbody fusion device, nanotextured surface	2 New Technology Group 2
4 Cervicothoracic Vertebral Joint	0 Open	F Interbody fusion device, radiolucent porous	3 New Technology Group 3
6 Thoracic Vertebral Joint	0 Open	9 Interbody fusion device, nanotextured surface	2 New Technology Group 2
6 Thoracic Vertebral Joint	0 Open	F Interbody fusion device, radiolucent porous	3 New Technology Group 3
7 Thoracic Vertebral Joints, 2 to 7	0 Open	9 Interbody fusion device, nanotextured surface	2 New Technology Group 2
7 Thoracic Vertebral Joints, 2 to 7	0 Open	F Interbody fusion device, radiolucent porous	3 New Technology Group 3

continued ⇨

© 2018 Channel Publishing, Ltd.

X R G FUSION – *continued*

Body Part – 4TH	Approach – 5TH	Device/Substance/ Technology – 6TH	Qualifier – 7TH
8 Thoracic Vertebral Joints, 8 or more	0 Open	9 Interbody fusion device, nanotextured surface	2 New Technology Group 2
8 Thoracic Vertebral Joints, 8 or more	0 Open	F Interbody fusion device, radiolucent porous	3 New Technology Group 3
A Thoracolumbar Vertebral Joint	0 Open	9 Interbody fusion device, nanotextured surface	2 New Technology Group 2
A Thoracolumbar Vertebral Joint	0 Open	F Interbody fusion device, radiolucent porous	3 New Technology Group 3
B Lumbar Vertebral Joint	0 Open	9 Interbody fusion device, nanotextured surface	2 New Technology Group 2
B Lumbar Vertebral Joint	0 Open	F Interbody fusion device, radiolucent porous	3 New Technology Group 3
C Lumbar Vertebral Joints, 2 or more	0 Open	9 Interbody fusion device, nanotextured surface	2 New Technology Group 2
C Lumbar Vertebral Joints, 2 or more	0 Open	F Interbody fusion device, radiolucent porous	3 New Technology Group 3
D Lumbosacral Joint	0 Open	9 Interbody fusion device, nanotextured surface	2 New Technology Group 2
D Lumbosacral Joint	0 Open	F Interbody fusion device, radiolucent porous	3 New Technology Group 3

© 2018 Channel Publishing, Ltd.

1ST - X New Technology
2ND - V Male Reproductive System
3RD - 5 DESTRUCTION

DESTRUCTION: Physical eradication of all or a portion of a body part by the direct use of energy, force, or a destructive agent.

Explanation: None of the body part is physically taken out
Examples: Robotic waterjet ablation – CMS Ex: Fulguration rectal polyp

Body Part – 4TH	Approach – 5TH	Device/Substance/ Technology – 6TH	Qualifier – 7TH
0 Prostate	8 Via natural or artificial opening endoscopic	A Robotic waterjet ablation	4 New Technology Group 4

1ST - X New Technology
2ND - W Anatomical Regions
3RD - 0 INTRODUCTION

INTRODUCTION: Putting in or on a therapeutic, diagnostic, nutritional, physiological, or prophylactic substance except blood or blood products.

Explanation: Substances other than blood and cleansing
Example: Infusion substance

Body Part – 4TH	Approach - 5TH	Device/Substance/ Technology – 6TH	Qualifier – 7TH
3 Peripheral Vein	3 Percutaneous	2 Ceftazidime-avibactam anti-infective 3 Idarucizumab, Dabigatran reversal agent 4 Isavuconazole anti-infective 5 Blinatumomab antineoplastic immunotherapy	1 New Technology Group 1
3 Peripheral Vein	3 Percutaneous	7 Andexanet alfa, Factor Xa inhibitor reversal agent 9 Defibrotide sodium anticoagulant	2 New Technology Group 2
3 Peripheral Vein	3 Percutaneous	A Bezlotoxumab monoclonal antibody B Cytarabine and daunorubicin liposome antineoplastic C Engineered autologous chimeric antigen receptor T-cell immunotherapy F Other new technology therapeutic substance	3 New Technology Group 3
3 Peripheral Vein	3 Percutaneous	G Plazomicin anti-infective H Synthetic human angiotensin II	4 New Technology Group 4
4 Central Vein	3 Percutaneous	2 Ceftazidime-avibactam anti-infective 3 Idarucizumab, Dabigatran reversal agent 4 Isavuconazole anti-infective 5 Blinatumomab antineoplastic immunotherapy	1 New Technology Group 1
4 Central Vein	3 Percutaneous	7 Andexanet alfa, Factor Xa inhibitor reversal agent 9 Defibrotide sodium anticoagulant	2 New Technology Group 2
4 Central Vein	3 Percutaneous	A Bezlotoxumab monoclonal antibody B Cytarabine and daunorubicin liposome antineoplastic C Engineered autologous chimeric antigen receptor T-cell immunotherapy F Other new technology therapeutic substance	3 New Technology Group 3
4 Central Vein	3 Percutaneous	G Plazomicin anti-infective H Synthetic human angiotensin II	4 New Technology Group 4
D Mouth and Pharynx	X External	8 Uridine triacetate	2 New Technology Group 2

© 2018 Channel Publishing, Ltd.

1ST - X New Technology
2ND - Y Extracorporeal
3RD - 0 INTRODUCTION

INTRODUCTION: Putting in or on a therapeutic, diagnostic, nutritional, physiological, or prophylactic substance except blood or blood products.

Explanation: Substances other than blood and cleansing
Example: Infusion substance

Body Part – 4TH	Approach – 5TH	Device/Substance/ Technology – 6TH	Qualifier – 7TH
V Vein Graft	X External	8 Endothelial damage inhibitor	3 New Technology Group 3

APPENDIX A
ROOT OPERATIONS OF THE MEDICAL AND SURGICAL SECTION

APPENDIX A contains the following parts:
PART 1: Groups of Similar Root Operations (Medical and Surgical Section)
PART 2: Alphabetic Listing of Root Operations (Medical and Surgical Section)

PART 1: Groups of Similar Root Operations (Medical and Surgical Section)

The Root Operations of the Medical and Surgical section are divided into logical groups that share similar attributes. Each root operation chart group includes: root operation name, objective of the procedure, site of the procedure, and an example of that root operation. These root operation chart groups are:

- Root operations that take out some or all of a body part
- Root operations that take out solids/fluids/gases from a body part
- Root operations involving cutting or separation only
- Root operations that put in/put back or move some/all of a body part
- Root operations that alter the diameter/route of a tubular body part
- Root operations that always involve a device
- Root operations involving examination only
- Root operations that define other repairs
- Root operations that define other objectives

Bold word(s) within each chart identify the concept that help differentiate it from other root operations within that chart.

Root operations that take out some or all of a body part

Root Operation	Objective of Procedure	Site of Procedure	Example
Excision	Cutting out/off without replacement	**Some** of a body part	Breast lumpectomy
Resection	Cutting out/off without replacement	**All** of a body part	Total mastectomy
Detachment	Cutting out/off without replacement	**Extremity only**, any level	Amputation above elbow
Destruction	**Eradicating** without replacement	Some/all of a body part	Fulguration of endometrium
Extraction	**Pulling out** or off without replacement	Some/all of a body part	Suction D&C

© 2018 Channel Publishing, Ltd.

Root operations that take out solids/fluids/gases from a body part

Root Operation	Objective of Procedure	Site of Procedure	Example
Drainage	Taking/letting out **fluids/gases**	Within a body part	Incision and drainage
Extirpation	Taking/cutting out **solid matter**	Within a body part	Thrombectomy
Fragmentation	**Breaking** solid matter into pieces	Within a body part	Lithotripsy

Root operations involving cutting or separation only

Root Operation	Objective of Procedure	Site of Procedure	Example
Division	Cutting into/**separating** a body part	Within a body part	Neurotomy
Release	**Freeing** a body part from constraint	Around a body part	Adhesiolysis

Root operations that put in/put back or move some/all of a body part

Root Operation	Objective of Procedure	Site of Procedure	Example
Transplantation	**Putting in** a living body part from a person/animal	Some/all of a body part	Kidney transplant
Reattachment	**Putting back** a detached body part	Some/all of a body part	Reattach finger
Transfer	**Moving** a body part to **function for** a similar body part	Some/all of a body part	Skin transfer flap
Reposition	**Moving** a body part to **normal** or other suitable location	Some/all of a body part	Move undescended testicle

Root operations that alter the diameter/route of a tubular body part

Root Operation	Objective of Procedure	Site of Procedure	Example
Restriction	**Partially** closing orifice/lumen	Tubular body part	Gastroesophageal fundoplication
Occlusion	**Completely** closing orifice/lumen	Tubular body part	Fallopian tube ligation
Dilation	**Expanding** orifice/lumen	Tubular body part	Percutaneous transluminal coronary angioplasty (PTCA)
Bypass	**Altering route** of passage	Tubular body part	Coronary artery bypass graft (CABG)

Root operations that always involve a device

Root Operation	Objective of Procedure	Site of Procedure	Example
Insertion	Putting in **non-biological** device	In/on a body part	Central line insertion
Replacement	Putting in device that **replaces** a body part	Some/all of a body part	Total hip replacement
Supplement	Putting in device that **reinforces** or augments a body part	In/on a body part	Abdominal wall hernior-rhaphy using mesh
Change	**Exchanging** device without cutting/puncturing	In/on a body part	Drainage tube change
Removal	**Taking out** device	In/on a body part	Central line removal
Revision	**Correcting** a malfunctioning/displaced device	In/on a body part	Revision of pacemaker in-sertion

© 2018 Channel Publishing, Ltd.

Root operations involving examination only

Root Operation	Objective of Procedure	Site of Procedure	Example
Inspection	Visual/manual **exploration**	Some/all of a body part	Diagnostic cystoscopy
Map	**Locating** electrical impulses/functional areas	Brain/cardiac conduction mechanism	Cardiac mapping

Root operations that define other repairs

Root Operation	Objective of Procedure	Site of Procedure	Example
Control	Stopping/attempting to stop **postprocedural bleeding**	Anatomical region	Post-prostatectomy bleeding control
Repair	**Restoring** body part to its normal structure	Some/all of a body part	Suture laceration

Root operations that define other objectives

Root Operation	Objective of Procedure	Site of Procedure	Example
Fusion	Rendering joint **immobile**	Joint	Spinal fusion
Alteration	**Modifying** body part for cosmetic purposes without affecting function	Some/all of a body part	Face lift
Creation	**Forming** a new body part to replicate the function of an absent body part	Some/all of a body part	Artificial vagina/penis

© 2018 Channel Publishing, Ltd.

PART 2: Alphabetic Listing of Root Operations (Medical and Surgical Section)

The Root Operations of the Medical and Surgical section are listed below in alphabetic order and include information detailing each root operation. Each root operation chart includes:

- Root Operation value and title
- Definition
- Explanation
- Examples

0 ALTERATION	DEFINITION: Modifying the anatomic structure of a body part without affecting the function of the body part
EXPLANATION:	Principal purpose is to improve appearance
EXAMPLES:	Face lift, breast augmentation

1 BYPASS	DEFINITION: Altering the route of passage of the contents of a tubular body part
EXPLANATION:	Rerouting contents of a body part to a downstream area of the normal route, to a similar route and body part, or to an abnormal route and dissimilar body part. Includes one or more anastomoses, with or without the use of a device
EXAMPLES:	Coronary artery bypass, colostomy formation

2 CHANGE	DEFINITION: Taking out or off a device from a body part and putting back an identical or similar device in or on the same body part without cutting or puncturing the skin or a mucous membrane
EXPLANATION:	All CHANGE procedures are coded using the approach EXTERNAL
EXAMPLES:	Urinary catheter change, gastrostomy tube change

3 CONTROL	DEFINITION: Stopping, or attempting to stop, postprocedural bleeding or other acute bleeding
EXPLANATION:	The site of the bleeding is coded as an anatomical region and not to a specific body part
EXAMPLES:	Control of post-prostatectomy hemorrhage, control of intracranial subdural hemorrhage, control of bleeding duodenal ulcer, control of retroperitoneal hemorrhage

4 CREATION	DEFINITION: Putting in or on biological or synthetic material to form a new body part that to the extent possible replicates the anatomic structure or function of an absent body part
EXPLANATION:	Used for gender reassignment surgery and corrective procedures in individuals with congenital anomalies
EXAMPLES:	Creation of vagina in a male, creation of right and left atrioventricular valve from common atrioventricualr valve

© 2018 Channel Publishing, Ltd.

5 DESTRUCTION

DEFINITION:	Physical eradication of all or a portion of a body part by the direct use of energy, force, or a destructive agent
EXPLANATION:	None of the body part is physically taken out
EXAMPLES:	Fulguration of rectal polyp, cautery of skin lesion

6 DETACHMENT

DEFINITION:	Cutting off all or portion of the upper or lower extremities
EXPLANATION:	The body part value is the site of the detachment, with a qualifier if applicable to further specify the level where the extremity was detached
EXAMPLES:	Below knee amputation, disarticulation of shoulder

7 DILATION

DEFINITION:	Expanding an orifice or the lumen of a tubular body part
EXPLANATION:	The orifice can be a natural orifice or an artificially created orifice. Accomplished by stretching a tubular body part using intraluminal pressure or by cutting part of the orifice or wall of the tubular body part.
EXAMPLES:	Percutaneous transluminal angioplasty, internal urethrotomy

8 DIVISION

DEFINITION:	Cutting into a body part, without draining fluids and/or gases from the body part, in order to separate or transect a body part
EXPLANATION:	All or a portion of the body part is separated into two or more portions
EXAMPLES:	Spinal cordotomy, osteotomy

9 DRAINAGE

DEFINITION:	Taking or letting out fluids and/or gases from a body part
EXPLANATION:	The qualifier DIAGNOSTIC is used to identify drainage procedures that are biopsies
EXAMPLES:	Thoracentesis, incision and drainage

B EXCISION

DEFINITION:	Cutting out or off, without replacement, a portion of a body part
EXPLANATION:	The qualifier DIAGNOSTIC is used to identify excision procedures that are biopsies
EXAMPLES:	Partial nephrectomy, liver biopsy

C EXTIRPATION

DEFINITION:	Taking or cutting out solid matter from a body part
EXPLANATION:	The solid matter may be an abnormal byproduct of a biological function or a foreign body; it may be imbedded in a body part or in the lumen of a tubular body part. The solid matter may or may not have been previously broken into pieces.
EXAMPLES:	Thrombectomy, choledocholithotomy

© 2018 Channel Publishing, Ltd.

D EXTRACTION	DEFINITION: Pulling or stripping out or off all or a portion of a body part by the use of force
EXPLANATION:	The qualifier DIAGNOSTIC is used to identify extraction procedures that are biopsies
EXAMPLES:	Dilation and curettage, vein stripping

F FRAGMENTATION	DEFINITION: Breaking solid matter in a body part into pieces
EXPLANATION:	Physical force (e.g., manual, ultrasonic) applied directly or indirectly is used to break the solid matter into pieces. The solid matter may be an abnormal byproduct of a biological function or a foreign body. The pieces of solid matter are not taken out.
EXAMPLES:	Extracorporeal shockwave lithotripsy, transurethral lithotripsy

G FUSION	DEFINITION: Joining together portions of an articular body part rendering the articular body part immobile
EXPLANATION:	The body part is joined together by fixation device, bone graft, or other means
EXAMPLES:	Spinal fusion, ankle arthrodesis

H INSERTION	DEFINITION: Putting in a nonbiological appliance that monitors, assists, performs or prevents a physiological function but does not physically take the place of a body part
EXPLANATION:	None
EXAMPLES:	Insertion of radioactive implant, insertion of central venous catheter

J INSPECTION	DEFINITION: Visually and/or manually exploring a body part
EXPLANATION:	Visual exploration may be performed with or without optical instrumentation. Manual exploration may be performed directly or through intervening body layers
EXAMPLES:	Diagnostic arthroscopy, exploratory laparotomy

K MAP	DEFINITION: Locating the route of passage of electrical impulses and/or locating functional areas in a body part
EXPLANATION:	Applicable only to the cardiac conduction mechanism and the central nervous system
EXAMPLES:	Cardiac mapping, cortical mapping

L OCCLUSION	DEFINITION: Completely closing an orifice or the lumen of a tubular body part
EXPLANATION:	The orifice can be a natural orifice or an artificially created orifice
EXAMPLES:	Fallopian tube ligation, ligation of inferior vena cava

© 2018 Channel Publishing, Ltd.

M REATTACHMENT	DEFINITION: Putting back in or on all or a portion of a separated body part to its normal location or other suitable location
EXPLANATION:	Vascular circulation and nervous pathways may or may not be reestablished
EXAMPLES:	Reattachment of hand, reattachment of avulsed kidney

N RELEASE	DEFINITION: Freeing a body part from an abnormal physical constraint by cutting or by the use of force
EXPLANATION:	Some of the restraining tissue may be taken out but none of the body part is taken out
EXAMPLES:	Adhesiolysis, carpal tunnel release

P REMOVAL	DEFINITION: Taking out or off a device from a body part
EXPLANATION:	If a device is taken out and a similar device put in without cutting or puncturing the skin or mucous membrane, the procedure is coded to the root operation CHANGE. Otherwise, the procedure for taking out a device is coded to the root operation REMOVAL.
EXAMPLES:	Drainage tube removal, cardiac pacemaker removal

Q REPAIR	DEFINITION: Restoring, to the extent possible, a body part to its normal anatomic structure and function
EXPLANATION:	Used only when the method to accomplish the repair is not one of the other root operations
EXAMPLES:	Colostomy takedown, suture of laceration

R REPLACEMENT	DEFINITION: Putting in or on biological or synthetic material that physically takes the place and/or function of all or a portion of a body part
EXPLANATION:	The body part may have been taken out or replaced, or may be taken out, physically eradicated, or rendered non-functional during the REPLACEMENT procedure. A REMOVAL procedure is coded for taking out the device used in a previous replacement procedure.
EXAMPLES:	Total hip replacement, bone graft, free skin graft

S REPOSITION	DEFINITION: Moving to its normal location, or other suitable location, all or a portion of a body part
EXPLANATION:	The body part is moved to a new location from an abnormal location, or from a normal location where it is not functioning correctly. The body part may or may not be cut out or off to be moved to the new location.
EXAMPLES:	Reposition of undescended testicle, fracture reduction

T RESECTION	DEFINITION: Cutting out or off, without replacement, all of a body part
EXPLANATION:	None
EXAMPLES:	Total nephrectomy, total lobectomy of lung

© 2018 Channel Publishing, Ltd.

V RESTRICTION	DEFINITION: Partially closing an orifice or the lumen of a tubular body part
EXPLANATION:	The orifice can be a natural orifice or an artificially created orifice
EXAMPLES:	Esophagogastric fundoplication, cervical cerclage

W REVISION	DEFINITION: Correcting, to the extent possible, a portion of a malfunctioning device or the position of a displaced device
EXPLANATION:	Revision can include correcting a malfunctioning or displaced device by taking out or putting in components of the device such as a screw or pin
EXAMPLES:	Adjustment of position of pacemaker lead, recementing of hip prosthesis

U SUPPLEMENT	DEFINITION: Putting in or on biologic or synthetic material that physically reinforces and/or augments the function of a portion of a body part
EXPLANATION:	The biological material is non-living, or is living and from the same individual. The body part may have been previously replaced, and the Supplement procedure is performed to physically reinforce and/or augment the function of the replaced body part.
EXAMPLES:	Herniorrhaphy using mesh, free nerve graft, mitral valve ring annuloplasty, put a new acetabular liner in a previous hip replacement

X TRANSFER	DEFINITION: Moving, without taking out, all or a portion of a body part to another location to take over the function of all or a portion of a body part
EXPLANATION:	The body part transferred remains connected to its vascular and nervous supply
EXAMPLES:	Tendon transfer, skin pedicle flap transfer

Y TRANSPLANTATION	DEFINITION: Putting in or on all or a portion of a living body part taken from another individual or animal to physically take the place and/or function of all or a portion of a similar body part
EXPLANATION:	The native body part may or may not be taken out, and the transplanted body part may take over all or a portion of its function
EXAMPLES:	Kidney transplant, heart transplant

© 2018 Channel Publishing, Ltd.

Root operation/type definitions, explanations, and examples of the Medical- and Surgical-Related Section and the Ancillary Section are found at the specific code tables in their respective sections.

APPENDIX B
APPROACH DEFINITIONS OF THE MEDICAL AND SURGICAL SECTION

0 OPEN	DEFINITION: Cutting through the skin or mucous membrane and any other body layers necessary to expose the site of the procedure
EXPLANATION:	Includes "laparoscopic-assisted" open approach procedures
EXAMPLES:	Kidney tranplant, laparoscopic-assisted sigmoidectomy

3 PERCUTANEOUS	DEFINITION: Entry, by puncture or minor incision, of instrumentation through the skin or mucous membrane and any other body layers necessary to reach the site of the procedure
EXPLANATION:	Includes procedures performed percutaneously via device placed for the procedure
EXAMPLES:	Needle biopsy of liver, fragmentation of kidney stone performed via percutaneous nephrostomy

4 PERCUTANEOUS ENDOSCOPIC	DEFINITION: Entry, by puncture or minor incision, of instrumentation through the skin or mucous membrane and any other body layers necessary to reach and visualize the site of the procedure
EXPLANATION:	Percutaneous procedures using visualization
EXAMPLES:	Laparoscopic cholecystectomy, arthroscopy

7 VIA NATURAL OR ARTIFICIAL OPENING	DEFINITION: Entry of instrumentation through a natural or artificial external opening to reach the site of the procedure
EXPLANATION:	Access entry through natural or artificial external opening WITHOUT visualization
EXAMPLES:	Insertion of urinary catheter, insertion of endotracheal tube

8 VIA NATURAL OR ARTIFICIAL OPENING ENDOSCOPIC	DEFINITION: Entry of instrumentation through a natural or artificial external opening to reach and visualize the site of the procedure
EXPLANATION:	Access entry through natural or artificial external opening using visualization
EXAMPLES:	Bronchoscopy, colonoscopy with biopsy

F VIA NATURAL OR ARTIFICIAL OPENING WITH PERCUTANEOUS ENDOSCOPIC ASSISTANCE	DEFINITION: Entry of instrumentation through a natural or artificial external opening and entry, by puncture or minor incision, of instrumentation through the skin or mucous membrane and any other body layers necessary to aid in the performance of the procedure
EXPLANATION:	Access entry through natural or artificial external opening AND using a separate percutaneous visualization
EXAMPLES:	Laparoscopic-assisted vaginal hysterectomy

X EXTERNAL	DEFINITION: Procedures performed directly on the skin or mucous membrane and procedures performed indirectly by the application of external force through the skin or mucous membrane
EXPLANATION:	Includes procedures performed within an orifice on structures that are visible without the aid of any instrumentation
EXAMPLES:	Closed reduction of fracture, suture of laceration, tonsillectomy

© 2018 Channel Publishing, Ltd.

NOTES

© 2018 Channel Publishing, Ltd.

BODY PART	USE:
Biceps brachii muscle	*use* Upper Arm Muscle, Left/Right
Biceps femoris muscle	*use* Upper Leg Muscle, Left/Right
Bicipital aponeurosis	*use* Subcutaneous Tissue and Fascia, Lower Arm, Left/Right
Bicuspid valve	*use* Mitral Valve
Body of femur	*use* Femoral Shaft, Left/Right
Body of fibula	*use* Fibula, Left/Right
Bony labyrinth	*use* Inner Ear, Left/Right
Bony orbit	*use* Orbit, Left/Right
Bony vestibule	*use* Inner Ear, Left/Right
Botallo's duct	*use* Pulmonary Artery, Left
Brachial (lateral) lymph node	*use* Lymphatic, Axillary, Left/Right
Brachialis muscle	*use* Upper Arm Muscle, Left/Right
Brachiocephalic artery Brachiocephalic trunk	*use* Innominate Artery
Brachiocephalic vein	*use* Innominate Vein, Left/Right
Brachioradialis muscle	*use* Lower Arm and Wrist Muscle, Left/Right
Broad ligament	*use* Uterine Supporting Structure
Bronchial artery	*use* Upper Artery
Bronchus intermedius	*use* Main Bronchus, Right
Buccal gland	*use* Buccal Mucosa
Buccinator lymph node	*use* Lymphatic, Head
Buccinator muscle	*use* Facial Muscle
Bulbospongiosus muscle	*use* Perineum Muscle
Bulbourethral (Cowper's) gland	*use* Urethra
Bundle of His Bundle of Kent	*use* Conduction Mechanism
Calcaneocuboid joint	*use* Tarsal Joint, Left/Right
Calcaneocuboid ligament	*use* Foot Bursa and Ligament, Left/Right
Calcaneofibular ligament	*use* Ankle Bursa and Ligament, Left/Right
Calcaneus	*use* Tarsal, Left/Right
Capitate bone	*use* Carpal, Left/Right
Cardia	*use* Esophagogastric Junction
Cardiac plexus	*use* Thoracic Sympathetic Nerve
Cardioesophageal junction	*use* Esophagogastric Junction
Caroticotympanic artery	*use* Internal Carotid Artery, Left/Right
Carotid glomus	*use* Carotid Body, Bilateral/Left/Right
Carotid sinus	*use* Internal Carotid Artery, Left/Right
Carotid sinus nerve	*use* Glossopharyngeal Nerve
Carpometacarpal ligament	*use* Hand Bursa and Ligament, Left/Right
Cauda equina	*use* Lumbar Spinal Cord
Cavernous plexus	*use* Head and Neck Sympathetic Nerve
Celiac (solar) plexus Celiac ganglion	*use* Abdominal Sympathetic Nerve
Celiac lymph node	*use* Lymphatic, Aortic
Celiac trunk	*use* Celiac Artery

BODY PART	USE:
Central axillary lymph node	*use* Lymphatic, Axillary, Left/Right
Cerebral aqueduct (Sylvius)	*use* Cerebral Ventricle
Cerebrum	*use* Brain
Cervical esophagus	*use* Esophagus, Upper
Cervical facet joint	*use* Cervical Vertebral Joint(s)
Cervical ganglion	*use* Head and Neck Sympathetic Nerve
Cervical interspinous ligament Cervical intertransverse ligament Cervical ligamentum flavum	*use* Head and Neck Bursa and Ligament
Cervical lymph node	*use* Lymphatic, Neck, Left/Right
Cervicothoracic facet joint	*use* Cervicothoracic Vertebral Joint
Choana	*use* Nasopharynx
Chondroglossus muscle	*use* Tongue, Palate, Pharynx Muscle
Chorda tympani	*use* Facial Nerve
Choroid plexus	*use* Cerebral Ventricle
Ciliary body	*use* Eye, Left/Right
Ciliary ganglion	*use* Head and Neck Sympathetic Nerve
Circle of Willis	*use* Intracranial Artery
Circumflex iliac artery	*use* Femoral Artery, Left/Right
Claustrum	*use* Basal Ganglia
Coccygeal body	*use* Coccygeal Glomus
Coccygeus muscle	*use* Trunk Muscle, Left/Right
Cochlea	*use* Inner Ear, Left/Right
Cochlear nerve	*use* Acoustic Nerve
Columella	*use* Nasal Mucosa and Soft Tissue
Common digital vein	*use* Foot Vein, Left/Right
Common facial vein	*use* Face Vein, Left/Right
Common fibular nerve	*use* Peroneal Nerve
Common hepatic artery	*use* Hepatic Artery
Common iliac (subaortic) lymph node	*use* Lymphatic, Pelvis
Common interosseous artery	*use* Ulnar Artery, Left/Right
Common peroneal nerve	*use* Peroneal Nerve
Condyloid process	*use* Mandible, Left/Right
Conus arteriosus	*use* Ventricle, Right
Conus medullaris	*use* Lumbar Spinal Cord
Coracoacromial ligament	*use* Shoulder Bursa and Ligament, Left/Right
Coracobrachialis muscle	*use* Upper Arm Muscle, Left/Right
Coracoclavicular ligament Coracohumeral ligament	*use* Shoulder Bursa and Ligament, Left/Right
Coracoid process	*use* Scapula, Left/Right
Corniculate cartilage	*use* Larynx
Corpus callosum	*use* Brain
Corpus cavernosum Corpus spongiosum	*use* Penis

APPENDIX C

© 2018 Channel Publishing, Ltd.

BODY PART	USE:
Corpus striatum	*use* Basal Ganglia
Corrugator supercilii muscle	*use* Facial Muscle
Costocervical trunk	*use* Subclavian Artery, Left/Right
Costoclavicular ligament	*use* Shoulder Bursa and Ligament, Left/Right
Costotransverse joint	*use* Thoracic Vertebral Joint
Costotransverse ligament	*use* Rib(s) Bursa and Ligament
Costovertebral joint	*use* Thoracic Vertebral Joint
Costoxiphoid ligament	*use* Sternum Bursa and Ligament
Cowper's (bulbourethral) gland	*use* Urethra
Cremaster muscle	*use* Perineum Muscle
Cribriform plate	*use* Ethmoid Bone, Left/Right
Cricoid cartilage	*use* Trachea
Cricothyroid artery	*use* Thyroid Artery, Left/Right
Cricothyroid muscle	*use* Neck Muscle, Left/Right
Crural fascia	*use* Subcutaneous Tissue and Fascia, Upper Leg, Left/Right
Cubital lymph node	*use* Lymphatic, Upper Extremity, Left/Right
Cubital nerve	*use* Ulnar Nerve
Cuboid bone	*use* Tarsal, Left/Right
Cuboideonavicular joint	*use* Tarsal Joint, Left/Right
Culmen	*use* Cerebellum
Cuneiform cartilage	*use* Larynx
Cuneonavicular joint	*use* Tarsal Joint, Left/Right
Cuneonavicular ligament	*use* Foot Bursa and Ligament, Left/Right
Cutaneous (transverse) cervical nerve	*use* Cervical Plexus
Deep cervical fascia	*use* Subcutaneous Tissue and Fascia, Neck, Left/Right
Deep cervical vein	*use* Vertebral Vein, Left/Right
Deep circumflex iliac artery	*use* External Iliac Artery, Left/Right
Deep facial vein	*use* Face Vein, Left/Right
Deep femoral artery	*use* Femoral Artery, Left/Right
Deep femoral (profunda femoris) vein	*use* Femoral Vein, Left/Right
Deep palmar arch	*use* Hand Artery, Left/Right
Deep transverse perineal muscle	*use* Perineum Muscle
Deferential artery	*use* Internal Iliac Artery, Left/Right
Deltoid fascia	*use* Subcutaneous Tissue and Fascia, Upper Arm, Left/Right
Deltoid ligament	*use* Ankle Bursa and Ligament, Left/Right
Deltoid muscle	*use* Shoulder Muscle, Left/Right
Deltopectoral (infraclavicular) lymph node	*use* Lymphatic, Upper Extremity, Left/Right

BODY PART	USE:
Dens	*use* Cervical Vertebra
Denticulate (dentate) ligament	*use* Spinal Meninges
Depressor anguli oris muscle Depressor labii inferioris muscle Depressor septi nasi muscle Depressor supercilii muscle	*use* Facial Muscle
Dermis	*use* Skin
Descending genicular artery	*use* Femoral Artery, Left/Right
Diaphragma sellae	*use* Dura Mater
Distal humerus	*use* Humeral Shaft, Left/Right
Distal humerus, involving joint	*use* Elbow Joint, Left/Right
Distal radioulnar joint	*use* Wrist Joint, Left/Right
Dorsal digital nerve	*use* Radial Nerve
Dorsal metacarpal vein	*use* Hand Vein, Left/Right
Dorsal metatarsal artery	*use* Foot Artery, Left/Right
Dorsal metatarsal vein	*use* Foot Vein, Left/Right
Dorsal scapular artery	*use* Subclavian Artery, Left/Right
Dorsal scapular nerve	*use* Brachial Plexus
Dorsal venous arch	*use* Foot Vein, Left/Right
Dorsalis pedis artery	*use* Anterior Tibial Artery, Left/Right
Duct of Santorini	*use* Pancreatic Duct, Accessory
Duct of Wirsung	*use* Pancreatic Duct
Ductus deferens	*use* Vas Deferens, Bilateral/Left/Right
Duodenal ampulla	*use* Ampulla of Vater
Duodenojejunal flexure	*use* Jejunum
Dura mater, intracranial	*use* Dura Mater
Dura mater, spinal	*use* Spinal Meninges
Dural venous sinus	*use* Intracranial Vein
Earlobe	*use* External Ear, Bilateral/Left/Right
Eighth cranial nerve	*use* Acoustic Nerve
Ejaculatory duct	*use* Vas Deferens, Bilateral/Left/Right
Eleventh cranial nerve	*use* Accessory Nerve
Encephalon	*use* Brain
Ependyma	*use* Cerebral Ventricle
Epidermis	*use* Skin
Epidural space, spinal	*use* Spinal Canal
Epiploic foramen	*use* Peritoneum
Epithalamus	*use* Thalamus
Epitrochlear lymph node	*use* Lymphatic, Upper Extremity, Left/Right
Erector spinae muscle	*use* Trunk Muscle, Left/Right
Esophageal artery	*use* Upper Artery
Esophageal plexus	*use* Thoracic Sympathetic Nerve
Ethmoidal air cell	*use* Ethmoid Sinus, Left/Right

© 2018 Channel Publishing, Ltd.

BODY PART	USE:
Extensor carpi radialis muscle Extensor carpi ulnaris muscle	*use* Lower Arm and Wrist Muscle, Left/Right
Extensor digitorum brevis muscle	*use* Foot Muscle, Left/Right
Extensor digitorum longus muscle	*use* Lower Leg Muscle, Left/Right
Extensor hallucis brevis muscle	*use* Foot Muscle, Left/Right
Extensor hallucis longus muscle	*use* Lower Leg Muscle, Left/Right
External anal sphincter	*use* Anal Sphincter
External auditory meatus	*use* External Auditory Canal, Left/Right
External maxillary artery	*use* Face Artery
External naris	*use* Nasal Mucosa and Soft Tissue
External oblique aponeurosis	*use* Subcutaneous Tissue and Fascia, Trunk
External oblique muscle	*use* Abdomen Muscle, Left/Right
External popliteal nerve	*use* Peroneal Nerve
External pudendal artery	*use* Femoral Artery, Left/Right
External pudendal vein	*use* Saphenous Vein, Left/Right
External urethral sphincter	*use* Urethra
Extradural space, intracranial	*use* Epidural Space, Intracranial
Extradural space, spinal	*use* Spinal Canal
Facial artery	*use* Face Artery
False vocal cord	*use* Larynx
Falx cerebri	*use* Dura Mater
Fascia lata	*use* Subcutaneous Tissue and Fascia, Upper Leg, Left/Right
Femoral head	*use* Upper Femur, Left/Right
Femoral lymph node	*use* Lymphatic, Lower Extremity, Left/Right
Femoropatellar joint	*use* Knee Joint, Left/Right *use* Knee Joint, Femoral Surface, Left/Right
Femorotibial joint	*use* Knee Joint, Left/Right *use* Knee Joint, Tibial Surface, Left/Right
Fibular artery	*use* Peroneal Artery, Left/Right
Fibularis brevis muscle Fibularis longus muscle	*use* Lower Leg Muscle, Left/Right
Fifth cranial nerve	*use* Trigeminal Nerve
Filum terminale	*use* Spinal Meninges
First cranial nerve	*use* Olfactory Nerve
First intercostal nerve	*use* Brachial Plexus
Flexor carpi radialis muscle Flexor carpi ulnaris muscle	*use* Lower Arm and Wrist Muscle, Left/Right

BODY PART	USE:
Flexor digitorum brevis muscle	*use* Foot Muscle, Left/Right
Flexor digitorum longus muscle	*use* Lower Leg Muscle, Left/Right
Flexor hallucis brevis muscle	*use* Foot Muscle, Left/Right
Flexor hallucis longus muscle	*use* Lower Leg Muscle, Left/Right
Flexor pollicis longus muscle	*use* Lower Arm and Wrist Muscle, Left/Right
Foramen magnum	*use* Occipital Bone
Foramen of Monro (intraventricular)	*use* Cerebral Ventricle
Foreskin	*use* Prepuce
Fossa of Rosenmuller	*use* Nasopharynx
Fourth cranial nerve	*use* Trochlear Nerve
Fourth ventricle	*use* Cerebral Ventricle
Fovea	*use* Retina, Left/Right
Frenulum labii inferioris	*use* Lower Lip
Frenulum labii superioris	*use* Upper Lip
Frenulum linguae	*use* Tongue
Frontal lobe	*use* Cerebral Hemisphere
Frontal vein	*use* Face Vein, Left/Right
Fundus uteri	*use* Uterus
Galea aponeurotica	*use* Subcutaneous Tissue and Fascia, Scalp
Ganglion impar (ganglion of Walther)	*use* Sacral Sympathetic Nerve
Gasserian ganglion	*use* Trigeminal Nerve
Gastric lymph node	*use* Lymphatic, Aortic
Gastric plexus	*use* Abdominal Sympathetic Nerve
Gastrocnemius muscle	*use* Lower Leg Muscle, Left/Right
Gastrocolic ligament Gastrocolic omentum	*use* Omentum
Gastroduodenal artery	*use* Hepatic Artery
Gastroesophageal (GE) junction	*use* Esophagogastric Junction
Gastrohepatic omentum Gastrophrenic ligament Gastrosplenic ligament	*use* Omentum
Gemellus muscle	*use* Hip Muscle, Left/Right
Geniculate ganglion	*use* Facial Nerve
Geniculate nucleus	*use* Thalamus
Genioglossus muscle	*use* Tongue, Palate, Pharynx Muscle
Genitofemoral nerve	*use* Lumbar Plexus
Glans penis	*use* Prepuce
Glenohumeral joint	*use* Shoulder Joint, Left/Right
Glenohumeral ligament	*use* Shoulder Bursa and Ligament, Left/Right
Glenoid fossa (of scapula)	*use* Glenoid Cavity, Left/Right
Glenoid ligament (labrum)	*use* Shoulder Joint, Left/Right
Globus pallidus	*use* Basal Ganglia
Glossoepiglottic fold	*use* Epiglottis

© 2018 Channel Publishing, Ltd.

BODY PART	USE:
Glottis	*use* Larynx
Gluteal lymph node	*use* Lymphatic, Pelvis
Gluteal vein	*use* Hypogastric Vein, Left/Right
Gluteus maximus muscle Gluteus medius muscle Gluteus minimus muscle	*use* Hip Muscle, Left/Right
Gracilis muscle	*use* Upper Leg Muscle, Left/Right
Great auricular nerve	*use* Cervical Plexus
Great cerebral vein	*use* Intracranial Vein
Great(er) saphenous vein	*use* Saphenous Vein, Left/Right
Greater alar cartilage	*use* Nasal Mucosa and Soft Tissue
Greater occipital nerve	*use* Cervical Nerve
Greater omentum	*use* Omentum
Greater splanchnic nerve	*use* Thoracic Sympathetic Nerve
Greater superficial petrosal nerve	*use* Facial Nerve
Greater trochanter	*use* Upper Femur, Left/Right
Greater tuberosity	*use* Humeral Head, Left/Right
Greater vestibular (Bartholin's) gland	*use* Vestibular Gland
Greater wing	*use* Sphenoid Bone
Hallux	*use* 1st Toe, Left/Right
Hamate bone	*use* Carpal, Left/Right
Head of fibula	*use* Fibula, Left/Right
Helix	*use* External Ear, Bilateral/Left/Right
Hepatic artery proper	*use* Hepatic Artery
Hepatic flexure	*use* Transverse Colon
Hepatic lymph node	*use* Lymphatic, Aortic
Hepatic plexus	*use* Abdominal Sympathetic Nerve
Hepatic portal vein	*use* Portal Vein
Hepatogastric ligament	*use* Omentum
Hepatopancreatic ampulla	*use* Ampulla of Vater
Humeroradial joint Humeroulnar joint	*use* Elbow Joint, Left/Right
Humerus, distal	*use* Humeral Shaft, Left/Right
Hyoglossus muscle	*use* Tongue, Palate, Pharynx Muscle
Hyoid artery	*use* Thyroid Artery, Left/Right
Hypogastric artery	*use* Internal Iliac Artery, Left/Right
Hypopharynx	*use* Pharynx
Hypophysis	*use* Pituitary Gland
Hypothenar muscle	*use* Hand Muscle, Left/Right
Ileal artery Ileocolic artery	*use* Superior Mesenteric Artery
Ileocolic vein	*use* Colic Vein
Iliac crest	*use* Pelvic Bone, Left/Right
Iliac fascia	*use* Subcutaneous Tissue and Fascia, Upper Leg, Left/Right
Iliac lymph node	*use* Lymphatic, Pelvis
Iliacus muscle	*use* Hip Muscle, Left/Right
Iliofemoral ligament	*use* Hip Bursa and Ligament, Left/Right
Iliohypogastric nerve Ilioinguinal nerve	*use* Lumbar Plexus

BODY PART	USE:
Iliolumbar artery	*use* Internal Iliac Artery, Left/Right
Iliolumbar ligament	*use* Lower Spine Bursa and Ligament
Iliotibial tract (band)	*use* Subcutaneous Tissue and Fascia, Upper Leg, Left/Right
Ilium	*use* Pelvic Bone, Left/Right
Incus	*use* Auditory Ossicle, Left/Right
Inferior cardiac nerve	*use* Thoracic Sympathetic Nerve
Inferior cerebellar vein Inferior cerebral vein	*use* Intracranial Vein
Inferior epigastric artery	*use* External Iliac Artery, Left/Right
Inferior epigastric lymph node	*use* Lymphatic, Pelvis
Inferior genicular artery	*use* Popliteal Artery, Left/Right
Inferior gluteal artery	*use* Internal Iliac Artery, Left/Right
Inferior gluteal nerve	*use* Sacral Plexus
Inferior hypogastric plexus	*use* Abdominal Sympathetic Nerve
Inferior labial artery	*use* Face Artery
Inferior longitudinal muscle	*use* Tongue, Palate, Pharynx Muscle
Inferior mesenteric ganglion	*use* Abdominal Sympathetic Nerve
Inferior mesenteric lymph node	*use* Lymphatic, Mesenteric
Inferior mesenteric plexus	*use* Abdominal Sympathetic Nerve
Inferior oblique muscle	*use* Extraocular Muscle, Left/Right
Inferior pancreatico-duodenal artery	*use* Superior Mesenteric Artery
Inferior phrenic artery	*use* Abdominal Aorta
Inferior rectus muscle	*use* Extraocular Muscle, Left/Right
Inferior suprarenal artery	*use* Renal Artery, Left/Right
Inferior tarsal plate	*use* Lower Eyelid, Left/Right
Inferior thyroid vein	*use* Innominate Vein, Left/Right
Inferior tibiofibular joint	*use* Ankle Joint, Left/Right
Inferior turbinate	*use* Nasal Turbinate
Inferior ulnar collateral artery	*use* Brachial Artery, Left/Right
Inferior vesical artery	*use* Internal Iliac Artery, Left/Right
Infraauricular lymph node	*use* Lymphatic, Head
Infraclavicular (delto-pectoral) lymph node	*use* Lymphatic, Upper Extremity, Left/Right
Infrahyoid muscle	*use* Neck Muscle, Left/Right
Infraparotid lymph node	*use* Lymphatic, Head
Infraspinatus fascia	*use* Subcutaneous Tissue and Fascia, Upper Arm, Left/Right
Infraspinatus muscle	*use* Shoulder Muscle, Left/Right
Infundibulopelvic ligament	*use* Uterine Supporting Structure
Inguinal canal Inguinal triangle	*use* Inguinal Region, Bilateral/Left/Right
Interatrial septum	*use* Atrial Septum
Intercarpal joint	*use* Carpal Joint, Left/Right
Intercarpal ligament	*use* Hand Bursa and Ligament, Left/Right

© 2018 Channel Publishing, Ltd.

BODY PART	USE:
Interclavicular ligament	*use* Shoulder Bursa and Ligament, Left/Right
Intercostal lymph node	*use* Lymphatic, Thorax
Intercostal muscle	*use* Thorax Muscle, Left/Right
Intercostal nerve Intercostobrachial nerve	*use* Thoracic Nerve
Intercuneiform joint	*use* Tarsal Joint, Left/Right
Intercuneiform ligament	*use* Foot Bursa and Ligament, Left/Right
Intermediate bronchus	*use* Main Bronchus, Right
Intermediate cuneiform bone	*use* Tarsal, Left/Right
Internal (basal) cerebral vein	*use* Intracranial Vein
Internal anal sphincter	*use* Anal Sphincter
Internal carotid artery, intracranial portion	*use* Intracranial Artery
Internal carotid plexus	*use* Head and Neck Sympathetic Nerve
Internal iliac vein	*use* Hypogastric Vein, Left/Right
Internal maxillary artery	*use* External Carotid Artery, Left/Right
Internal naris	*use* Nasal Mucosa and Soft Tissue
Internal oblique muscle	*use* Abdomen Muscle, Left/Right
Internal pudendal artery	*use* Internal Iliac Artery, Left/Right
Internal pudendal vein	*use* Hypogastric Vein, Left/Right
Internal thoracic artery	*use* Internal Mammary Artery, Left/Right Subclavian Artery, Left/Right
Internal urethral sphincter	*use* Urethra
Interphalangeal (IP) joint	*use* Finger Phalangeal Joint, Left/Right Toe Phalangeal Joint, Left/Right
Interphalangeal ligament	*use* Hand Bursa and Ligament, Left/Right Foot Bursa and Ligament, Left/Right
Interspinalis muscle	*use* Trunk Muscle, Left/Right
Interspinous ligament, cervical	*use* Head and Neck Bursa and Ligament
Interspinous ligament, lumbar	*use* Lower Spine Bursa and Ligament
Interspinous ligament, thoracic	*use* Upper Spine Bursa and Ligament
Intertransversarius muscle	*use* Trunk Muscle, Left/Right
Intertransverse ligament, cervical	*use* Head and Neck Bursa and Ligament
Intertransverse ligament, lumbar	*use* Lower Spine Bursa and Ligament
Intertransverse ligament, thoracic	*use* Upper Spine Bursa and Ligament
Interventricular foramen (Monro)	*use* Cerebral Ventricle
Interventricular septum	*use* Ventricular Septum

BODY PART	USE:
Intestinal lymphatic trunk	*use* Cisterna Chyli
Ischiatic nerve	*use* Sciatic Nerve
Ischiocavernosus muscle	*use* Perineum Muscle
Ischiofemoral ligament	*use* Hip Bursa and Ligament, Left/Right
Ischium	*use* Pelvic Bone, Left/Right
Jejunal artery	*use* Superior Mesenteric Artery
Jugular body	*use* Glomus Jugulare
Jugular lymph node	*use* Lymphatic, Neck, Left/Right
Labia majora Labia minora	*use* Vulva
Labial gland	*use* Upper Lip, Lower Lip
Lacrimal canaliculus Lacrimal punctum Lacrimal sac	*use* Lacrimal Duct, Left/Right
Laryngopharynx	*use* Pharynx
Lateral (brachial) lymph node	*use* Lymphatic, Axillary, Left/Right
Lateral canthus	*use* Upper Eyelid, Left/Right
Lateral collateral ligament (LCL)	*use* Knee Bursa and Ligament, Left/Right
Lateral condyle of femur	*use* Lower Femur, Left/Right
Lateral condyle of tibia	*use* Tibia, Left/Right
Lateral cuneiform bone	*use* Tarsal, Left/Right
Lateral epicondyle of femur	*use* Lower Femur, Left/Right
Lateral epicondyle of humerus	*use* Humeral Shaft, Left/Right
Lateral femoral cutaneous nerve	*use* Lumbar Plexus
Lateral malleolus	*use* Fibula, Left/Right
Lateral meniscus	*use* Knee Joint, Left/Right
Lateral nasal cartilage	*use* Nasal Mucosa and Soft Tissue
Lateral plantar artery	*use* Foot Artery, Left/Right
Lateral plantar nerve	*use* Tibial Nerve
Lateral rectus muscle	*use* Extraocular Muscle, Left/Right
Lateral sacral artery	*use* Internal Iliac Artery, Left/Right
Lateral sacral vein	*use* Hypogastric Vein, Left/Right
Lateral sural cutaneous nerve	*use* Peroneal Nerve
Lateral tarsal artery	*use* Foot Artery, Left/Right
Lateral temporo-mandibular ligament	*use* Head and Neck Bursa and Ligament
Lateral thoracic artery	*use* Axillary Artery, Left/Right
Latissimus dorsi muscle	*use* Trunk Muscle, Left/Right
Least splanchnic nerve	*use* Thoracic Sympathetic Nerve
Left ascending lumbar vein	*use* Hemiazygos Vein
Left atrioventricular valve	*use* Mitral Valve
Left auricular appendix	*use* Atrium, Left
Left colic vein	*use* Colic Vein
Left coronary sulcus	*use* Heart, Left
Left gastric artery	*use* Gastric Artery

© 2018 Channel Publishing, Ltd.

BODY PART	USE:
Left gastroepiploic artery	*use* Splenic Artery
Left gastroepiploic vein	*use* Splenic Vein
Left inferior phrenic vein	*use* Renal Vein, Left
Left inferior pulmonary vein	*use* Pulmonary Vein, Left
Left jugular trunk	*use* Thoracic Duct
Left lateral ventricle	*use* Cerebral Ventricle
Left ovarian vein Left second lumbar vein	*use* Renal Vein, Left
Left subclavian trunk	*use* Thoracic Duct
Left subcostal vein	*use* Hemiazygos Vein
Left superior pulmonary vein	*use* Pulmonary Vein, Left
Left suprarenal vein Left testicular vein	*use* Renal Vein, Left
Leptomeninges, intracranial	*use* Cerebral Meninges
Leptomeninges, spinal	*use* Spinal Meninges
Lesser alar cartilage	*use* Nasal Mucosa and Soft Tissue
Lesser occipital nerve	*use* Cervical Plexus
Lesser omentum	*use* Omentum
Lesser saphenous vein	*use* Saphenous Vein, Left/Right
Lesser splanchnic nerve	*use* Thoracic Sympathetic Nerve
Lesser trochanter	*use* Upper Femur, Left/Right
Lesser tuberosity	*use* Humeral Head, Left/Right
Lesser wing	*use* Sphenoid Bone
Levator anguli oris muscle	*use* Facial Muscle
Levator ani muscle	*use* Perineum Muscle
Levator labii superioris alaeque nasi muscle Levator labii superioris muscle	*use* Facial Muscle
Levator palpebrae superioris muscle	*use* Upper Eyelid, Left/Right
Levator scapulae muscle	*use* Neck Muscle, Left/Right
Levator veli palatini muscle	*use* Tongue, Palate, Pharynx Muscle
Levatores costarum muscle	*use* Thorax Muscle, Left/Right
Ligament of head of fibula	*use* Knee Bursa and Ligament, Left/Right
Ligament of the lateral malleolus	*use* Ankle Bursa and Ligament, Left/Right
Ligamentum flavum, cervical	*use* Head and Neck Bursa and Ligament
Ligamentum flavum, lumbar	*use* Lower Spine Bursa and Ligament
Ligamentum flavum, thoracic	*use* Upper Spine Bursa and Ligament
Lingual artery	*use* External Carotid Artery, Left/Right
Lingual tonsil	*use* Pharynx
Locus ceruleus	*use* Pons
Long thoracic nerve	*use* Brachial Plexus

BODY PART	USE:
Lumbar artery	*use* Abdominal Aorta
Lumbar facet joint	*use* Lumbar Vertebral Joint
Lumbar ganglion	*use* Lumbar Sympathetic Nerve
Lumbar lymph node	*use* Lymphatic, Aortic
Lumbar lymphatic trunk	*use* Cisterna Chyli
Lumbar splanchnic nerve	*use* Lumbar Sympathetic Nerve
Lumbosacral facet joint	*use* Lumbosacral Joint
Lumbosacral trunk	*use* Lumbar Nerve
Lunate bone	*use* Carpal, Left/Right
Lunotriquetral ligament	*use* Hand Bursa and Ligament, Left/Right
Macula	*use* Retina, Left/Right
Malleus	*use* Auditory Ossicle, Left/Right
Mammary duct Mammary gland	*use* Breast, Bilateral/Left/Right
Mammillary body	*use* Hypothalamus
Mandibular nerve	*use* Trigeminal Nerve
Mandibular notch	*use* Mandible, Left/Right
Manubrium	*use* Sternum
Masseter muscle	*use* Head Muscle
Masseteric fascia	*use* Subcutaneous Tissue and Fascia, Face
Mastoid air cells	*use* Mastoid Sinus, Left/Right
Mastoid (postauricular) lymph node	*use* Lymphatic, Neck, Left/Right
Mastoid process	*use* Temporal Bone, Left/Right
Maxillary artery	*use* External Carotid Artery, Left/Right
Maxillary nerve	*use* Trigeminal Nerve
Medial canthus	*use* Lower Eyelid, Left/Right
Medial collateral ligament (MCL)	*use* Knee Bursa and Ligament, Left/Right
Medial condyle of femur	*use* Lower Femur, Left/Right
Medial condyle of tibia	*use* Tibia, Left/Right
Medial cuneiform bone	*use* Tarsal, Left/Right
Medial epicondyle of femur	*use* Lower Femur, Left/Right
Medial epicondyle of humerus	*use* Humeral Shaft, Left/Right
Medial malleolus	*use* Tibia, Left/Right
Medial meniscus	*use* Knee Joint, Left/Right
Medial plantar artery	*use* Foot Artery, Left/Right
Medial plantar nerve Medial popliteal nerve	*use* Tibial Nerve
Medial rectus muscle	*use* Extraocular Muscle, Left/Right
Medial sural cutaneous nerve	*use* Tibial Nerve
Median antebrachial vein Median cubital vein	*use* Basilic Vein, Left/Right
Median sacral artery	*use* Abdominal Aorta
Mediastinal cavity	*use* Mediastinum
Mediastinal lymph node	*use* Lymphatic, Thorax
Mediastinal space	*use* Mediastinum
Meissner's (submucous) plexus	*use* Abdominal Sympathetic Nerve

© 2018 Channel Publishing, Ltd.

BODY PART	USE:
Membranous urethra	*use* Urethra
Mental foramen	*use* Mandible, Left/Right
Mentalis muscle	*use* Facial Muscle
Mesoappendix Mesocolon	*use* Mesentery
Metacarpal ligament Metacarpophalangeal ligament	*use* Hand Bursa and Ligament, Left/Right
Metatarsal ligament	*use* Foot Bursa and Ligament, Left/Right
Metatarsophalangeal (MTP) joint	*use* Metatarsal-Phalangeal Joint, Left/Right
Metatarsophalangeal ligament	*use* Foot Bursa and Ligament, Left/Right
Metathalamus	*use* Thalamus
Midcarpal joint	*use* Carpal Joint, Left/Right
Middle cardiac nerve	*use* Thoracic Sympathetic Nerve
Middle cerebral artery	*use* Intracranial Artery
Middle cerebral vein	*use* Intracranial Vein
Middle colic vein	*use* Colic Vein
Middle genicular artery	*use* Popliteal Artery, Left/Right
Middle hemorrhoidal vein	*use* Hypogastric Vein, Left/Right
Middle rectal artery	*use* Internal Iliac Artery, Left/Right
Middle suprarenal artery	*use* Abdominal Aorta
Middle temporal artery	*use* Temporal Artery, Left/Right
Middle turbinate	*use* Nasal Turbinate
Mitral annulus	*use* Mitral Valve
Molar gland	*use* Buccal Mucosa
Musculocutaneous nerve	*use* Brachial Plexus
Musculophrenic artery	*use* Internal Mammary Artery, Left/Right
Musculospiral nerve	*use* Radial Nerve
Myelencephalon	*use* Medulla Oblongata
Myenteric (Auerbach's) plexus	*use* Abdominal Sympathetic Nerve
Myometrium	*use* Uterus
Nail bed, Nail plate	*use* Finger Nail, Toe Nail
Nasal cavity	*use* Nasal Mucosa and Soft Tissue
Nasal concha	*use* Nasal Turbinate
Nasalis muscle	*use* Facial Muscle
Nasolacrimal duct	*use* Lacrimal Duct, Left/Right
Navicular bone	*use* Tarsal, Left/Right
Neck of femur	*use* Upper Femur, Left/Right
Neck of humerus (anatomical) (surgical)	*use* Humeral Head, Left/Right
Nerve to the stapedius	*use* Facial Nerve
Neurohypophysis	*use* Pituitary Gland
Ninth cranial nerve	*use* Glossopharyngeal Nerve
Nostril	*use* Nasal Mucosa and Soft Tissue
Obturator artery	*use* Internal Iliac Artery, Left/Right
Obturator lymph node	*use* Lymphatic, Pelvis
Obturator muscle	*use* Hip Muscle, Left/Right
Obturator nerve	*use* Lumbar Plexus
Obturator vein	*use* Hypogastric Vein, Left/Right

BODY PART	USE:
Obtuse margin	*use* Heart, Left
Occipital artery	*use* External Carotid Artery, Left/Right
Occipital lobe	*use* Cerebral Hemisphere
Occipital lymph node	*use* Lymphatic, Neck, Left/Right
Occipitofrontalis muscle	*use* Facial Muscle
Odontoid process	*use* Cervical Vertebra
Olecranon bursa	*use* Elbow Bursa and Ligament, Left/Right
Olecranon process	*use* Ulna, Left/Right
Olfactory bulb	*use* Olfactory Nerve
Ophthalmic artery	*use* Intracranial Artery
Ophthalmic nerve	*use* Trigeminal Nerve
Ophthalmic vein	*use* Intracranial Vein
Optic chiasma	*use* Optic Nerve
Optic disc	*use* Retina, Left/Right
Optic foramen	*use* Sphenoid Bone
Orbicularis oculi muscle	*use* Upper Eyelid, Left/Right
Orbicularis oris muscle	*use* Facial Muscle
Orbital fascia	*use* Subcutaneous Tissue and Fascia, Face
Orbital portion of: ethmoid bone, frontal bone, lacrimal bone, maxilla, palatine bone, sphenoid bone, zygomatic bone	*use* Orbit, Left/Right
Oropharynx	*use* Pharynx
Otic ganglion	*use* Head and Neck Sympathetic Nerve
Oval window	*use* Middle Ear, Left/Right
Ovarian artery	*use* Abdominal Aorta
Ovarian ligament	*use* Uterine Supporting Structure
Oviduct	*use* Fallopian Tube, Left/Right
Palatine gland	*use* Buccal Mucosa
Palatine tonsil	*use* Tonsils
Palatine uvula	*use* Uvula
Palatoglossal muscle Palatopharyngeal muscle	*use* Tongue, Palate, Pharynx Muscle
Palmar cutaneous nerve	*use* Median Nerve, Radial Nerve
Palmar fascia (aponeurosis)	*use* Subcutaneous Tissue and Fascia, Hand, Left/Right
Palmar interosseous muscle	*use* Hand Muscle, Left/Right
Palmar ulnocarpal ligament	*use* Wrist Bursa and Ligament, Left/Right
Palmar (volar) digital vein Palmar (volar) metacarpal vein	*use* Hand Vein, Left/Right
Palmaris longus muscle	*use* Lower Arm and Wrist Muscle, Left/Right
Pancreatic artery	*use* Splenic Artery
Pancreatic plexus	*use* Abdominal Sympathetic Nerve
Pancreatic vein	*use* Splenic Vein

© 2018 Channel Publishing, Ltd.

BODY PART	USE:
Pancreaticosplenic lymph node Paraaortic lymph node	*use* Lymphatic, Aortic
Pararectal lymph node	*use* Lymphatic, Mesenteric
Parasternal lymph node Paratracheal lymph node	*use* Lymphatic, Thorax
Paraurethral (Skene's) gland	*use* Vestibular Gland
Parietal lobe	*use* Cerebral Hemisphere
Parotid lymph node	*use* Lymphatic, Head
Parotid plexus	*use* Facial Nerve
Pars flaccida	*use* Tympanic Membrane, Left/Right
Patellar ligament	*use* Knee Bursa and Ligament, Left/Right
Patellar tendon	*use* Knee Tendon, Left/Right
Patellofemoral joint	*use* Knee Joint, Left/Right *use* Knee Joint, Femoral Surface, Left/Right
Pectineus muscle	*use* Upper Leg Muscle, Left/Right
Pectoral (anterior) lymph node	*use* Lymphatic, Axillary, Left/Right
Pectoral fascia	*use* Subcutaneous Tissue and Fascia, Chest
Pectoralis major muscle Pectoralis minor muscle	*use* Thorax Muscle, Left/Right
Pelvic splanchnic nerve	*use* Abdominal Sympathetic Nerve Sacral Sympathetic Nerve
Penile urethra	*use* Urethra
Pericardiophrenic artery	*use* Internal Mammary Artery, Left/Right
Perimetrium	*use* Uterus
Peroneus brevis muscle Peroneus longus muscle	*use* Lower Leg Muscle, Left/Right
Petrous part of temporal bone	*use* Temporal Bone, Left/Right
Pharyngeal constrictor muscle	*use* Tongue, Palate, Pharynx Muscle
Pharyngeal plexus	*use* Vagus Nerve
Pharyngeal recess	*use* Nasopharynx
Pharyngeal tonsil	*use* Adenoids
Pharyngotympanic tube	*use* Eustachian Tube, Left/Right
Pia mater, intracranial	*use* Cerebral Meninges
Pia mater, spinal	*use* Spinal Meninges
Pinna	*use* External Ear, Bilateral/Left/Right
Piriform recess (sinus)	*use* Pharynx
Piriformis muscle	*use* Hip Muscle, Left/Right
Pisiform bone	*use* Carpal, Left/Right
Pisohamate ligament Pisometacarpal ligament	*use* Hand Bursa and Ligament, Left/Right
Plantar digital vein	*use* Foot Vein, Left/Right
Plantar fascia (aponeurosis)	*use* Subcutaneous Tissue and Fascia, Foot, Left/Right
Plantar metatarsal vein Plantar venous arch	*use* Foot Vein, Left/Right

BODY PART	USE:
Platysma muscle	*use* Neck Muscle, Left/Right
Plica semilunaris	*use* Conjunctiva, Left/Right
Pneumogastric nerve	*use* Vagus Nerve
Pneumotaxic center Pontine tegmentum	*use* Pons
Popliteal ligament	*use* Knee Bursa and Ligament, Left/Right
Popliteal lymph node	*use* Lymphatic, Lower Extremity, Left/Right
Popliteal vein	*use* Femoral Vein, Left/Right
Popliteus muscle	*use* Lower Leg Muscle, Left/Right
Postauricular (mastoid) lymph node	*use* Lymphatic, Neck, Left/Right
Postcava	*use* Inferior Vena Cava
Posterior (subscapular) lymph node	*use* Lymphatic, Axillary, Left/Right
Posterior auricular artery	*use* External Carotid Artery, Left/Right
Posterior auricular nerve	*use* Facial Nerve
Posterior auricular vein	*use* External Jugular Vein, Left/Right
Posterior cerebral artery	*use* Intracranial Artery
Posterior chamber	*use* Eye, Left/Right
Posterior circumflex humeral artery	*use* Axillary Artery, Left/Right
Posterior communicating artery	*use* Intracranial Artery
Posterior cruciate ligament (PCL)	*use* Knee Bursa and Ligament, Left/Right
Posterior facial (retro-mandibular) vein	*use* Face Vein, Left/Right
Posterior femoral cutaneous nerve	*use* Sacral Plexus
Posterior inferior cerebellar artery (PICA)	*use* Intracranial Artery
Posterior interosseous nerve	*use* Radial Nerve
Posterior labial nerve Posterior scrotal nerve	*use* Pudendal Nerve
Posterior spinal artery	*use* Vertebral Artery, Left/Right
Posterior tibial recurrent artery	*use* Anterior Tibial Artery, Left/Right
Posterior ulnar recurrent artery	*use* Ulnar Artery, Left/Right
Posterior vagal trunk	*use* Vagus Nerve
Preauricular lymph node	*use* Lymphatic, Head
Precava	*use* Superior Vena Cava
Prepatellar bursa	*use* Knee Bursa and Ligament, Left/Right
Pretracheal fascia Prevertebral fascia	*use* Subcutaneous Tissue and Fascia, Neck, Left/Right
Princeps pollicis artery	*use* Hand Artery, Left/Right
Procerus muscle	*use* Facial Muscle
Profunda brachii	*use* Brachial Artery, Left/Right
Profunda femoris (deep femoral) vein	*use* Femoral Vein, Left/Right

© 2018 Channel Publishing, Ltd.

BODY PART	USE:
Pronator quadratus muscle Pronator teres muscle	*use* Lower Arm and Wrist Muscle, Left/Right
Prostatic urethra	*use* Urethra
Proximal radioulnar joint	*use* Elbow Joint, Left/Right
Psoas muscle	*use* Hip Muscle, Left/Right
Pterygoid muscle	*use* Head Muscle
Pterygoid process	*use* Sphenoid Bone
Pterygopalatine (spheno-palatine) ganglion	*use* Head and Neck Sympathetic Nerve
Pubis	*use* Pelvic Bone, Left/Right
Pubofemoral ligament	*use* Hip Bursa and Ligament, Left/Right
Pudendal nerve	*use* Sacral Plexus
Pulmoaortic canal	*use* Pulmonary Artery, Left
Pulmonary annulus	*use* Pulmonary Valve
Pulmonary plexus	*use* Vagus Nerve/Thoracic Sympathetic Nerve
Pulmonic valve	*use* Pulmonary Valve
Pulvinar	*use* Thalamus
Pyloric antrum Pyloric canal Pyloric sphincter	*use* Stomach, Pylorus
Pyramidalis muscle	*use* Abdomen Muscle, Left/Right
Quadrangular cartilage	*use* Nasal Septum
Quadrate lobe	*use* Liver
Quadratus femoris muscle	*use* Hip Muscle, Left/Right
Quadratus lumborum muscle	*use* Trunk Muscle, Left/Right
Quadratus plantae muscle	*use* Foot Muscle, Left/Right
Quadriceps (femoris)	*use* Upper Leg Muscle, Left/Right
Radial collateral carpal ligament	*use* Wrist Bursa and Ligament, Left/Right
Radial collateral ligament	*use* Elbow Bursa and Ligament, Left/Right
Radial notch	*use* Ulna, Left/Right
Radial recurrent artery	*use* Radial Artery, Left/Right
Radial vein	*use* Brachial Vein, Left/Right
Radialis indicis	*use* Hand Artery, Left/Right
Radiocarpal joint	*use* Wrist Joint, Left/Right
Radiocarpal ligament Radioulnar ligament	*use* Wrist Bursa and Ligament, Left/Right
Rectosigmoid junction	*use* Sigmoid Colon
Rectus abdominis muscle	*use* Abdomen Muscle, Left/Right
Rectus femoris muscle	*use* Upper Leg Muscle, Left/Right
Recurrent laryngeal nerve	*use* Vagus Nerve
Renal calyx Renal capsule Renal cortex	*use* Kidney, Bilateral/Left/Right
Renal plexus	*use* Abdominal Sympathetic Nerve
Renal segment	*use* Kidney, Bilateral/Left/Right
Renal segmental artery	*use* Renal Artery, Left/Right

BODY PART	USE:
Retroperitoneal cavity	*use* Retroperitoneum
Retroperitoneal lymph node	*use* Lymphatic, Aortic
Retroperitoneal space	*use* Retroperitoneum
Retropharyngeal lymph node	*use* Lymphatic, Neck, Left/Right
Retropubic space	*use* Pelvic Cavity
Rhinopharynx	*use* Nasopharynx
Rhomboid major muscle Rhomboid minor muscle	*use* Trunk Muscle, Left/Right
Right ascending lumbar vein	*use* Azygos Vein
Right atrioventricular valve	*use* Tricuspid Valve
Right auricular appendix	*use* Atrium, Right
Right colic vein	*use* Colic Vein
Right coronary sulcus	*use* Heart, Right
Right gastric artery	*use* Gastric Artery
Right gastroepiploic vein	*use* Superior Mesenteric Vein
Right inferior phrenic vein	*use* Inferior Vena Cava
Right inferior pulmonary vein	*use* Pulmonary Vein, Right
Right jugular trunk	*use* Lymphatic, Right Neck
Right lateral ventricle	*use* Cerebral Ventricle
Right lymphatic duct	*use* Lymphatic, Right Neck
Right ovarian vein Right second lumbar vein	*use* Inferior Vena Cava
Right subclavian trunk	*use* Lymphatic, Right Neck
Right subcostal vein	*use* Azygos Vein
Right superior pulmonary vein	*use* Pulmonary Vein, Right
Right suprarenal vein Right testicular vein	*use* Inferior Vena Cava
Rima glottidis	*use* Larynx
Risorius muscle	*use* Facial Muscle
Round ligament of uterus	*use* Uterine Supporting Structure
Round window	*use* Inner Ear, Left/Right
Sacral ganglion	*use* Sacral Sympathetic Nerve
Sacral lymph node	*use* Lymphatic, Pelvis
Sacral splanchnic nerve	*use* Sacral Sympathetic Nerve
Sacrococcygeal ligament	*use* Lower Spine Bursa and Ligament
Sacrococcygeal symphysis	*use* Sacrococcygeal Joint
Sacroiliac ligament Sacrospinous ligament Sacrotuberous ligament	*use* Lower Spine Bursa and Ligament
Salpingopharyngeus muscle	*use* Tongue, Palate, Pharynx Muscle
Salpinx	*use* Fallopian Tube, Left/Right
Saphenous nerve	*use* Femoral Nerve
Sartorius muscle	*use* Upper Leg Muscle, Left/Right
Scalene muscle	*use* Neck Muscle, Left/Right
Scaphoid bone	*use* Carpal, Left/Right

© 2018 Channel Publishing, Ltd.

BODY PART	USE:
Scapholunate ligament Scaphotrapezium ligament	*use* Hand Bursa and Ligament, Left/Right
Scarpa's (vestibular) ganglion	*use* Acoustic Nerve
Sebaceous gland	*use* Skin
Second cranial nerve	*use* Optic Nerve
Sella turcica	*use* Sphenoid Bone
Semicircular canal	*use* Inner Ear, Left/Right
Semimembranosus muscle Semitendinosus muscle	*use* Upper Leg Muscle, Left/Right
Septal cartilage	*use* Nasal Septum
Serratus anterior muscle	*use* Thorax Muscle, Left/Right
Serratus posterior muscle	*use* Trunk Muscle, Left/Right
Seventh cranial nerve	*use* Facial Nerve
Short gastric artery	*use* Splenic Artery
Sigmoid artery	*use* Inferior Mesenteric Artery
Sigmoid flexure	*use* Sigmoid Colon
Sigmoid vein	*use* Inferior Mesenteric Vein
Sinoatrial node	*use* Conduction Mechanism
Sinus venosus	*use* Atrium, Right
Sixth cranial nerve	*use* Abducens Nerve
Skene's (paraurethral) gland	*use* Vestibular Gland
Small saphenous vein	*use* Saphenous Vein, Left/Right
Solar (celiac) plexus	*use* Abdominal Sympathetic Nerve
Soleus muscle	*use* Lower Leg Muscle, Left/Right
Sphenomandibular ligament	*use* Head and Neck Bursa and Ligament
Sphenopalatine (pterygo-palatine) ganglion	*use* Head and Neck Sympathetic Nerve
Spinal nerve, cervical	*use* Cervical Nerve
Spinal nerve, lumbar	*use* Lumbar Nerve
Spinal nerve, sacral	*use* Sacral Nerve
Spinal nerve, thoracic	*use* Thoracic Nerve
Spinous process	*use* Cervical, Thoracic, Lumbar Vertebra
Spiral ganglion	*use* Acoustic Nerve
Splenic flexure	*use* Transverse Colon
Splenic plexus	*use* Abdominal Sympathetic Nerve
Splenius capitis muscle	*use* Head Muscle
Splenius cervicis muscle	*use* Neck Muscle, Left/Right
Stapes	*use* Auditory Ossicle, Left/Right
Stellate ganglion	*use* Head and Neck Sympathetic Nerve
Stensen's duct	*use* Parotid Duct, Left/Right
Sternoclavicular ligament	*use* Shoulder Bursa and Ligament, Left/Right
Sternocleidomastoid artery	*use* Thyroid Artery, Left/Right
Sternocleidomastoid muscle	*use* Neck Muscle, Left/Right
Sternocostal ligament	*use* Sternum Bursa and Ligament

BODY PART	USE:
Styloglossus muscle	*use* Tongue, Palate, Pharynx Muscle
Stylomandibular ligament	*use* Head and Neck Bursa and Ligament
Stylopharyngeus muscle	*use* Tongue, Palate, Pharynx Muscle
Subacromial bursa	*use* Shoulder Bursa and Ligament, Left/Right
Subaortic (common iliac) lymph node	*use* Lymphatic, Pelvis
Subarachnoid space, spinal	*use* Spinal Canal
Subclavicular (apical) lymph node	*use* Lymphatic, Axillary, Left/Right
Subclavius muscle	*use* Thorax Muscle, Left/Right
Subclavius nerve	*use* Brachial Plexus
Subcostal artery	*use* Upper Artery
Subcostal muscle	*use* Thorax Muscle, Left/Right
Subcostal nerve	*use* Thoracic Nerve
Subdural space, spinal	*use* Spinal Canal
Submandibular ganglion	*use* Facial Nerve Head and Neck Sympathetic Nerve
Submandibular gland	*use* Submaxillary Gland, Left/Right
Submandibular lymph node	*use* Lymphatic, Head
Submaxillary ganglion	*use* Head and Neck Sympathetic Nerve
Submaxillary lymph node	*use* Lymphatic, Head
Submental artery	*use* Face Artery
Submental lymph node	*use* Lymphatic, Head
Submucous (Meissner's) plexus	*use* Abdominal Sympathetic Nerve
Suboccipital nerve	*use* Cervical Nerve
Suboccipital venous plexus	*use* Vertebral Vein, Left/Right
Subparotid lymph node	*use* Lymphatic, Head
Subscapular aponeurosis	*use* Subcutaneous Tissue and Fascia, Upper Arm, Left/Right
Subscapular artery	*use* Axillary Artery, Left/Right
Subscapular (posterior) lymph node	*use* Lymphatic, Axillary, Left/Right
Subscapularis muscle	*use* Shoulder Muscle, Left/Right
Substantia nigra	*use* Basal Ganglia
Subtalar (talocalcaneal) joint	*use* Tarsal Joint, Left/Right
Subtalar ligament	*use* Foot Bursa and Ligament, Left/Right
Subthalamic nucleus	*use* Basal Ganglia
Superficial circumflex iliac vein	*use* Saphenous Vein, Left/Right
Superficial epigastric artery	*use* Femoral Artery, Left/Right
Superficial epigastric vein	*use* Saphenous Vein, Left/Right

© 2018 Channel Publishing, Ltd.

BODY PART	USE:
Superficial palmar arch	*use* Hand Artery, Left/Right
Superficial palmar venous arch	*use* Hand Vein, Left/Right
Superficial temporal artery	*use* Temporal Artery, Left/Right
Superficial transverse perineal muscle	*use* Perineum Muscle
Superior cardiac nerve	*use* Thoracic Sympathetic Nerve
Superior cerebellar vein **Superior cerebral vein**	*use* Intracranial Vein
Superior clunic (cluneal) nerve	*use* Lumbar Nerve
Superior epigastric artery	*use* Internal Mammary Artery, Left/Right
Superior genicular artery	*use* Popliteal Artery, Left/Right
Superior gluteal artery	*use* Internal Iliac Artery, Left/Right
Superior gluteal nerve	*use* Lumbar Plexus
Superior hypogastric plexus	*use* Abdominal Sympathetic Nerve
Superior labial artery	*use* Face Artery
Superior laryngeal artery	*use* Thyroid Artery, Left/Right
Superior laryngeal nerve	*use* Vagus Nerve
Superior longitudinal muscle	*use* Tongue, Palate, Pharynx Muscle
Superior mesenteric ganglion	*use* Abdominal Sympathetic Nerve
Superior mesenteric lymph node	*use* Lymphatic, Mesenteric
Superior mesenteric plexus	*use* Abdominal Sympathetic Nerve
Superior oblique muscle	*use* Extraocular Muscle, Left/Right
Superior olivary nucleus	*use* Pons
Superior rectal artery	*use* Inferior Mesenteric Artery
Superior rectal vein	*use* Inferior Mesenteric Vein
Superior rectus muscle	*use* Extraocular Muscle, Left/Right
Superior tarsal plate	*use* Upper Eyelid, Left/Right
Superior thoracic artery	*use* Axillary Artery, Left/Right
Superior thyroid artery	*use* External Carotid Artery, Left/Right Thyroid Artery, Left/Right
Superior turbinate	*use* Nasal Turbinate
Superior ulnar collateral artery	*use* Brachial Artery, Left/Right
Supraclavicular (Virchow's) lymph node	*use* Lymphatic, Neck, Left/Right
Supraclavicular nerve	*use* Cervical Plexus
Suprahyoid lymph node	*use* Lymphatic, Head
Suprahyoid muscle	*use* Neck Muscle, Left/Right
Suprainguinal lymph node	*use* Lymphatic, Pelvis
Supraorbital vein	*use* Face Vein, Left/Right
Suprarenal gland	*use* Adrenal Gland, Bilateral/Left/Right
Suprarenal plexus	*use* Abdominal Sympathetic Nerve
Suprascapular nerve	*use* Brachial Plexus
Supraspinatus fascia	*use* Subcutaneous Tissue and Fascia, Upper Arm, Left/Right
Supraspinatus muscle	*use* Shoulder Muscle, Left/Right
Supraspinous ligament	*use* Lower Spine Bursa and Ligament *use* Upper Spine Bursa and Ligament
Suprasternal notch	*use* Sternum
Supratrochlear lymph node	*use* Lymphatic, Upper Extremity, Left/Right
Sural artery	*use* Popliteal Artery, Left/Right
Sweat gland	*use* Skin
Talocalcaneal (subtalar) joint	*use* Tarsal Joint, Left/Right
Talocalcaneal ligament	*use* Foot Bursa and Ligament, Left/Right
Talocalcaneonavicular joint	*use* Tarsal Joint, Left/Right
Talocalcaneonavicular ligament	*use* Foot Bursa and Ligament, Left/Right
Talocrural joint	*use* Ankle Joint, Left/Right
Talofibular ligament	*use* Ankle Bursa and Ligament, Left/Right
Talus bone	*use* Tarsal, Left/Right
Tarsometatarsal ligament	*use* Foot Bursa and Ligament, Left/Right
Temporal lobe	*use* Cerebral Hemisphere
Temporalis muscle **Temporoparietalis muscle**	*use* Head Muscle
Tensor fasciae latae muscle	*use* Hip Muscle, Left/Right
Tensor veli palatini muscle	*use* Tongue, Palate, Pharynx Muscle
Tenth cranial nerve	*use* Vagus Nerve
Tentorium cerebelli	*use* Dura Mater
Teres major muscle **Teres minor muscle**	*use* Shoulder Muscle, Left/Right
Testicular artery	*use* Abdominal Aorta
Thenar muscle	*use* Hand Muscle, Left/Right
Third cranial nerve	*use* Oculomotor Nerve
Third occipital nerve	*use* Cervical Nerve
Third ventricle	*use* Cerebral Ventricle
Thoracic aortic plexus	*use* Thoracic Sympathetic Nerve
Thoracic esophagus	*use* Esophagus, Middle
Thoracic facet joint	*use* Thoracic Vertebral Joint
Thoracic ganglion	*use* Thoracic Sympathetic Nerve
Thoracoacromial artery	*use* Axillary Artery, Left/Right
Thoracolumbar facet joint	*use* Thoracolumbar Vertebral Joint
Thymus gland	*use* Thymus
Thyroarytenoid muscle	*use* Neck Muscle, Left/Right
Thyrocervical trunk	*use* Thyroid Artery, Left/Right
Thyroid cartilage	*use* Larynx
Tibialis anterior muscle **Tibialis posterior muscle**	*use* Lower Leg Muscle, Left/Right
Tibiofemoral joint	*use* Knee Joint, Left/Right *use* Knee Joint, Tibial Surface, Left/Right

© 2018 Channel Publishing, Ltd.

BODY PART	USE:
Tongue, base of	*use* Pharynx
Tracheobronchial lymph node	*use* Lymphatic, Thorax
Tragus	*use* External Ear, Bilateral/Left/Right
Transversalis fascia	*use* Subcutaneous Tissue and Fascia, Trunk
Transverse (cutaneous) cervical nerve	*use* Cervical Plexus
Transverse acetabular ligament	*use* Hip Bursa and Ligament, Left/Right
Transverse facial artery	*use* Temporal Artery, Left/Right
Transverse foramen	*use* Cervical Vertebra
Transverse humeral ligament	*use* Shoulder Bursa and Ligament, Left/Right
Transverse ligament of atlas	*use* Head and Neck Bursa and Ligament
Transverse process	*use* Cervical, Thoracic, Lumbar Vertebra
Transverse scapular ligament	*use* Shoulder Bursa and Ligament, Left/Right
Transverse thoracis muscle	*use* Thorax Muscle, Left/Right
Transversospinalis muscle	*use* Trunk Muscle, Left/Right
Transversus abdominis muscle	*use* Abdomen Muscle, Left/Right
Trapezium bone	*use* Carpal, Left/Right
Trapezius muscle	*use* Trunk Muscle, Left/Right
Trapezoid bone	*use* Carpal, Left/Right
Triceps brachii muscle	*use* Upper Arm Muscle, Left/Right
Tricuspid annulus	*use* Tricuspid Valve
Trifacial nerve	*use* Trigeminal Nerve
Trigone of bladder	*use* Bladder
Triquetral bone	*use* Carpal, Left/Right
Trochanteric bursa	*use* Hip Bursa and Ligament, Left/Right
Twelfth cranial nerve	*use* Hypoglossal Nerve
Tympanic cavity	*use* Middle Ear, Left/Right
Tympanic nerve	*use* Glossopharyngeal Nerve
Tympanic part of temporal bone	*use* Temporal Bone, Left/Right
Ulnar collateral carpal ligament	*use* Wrist Bursa and Ligament, Left/Right
Ulnar collateral ligament	*use* Elbow Bursa and Ligament, Left/Right
Ulnar notch	*use* Radius, Left/Right
Ulnar vein	*use* Brachial Vein, Left/Right
Umbilical artery	*use* Internal Iliac Artery, Left/Right *use* Lower Artery
Ureteral orifice	*use* Ureter, Bilateral/Left/Right
Ureteropelvic junction (UPJ)	*use* Kidney Pelvis, Left/Right
Ureterovesical orifice	*use* Ureter, Bilateral/Left/Right
Uterine artery	*use* Internal Iliac Artery, Left/Right
Uterine cornu	*use* Uterus
Uterine tube	*use* Fallopian Tube, Left/Right
Uterine vein	*use* Hypogastric Vein, Left/Right
Vaginal artery	*use* Internal Iliac Artery, Left/Right
Vaginal vein	*use* Hypogastric Vein, Left/Right
Vastus intermedius muscle **Vastus lateralis muscle** **Vastus medialis muscle**	*use* Upper Leg Muscle, Left/Right
Ventricular fold	*use* Larynx
Vermiform appendix	*use* Appendix
Vermilion border	*use* Upper Lip, Lower Lip
Vertebral arch **Vertebral body**	*use* Cervical, Thoracic, Lumbar Vertebra
Vertebral canal	*use* Spinal Canal
Vertebral foramen **Vertebral lamina** **Vertebral pedicle**	*use* Cervical, Thoracic, Lumbar Vertebra
Vesical vein	*use* Hypogastric Vein, Left/Right
Vestibular nerve **Vestibular (Scarpa's) ganglion** **Vestibulocochlear nerve**	*use* Acoustic Nerve
Virchow's (supraclavicular) lymph node	*use* Lymphatic, Neck, Left/Right
Vitreous body	*use* Vitreous, Left/Right
Vocal fold	*use* Vocal Cord, Left/Right
Volar (palmar) digital vein **Volar (palmar) metacarpal vein**	*use* Hand Vein, Left/Right
Vomer bone	*use* Nasal Septum
Vomer of nasal septum	*use* Nasal Bone
Xiphoid process	*use* Sternum
Zonule of Zinn	*use* Lens, Left/Right
Zygomatic process of frontal bone	*use* Frontal Bone
Zygomatic process of temporal bone	*use* Temporal Bone, Left/Right
Zygomaticus muscle	*use* Facial Muscle

© 2018 Channel Publishing, Ltd.

DEVICE	USE:
3f (Aortic) Bioprosthesis valve	*use* Zooplastic Tissue in Heart and Great Vessels
AbioCor® Total Replacement Heart	*use* Synthetic Substitute
Absolute Pro Vascular (OTW) Self-Expanding Stent System	*use* Intraluminal Device
Acculink (RX) Carotid Stent System	*use* Intraluminal Device
Acellular Hydrated Dermis	*use* Nonautologous Tissue Substitute
Acetabular cup	*use* Liner in Lower Joints
Activa PC neurostimulator	*use* Stimulator Generator, Multiple Array for Insertion in Subcutaneous Tissue and Fascia
Activa RC neurostimulator	*use* Stimulator Generator, Multiple Array Rechargeable for Insertion in Subcutaneous Tissue and Fascia
Activa SC neurostimulator	*use* Stimulator Generator, Single Array for Insertion in Subcutaneous Tissue and Fascia
ACUITY™ Steerable Lead	*use* Cardiac Lead, Pacemaker for Insertion in Heart and Great Vessels Cardiac Lead, Defibrillator for Insertion in Heart and Great Vessels
Advisa (MRI)	*use* Pacemaker, Dual Chamber for Insertion in Subcutaneous Tissue and Fascia
AFX® Endovascular AAA System	*use* Intraluminal Device
AMPLATZER® Muscular VSD Occluder	*use* Synthetic Substitute
AMS 800® Urinary Control System	*use* Artificial Sphincter in Urinary System
AneuRx® AAA Advantage®	*use* Intraluminal Device
Annuloplasty ring	*use* Synthetic Substitute
Articulating spacer (antibiotic)	*use* Articulating Spacer in Lower Joints
Artificial anal sphincter (AAS)	*use* Artificial Sphincter in Gastrointestinal System
Artificial bowel sphincter (neosphincter)	*use* Artificial Sphincter in Gastrointestinal System
Artificial urinary sphincter (AUS)	*use* Artificial Sphincter in Urinary System
Ascenda Intrathecal Catheter	*use* Infusion Device
Assurant (Cobalt) stent	*use* Intraluminal Device
AtriClip LAA Exclusion System	*use* Extraluminal Device
Attain Ability® lead	*use* Cardiac Lead, Pacemaker for Insertion in Heart and Great Vessels Cardiac Lead, Defibrillator for Insertion in Heart and Great Vessels
Attain StarFix® (OTW) lead	*use* Cardiac Lead, Pacemaker for Insertion in Heart and Great Vessels Cardiac Lead, Defibrillator for Insertion in Heart and Great Vessels
Autograft	*use* Autologous Tissue Substitute
Autologous artery graft	*use* Autologous Arterial Tissue in Heart and Great Vessels Autologous Arterial Tissue in Upper Arteries, Lower Arteries Autologous Arterial Tissue in Upper Veins, Lower Veins
Autologous vein graft	*use* Autologous Venous Tissue in Heart and Great Vessels Autologous Venous Tissue in Upper Arteries, Lower Arteries Autologous Venous Tissue in Upper Veins, Lower Veins
Axial Lumbar Interbody Fusion System	*use* Interbody Fusion Device in Lower Joints
AxiaLIF® System	*use* Interbody Fusion Device in Lower Joints
BAK/C® Interbody Cervical Fusion System	*use* Interbody Fusion Device in Upper Joints
Bard® Composix® (E/X)(LP) mesh	*use* Synthetic Substitute
Bard® Composix® Kugel® patch	*use* Synthetic Substitute
Bard® Dulex™ mesh	*use* Synthetic Substitute
Bard® Ventralex™ hernia patch	*use* Synthetic Substitute
Baroreflex Activation Therapy® (BAT®)	*use* Stimulator Lead in Upper Arteries Stimulator Generator in Subcutaneous Tissue and Fascia
Berlin Heart Ventricular Assist Device	*use* Implantable Heart Assist System in Heart and Great Vessels
Bioactive embolization coil(s)	*use* Intraluminal Device, Bioactive in Upper Arteries
Biventricular external heart assist system	*use* Short-term External Heart Assist System in Heart and Great Vessels
Blood glucose monitoring system	*use* Monitoring Device
Bone anchored hearing device	*use* Hearing Device, Bone Conduction for Insertion in Ear, Nose, Sinus Hearing Device in Head and Facial Bones

© 2018 Channel Publishing, Ltd.

DEVICE	USE:
Bone bank bone graft	*use* Nonautologous Tissue Substitute
Bone screw (interlocking) (lag) (pedicle) (recessed)	*use* Internal Fixation Device in Head and Facial Bones, Upper Bones, Lower Bones
Bovine pericardial valve	*use* Zooplastic Tissue in Heart and Great Vessels
Bovine pericardium graft	*use* Zooplastic Tissue in Heart and Great Vessels
Brachytherapy seeds	*use* Radioactive Element
BRYAN® Cervical Disc System	*use* Synthetic Substitute
BVS 5000 Ventricular Assist Device	*use* Short-term External Heart Assist System in Heart and Great Vessels
Cardiac contractility modulation lead	*use* Cardiac Lead in Heart and Great Vessels
Cardiac event recorder	*use* Monitoring Device
Cardiac resynchronization therapy (CRT) lead	*use* Cardiac Lead, Pacemaker for Insertion in Heart and Great Vessels Cardiac Lead, Defibrillator for Insertion in Heart and Great Vessels
CardioMEMS® pressure sensor	*use* Monitoring Device, Pressure Sensor for Insertion in Heart and Great Vessels
Carotid (artery) sinus (baroreceptor) lead	*use* Stimulator Lead in Upper Arteries
Carotid WALLSTENT® Monorail® Endoprosthesis	*use* Intraluminal Device
Centrimag® Blood Pump	*use* Short-term External Heart Assist System in Heart and Great Vessels
Ceramic on ceramic bearing surface	*use* Synthetic Substitute, Ceramic for Replacement in Lower Joints
Cesium-131 Collagen Implant	*use* Radioactive Element, Cesium-131 Collagen Implant for Insertion in Central Nervous System and Cranial Nerves
Clamp and rod internal fixation system (CRIF)	*use* Internal Fixation Device in Upper Bones, Lower Bones
COALESCE® Radiolucent interbody fusion device	*use* Interbody Fusion Device, Radiolucent Porous in New Technology
CoAxia NeuroFlo catheter	*use* Intraluminal Device
Cobalt/chromium head and polyethylene socket	*use* Synthetic Substitute, Metal on Polyethylene for Replacement in Lower Joints
Cobalt/chromium head and socket	*use* Synthetic Substitute, Metal for Replacement in Lower Joints
Cochlear implant (CI), multiple channel (electrode)	*use* Hearing Device, Multiple Channel Cochlear Prosthesis for Insertion in Ear, Nose, Sinus
Cochlear implant (CI), single channel (electrode)	*use* Hearing Device, Single Channel Cochlear Prosthesis for Insertion in Ear, Nose, Sinus
COGNIS® CRT-D	*use* Cardiac Resynchronization Defibrillator Pulse Generator for Insertion in Subcutaneous Tissue and Fascia
COHERE® Radiolucent interbody fusion device	*use* Interbody Fusion Device, Radiolucent Porous in New Technology
Colonic Z-Stent®	*use* Intraluminal Device
Complete (SE) stent	*use* Intraluminal Device
Concerto II CRT-D	*use* Cardiac Resynchronization Defibrillator Pulse Generator for Insertion in Subcutaneous Tissue and Fascia
CONSERVE® PLUS Total Resurfacing Hip System	*use* Resurfacing Device in Lower Joints
Consulta CRT-D	*use* Cardiac Resynchronization Defibrillator Pulse Generator for Insertion in Subcutaneous Tissue and Fascia
Consulta CRT-P	*use* Cardiac Resynchronization Pacemaker Pulse Generator for Insertion in Subcutaneous Tissue and Fascia
CONTAK RENEWAL® 3 RF (HE) CRT-D	*use* Cardiac Resynchronization Defibrillator Pulse Generator for Insertion in Subcutaneous Tissue and Fascia
Contegra Pulmonary Valved Conduit	*use* Zooplastic Tissue in Heart and Great Vessels
Continuous Glucose Monitoring (CGM) device	*use* Monitoring Device
Cook Biodesign® Fistula Plug(s)	*use* Nonautologous Tissue Substitute
Cook Biodesign® Hernia Graft(s)	*use* Nonautologous Tissue Substitute
Cook Biodesign® Layered Graft(s)	*use* Nonautologous Tissue Substitute
Cook Zenapro™ Layered Graft(s)	*use* Nonautologous Tissue Substitute
Cook Zenith AAA Endovascular Graft	*use* Intraluminal Device, Branched or Fenestrated, One or Two Arteries for Restriction in Lower Arteries *use* Intraluminal Device, Branched or Fenestrated, Three or More Arteries for Restriction in Lower Arteries *use* Intraluminal Device
CoreValve transcatheter aortic valve	*use* Zooplastic Tissue in Heart and Great Vessels

© 2018 Channel Publishing, Ltd.

DEVICE	USE:
Cormet Hip Resurfacing System	*use* Resurfacing Device in Lower Joints
CoRoent® XL	*use* Interbody Fusion Device in Lower Joints
Corox (OTW) Bipolar Lead	*use* Cardiac Lead, Pacemaker for Insertion in Heart and Great Vessels Cardiac Lead, Defibrillator for Insertion in Heart and Great Vessels
Cortical strip neurostimulator lead	*use* Neurostimulator Lead in Central Nervous System and Cranial Nerves
Cultured epidermal cell autograft	*use* Autologous Tissue Substitute
CYPHER® Stent	*use* Intraluminal Device, Drug-eluting in Heart and Great Vessels
Cystostomy tube	*use* Drainage Device
DBS lead	*use* Neurostimulator Lead in Central Nervous System and Cranial Nerves
DeBakey Left Ventricular Assist Device	*use* Implantable Heart Assist System in Heart and Great Vessels
Deep brain neurostimulator lead	*use* Neurostimulator Lead in Central Nervous System and Cranial Nerves
Delta frame external fixator	*use* External Fixation Device, Hybrid for Insertion in Upper Bones, Lower Bones External Fixation Device, Hybrid for Reposition in Upper Bones, Lower Bones
Delta III Reverse shoulder prosthesis	*use* Synthetic Substitute, Reverse Ball and Socket for Replacement in Upper Joints
Diaphragmatic pacemaker generator	*use* Stimulator Generator in Subcutaneous Tissue and Fascia
Direct Lateral Interbody Fusion (DLIF) device	*use* Interbody Fusion Device in Lower Joints
Driver stent (RX) (OTW)	*use* Intraluminal Device
DuraHeart Left Ventricular Assist System	*use* Implantable Heart Assist System in Heart and Great Vessels
Durata® Defibrillation Lead	*use* Cardiac Lead, Defibrillator for Insertion in Heart and Great Vessels
Dynesys® Dynamic Stabilization System	*use* Spinal Stabilization Device, Pedicle-Based for Insertion in Upper Joints, Lower Joints
E-Luminexx™ (Biliary) (Vascular) Stent	*use* Intraluminal Device
EDWARDS INTUITY Elite valve system	*use* Zooplastic Tissue, Rapid Deployment Technique in New Technology
Electrical bone growth stimulator (EBGS)	*use* Bone Growth Stimulator in Head and Facial Bones, Upper Bones, Lower Bones
Electrical muscle stimulation (EMS) lead	*use* Stimulator Lead in Muscles
Electronic muscle stimulator lead	*use* Stimulator Lead in Muscles
Embolization coil(s)	*use* Intraluminal Device
Endeavor® (III) (IV) (Sprint) Zotarolimus-eluting Coronary Stent System	*use* Intraluminal Device, Drug-eluting in Heart and Great Vessels
Endologix AFX® Endovascular AAA System	*use* Intraluminal Device
EndoSure® sensor	*use* Monitoring Device, Pressure Sensor for Insertion in Heart and Great Vessels
ENDOTAK RELIANCE® (G) Defibrillation Lead	*use* Cardiac Lead, Defibrillator for Insertion in Heart and Great Vessels
Endotracheal tube (cuffed) (double-lumen)	*use* Intraluminal Device, Endotracheal Airway in Respiratory System
Endurant® Endovascular Stent Graft	*use* Intraluminal Device
Endurant® II AAA stent graft system	*use* Intraluminal Device
EnRhythm	*use* Pacemaker, Dual Chamber for Insertion in Subcutaneous Tissue and Fascia
Enterra gastric neurostimulator	*use* Stimulator Generator, Multiple Array for Insertion in Subcutaneous Tissue and Fascia
Epic™ Stented Tissue Valve (aortic)	*use* Zooplastic Tissue in Heart and Great Vessels
Epicel® cultured epidermal autograft	*use* Autologous Tissue Substitute
Esophageal obturator airway (EOA)	*use* Intraluminal Device, Airway in Gastrointestinal System
Esteem® implantable hearing system	*use* Hearing Device in Ear, Nose, Sinus
Evera (XT) (S) (DR/VR)	*use* Defibrillator Generator for Insertion in Subcutaneous Tissue and Fascia
Everolimus-eluting coronary stent	*use* Intraluminal Device, Drug-eluting in Heart and Great Vessels
Ex-PRESS™ mini glaucoma shunt	*use* Synthetic Substitute
EXCLUDER® AAA Endoprothesis	*use* Intraluminal Device, Branched or Fenestrated, One or Two Arteries for Restriction in Lower Arteries *use* Intraluminal Device, Branched or Fenestrated, Three or More Arteries for Restriction in Lower Arteries *use* Intraluminal Device
EXCLUDER® IBE Endoprothesis	*use* Intraluminal Device, Branched or Fenestrated, One or Two Arteries for Restriction in Lower Arteries

© 2018 Channel Publishing, Ltd.

DEVICE	USE:
Express® (LD) Premounted Stent System	*use* Intraluminal Device
Express® Biliary SD Monorail® Premounted Stent System	*use* Intraluminal Device
Express® SD Renal Monorail® Premounted Stent System	*use* Intraluminal Device
External fixator	*use* External Fixation Device in Head and Facial Bones, Upper Bones, Lower Bones, Upper Joints, Lower Joints
EXtreme Lateral Interbody Fusion (XLIF) device	*use* Interbody Fusion Device in Lower Joints
Facet replacement spinal stabilization device	*use* Spinal Stabilization Device, Facet Replacement for Insertion in Upper Joints, Lower Joints
FLAIR® Endovascular Stent Graft	*use* Intraluminal Device
Flexible Composite Mesh	*use* Synthetic Substitute
Foley catheter	*use* Drainage Device
Formula™ Balloon-Expandable Renal Stent System	*use* Intraluminal Device
Freestyle (Stentless) Aortic Root Bioprosthesis	*use* Zooplastic Tissue in Heart and Great Vessels
Fusion screw (compression) (lag) (locking)	*use* Internal Fixation Device in Upper Joints, Lower Joints
GammaTile™	*use* Radioactive Element, Cesium-131 Collagen Implant for Insertion in Central Nervous System and Cranial Nerves
Gastric electrical stimulation (GES) lead	*use* Stimulator Lead in Gastrointestinal System
Gastric pacemaker lead	*use* Stimulator Lead in Gastrointestinal System
GORE® DUALMESH®	*use* Synthetic Substitute
GORE EXCLUDER® AAA Endoprothesis	*use* Intraluminal Device, Branched or Fenestrated, One or Two Arteries for Restriction in Lower Arteries *use* Intraluminal Device, Branched or Fenestrated, Three or More Arteries for Restriction in Lower Arteries *use* Intraluminal Device
GORE EXCLUDER® IBE Endoprothesis	*use* Intraluminal Device, Branched or Fenestrated, One or Two Arteries for Restriction in Lower Arteries
GORE TAG® Thoracic Endoprothesis	*use* Intraluminal Device
Guedel airway	*use* Intraluminal Device, Airway in Mouth and Throat
Hancock Bioprosthesis (aortic) (mitral) valve	*use* Zooplastic Tissue in Heart and Great Vessels
Hancock Bioprosthetic Valved Conduit	*use* Zooplastic Tissue in Heart and Great Vessels
HeartMate 3™ LVAS	*use* Implantable Heart Assist System in Heart and Great Vessels
HeartMate II® Left Ventricular Assist Device (LVAD)	*use* Implantable Heart Assist System in Heart and Great Vessels
HeartMate XVE® Left Ventricular Assist Device (LVAD)	*use* Implantable Heart Assist System in Heart and Great Vessels
Herculink (RX) Elite Renal Stent System	*use* Intraluminal Device
Hip (joint) liner	*use* Liner in Lower Joints
Holter valve ventricular shunt	*use* Synthetic Substitute
Ilizarov external fixator	*use* External Fixation Device, Ring for Insertion in Upper Bones, Lower Bones External Fixation Device, Ring for Reposition in Upper Bones, Lower Bones
Ilizarov-Vecklich device	*use* External Fixation Device, Limb Lengthening for Insertion in Upper Bones, Lower Bones
Impella® Heart Pump	*use* Short-term External Heart Assist System in Heart and Great Vessels
Implantable cardioverter-defibrillator (ICD)	*use* Defibrillator Generator for Insertion in Subcutaneous Tissue and Fascia
Implantable drug infusion pump (anti-spasmodic) (chemotherapy) (pain)	*use* Infusion Device, Pump in Subcutaneous Tissue and Fascia
Implantable glucose monitoring device	*use* Monitoring Device
Implantable hemodynamic monitor (IHM)	*use* Monitoring Device, Hemodynamic for Insertion in Subcutaneous Tissue and Fascia
Implantable hemodynamic monitoring system (IHMS)	*use* Monitoring Device, Hemodynamic for Insertion in Subcutaneous Tissue and Fascia
Implantable Miniature Telescope™ (IMT)	*use* Synthetic Substitute, Intraocular Telescope for Replacement in Eye
Implanted (venous) (access) port	*use* Vascular Access Device, Totally Implantable in Subcutaneous Tissue and Fascia
InDura, intrathecal catheter (1P) (spinal)	*use* Infusion Device

© 2018 Channel Publishing, Ltd.

DEVICE	USE:
Injection reservoir, port	*use* Vascular Access Device, Totally Implantable in Subcutaneous Tissue and Fascia
Injection reservoir, pump	*use* Infusion Device, Pump in Subcutaneous Tissue and Fascia
Interbody fusion (spine) cage	*use* Interbody Fusion Device in Upper Joints, Lower Joints
Interspinous process spinal stabilization device	*use* Spinal Stabilization Device, Interspinous Process for Insertion in Upper Joints, Lower Joints
InterStim® Therapy lead	*use* Neurostimulator Lead in Peripheral Nervous System
InterStim® Therapy neurostimulator	*use* Stimulator Generator, Single Array for Insertion in Subcutaneous Tissue and Fascia
Intramedullary (IM) rod (nail)	*use* Internal Fixation Device, Intramedullary in Upper Bones, Lower Bones
Intramedullary skeletal kinetic distractor (ISKD)	*use* Internal Fixation Device, Intramedullary in Upper Bones, Lower Bones
Intrauterine device (IUD)	*use* Contraceptive Device in Female Reproductive System
INTUITY Elite valve system, EDWARDS	*use* Zooplastic Tissue, Rapid Deployment Technique in New Technology
Itrel (3) (4) neurostimulator	*use* Stimulator Generator, Single Array for Insertion in Subcutaneous Tissue and Fascia
Joint fixation plate	*use* Internal Fixation Device in Upper Joints, Lower Joints
Joint liner (insert)	*use* Liner in Lower Joints
Joint spacer (antibiotic)	*use* Spacer in Upper Joints, Lower Joints
Kappa	*use* Pacemaker, Dual Chamber for Insertion in Subcutaneous Tissue and Fascia
Kirschner wire (K-wire)	*use* Internal Fixation Device in Head and Facial Bones, Upper Bones, Lower Bones, Upper Joints, Lower Joints
Knee (implant) insert	*use* Liner in Lower Joints
Kuntscher nail	*use* Internal Fixation Device, Intramedullary in Upper Bones, Lower Bones
LAP-BAND® adjustable gastric banding system	*use* Extraluminal Device
LifeStent® (Flexstar) (XL) Vascular Stent System	*use* Intraluminal Device
LIVIAN™ CRT-D	*use* Cardiac Resynchronization Defibrillator Pulse Generator for Insertion in Subcutaneous Tissue and Fascia
Loop recorder, implantable	*use* Monitoring Device
MAGEC® Spinal Bracing and Distraction System	*use* Magnetically Controlled Growth Rod(s) in New Technology
Mark IV Breathing Pacemaker System	*use* Stimulator Generator in Subcutaneous Tissue and Fascia
Maximo II DR (VR)	*use* Defibrillator Generator for Insertion in Subcutaneous Tissue and Fascia
Maximo II DR CRT-D	*use* Cardiac Resynchronization Defibrillator Pulse Generator for Insertion in Subcutaneous Tissue and Fascia
Medtronic Endurant® II AAA stent graft system	*use* Intraluminal Device
Melody® transcatheter pulmonary valve	*use* Zooplastic Tissue in Heart and Great Vessels
Metal on metal bearing surface	*use* Synthetic Substitute, Metal for Replacement in Lower Joints
Micro-Driver stent (RX) (OTW)	*use* Intraluminal Device
MicroMed HeartAssist	*use* Implantable Heart Assist System in Heart and Great Vessels
Micrus CERECYTE microcoil	*use* Intraluminal Device, Bioactive in Upper Arteries
MIRODERM™ Biologic Wound Matrix	*use* Skin Substitute, Porcine Liver Derived in New Technology
MitraClip valve repair system	*use* Synthetic Substitute
Mitroflow® Aortic Pericardial Heart Valve	*use* Zooplastic Tissue in Heart and Great Vessels
Mosaic Bioprosthesis (aortic) (mitral) valve	*use* Zooplastic Tissue in Heart and Great Vessels
MULTI-LINK (VISION) (MINI-VISION) (ULTRA) Coronary Stent System	*use* Intraluminal Device
nanoLOCK™ interbody fusion device	*use* Interbody Fusion Device, Nanotextured Surface in New Technology
Nasopharyngeal airway (NPA)	*use* Intraluminal Device, Airway in Ear, Nose, Sinus
Neuromuscular electrical stimulation (NEMS) lead	*use* Stimulator Lead in Muscles
Neurostimulator generator, multiple channel	*use* Stimulator Generator, Multiple Array for Insertion in Subcutaneous Tissue and Fascia
Neurostimulator generator, multiple channel rechargeable	*use* Stimulator Generator, Multiple Array Rechargeable for Insertion in Subcutaneous Tissue and Fascia
Neurostimulator generator, single channel	*use* Stimulator Generator, Single Array for Insertion in Subcutaneous Tissue and Fascia
Neurostimulator generator, single channel rechargeable	*use* Stimulator Generator, Single Array Rechargeable for Insertion in Subcutaneous Tissue and Fascia

© 2018 Channel Publishing, Ltd.

DEVICE	USE:
Neutralization plate	*use* Internal Fixation Device in Head and Facial Bones, Upper Bones, Lower Bones
Nitinol framed polymer mesh	*use* Synthetic Substitute
Non-tunneled central venous catheter	*use* Infusion Device
Novacor Left Ventricular Assist Device	*use* Implantable Heart Assist System in Heart and Great Vessels
Novation® Ceramic AHS® (Articulation Hip System)	*use* Synthetic Substitute, Ceramic for Replacement in Lower Joints
Omnilink Elite Vascular Balloon Expandable Stent System	*use* Intraluminal Device
Open Pivot Aortic Valve Graft (AVG)	*use* Synthetic Substitute
Open Pivot (mechanical) valve	*use* Synthetic Substitute
Optimizer™ III implantable pulse generator	*use* Contractility Modulation Device for Insertion in Subcutaneous Tissue and Fascia
Oropharyngeal airway (OPA)	*use* Intraluminal Device, Airway in Mouth and Throat
Ovatio™ CRT-D	*use* Cardiac Resynchronization Defibrillator Pulse Generator for Insertion in Subcutaneous Tissue and Fascia
OXINIUM	*use* Synthetic Substitute, Oxidized Zirconium on Polyethylene for Replacement in Lower Joints
Paclitaxel-eluting coronary stent	*use* Intraluminal Device, Drug-eluting in Heart and Great Vessels
Paclitaxel-eluting peripheral stent	*use* Intraluminal Device, Drug-eluting in Upper Arteries, Lower Arteries
Partially absorbable mesh	*use* Synthetic Substitute
Pedicle-based dynamic stabilization device	*use* Spinal Stabilization Device, Pedicle-Based for Insertion in Upper Joints, Lower Joints
Perceval sutureless valve	*use* Zooplastic Tissue, Rapid Deployment Technique in New Technology
Percutaneous endoscopic gastrojejunostomy (PEG/J) tube	*use* Feeding Device in Gastrointestinal System
Percutaneous endoscopic gastrostomy (PEG) tube	*use* Feeding Device in Gastrointestinal System
Percutaneous nephrostomy catheter	*use* Drainage Device
Peripherally inserted central catheter (PICC)	*use* Infusion Device
Pessary ring	*use* Intraluminal Device, Pessary in Female Reproductive System
Phrenic nerve stimulator generator	*use* Stimulator Generator in Subcutaneous Tissue and Fascia
Phrenic nerve stimulator lead	*use* Diaphragmatic Pacemaker Lead in Respiratory System
PHYSIOMESH™ Flexible Composite Mesh	*use* Synthetic Substitute
Pipeline™ Embolization device (PED)	*use* Intraluminal Device
Polyethylene socket	*use* Synthetic Substitute, Polyethylene for Replacement in Lower Joints
Polymethylmethacrylate (PMMA)	*use* Synthetic Substitute
Polypropylene mesh	*use* Synthetic Substitute
Porcine (bioprosthetic) valve	*use* Zooplastic Tissue in Heart and Great Vessels
PRESTIGE® Cervical Disc	*use* Synthetic Substitute
PrimeAdvanced neurostimulator (SureScan) (MRI Safe)	*use* Stimulator Generator, Multiple Array for Insertion in Subcutaneous Tissue and Fascia
PROCEED™ Ventral Patch	*use* Synthetic Substitute
Prodisc-C	*use* Synthetic Substitute
Prodisc-L	*use* Synthetic Substitute
PROLENE Polypropylene Hernia System (PHS)	*use* Synthetic Substitute
Protecta XT CRT-D	*use* Cardiac Resynchronization Defibrillator Pulse Generator for Insertion in Subcutaneous Tissue and Fascia
Protecta XT DR (XT VR)	*use* Defibrillator Generator for Insertion in Subcutaneous Tissue and Fascia
Protégé® RX Carotid Stent System	*use* Intraluminal Device
Pump reservoir	*use* Infusion Device, Pump in Subcutaneous Tissue and Fascia
REALIZE® Adjustable Gastric Band	*use* Extraluminal Device
Rebound HRD® (Hernia Repair Device)	*use* Synthetic Substitute
RestoreAdvanced neurostimulator (SureScan) (MRI Safe)	*use* Stimulator Generator, Multiple Array Rechargeable for Insertion in Subcutaneous Tissue and Fascia
RestoreSensor neurostimulator (SureScan) (MRI Safe)	*use* Stimulator Generator, Multiple Array Rechargeable for Insertion in Subcutaneous Tissue and Fascia
RestoreUltra neurostimulator (SureScan) (MRI Safe)	*use* Stimulator Generator, Multiple Array Rechargeable for Insertion in Subcutaneous Tissue and Fascia

© 2018 Channel Publishing, Ltd.

DEVICE	USE:
Reveal (DX) (XT)	*use* Monitoring Device
Reverse® Shoulder Prosthesis	*use* Synthetic Substitute, Reverse Ball and Socket for Replacement in Upper Joints
Revo MRI™ SureScan® pacemaker	*use* Pacemaker, Dual Chamber for Insertion in Subcutaneous Tissue and Fascia
Rheos® System device	*use* Stimulator Generator in Subcutaneous Tissue and Fascia
Rheos® System lead	*use* Stimulator Lead in Upper Arteries
RNS System lead	*use* Neurostimulator Lead in Central Nervous System and Cranial Nerves
RNS system neurostimulator generator	*use* Neurostimulator Generator in Head and Facial Bones
Sacral nerve modulation (SNM) lead	*use* Stimulator Lead in Urinary System
Sacral neuromodulation lead	*use* Stimulator Lead in Urinary System
SAPIEN transcatheter aortic valve	*use* Zooplastic Tissue in Heart and Great Vessels
Secura (DR) (VR)	*use* Defibrillator Generator for Insertion in Subcutaneous Tissue and Fascia
Sheffield hybrid external fixator	*use* External Fixation Device, Hybrid for Insertion in Upper Bones, Lower Bones External Fixation Device, Hybrid for Reposition in Upper Bones, Lower Bones
Sheffield ring external fixator	*use* External Fixation Device, Ring for Insertion in Upper Bones, Lower Bones External Fixation Device, Ring for Reposition in Upper Bones, Lower Bones
Single lead pacemaker (atrium) (ventricle)	*use* Pacemaker, Single Chamber for Insertion in Subcutaneous Tissue and Fascia
Single lead rate responsive pacemaker (atrium) (ventricle)	*use* Pacemaker, Single Chamber Rate Responsive for Insertion in Subcutaneous Tissue and Fascia
Sirolimus-eluting coronary stent	*use* Intraluminal Device, Drug-eluting in Heart and Great Vessels
SJM Biocor® Stented Valve System	*use* Zooplastic Tissue in Heart and Great Vessels
Spacer, articulating (antibiotic)	*use* Articulating Spacer in Lower Joints
Spacer, static (antibiotic)	*use* Spacer in Lower Joints
Spinal cord neurostimulator lead	*use* Neurostimulator Lead in Central Nervous System and Cranial Nerves
Spinal growth rod(s), magnetically controlled	*use* Magnetically Controlled Growth Rod(s) in New Technology
Spiration IBV™ Valve System	*use* Intraluminal Device, Endobronchial Valve in Respiratory System
Static spacer (antibiotic)	*use* Spacer in Lower Joints
Stent, intraluminal (cardiovascular) (gastrointestinal) (hepatobiliary) (urinary)	*use* Intraluminal Device
Stented tissue valve	*use* Zooplastic Tissue in Heart and Great Vessels
Stratos LV	*use* Cardiac Resynchronization Pacemaker Pulse Generator for Insertion in Subcutaneous Tissue and Fascia
Subcutaneous injection reservoir, port	*use* Vascular Access Device, Totally Implantable in Subcutaneous Tissue and Fascia
Subcutaneous injection reservoir, pump	*use* Infusion Device, Pump in Subcutaneous Tissue and Fascia
Subdermal progesterone implant	*use* Contraceptive Device in Subcutaneous Tissue and Fascia
Sutureless valve, Perceval	*use* Zooplastic Tissue, Rapid Deployment Technique in New Technology
SynCardia Total Artificial Heart	*use* Synthetic Substitute
Synchra CRT-P	*use* Cardiac Resynchronization Pacemaker Pulse Generator for Insertion in Subcutaneous Tissue and Fascia
SynchroMed pump	*use* Infusion Device, Pump in Subcutaneous Tissue and Fascia
Talent® Converter	*use* Intraluminal Device
Talent® Occluder	*use* Intraluminal Device
Talent® Stent Graft (abdominal) (thoracic)	*use* Intraluminal Device
TandemHeart® System	*use* Short-term External Heart Assist System in Heart and Great Vessels
TAXUS® Liberté® Paclitaxel-eluting Coronary Stent System	*use* Intraluminal Device, Drug-eluting in Heart and Great Vessels
Therapeutic occlusion coil(s)	*use* Intraluminal Device
Thoracostomy tube	*use* Drainage Device
Thoratec IVAD (Implantable Ventricular Assist Device)	*use* Implantable Heart Assist System in Heart and Great Vessels
Thoratec Paracorporeal Ventricular Assist Device	*use* Short-term External Heart Assist System in Heart and Great Vessels
Tibial insert	*use* Liner in Lower Joints
Tissue bank graft	*use* Nonautologous Tissue Substitute
Tissue expander (inflatable) (injectable)	*use* Tissue Expander in Skin and Breast Tissue Expander in Subcutaneous Tissue and Fascia

© 2018 Channel Publishing, Ltd.

DEVICE	USE:
Titanium Sternal Fixation System (TSFS)	*use* Internal Fixation Device, Rigid Plate for Insertion in Upper Bones Internal Fixation Device, Rigid Plate for Reposition in Upper Bones
Total artificial (replacement) heart	*use* Synthetic Substitute
Tracheostomy tube	*use* Tracheostomy Device in Respiratory System
Trifecta™ Valve (aortic)	*use* Zooplastic Tissue in Heart and Great Vessels
Tunneled central venous catheter	*use* Vascular Access Device, Tunneled in Subcutaneous Tissue and Fascia
Tunneled spinal (intrathecal) catheter	*use* Infusion Device
Two lead pacemaker	*use* Pacemaker, Dual Chamber for Insertion in Subcutaneous Tissue and Fascia
Ultraflex™ Precision Colonic Stent System	*use* Intraluminal Device
ULTRAPRO Hernia System (UHS)	*use* Synthetic Substitute
ULTRAPRO Partially Absorbable Lightweight Mesh	*use* Synthetic Substitute
ULTRAPRO Plug	*use* Synthetic Substitute
Ultrasonic osteogenic stimulator	*use* Bone Growth Stimulator in Head and Facial Bones, Upper Bones, Lower Bones
Ultrasound bone healing system	*use* Bone Growth Stimulator in Head and Facial Bones, Upper Bones, Lower Bones
Uniplanar external fixator	*use* External Fixation Device, Monoplanar for Insertion in Upper Bones, Lower Bones External Fixation Device, Monoplanar for Reposition in Upper Bones, Lower Bones
Urinary incontinence stimulator lead	*use* Stimulator Lead in Urinary System
Vaginal pessary	*use* Intraluminal Device, Pessary in Female Reproductive System
Valiant Thoracic Stent Graft	*use* Intraluminal Device
Vectra® Vascular Access Graft	*use* Vascular Access Device, Tunneled in Subcutaneous Tissue and Fascia
Ventrio™ Hernia Patch	*use* Synthetic Substitute
Versa	*use* Pacemaker, Dual Chamber for Insertion in Subcutaneous Tissue and Fascia
Virtuoso (II) (DR) (VR)	*use* Defibrillator Generator for Insertion in Subcutaneous Tissue and Fascia
Viva (XT) (S)	*use* Cardiac Resynchronization Defibrillator Pulse Generator for Insertion in Subcutaneous Tissue and Fascia
WALLSTENT® Endoprosthesis	*use* Intraluminal Device
X-STOP® Spacer	*use* Spinal Stabilization Device, Interspinous Process for Insertion in Upper Joints, Lower Joints
Xact Carotid Stent System	*use* Intraluminal Device
Xenograft	*use* Zooplastic Tissue in Heart and Great Vessels
XIENCE Everolimus Eluting Coronary Stent System	*use* Intraluminal Device, Drug-eluting in Heart and Great Vessels
XLIF® System	*use* Interbody Fusion Device in Lower Joints
Zenith AAA Endovascular Graft	*use* Intraluminal Device, Branched or Fenestrated, One or Two Arteries for Restriction in Lower Arteries *use* Intraluminal Device, Branched or Fenestrated, Three or More Arteries for Restriction in Lower Arteries *use* Intraluminal Device
Zenith Flex® AAA Endovascular Graft	*use* Intraluminal Device
Zenith TX2® TAA Endovascular Graft	*use* Intraluminal Device
Zenith® Renu™ AAA Ancillary Graft	*use* Intraluminal Device
Zilver® PTX® (paclitaxel) Drug-Eluting Peripheral Stent	*use* Intraluminal Device, Drug-eluting in Upper Arteries, Lower Arteries
Zimmer® NexGen® LPS Mobile Bearing Knee	*use* Synthetic Substitute
Zimmer® NexGen® LPS-Flex Mobile Knee	*use* Synthetic Substitute
Zotarolimus-eluting coronary stent	*use* Intraluminal Device, Drug-eluting in Heart and Great Vessels

© 2018 Channel Publishing, Ltd.

Specific Device	Operation	In Body System	General Device
Autologous Arterial Tissue	All applicable	Heart and Great Vessels Lower Arteries, Lower Veins Upper Arteries, Upper Veins	Autologous Tissue Substitute
Autologous Venous Tissue	All applicable	Heart and Great Vessels Lower Arteries, Lower Veins Upper Arteries, Upper Veins	Autologous Tissue Substitute
Cardiac Lead, Defibrillator	Insertion	Heart and Great Vessels	Cardiac Lead
Cardiac Lead, Pacemaker	Insertion	Heart and Great Vessels	Cardiac Lead
Cardiac Resynchronization Defibrillator Pulse Generator	Insertion	Subcutaneous Tissue/Fascia	Cardiac Rhythm Related Device
Cardiac Resynchronization Pacemaker Pulse Generator	Insertion	Subcutaneous Tissue/Fascia	Cardiac Rhythm Related Device
Contractility Modulation Device	Insertion	Subcutaneous Tissue/Fascia	Cardiac Rhythm Related Device
Defibrillator Generator	Insertion	Subcutaneous Tissue/Fascia	Cardiac Rhythm Related Device
Epiretinal Visual Prosthesis	All applicable	Eye	Synthetic Substitute
External Fixation Device, Hybrid	Insertion	Lower Bones, Upper Bones	External Fixation Device
External Fixation Device, Hybrid	Reposition	Lower Bones, Upper Bones	External Fixation Device
External Fixation Device, Limb Lengthening	Insertion	Lower Bones, Upper Bones	External Fixation Device
External Fixation Device, Monoplanar	Insertion	Lower Bones, Upper Bones	External Fixation Device
External Fixation Device, Monoplanar	Reposition	Lower Bones, Upper Bones	External Fixation Device
External Fixation Device, Ring	Insertion	Lower Bones, Upper Bones	External Fixation Device
External Fixation Device, Ring	Reposition	Lower Bones, Upper Bones	External Fixation Device
Hearing Device, Bone Conduction	Insertion	Ear, Nose, Sinus	Hearing Device
Hearing Device, Multiple Channel Cochlear Prosthesis	Insertion	Ear, Nose, Sinus	Hearing Device
Hearing Device, Single Channel Cochlear Prosthesis	Insertion	Ear, Nose, Sinus	Hearing Device
Internal Fixation Device, Intramedullary	All applicable	Lower Bones, Upper Bones	Internal Fixation Device
Internal Fixation Device, Rigid Plate	Insertion	Upper Bones	Internal Fixation Device
Internal Fixation Device, Rigid Plate	Reposition	Upper Bones	Internal Fixation Device
Intraluminal Device, Airway	All applicable	Ear, Nose, Sinus Gastrointestinal System Mouth and Throat	Intraluminal Device
Intraluminal Device, Bioactive	All applicable	Upper Arteries	Intraluminal Device
Intraluminal Device, Branched or Fenestrated, One or Two Arteries	Restriction	Heart and Great Vessels Lower Arteries	Intraluminal Device
Intraluminal Device, Branched or Fenestrated, Three or More Arteries	Restriction	Heart and Great Vessels Lower Arteries	Intraluminal Device
Intraluminal Device, Drug-eluting	All applicable	Heart and Great Vessels Lower Arteries, Upper Arteries	Intraluminal Device
Intraluminal Device, Drug-eluting, Four or More	All applicable	Heart and Great Vessels Lower Arteries, Upper Arteries	Intraluminal Device
Intraluminal Device, Drug-eluting, Three	All applicable	Heart and Great Vessels Lower Arteries, Upper Arteries	Intraluminal Device
Intraluminal Device, Drug-eluting, Two	All applicable	Heart and Great Vessels Lower Arteries, Upper Arteries	Intraluminal Device
Intraluminal Device, Endobronchial Valve	All applicable	Respiratory System	Intraluminal Device
Intraluminal Device, Endotracheal Airway	All applicable	Respiratory System	Intraluminal Device
Intraluminal Device, Four or More	All applicable	Heart and Great Vessels Lower Arteries, Upper Arteries	Intraluminal Device
Intraluminal Device, Pessary	All applicable	Female Reproductive System	Intraluminal Device
Intraluminal Device, Radioactive	All applicable	Heart and Great Vessels	Intraluminal Device
Intraluminal Device, Three	All applicable	Heart and Great Vessels Lower Arteries, Upper Arteries	Intraluminal Device
Intraluminal Device, Two	All applicable	Heart and Great Vessels Lower Arteries, Upper Arteries	Intraluminal Device
Monitoring Device, Hemodynamic	Insertion	Subcutaneous Tissue/Fascia	Monitoring Device
Monitoring Device, Pressure Sensor	Insertion	Heart and Great Vessels	Monitoring Device

© 2018 Channel Publishing, Ltd.

Specific Device	Operation	In Body System	General Device
Pacemaker, Dual Chamber	Insertion	Subcutaneous Tissue/Fascia	Cardiac Rhythm Related Device
Pacemaker, Single Chamber	Insertion	Subcutaneous Tissue/Fascia	Cardiac Rhythm Related Device
Pacemaker, Single Chamber Rate Responsive	Insertion	Subcutaneous Tissue/Fascia	Cardiac Rhythm Related Device
Spinal Stabilization Device, Facet Replacement	Insertion	Lower Joints, Upper Joints	Internal Fixation Device
Spinal Stabilization Device, Interspinous Process	Insertion	Lower Joints, Upper Joints	Internal Fixation Device
Spinal Stabilization Device, Pedicle-Based	Insertion	Lower Joints, Upper Joints	Internal Fixation Device
Stimulator Generator, Multiple Array	Insertion	Subcutaneous Tissue/Fascia	Stimulator Generator
Stimulator Generator, Multiple Array Rechargeable	Insertion	Subcutaneous Tissue/Fascia	Stimulator Generator
Stimulator Generator, Single Array	Insertion	Subcutaneous Tissue/Fascia	Stimulator Generator
Stimulator Generator, Single Array Rechargeable	Insertion	Subcutaneous Tissue/Fascia	Stimulator Generator
Synthetic Substitute, Ceramic	Replacement	Lower Joints	Synthetic Substitute
Synthetic Substitute, Ceramic on Polyethylene	Replacement	Lower Joints	Synthetic Substitute
Synthetic Substitute, Intraocular Telescope	Replacement	Eye	Synthetic Substitute
Synthetic Substitute, Metal	Replacement	Lower Joints	Synthetic Substitute
Synthetic Substitute, Metal on Polyethylene	Replacement	Lower Joints	Synthetic Substitute
Synthetic Substitute, Oxidized Zirconium on Polyethylene	Replacement	Lower Joints	Synthetic Substitute
Synthetic Substitute, Polyethylene	Replacement	Lower Joints	Synthetic Substitute
Synthetic Substitute, Reverse Ball and Socket	Replacement	Upper Joints	Synthetic Substitute

© 2018 Channel Publishing, Ltd.

APPENDIX F – QUALIFIER KEY
PHYSICAL REHABILITATION AND DIAGNOSTIC AUDIOLOGY

Acoustic Reflex Decay	Definition: Measures reduction in size/strength of acoustic reflex over time Includes/Examples: Includes site of lesion test
Acoustic Reflex Patterns	Definition: Defines site of lesion based upon presence/absence of acoustic reflexes with ipsilateral vs. contralateral stimulation
Acoustic Reflex Threshold	Definition: Determines minimal intensity that acoustic reflex occurs with ipsilateral and/or contralateral stimulation
Aerobic Capacity and Endurance	Definition: Measures autonomic responses to positional changes; perceived exertion, dyspnea or angina during activity; performance during exercise protocols; standard vital signs; and blood gas analysis or oxygen consumption
Alternate Binaural or Monaural Loudness Balance	Definition: Determines auditory stimulus parameter that yields the same objective sensation. Includes/Examples: Sound intensities that yield same loudness perception
Anthropometric Characteristics	Definition: Measures edema, body fat composition, height, weight, length and girth
Aphasia (Assessment)	Definition: Measures expressive and receptive speech and language function including reading and writing
Aphasia (Treatment)	Definition: Applying techniques to improve, augment, or compensate for receptive/expressive language impairments
Articulation/Phonology (Assessment)	Definition: Measures speech production
Articulation/Phonology (Treatment)	Definition: Applying techniques to correct, improve, or compensate for speech productive impairment
Assistive Listening Device	Definition: Assists in use of effective and appropriate assistive listening device/system
Assistive Listening System/Device Selection	Definition: Measures the effectiveness and appropriateness of assistive listening systems/devices
Assistive, Adaptive, Supportive or Protective Devices	Explanation: Devices to facilitate or support achievement of a higher level of function in wheelchair mobility; bed mobility; transfer or ambulation ability; bath and showering ability; dressing; grooming; personal hygiene; play or leisure
Auditory Evoked Potentials	Definition: Measures electric responses produced by the VIIIth cranial nerve and brainstem following auditory stimulation
Auditory Processing (Assessment)	Definition: Evaluates ability to receive and process auditory information and comprehension of spoken language
Auditory Processing (Treatment)	Definition: Applying techniques to improve the receiving and processing of auditory information and comprehension of spoken language
Augmentative/Alternative Communication System (Assessment)	Definition: Determines the appropriateness of aids, techniques, symbols, and/or strategies to augment or replace speech and enhance communication Includes/Examples: Includes the use of telephones, writing equipment, emergency equipment, and TDD
Augmentative/Alternative Communication System (Treatment)	Includes/Examples: Includes augmentative communication devices and aids
Aural Rehabilitation	Definition: Applying techniques to improve the communication abilities associated with hearing loss
Aural Rehabilitation Status	Definition: Measures impact of a hearing loss including evaluation of receptive and expressive communication skills
Bathing/Showering	Includes/Examples: Includes obtaining and using supplies; soaping, rinsing, and drying body parts; maintaining bathing position; and transferring to and from bathing positions
Bathing/Showering Techniques	Definition: Activities to facilitate obtaining and using supplies, soaping, rinsing and drying body parts, maintaining bathing position, and transferring to and from bathing positions
Bed Mobility (Assessment)	Definition: Transitional movement within bed
Bed Mobility (Treatment)	Definition: Exercise or activities to facilitate transitional movements within bed
Bedside Swallowing and Oral Function	Includes/Examples: Bedside swallowing includes assessment of sucking, masticating, coughing, and swallowing. Oral function includes assessment of musculature for controlled movements, structures and functions to determine coordination and phonation

© 2018 Channel Publishing, Ltd.

Bekesy Audiometry	Definition: Uses an instrument that provides a choice of discrete or continuously varying pure tones; choice of pulsed or continuous signal
Binaural Electroacoustic Hearing Aid Check	Definition: Determines mechanical and electroacoustic function of bilateral hearing aids using hearing aid test box
Binaural Hearing Aid (Assessment)	Definition: Measures the candidacy, effectiveness, and appropriateness of hearing aids. Explanation: Measures bilateral fit
Binaural Hearing Aid (Treatment)	Explanation: Assists in achieving maximum understanding and performance
Bithermal, Binaural Caloric Irrigation	Definition: Measures the rhythmic eye movements stimulated by changing the temperature of the vestibular system
Bithermal, Monaural Caloric Irrigation	Definition: Measures the rhythmic eye movements stimulated by changing the temperature of the vestibular system in one ear
Brief Tone Stimuli	Definition: Measures specific central auditory process
Cerumen Management	Definition: Includes examination of external auditory canal and tympanic membrane and removal of cerumen from external ear canal
Cochlear Implant	Definition: Measures candidacy for cochlear implant
Cochlear Implant Rehabilitation	Definition: Applying techniques to improve the communication abilities of individuals with cochlear implant; includes programming the device, providing patients/families with information
Communicative/Cognitive Integration Skills (Assessment)	Definition: Measures ability to use higher cortical functions Includes/Examples: Includes orientation, recognition, attention span, initiation and termination of activity, memory, sequencing, categorizing, concept formation, spatial operations, judgment, problem solving, generalization and pragmatic communication
Communicative/Cognitive Integration Skills (Treatment)	Definition: Activities to facilitate the use of higher cortical functions Includes/Examples: Includes level of arousal, orientation, recognition, attention span, initiation and termination of activity, memory sequencing, judgment and problem solving, learning and generalization, and pragmatic communication
Computerized Dynamic Posturography	Definition: Measures the status of the peripheral and central vestibular system and the sensory/motor component of balance; evaluates the efficacy of vestibular rehabilitation
Conditioned Play Audiometry	Definition: Behavioral measures using nonspeech and speech stimuli to obtain frequency-specific and ear-specific information on auditory status from the patient Explanation: Obtains speech reception threshold by having patient point to pictures of spondaic words
Coordination/Dexterity (Assessment)	Definition: Measures large and small muscle groups for controlled goal-directed movements Explanation: Dexterity includes object manipulation
Coordination/Dexterity (Treatment)	Definition: Exercise or activities to facilitate gross coordination and fine coordination
Cranial Nerve Integrity	Definition: Measures cranial nerve sensory and motor functions, including tastes, smell and facial expression
Dichotic Stimuli	Definition: Measures specific central auditory process
Distorted Speech	Definition: Measures specific central auditory process
Dix-Hallpike Dynamic	Definition: Measures nystagmus following Dix-Hallpike maneuver
Dressing	Includes/Examples: Includes selecting clothing and accessories, obtaining clothing from storage, dressing and, fastening and adjusting clothing and shoes, and applying and removing personal devices, prosthesis or orthosis
Dressing Techniques	Definition: Activities to facilitate selecting clothing and accessories, dressing and undressing, adjusting clothing and shoes, applying and removing devices, prostheses or orthoses
Dynamic Orthosis	Includes/Examples: Includes customized and prefabricated splints, inhibitory casts, spinal and other braces, and protective devices; allows motion through transfer of movement from other body parts or by use of outside forces
Ear Canal Probe Microphone	Definition: Real ear measures
Ear Protector Attentuation	Definition: Measures ear protector fit and effectiveness
Electrocochleography	Definition: Measures the VIIIth cranial nerve action potential
Environmental, Home and Work Barriers	Definition: Measures current and potential barriers to optimal function, including safety hazards, access problems and home or office design

© 2018 Channel Publishing, Ltd.

Ergonomics and Body Mechanics	Definition: Ergonomic measurement of job tasks, work hardening or work conditioning needs; functional capacity; and body mechanics
Eustachian Tube Function	Definition: Measures eustachian tube function and patency of eustachian tube
Evoked Otoacoustic Emissions, Diagnostic	Definition: Measures auditory evoked potentials in a diagnostic format
Evoked Otoacoustic Emissions, Screening	Definition: Measures auditory evoked potentials in a screening format
Facial Nerve Function	Definition: Measures electrical activity of the VIIth cranial nerve (facial nerve)
Feeding/Eating (Assessment)	Includes/Examples: Includes setting up food, selecting and using utensils and tableware, bringing food or drink to mouth, cleaning face, hands, and clothing, and management of alternative methods of nourishment
Feeding/Eating (Treatment)	Definition: Exercise or activities to facilitate setting up food, selecting and using utensils and tableware, bringing food or drink to mouth, cleaning face, hands, and clothing, and management of alternative methods of nourishment
Filtered Speech	Definition: Uses high or low pass filtered speech stimuli to assess central auditory processing disorders, site of lesion testing
Fluency (Assessment)	Definition: Measures speech fluency or stuttering
Fluency (Treatment)	Definition: Applying techniques to improve and augment fluent speech
Gait and/or Balance	Definition: Measures biomechanical, arthrokinematic and other spatial and temporal characteristics of gait and balance
Gait Training/Functional Ambulation	Definition: Exercise or activities to facilitate ambulation on a variety of surfaces and in a variety of environments
Grooming/Personal Hygiene (Assessment)	Includes/Examples: Includes ability to obtain and use supplies in a sequential fashion, general grooming, oral hygiene, toilet hygiene, personal care devices, including care for artificial airways
Grooming/Personal Hygiene (Treatment)	Definition: Activities to facilitate obtaining and using supplies in a sequential fashion: general grooming, oral hygiene, toilet hygiene, cleaning body, and personal care devices, including artificial airways
Hearing and Related Disorders Counseling	Definition: Provides patients/families/caregivers with information, support, referrals to facilitate recovery from a communication disorder Includes/Examples: Includes strategies for psychosocial adjustment to hearing loss for clients and families/caregivers
Hearing and Related Disorders Prevention	Definition: Provides patients/families/caregivers with information and support to prevent communication disorders
Hearing Screening	Definition: Pass/refer measures designed to identify need for further audiologic assessment
Home Management (Assessment)	Definition: Obtaining and maintaining personal and household possessions and environment Includes/Examples: Includes clothing care, cleaning, meal preparation and cleanup, shopping, money management, household maintenance, safety procedures, and childcare/parenting
Home Management (Treatment)	Definition: Activities to facilitate obtaining and maintaining personal household possessions and environment Includes/Examples: Includes clothing care, cleaning, meal preparation and clean-up, shopping, money management, household maintenance, safety procedures, childcare/parenting
Instrumental Swallowing and Oral Function	Definition: Measures swallowing function using instrumental diagnostic procedures Explanation: Methods include videofluoroscopy, ultrasound, manometry, endoscopy
Integumentary Integrity	Includes/Examples: Includes burns, skin conditions, ecchymosis, bleeding, blisters, scar tissue, wounds and other traumas, tissue mobility, turgor and texture
Manual Therapy Techniques	Definition: Techniques in which the therapist uses his/her hands to administer skilled movements. Includes/Examples: Includes connective tissue massage, joint mobilization and manipulation, manual lymph drainage, manual traction, soft tissue mobilization and manipulation
Masking Patterns	Definition: Measures central auditory processing status
Monaural Electroacoustic Hearing Aid Check	Definition: Determines mechanical and electroacoustic function of one hearing aid using hearing aid test box

© 2018 Channel Publishing, Ltd.

Monaural Hearing Aid (Assessment)	Definition: Measures the candidacy, effectiveness, and appropriateness of a hearing aid Explanation: Measures unilateral fit
Monaural Hearing Aid (Treatment)	Explanation: Assists in achieving maximum understanding and performance
Motor Function (Assessment)	Definition: Measures the body's functional and versatile movement patterns Includes/Examples: Includes motor assessment scales, analysis of head, trunk and limb movement, and assessment of motor learning
Motor Function (Treatment)	Definition: Exercise or activities to facilitate crossing midline, laterality, bilateral integration, praxis, neuromuscular relaxation, inhibition, facilitation, motor function and motor learning
Motor Speech (Assessment)	Definition: Measures neurological motor aspects of speech production
Motor Speech (Treatment)	Definition: Applying techniques to improve and augment the impaired neurological motor aspects of speech production
Muscle Performance (Assessment)	Definition: Measures muscle strength, power and endurance using manual testing, dynamometry or computer-assisted electromechanical muscle test; functional muscle strength, power and endurance; muscle pain, tone, or soreness; or pelvic-floor musculature. Explanation: Muscle endurance refers to the ability to contract a muscle repeatedly over time
Muscle Performance (Treatment)	Definition: Exercise or activities to increase the capacity of a muscle to do work in terms of strength, power, and/or endurance. Explanation: Muscle strength is the force exerted to overcome resistance in one maximal effort. Muscle power is work produced per unit of time, or the product of strength and speed. Muscle endurance is the ability to contract a muscle repeatedly over time
Neuromotor Development	Definition: Measures motor development, righting and equilibrium reactions, and reflex and equilibrium reactions
Non-invasive Instrumental Status	Definition: Instrumental measures of oral, nasal, vocal, and velopharyngeal functions as they pertain to speech production
Nonspoken Language (Assessment)	Definition: Measures nonspoken language (print, sign, symbols) for communication
Nonspoken Language (Treatment)	Definition: Applying techniques that improve, augment, or compensate spoken communication
Oral Peripheral Mechanism	Definition: Structural measures of face, jaw, lips, tongue, teeth, hard and soft palate, pharynx as related to speech production
Orofacial Myofunctional (Assessment)	Definition: Measures orofacial myofunctional patterns for speech and related functions
Orofacial Myofunctional (Treatment)	Definition: Applying techniques to improve, alter, or augment impaired orofacial myofunctional patterns and related speech production errors
Oscillating Tracking	Definition: Measures ability to visually track
Pain	Definition: Measures muscle soreness, pain and soreness with joint movement, and pain perception Includes/Examples: Includes questionnaires, graphs, symptom magnification scales or visual analog scales
Perceptual Processing (Assessment)	Definition: Measures stereognosis, kinesthesia, body schema, right-left discrimination, form constancy, position in space, visual closure, figure-ground, depth perception, spatial relations and topographical orientation
Perceptual Processing (Treatment)	Definition: Exercise and activities to facilitate perceptual processing Explanation: Includes stereognosis, kinesthesia, body schema, right-left discrimination, form constancy, position in space, visual closure, figure-ground, depth perception, spatial relations, and topographical orientation Includes/Examples: Includes stereognosis, kinesthesia, body schema, right-left discrimination, form constancy, position in space, visual closure, figure-ground, depth perception, spatial relations, and topographical orientation
Performance Intensity Phonetically Balanced Speech Discrimination	Definition: Measures word recognition over varying intensity levels
Postural Control	Definition: Exercise or activities to increase postural alignment and control
Prosthesis	Definition: Artificial substitutes for missing body parts that augment performance or function. Includes/Examples: Limb prosthesis, ocular prosthesis

© 2018 Channel Publishing, Ltd.

Psychosocial Skills (Assessment)	Definition: The ability to interact in society and to process emotions Includes/Examples: Includes psychological (values, interests, self-concept); social (role performance, social conduct, interpersonal skills, self expression); self-management (coping skills, time management, self-control)
Psychosocial Skills (Treatment)	Definition: The ability to interact in society and to process emotions Includes/Examples: Includes psychological (values, interests, self-concept); social (role performance, social conduct, interpersonal skills, self expression); self-management (coping skills, time management, self-control)
Pure Tone Audiometry, Air	Definition: Air-conduction pure tone threshold measures with appropriate masking
Pure Tone Audiometry, Air and Bone	Definition: Air-conduction and bone-conduction pure tone threshold measures with appropriate masking
Pure Tone Stenger	Definition: Measures unilateral nonorganic hearing loss based on simultaneous presentation of pure tones of differing volume
Range of Motion and Joint Integrity	Definition: Measures quantity, quality, grade, and classification of joint movement and/or mobility Explanation: Range of Motion is the space, distance or angle through which movement occurs at a joint or series of joints. Joint integrity is the conformance of joints to expected anatomic, biomechanical and kinematic norms
Range of Motion and Joint Mobility	Definition: Exercise or activities to increase muscle length and joint mobility
Receptive/Expressive Language (Assessment)	Definition: Measures receptive and expressive language
Receptive/Expressive Language (Treatment)	Definition: Applying techniques to improve and augment receptive/expressive language
Reflex Integrity	Definition: Measures the presence, absence, or exaggeration of developmentally appropriate, pathologic or normal reflexes
Select Picture Audiometry	Definition: Establishes hearing threshold levels for speech using pictures
Sensorineural Acuity Level	Definition: Measures sensorineural acuity masking presented via bone conduction
Sensory Aids	Definition: Determines the appropriateness of a sensory prosthetic device, other than a hearing aid or assistive listening system/device
Sensory Awareness/Processing/Integrity	Includes/Examples: Includes light touch, pressure, temperature, pain, sharp/dull, proprioception, vestibular, visual, auditory, gustatory, and olfactory
Short Increment Sensitivity Index	Definition: Measures the ear's ability to detect small intensity changes; site of lesion test requiring a behavioral response
Sinusoidal Vertical Axis Rotational	Definition: Measures nystagmus following rotation
Somatosensory Evoked Potentials	Definition: Measures neural activity from sites throughout the body
Speech and/or Language Screening	Definition: Identifies need for further speech and/or language evaluation
Speech Threshold	Definition: Measures minimal intensity needed to repeat spondaic words
Speech-Language Pathology and Related Disorders Counseling	Definition: Provides patients/families with information, support, referrals to facilitate recovery from a communication disorder
Speech-Language Pathology and Related Disorders Prevention	Definition: Applying techniques to avoid or minimize onset and/or development of a communication disorder
Speech/Word Recognition	Definition: Measures ability to repeat/identify single syllable words; scores given as a percentage; includes word recognition/speech discrimination
Staggered Spondaic Word	Definition: Measures central auditory processing site of lesion based upon dichotic presentation of spondaic words
Static Orthosis	Includes/Examples: Includes customized and prefabricated splints, inhibitory casts, spinal and other braces, and protective devices; has no moving parts, maintains joint(s) in desired position
Stenger	Definition: Measures unilateral nonorganic hearing loss based on simultaneous presentation of signals of differing volume
Swallowing Dysfunction	Definition: Activities to improve swallowing function in coordination with respiratory function Includes/Examples: Includes function and coordination of sucking, mastication, coughing, swallowing
Synthetic Sentence Identification	Definition: Measures central auditory dysfunction using identification of third order approximations of sentences and competing messages

© 2018 Channel Publishing, Ltd.

Temporal Ordering of Stimuli	Definition: Measures specific central auditory process
Therapeutic Exercise	Definition: Exercise or activities to facilitate sensory awareness, sensory processing, sensory integration, balance training, conditioning, reconditioning Includes/Examples: Includes developmental activities, breathing exercises, aerobic endurance activities, aquatic exercises, stretching and ventilatory muscle training
Tinnitus Masker (Assessment)	Definition: Determines candidacy for tinnitus masker
Tinnitus Masker (Treatment)	Explanation: Used to verify physical fit, acoustic appropriateness, and benefit; assists in achieving maximum benefit
Tone Decay	Definition: Measures decrease in hearing sensitivity to a tone; site of lesion test requiring a behavioral response
Transfer	Definition: Transitional movement from one surface to another
Transfer Training	Definition: Exercise or activities to facilitate movement from one surface to another
Tympanometry	Definition: Measures the integrity of the middle ear; measures ease at which sound flows through the tympanic membrane while air pressure against the membrane is varied
Unithermal Binaural Screen	Definition: Measures the rhythmic eye movements stimulated by changing the temperature of the vestibular system in both ears using warm water, screening format
Ventilation, Respiration and Circulation	Definition: Measures ventilatory muscle strength, power and endurance, pulmonary function and ventilatory mechanics. Includes/Examples: Includes ability to clear airway, activities that aggravate or relieve edema, pain, dyspnea or other symptoms, chest wall mobility, cardiopulmonary response to performance of ADL and IAD, cough and sputum, standard vital signs
Vestibular	Definition: Applying techniques to compensate for balance disorders; includes habituation, exercise therapy, and balance retraining
Visual Motor Integration (Assessment)	Definition: Coordinating the interaction of information from the eyes with body movement during activity
Visual Motor Integration (Treatment)	Definition: Exercise or activities to facilitate coordinating the interaction of information from eyes with body movement during activity
Visual Reinforcement Audiometry	Definition: Behavioral measures using nonspeech and speech stimuli to obtain frequency/ear-specific information on auditory status Includes/Examples: Includes a conditioned response of looking toward a visual reinforcer (e.g., lights, animated toy) every time auditory stimuli are heard
Vocational Activities and Functional Community or Work Reintegration Skills (Assessment)	Definition: Measures environmental, home, work (job/school/play) barriers that keep patients from functioning optimally in their environment. Includes/Examples: Includes assessment of vocational skill and interests, environment of work (job/school/play), injury potential and injury prevention or reduction, ergonomic stressors, transportation skills, and ability to access and use community resources
Vocational Activities and Functional Community or Work Reintegration Skills (Treatment)	Definition: Activities to facilitate vocational exploration, body mechanics training, job acquisition, and environmental or work (job/school/play) task adaptation Includes/Examples: Includes injury prevention and reduction, ergonomic stressor reduction, job coaching and simulation, work hardening and conditioning, driving training, transportation skills, and use of community resources
Voice (Assessment)	Definition: Measures vocal structure, function and production
Voice (Treatment)	Definition: Applying techniques to improve voice and vocal function
Voice Prosthetic (Assessment)	Definition: Determines the appropriateness of voice prosthetic/adaptive device to enhance or facilitate communication
Voice Prosthetic (Treatment)	Includes/Examples: Includes electrolarynx, and other assistive, adaptive, supportive devices
Wheelchair Mobility (Assessment)	Definition: Measures fit and functional abilities within wheelchair in a variety of environments
Wheelchair Mobility (Treatment)	Definition: Management, maintenance and controlled operation of a wheelchair, scooter or other device, in and on a variety of surfaces and environments
Wound Management	Includes/Examples: Includes non-selective and selective debridement (enzymes, autolysis, sharp debridement), dressings (wound coverings, hydrogel, vacuum-assisted closure), topical agents, etc.

© 2018 Channel Publishing, Ltd.

APPENDIX G – QUALIFIER KEY FOR MENTAL HEALTH

Behavioral	Definition: Primarily to modify behavior Includes/Examples: Includes modeling and role playing, positive reinforcement of target behaviors, response cost, and training of self-management skills
Cognitive	Definition: Primarily to correct cognitive distortions and errors
Cognitive-Behavioral	Definition: Combining cognitive and behavioral treatment strategies to improve functioning. Explanation: Maladaptive responses are examined to determine how cognitions relate to behavior patterns in response to an event. Uses learning principles and information-processing models
Developmental	Definition: Age-normed developmental status of cognitive, social and adaptive behavior skills
Intellectual and Psychoeducational	Definition: Intellectual abilities, academic achievement and learning capabilities (including behaviors and emotional factors affecting learning)
Interactive	Definition: Uses primarily physical aids and other forms of non-oral interaction with a patient who is physically, psychologically or developmentally unable to use ordinary language for communication Includes/Examples: Includes the use of toys in symbolic play
Interpersonal	Definition: Helps an individual make changes in interpersonal behaviors to reduce psychological dysfunction Includes/Examples: Includes exploratory techniques, encouragement of affective expression, clarification of patient statements, analysis of communication patterns, use of therapy relationship and behavior change techniques
Neurobehavioral and Cognitive Status	Definition: Includes neurobehavioral status exam, interview(s), and observation for the clinical assessment of thinking, reasoning and judgment, acquired knowledge, attention, memory, visual spatial abilities, language functions, and planning
Neuropsychological	Definition: Thinking, reasoning and judgment, acquired knowledge, attention, memory, visual spatial abilities, language functions, planning
Personality and Behavioral	Definition: Mood, emotion, behavior, social functioning, psychopathological conditions, personality traits and characteristics
Psychoanalysis	Definition: Methods of obtaining a detailed account of past and present mental and emotional experiences to determine the source and eliminate or diminish the undesirable effects of unconscious conflicts Explanation: Accomplished by making the individual aware of their existence, origin, and inappropriate expression in emotions and behavior
Psychodynamic	Definition: Exploration of past and present emotional experiences to understand motives and drives using insight-oriented techniques to reduce the undesirable effects of internal conflicts on emotions and behavior Explanation: Techniques include empathetic listening, clarifying self-defeating behavior patterns, and exploring adaptive alternatives
Psychophysiological	Definition: Monitoring and alteration of physiological processes to help the individual associate physiological reactions combined with cognitive and behavioral strategies to gain improved control of these processes to help the individual cope more effectively
Supportive	Definition: Formation of therapeutic relationship primarily for providing emotional support to prevent further deterioration in functioning during periods of particular stress. Explanation: Often used in conjunction with other therapeutic approaches
Vocational	Definition: Exploration of vocational interests, aptitudes and required adaptive behavior skills to develop and carry out a plan for achieving a successful vocational placement. Includes/Examples: Includes enhancing work related adjustment and/or pursuing viable options in training education or preparation

© 2018 Channel Publishing, Ltd.

SUBSTANCE	USE:
AIGISRx Antibacterial Envelope Antimicrobial envelope	*use* Anti-Infective Envelope
Angiotensin II	*use* Synthetic Human Angiotensin II
Axicabtagene Ciloeucel	*use* Engineered Autologous Chimeric Antigen Receptor T-cell Immunotherapy
Bone morphogenetic protein 2 (BMP 2)	*use* Recombinant Bone Morphogenetic Protein
CBMA (Concentrated Bone Marrow Aspirate)	*use* Concentrated Bone Marrow Aspirate
Clolar	*use* Clofarabine
Defitelio	*use* Defibrotide Sodium Anticoagulant
DuraGraft® Endothelial Damage Inhibitor	*use* Endothelial Damage Inhibitor
Factor Xa Inhibitor Reversal Agent, Andexanet Alfa	*use* Andexanet Alfa, Factor Xa Inhibitor Reversal Agent
GIAPREZA™ Human angiotensin II, synthetic	*use* Synthetic Human Angiotensin II *use* Synthetic Human Angiotensin II
Kcentra	*use* 4-Factor Prothrombin Complex Concentrate
KYMRIAH	*use* Engineered Autologous Chimeric Antigen Receptor T-cell Immunotherapy
Nesiritide	*use* Human B-type Natriuretic Peptide
rhBMP-2	*use* Recombinant Bone Morphogenetic Protein
Seprafilm	*use* Adhesion Barrier
STELARA®	*use* Other New Technology Therapeutic Substance
Tisagenlecleucel	*use* Engineered Autologous Chimeric Antigen Receptor T-cell Immunotherapy
Tissue Plasminogen Activator (tPA) (r-tPA)	*use* Other Thrombolytic
Ustekinumab	*use* Other New Technology Therapeutic Substance
Vistogard®	*use* Uridine Triacetate
Voraxaze	*use* Glucarpidase
VYXEOS™	*use* Cytarabine and Daunorubicin Liposome Antineoplastic
ZINPLAVA™	*use* Bezlotoxumab Monoclonal Antibody
Zyvox	*use* Oxazolidinones

APPENDIX I – NEW TECHNOLOGY DEVICE KEY

DEVICE	USE:
COALESCE® radiolucent interbody fusion device	*use* Interbody Fusion Device, Radiolucent Porous in New Technology
COHERE® radiolucent interbody fusion device	*use* Interbody Fusion Device, Radiolucent Porous in New Technology
EDWARDS INTUITY Elite valve system	*use* Zooplastic Tissue, Rapid Deployment Technique in New Technology
INTUITY Elite valve system, EDWARDS	*use* Zooplastic Tissue, Rapid Deployment Technique in New Technology
MAGEC® Spinal Bracing and Distraction System	*use* Magnetically Controlled Growth Rod(s) in New Technology
MIRODERM™ Biologic Wound Matrix	*use* Skin Substitute, Porcine Liver Derived in New Technology
nanoLOCK™ interbody fusion device	*use* Interbody Fusion Device, Nanotextured Surface in New Technology
Perceval sutureless valve	*use* Zooplastic Tissue, Rapid Deployment Technique in New Technology
Spinal growth rod(s), magnetically controlled	*use* Magnetically Controlled Growth Rod(s) in New Technology
Sutureless valve, Perceval	*use* Zooplastic Tissue, Rapid Deployment Technique in New Technology

© 2018 Channel Publishing, Ltd.